MW00999957

Musculoskeletal Interventions

Notice

Medicine is an ever-changing science. As new research and clinical experience broaden our knowledge, changes in treatment and drug therapy are required. The authors and the publisher of this work have checked with sources believed to be reliable in their efforts to provide information that is complete and generally in accord with the standards accepted at the time of publication. However, in view of the possibility of human error or changes in medical sciences, neither the authors nor the publisher nor any other party who has been involved in the preparation or publication of this work warrants that the information contained herein is in every respect accurate or complete, and they disclaim all responsibility for any errors or omissions or for the results obtained from use of the information contained in this work. Readers are encouraged to confirm the information contained herein with other sources. For example and in particular, readers are advised to check the product information sheet included in the package of each drug they plan to administer to be certain that the information contained in this work is accurate and that changes have not been made in the recommended dose or in the contraindications for administration. This recommendation is of particular importance in connection with the new or infrequently used drugs.

Third Edition

Musculoskeletal Interventions

Techniques for Therapeutic Exercise

Barbara J. Hoogenboom, EdD, PT, SCS, ATC
Professor
Department of Physical Therapy
Grand Valley State University
Grand Rapids, Michigan

Michael L. Voight, DHSc, PT, OCS, SCS, ATC, CSCS, FAPTA
Professor
School of Physical Therapy
Belmont University
Nashville, Tennessee

William E. Prentice, PhD, PT, ATC, FNATA
Professor
Coordinator of Sports Medicine Specialization
Department of Exercise and Sport Science
University of North Carolina at Chapel Hill
Chapel Hill, North Carolina

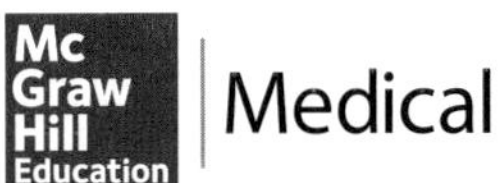

New York Chicago San Francisco Athens London Madrid
Mexico City Milan New Delhi Singapore Sydney Toronto

MUSCULOSKELETAL INTERVENTIONS: TECHNIQUES FOR THERAPEUTIC EXERCISE, THIRD EDITION

1 2 3 4 5 6 7 8 9 0 CTP/CTP 19 18 17 16 15 14

ISBN 978-0-07-179369-8
MHID 0-07-179369-0

This book was set in Utopia by Thomson Digital.
The editors were Michael Weitz and Brian Kearns.
The production supervisor was Catherine Saggese.
The illustration manager was Armen Ovsepyan.
Project management was provided by Ritu Joon, Thomson Digital.
The designer was Mary Young/EPS Studios; the cover designer was Thomas De Pierro.
Cover Photo Credit: © Creasource/Corbis.
China Translation & Printing Services, Ltd. was printer and binder.

This book is printed on acid-free paper.

Catalog-in-Publication Data is on file for this title at the Library of Congress.

International Edition ISBN 978-1-25-925143-6; MHID 1-25-925143-8.

Contents

PART 4 Intervention Strategies for Specific Injuries

PART 5 Special Consideration for Specific Patient Populations

Contributors

Jeanine Beasley, EdD, OTR, CHT, FAOTA
Associate Professor
Certified Hand Therapist
Department of Occupational Therapy
Grand Valley State University
Mary Free Bed Rehabilitation Hospital
Rockford, Michigan

Jolene L. Bennett, MA, PT, OCS, ATC, CertMDT
Clinical Specialist for Orthopedics and Sports Medicine
Spectrum Health Rehabilitation and Sports Medicine
Visser Family YMCA
Grandville, Michigan

Turner A. Blackburn, Jr., MEd, PT, ATC
Vice President
Clemson Sports Medicine and Rehabilitation
Manchester, Georgia

David Carfagno, DO
Board Certified Internal Medicine and Sports Medicine Physician
Scottsdale Sports Medicine
Scottsdale, Arizona

Mark De Carlo, PT, DPT, MHA, SCS, ATC
Director of Research and Clinical Education
Accelerated Rehabilitation Centers
Carmel, Indiana

Mike Clark, DPT, MS, CES, PES
Chairman, Founder, Chief Science Officer
Fusionetics
Alpharetta, Georgia

Gray Cook, MSPT, OCS, CSCS
Clinical Director
Orthopedic and Sports Physical Therapy
Danville, Virginia

Craig R. Denegar, PhD, PT, ATC, FNATA
Director of Physical Therapy Program
Professor of Kinesiology
Department of Physical Therapy
University of Connecticut
Storrs, Connecticut

Todd S. Ellenbecker, DPT, MS, SCS, OCS, CSCS
Senior Director of Medical Services
National Director of Clinical Research
Physiotherapy Associates Scottsdale Sports Clinic
Physiotherapy Associates
Scottsdale, Arizona

Terry L. Grindstaff, PhD, PT, ATC, SCS, CSCS
Assistant Professor
Department of Physical Therapy
Creighton University
Omaha, Nebraska

John A. Guido, Jr., DPT, ATC
Sports Therapist
Department of Outpatient Physical Therapy
Ochsner Hospital
New Orleans, Louisiana

Kevin M. Guskiewicz, PhD, ATC, FNATA, FACSM
Senior Associate Dean, College of Arts and Sciences
Professor
Department of Exercise and Sport Science
University of North Carolina
Chapel Hill, North Carolina

John S. Halle, PT, PhD, ECS
Professor
School of Physical Therapy
School of Physical Therapy, Belmont University
Nashville, Tennessee

Christopher J. Hirth, MSPT, PT, ATC
Director of Rehabilitation
Physical Therapist/Athletic Trainer
Campus Health Service
University of North Carolina
Chapel Hill, North Carolina

Barbara J. Hoogenboom, EdD, PT, SCS, ATC
Professor
Department of Physical Therapy
Grand Valley State University
Grand Rapids, Michigan

Daniel N. Hooker, PhD, PT, ATC, SCS
Physical Therapist/ Athletic Trainer, Retired
Division of Sports Medicine
University of North Carolina
Chapel Hill, North Carolina

Stuart L. (Skip) Hunter, PT, ATC
Owner
Clemson Sports Medicine
Clemson, South Carolina

B.J. Lehecka, DPT
Assistant Professor
Department of Physical Therapy/ Outpatient Orthopedic Physical Therapy
Wichita State University/Via Christi Health
Wichita, Kansas

Nancy E. Lomax, PT
Staff Physical Therapist
Spectrum Health Rehabilitation and Sports Medicine Services
Visser Family YMCA
Grandville, Michigan

Dianna Lunsford, OTD, MEd, OTR/L, CHT
Assistant Professor
Department of Occupational Therapy
Grand Valley State University
Grand Rapids, Michigan

Eric M. Magrum, DPT, OCS, FAAOMPT
Senior Physical Therapist and Director of Orthopedic Residency Program
University of Virginia/Healthsouth Outpatient Sports Medicine
Charlottesville, Virginia

Robert C. Manske, DPT, PT, MEd, SCS, ATC, CSCS
Professor and Chair
Department of Physical Therapy/Outpatient Orthopedic Physical Therapy
Wichita State University/Via Christi Health
Wichita, Kansas

Ryan McDivitt, PT, DPT, ATC
Facility Manager
Accelerated Rehabilitation Centers
Avon, Indiana

Scott Miller, MS, PT, SCS, CSCS
Director of Clinical Operations
Agility Health Physical Therapy and Sports Performance
Portage, Michigan

Joseph Myers, PhD, ATC
Associate Professor
Department of Exercise and Sport Science
University of North Carolina at Chapel Hill
Chapel Hill, North Carolina

Phil Page, PhD, PT, ATC, CSCS, FACSM
Director of Research and Education
Performance Health
Baton Rouge, Louisiana

Tad E. Pieczynski, PT, MS, CSCS
Assistant Clinic Director
Physiotherapy Associates
Scottsdale Sports Clinic
Scottsdale, Arizona

William E. Prentice, PhD, PT, ATC, FNATA
Professor
Coordinator of Sports Medicine Specialization
Department of Exercise and Sport Science
University of North Carolina at Chapel Hill
Chapel Hill, North Carolina

Greg Rose, DC
Co-Founder
Titleist Performance Institute
Oceanside, California

Terri Jo Rucinski, MA, PT, ATC
Physical Therapist/Athletic Trainer
Campus Health Service
Division of Sports Medicine
University of North Carolina at Chapel Hill
Chapel Hill, North Carolina

Rob Schneider, MSPT, PT, ATC, SCS
Director
Proaxis Therapy
Carrboro, North Carolina

Teresa L. Schuemann, PT, SCS, ATC
Program Director
Evidence in Motion, Sports Physical Therapy Residency
Proaxis Physical Therapy
Fort Collins, Colorado

Patrick D. Sells, DA, ACSM
Assistant Professor
School of Physical Therapy
Belmont University
Nashville, Tennessee

Michael J. Shoemaker, PT, DPT, GCS
Assistant Professor
Department of Physical Therapy
Grand Valley State University Program in Physical Therapy
Cook-DeVos Center for Health Sciences
Grand Rapids, Michigan

Robyn K. Smith, MS, PT, SCS
Staff Physical Therapist
Center for Physical Rehabilitation
Belmont, Michigan

Stephanie M. Squitieri, DPT, CSCS
Senior Physical Therapist
PRO Sports Physical Therapy of Westchester
Scarsdale, New York

Gregory C. Thomas, DPT, CSCS
PRO Sports Physical Therapy
Scarsdale, New York

Steven R. Tippett, PhD, PT, SCS, ATC
Professor and Chair
Department of Physical Therapy and Health Science
Bradley University
Peoria, Illinois

Timothy F. Tyler, MSPT, ATC
Clinical Research Associate
PRO Sports Physical Therapy of Westchester
Nicholas Institute for Sports Medicine and Athletic Trauma (NISMAT)
Lenox Hill Hospital
Scarsdale, New York

Michael L. Voight, DHSc, PT, OCS, SCS, ATC, FAPTA
Professor
School of Physical Therapy
Belmont University
Nashville, Tennessee

Preface

Movement is an integral part of human experience. Functional movement is necessary for participation in all aspects of life, including activities of daily living, work, occupation, avocation, and sport. This philosophy is evident in the new Vision Statement that was adopted by the American Physical Therapy Association House of Delegates in June 2013:

"Transforming society by optimizing movement to improve the human experience."

In the 7 years since the last edition of the textbook, the focus of rehabilitation has become increasingly related to human movement. The editors and authors who have contributed to this textbook have been on this path for years. Together, we offer decades of highly variant experience in order to produce a textbook that offers a movement-based, functional perspective to the treatment of musculoskeletal dysfunction and injury. The art and science of caring for a patient or client is rooted in evidence-based practice, but requires knowledge of foundational sciences, application of theory, as well as skill, creativity, and innovation; however, above all we believe, it relates to movement. Several areas within the current 31-chapter edition have been expanded to best reflect the contemporary practice of physical therapy including clinical decision-making, algorithmic thinking, the neuromuscular scanning examination, functional movement screening, and the essentials of functional exercise.

The purpose of this text is to provide a comprehensive guide to assist practitioners in the design, implementation, and progression of rehabilitation programs for patients with musculoskeletal dysfunction. This includes dysfunction that occurs due to imbalance, overuse, injury, as well as postoperatively. It is intended for use in musculoskeletal intervention courses that teach students the application of theory, decision-making in therapeutic interventions, and rehabilitation progressions. However, it is equally well-suited for the practicing physical therapist looking for novel ideas for therapeutic interventions. The contributing authors have attempted to use our collective expertise, creativity, and knowledge to produce a textbook that encompasses many aspects of musculoskeletal rehabilitation and positively affects approaches to intervention, with a focus on function!

Organization

The text is divided into the same five parts as the previous edition. In Part 1: The Foundations of the Rehabilitation Process a revised chapter has been provided (Chapter 1) that summarizes *The Guide to Physical Therapist Practice*, as well as the important skill of clinical decision-making, highlighted by the use of algorithmic thinking. The other two chapters on tissue healing (Chapter 2) and the Neuromuscular Scan Examination (Chapter 3) complete the foundational concepts portion of the text that provides the basis for each of the upcoming sections. Very little time is spent on the process of examination in musculoskeletal practice, as the focus of this text is intervention.

Part 2: Treating Physiologic Impairments During Rehabilitation provides in-depth information about the general impairments that may need to be addressed throughout all phases of rehabilitation. These chapters include information about the management of pain (Chapter 4); an updated chapter on posture and function (Chapter 5); muscle performance

(Chapter 6); endurance and aerobic capacity (Chapter 7); mobility and range of motion (Chapter 8); and neuromuscular function (Chapter 9). Each of these introductory chapters highlights both methods for managing impairments described in the subsequent chapters, as well as new "clinical pearl" boxes to highlight the authors experience with regard to interventions.

Part 3: The Tools of Rehabilitation provides the reader with an overview of rehabilitation "tools" that can be used during the rehabilitation of many types of patients or clients. It provides the reader with detailed information on how each tool can be applied throughout the rehabilitation process in order to achieve high-level outcomes that are functionally relevant. The tools of rehabilitation covered in this part include: plyometric exercise (Chapter 10); open- and closed-kinetic chain interventions (Chapter 11); proprioceptive neuromuscular facilitation techniques (Chapter 12); joint mobilization (Chapter 13); postural stability and balance interventions (Chapter 14); core stabilization training (Chapter 15); aquatic therapy (Chapter 16); functional movement screening (Chapter 17); functional exercise and progressions (Chapter 18); and the essentials of functional exercise interventions, including a novel exercise prescription and progression matrix (Chapter 19). Of note are the updated chapters on functional movement screening and functional intervention, reflecting paradigm shifts in practice.

The fourth part of the text uses a regional approach to address specific application of intervention throughout the body. Part 4: Interventions for Specific Injuries builds upon the varied information presented in Part 3, by offering applications of techniques and interventions related to common overuse, traumatic, and postoperative musculoskeletal dysfunction. Included are detailed rehabilitation suggestions for conditions common to the shoulder complex (Chapter 20); the elbow (Chapter 21); the wrist, hand, and digits (Chapter 22); the groin, hip, and thigh (Chapter 23); the knee (Chapter 24), the lower leg (Chapter 25); the ankle and foot (Chapter 26); the cervical and thoracic spines (Chapter 27); and the lumbar spine (Chapter 28). Of note is the addition of the comprehensive chapter on the cervical and thoracic region. Each of these regionally based chapters provides in-depth discussion of pathomechanics and injury mechanisms while focusing on rehabilitation strategies and concerns for specific injuries and providing example protocols. As the title indicates, this is a textbook dedicated to intervention. Thus, it should be noted that detailed examination strategies and special test procedures are not a part of these regional chapters; therefore, it is likely that this text will accompany a text on examination, differential diagnosis, evaluation, and prognosis.

The fifth part of the text, Part 5: Special Considerations for Specific Populations, provides application of all the previous intervention strategies and how these may need to be selected, adapted, and utilized in three unique groups of patients: the geriatric patient (Chapter 29), the pediatric patient (Chapter 30), and the physically active female (Chapter 31). The editors and authors believe that these groups of patients deserve special consideration and attention during the rehabilitation process.

Updated, Evidence-based Intervention Strategies

Musculoskeletal Interventions: Techniques for Therapeutic Exercise, 3rd ed, offers a state-of-the art comprehensive collection of rehabilitation techniques and strategies for the physical therapist who intervenes with patients of all ages, abilities, and functional levels. The contributing authors have made every attempt to provide the reader with updated, evidence-based strategies for patient management, while reflecting our unique experience and creativity. The editors have assembled a group of experienced and well-respected clinicians, researchers, and academics/educators in order to cover all aspects of musculoskeletal rehabilitation. All updates were submitted to critical editorial review to ensure accuracy and relevancy.

Learning Aids

The learning aids provided in this text include:

Objectives—provided at the beginning of each chapter presented to identify critical concepts presented within each chapter.
Tables—for presentation of concepts and organization of complex information.
Figures—updated full-color illustrations and figures are a feature of the third edition!
"Clinical Pearls," new to this edition to assist the reader in application of concepts and offer insights or connections between information, as provided by the authors of chapters.
Summary points provided at the end of each chapter outlining major points within, for the reader to determine their level of comprehension.
End of Chapter Treatment Guidelines—present in the regionally organized chapters to illustrate a possible sequence of interventions or a postoperative protocol.
References—a comprehensive, updated list of references is provided with each chapter.

Instructor Resources

Power Points—Tables and photographs in the text will be available as PowerPoints to professors who adopt the text
Videos—Videos of critical skills in the text will be available to professors who adopt the text and a larger selection of the video library will be available to AccessPhysiotherapy subscribers
Enhanced Ebook—This third edition will also be offered as an enhanced ebook, which will incorporate videos and include interactive quizzes.

Acknowledgments

This textbook is all about movement: movement within the profession of physical therapy, movement as a part of human function, and movement in personal goals, dreams, and career paths that occur during a lifetime. The process of preparing and editing the 31 chapter manuscripts for this textbook was daunting in the face of all of the other activities and demands of life. The collaborative dedication of three editors with a common goal of producing a unique, relevant, and current textbook on musculoskeletal intervention made this revision possible. The three editors of this text each bring a unique perspective regarding writing, therapeutic exercise, clinical interventions, and the process of rehabilitation. Even amid our differences we were able to work together, achieve a common vision, and have this updated textbook to show for it!

We would like to personally thank each of the amazing contributing authors. They were asked to contribute to this text because we have tremendous respect for them personally and professionally. These individuals have distinguished themselves as educators, clinicians, and researchers, dedicated to the rehabilitation of a wide variety of individuals of all abilities, ages, and walks of life. We are exceedingly grateful for their input and willingness to share their ideas in writing and pictures.

Finally, we would collectively like to thank people important to us throughout our careers and the process of revising and editing this textbook. To our many friends and colleagues who have contributed to "who we are today" with creative thinking, intellectual challenges, and mentorship; you have shaped and influenced us, for that we are grateful. You have instilled in each of us the desire to continue learning, to challenge others to learn, grow, be change agents, and to seek continued improvement in the practice of physical therapy. These same friends and colleagues constantly keep us growing (older), laughing, loving life, and enjoying the many blessings of careers in rehabilitation.

Barb would like thank her great family; Dave, Lindsay, and Matthew—who continually support her during her crazy adventures; which often equate to time away from home. Barb would also like to thank her parents for their guidance, encouragement, and love of education and writing. Their examples have shaped a lifetime of goals and dreams. Finally, thanks to her sports physical therapy colleagues and the DPT students at Grand Valley State University who keep her moving, learning, and growing every day.

Mike would like to give special thanks to several individuals. First to his co-editors/authors, Barb and Bill who put up with countless rewrites and missed deadlines while at the same time constantly changing things—thanks, I owe both of them an extreme debt of gratitude; secondly, to John Halle and his colleagues at Belmont University. They have provided him the academic freedom and time to pursue this project. They challenge him every day to seek excellence. And lastly, to his close family; his parents who started him down the right path and gave him educational freedom; to his mentor Tab Blackburn, who has continued to give him professional direction; and finally to his wife Cissy, who has had to pay the price for his passion for excellence while at the same time providing inspiring wisdom and endless support to help sustain his passion for being an educator.

Bill would like to thank his family—Tena, Brian, and Zachary—who make an effort such as this worthwhile. They keep him grounded and help to maintain his focus in both his personal and professional life.

Thank-you to all—we enjoyed the ride and hope you enjoy the outcome!

Barbara J. Hoogenboom
Michael L. Voight
William E. Prentice

1

Introduction to the Therapeutic Interventions

The Guide to Physical Therapist Practice, Clinical Reasoning, and an Algorithmic-Approach to Intervention

Barbara J. Hoogenboom and Michael L. Voight

OBJECTIVES **After completion of this chapter, the physical therapist should be able to do the following:**

- Describe components of *The Guide to Physical Therapist Practice,* and its relationship to the 4 elements of the disablement model as described by Saad Nagi.
- Compare and contrast the disablement model, the medical model, and a functional movement model of dealing with the effects of injury and dysfunction.
- Identify the components of the examination process as defined by *The Guide*.
- Describe the components of and sequence of steps in the clinical decision-making process related to evaluation, diagnosis, prognosis, and intervention.
- Contrast novice and expert clinical reasoning and decision making in physical therapist practice.
- Relate clinical reasoning to quality provision of physical therapy, in terms of both diagnosis and selection of interventions.

(*continued*)

OBJECTIVES *(continued)*

- Relate evidence-based practice to clinical reasoning.
- Describe the algorithmic approach to clinical reasoning for intervention selection.
- Use sample basic algorithms to examine clinical reasoning for each of the 4 phases of rehabilitation (acute, intermediate, advanced, and return to function).
- Describe a basic algorithmic decision-making process based upon results of the examination.
- Articulate a movement-based philosophy upon which to construct plans for intervention in physical therapy practice.

Physical therapists play an exciting and vital role in the provision of health care. As a profession, physical therapists contribute in a variety of ways to the health care system. No longer are physical therapists seen only as providers of rehabilitation, but also as participants in the processes of patient education, disease prevention, and promotion of health and wellness. Physical therapists of the 21st century must have a united voice with regard to our scope of practice, our models of health care delivery, and the types of patients and clients we serve, as well as the types of examination measures and interventions we use to remedy or prevent impairments, functional limitations, and disabilities in our patients and clients. We must be active, knowledgeable educators of the public, other health care providers, third-party payers, and health policy makers as we advocate for the profession of physical therapy.

The Guide to Physical Therapist Practice

The Guide to Physical Therapist Practice (*The Guide*) was first published in the November 1997 issue of *Physical Therapy* as a document to describe the practice of physical therapy.[1] It was developed by consensus of an expert clinician panel, whose members were chosen from across the United States and who represented perspectives from a variety of practice settings. Prior to its publication, the document underwent extensive clinician review and repeated edits. *The Guide* is not a static document, rather it is a "living" document that is intended to grow and change with the profession of physical therapy. A revision to the original *The Guide* was published in 2001.[2] This evolution represented the culmination of input from the panels, educators, and clinicians, and attempted to improve the utility of *The Guide*. Subsequently, in 2003, *The Interactive Guide to Physical Therapist Practice* was released on CD-ROM, allowing access to a digital version of *The Guide*, search capabilities, and cross-referencing, as well as an index of tests and measures with hyperlinks to reliability and validity studies and citations.[3] Next, *The Guide* is anticipated to be updated to include the World Health Organization International Classification of Functioning, Disability, and Health (ICF) model.

The Guide is not a cookbook. It provides a framework for physical therapy practice, but does not provide clinical guidelines or protocols for intervention. Clinical guidelines must be developed based upon evidence, whereas the preferred practice patterns contained in *The Guide* are merely patterns considered by *The Guide* developers as most commonly used or most appropriate patterns of patient and client intervention.[7] Likewise, there is neither a recommended fee structure in *The Guide* nor any direct connection to current procedural terminology codes. Although some (International Classification of Diseases) ICD-9 codes are listed and referred to in Part 2, they should not be used to code for billing purposes. *The Guide* does not specify the site of care; rather, it uses the *episode of care* concept that crosses all rehabilitation settings related to each episode. *The Guide* also does not address the state-to-state variances in the scope of practice.

Disablement Model

The Guide was developed based upon the disablement model developed by Saad Nagi in 1969.[22] It was designed to describe the effects of disease and injury at both the personal and societal levels as well as their functional consequences. The disablement model emphasizes the functional and health status of individuals, with intervention based on improving these aspects of the patient's condition.[1-3] The model has 4 elements:

Pathology ↔ *Impairment* ↔ *Functional limitation* ↔ *Disability*

Pathology is the interruption of the normal cellular processes from a biomechanical, physiologic, or anatomic perspective.[1-3] The body often responds to an injury or pathology with a defensive reaction in order to restore the normal state. Examples of this include hemarthrosis in the case of ligament rupture, or the inflammatory process in response to connective tissue damage (tear/stretch). Intervention at this level is generally handled by physicians and is often pharmacologic and/or surgical in nature.

Impairment is any loss or abnormality of physiologic, psychological, or anatomic structure or function at the level of organs and body systems.[1-3] Physical therapists typically measure the signs and symptoms that present in conjunction with an injury, illness, or pathology, and identify the subsequent impairments. Physical therapists often intervene trying to attempt correctly identified impairments. Examples of physiologic impairments include muscle weakness, range-of-motion loss, pain, and abnormal joint play. Anatomic impairments include structural conditions such as genu recurvatum, scoliosis, femoral anteversion, and alterations in foot alignment.

Functional limitation is a deviation from the normal behavior in performing tasks and activities from that which would be considered traditional or expected for an individual.[1-3] Functional limitations are tasks or activities that are not performed in the usual efficient or skilled fashion. Problems with transfers, standing, walking, running, and climbing stairs are all examples of functional limitations.

Disability is the incapacity in performing a broad range of tasks and activities that are usually expected in specific social roles.[1-3] Inability to function as a spouse, student, parent, or worker (in the home or outside of the home) constitutes a disability.

The scope of physical therapist practice overlaps with many portions of the disablement model, as shown in Figure 1-1.

The disablement process is a 2-way continuum affected by intraindividual and extraindividual risk factors (Figure 1-2). Intraindividual factors include habits, lifestyle, behavior, psychosocial characteristics, age and sex, educational level and income, weight, and family history. Extraindividual factors comprise the medical care received, the pharmacologic and other therapies available, the physical environment, and any external supports. The relationship between these aspects will vary between individuals and will ultimately determine the impact of the disease or injury.

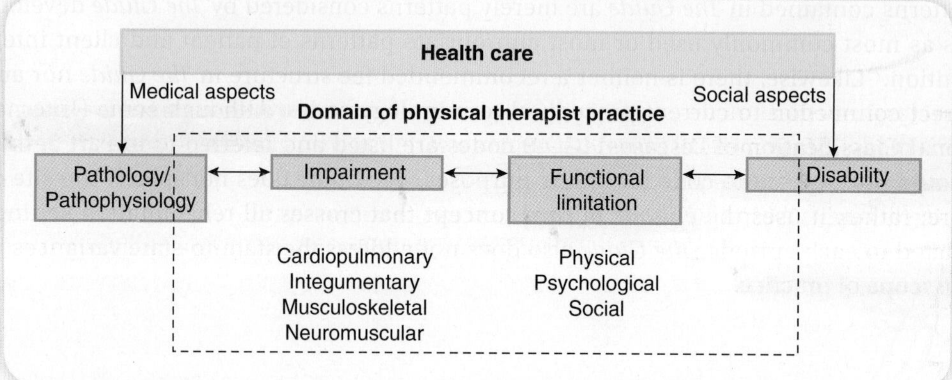

Figure 1-1

The scope of physical therapist practice within the continuum of health care services and the context of the disablement model. (Reproduced, with permission, from the American Physical Therapy Association [APTA]. The guide to physical therapist practice. 2nd ed. *Phys Ther*. 2001;81(1):9-738.)

Most physical therapists have treated patients who had significant impairments but remained extremely functional. Most have also treated patients who were disabled by what seemed to be minor impairments or functional limitations. Unfortunately, there are few studies in the literature to show a direct cause-and-effect relationship between impairments, functional limitations, and disability. In addition to the Nagi model, *The Guide* is also strongly influenced by 2 additional conceptual frameworks: the integration of prevention and wellness strategies and the patient/client management model. These influential frameworks are discussed further in subsequent sections.

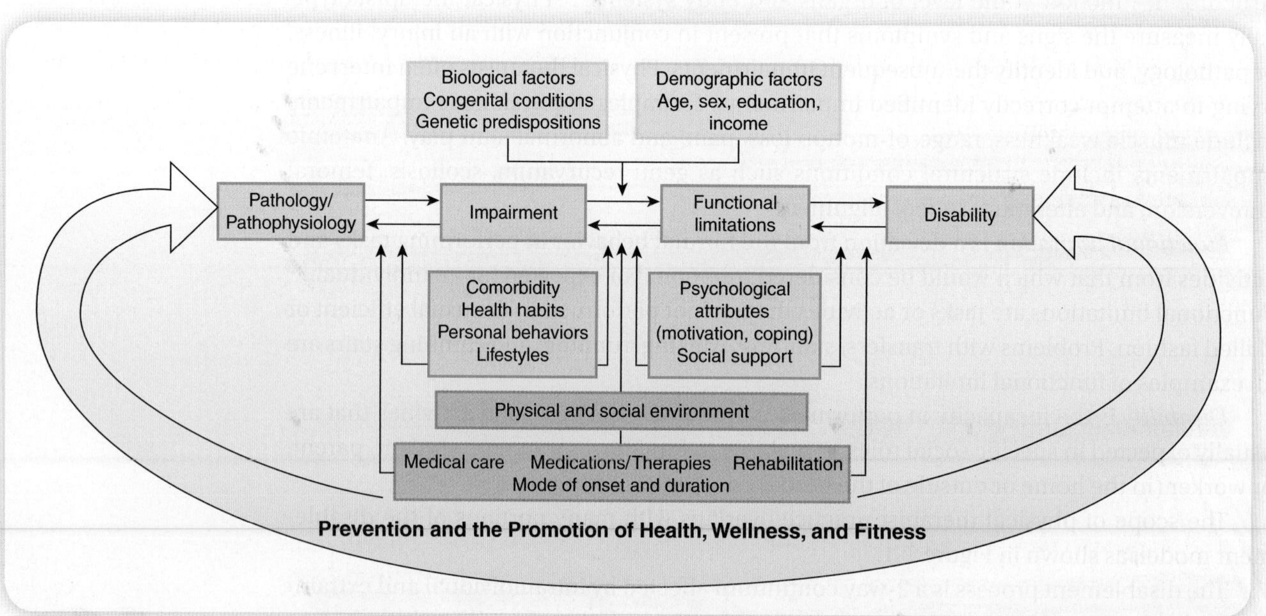

Figure 1-2

An expanded disablement model showing interactions among individual and environmental factors, prevention, and the promotion of health, wellness, and fitness. (Reproduced, with permission, from the APTA. The guide to physical therapist practice. 2nd ed. *Phys Ther*. 2001;81(1):9-738.)

Other Models of Patient Management

The classic medical model of patient management is distinctly different from the disablement model. Many medical providers address a wide variety of disease processes, illnesses, or injuries that patients present with, using the medical patient management model. This typically begins with the history and physical examination (not unlike that which occurs during the disablement model), which is typically followed by some type of additional invasive tests or measures such as lab work or diagnostic imaging. The combination of the history and physical and additional tests allow the practitioner to arrive at a cellular, structural, or systems level diagnosis. Typically, pharmacologic or other medical management is utilized, or the patient or client is referred to surgery, with the ultimate goal being cure or repair of the tissue, system, or structure. In this model, referral to other practitioners may also accompany treatment, with the goal remaining cure or repair of the errant tissue, system, or structure.

Finally, a new functional movement model is emerging in physical therapist practice. This model uses the analysis of basic functional movements in order to determine if a movement dysfunction is present, as compared to attempting to describe dysfunction at the impairment level. The strength of using this model is that the practitioner can work algorithmically "backward" in order to determine the actual cause of the movement impairment. Through the use of systematic examination procedures and algorithmic thinking, the clinician is able to arrive at the specific impairment and then begin functionally based interventions that assist the patient or client in return to optimal function. Algorithms are discussed in the Introduction to Algorithm section of this chapter, while functional movement assessment and intervention is covered thoroughly in Chapters 19 and 20.

Overview of *The Guide:* Part 1

The original purpose of *The Guide* was to improve the quality of physical therapy, promote appropriate use of services, enhance customer satisfaction, and reduce unwarranted variations in physical therapy management. Prevention and wellness initiatives are also stressed and will help decrease the need for services.[1-3]

Chapter 1 provides a description of "who" physical therapists are and "what" they do. This description includes the various practice settings in which a physical therapist may practice, including some less traditional ones like corporate or industrial health centers and fitness centers. In this chapter, the terms "patients" and "clients" are defined as

- **Patients** are "individuals who are the recipients of physical therapy examination, evaluation, diagnosis, prognosis, and intervention and who have a disease, disorder, condition impairment, functional limitation, or disability" (Ref. 2, p. 689)
- **Clients** are "individuals who engage the services of a physical therapist and who can benefit from the physical therapist's consultation, interventions, professional advice, health promotion, fitness, wellness, or prevention services" (Ref. 2, p. 685). Clients are also businesses, school systems, and others to whom physical therapists provide services.[1-3]

The chapter continues with a general discussion of the scope of practice for physical therapists, acknowledging that this varies by state. Physical therapists provide direct services to patients as well as interact with other professionals, provide prevention and wellness services, consult, engage in critical inquiry (research), educate, administrate, and supervise support personnel.

Physical therapy is an integral part of secondary and tertiary rehabilitative care. Chapter 1 of *The Guide* expands on this model with a discussion of the physical therapist's role in primary care and in wellness. The concepts of primary care and wellness involve restoring health, alleviating pain, and preventing the onset of impairments, functional limitations, disabilities, or changes in physical function and health status resulting from injury, disease, or other causes.[1,2] Physical therapists play major roles in secondary and tertiary care of those with conditions of the musculoskeletal, neuromuscular, cardiovascular/pulmonary, and integumentary systems that may have been treated primarily by another practitioner. Often, secondary care is provided in acute care and rehabilitation hospitals as well as outpatient clinics, home health settings, and within school systems.[2,3] Tertiary care is often provided by physical therapists in more specialized, comprehensive, technologically advanced settings in response to another health care practitioners' request for consultation and specialized services offered by the therapist.[1-3]

The clinical decision-making process presented in *The Guide* comprises the 5 elements of the patient/client management model (Figure 1-3): examination, evaluation, diagnosis, prognosis, and intervention. This clinical decision-making model is explored in greater depth later in this chapter in the section titled Clinical Reasoning and Decision Making.

The physical therapist begins with a thorough *examination*. Because the focus of this text is intervention, the examination process will not be described in detail.

The next 3 steps in the process involve ***decision making***. Using the information gathered through the examination, the physical therapist formulates an *evaluation*. This is the clinical judgement that results from assessing the situation in its entirety from multiple points of view. Factors such as loss of function or presence of dysfunctional movement patterns, social considerations, and health status are taken into consideration when developing a *diagnosis* (cluster of signs and symptoms) and *prognosis* (optimal level of improvement and time to get there), which guides the interventions that are chosen and performed during comprehensive management of the patient.[1]

Intervention describes the skilled interaction of the physical therapist when performing the therapeutic techniques and/or delegating and overseeing services. The goal is to produce a positive change in the condition or functional performance of the patient. Intervention strategies should be constantly evaluated and reevaluated for their effectiveness with goals of remediation of impairments, improvement in functional outcomes, as well as secondary and tertiary prevention and the goal of long-term wellness. Continued care is based on the patient's response and progress toward the determined goals.[1-3]

There are 3 important components to the intervention: (a) coordination, communication, and documentation; (b) patient/client-related instruction (education); and (c) procedural interventions. Management of every patient will include some aspect of the first 2 intervention components and often 1 or more procedural interventions. There are 9 procedural interventions, listed by level of importance and utilization in the practice of physical therapy:

- Therapeutic exercise (the focus of this textbook)
- Functional training in self-care and home management
- Functional training in work, community, and leisure integration or reintegration
- Manual therapy techniques, including mobilization/manipulation
- Prescription, application, and, as appropriate, fabrication of devices and equipment
- Airway clearance techniques
- Integumentary repair and protective techniques
- Electrotherapeutic modalities
- Physical agents and mechanical modalities

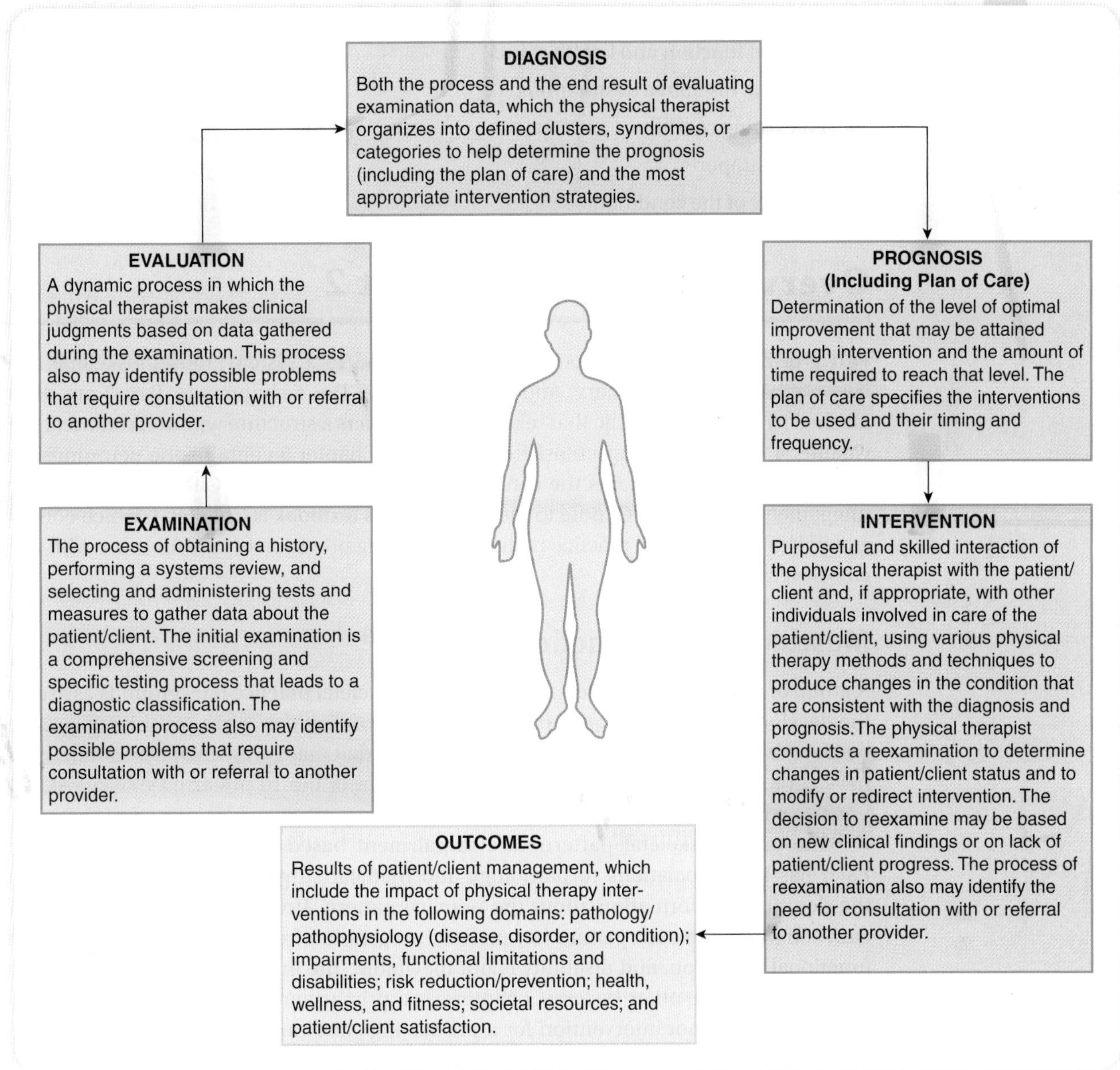

Figure 1-3 The patient/client management model

An expanded disablement model showing interactions among individual and environmental factors, prevention, and the promotion of health, wellness, and fitness. (Reproduced, with permission, from the APTA. The guide to physical therapist practice. 2nd ed. *Phys Ther*. 2001;81(1):9-738.)

Examination findings, the evaluation, diagnosis, and prognosis and any available research evidence should support the choice of intervention. Factors that might influence the choice of interventions as well as the prognosis include[1]:

- Chronicity or severity of current condition
- Level of current impairment
- Functional limitation or disability
- Living environment

- Multisite or multisystem involvement
- Physical function and health status
- Potential discharge destinations
- Preexisting conditions or diseases
- Social supports
- Stability of the condition(s)

Overview of *The Guide*: Part 2

Part 2 of *The Guide* has 4 sections, each dedicated to a system: musculoskeletal, neuromuscular, cardiopulmonary, and integumentary. The 4 chapters in Part 2 are distinguished by a specific graphic that relates to and depicts a structure within the content area. Chapter 4 contains the musculoskeletal patterns, Chapter 5 contains the neuromuscular patterns, Chapter 6 contains the cardiopulmonary patterns, and Chapter 7 contains the integumentary patterns. Of note to the reader of this textbook is Chapter 4, which contains general information and practice patterns describing provision of care for those with musculoskeletal dysfunction.

Musculoskeletal Practice Patterns[1-3]

A group of experts from a wide variety of musculoskeletal practice backgrounds assisted in the development of the practice patterns. Patterns of disorders were considered, grouped because of their similarities, and it was determined that many were managed similarly and have comparable outcomes. Thus, the development of the 10 preferred musculoskeletal practice patterns occurred.

The musculoskeletal patterns are impairment based and their titles reflect this. Each has key associations to pathology and medical/surgical diagnoses noted within the descriptive information about the practice pattern. Primary prevention is a significant component to each pattern because the progression from pathology to impairment, functional limitation, and disability is not inevitable. The first preferred practice pattern, like the first in the other systems' chapters, is a primary prevention pattern. The aim of such a pattern is not intervention for a preexisting condition, impairment, or functional limitation, rather prevention of each of these conditions. The rest of the patterns are for intervention in conditions that fit into the cluster of signs and symptoms that form the movement-based diagnosis. The following is a description of each pattern, the purpose of which is to get a sense of which patients and diagnoses would fall within this category of practice patterns[1-3]:

4A. Primary prevention/risk reduction for skeletal demineralization

4B. Impaired posture

4C. Impaired muscle performance

4D. Impaired joint mobility, motor function, muscle performance, and range of motion associated with connective tissue dysfunction

4E. Impaired joint mobility, motor function, muscle performance, and range of motion associated with localized inflammation

4F. Impaired joint mobility, motor function, muscle performance, range of motion, and reflex integrity associated with spinal disorders

4G. Impaired joint mobility, motor function, muscle performance, and range of motion associated with fracture

4H. Impaired joint mobility, motor function, muscle performance, and range of motion associated with joint arthroplasty

4I. Impaired joint mobility, motor function, muscle performance, and range of motion associated with bony or soft tissue surgery

4J. Impaired joint mobility, motor function, muscle performance, gait, locomotion, and balance associated with amputation

Clinical Pearl

Note that many of the first descriptive words in Musculoskeletal Practice Patterns 4D-4J are the same! They describe impairments and movement dysfunction commonly seen and predictably related in similar diagnostic groups.

The original *The Guide* had areas of musculoskeletal practice not covered by the preferred practice patterns. For instance, there was no pattern dealing with the management of patients with impairments caused by upper-extremity amputations. Because *The Guide* is a fluid document and is subject to updating and evolution, the second edition of *The Guide* included amputations of both the upper and the lower extremities. It is likely that other diagnoses will be added to or placed in different practice patterns on a regular basis as practice evolves and *The Guide* continues to evolve.

Overview of *The Guide*: Parts 3 and 4

When the second edition and revision of *The Guide* was initiated, a task force of expert clinicians and researchers was assembled to identify the vast array of test and measures used in examinations by a physical therapist and to collect the pertinent information on the reliability and validity of the tests or measures, as available in the peer-reviewed literature. Concomitantly, a second task force was convened to identify outcome measures relevant to physical therapist practice and provide similar documentation. The work of both groups was released on the CD-ROM version of *The Guide* as the *Catalog of Tests and Measures*.[3] These task forces also helped to create the outline of a minimal data set for initial examination and several templates for documentation, which can also be found in the second edition of *The Guide*. Because the focus of this textbook is intervention, the reader is directed to other comprehensive texts that exist regarding examination in physical therapy for additional information.

The impact of *The Guide to Physical Therapist Practice* on the profession of physical therapy is evident, although its utilization clinically and in academic institutions varies. Ongoing incorporation of *The Guide* into the practice of physical therapy will facilitate dialogue and improved understanding of how clinicians classify patients, develop clinical diagnoses, and determine prognoses for common groups of patients and clients. This document will continue to be a part of the professional landscape will continue to influence both the practice of and public understanding of physical therapy in positive ways.

Clinical Reasoning and Decision Making

Physical therapists make decisions related to examination, evaluation, diagnosis, prognosis, and intervention on a daily basis. Independent decision making is one of the hallmarks of an autonomous profession, a status for which the profession of physical therapy is striving.[6] To make reasoned, independent decisions, the physical therapist must use refined, well-developed, clinical reasoning skills. Higgs and Jones have defined clinical reasoning as the practice used by the therapist to *structure* the health care process.[12] Knowledge, clinical data, patient preferences, and professional judgment all play a role in clinical reasoning. Clinical reasoning can also be described as the progression used by practitioners to plan, direct, carry out, and reflect on patient care. Clearly clinical reasoning is not a simple process; rather, it is a complex and multifaceted process of analysis and synthesis. Such a process enables therapists to view the client and their rehabilitation with depth and breadth of understanding.

Clinical reasoning is described by Edwards et al as "a way of thinking and taking action within clinical practice" (Ref. 6, p. 322). Clinical reasoning is often first utilized in the examination process and has both diagnostic and narrative components.[6] The construct known as clinical reasoning has also been discussed in Chapter 3 in relationship to the scanning examination. Once again, it is important to note that the clinical reasoning process cannot be separated from knowledge. If insufficient knowledge is present, it is likely that diagnoses and decisions based on such knowledge will provide faulty conclusions. In other words, the clinical reasoning process is only as strong and viable as the knowledge base from which the diagnosis or clinical decision is rendered.

Good clinical decision making is key to effective patient/client management. Physical therapists play a critical role in assessing neuromusculoskeletal problems, formulating a comprehensive picture of the problem(s), and choosing interventions to efficiently manage the problem. As more patients enter the physical therapy system directly or via the general practitioner, the ability of the therapist to skillfully assess patients and determine the need for care is paramount. Many patients present or are referred to therapy without a clear diagnosis, especially in the realm of musculoskeletal practice. At the most basic level, the therapist must be able to make the crucial "keep–refer" decision regarding whether the treatment needed is within their scope of practice. If the choice is made to refer, the therapist must know how to do so in order to get the best care for the patient.

Skillful clinical decision making requires foundational knowledge of anatomy, kinesiology, and biomechanics that is applied to each patient. The use of such knowledge is critical to assessing normal and abnormal movement, as well as understanding both the pathologic and normal healing processes. Together, this frame of reference helps the therapist determine the diagnosis, prognosis, and plan of care.

Tacit knowledge combined with accumulated clinical experience contributes to the art of the practice of physical therapy. Bruning, Schraw, and Ronning describe *schemata* as the complex representations of phenomenon by which individuals receive, store, and organize information.[4] As schemata help therapists to organize and retrieve knowledge, scripts or procedural rules help to guide thinking and organize common occurrences or events. Both of these strategies support effective processing of information by providing efficient mental frameworks for handling complex information.

There are few certainties in patient care. Rather, biologic, physiologic, and psychological events occur in uncertain, but often in predictable patterns. Every problem solved or decision made by a clinician is probabilistic[11] and involves a combination of hypothesis testing and pattern recognition. Hypothetic deductive reasoning and early hypothesis generation can occur with a limited database and is a way to structure the clinical examination and thinking process. A hypothesis is really a clinical impression based on an assumption of causality. By definition, "a hypothesis is a testable idea—a tentative, but best, estimate that only time can prove correct" (Ref. 20, p. 1391). Hence, clinicians apply the clinical reasoning process to the clinical decision-making process for examination and diagnosis as well as selection of interventions.

Clinical Pearl

Effective decision-making about evaluation, diagnosis, and prognosis requires approaching the problem in a systematic and orderly fashion, and this approach can also carry over into decisions about therapeutic interventions.

Clearly, reasoning does not occur in a "clinician induced vacuum." Multiple factors play a role in the clinical reasoning process, not the least of which is the identified problem as it is seen and described by the patient. Narrative reasoning involves the ability to collect and attempt to understand patients' "stories,"[6] experiences, perspectives, contexts, cultural backgrounds, and beliefs. It is important to remember that the patient's personal descriptive traits and characteristics, culture, past experiences and history, comorbidities, life situation, and personal beliefs all strongly affect the process of clinical reasoning. Vital to the process of treatment planning is taking into account the problems as they are *seen by the patient*, named the patient-identified problems, as well as the non–patient-identified problems.[19] Non–patient-identified problems are problems not identified by the patient that may have been preexisting, unknown to a patient, or identified by the therapist or another. Identification of non–patient-identified problems are especially important for excellent care as well as a prevention- and wellness-orientated practice of physical therapy as described in *The Guide to Physical Therapist Practice* (Table 1-1).[1]

The second application of clinical reasoning is during the treatment planning and intervention selection process. Edwards[8] describes 6 types of reasoning that comprise decisions made regarding management of patients and clients. These are procedural or intervention reasoning, interactive patient–therapist rapport building reasoning, collaborative patient–therapist reasoning, instructional reasoning, predictive reasoning, and ethical reasoning. The prior-listed clinical reasoning strategies are often used in combination. An emergent

Table 1-1 HOAC II Definitions of Problems

Type of Problem	Definition	Examples
PIPs	Impairments, functional limitations, and disabilities, easily identified by the patient	Pain, loss of ROM about a joint, loss of strength, impaired gait, impaired ADLs
NPIPs	Problems identified by someone other than the patient such as a health care provider, caregiver or family member	Postural impairments, respiratory dysfunction, general deconditioning, musculoskeletal imbalances
Anticipated problems	Problems that do not exist at the current time, but may develop related to existing problems (both PIPs and NPIPs); can be prevented with proper management	Secondary shortening of muscles because of poor posture or gait deviations

ADL, Activities of daily living; NPIPs, non–patient-identified problems; PIPs, patient-identified problems; ROM, range of motion.

Data from Rothstein J, Echternach J, Riddle D. The Hypothesis-Oriented Algorithm for Clinicians II (HOAC II): a guide for patient management. *Phys Ther*. 2003;83:455-470.

dialectical model of clinical reasoning that includes cognitive and decision-making processes (hypothetic-deductive reasoning), as well as reasoning skills necessary to interact with patients in their individual unique scaffold of experience, personality, and assumptions (narrative or communicative reasoning), has been reported in the literature.[2,6,7,11,12] Although each individual must ultimately construct their own schemata and procedural rules for clinical reasoning, tools exist that may assist practitioners to develop expert skills.[20]

Expert Versus Novice Decision Making

There is a well-developed body of literature about how experts make decisions.[7,8,11,17] Experienced clinicians use a well-developed collection of clinical experiences for their reasoning, while novice clinicians rely on clear-cut patterns and clues. Experts see meaningful patterns, solve problems quickly, and rely on self-monitoring (reflection).[12]

May and Dennis stated: "Experts, when compared with novices in the same field, exhibit a superior structuring of knowledge into clinically relevant patterns that are unlocked by key cues in the decision environment. Patterns stored in memory enable the expert to recognize meaningful relationships and generate likely hypotheses" (Ref. 17, p. 191). In research across many health professions, experts have been shown to excel within their specific knowledge domains, are able to see relationships, possess enhanced memory (relates to banked experience), are skilled in qualitative analysis, and have well-developed reflection skills.[12]

Likewise, researchers agree that novice decision makers function differently than their expert counterparts. They tend to value quantitative data, likely have more error during the process, and are slower in problem solving.[12]

How then do novices develop into competent decision makers and experts? Although experience is necessary for the contextual problem-solving process used by experts, less is known about the process of how problem-solving expertise is developed.[13] A major distinction that has been described between expert and novice problem solvers is that experts use *forward reasoning* rather than the *backward reasoning* or hypothetic-deductive process used by novices.[7,8] Forward reasoning is the application of a number of "if-then" rules to a problem to move forward from data to diagnosis or treatment intervention. An algorithmic approach seeks to use a number of "if-then" decisions to assist in problem solving. As previously noted, any problem-solving model that attempts to assist novices and developing clinicians must take into account the knowledge base and organizational skills of the individual. Practitioners with "high knowledge" make more inferences from prior knowledge than novices and intermediate level practioners.[8] Interestingly, experts often seem to do less problem solving than novices because they have a depth and breadth of previously stored solutions to clinical problems that they recall and use.[14] It should be noted, however, that experience alone does not always provide *accurate* solutions to problems or enable clinicians to make efficient, reasoned diagnoses. Although novices tend to solve problems incorrectly or simplistically, experts can also develop patterned thinking and rely too heavily on experience and make premature diagnoses without fully examining subtle possibilities and varied data.[15]

Problem Solving, Clinical Decision Making, and the Use of Evidence-Based Practice

Being a good problem solver is not sufficient in this day and age. According to Miller, Nyland, and Wormal, "rehabilitation clinicians must be creative problem solvers who can translate relevant research into functional interventions" (Ref. 18, p. 453). It is important to remember that in contemporary physical therapy practice, decisions related to clinical practice should be based on the best available evidence whenever possible.

Clinicians should use the available literature to determine the best treatment(s) for their patients. Evidence-based practice has been defined as "the conscientious and judicious use of current best evidence in making decisions about the care of individual patients."[21,25] Implicit in this definition is the need for a method of determining what constitutes the "best" evidence. Before evidence can be integrated into the management of patients, an appraisal of the quality of the evidence must be completed. A major problem in the appraisal process is that of deciding whether the evidence is definitive enough to indicate an effect other than chance. The ability to judge and interpret the evidence for intervention techniques is a skill that must be developed if a clinician wishes to become evidenced based in their practice. Therefore, the ability to interpret and evaluate the evidence becomes an integral part in the clinical decision-making process. The standard for the assessment of the efficacy and value of intervention is the clinical trial. Most desirable is the prospective study, which assesses the effect and value of an intervention against those found in a control group, using human subjects.[9] Unfortunately, many of the studies in the literature that address physical therapy topics are not clinical trials, as there is no control to judge efficacy of the intervention and there are no interventions from which to draw comparisons.[3] In addition to a control group, the ideal clinical trial uses a blinded, randomized design, both for subject assignment to groups and for assessment of outcomes (Table 1-2).[5] The control can be a current standard practice, a placebo, or no active intervention.[9] Clinicians must constantly remind themselves that without information gathered from controlled clinical trials, they have limited scientific basis for their interventions. Many interventions offered by physical therapists use low levels of evidence or worse, personal testimony for the rationale behind their use. As the profession grows and the evidence base from which physical therapists can glean information

Table 1-2 Levels of Evidence for Research

Level of Evidence	Types of Studies
Level	• High-quality randomized controlled trials • Systematic review of level I randomized controlled trials • Prospective studies (all patients enrolled at the same point in their pathology with >80% follow-up of enrolled patients)
Level II	• Prospective cohort studies • Poor-quality randomized controlled trial (eg, no blinding, or improper randomization, <80% follow-up) • Systematic review of level II studies • Retrospective study • Study of untreated controls from a previous randomized controlled trial
Level III	• Case-control studies • Retrospective cohort studies • Systematic review of level III studies
Level IV	• Case series (no, or historical, control group)
Level V	• Expert opinion

Data from the *J Bone Joint Surg*, instructions for Authors.

increases, the correctness, defensibility, and ultimately the effectiveness of chosen interventions can only increase.

Evidence-based practice is the standard to which physical therapists must strive for direction in clinical decision-making and problem solving related to both diagnosis and selection of interventions. Frequent, speedy use of evidence to answer clinical questions, base decisions, or solve problems is mandatory as the profession of physical therapy continues to develop and grow.

Introduction to Algorithms

Algorithms are tools that assist practitioners in the development of expert skills. *Encyclopedia Britannica* defines an algorithm as "systematic procedure that produces—in a finite number of steps—the answer to a question or the solution of a problem."[10] An algorithm provides a graphic, step-by-step procedure for guiding decision making. Alternately, algorithms have been described as decision trees. In medical fields, algorithms are developed and used for clinical decision making related to the diagnostic process and management of cases. Algorithms can provide structured care pathways and a systematic approach to the selection of therapeutic interventions. Because algorithms are *not* prescriptive or protocol driven, they allow for clinical decisions and adjustments to be made during the clinical reasoning and decision-making processes. Algorithmic thinking and the associated graphic structure seems to fit the forward reasoning process previously described as being used by experts. An algorithm is simply a decision tree filled with "if–then" decisions related to examination and intervention planning. Rothstein and Echternach[24] described a conceptual scheme for problem solving in physical therapy that they named the *hypothesis-oriented algorithm for clinicians* (HOAC). This algorithm-based scheme was designed to guide the therapist from evaluation to intervention planning with a logical sequence of activities. The HOAC requires the therapist to define goals for patient intervention and determine if they have been met, thereby assisting in clinical decision making. It also requires that the therapist generate hypotheses early in the examination process regarding the underlying cause(s) of functional limitations. Such a strategy is often used by expert physicians and therapists.

The first part of the HOAC is a sequential guide to examination and planning of interventions. The second part of the HOAC is a branching diagram (algorithm) that relates to clinical decisions that must be made throughout the patient care interventions. The HOAC requires that the therapist relate all interventions to hypotheses, thereby forcing justification of all aspects of interventions. Use of such an algorithm-based approach should promote use of suitable, evidence-based interventions and discourage the use of "popular" or routine interventions. In response to changes in the health care system and the practice of physical therapy, the HOAC was revised and became the HOAC II (Figures 1-4 to 1-7).[19] The authors of the HOAC II contend that it links the use of evidence in decision making and documentation of the type and scope of evidence used in the examination and intervention processes. Such a linkage or connection between evidence and intervention selection and planning is important in the current climate of health care. Physical therapists must justify and provide evidence for selected interventions whenever possible. The HOAC II also provides the physical therapist with a tool for planning and evaluating activities intended for prevention. Like the original HOAC, the second part of the HOAC II is an algorithm that covers intervention, monitoring of intervention effects, and altering the plan of care appropriately to progress toward desired outcomes. Although a detailed discussion of the HOAC and the HOAC II is beyond the scope of this chapter, both are valuable tools that have influenced the current authors thinking about use of algorithms in treatment planning and intervention selection.

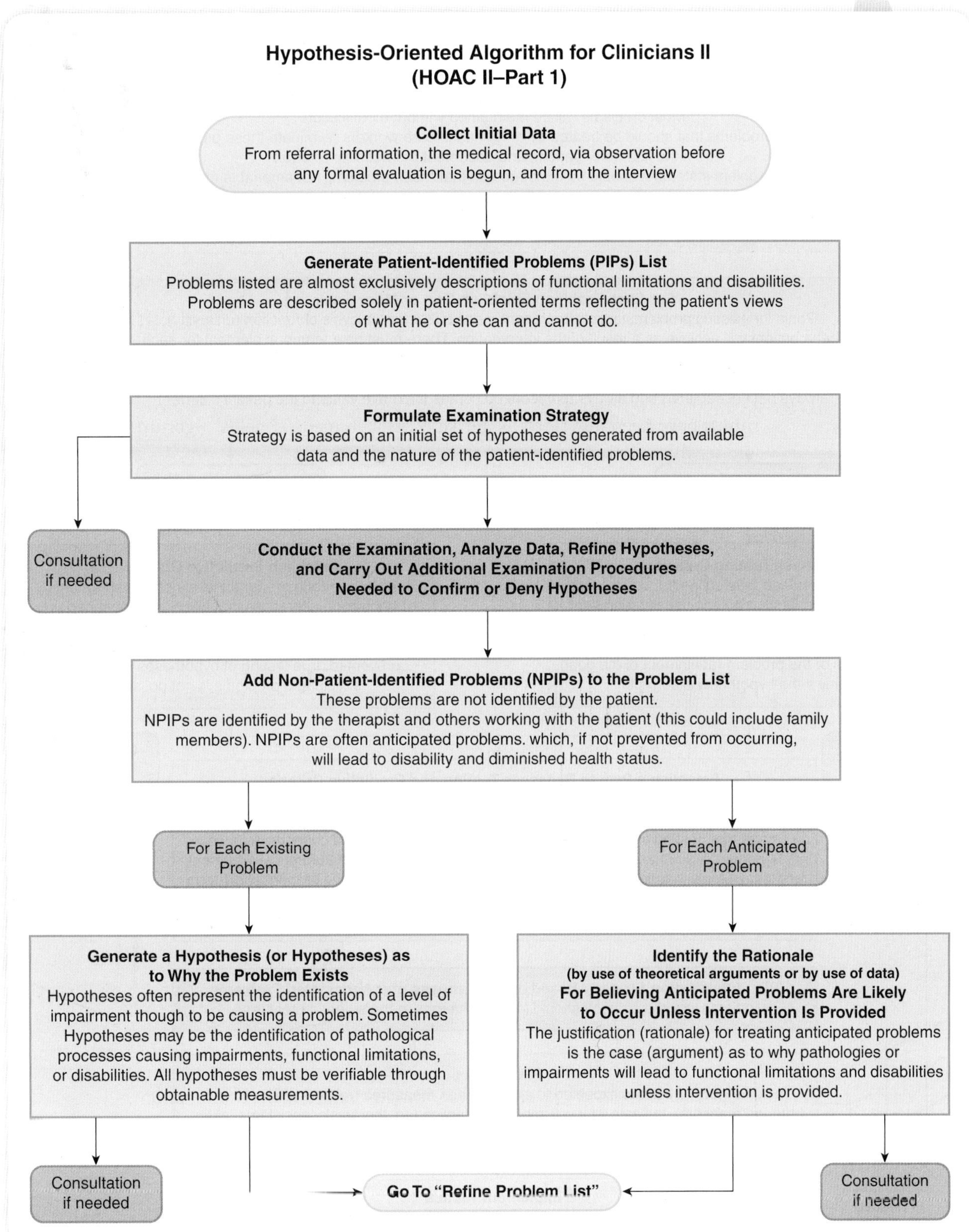

Figure 1-4 **HOAC II diagram 1**

The initial steps of part 1 of the HOAC II. (Reproduced, with permission, from the APTA, from Rothstein J, Echternach J, Riddle D. The Hypothesis-Oriented Algorithm for Clinicians II (HOAC II): a guide for patient management. *Phys Ther*. 2003;83:455-470.)

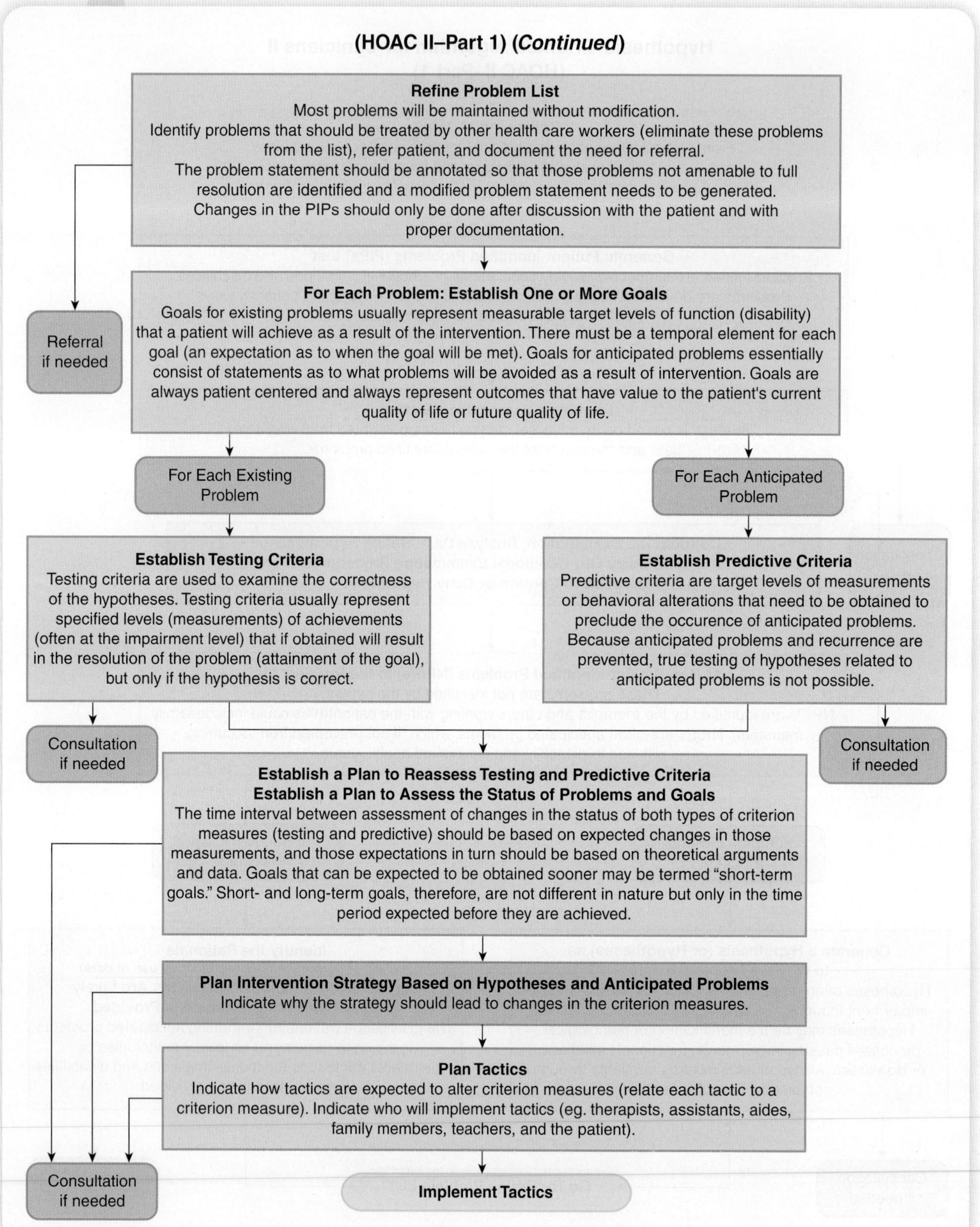

Figure 1-5 **HOAC II diagram 2**

The final steps of Part 1 of the HOAC II. (Reproduced, with permission, from the APTA, from Rothstein J, Echternach J, Riddle D. The Hypothesis-Oriented Algorithm for Clinicians II (HOAC II): a guide for patient management. *Phys Ther*. 2003;83:455-470.)

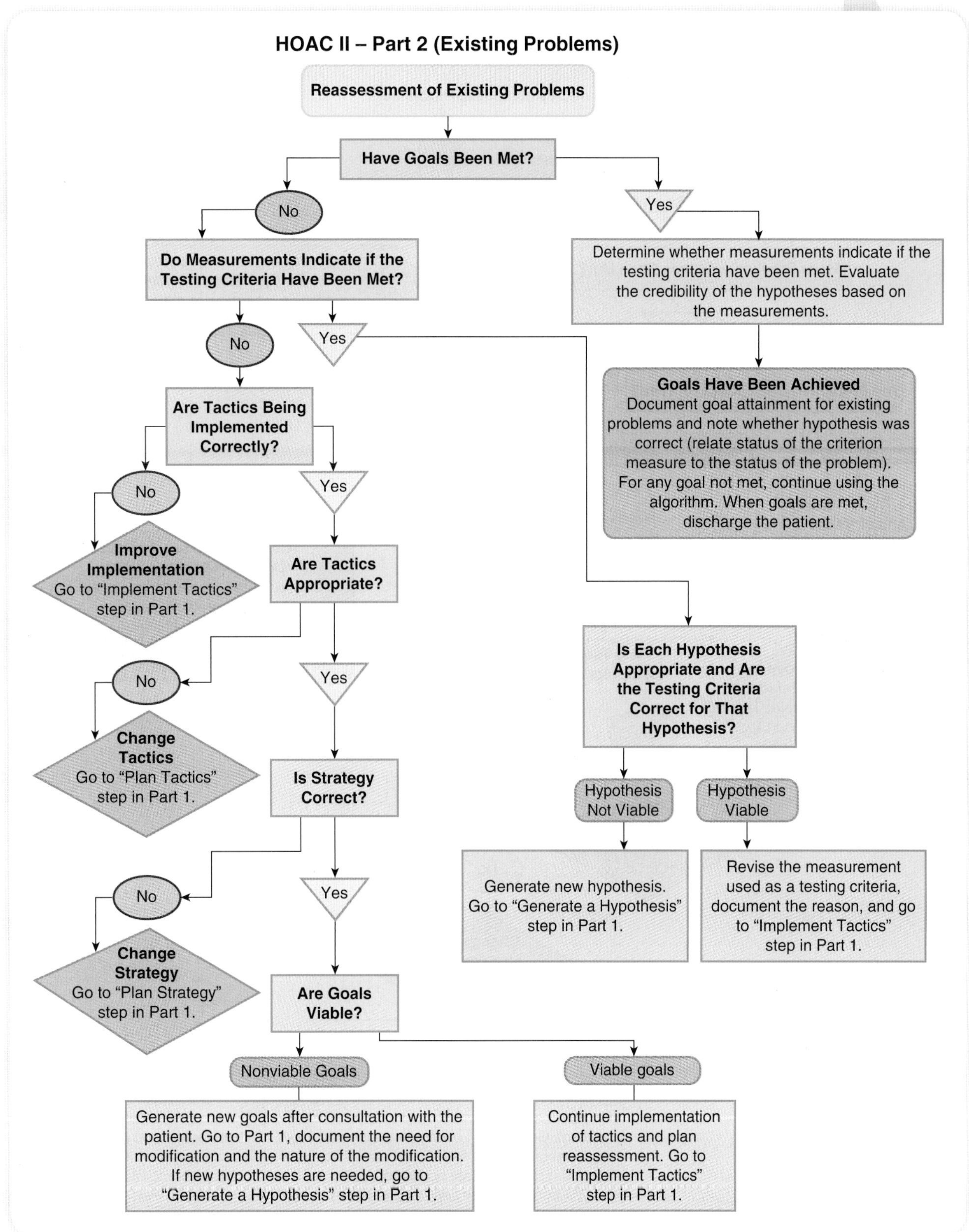

Figure 1-6 **HOAC II diagram 3**

The algorithm for reassessment of existing problems in part 2 of the HOAC II. (Reproduced, with permission, from the APTA, from Rothstein J, Echternach J, Riddle D. The Hypothesis-Oriented Algorithm for Clinicians II (HOAC II): a guide for patient management. *Phys Ther*. 2003;83:455-470.)

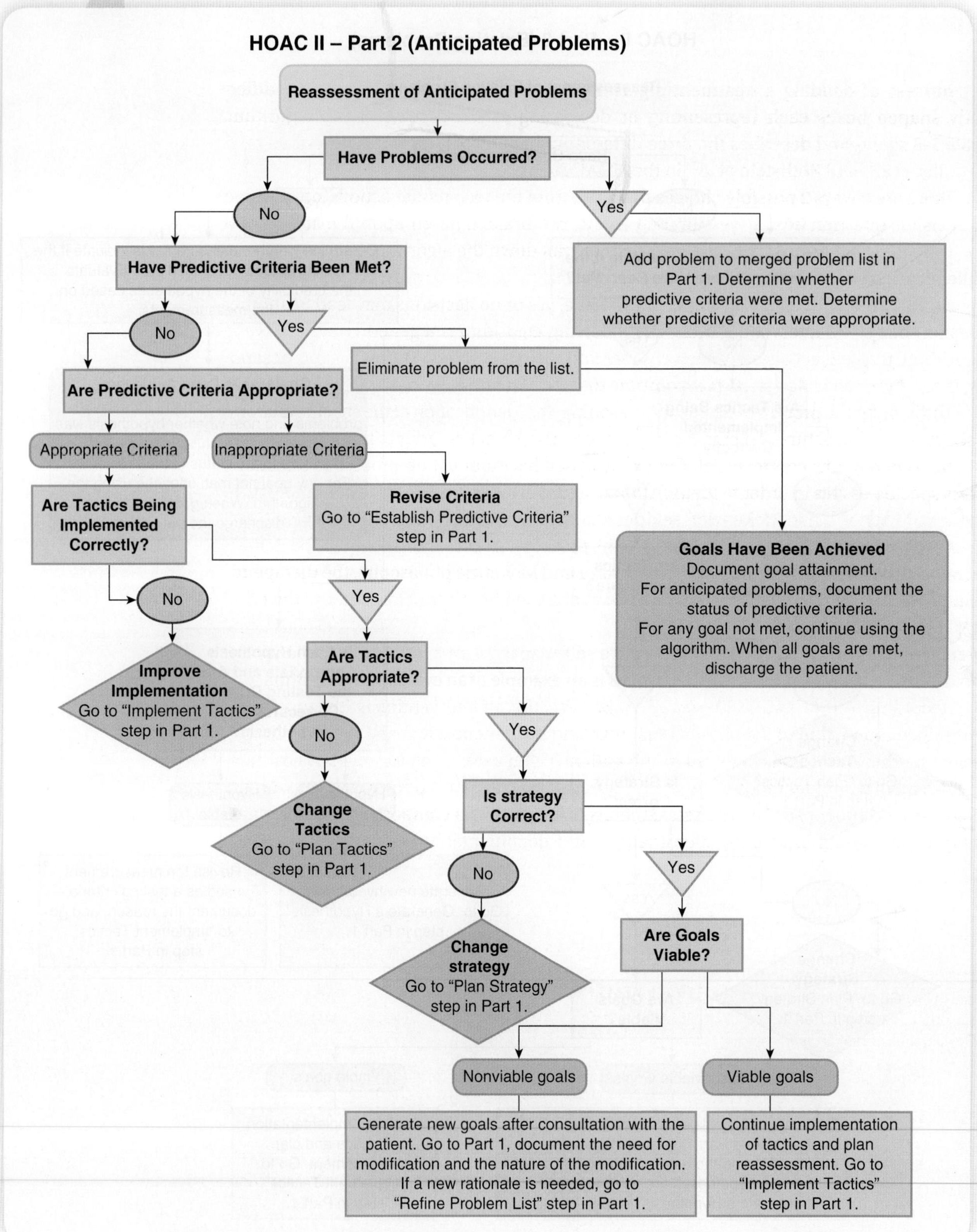

Figure 1-7 **HOAC II diagram 4**

The algorithm for reassessment of anticipated problems in part 2 of the HOAC II. (Reproduced, with permission, from the APTA, from Rothstein J, Echternach J, Riddle D. The Hypothesis-Oriented Algorithm for Clinicians II (HOAC II): a guide for patient management. *Phys Ther*. 2003;83:455-470.)

How to Construct an Algorithm

The process of building a treatment algorithm is not complex. It involves using differently shaped boxes each representing or describing varied aspects of the algorithm. Table 1-3 shows and describes the three differently shaped open forms, as described both by Miller et al[21] and Rothstein et al[23] in the HOAC II-Part 2.

There are always 2 possible choices that arise from the rectangular action/intervention or decision/question box: a "yes" branch and a "no" branch. Based upon the answer to a yes or no decision or question, the next path or trail down the algorithm is chosen. In the Miller et al[21] scheme, the yes or no treatment options for each path must be provided in the algorithm, whereas in the Rothstein et al[23] scheme, yes or no decisions may lead to another question box or an intervention box. The following algorithm is a generic example of the algorithms that will accompany each chapter and assist the reader in making and describing the many clinical decisions that combine to form a cohesive therapeutic intervention.

Throughout the process of diagnostic reasoning, the identification of the specific anatomical structure or structures causing the impairment or dysfunction prior to the initiation of an intervention remains controversial. Cyriax[7] designed his examination process to selectively stress specific tissues in order to identify the structure involved and its stage of pathology. In contrast, Maitland[18] and McKenzie[19] seldom identify the involved structure, believing that it is not always possible, or even necessary, for the prescription and safe delivery of appropriate therapeutic interventions. Based on the Maitland and McKenzie philosophy, the therapeutic strategy is determined solely from the responses obtained from tissue loading and the effect that loading has on symptoms. Once these responses have been determined, the focus of the intervention is to provide sound and effective self-management strategies for patients that avoid harmful tissue overloading.[16] Figure 1-8 is an example of an evaluation algorithm.

According to *The Guide to Physical Therapist Practice*, an intervention is "the purposeful and skilled interaction of the physical therapist and the patient/client and, when appropriate, with other individuals involved in the patient/client care, using various physical therapy procedures and techniques to produce changes in the condition consistent with the diagnosis and prognosis."[1] The physical therapy intervention is composed of 3 interrelated components: communication, coordination, and documentation; patient/client-related

Table 1-3 **Shapes and Descriptions of Algorithm Components**

Physical Representation of Algorithm Shape	Description of Form Contents (Miller et al[21])	Alternate Use of Forms (Rothstein et al[23,24])
Oval	The oval represents a clinical problem or entity.	The oval represents an assessment of an existing problem.
Rectangle	The rectangle represents an action to be taken or an intervention to be provided.	The rectangle represents a decision or clinical question.
Hexagon / Diamond	The hexagon represents a clinical question that has become apparent, which leads to a decision based upon evidence, whenever possible.	The diamond represents interventions, changes in strategy or actions.

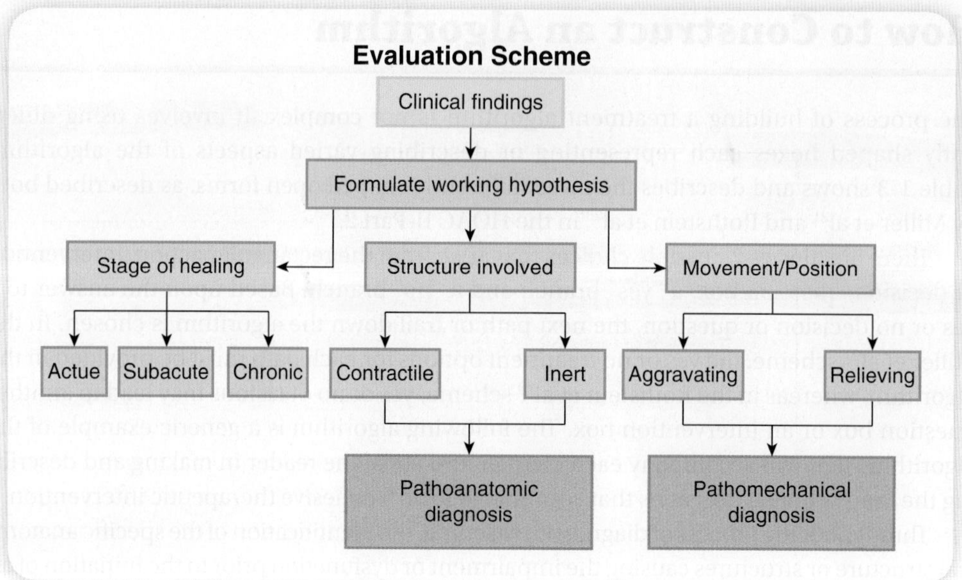

Figure 1-8 General evaluation scheme algorithm

instruction; and procedural interventions. As previously discussed, the patient/client management model provides a structure within which interventions are chosen in relationship to a movement-based categorization of signs and symptoms or a movement-based diagnosis (named in a preferred practice pattern).

Choices related to physical therapy procedural interventions are most effectively addressed from a problem-oriented approach, based on the knowledge of anatomy and biomechanics, the evaluation, the patient's functional needs, and mutually agreed upon goals.[1] Decisions regarding the specific interventions chosen are made in order to most effectively improve the patients' ability to return to the previous level of function. The most successful intervention programs are those that are custom designed from a blend of clinical experience and scientific data (see Chapter 19 for more information on creating exercise programs), with the level of improvement achieved related to goal setting and the attainment of those goals.

Introduction to the 4-Phase Approach to Rehabilitation

A number of principles should guide the intervention through the various stages of healing and return to function. The comprehensive intervention usually follows a 4-tiered approach, beginning initially in the acute phase and progressing to subacute or intermediate phase, then the advanced phase, and finally, the return to function. Within the 4-phase approach, general intervention principles are applied. These are not listed in order of importance, but instead reflect the sequence of application.

Acute Phase (Figure 1-9)

Control of Pain and Inflammation

Soft-tissue injuries are common in the general population and often are a reason for referral to physical therapy. The results of most soft-tissue injuries include conditions of pain, inflammation, and edema. Pain serves as the body's protective mechanism, giving an

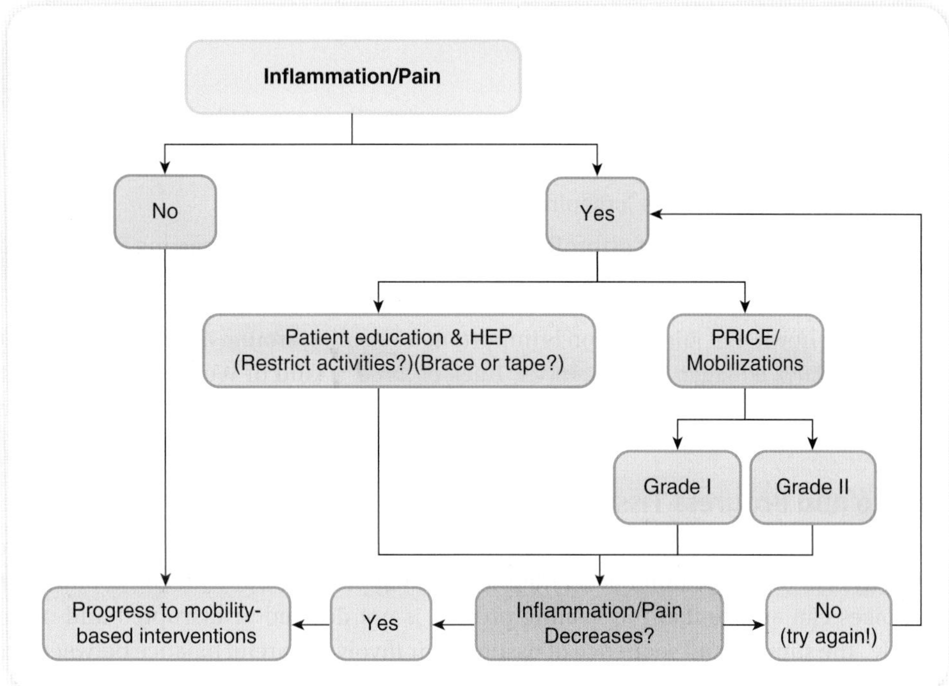

Figure 1-9 **Inflammation/pain algorithm**

HEP, home exercise program.

individual cues as to protect the area from additional tissue damage. At the simplest level, the transmission of information relating to pain from the periphery to the central nervous system depends upon integration at 3 levels: the spinal cord, the brainstem, and forebrain. (Refer to Chapter 4 for an in-depth discussion of pain.)

Inflammation and edema occur as a part of the healing process. The inflammatory response is a necessary initial response to an injury. Edema is a subsequent condition that occurs as a result of the inflammatory response, which may inhibit healing and return to function. Consequently, the goals during this initial phase of intervention for an acute injury are to decrease pain, control inflammation and edema, and protect the damaged structures from further damage, while concurrently attempting to increase the range of motion (ROM) and function. During the acute phase of healing, the principles of PRICE (protection, rest, ice, compression, and elevation) are recommended. In addition, manual therapy and early motion are introduced to the rehabilitation process. Chapters 8 and 13 provide further information on ROM and manual techniques, respectively.

The controlled application of a variety of techniques for control of pain, inflammation, and edema can have many therapeutic benefits. These benefits are theoretically achieved through:

- Mechanical stimulation of large-fiber joint afferents of the joint capsule, soft tissue, and other structures that assists in pain reduction
- Stimulation of endogenous endorphins and enkephalins, which aid in pain reduction,
- Decrease of intraarticular pressure, which aids in pain reduction
- Mechanical effects, which may improve joint mobility
- Positive effects on remodeling of local connective tissue
- Effective gliding of tendons within their sheaths
- Increased joint lubrication, important for nourishment of articular cartilage.

Application of Interventions to Provide Early Motion

Early motion is important for:

- Reduction of the muscle atrophy that occurs primarily in type I fibers
- Maintenance of joint function
- Prevention of ligamentous "creeping"
- Reduction of the chance of arthrofibrosis or excessive soft tissue scarring
- Enhancement of cartilage nutrition and vascularization, crucial for healing.

Research has shown that joint motion is important for healing around a joint and early joint motion stimulates collagen healing in the lines of force, a kind of Wolff law of ligaments. Early ROM exercises may be performed actively or passively while protecting the healing tissues.

Promote and Progress Tissue Healing

Tissue repair follows a predictable course in response to both internal and external processes. Physical therapy cannot accelerate the healing process, but with correct intervention choices can ensure that the healing process is not delayed or disrupted and occurs optimally. The support and sequence of tissue repair involve a careful balance between protection and controlled application of functional stresses to the healing tissue.

Clearly, the rehabilitation interventions used to assist during the repair process differ, depending on the degree/extent of the damage, the tissue involved, and stage of healing. Most tissues heal in a predictable manner, with equally predictable markers. These markers inform the clinician as to the stage of the repair that the tissue is in. Awareness of the various stages of healing is essential for determining the intensity of a particular intervention in order for clinician to avoid damaging healing tissues. Decisions to advance or change the rehabilitative process need to be based on the recognition of these signs and symptoms, and on an awareness of the time frames associated with each of the phases. For additional information on the phases of issue healing, refer to Chapter 2.

Intermediate Phase (Figure 1-10)

Therapeutic exercise is the foundation of physical therapy and a primary component of the bulk of interventions. In fact, *The Guide to Physical Therapist Practice* lists therapeutic exercise as one of the 3 categories of procedural interventions that forms the core of most physical therapy plans of care.[1] Prescribed appropriately, therapeutic exercise can be used to regain, maintain, and advance a patient's functional status by increasing ROM and mobility (flexibility), muscle performance (strength, power, and endurance), and motor performance (neuromuscular skill).

Therefore, as appropriate, it is the responsibility of the therapist to choose therapeutic interventions and instruct the patient on a supplemental exercise program that

- *Restores full and pain-free ROM.* All clinicians would agree that the restoration of, or improvement in, ROM is an important goal of the rehabilitation program. ROM may be viewed as a combination of the amount of joint motion, joint play, and the degree of extensibility of the periarticular and connective tissues that cross the joint, termed *flexibility*.

Prior to intervention with aggressive ROM exercises, joint play must be normalized in order to prevent complications that are likely to occur if abnormal osteo- and arthrokinematics during active and passive motion are present. In addition to general information available in Chapters 8 and 13, each regional chapter has specific mobilization techniques included.

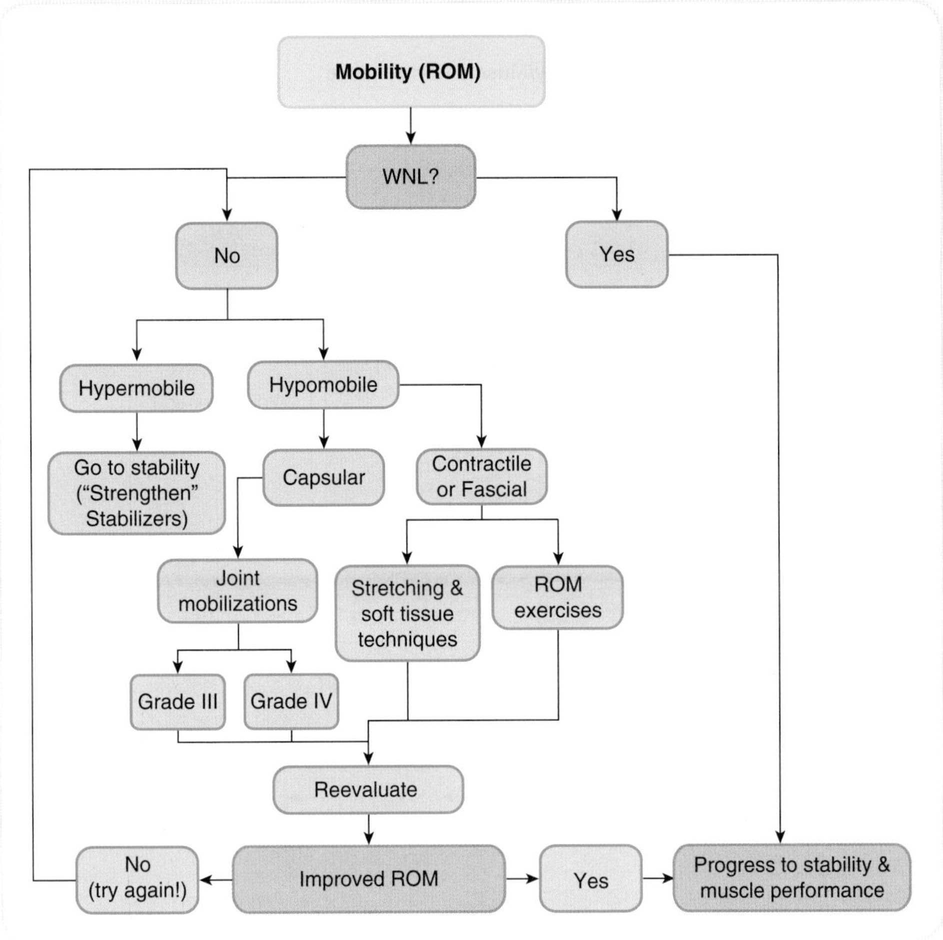

Figure 1-10 **ROM algorithm**

WNL, within normal limits.

A hierarchy exists for ROM during the subacute phase of healing to ensure that any progression is performed in a safe and controlled fashion. The hierarchy for the ROM exercises is as follows:

- Passive ROM
- Active-assisted ROM
- Active ROM

Advanced Phase (Figure 1-11)

In this phase of rehabilitation, the therapeutic exercise program must be progressed (both in the clinic and at home), selecting interventions that

- *Restore muscular strength, power, and endurance.* Like ROM, adequate muscular strength, power, and endurance are prerequisites for function. A wide variety of interventions exist that address deficits of muscle performance, and the individual therapist must decide what is the best intervention based upon a variety of patient factors and characteristics. Physical therapists should be experts in selective exercise prescription in order to increase all facets of muscle performance. Chapter 6 provides the foundation for choices of therapeutic interventions for development of muscular strength, power, and endurance.

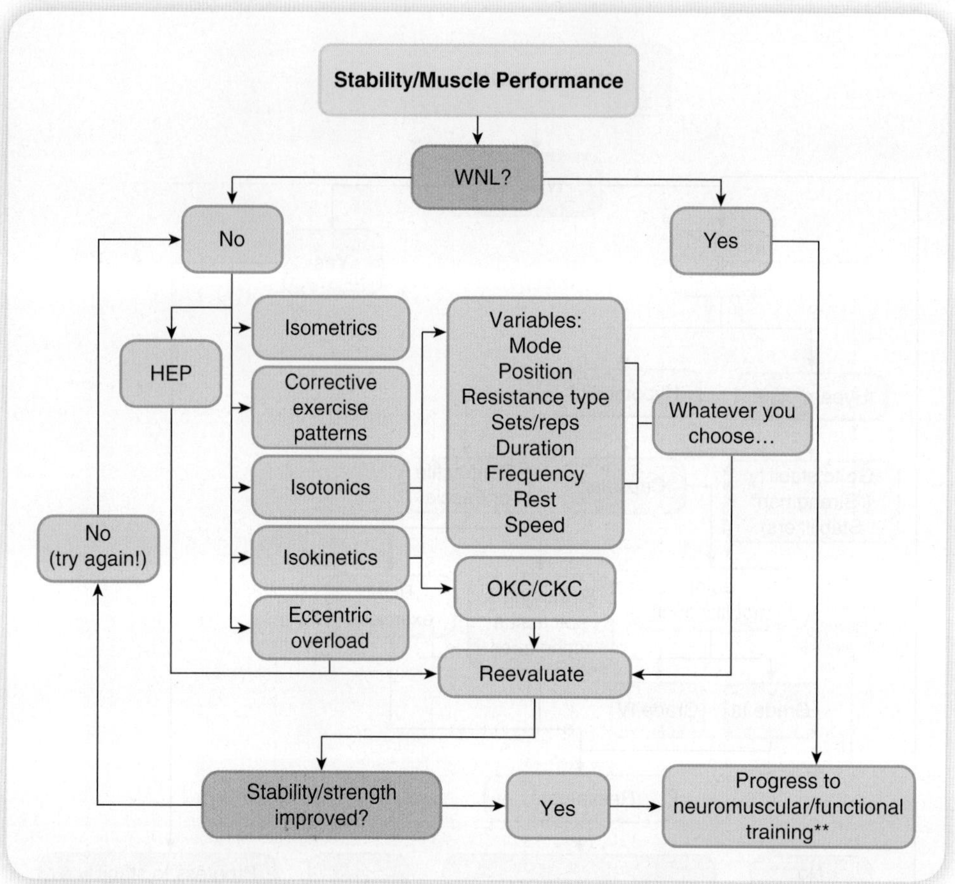

Figure 1-11 Muscular strength, power, and endurance algorithm

**Note, neuromuscular and functional activities may be addressed during some of the activities included in this phase. (CKC, closed kinetic chain; HEP, home exercise program; OKC, open kinetic chain; WNL, within normal limits.)

The hierarchy for the progression of resistive exercises for restoration of muscle performance impairments is

- Single-angle, submaximal isometrics performed in the neutral position
- Multiple-angle, submaximal isometrics performed at various angles of the range
- Multiple-angle maximal isometrics
- Submaximal, short arc, isotonic exercises
- Submaximal, full ROM isotonic exercise
- Maximal short arc isotonic exercise, progressing to full ROM maximal isotonics
- Open- and closed-kinetic chain exercises in the isotonic mode (refer to Chapter 11 for more details on these topics)
- Isokinetics

Gentle resistive exercises can be introduced very early in the rehabilitative process. At regular intervals, the clinician should ensure that

- The patient is being compliant with the patient's exercise program at home
- The patient is aware of the rationale behind the exercise program
- The patient is performing the exercise program correctly and at the appropriate intensity

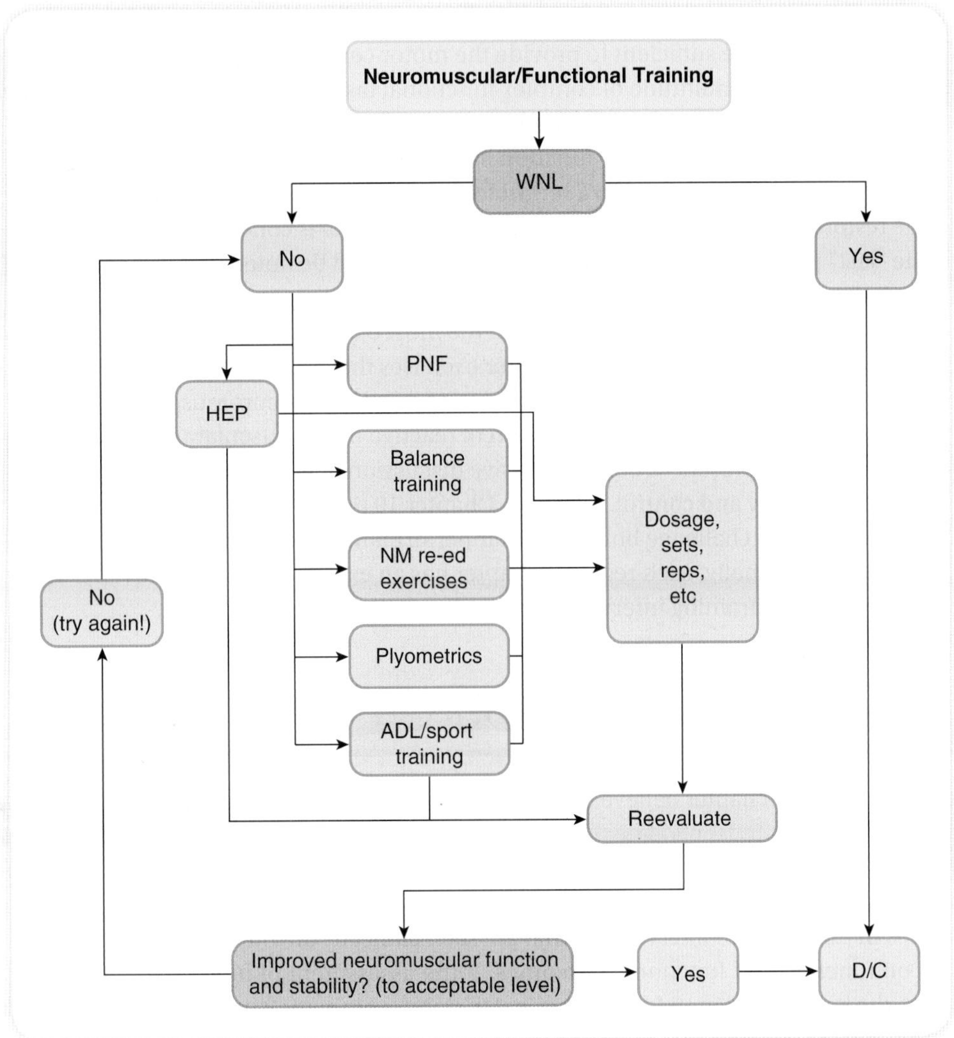

Figure 1-12 **Neuromuscular efficiency/functional return algorithm**

ADL, activities of daily living; D/C, discharge; HEP, home exercise program; NM, neuromuscular; PNF, proprioceptive neuromuscular facilitation; Re-Ed, Re-education; WNL, within normal limits.

- The patient's exercise program is being updated and appropriately based on clinical findings and patient response.

Each regional chapter in this text also has many excellent suggestions for specific therapeutic exercises for the advanced phase of rehabilitation where the focus tends to be on muscular performance enhancement.

Return to Function Phase (Figure 1-12)

Assuming proper ROM and muscle performance, the final phase of rehabilitation involves restoration of function. In this phase, interventions are chosen that

- *Restore neuromuscular efficiency and improve the overall fitness and functional outcome of the patient.* Restoration of neuromuscular control and efficiency is vital to the function of the patient. Complete ROM and flexibility about a joint is not enough for normal function. Likewise, isolated muscular strengthening in any mode or motion may not be sufficient to provide the motor control and motor performance necessary for the multitude of complex functional tasks in which patients participate. Therefore, the final step of the rehabilitation process is the introduction of activities that challenge neuromuscular function in specific motions, patterns, and tasks, thereby assisting the patient to a return to the highest level of function. Although the restoration of neuromuscular efficiency and control is conceptually viewed as the "last" part of the rehabilitation algorithm, it should be noted that techniques to challenge the neuromuscular control system are present in several previous intervention algorithms. For example, at the most basic level, active ROM challenges the proprioceptive control system. Other exercises that are viewed primarily for strengthening can also have a dual purpose of developing neuromuscular control. Chapter 9 presents a detailed discussion of reactive neuromuscular training, and Chapter 14 presents a comprehensive discussion of techniques to regain postural stability and control. Likewise, Chapter 10 presents options for plyometric interventions to challenge both muscular performance and neuromuscular control. Additionally, each regional chapter has an excellent variety of advanced, neuromuscular training interventions specific to the region.

Functional Movement-Based Thinking

The authors of this chapter believe firmly in the necessity of "forward" or progressive functional thinking that must pervade the examination and rehabilitation process of all patients and clients. This will be further addressed in the application of the concepts of mobility and stability to both examination and intervention paradigms. Although perhaps obvious, the gaps in examination intervention that are seen clinically are often a result of the lack of focus on function and functional outcomes. If the assessment of functional movement is used as the basic foundation for the physical therapy examination, it becomes easier to isolate the specific impairments that contribute to the dysfunction. Thus, philosophically, the authors adhere to a functionally focused examination (presented in Chapter 17). Throughout the text, the reader will notice the strong focus on function in the general intervention sections, as well as in the regional intervention chapters. This functional focus is specifically applied with regard to intervention, progression of intervention, and testing for return to activities in Chapters 18 and 19.

Conclusion

Physical therapist practice changes rapidly. Techniques, skills, and patterns of practice are constantly evolving and changing. The best physical therapists are those who grow and change as practice changes, rely upon evidence-based practice, but maintain a systematic, functional approach to examination and intervention.

Clinical reasoning and decision-making are important to the efficient and effective treatment of patients. These constructs develop over time, and can be enhanced by the use of available models such as the patient-client management model described in *The Guide.*

Algorithms are one way to illustrate the process of clinical reasoning. They are a graphic representation of a series of "if/then" decisions that may assist clinicians in developing diagnoses and selecting interventions. They serve to structure the process of clinical reasoning and illustrate the sequential nature of the clinical reasoning process used by therapists with experience and expertise. Finally, because evidence in physical therapy is constantly developing and changing, algorithms should not be viewed as static, rigid, or prescriptive decision-making tools. The clinical reasoning process is a complex, nonlinear process that requires a sufficient knowledge base and application of that knowledge in relation to an ever-changing base of evidence.

SUMMARY

1. *The Guide to Physical Therapist Practice* was published to describe the practice of physical therapy.
2. Subsequent revisions have made updates, improvements, and changes in the content of *The Guide*.
3. *The Guide* is not a cookbook for provision care, but rather a document to describe examination, evaluation, and intervention possibilities, as well as to use clinical decision-making to improve the quality of physical therapy services.
4. The preferred practice patterns are structured with diagnostic labels that are based upon impairments.
5. The quality of physical therapy provision, in terms of both diagnostic reasoning and selection of interventions, may be impacted by the use of algorithms.
6. Clinical reasoning skills are strongly related to experience and develop over a career.
7. Clinical decision processes of experts and novices differ. Algorithms may be a tool to enhance the process in novices and progress their skills toward that of experts.
8. All clinical reasoning should be an application of evidence-based practice.
9. The algorithmic approach to clinical reasoning may be used to guide intervention selection, in broad terms however, sufficient evidence does not yet exist to allow them to specifically direct clinical intervention decisions.
10. Algorithmic thinking can be applied to all subsequent chapters and is useful in the 4-phased rehabilitation model which includes:
    - Acute phase
    - Intermediate phase
    - Advanced phase
    - Return to function

REFERENCES

1. American Physical Therapy Association. The guide to physical therapist practice. *Phys Ther.* 1997;77: 1163-1650.
2. American Physical Therapy Association. The Guide to Physical Therapist Practice. 2nd ed. *Phys Ther.* 2001;81(1):9-738.
3. American Physical Therapy Association. *The Interactive Guide to Physical Therapist Practice, with Catalog of Tests and Measures.* Version 1.1. Alexandria, VA: American Physical Therapy Association; 2003.
4. Arocha J, Patel V, Patel Y. Hypothesis generation and the coordination of theory and evidence in novice diagnostic reasoning. *Med Decis Making.* 1993;13:198-211.
5. Bloch R. Methodology in clinical back pain trials. *Spine.* 1987;12:430-432.
6. Bruning R, Schraw G, Ronning R. *Cognitive Psychology.* 3rd ed. Upper Saddle River, NJ: Merrill; 1999.
7. Cyriax J. The diagnosis of soft tissue lesions. In: Cyriax J, ed. *Textbook of Orthopaedic Medicine.* London, UK: Spottis-Woode Ballantyne; 1978.

8. Edwards I, Jones M, Carr J, Baunack-Mayer A, Jensen G. Clinical reasoning strategies in physical therapy. *Phys Ther.* 2004;84(4):312-330.
9. Elstein A, Schwarz A. Evidence base of clinical diagnosis: clinical problem solving and diagnostic decision making—selective review of the cognitive literature. *BMJ.* 2002;324:729-732.
10. Elstein A, Shulman L, Sprafka S. Medical problem solving: a ten-year retrospective. *Eval Health Prof.* 1990;13:5-36.
11. Friedman LM, Furberg CD, DeMets DL. Fundamentals of clinical trials. St. Louis, MO: Mosby-Year Books; 1985.
12. http://www.britannica.com/eb/article-9005707?query=algorithm&ct=. Accessed on August 15, 2012.
13. Hack L. Foundations for modalities as procedural interventions: principles of clinical decision making. In: Michlovitz SL, Nolan TP, ed. *Modalities for Therapeutic Intervention.* 4th ed. Philadelphia, PA: FA Davis; 2005.
14. Higgs J, Jones M. Clinical reasoning in the health professions. In: Higgs J, Jones M, eds. *Clinical Reasoning in the Health Professions.* 2nd ed. Boston, MA: Butterworth-Heinemann; 2000.
15. Jensen G, Shepard K, Gwyer J, Hack L. Attribute dimensions that distinguish master and novice physical therapy clinicians in orthopedic settings. *Phys Ther.* 1992;72:711-722.
16. Jette A. Physical disablement concepts for physical therapy research and practice. *Phys Ther.* 1994;74:375-382.
17. Kahney H. *Problem Solving: Current Issues.* Buckingham, UK: Open University Press; 1993.
18. Maitland GD. *Maitland's Vertebral Manipulation.* 6th ed. Oxford, UK: Butterworth Heinemann; 2001.
19. McKenzie RA. *The Lumbar Spine: Mechanical Diagnosis and Therapy.* Waikanae, New Zealand: Spinal Publications; 1989.
20. May B, Dennis J. Expert decision making in physical therapy: a survey of practitioners. *Phys Ther.* 1991;71:190-216.
21. Miller T, Nyland J, Wormal W. Therapeutic exercise program design considerations: "Putting it all together." In: Nyland J, ed. *Clinical Decisions in Therapeutic Exercise.* Upper Saddle River, NJ: Pearson Education; 2006.
22. Nagi SZ. *Disability and Rehabilitation.* Columbus, OH: Ohio State University Press; 1969.
23. Rothstein J, Echternach J, Riddle D. The hypothesis-oriented algorithm for clinicians II (HOAC II): a guide for patient management. *Phys Ther.* 2003;83:455-470.
24. Rothstein J, Echternach J. The hypothesis-oriented algorithm for clinicians: a method for evaluation and treatment planning. *Phys Ther.* 1986;66:1388-1394.
25. Sackett DL, Rosenberg WM, Gray JA, et al. Evidence-based medicine: what it is and what it isn't. *BMJ.* 1996;312:71-72.

2

Understanding and Managing the Healing Process Through Rehabilitation

William E. Prentice

OBJECTIVES

After completion of this chapter, the physical therapist should be able to do the following:

- Describe the pathophysiology of the healing process.
- Identify the factors that can impede the healing process.
- Discuss the etiology and pathology of various musculoskeletal injuries associated with various types of tissues.
- Compare healing processes relative to specific musculoskeletal structures.
- Explain the importance of initial first aid and injury management of these injuries and their impact on the rehabilitation process.
- Discuss the use of various analgesics, antiinflammatories, and antipyretics in facilitating the healing process during a rehabilitation program.

Injury rehabilitation requires sound knowledge and understanding of the etiology and pathology involved in various musculoskeletal injuries that may occur.[24,84,93] When injury occurs, the therapist is charged with designing, implementing, and supervising the rehabilitation program. Rehabilitation protocols and progressions must be based primarily on the physiologic responses of the tissues to injury and on an understanding of how various tissues heal.[39,43,46] Thus the therapist must understand the healing process to effectively supervise the rehabilitative process. This chapter discusses the healing process relative to the various musculoskeletal injuries that may be encountered by an therapist.

Understanding the Healing Process

Rehabilitation programs must be based on the cycle of the healing process (Figure 2-1). The therapist must have a sound understanding of the sequence of the various phases of the healing process.[31] The physiologic responses of the tissues to trauma follow a predictable sequence and time frame.[41] Decisions on how and when to alter and progress a rehabilitation program should be primarily based on recognition of signs and symptoms, as well as on an awareness of the time frames associated with the various phases of healing.[57,72]

The healing process consists of the inflammatory response phase, the fibroblastic repair phase, and the maturation remodeling phase. It must be stressed that although the phases

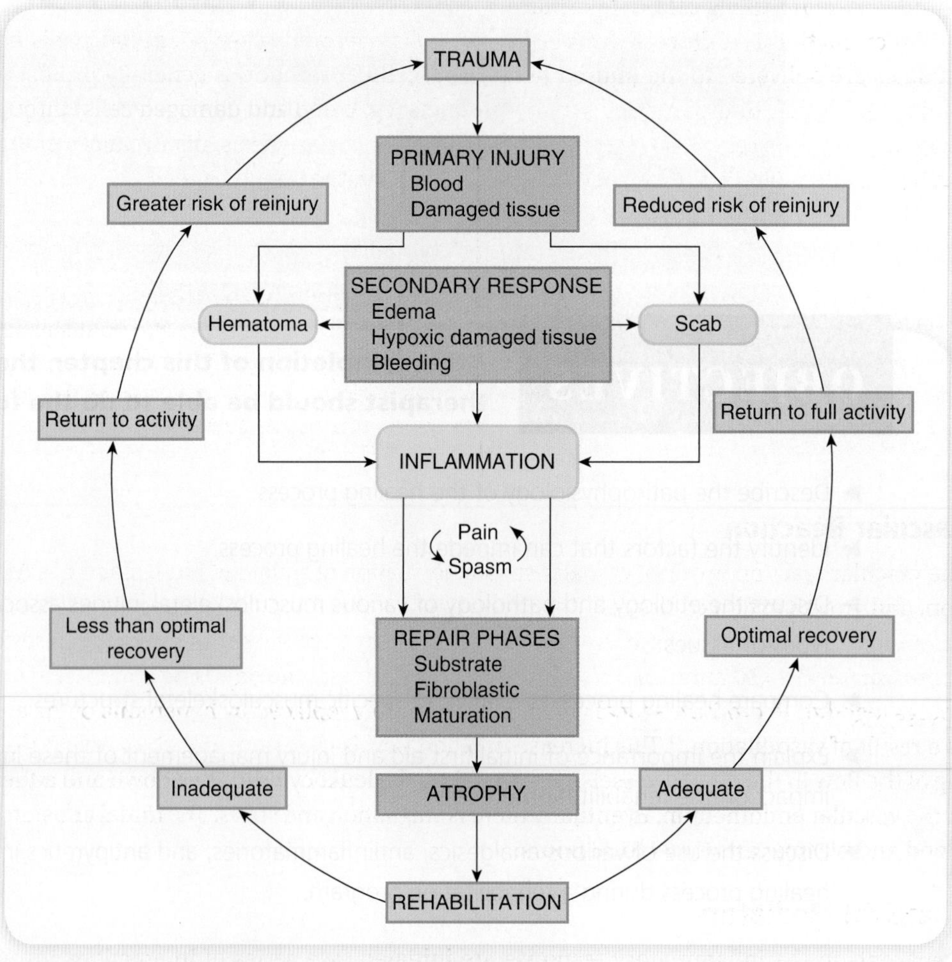

Figure 2-1 **A cycle of sport-related injury**

(From Booher and Thibadeau. *Athletic Injury Assessment*. Mosby; 1994.)

of healing are presented as 3 separate entities, the healing process is a continuum. Phases of the healing process overlap one another and have no definitive beginning or end points.[73]

Primary Injury

Primary injuries are almost always described as being either chronic or acute in nature, resulting from macrotraumatic or microtraumatic forces. Injuries classified as macrotraumatic occur as a result of acute trauma and produce immediate pain and disability. Macrotraumatic injuries include fractures, dislocations, subluxations, sprains, strains, and contusions. Microtraumatic injuries are most often called overuse injuries and result from repetitive overloading or incorrect mechanics associated with repeated motion.[59] Microtraumatic injuries include tendinitis, tenosynovitis, bursitis, etc. A secondary injury is essentially the inflammatory or hypoxia response that occurs with the primary injury.

Inflammatory Response Phase

Once a tissue is injured, the process of healing begins immediately (Figure 2-2*A*).[16] The destruction of tissue produces direct injury to the cells of the various soft tissues.[35] Cellular injury results in altered metabolism and the liberation of materials that initiate the inflammatory response. It is characterized symptomatically by redness, swelling, tenderness, and increased temperature.[18,54] This initial inflammatory response is critical to the entire healing process.[14] If this response does not accomplish what it is supposed to or if it does not subside, normal healing cannot take place.[37]

Inflammation is a process through which leukocytes and other phagocytic cells and exudates are delivered to the injured tissue. This cellular reaction is generally protective, tending to localize or dispose of injury by-products (eg, blood and damaged cells) through phagocytosis, thus setting the stage for repair. Local vascular effects, disturbances of fluid exchange, and migration of leukocytes from the blood to the tissues occur.[38]

Clinical Pearl

Immediate action to control swelling can expedite the healing process. The therapist should first provide compression and elevation. Applying ice, which decreases the metabolic demands of the uninjured cells, can prevent secondary hypoxic injury. Ice also slows nerve conduction velocity, which will decrease pain and thus limit muscle guarding.

Vascular Reaction

The vascular reaction involves vascular spasm, formation of a platelet plug, blood coagulation, and growth of fibrous tissue.[77] The immediate response to tissue damage is a vasoconstriction of the vascular walls in the vessels leading away from the site of injury that lasts for approximately 5 to 10 minutes. This vasoconstriction presses the opposing endothelial wall linings together to produce a local anemia that is rapidly replaced by hyperemia of the area as a result of vasodilation.[1] This increase in blood flow is transitory and gives way to slowing of the flow in the dilated vessels, thus enabling the leukocytes to slow down and adhere to the vascular endothelium. Eventually there is stagnation and stasis. The initial effusion of blood and plasma lasts for 24 to 36 hours.

Chemical Mediators

The events in the inflammatory response are initiated by a series of interactions involving several chemical mediators. Some of these chemical mediators are derived from the invading organism, some are released by the damaged tissue, others are generated by several plasma enzyme systems, and still others are products of various white blood cells

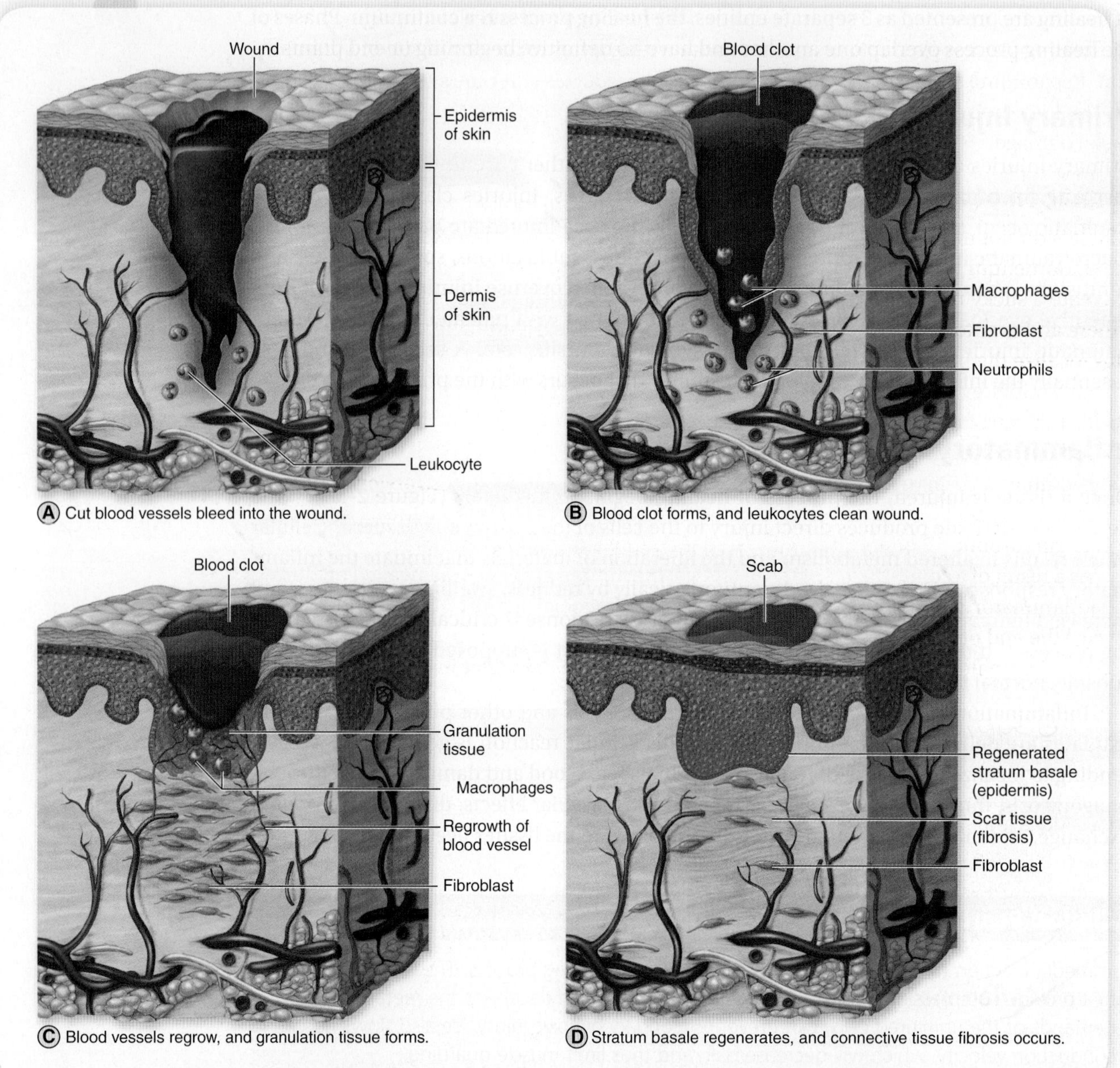

Figure 2-2 Initial injury and inflammatory response phase of the healing process

A. Cut blood vessels bleed into the wound. **B.** Blood clot forms, and leukocytes clean the wound. **C.** Blood vessels regrow, and granulation tissue forms in the fibroblastic repair phase of the healing process. **D.** Epithelium regenerates, and connective tissue fibrosis occurs in the maturation-remodeling phase of the healing process. (Reproduced with permission from Prentice. *Principles of Athletic Training*. 14th ed. New York: McGraw-Hill; 2011.)

participating in the inflammatory response. Three chemical mediators—histamine, leukotrienes, and cytokines—are important in limiting the amount of exudate, and thus swelling, after injury. Histamine, released from the injured mast cells, causes vasodilation and increased cell permeability, owing to a swelling of endothelial cells and then separation between the cells. Leukotrienes and prostaglandins are responsible for margination, in which leukocytes (neutrophils and macrophages) adhere along the cell walls. They also increase cell permeability locally, thus affecting the passage of the fluid and white blood cells through cell walls via diapedesis to form exudate. Consequently, vasodilation and active hyperemia are important in exudate (plasma) formation and in supplying leukocytes to the injured area. Cytokines, in particular chemokines and interleukin, are the major regulators of leukocyte traffic and help to attract leukocytes to the actual site of inflammation. Responding to the presence of chemokines, phagocytes enter the site of inflammation within a few hours. The amount of swelling that occurs is directly related to the extent of vessel damage.

Formation of a Clot

Platelets do not normally adhere to the vascular wall. However, injury to a vessel disrupts the endothelium and exposes the collagen fibers. Platelets adhere to the collagen fibers to create a sticky matrix on the vascular wall, to which additional platelets and leukocytes adhere and eventually form a plug. These plugs obstruct local lymphatic fluid drainage and thus localize the injury response (see Figure 2-2*B*).

The initial event that precipitates clot formation is the conversion of fibrinogen to fibrin. This transformation occurs because of a cascading effect, beginning with the release of a protein molecule called *thromboplastin* from the damaged cell. Thromboplastin causes prothrombin to be changed into thrombin, which, in turn, causes the conversion of fibrinogen into a very sticky fibrin clot that shuts off blood supply to the injured area. Clot formation begins around 12 hours after injury and is completed within 48 hours.

As a result of a combination of these factors, the injured area becomes walled off during the inflammatory stage of healing. The leukocytes phagocytize most of the foreign debris toward the end of the inflammatory phase, setting the stage for the fibroblastic phase. This initial inflammatory response lasts for approximately 2 to 4 days after initial injury.

Clinical Pearl

It can take up to 3 or 4 days for the inflammatory response to subside. During this time, the muscle is initializing repair by containing the injury by clot formation. Too much stress during this time could increase the time it takes the muscle to heal. After that, it may take a couple of weeks before fibroblastic and myoblastic activity has restored tissue strength to a point where the tissue can withstand the stresses of exercise.

Chronic Inflammation

A distinction must be made between the acute inflammatory response as previously described and chronic inflammation. Chronic inflammation occurs when the acute inflammatory response does not respond sufficiently to eliminate the injuring agent and restore tissue to its normal physiologic state. Thus, only low concentrations of the chemical mediators are present. The neutrophils that are normally present during acute inflammation are replaced by macrophages, lymphocytes, fibroblasts, and plasma cells. As this low-grade inflammation persists, damage occurs to connective tissue, resulting in tissue necrosis and fibrosis prolonging the healing process. Chronic inflammation involves the production of granulation tissue and fibrous connective tissue. These cells accumulate in a highly vascularized and innervated loose connective tissue matrix in the area of injury.[53] The specific mechanisms that cause an insufficient acute inflammatory response are unknown, but they appear to be related to situations that involve overuse or overload with cumulative microtrauma to a particular structure.[28,53] There is no specific time frame in which the acute inflammation transitions to chronic inflammation. It does appear that chronic inflammation is resistant to both physical and pharmacologic treatments.[44]

Use of Antiinflammatory Medications

A physician will routinely prescribe nonsteroidal antiinflammatory drugs (NSAIDs) for a patient who has sustained an injury.[2] These medications are certainly effective in minimizing pain and swelling associated with inflammation and can enhance return to normal activity. However, there are some concerns that the use of NSAIDs acutely following injury might actually interfere with inflammation, thus delaying the healing process.

Fibroblastic Repair Phase

During the fibroblastic phase of healing, proliferative and regenerative activity leading to scar formation and repair of the injured tissue follows the vascular and exudative phenomena of inflammation (see Figure 2-2*C*).[41] The period of scar formation referred to as fibroplasia begins within the first few hours after injury and can last as long as 4 to 6 weeks. During this period, many of the signs and symptoms associated with the inflammatory response subside. The patient might still indicate some tenderness to touch and will usually complain of pain when particular movements stress the injured structure. As scar formation progresses, complaints of tenderness or pain gradually disappear.[39]

During this phase, growth of endothelial capillary buds into the wound is stimulated by a lack of oxygen, after which the wound is capable of healing aerobically.[18] Along with increased oxygen delivery comes an increase in blood flow, which delivers nutrients essential for tissue regeneration in the area.[18]

The formation of a delicate connective tissue called *granulation tissue* occurs with the breakdown of the fibrin clot. Granulation tissue consists of fibroblasts, collagen, and capillaries. It appears as a reddish granular mass of connective tissue that fills in the gaps during the healing process.

As the capillaries continue to grow into the area, fibroblasts accumulate at the wound site, arranging themselves parallel to the capillaries. Fibroblastic cells begin to synthesize an extracellular matrix that contains protein fibers of collagen and elastin, a ground substance that consists of nonfibrous proteins called proteoglycans, glycosaminoglycans, and fluid. On about day 6 or 7, fibroblasts also begin producing collagen fibers that are deposited in a random fashion throughout the forming scar. As the collagen continues to proliferate, the tensile strength of the wound rapidly increases in proportion to the rate of collagen synthesis. As the tensile strength increases, the number of fibroblasts diminishes, signaling the beginning of the maturation phase.

This normal sequence of events in the repair phase leads to the formation of minimal scar tissue. Occasionally, a persistent inflammatory response and continued release of inflammatory products can promote extended fibroplasia and excessive fibrogenesis, which can lead to irreversible tissue damage.[97] Fibrosis can occur in synovial structures, as with adhesive capsulitis in the shoulder, in extraarticular tissues including tendons and ligaments, in bursa, or in muscle.

Clinical Pearl

Muscle healing generally takes longer than ligament. While fibroblasts are laying down new collagen for connective tissue repair, myoblasts are working to replace the contractile tissue.

The Importance of Collagen

Collagen is a major structural protein that forms strong, flexible, inelastic structures that hold connective tissue together. There are at least 16 types of collagen, but 80% to 90% of the collagen in the body consists of types I, II, and III. Type I collagen is found in skin, fascia, tendon, bone, ligaments, cartilage, and interstitial tissues; type II can be found in hyaline cartilage and vertebral disks; and type III is found in skin, smooth muscle, nerves, and blood vessels. Type III collagen has less tensile strength than does type I, and tends to be found more in the fibroblastic repair phase. Collagen enables a tissue to resist mechanical forces and deformation. Elastin, however, produces highly elastic tissues that assist in recovery from deformation. Collagen fibrils are the loadbearing elements of connective tissue. They are arranged to accommodate tensile stress, but are not as capable of resisting shear or compressive stress. Consequently, the direction of orientation of collagen fibers is along lines of tensile stress.[93]

Collagen has several mechanical and physical properties that allow it to respond to loading and deformation, permitting it to withstand high tensile stress. The mechanical properties of collagen include elasticity, which is the capability to recover normal length after elongation; viscoelasticity, which allows for a slow return to normal length and shape after deformation; and plasticity, which allows for permanent change or deformation. The physical properties include force relaxation, which indicates the decrease in the amount of force needed to maintain a tissue at a set amount of displacement or deformation over time; creep response, which is the ability of a tissue to deform over time while a constant load is imposed; and hysteresis, which is the amount of relaxation a tissue has undergone during deformation and displacement. Injury results when the mechanical and physical limitations of connective tissue are exceeded.[103]

Maturation Remodeling Phase

The maturation remodeling phase of healing is a long-term process (see Figure 2-2*D*). This phase features a realignment or remodeling of the collagen fibers that make up scar tissue according to the tensile forces to which that scar is subjected. Ongoing breakdown and synthesis of collagen occur with a steady increase in the tensile strength of the scar matrix. With increased stress and strain, the collagen fibers realign in a position of maximum efficiency parallel to the lines of tension.[21] The tissue gradually assumes normal appearance and function, although a scar is rarely as strong as the normal injured tissue. Usually by the end of approximately 3 weeks, a firm, strong, contracted, nonvascular scar exists. The maturation phase of healing might require several years to be totally complete.

Role of Progressive Controlled Mobility During the Healing Process

The Wolff law states that bone and soft tissue will respond to the physical demands placed on them, causing them to remodel or realign along lines of tensile force.[101] Consequently, it is critical that injured structures be exposed to progressively increasing loads throughout the rehabilitative process.[73]

In animal models, controlled mobilization is superior to immobilization for scar formation, revascularization, muscle regeneration, and reorientation of muscle fibers and tensile properties.[71] However, a brief period of immobilization of the injured tissue during the inflammatory response phase is recommended and will likely facilitate the process of healing by controlling inflammation, thus reducing clinical symptoms. As healing progresses to the repair phase, controlled activity directed toward return to normal flexibility and strength should be combined with protective support or bracing.[50] Generally, clinical signs and symptoms disappear at the end of this phase.

As the remodeling phase begins, aggressive active range-of-motion and strengthening exercises should be incorporated to facilitate tissue remodeling and realignment. To a great extent, pain will dictate rate of progression. With initial injury, pain is intense; it tends to decrease and eventually subside altogether as healing progresses. Any exacerbation of pain, swelling, or other clinical symptoms during or after a particular exercise or activity indicate that the load is too great for the level of tissue repair or remodeling. The therapist must be aware of the time required for the healing process and realize that being overly aggressive can interfere with that process.

> **Clinical Pearl**
>
> Once an injured structure has progressed through the inflammatory phase and repair has begun, sufficient tensile stress should be provided to ensure optimal repair and positioning of the new fibers (according to the Wolff law). Efforts should be made right away to avoid the strength loss that comes with immobility because of pain.

Factors That Impede Healing

Extent of Injury

The nature of the inflammatory response is determined by the extent of the tissue injury. Microtears or soft tissue involve only minor damage and are most often associated with overuse. Macrotears involve significantly greater destruction of soft tissue and result in clinical symptoms and functional alterations. Macrotears are generally caused by acute trauma.[19]

Edema

The increased pressure caused by swelling retards the healing process, causes separation of tissues, inhibits neuromuscular control, produces reflexive neurologic changes, and impedes nutrition in the injured part. Edema is best controlled and managed during the initial first-aid management period, as described previously.[17]

Hemorrhage

Bleeding occurs with even the smallest amount of damage to the capillaries. Bleeding produces the same negative effects on healing as does the accumulation of edema, and its presence produces additional tissue damage and thus exacerbation of the injury.[67]

Poor Vascular Supply

Injuries to tissues with a poor vascular supply heal poorly and at a slow rate. This response is likely related to a failure in the initial delivery of phagocytic cells and fibroblasts necessary for scar formation.[67]

Separation of Tissue

Mechanical separation of tissue can significantly impact the course of healing. A wound that has smooth edges in good apposition will tend to heal by primary intention with minimal scarring. Conversely, a wound that has jagged, separated edges must heal by secondary intention, with granulation tissue filling the defect, and excessive scarring.[76]

Muscle Spasm

Muscle spasm causes traction on the torn tissue, separates the 2 ends, and prevents approximation. Local and generalized ischemia can result from spasm.

Atrophy

Wasting away of muscle tissue begins immediately with injury. Strengthening and early mobilization of the injured structure retard atrophy.

Corticosteroids

Use of corticosteroids in the treatment of inflammation is controversial. Steroid use in the early stages of healing has been demonstrated to inhibit fibroplasia, capillary proliferation, collagen synthesis, and increases in tensile strength of the healing scar. Their use in the later stages of healing and with chronic inflammation is debatable.

Keloids and Hypertrophic Scars

Keloids occur when the rate of collagen production exceeds the rate of collagen breakdown during the maturation phase of healing. This process leads to hypertrophy of scar tissue, particularly around the periphery of the wound.

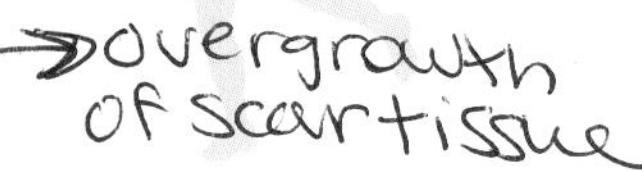

Infection

The presence of bacteria in the wound can delay healing, causes excessive granulation tissue, and frequently causes large, deformed scars.[12]

Humidity, Climate, and Oxygen Tension

Humidity significantly influences the process of epithelization. Occlusive dressing stimulates the epithelium to migrate twice as fast without crust or scab formation. The formation of a scab occurs with dehydration of the wound and traps wound drainage, which promotes infection. Keeping the wound moist provides an advantage for the necrotic debris to go to the surface and be shed.

Oxygen tension relates to the neovascularization of the wound, which translates into optimal saturation and maximal tensile strength development. Circulation to the wound can be affected by ischemia, venous stasis, hematomas, and vessel trauma.

Health, Age, and Nutrition

The elastic qualities of the skin decrease with age. Degenerative diseases, such as diabetes and arteriosclerosis, also become a concern of the older patient and can affect wound healing. Nutrition is important for wound healing—in particular, vitamins C (for collagen synthesis and immune system), K (for clotting), and A (for the immune system); zinc (for the enzyme systems) and amino acids play critical roles in the healing process.

Injuries to Articular Structures

Before discussing injuries to the various articular structures, a review of joint structure is in order (Figure 2-3).[66] All synovial joints are composed of 2 or more bones that articulate with one another to allow motion in 1 or more places. The articulating surfaces of the bone are lined with a very thin, smooth, cartilaginous covering called a *hyaline cartilage*. All joints are entirely surrounded by a thick, ligamentous joint capsule. The inner surface of this joint capsule is lined by a very thin synovial membrane that is highly vascularized and innervated. The synovial membrane produces synovial fluid, the functions of which include lubrication, shock absorption, and nutrition of the joint.[89]

Some joints contain a thick fibrocartilage called a *meniscus*. The knee joint, for example, contains 2 wedge-shaped menisci that deepen the articulation and provide shock absorption in that joint. Finally, the main structural support and joint stability is provided by the ligaments, which may be either thickened portions of a joint capsule or totally separate bands.

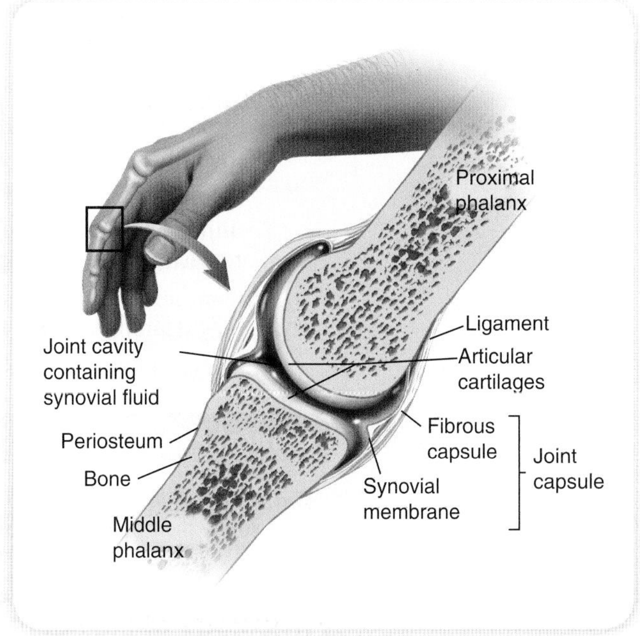

Figure 2-3 General anatomy of a synovial joint

(Reproduced with permission from Prentice. *Principles of Athletic Training.* 14th ed. New York: McGraw-Hill; 2011.)

Ligament Sprains

Ligaments are composed of dense connective tissue arranged in parallel bundles of collagen composed of rows of fibroblasts. Although bundles are arranged in

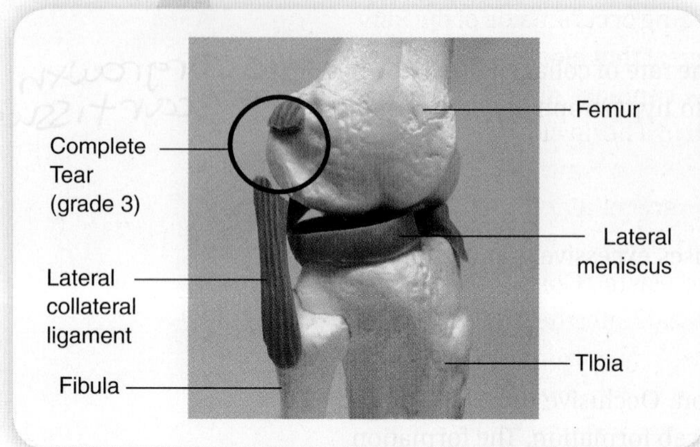

Figure 2-4 **Grade 3 ligament sprain in the knee joint**

(Reproduced with permission from Prentice. *Principles of Athletic Training*. 14th ed. New York: McGraw-Hill; 2011.)

parallel, not all collagen fibers are arranged in parallel. Ligaments and tendons are very similar in structure. However, ligaments are usually more flattened than tendons, and collagen fibers in ligaments are more compact. The anatomical positioning of the ligaments determines in part what motions a joint can make.

A sprain involves damage to a ligament that provides support to a joint. A ligament is a tough, relatively inelastic band of tissue that connects one bone to another. A ligament's primary function is threefold: to provide stability to a joint, to provide control of the position of one articulating bone to another during normal joint motion, and to provide proprioceptive input or a sense of joint position through the function of free nerve endings or mechanoreceptors located within the ligament.

If stress is applied to a joint that forces motion beyond its normal limits or planes of movement, injury to the ligament is likely (Figure 2-4).[34] The severity of damage to the ligament is classified in many different ways; however, the most commonly used system involves 3 grades (degrees) of ligamentous sprain:

Grade 1 sprain: There is some stretching or perhaps tearing of the ligamentous fibers, with little or no joint instability. Mild pain, little swelling, and joint stiffness might be apparent.

Grade 2 sprain: There is some tearing and separation of the ligamentous fibers and moderate instability of the joint. Moderate-to-severe pain, swelling, and joint stiffness should be expected.

Clinical Pearl

The presence of gross laxity would suggest a grade 3 sprain. The patient be referred to the physician for further evaluation.

Grade 3 sprain: There is total rupture of the ligament, manifested primarily by gross instability of the joint. Severe pain might be present initially, followed by little or no pain because of total disruption of nerve fibers. Swelling might be profuse, and thus the joint tends to become very stiff some hours after the injury. A third-degree sprain with marked instability usually requires some form of immobilization lasting several weeks. Frequently, the force producing the ligament injury is so great that other ligaments or structures surrounding the joint are also injured. With cases in which there is injury to multiple joint structures, surgical repair reconstruction may be necessary to correct an instability.

Clinical Pearl

In a complete ligament tear, it is likely that the nerves in that structure will also be completely disrupted. Therefore, no pain signals can be transmitted.

Physiology of Ligament Healing

The healing process in the sprained ligament follows the same course of repair as with other vascular tissues. Immediately after injury and for approximately 72 hours there is a loss of blood from damaged vessels and attraction of inflammatory cells into the injured area. If a ligament is sprained outside of a joint capsule (extraarticular ligament), bleeding occurs in a subcutaneous space. If an intraarticular ligament is injured, bleeding occurs inside of the joint capsule until either clotting occurs or the pressure becomes so great that bleeding ceases.

During the next 6 weeks, vascular proliferation with new capillary growth begins to occur along with fibroblastic activity, resulting in the formation of a fibrin clot. It is essential that the torn ends of the ligament be reconnected by bridging this clot. Synthesis of collagen and ground substance of proteoglycan as constituents of an intracellular matrix contributes to the proliferation of the scar that bridges between the torn ends of the ligament. This scar initially is soft and viscous but eventually becomes more elastic. Collagen fibers are arranged in a random woven pattern with little organization. Gradually there is a decrease in fibroblastic activity, a decrease in vascularity, and an increase to a maximum in collagen density of the scar.[4] Failure to produce enough scar and failure to reconnect the ligament to the appropriate location on a bone are the two reasons why ligaments are likely to fail.

Over the next several months the scar continues to mature, with the realignment of collagen occurring in response to progressive stresses and strains. The maturation of the scar may require as long as 12 months to complete.[4] The exact length of time required for maturation depends on mechanical factors such as apposition of torn ends and length of the period of immobilization.

Factors Affecting Ligament Healing

Surgically repaired extraarticular ligaments have healed with decreased scar formation and are generally stronger than unrepaired ligaments initially, although this strength advantage might not be maintained as time progresses. Unrepaired ligaments heal by fibrous scarring effectively lengthening the ligament and producing some degree of joint instability. With intraarticular ligament tears, the presence of synovial fluid dilutes the hematoma, thus preventing formation of a fibrin clot and spontaneous healing.[42]

Several studies show that actively exercised ligaments are stronger than those that are immobilized. Ligaments that are immobilized for periods of several weeks after injury tend to decrease in tensile strength and also exhibit weakening of the insertion of the ligament to bone.[72] Thus it is important to minimize periods of immobilization and progressively stress the injured ligaments while exercising caution relative to biomechanical considerations for specific ligaments.[4,68]

It is not likely that the inherent stability of the joint provided by the ligament before injury will be regained. Thus, to restore stability to the joint, the other structures that surround that joint, primarily muscles and their tendons, must be strengthened. The increased muscle tension provided by resistance training can improve stability of the injured joint.[68,88]

Cartilage Damage

Cartilage is a type of rigid connective tissue that provides support and acts as a framework in many structures. It is composed of chondrocyte cells contained in small chambers called *lacunae*, surrounded completely by an intracellular matrix. The matrix consists of varying ratios of collagen and elastin and a ground substance made of proteoglycans and glycosaminoglycans, which are nonfibrous protein molecules. These proteoglycans act as sponges and trap large quantities of water, which allow cartilage to spring back after being compressed.[96] Cartilage has a poor blood supply, thus healing after injury is very slow. There are 3 types of cartilage. *Hyaline cartilage* is found on the articulating surfaces of bone and in the soft part of the nose. It contains large quantities of collagen and proteoglycan. *Fibrocartilage* forms the intervertebral disk and menisci located in several joint spaces. It has greater amounts of collagen than proteoglycan and is capable of withstanding a great deal of pressure. *Elastic cartilage* is found in the auricle of the ear and the larynx. It is more flexible than the other types of cartilage and consists of collagen, proteoglycan, and elastin.[79]

Osteoarthrosis is a degenerative condition of bone and cartilage in and about the joint. Arthritis should be defined as primarily an inflammatory condition with possible secondary destruction.[6] Arthrosis is primarily a degenerative process with destruction of cartilage, remodeling of bone, and possible secondary inflammatory components.

Cartilage fibrillates, that is, releases fibers or groups of fibers and ground substance into the joint.[29] Peripheral cartilage that is not exposed to weightbearing or compression-decompression mechanisms is particularly likely to fibrillate. Fibrillation is typically found in the degenerative process associated with poor nutrition or disuse. This process can then extend even to weightbearing areas, with progressive destruction of cartilage proportional to stresses applied on it. When forces are increased, thus increasing stress, osteochondral or subchondral fractures can occur. Concentration of stress on small areas can produce pressures that overwhelm the tissue's capabilities. Typically, lower-limb joints have to handle greater stresses, but their surface area is usually larger than the surface area of upper limbs. The articular cartilage is protected to some extent by the synovial fluid, which acts as a lubricant. It is also protected by the subchondral bone, which responds to stresses in an elastic fashion. It is more compliant than compact bone, and microfractures can be a means of force absorption. Trabeculae might fracture or might be displaced due to pressures applied on the subchondral bone. In compact bone, fracture can be a means of defense to dissipate force. In the joint, forces might be absorbed by joint movement and eccentric contraction of muscles.[27]

In the majority of joints where the surfaces are not congruent, the applied forces tend to concentrate in certain areas, which increases joint degeneration. Osteophytosis occurs as a bone attempts to increase its surface area to decrease contact forces. People typically describe this growth as "bone spurs." Chondromalacia is the nonprogressive transformation of cartilage with irregular surfaces and areas of softening. It typically occurs first in non-weightbearing areas and may progress to areas of excessive stress.[26]

In physically active individuals, certain joints maybe more susceptible to a response resembling osteoarthrosis.[70] The proportion of body weight resting on the joint, the pull of the musculotendinous unit, and any significant external force applied to the joint are predisposing factors. Altered joint mechanics caused by laxity or previous trauma are also factors that come into play.[45] The intensity of forces can be great, as in the hip, where the previously mentioned factors can produce pressures or forces 4 times that of body weight and up to 10 times that of body weight on the knee.

Typically, muscle forces generate more stress than body weight itself. Particular injuries are conducive to osteoarthritic changes such as subluxation and dislocation of the patella, osteochondritis dissecans, recurrent synovial effusion, and hemarthrosis. Also, ligamentous injuries can bring about a disruption of proprioceptive mechanisms, loss of adequate joint alignment, and meniscal damage in the knees with removal of the injured meniscus.[40] Other factors that have an impact are loss of full range of motion, poor muscular power and strength, and altered biomechanics of the joint. Spurring and spiking of bone are not synonymous with osteoarthrosis if the joint space is maintained and the cartilage lining is intact. It may simply be an adaptation to the increased stress of physical activity.[29]

Physiology of Cartilage Healing

Cartilage has a relatively limited healing capacity. When chondrocytes are destroyed and the matrix is disrupted, the course of healing is variable, depending on whether damage is to cartilage alone or also to subchondral bone. Injuries to the articular cartilage alone fail to elicit clot formation or a cellular response. For the most part the chondrocytes adjacent to the injury are the only cells that show any signs of proliferation and synthesis of matrix. Thus the defect fails to heal, although the extent of the damage tends to remain the same.[33,58]

If subchondral bone is also affected, inflammatory cells enter the damaged area and formulate granulation tissue. In this case, the healing process proceeds normally, with differentiation of granulation tissue cells into chondrocytes occurring in approximately 2 weeks. At approximately 2 months, normal collagen has been formed.

Injuries to the knee articular cartilage are extremely common, and until recently, methods for treatment did not produce good long-term results.[102] A better understanding of how articular cartilage responds to injury has produced various techniques that hold promise for long-term success.[91] One such technique is autologous chondrocyte implantation, in which a patient's own cartilage cells are harvested, grown ex vivo, and reimplanted in a full-thickness articular surface defect. Results are available with up to 10 years of follow-up, and more than 80% of patients have shown improvement with relatively few complications.

Injuries to Bone

Bone is a type of connective tissue consisting of both living cells and minerals deposited in a matrix (Figure 2-5). Each bone consists of 3 major components. The epiphysis is an expanded portion at each end of the bone that articulates with another bone. Each articulating surface is covered by an articular, or hyaline, cartilage. The diaphysis is the shaft of the bone. The epiphyseal or growth plate is the major site of bone growth and elongation. Once bone growth ceases, the plate ossifies and forms the epiphyseal line. With the exception of the articulating surfaces, the bone is completely enclosed by the periosteum, a tough, highly vascularized and innervated fibrous tissue.[55]

The 2 types of bone material are cancellous, or spongy, bone and cortical, or compact, bone. Cancellous bone contains a series of air spaces referred to as trabeculae, whereas cortical bone is relatively solid. Cortical bone in the diaphysis forms a hollow medullary canal in long bone, which is lined with endosteum and filled with bone marrow. Bone has rich blood supply that certainly facilitates the healing process after injury. Bone has the functions of support, movement, and protection. Furthermore, bone stores and releases calcium into the bloodstream and manufactures red blood cells.[93]

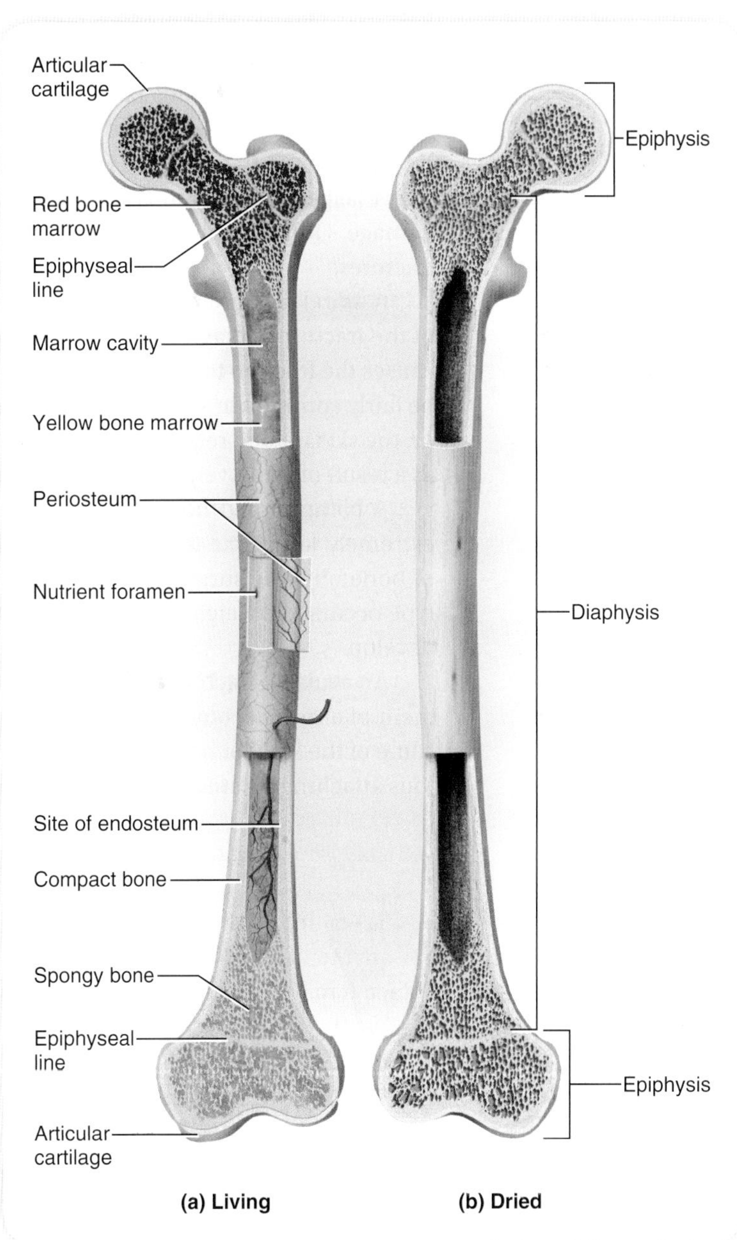

Figure 2-5 The gross structure of the long bones includes the diaphysis, epiphysis, articular cartilage, and periosteum

(Reproduced with permission from Saladin. *Anatomy and physiology*. 5th ed. Dubuque, IA: McGraw-Hill; 2010.)

Fractures

Fractures are extremely common injuries among the athletic population. They can be generally classified as being either open or closed. A closed fracture involves little or no displacement of bones and thus little or no soft-tissue disruption. An open fracture involves enough displacement of the fractured ends that the bone actually disrupts the cutaneous layers and breaks through the skin. Both fractures can be relatively serious if not managed properly, but an increased possibility of infection exists in an open fracture. Fractures may also be considered complete, in which the bone is broken into at least 2 fragments, or incomplete, where the fracture does not extend completely across the bone.

The varieties of fractures that can occur include greenstick, transverse, oblique, spiral, comminuted, avulsion, and stress. A greenstick fracture (Figure 2-6*A*) occurs most often in children whose bones are still growing and have not yet had a chance to calcify and harden. It is called a greenstick fracture because of the resemblance to the splintering that occurs to a tree twig that is bent to the point of breaking. Because the twig is green, it splinters but can be bent without causing an actual break.

A transverse fracture (see Figure 2-6*B*) involves a crack perpendicular to the longitudinal axis of the bone that goes all the way through the bone. Displacement might occur; however, because of the shape of the fractured ends, the surrounding soft tissue (eg, muscles, tendons, and fat) sustains relatively little damage.

A linear fracture runs parallel to the long axis of a bone and is similar in severity to a transverse fracture (see Figure 2-6*C*).

An oblique fracture (see Figure 2-6*D*) results in a diagonal crack across the bone and 2 very jagged, pointed ends that, if displaced, can potentially cause a good bit of soft-tissue damage. Oblique and spiral fractures are the 2 types most likely to result in compound fractures.

A spiral fracture (see Figure 2-6*E*) is similar to an oblique fracture in that the angle of the fracture is diagonal across the bone. In addition, an element of twisting or rotation causes the fracture to spiral along the longitudinal axis of the bone. Spiral fractures used to be fairly common in ski injuries occurring just above the top of the boot when the bindings on the ski failed to release when the foot was rotated. These injuries are now less common as a result of improvements in equipment design.

A comminuted fracture (see Figure 2-6*F*) is a serious problem that can require an extremely long time for rehabilitation. In the comminuted fracture, multiple fragments of bone must be surgically repaired and fixed with screws and wires. If a fracture of this type occurs to a weightbearing bone in the leg, a permanent discrepancy in leg length can develop.

An avulsion fracture occurs when a fragment of bone is pulled away at the bony attachment of a muscle, tendon, or ligament. Avulsion fractures are common in the fingers and some of the smaller bones but can also occur in larger bones where tendinous or ligamentous attachments are subjected to a large amount of force.

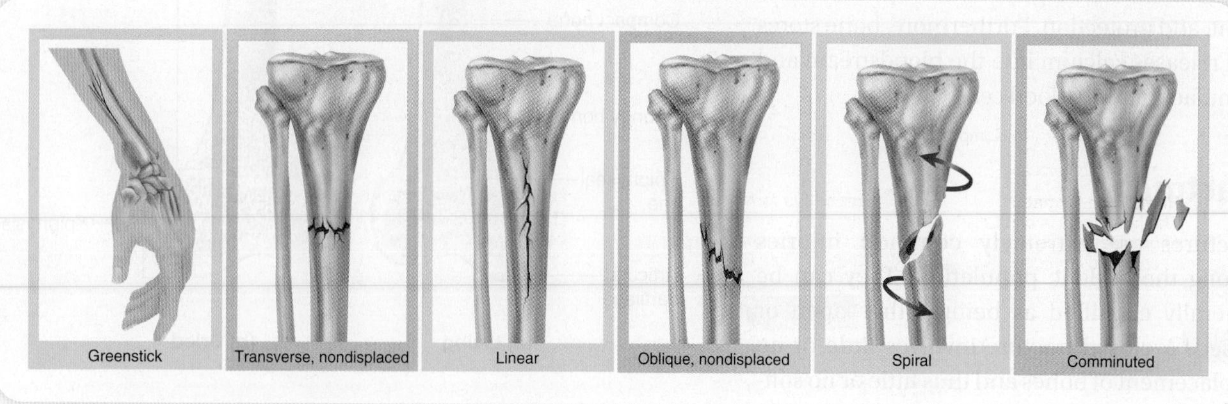

Figure 2-6 **Fractures of bone**

A. Greenstick. **B.** Transverse. **C.** Linear. **D.** Oblique. **E.** Spiral. **F.** Comminuted. (Reproduced with permission from Prentice. *Essentials of Athletic Injury Management*. 9th ed. New York: McGraw-Hill; 2013.)

Perhaps the most common fracture resulting from physical activity is the stress fracture. Unlike the other types of fractures that have been discussed, the stress fracture results from overuse or fatigue rather than acute trauma.[49] Common sites for stress fractures include the weightbearing bones of the leg and foot. In either case, repetitive forces transmitted through the bones produce irritations and microfractures at a specific area in the bone. The pain usually begins as a dull ache that becomes progressively more painful day after day. Initially, pain is most severe during activity. However, when a stress fracture actually develops, pain tends to become worse after the activity is stopped.[80]

The biggest problem with a stress fracture is that often it does not show up on an X-ray film until the osteoblasts begin laying down subperiosteal callus or bone, at which point a small white line, or a callus, appears. However, a bone scan might reveal a potential stress fracture in as little as 2 days after onset of symptoms. If a stress fracture is suspected, the patient should stop any activity that produces added stress or fatigue to the area for a minimum of 14 days. Stress fractures do not usually require casting but might become normal fractures that must be immobilized if handled incorrectly.[92] If a fracture occurs, it should be managed and rehabilitated by a qualified orthopedist and physical therapist.

Physiology of Bone Healing

Healing of injured bone tissue is similar to soft-tissue healing in that all phases of the healing process can be identified, although bone regeneration capabilities are somewhat limited. However, the functional elements of healing differ significantly from those of soft tissue. Tensile strength of the scar is the single most critical factor in soft-tissue healing, whereas bone has to contend with a number of additional forces, including torsion, bending, and compression.[46] Trauma to bone can vary from contusions of the periosteum to closed, nondisplaced fractures to severely displaced open fractures that also involve significant soft-tissue damage. When a fracture occurs, blood vessels in the bone and the periosteum are damaged, resulting in bleeding and subsequent clot formation (Figure 2-7). Hemorrhaging from the marrow is contained by the periosteum and the surrounding soft tissue in the

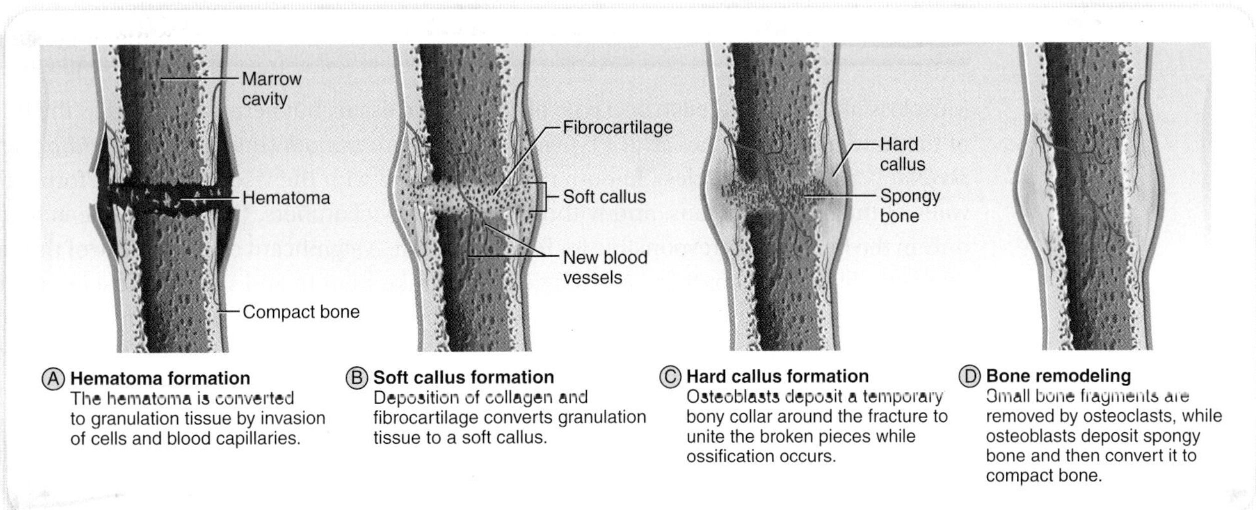

Figure 2-7 The healing of a fracture

A. Blood vessels are broken at the fracture line; the blood clots and forms a fracture hematoma. **B.** Blood vessels grow into the fracture and a fibrocartilage soft callus forms. **C.** The fibrocartilage becomes ossified and forms a bony callus made of spongy bone. **D.** Osteoclasts remove excess tissue from the bony callus and the bone eventually resembles its original appearance. (Reproduced with permission from Prentice. *Principles of Athletic Training*. 14th ed. New York: McGraw-Hill; 2011.)

region of the fracture. In approximately 1 week, fibroblasts begin laying down a fibrous collagen network. The fibrin strands within the clot serve as the framework for proliferating vessels. Chondroblast cells begin producing fibrocartilage, creating a callus between the broken bones. At first, the callus is soft and firm because it is composed primarily of collagenous fibrin. The callus becomes firm and more rubbery as cartilage beings to predominate. Bone-producing cells called osteoblasts begin to proliferate and enter the callus, forming cancellous bone trabeculae, which eventually replace the cartilage. Finally the callus crystallizes into bone, at which point remodeling of the bone begins. The callus can be divided into two portions, the external callus located around the periosteum on the outside of the fracture and the internal callus found between the bone fragments. The size of the callus is proportional both to the damage and to the amount of irritation to the fracture site during the healing process. Also during this time osteoclasts begin to appear in the area to resorb bone fragments and clean up debris.[42,46,83]

The remodeling process is similar to the growth process of bone in that the fibrous cartilage is gradually replaced by fibrous bone and then by more structurally efficient lamellar bone. Remodeling involves an ongoing process during which osteoblasts lay down new bone and osteoclasts remove and break down bone according to the forces placed upon the healing bone.[62] The Wolff law maintains that a bone will adapt to mechanical stresses and strains by changing size, shape, and structure. Therefore, once the cast is removed, the bone must be subjected to normal stresses and strains so that tensile strength can be regained before the healing process is complete.[36,90]

The time required for bone healing is variable and based on a number of factors, such as severity of the fracture, site of the fracture, extensiveness of the trauma, and age of the patient. Normal periods of immobilization range from as short as 3 weeks for the small bones in the hands and feet to as long as 8 weeks for the long bones of the upper and lower extremities. In some instances, such as fractures in the 4 small toes, immobilization might not be required for healing. The healing process is certainly not complete when the splint or cast is removed. Osteoblastic and osteoclastic activity might continue for 2 to 3 years after severe fractures.[49,62]

Injuries to Musculotendinous Structures

Muscle is often considered to be a type of connective tissue, but here it is treated as the third of the fundamental tissues. The 3 types of muscles are *smooth* (involuntary), *cardiac,* and *skeletal* (voluntary) muscles. Smooth muscle is found with the viscera, where it forms the walls of the internal organs, and within many hollow chambers. Cardiac muscle is found only in the heart and is responsible for its contraction. A significant characteristic of the cardiac muscle is that it contracts as a single fiber, unlike smooth and skeletal muscles, which contract as separate units. This characteristic forces the heart to work as a single unit continuously; therefore, if one portion of the muscle should die (as in myocardial infarction), contraction of the heart does not cease.[79]

Skeletal muscle is the striated muscle within the body, responsible for the movement of bony levers (Figure 2-8). Skeletal muscle consists of 2 portions: (a) the muscle belly, and (b) its tendons, which are collectively referred to as a musculotendinous unit. The muscle belly is composed of separate, parallel elastic fibers called *myofibrils.* Myofibrils are composed of thousands of small sarcomeres, which are the functional units of the muscle. Sarcomeres contain the contractile elements of the muscle, as well as a substantial amount of connective tissue that holds the fibers together. Myofilaments are small contractile elements of protein within the sarcomere. There are 2 distinct types of myofilaments: thin *actin myofilaments* and thicker *myosin myofilaments.* Fingerlike projections, or crossbridges, connect

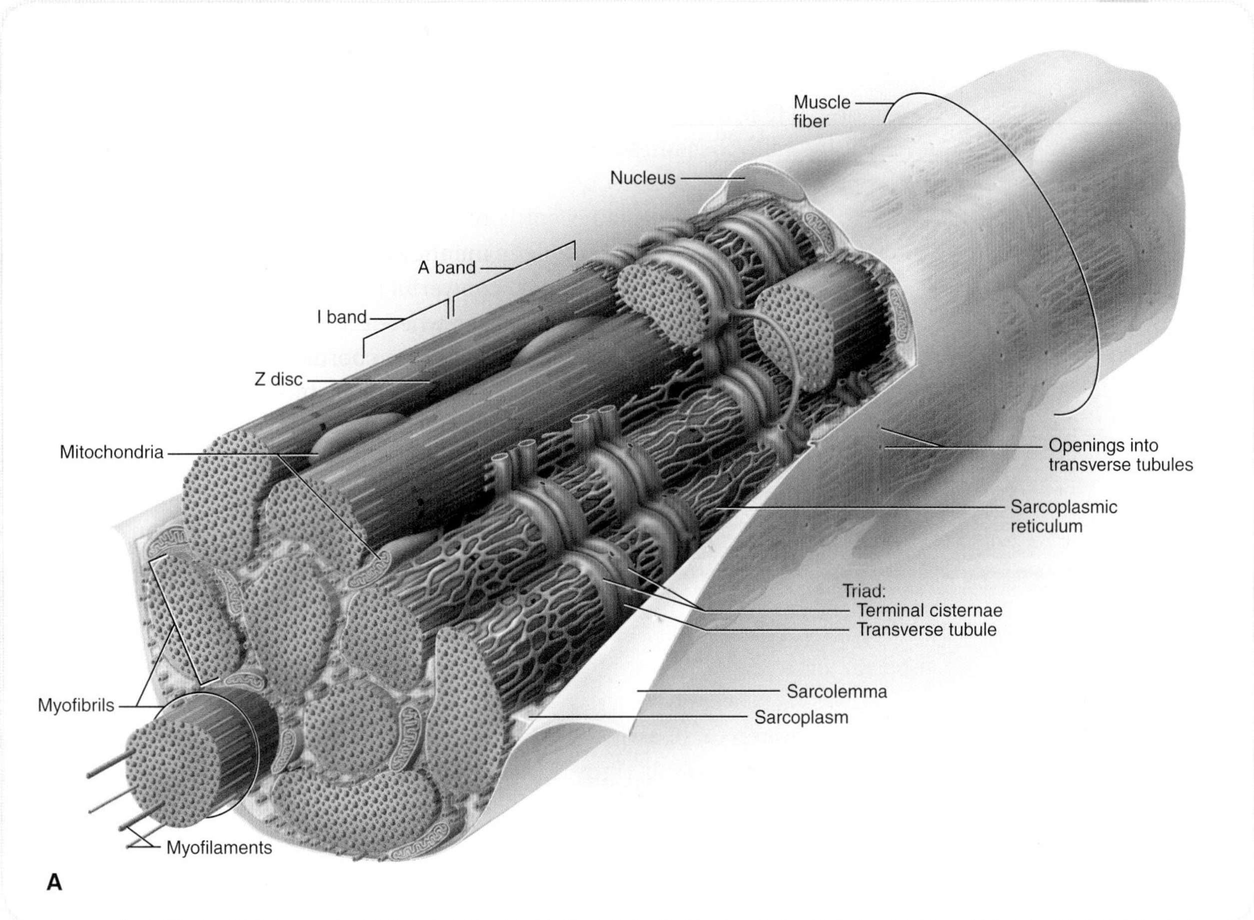

Figure 2-8 Parts of a muscle

A. Muscle is composed of individual muscle fibers (muscle cells). Each muscle fiber contains myofibrils in which the banding patterns of the sarcomeres are seen. **B.** The myofibrils are composed of actin myofilament and myosin myofilaments, which are formed from thousands of individual actin and myosin molecules. (Reproduced with permission from Saladin. *Anatomy and Physiology*. 6th ed. New York: McGraw-Hill; 2012.)

the actin and myosin myofilaments.[83] When a muscle is stimulated to contract, the cross-bridges pull the myofilaments closer together, thus shortening the muscle and producing movement at the joint that the muscle crosses.[25]

The muscle tendon attaches the muscle directly to the bone. The muscle tendon is composed primarily of collagen fibers and a matrix of proteoglycan, which is produced by the tenocyte cell. The collagen fibers are grouped together into primary bundles. Groups of primary bundles join together to form hexagonal-shaped secondary bundles. Secondary bundles are held together by intertwined loose connective tissue containing elastin, called the *endotenon*. The entire tendon is surrounded by a connective tissue layer, called the *epitenon*. The outermost layer of the tendon is the paratenon, which is a double-layer connective tissue sheath lined on the inside with synovial membrane (Figure 2-9).[56]

All skeletal muscles exhibit 4 characteristics: (a) elasticity, the ability to change in length or stretch; (b) extensibility, the ability to shorten and return to normal length; (c) excitability, the ability to respond to stimulation from the nervous system; and (d) contractility, the ability to shorten and contract in response to some neural command.[55]

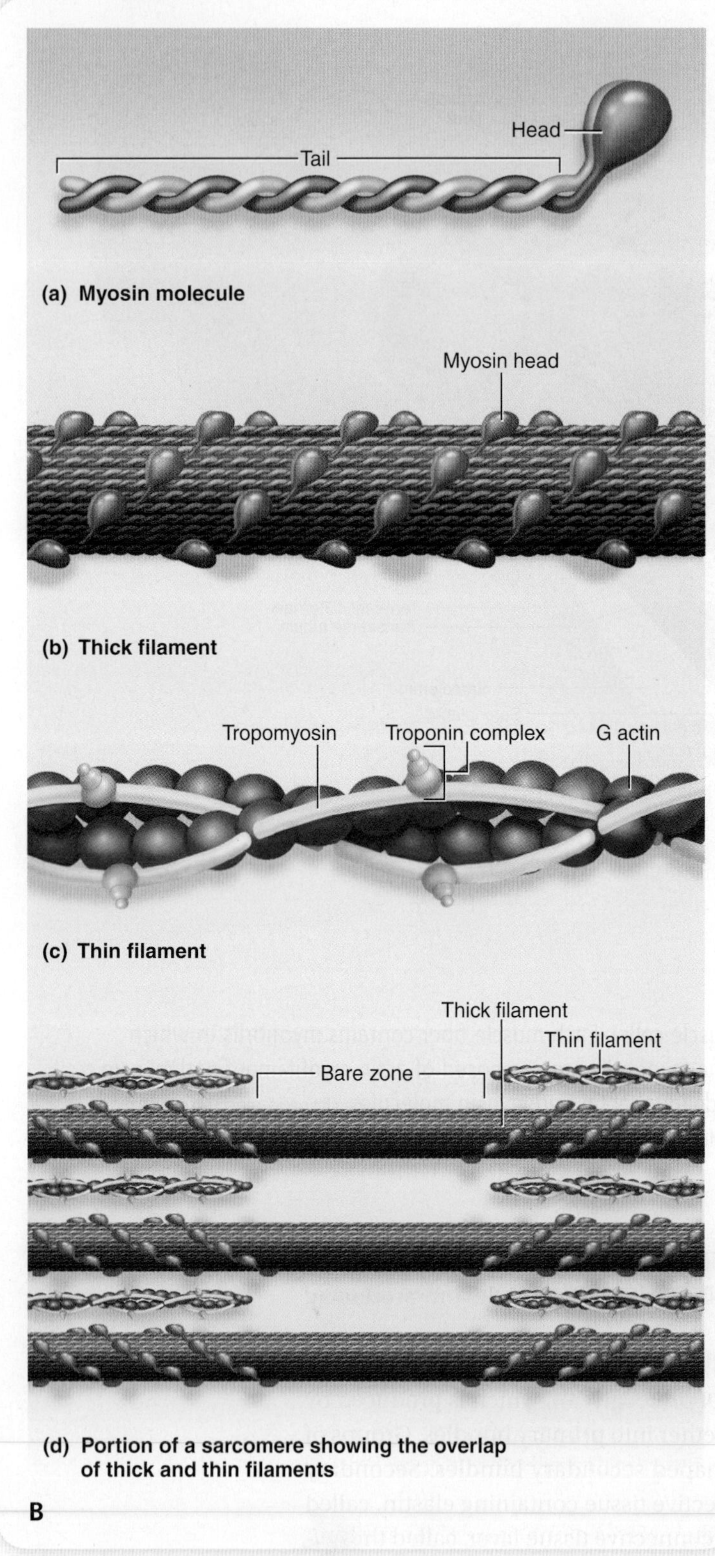

Figure 2-8 *(Continued)*

Skeletal muscles show considerable variation in size and shape. Large muscles generally produce gross motor movements at large joints, such as knee flexion produced by contraction of the large, bulky hamstring muscles. Smaller skeletal muscles, such as the long flexors of the fingers, produce fine motor movements. Muscles producing movements that are powerful in nature are usually thicker and longer, whereas those producing finer movements requiring coordination are thin and relatively shorter. Other muscles may be flat, round, or fan-shaped.[42,83] Muscles may be connected to a bone by a single tendon or by 2 or 3 separate tendons at either end. Muscles that have 2 separate muscle and tendon attachments are called biceps, and muscles with 3 separate muscle and tendon attachments are called triceps.

Muscles contract in response to stimulation by the central nervous system. An electrical impulse transmitted from the central nervous system through a single motor nerve to a group of muscle fibers causes a depolarization of those fibers. The motor nerve and the group of muscle fibers that it innervates are collectively referred to as a motor unit. An impulse coming from the central nervous system and traveling to a group of fibers through a particular motor nerve causes all the muscle fibers in that motor unit to depolarize and contract. This is referred to as the all-or-none response and applies to all skeletal muscles in the body.[42]

Muscle Strains

If a musculotendinous unit is overstretched or forced to contract against too much resistance, exceeding the extensibility limits or the tensile capabilities of the weakest component within the unit, damage can occur to the muscle fibers, at the musculotendinous juncture, in the tendon, or at the tendinous attachment to the bone.[34] Any of these injuries may be referred to as a strain (Figure 2-10). Muscle strains, like ligament sprains, are subject to various classification systems. The following is a simple system of classification of muscle strains:

Grade 1 strain: Some muscle or tendon fibers have been stretched or actually torn. Active motion produces some tenderness and pain. Movement is painful, but full range of motion is usually possible.

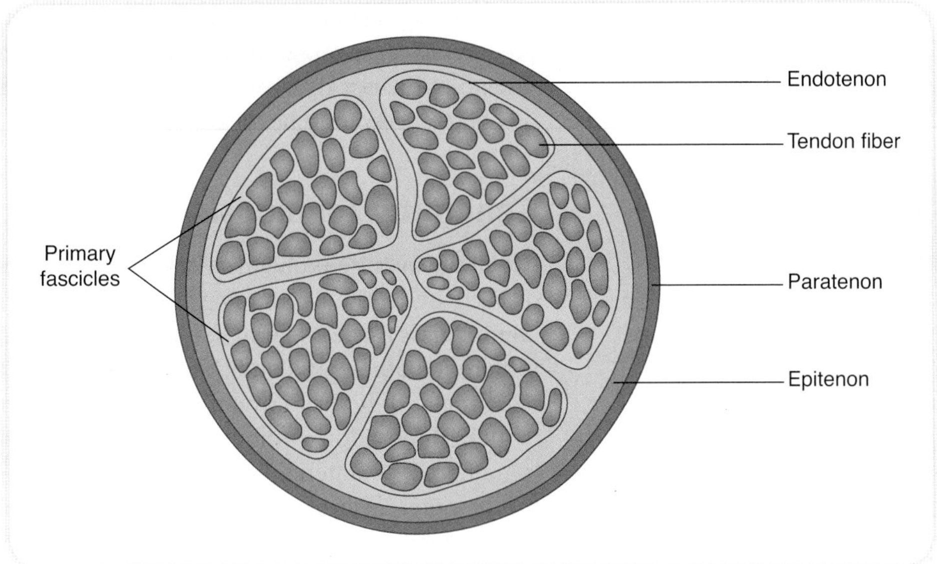

Figure 2-9 **Structure of a tendon**

Grade 2 strain: Some muscle or tendon fibers have been torn and active contraction of the muscle is extremely painful. Usually a palpable depression or divot exists somewhere in the muscle belly at the spot where the muscle fibers have been torn. Some swelling might occur because of capillary bleeding.

Grade 3 strain: There is a complete rupture of muscle fibers in the muscle belly, in the area where the muscle becomes tendon, or at the tendinous attachment to the bone. The patient has significant impairment to, or perhaps total loss of, movement. Pain is intense initially but diminishes quickly because of complete separation of the nerve fibers. Musculotendinous ruptures are most common in the biceps tendon of the upper arm or in the Achilles heel cord in the back of the calf. When either of these tendons rupture, the muscle tends to bunch toward its proximal attachment. With the exception of an Achilles rupture, which is frequently surgically repaired, the majority of third-degree strains are treated conservatively with some period of immobilization.

Physiology of Muscle Healing

Injuries to muscle tissue involve similar processes of healing and repair as discussed for other tissues. Initially there will be hemorrhage and edema followed almost immediately by phagocytosis to clear debris. Within a few days there is a proliferation of ground substance, and fibroblasts begin producing a gel-type matrix that surrounds the connective tissue, leading to fibrosis and scarring. At the same time, myoblastic cells form in the area of injury, which will eventually lead to regeneration or new myofibrils. Thus regeneration of both connective tissue and muscle tissue begins.[13]

Collagen fibers undergo maturation and orient themselves along lines of tensile force according to the Wolff law. Active contraction of the muscle is critical in regaining normal tensile strength.[5,50]

Regardless of the severity of the strain, the time required for rehabilitation is fairly lengthy. In many instances, rehabilitation time for a muscle strain is longer than that for a ligament sprain. These incapacitating muscle strains occur most frequently in the large, force-producing hamstring and quadriceps muscles of the lower extremity. The treatment of hamstring strains requires a healing period of at least 5 to 8 weeks and a considerable amount

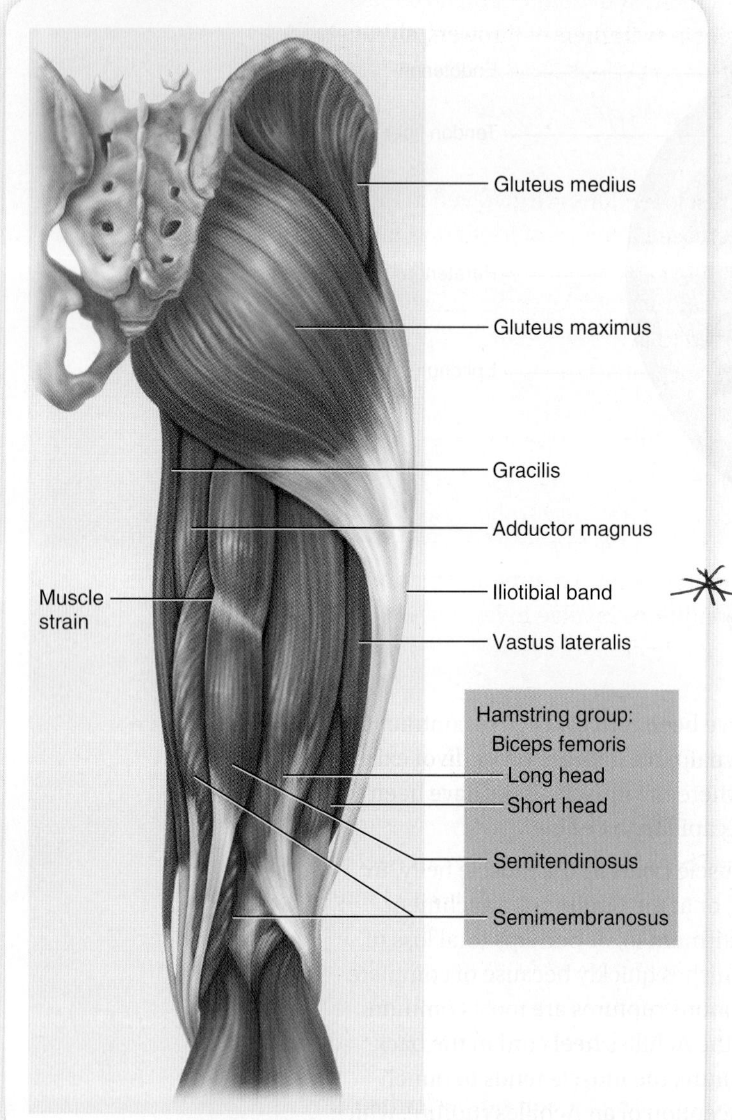

Figure 2-10 A muscle strain results in tearing or separation of fibers

(Reproduced with permission from Prentice. *Principles of Athletic Training*. 14th ed. New York: McGraw-Hill; 2011.)

of patience. Attempts to return to activity too soon frequently cause reinjury to the area of the musculotendinous unit that has been strained, and the healing process must begin again.[60]

Tendinitis/Tendinosis

Of all the overuse problems associated with physical activity, tendinitis is among the most common.[48] Tendinitis is a catchall term that can describe many different pathologic conditions for a tendon. It essentially describes any inflammatory response within the tendon without inflammation of the paratenon.[87] Paratenonitis involves inflammation of the outer layer of the tendon only, and usually occurs when the tendon rubs over a bony prominence. Tendinosis describes a tendon that has significant degenerative changes with no clinical or histologic signs of an inflammatory response.[20]

In cases of what is most often called chronic tendinitis, there is evidence of significant tendon degeneration, loss of normal collagen structure, loss of cellularity in the area, but absolutely no inflammatory cellular response in the tendon.[81] The inflammatory process is an essential part of healing. Inflammation is supposed to be a brief process with an end point after its function in the healing process has been fulfilled. The point or the cause in the pathologic process where the acute inflammatory cellular response terminates and the chronic degeneration begins is difficult to determine.[23] As mentioned previously, with chronic tendinitis the cellular response involves a replacement of leukocytes with macrophages and plasma cells.[99]

During muscle activity a tendon must move or slide on other structures around it whenever the muscle contracts. If a particular movement is performed repeatedly, the tendon becomes irritated and inflamed. This inflammation is manifested by pain on movement, swelling, possibly some warmth, and usually crepitus. Crepitus is a crackling sound similar to the sound produced by rolling hair between the fingers by the ear. Crepitus is usually caused by the adherence of the paratenon to the surrounding structures as it slides back and forth. This adhesion is caused primarily by the chemical products of inflammation that accumulate on the irritated tendon.[20]

The key to treating tendinitis is rest. If the repetitive motion causing irritation to the tendon is eliminated, chances are that the inflammatory process will allow the tendon to heal.[65] Unfortunately, a patient who is seriously involved with some physical activity might have difficulty in resting for 2 weeks or more while the tendinitis subsides. Antiinflammatory medications and therapeutic modalities are also helpful in reducing the inflammatory responses. An alternative activity, such as bicycling or swimming, is necessary to maintain fitness levels to a certain degree, while allowing the tendon a chance to heal.[30]

Tendinitis most commonly occurs in the Achilles tendon in the back of the lower leg in runners or in the rotator cuff tendons of the shoulder joint in swimmers or throwers, although it can certainly flare up in any tendon in which overuse and repetitive movements occur.

Tenosynovitis

Tenosynovitis is very similar to tendinitis in that the muscle tendons are involved in inflammation. However, many tendons are subject to an increased amount of friction as a result of the tightness of the space through which they must move. In these areas of high friction, tendons are usually surrounded by synovial sheaths that reduce friction on movement. If the tendon sliding through a synovial sheath is subjected to overuse, inflammation is likely to occur. The inflammatory process produces by-products that are "sticky" and tend to cause the sliding tendon to adhere to the synovial sheath surrounding it.[51]

Symptomatically, tenosynovitis is very similar to tendinitis, with pain on movement, tenderness, swelling, and crepitus. Movement may be more limited with tenosynovitis because the space provided for the tendon and its synovial covering is more limited. Tenosynovitis occurs most commonly in the long flexor tendons of the fingers as they cross over the wrist joint and in the biceps tendon around the shoulder joint. Treatment for tenosynovitis is the same as that for tendinitis. Because both conditions involve inflammation, mild antiinflammatory drugs, such as aspirin, might be helpful in chronic cases.[51]

Physiology of Tendon Healing

Unlike most soft-tissue healing, tendon injuries pose a particular problem in rehabilitation.[40] The injured tendon requires dense fibrous union of the separated ends and both extensibility and flexibility at the site of attachment. Thus an abundance of collagen is required to achieve good tensile strength. Unfortunately, collagen synthesis can become excessive, resulting in fibrosis, in which adhesions form in surrounding tissues and interfere with the gliding that is essential for smooth motion. Fortunately, over a period of time the scar tissue of the surrounding tissues becomes elongated in its structure because of a breakdown in the crosslinks between fibrin units and thus allows the necessary gliding motion. A tendon injury that occurs where the tendon is surrounded by a synovial sheath can be potentially devastating.

A typical time frame for tendon healing would be that during the second week when the healing tendon adheres to the surrounding tissue to form a single mass and during the third week when the tendon separates to varying degrees from the surrounding tissues. However, the tensile strength is not sufficient to permit a strong pull on the tendon for at least 4 to 5 weeks, the danger being that a strong contraction can pull the tendon ends apart.[85]

Injuries to Nerve Tissue

The final fundamental tissue is nerve tissue (Figure 2-11). This tissue provides sensitivity and communication from the central nervous system (brain and spinal cord) to the muscles, sensory organs, various systems, and the periphery. The basic nerve cell is the neuron. The neuron cell body contains a large nucleus and branched extensions called *dendrites*, which respond to neurotransmitter substances released from other nerve cells. From each nerve cell arises a single axon, which conducts the nerve impulses. Large axons found in peripheral nerves are enclosed in sheaths composed of Schwann cells, which are tightly wound around the axon. A nerve is a bundle of nerve cells held together by some connective tissue, usually a lipid-protein layer called the *myelin sheath*, on the outside of the axon.[93] Neurology is an extremely complex science, and only a brief presentation of its relevance to musculoskeletal injuries is made here.[16]

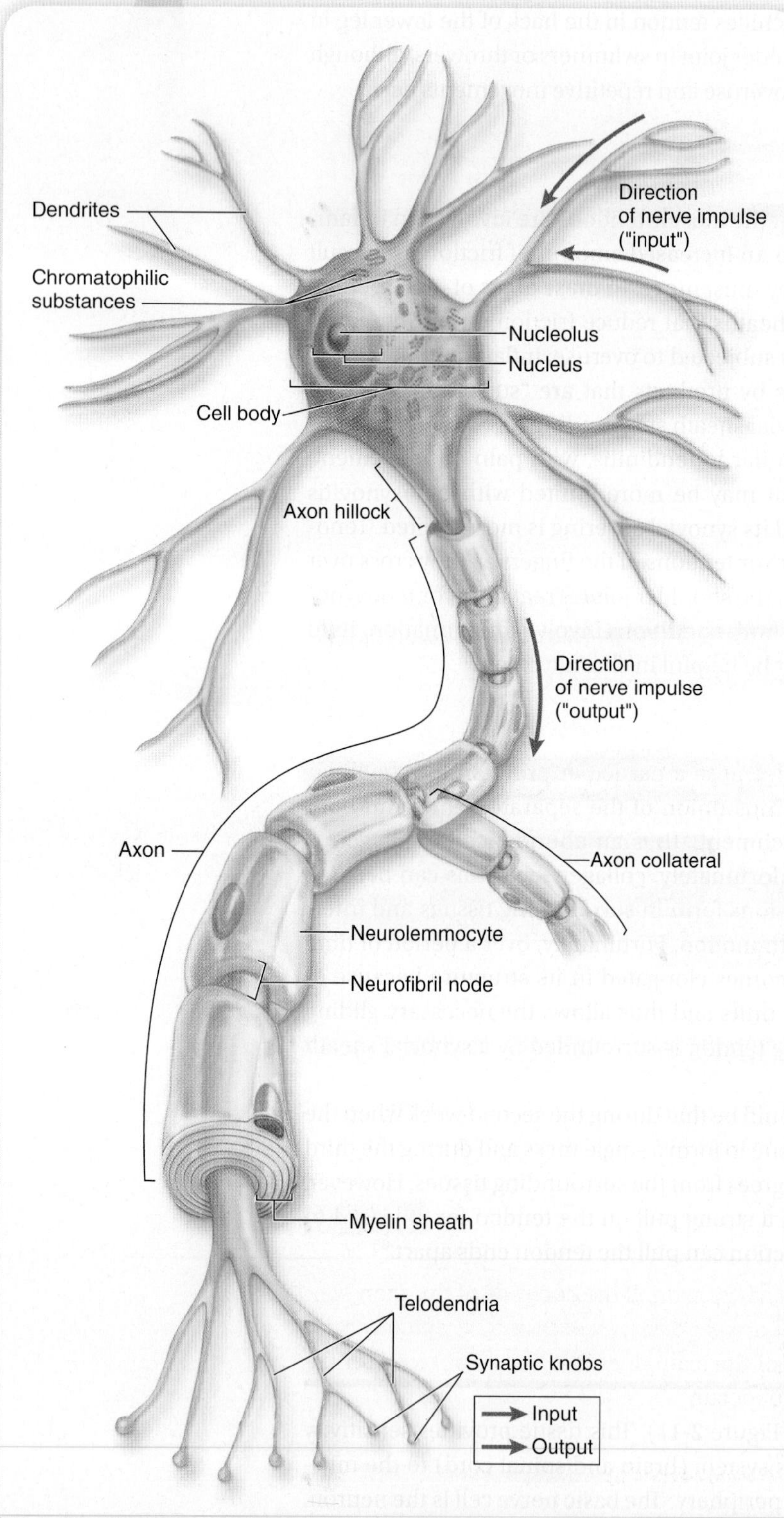

Figure 2-11 Structural features of a nerve cell

(Reproduced with permission from Prentice. *Principles of Athletic Training*. 14th ed. New York: McGraw-Hill; 2011.)

Nerve injuries usually involve either contusions or inflammations. More serious injuries involve the crushing of a nerve or complete division (severing). This type of injury can produce lifelong physical disability, such as paraplegia or quadriplegia, and thus should not be overlooked in any circumstance.

Of critical concern to the therapist is the importance of the nervous system in proprioception and neuromuscular control of movement as an integral part of a rehabilitation program. Chapter 4 discusses this in great detail.

Physiology of Nerve Healing

Nerve cell tissue is specialized and cannot regenerate once the nerve cell dies. In an injured peripheral nerve, however, the nerve fiber can regenerate significantly if the injury does not affect the cell body (Figure 2-12). The proximity of the axonal injury to the cell body can significantly affect the time required for healing. The closer an injury is to the cell body, the more difficult is the regenerative process. In the case of severed nerve, surgical intervention can markedly enhance regeneration.[79]

For regeneration to occur, an optimal environment for healing must exist. When a nerve is cut, several degenerative changes occur that interfere with the neural pathways (see Figure 2-12). Within the first 3 to 5 days the portion of the axon distal to the cut begins to degenerate and breaks into irregular segments. There is also a concomitant increase in metabolism and protein production by the nerve cell body to facilitate the regenerative process. The neuron in the cell body contains the genetic material and produces chemicals necessary for maintenance of the axon. These substances cannot be transmitted to the distal part of the axon, and eventually there will be complete degeneration.[83]

In addition, the myelin portion of the Schwann cells around the degenerating axon also degenerates, and the myelin is phagocytized. The Schwann

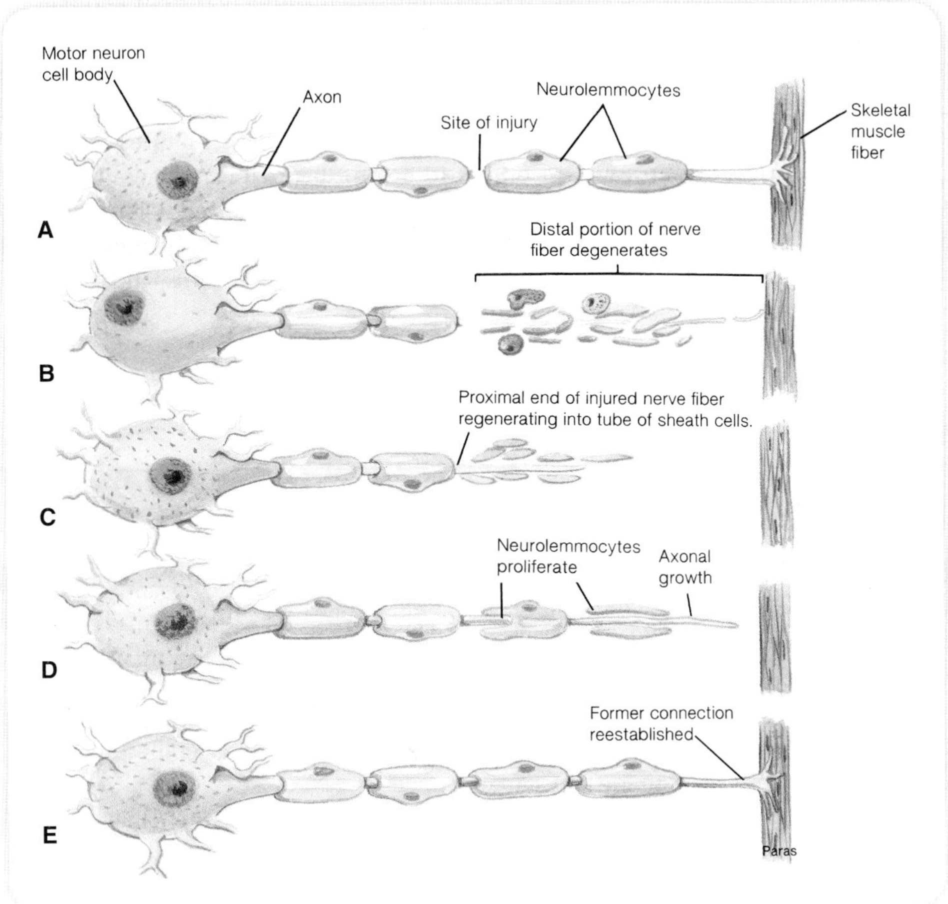

Figure 2-12 Neuron regeneration

A. If a neuron is severed through a myelinated axon, the proximal portion may survive, but (**B**) the distal portion will degenerate through phagocytosis. **C** and **D.** The myelin layer provides a pathway for regeneration of the axon, and (**E**) innervation is restored. (Reproduced with permission from Prentice. *Principles of Athletic Training*. 14th ed. New York: McGraw-Hill; 2011.)

cells divide, forming a column of cells in place of the axon. If the cut ends of the axon contact this column of Schwann cells, the chances are good that an axon may eventually reinnervate distal structures. If the proximal end of the axon does not make contact with the column of Schwann cells, reinnervation will not occur.

Clinical Pearl

Peripheral nerves are likely to regenerate if the cell body has not been damaged. The closer the injury is to the cell body, the more difficult the healing process is. If a nerve is severed, surgical intervention can significantly improve chances of regeneration.

The axon proximal to the cut has minimal degeneration initially and then begins the regenerative process with growth from the proximal axon. Bulbous enlargements and several axon sprouts form at the end of the proximal axon. Within approximately 2 weeks, these sprouts grow across the scar that has developed in the area of the cut and enter the column of Schwann cells. Only one of these sprouts will form the new axon, while the others will degenerate. Once the axon grows through the Schwann cell columns, remaining Schwann cells proliferate along the length of the degenerating fiber and form new myelin around the growing axon, which will eventually reinnervate distal structures.[42]

Regeneration is slow, at a rate of only 3 to 4 mm/day. Axon regeneration can be obstructed by scar formation caused by excessive fibroplasia. Damaged nerves within the central nervous system regenerate very poorly compared to nerves in the peripheral nervous system. Central nervous system axons lack connective tissue sheaths, and the myelin-producing Schwann cells fail to proliferate.[42,83]

Additional Musculoskeletal Injuries

Dislocations and Subluxations

A dislocation occurs when at least 1 bone in an articulation is forced out of its normal and proper alignment and stays out until it is either manually or surgically put back into place or reduced.[10] Dislocations most commonly occur in the shoulder joint, elbow, and fingers, but they can occur wherever 2 bones articulate.[15,64,82]

A subluxation is like a dislocation except that in this situation a bone pops out of its normal articulation but then goes right back into place. Subluxations most commonly occur in the shoulder joint, as well as in the kneecap in females.

Dislocations should never be reduced immediately, regardless of where they occur. The patient should have an X-ray to rule out fractures or other problems before reduction. Inappropriate techniques of reduction might only exacerbate the problem. Return to activity after dislocation or subluxation is largely dependent on the degree of soft-tissue damage.[15]

Bursitis

In many areas, particularly around joints, friction occurs between tendons and bones, skin and bone, or 2 muscles. Without some mechanism of protection in these high-friction areas, chronic irritation would be likely.[93]

Bursae are essentially pieces of synovial membrane that contain small amounts of synovial fluid. This presence of synovium permits motion of surrounding structures without friction. If excessive movement or perhaps some acute trauma occurs around these bursae, they become irritated and inflamed and begin producing large amounts of synovial fluid. The longer the irritation continues or the more severe the acute trauma, the more fluid is produced. As the fluid continues to accumulate in a limited space, pressure tends to increase and causes irritation of the pain receptors in the area.

Bursitis can be extremely painful and can severely restrict movement, especially if it occurs around a joint. Synovial fluid continues to be produced until the movement or trauma producing the irritation is eliminated.

A bursa that occasionally completely surrounds a tendon to allow more freedom of movement in a tight area is referred to as a synovial sheath. Irritation of this synovial sheath may restrict tendon motion.

All joints have many bursae surrounding them. Perhaps the 3 bursae most commonly irritated as a result of various types of physical activity are the subacromial bursa in the shoulder joint, the olecranon bursa on the tip of the elbow, and the prepatellar bursa on the front surface of the patella. All 3 of these bursae have produced large amounts of synovial fluid, affecting motion at their respective joints.

Muscle Soreness

Overexertion in strenuous muscular exercise often results in muscular pain. At one time or another, almost everyone has experienced muscle soreness, usually resulting from some physical activity to which we are unaccustomed.

There are 2 types of muscle soreness. The first type of muscle pain is acute and accompanies fatigue. It is transient and occurs during and immediately after exercise. The second type of soreness involves delayed muscle pain that appears approximately 12 hours after injury. It becomes most intense after 24 to 48 hours and then gradually subsides so that the muscle becomes symptom-free after 3 or 4 days. This second type of pain may best be described as a syndrome of delayed muscle pain, leading to increased muscle tension, edema formation, increased stiffness, and resistance to stretching.[61]

The cause of delayed-onset muscle soreness (DOMS) has been debated. Initially, it was hypothesized that soreness was caused by an excessive buildup of lactic acid in exercised muscles. However, recent evidence essentially rules out this theory.[1]

It has also been hypothesized that DOMS is caused by the tonic, localized spasm of motor units, varying in number with the severity of pain. This theory maintains that exercise causes varying degrees of ischemia in the working muscles. This ischemia causes pain, which results in reflex tonic muscle contraction that increases and prolongs the ischemia. Consequently a cycle of increasing severity is begun.[25] As with the lactic acid theory, the spasm theory has also been discounted.

Currently there are 2 schools of thought relative to the cause of DOMS. DOMS seems to occur from very small tears in the muscle tissue, which seem to be more likely with eccentric or isometric contractions.[1] It is generally believed that the initial damage caused by eccentric exercise is mechanical damage to either the muscular or the connective tissue. Edema accumulation and delays in the rate of glycogen repletion are secondary reactions to mechanical damage.[69]

DOMS might be caused by structural damage to the elastic components of connective tissue at the musculotendinous junction. This damage results in the presence of hydroxyproline, a protein by-product of collagen breakdown, in blood and urine.[19] It has also been documented that structural damage to the muscle fibers results in an increase in blood serum levels of various protein/enzymes, including creatine kinase. This increase indicates that there is likely some damage to the muscle fiber as a result of strenuous exercise.[1]

Muscle soreness can best be prevented by beginning at a moderate level of activity and gradually progressing the intensity of the exercise over time. Treatment of muscle soreness usually also involves some type of stretching activity.[39] As for other conditions discussed in this chapter, ice is important as a treatment for muscle soreness, particularly within the first 48 to 72 hours.

Contusions

Contusion is synonymous with bruise. The mechanism that produces a contusion is a blow from some external object that causes soft tissues (eg, skin, fat, muscle, ligaments, joint capsule) to be compressed against the hard bone underneath.[100] If the blow is hard enough, capillaries rupture and allow bleeding into the tissues. The bleeding, if superficial enough, causes a bluish-purple discoloration of the skin that persists for several days. The contusion may be very sore to the touch. If damage has occurred to muscle, pain may be elicited on active movement. In most cases the pain ceases within a few days, and discoloration disappears in usually 2 to 3 weeks.

The major problem with contusions occurs where an area is subjected to repeated blows. If the same area, or more specifically the same muscle, is bruised repeatedly, small calcium deposits might begin to accumulate in the injured area. These pieces of calcium might be found between several fibers in the muscle belly, or calcium might form a spur that projects from the underlying bone. These calcium formations, which can significantly impair movement, are referred to as myositis ossificans. In some cases myositis ossificans develops from a single trauma.[8]

The key to preventing myositis ossificans from occurring from repeated contusions is protection of the injured area by padding.[8] If the area is properly protected after the first contusion, myositis ossificans might never develop. Protection, along with rest, might allow the calcium to be reabsorbed and eliminate any need for surgical intervention. The 2 areas that seem to be the most vulnerable to repeated contusions during physical activity are the quadriceps muscle group on the front of the thigh and the biceps muscle on the front of the upper arm.[100] The formation of myositis ossificans in either of these or any other areas can be detected on radiograph films.

Incorporating Therapeutic Exercise to Affect the Healing Process

Rehabilitation exercise progressions can generally be subdivided into 3 phases, based primarily on the 3 stages of the healing process: phase 1, the acute phase; phase 2, the repair phase; and phase 3, the remodeling phase. Depending on the type and extent of injury and the individual response to healing, phases will usually overlap. Each phase must include carefully considered goals and criteria for progressing from one phase to another.[72]

Presurgical Exercise Phase

This phase would apply only to those patients who sustain injuries that require surgery. If surgery can be postponed, exercise may be used as a means to improve its outcome. By allowing the initial inflammatory response phase to resolve, by maintaining or, in some cases, increasing muscle strength and flexibility, levels of cardiorespiratory fitness, and improving neuromuscular control, the patient may be better prepared to continue the exercise rehabilitative program after surgery.

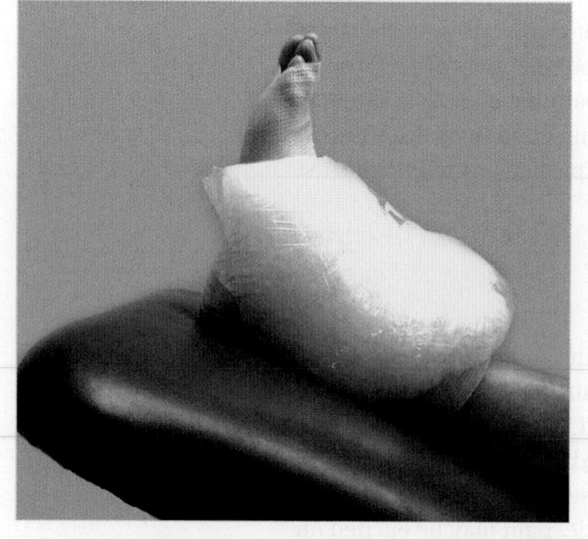

Figure 2-13

Musculoskeletal injuries should be treated initially with protection, restricted activity, ice, compression, and elevation.

Phase 1: The Acute Injury Phase

Phase 1 begins immediately when injury occurs and can last as long as 4 days following injury. During this phase, the inflammatory stage of the healing process is attempting to "clean up the mess," thus creating an environment that is conducive to the fibroblastic stage. As indicated in Chapter 1, the primary focus of rehabilitation during this stage is to control swelling and to modulate pain by using the PRICE (Protection, Restricted activity, Ice, Compression, and Elevation) technique immediately following injury. Ice, compression, and elevation should be used as much as possible during this phase (Figure 2-13).[73]

Rest of the injured part is critical during this phase. It is widely accepted that early mobility during rehabilitation is essential. However, if the therapist becomes overly aggressive during the first 48 hours following injury, and does not allow the injured part to be rested during the inflammatory stage of healing, the inflammatory process never really gets a chance to accomplish what it is supposed to. Consequently, the length of time required for inflammation might be extended. Therefore, immobility during the first 24 to 48 hours following injury is necessary to control inflammation. If the injury involves the lower extremity, the patient should be encouraged to be non-weightbearing for the first 24 hours and progressively bear more weight as pain permits.

By day 2 or 3, swelling begins to subside and eventually stops altogether. The injured area may feel warm to the touch, and some discoloration is usually apparent. The injury is still painful to the touch, and some pain is elicited on movement of the injured part.[98] Following injury there will almost always be some loss in range of motion. Acutely, that loss can be attributed primarily to pain and thus modalities (ie, ice, electrical stimulation) that modulate pain should be routinely incorporated into each treatment session. At this point the patient should begin active mobility exercises, working through a pain-free range of motion. In this phase, strengthening is less important than regaining range of motion, but should not be entirely ignored.

A physician may choose to have the patient take NSAIDs to help control swelling and inflammation. It is usually helpful to continue this medication throughout the rehabilitative process.[2]

Phase 2: The Repair Phase

Once the inflammatory response has subsided, the repair phase begins. During this stage of the healing process, fibroblastic cells are laying down a matrix of collagen fibers and forming scar tissue. This stage might begin as early as 2 days after the injury and can last for several weeks. At this point, swelling has stopped completely. The injury is still tender to the touch but is not as painful as it was during the previous stage. There is less pain on active and passive motion.[73]

As soon as inflammation is controlled, the therapist should immediately begin to incorporate into the rehabilitation program activities that can maintain levels of cardiorespiratory fitness, restore full range of motion, restore or increase strength, and reestablish neuromuscular control. The therapist should design exercises that simultaneously challenge the neural, muscular, and articular systems to help the patient regain neuromuscular control. As neuromuscular control improves strength will also improve. The patient very quickly "forgets" how to correctly execute even simple motor patterns such as walking, and the central nervous system must relearn how to integrate visual, proprioceptive, and kinematic information that collectively produces coordinated movement.

As in the acute phase, modalities should be used to control pain and swelling. Cryotherapy should still be used during the early portion of this phase to reduce the likelihood of swelling.[52] Electrical stimulating currents can help with controlling pain and improving strength and range of motion.[73]

Phase 3: The Remodeling Phase

The remodeling phase is the longest of the 3 phases and can last for several years, depending on the severity of the injury. The ultimate goal during this maturation stage of the healing process is return to activity. The injury is no longer painful to the touch, although some progressively decreasing pain might still be felt on motion. The collagen fibers must be realigned according to tensile stresses and strains placed upon them during functional exercises.

The focus during this phase should be on regaining functional skills. Functional training involves the repeated performance of movement or skill for the purpose of perfecting that skill. Strengthening exercises should progressively place on the injured structures stresses and strains that would normally be encountered during activity. Plyometric strengthening exercises can be used to improve muscle power and explosiveness.[40] Functional testing should be done to determine specific skill weaknesses that need to be addressed prior to normal activity return.

At this point some type of heating modality is beneficial to the healing process. The deep-heating modalities, ultrasound, or the diathermies should be used to increase circulation to the deeper tissues. Massage and gentle mobilization may also be used to reduce guarding, increase circulation, and reduce pain. Increased blood flow delivers the essential nutrients to the injured area to promote healing, and increased lymphatic flow assists in breakdown and removal of waste products.[73]

Using Medications to Affect the Healing Process

Medications are most commonly used in rehabilitation for pain relief. A patient may be continuously in pain that can be associated with even minor injury.

The over-the-counter nonnarcotic analgesics often used include aspirin (salicylate), acetaminophen, naproxen sodium ketoprofen, and ibuprofen. These belong to the group of drugs called NSAIDs. Aspirin is one of the most commonly used drugs in the world.[78] Because of its easy availability, it is also likely the most misused drug. Aspirin is a derivative of salicylic acid and is used for its analgesic, antiinflammatory, and antipyretic capabilities.

Analgesia can result from several mechanisms. Aspirin can interfere with the transmission of painful impulses in the thalamus.[78] Soft-tissue injury leads to tissue necrosis. This tissue injury causes the release of arachidonic acid from phospholipid cell walls. Oxygenation of arachidonic acid by cyclooxygenase produces a variety of prostaglandins, thromboxane, and prostacyclin that mediate the subsequent inflammatory reaction.[2] The predominant mechanism of action of aspirin and other NSAIDs is the inhibition of prostaglandin synthesis by blocking the cyclooxygenase pathway.[95] Pain and inflammation are reduced by the blockage of accumulation of proinflammatory prostaglandins in the synovium or cartilage.

Stabilization of the lysosomal membrane also occurs, preventing the efflux of destructive lysosomal enzymes into the joints.[47] Aspirin is the only NSAID that irreversibly inhibits cyclooxygenase; the other NSAIDs provide reversible inhibition. Aspirin can also reduce fever by altering sympathetic outflow from the hypothalamus, which produces increased vasodilation and heat loss through sweating.[22,47] Among the side effects of aspirin usage are gastric distress, heartburn, some nausea, tinnitus, headache, and diarrhea. More serious consequences can develop with prolonged use or high dosages.[3]

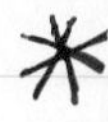

A patient should be very cautious about selecting aspirin as a pain reliever, for a number of reasons. Aspirin inhibits aggregation of platelets and thus impairs the clotting mechanism should injury occur.[3] Aspirin's irreversible inhibition of cyclooxygenase, which leads to reduced production of clotting factors, creates a bleeding risk not present with the other NSAIDs.[94] Prolonged bleeding at an injured site will increase the amount of swelling, which has a direct effect on the time required for rehabilitation.

Use of aspirin as an antiinflammatory medication should be recommended with caution. Other antiinflammatory medications do not produce as many undesirable side effects as aspirin. Generally prescription antiinflammatories are considered to be equally effective.

Aspirin sometimes produces gastric discomfort. Buffered aspirin is no less irritating to the stomach than regular aspirin, but enteric-coated tablets resist aspirin breakdown in the stomach and might minimize gastric discomfort. Regardless of the form of aspirin ingested, it should be taken with meals or with large quantities of water (8 to 10 oz/tablet) to reduce the likelihood of gastric irritation.

Ibuprofen is classified as an NSAID; however, it also has analgesic and antipyretic effects, including the potential for gastric irritation. It does not affect platelet aggregation as aspirin does. Ibuprofen administered at a dose of 200 mg does not require a prescription and at that dosage may be used for analgesia. At a dose of 400 mg, the effects are both analgesic and antiinflammatory.[9] Dosage forms greater than 200 mg require a prescription. For names and recommended doses of prescription NSAIDs, refer to Table 2-1.

Acetaminophen, like aspirin, has both analgesic and antipyretic effects, but it does not have significant antiinflammatory capabilities. Acetaminophen is indicated for relief

Table 2-1 Frequently Used NSAIDs

Generic Name	Drug/Trade Name	Dosage Range (mg) and Frequency	Maximum Daily Dose (mg)
Celecoxib	Celebrex	100–200 mg twice a day	200
Aspirin	Aspirin	325–650 mg every 4 hours	4,000
Diclofenac	Voltaren	50–75 mg twice a day	200
Diclofenac	Cataflam	50–75 mg twice a day	200
Diflunasil	Dolobid	500–1,000 mg followed by 250–500 mg 2 or 3 times a day	1,500
Fenoprofen	Nalfon	300–600 mg 3 or 4 times a day	3,200
Ibuprofen	Motrin	400–800 mg 3 or 4 times a day	3,200
Indomethacin	Indocin	5–150 mg a day in 3 or 4 divided doses	200
Ketoprofen	Orudis	75 mg 3 times a day or 50 mg 4 times a day	300
Mefenamic acid	Ponstel	500 mg followed by 250 mg every 6 hours	1,000
Naproxen	Naprosyn	250–500 mg twice a day	1,250
Naproxen	Anaprox	550 mg followed by 275 mg every 6 to 8 hours	1,375
Piroxicam	Feldene	20 mg a day	20
Sulindac	Clinoril	200 mg twice a day	400
Tolmetin	Tolectin	400 mg 3 or 4 times a day	1,800
Nabumatone	Relafen	1,000 mg once or twice a day	2,000
Flurbiprofen	Ansaid	50–100 mg 2 or 3 times a day	300
Keterolac	Toradol	10 mg every 4 to 6 hours for pain; *not to be used for more than 5 days*	40
Etudolac	Lodine	200–400 mg every 6 to 8 hours	1,200
Meloxicam	Mobic	7.5 mg once a day	15
Oxaprosin	Daypro	1,200 mg once a day	1,800

(Reproduced with permission from Prentice. *Principles of Athletic Training*. 14th ed. New York: McGraw-Hill; 2011.)

of mild somatic pain and fever reduction through mechanisms similar to those of aspirin.[3]

The primary advantage of acetaminophen is that it does not produce gastritis, irritation, or gastrointestinal bleeding. Likewise, it does not affect platelet aggregation and thus does not increase clotting time after an injury.[75]

For the patient who is not in need of an antiinflammatory medication but who requires some pain-relieving medication or an antipyretic, acetaminophen should be the drug of choice. If inflammation is a consideration, physician may elect to use a type of NSAID. Most NSAIDs are prescription medications that, like aspirin, have not only antiinflammatory but also analgesic and antipyretic effects.[47] They are effective for patients who cannot tolerate aspirin because of associated gastrointestinal distress. Patients who have the aspirin allergy triad of (a) nasal polyps, (b) associated bronchospasms/asthma, and (c) history of anaphylaxis should not receive any NSAID. Caution is advised when using NSAIDs in persons who might be subject to dehydration. NSAIDs inhibit prostaglandin synthesis and therefore can compromise the elaboration of prostaglandins within the kidney during salt and/or water deficits. This can lead to ischemia within the kidney.[47,63] Adequate hydration is essential to reduce the risk of renal toxicity in patients taking NSAIDs.

NSAID antiinflammatory capabilities are thought to be equal to those of aspirin, their advantages being that NSAIDs have fewer side effects and relatively longer duration of action. NSAIDs have analgesic and antipyretic capabilities; the short-acting over-the-counter NSAIDs may be used in cases of mild headache or increased body temperature in place of aspirin or acetaminophen. They can be used to relieve many other mildly to moderately painful somatic conditions like menstrual cramps and soft-tissue injury.[9]

It has been recommended that patients receiving long-acting NSAIDs have monitoring of liver function enzymes during the course of therapy because of case reports of hepatic failure associated with the use of long-acting NSAIDs.[74]

The NSAIDs are used primarily for reducing the pain, stiffness, swelling, redness, and fever associated with localized inflammation, most likely by inhibiting the synthesis of prostaglandins.[9] The therapist must be aware that inflammation is simply a response to some underlying trauma or condition and that the source of irritation must be corrected or eliminated for these antiinflammatory medications to be effective.[86] Both naproxen and ketoprofen (now available without a prescription) have been shown to provide additional benefit when administered concomitantly with physical therapy.[63]

Muscle guarding accompanies many musculoskeletal injuries. Elimination of this guarding should facilitate programs of rehabilitation. In many situations, centrally acting oral muscle relaxants are used to reduce guarding. However, to date the efficacy of using muscle relaxants has not been substantiated, and they do not appear to be superior to analgesics or sedatives in either acute or chronic conditions.[7]

Many analgesics and antiinflammatory products are available over the counter in combination products (ie, those containing 2 or more nonnarcotic analgesics with or without caffeine). Chronic use of analgesics containing aspirin and phenacetin or acetaminophen contributes to the development of papillary necrosis and analgesic-associated nephropathy. The presence of caffeine plays a role in dependency on these products leading to chronic use.

Rehabilitation Philosophy

The rehabilitation philosophy relative to inflammation and healing after injury is to assist the natural process of the body while doing no harm.[53] The course of rehabilitation chosen by therapist must focus on their knowledge of the healing process and its therapeutic modifiers to guide, direct, and stimulate the structural function and integrity of the injured part. The primary goal should be to have a positive influence on the inflammation and repair process to expedite recovery of function in terms of range of motion, muscular strength and endurance, neuromuscular control, and cardiorespiratory endurance.[29,32] The therapist must try to minimize the early effects of excessive inflammatory processes including pain modulation, edema control, and reduction of associated muscle spasm, which can produce loss of joint motion and contracture. Finally, the therapist should concentrate on preventing the recurrence of injury by influencing the structural ability of the injured tissue to resist future overloads by incorporating various therapeutic exercises.[53] The subsequent chapters of this book can serve as a guide for the therapist in using the many different rehabilitation tools available.

SUMMARY

1. The 3 phases of the healing process are the inflammatory response phase, the fibroblastic repair phase, and the maturation remodeling phase. These occur in sequence, but overlap one another in a continuum.
2. Factors that can impede the healing process include edema, hemorrhage, lack of vascular supply, separation of tissue, muscle spasm, atrophy, corticosteroids, hypertrophic scars, infection, climate and humidity, age, health, and nutrition.
3. Ligament sprains involve stretching or tearing the fibers that provide stability at the joint.
4. Fractures can be classified as greenstick, transverse, oblique, spiral, comminuted, impacted, avulsive, or stress.
5. Osteoarthritis involves degeneration of the articular cartilage or subchondral bone.
6. Muscle strains involve a stretching or tearing of muscle fibers and their tendons and cause impairment to active movement.
7. Tendinitis, an inflammation of a muscle tendon that causes pain on movement, usually occurs because of overuse.
8. Tenosynovitis is an inflammation of the synovial sheath through which a tendon must slide during motion.
9. Dislocations and subluxations involve disruption of the joint capsule and ligamentous structures surrounding the joint.
10. Bursitis is an inflammation of the synovial membranes located in areas where friction occurs between various anatomic structures.
11. Muscle soreness can be caused by spasm, connective tissue damage, muscle tissue damage, or some combination of these.
12. Repeated contusions can lead to the development of myositis ossificans.
13. All injuries should be initially managed with protection, rest, ice, compression, and elevation to control swelling and thus reduce the time required for rehabilitation.
14. A patient who requires an analgesic for pain relief should be given acetaminophen because aspirin may produce gastric upset and slow clotting time.
15. For treating inflammation, NSAIDs are recommended because they do not produce many of the side effects associated with aspirin use.

REFERENCES

1. Allen T. Exercise-induced muscle damage: mechanisms, prevention, and treatment. *Physiother Can.* 2004;56(2):67-79.
2. Almekinders LC. Anti-inflammatory treatment of muscular injuries in sport: an update of recent studies. *Sports Med.* 1999;28(6):383-388.
3. Alper B. Evidence-based medicine. Update: acetaminophen effective in osteoarthritis (NSAIDs more effective). *Clin Adv Nurse Pract.* 2004;7(12):98-99.
4. Arnoczky SP. Physiologic principles of ligament injuries and healing. In: Scott WN, ed. *Ligament and Extensor Mechanism Injuries of the Knee.* St. Louis, MO: Mosby; 1991:67-82.
5. Athanasiou KA, Shah AR, Hernandez RJ, LeBaron RG. Basic science of articular cartilage repair. *Clin Sports Med.* 2001;20(2):223-247.
6. Bandy W, Dunleavy K. Adaptability of skeletal muscle: Response to increased and decreased use. In: Zachazewski J, Magee D, Quillen W, eds. *Athletic Injuries and Rehabilitation.* Philadelphia, PA: WB Saunders; 1996:55-70.
7. Beebe F. A clinical and pharmacologic review of skeletal muscle relaxants for musculoskeletal conditions. *Am J Ther.* 2005;12(2):151-171.
8. Beiner J. Muscle contusion injury and myositis ossificans traumatica. *Clin Orthop Relat Res.* 2002;(403 Suppl): S110-S119.
9. Biederman R. Pharmacology in rehabilitation: non-steroidal anti-inflammatory agents. *J Orthop Sports Phys Ther.* 2005;35(6):356-367.
10. Bottoni C, Hart L. Recurrent shoulder dislocations after arthroscopic stabilization or nonoperative treatment. *Clin J Sport Med.* 2003;13(2):128-129.
11. Briggs J. Soft and bony tissues-injury, repair and treatment implications. In: Briggs J. ed. *Sports Therapy: Theoretical and Practical Thoughts and Considerations.* Chichester, UK: Corpus; 2001.
12. Booher JM, Thibodeau GA. *Athletic Injury Assessment.* 4th ed. St. Louis, MO: McGraw-Hill; 2000.
13. Brothers A. Basic clinical management of muscle strains and tears: Following appropriate treatment, most patients can return to sports activity. *J Musculoskelet Med.* 2003;20(6):303-307.
14. Bryant MW. Wound healing. *CIBA Clin Symp.* 1997; 29(3):2-36.
15. Burra G. Acute shoulder and elbow dislocations in the patient. *Orthop Clin North Am.* 2002;33(3):479-495.
16. Butler D. Nerve structure, function, and physiology. In: Zachazewski J, Magee D, Quillen W, eds. *Athletic Injuries and Rehabilitation.* Philadelphia, PA: WB Saunders; 1996:170-183.
17. Cailliet R. *Soft Tissue Pain and Disability.* 3rd ed. Philadelphia, PA: FA Davis; 1996.
18. Carrico TJ, Mehrhof AI, Cohen IK. Biology and wound healing. *Surg Clin North Am.* 1984;64(4):721-734.
19. Clancy W. Tendon trauma and overuse injuries. In: Leadbetter W, Buckwalter J, Gordon S, eds. *Sports-Induced Inflammation.* Park Ridge, IL: American Academy of Orthopaedic Surgeons; 1990:609-618.
20. Clarkson PM, Tremblay I. Exercise-induced muscle damage, repair and adaptation in humans. *J Appl Physiol.* 1988;65:1-6.
21. Cox D. Growth factors in wound healing. *J Wound Care.* 1993;2(6):339-342.
22. Curtis J. A group randomized trial to improve safe use of nonsteroidal anti-inflammatory drugs. *Am J Manag Care.* 2005;11(9):537-543.
23. Curwin S. Tendon injuries, pathophysiology and treatment. In: Zachazewski J, Magee D, Quillen W, eds. *Athletic Injuries and Rehabilitation.* Philadelphia, PA: WB Saunders; 1996:27-54.
24. Damjanov I. *Anderson's Pathology.* 10th ed. St. Louis, MO: Mosby; 1996.
25. deVries HA. Quantitative EMG investigation of spasm theory of muscle pain. *Am J Phys Med.* 1996;45:119-134.
26. Di Domenica F. Physical and rehabilitative approaches in osteoarthritis. *Semin Arthritis Rheum.* 2005;34(6; Suppl 2):62-69.
27. Dieppe P. Pathogenesis and management of pain in osteoarthritis. *Lancet.* 2005;365(9463):965-973.
28. Fantone J. Basic concepts in inflammation. In: Leadbetter W, Buckwalter J, Gordon S, eds. *Sports-Induced Inflammation.* Park Ridge, IL: American Academy of Orthopaedic Surgeons; 1990:25-54.
29. Felson D. Osteoarthritis. *Curr Opin Rheumatol.* 2005;17(5):624-656, 684-697.
30. Fitzgerald GK. Considerations for evaluation and treatment of overuse tendon injuries. *Athl Ther Today.* 2000;5(4): 14-19.
31. Frank C. Ligament injuries: Pathophysiology and healing. In: Zachazewski J, Magee D, Quillen W, eds. *Athletic Injuries and Rehabilitation.* Philadelphia, PA: WB Saunders; 1996:9-26.
32. Frank C, Shrive N, Hiraoka H, Nakamura N, Kaneda Y, Hart D. Optimization of the biology of soft tissue repair. *J Sci Med Sport.* 1990;2(3):190-210.
33. Gelberman R, Goldberg V, An K-N, et al. Soft tissue healing. In: Woo SL-Y, Buckwalter J, eds. *Injury and Repair of Musculoskeletal Soft Tissues.* Park Ridge, IL: American Academy of Orthopaedic Surgeons; 1988.
34. Glick JM. Muscle strains: prevention and treatment. *Phys Sportsmed.* 1980;8(11):73-77.
35. Goldenberg M. Wound care management: proper protocol differs from athletic trainers' perceptions. *J Athl Train.* 1996;31(1):12-16.

36. Gradisar IA. Fracture stabilization and healing. In: Gould JA, Davies GJ, eds. *Orthopaedic and Sports Physical Therapy*. St. Louis, MO: Mosby; 1985:118-134.
37. Gross A, Cutright DE, Bhaskar SN. Effectiveness of pulsating water jet lavage in treatment of contaminated crush wounds. *Am J Surg*. 1972;124:73-75.
38. Guyton AC, Hell J. *Pocket Companion to Textbook of Medical Physiology*. Philadelphia, PA: WB Saunders; 2006.
39. Hart L. Effects of stretching on muscle soreness and risk of injury: a meta-analysis. *Clin J Sport Med*. 2003;13(5):321-322.
40. Henning CE. Semilunar cartilage of the knee: function and pathology. In: Pandolf KB, ed. *Exercise and Sport Science Review*. New York, NY: Macmillan; 1988.
41. Hettinga DL. Inflammatory response of synovial joint structures. In: Gould JA, Davies GJ, eds. *Orthopaedic and Sports Physical Therapy*. St. Louis, MO: Mosby; 1985:87-117.
42. Hole J. Human Anatomy and Physiology. St. Louis, MO: McGraw-Hill; 2007.
43. Houglum P. Soft tissue healing and its impact on rehabilitation. *J Sport Rehabil*. 1992;1(1):19-39.
44. Hubbel S, Buschbacher R. Tissue injury and healing: Using medications, modalities, and exercise to maximize recovery. In: Bushbacher R, Branddom R, eds. *Sports Medicine and Rehabilitation: A Sport Specific Approach*. Philadelphia, PA: Hanley & Belfus; 1994.
45. James CB, Uhl TL. A review of articular cartilage pathology and the use of glucosamine sulfate. *J Athl Train*. 2001;39(4):413-419.
46. Junge T. Bone healing. *Surg Technol*. 2002;34(5):26-29.
47. Kaplan R. Current status of nonsteroidal anti-inflammatory drugs in physiatry: Balancing risks and benefits in pain management. *Am J Phys Med Rehabil*. 2005;84(11):885-894.
48. Khan KM, Cook JL, Taunton JE, Bonar F. Overuse tendinosis, not tendinitis. Part 1: a new paradigm for a difficult clinical problem. *Phys Sportsmed*. 2000;28(5): 38-43, 47-48.
49. Kelly A. Managing stress fractures in patients. *J Musculoskelet Med*. 2005;22(9):463-465, 468-470, 472.
50. Kibler WB. Concepts in exercise rehabilitation of athletic injury. In: Leadbetter W, Buckwalter J, Gordon S, eds. *Sports-Induced Inflammation*. Park Ridge, IL: American Academy of Orthopaedic Surgeons; 1990:759-780.
51. Kibler W. Current concepts in tendinopathy. *Clin Sports Med*. 2003;22(4):xi, xiii, 675-684.
52. Knight KL. *Cryotherapy in Sport Injury Management*. Champaign, IL: Human Kinetics; 1995.
53. Leadbetter W. Introduction to sports-induced soft-tissue inflammation. In: Leadbetter W, Buckwalter J, Gordon S, eds. *Sports-Induced Inflammation*. Park Ridge, IL: American Academy of Orthopaedic Surgeons; 1990:3-24.
54. Leadbetter W, Buckwalter J, Gordon S, eds. *Sports-Induced Inflammation*. Park Ridge, IL: American Academy of Orthopaedic Surgeons; 1990.
55. Loitz-Ramage B, Zernicke R. Bone biology and mechanics. In: Zachazewski J, Magee D, Quillen W, eds. *Athletic Injuries and Rehabilitation*. Philadelphia, PA: WB Saunders; 1996:99-119.
56. Maffulli N, Benazzo F. Basic science of tendons. *Sports Med Arthrosc Rev*. 2000;8(1):1-5.
57. Marchesi VT. Inflammation and healing. In: Kissane JM, ed. *Andersons' Pathology*. 9th ed. St. Louis, MO: Mosby; 1996.
58. Martinez-Hernanadez A, Amenta P. Basic concepts in wound healing. In: Leadbetter W, Buckwalter J, Gordon S, eds. *Sports-Induced Inflammation*. Park Ridge, IL: American Academy of Orthopaedic Surgeons; 1990.
59. Matheson G, MacIntyre J, Taunton J. Musculoskeletal injuries associated with physical activity in older adults. *Med Sci Sports Exerc*. 1989;21:379-385.
60. Malone T, Garrett W, Zachewski J. Muscle: deformation, injury and repair. In: Zachazewski J, Magee D, Quillen W, eds. *Athletic Injuries and Rehabilitation*. Philadelphia, PA: WB Saunders; 1996:71-91.
61. Malone T, McPhoil T, eds. *Orthopaedic and Sports Physical Therapy*. St. Louis, MO: Mosby; 1997.
62. Mayo Clinic. Fracture healing: what it takes to heal a break. *Mayo Clin Health Lett*. 2002;20(2):1-3.
63. McCormack K, Brune K. Toward defining the analgesic role of non-steroidal anti-inflammatory drugs in the management of acute and soft tissue injuries. *Sports Med*. 1993;3:106-117.
64. Mehta J. Elbow dislocations in adults and children. *Clin Sports Med*. 2004;23(4):609-627.
65. Murrell GA, Jang D, Lily E, Best T. The effects of immobilization and exercise on tendon healing-abstract. *J Sci Med Sport*. 1999;2(1 Suppl):40.
66. Levangie P, Norkin C. *Joint Structure and Function: A Comprehensive Analysis*. Philadelphia, PA: FA Davis; 2005.
67. Norris S, Provo B, Stotts N. Physiology of wound healing and risk factors that impede the healing process. *AACN Clin Issues Crit Care Nurs*. 1990;1(3):545-552.
68. Ng G. Ligament injury and repair: current concepts. *Hong Kong Physiother J*. 2002;20:22-29.
69. O'Reilly K, Warhol M, Fielding R, et al. Eccentric exercise induced muscle damage impairs muscle glycogen depletion. *J Appl Physiol*. 1987;63:252-256.
70. Panush RS, Brown DG. Exercise and arthritis. *Sports Med*. 1987;4:54-64.
71. Peterson L, Renstrom P. Injuries in musculoskeletal tissues. In: Peterson L, ed. *Sports Injuries: Their Prevention and Treatment*. 3rd ed. Champaign, IL: Human Kinetics; 2001.
72. Prentice W. *Principles of Athletic Training*. 15th ed. New York, NY: McGraw-Hill; 2013.
73. Prentice WE, ed. *Therapeutic Modalities in Rehabilitation*. New York, NY: McGraw-Hill; 2011.
74. Purdum P, Shelden S, Boyd J. Oxaprozin induced hepatitis. *Ann Pharmacother*. 1994;28:1159-1161.

75. Rahusen F. Nonsteroidal anti-inflammatory drugs and acetaminophen in the treatment of an acute muscle injury. *Am J Sports Med.* 2004;32(8):1856-1859.
76. Robbins SL, Cotran RS, Kumar V. *Pathologic Basis of Disease.* 3rd ed. New York, NY: Elsevier Science; 2004.
77. Rywlin AM. Hemopoietic system. In: Kissane JM, ed. *Andersons' Pathology.* 9th ed. St. Louis, MO: Mosby; 1996.
78. Sachs C. Oral analgesics for acute nonspecific pain. *Am Fam Physician.* 2005;71(5):913-918, 847-849.
79. Saladin K. *Anatomy and Physiology.* New York, NY: McGraw-Hill; 2011.
80. Sanderlin B. Common stress fractures. *Am Fam Physician.* 2003;68(8):1527-1532, 1478-1479.
81. Sandrey MA. Effects of acute and chronic pathomechanics on the normal histology and biomechanics of tendons: a review. *J Sport Rehabil.* 2000;9(4):339-352.
82. Schenck R. Classification of knee dislocations. *Oper Tech Sports Med.* 2003;11(3):193-198.
83. Seeley R, Stephens T, Tate P. *Anatomy and Physiology.* St. Louis, MO: McGraw-Hill; 2005.
84. Seller RH. *Differential Diagnosis of Common Complaints.* Philadelphia, PA: Elsevier Health Sciences; 2007.
85. Sharma P. Tendon injury and tendinopathy: healing and repair. *J Bone Joint Surg Am.* 2005;87(1):187-202.
86. Shrier I, Stovitz S. Best of the literature: do anti-inflammatory agents promote muscle healing? *Phys Sportsmed.* 2005;33(6):12.
87. Stanish WD, Curwin S, Mandell S. *Tendinitis: Its Etiology and Treatment.* Oxford, UK: Oxford University Press; 2000.
88. Soto-Quijano D. Work-related musculoskeletal disorders of the upper extremity. *Crit Rev Phys Rehabil Med.* 2005;17(1):65-82.
89. Stewart J. *Clinical Anatomy and Physiology.* Miami, FL: MedMaster; 2001.
90. Stone MH. Implications for connective tissue and bone alterations resulting from rest and exercise training. *Med Sci Sports Exerc.* 1988;20(5):S162-168.
91. Terry M, Fincher AL. Postoperative management of articular cartilage repair. *Athl Ther Today.* 2000;5(2):57-58.
92. Tuan K. Stress fractures in patients: risk factors, diagnosis, and management. *Orthopedics.* 2004;27(6):583-593.
93. Van de Graaff K. *Human Anatomy.* New York, NY: McGraw-Hill; 2006.
94. Vane J. Inhibition of prostaglandin synthesis as a mechanism of action for aspirin-like drugs. *Nat New Biol.* 1971;231:232-235.
95. Vane J. The evolution of nonsteroidal anti-inflammatory drugs and their mechanism of action. *Drugs.* 1987;33(1):18-27.
96. Walker J. Cartilage of human joints and related structures. In: Zachazewski J, Magee D, Quillen W, eds. *Athletic Injuries and Rehabilitation.* Philadelphia, PA: WB Saunders; 1996:120-151.
97. Wahl S, Renstrom P. Fibrosis in soft-tissue injuries. In: Leadbetter W, Buckwalter J, Gordon S, eds. *Sports-Induced Inflammation.* Park Ridge, IL: American Academy of Orthopaedic Surgeons; 1990:637-648.
98. Wells PE, Frampton V, Bowsher D. *Pain Management in Physical Therapy.* Norwalk, CT: Appleton & Lange; 1988.
99. Wilder R. Overuse injuries: tendinopathies, stress fractures, compartment syndrome, and shin splints. *Clin Sports Med.* 2004;23(1):55-81.
100. Wissen WT. An aggressive approach to managing quadriceps contusions. *Athl Ther Today.* 2000;5(1):36-37.
101. Woo SL-Y, Buckwalter J, eds. *Injury and Repair of Musculoskeletal Soft Tissues.* Park Ridge, IL: American Academy of Orthopaedic Surgeons; 1988.
102. Wroble RR. Articular cartilage injury and autologous chondrocyte implantation: which patients might benefit? *Phys Sportsmed.* 2000;28(11):43-49.
103. Zachezewski J. Flexibility for sports. In: Sanders B, ed. *Sports Physical Therapy.* Norwalk, CT: Appleton & Lange; 1990:201-238.

3

Neuromuscular Scan Examination

John S. Halle

OBJECTIVES

After completion of this chapter, the physical therapist should be able to do the following:

- List and discuss the basic purposes of a scan exam as outlined in this chapter.
- Describe how a scan exam is fundamentally different from an algorithm.
- Discuss the potential role of a prescreening questionnaire in a scan examination.
- Compare and contrast the basic elements of a scan examination to the "five elements of patient/client management," that are described in *The Guide to Physical Therapy Practice*.
- List the 5 elements of the scan examination outlined in this chapter, and summarize the key information that should be obtained from each of those topic areas.
- Describe the vital informational elements derived from each of the following items that are part of the patient history portion of the examination:
  - Age
  - Gender
  - Ethnic makeup
  - Morphology
  - Family history
  - Past medical history
  - Medications
  - Mechanism of injury
  - AM/PM pattern of pain
  - Nature of pain
  - Training history
- Within a scan examination, "clearing tests" are typically used. Explain the role and limitations associated with clearing tests.
- Explain what is meant by the terms, "yellow flags" and "red flags." Additionally, when a yellow or red flag finding is identified, discuss the response options available.

Purpose of a Scan Examination

Everyone has a concept in their mind about scanning a given situation. When driving and intersections are encountered, a system is employed that examines what is occurring off in the distance, as well as any potential issues that might be coming from the right and left. Attention is also paid to the existence of signs or traffic lights, any obstacles like parked cars or debris in the roadway, and anything out of the ordinary that could signal high risk, such as children playing with a ball. Additionally, in the back of the driver's mind, factors such as the amount of light available because of the time of day, the condition of the road, weather conditions, and the type of vehicle being driven, are all factored into the mix. With this information, the driver is able to successfully scan the intersection and make all needed adjustments to either stop and respond to a potential emergency or pass through this point in space.

The 2 most important elements that allow the scan described above to work time after time are the employment of a system and experience. When starting to drive, most individuals learn the rules of the road and know to obey traffic lights. When a light turns green, movement into the intersection is started, and, on a rare occasion, the car is broadsided. This accident occurs because even though the driver was obeying the rules of the road, the limited system of the typical neophyte driver does not take the time to additionally check that the other vehicles in their vicinity are also complying with the rules and not trying to push that yellow-red light that they have encountered. This comes with experience, and experience takes time and practice.

What does the above have to do with a scan examination performed on a patient? It is a metaphor that illustrates several important points. First, everyone is familiar with the concept of scanning something. A scan is an efficient and relatively quick appraisal of a situation that does not look for every fact, but works extremely hard to identify key facts and insure that all high-risk situations are identified and addressed. Second, the scan is based on a system. Without a system, holes will develop and some of the key facts identified in point number 1 will be missed. When put in the context of patient care, the potential lack of a system results in less-than-optimal care, and, on occasion, will result in a negative outcome for the patient. In situations like driving, these systems often develop over time with experience and are largely based on visual information. In the realm of patient care, the scan examination is biased to a heavier didactic base that requires the linkage of specific knowledge with pathologies/injuries. Although this improves with experience, the system should ideally be very tight from the beginning for the provision of competent medical care from the first patient seen to the most recently evaluated. This requires study and a system that is both simple enough to be implemented with all patients examined, and flexible enough that it allows modification based on the region of the body evaluated or on the specific situation. The information gained from this system will be used to develop a working hypothesis regarding what might be underlying cause of the patient's problem. Third, while a quick and nonexhaustive appraisal of the situation, the scan forms the foundational elements for a more detailed examination, either at the initial visit or during a follow-up visit. Fourth, implementation of a scan exam is an efficient way to gain an understanding of the reason that the patient is seeking care. The scan exam provides enough information to develop an excellent grasp of what the patient is seeking and whether or not they have come to the health care provider that is best suited to address the issue. Last, and perhaps most importantly, the scan examination looks for potential pathology that requires referral or immediate care, so that serious or life-threatening pathology is not missed. This key point goes directly to a point that is often (incorrectly) credited to the Hippocratic oath of "first, do no harm."[26] (While "do no harm" expresses some of the general sentiment of the Hippocratic oath and is a primary goal of all health care providers, the phrase is not included as part of the oath, but rather as part of another writing of Hippocrates.[26])

Purposes of the Scan Exam

- Used to develop a working hypothesis (assists with ruling potential causes "in" or "out").
- Is based on a system that is both manageable (simple) and adaptable.
- Provides the basis of why the patient has presented for care.
- Identifies pathologies/problems that require immediate care or referral (a key purpose of the scan exam!).

Caveats to Consider When Performing a Scan Exam

Prior to getting into the "the specific pieces" that makeup the typical scan exam, there are a few caveats that should be addressed. First, while a scan exam is by design quick and efficient, it is not another name for taking shortcuts. Whenever the responsibility for examining a patient is accepted, the patient deserves the health care practitioner's full attention and review in a way that will serve the patient properly.

This leads to the second caveat of having a system that is implemented *every time* a patient is examined. Only with a system will all the basic elements needed to scan the patient be included every time. The system also keeps the practitioner from being myopic; examining only what appears to be obvious. Instead, a system requires that outside possibilities involving other biologic systems be reviewed every time an evaluation is performed, and, occasionally, this is the truly important information.

Third, take notes or use a template while performing the scan exam. Research shows that health care providers do a better job of accurately summarizing what was observed during the examination if they record information once and do not try to reconstruct findings from memory at a later time.[88,97,99] If you are basing decisions on your evaluation, then you are obligated to take notes along the way to insure that the summary report is accurate.

Fourth, the scan examination is *not* an algorithm. Rather, it is a framework that has specific points that can be applied to a variety of situations. Because it is a framework, it is as adaptable as required and can be used for an upper-quarter evaluation, a lower-quarter evaluation, or as part of some other requirement. For the purposes of this description, most of the examples provided will be with either upper- or lower-quarter examinations, as they are the most common application of the scan examination process.

Last, physical examination procedures are used as part of the scan examination that are occasionally called "clearing tests." The basic purpose of these tests is to assist in ruling an area in or out, as a source of the patient's problem. An example in the upper-quarter screen is a foraminal encroachment (Spurling) test, which is intended to provoke symptoms in patients with a radiculopathy caused by an intervertebral foraminal stenosis (Figure 3-1). A positive foraminal encroachment test suggests that a working hypothesis of cervical radiculopathy is a viable consideration and that further tests should be performed to see if there is any collaborative evidence. Few practitioners have difficulty building on the results of a positive test. Negative findings for a test of this type are often interpreted as "ruling out" the cervical spine as a source of the patient's problem. This is where the caveat or warning needs to be stated. Because no physical exam test has absolute sensitivity or specificity (and many have only fair to good sensitivity and specificity), a negative finding is only one piece of collaborative information that needs to be viewed in light of all the information. Thus, in the presence of a negative foraminal encroachment test, the neck has not been ruled out. Rather, a clear-cut neck problem has not been demonstrated, but the entirety

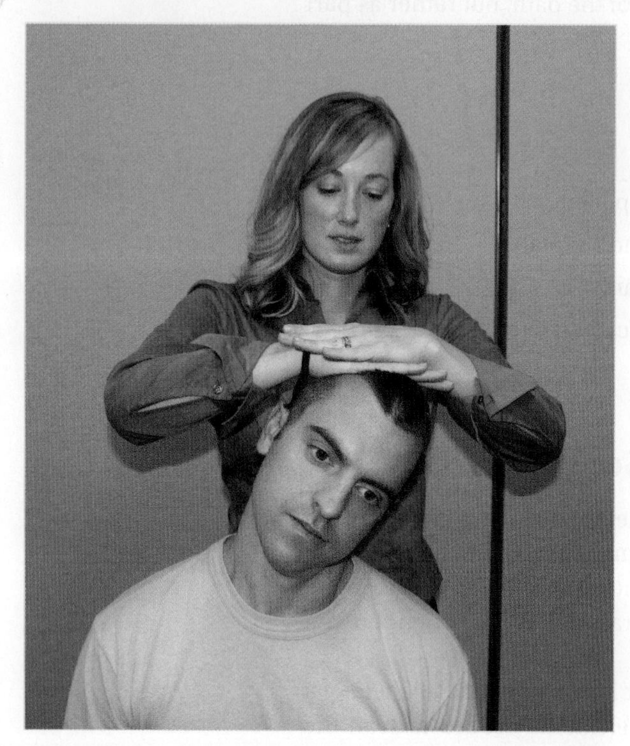

Figure 3-1 Example of a Spurling test (foraminal encroachment test)

of the information provided by the scan exam needs to be reviewed and patterns or tests that collaborate each other need to be identified, and applied to the working hypothesis.

Conceptual Similarities and Differences Between a Scan Exam and the "Five Elements of Patient/Client Management" That Are Described in *The Guide to Physical Therapy Practice*

Both the scan exam and the elements of patient/client management outlined in *The Guide to Physical Therapy Practice* (2nd ed. at p. 133),[6] are systemic ways of approaching a patient in an attempt to provide high quality care. Thus, these 2 systems are much more similar than they are different. The key difference is that the scan examination is an approach that is typically applied to patients presenting with neuromusculoskeletal complaints and it is performed as either an upper- or lower-quarter screen. *The Guide to Physical Therapy Practice (The Guide)*, on the other hand, has developed the 5 elements of patient/client management that can be used as a system to approach virtually any type of patient, ranging from a pediatric patient with a permanent neurologic condition to a patient with a serious injury to the integument, such as a burn patient. Thus, while the scan exam as outlined here is adaptable beyond the upper and lower quarter, those 2 regions are the primary focus of scan exams. In having that focus, the system built will probably have a little more specificity for patient's that fall into the neuromusculoskeletal realm, rather than *The Guide's* system that is applicable to all patient categories.

Additionally, small elements of the examination are handled a little differently by each of these approaches. Both systems begin the evaluation with a history and both also consider a wide range of possible reasons for the presenting problem. The scan exam typically has some built-in "systems review" questions that are part of the history, while *The Guide* outlines the "systems review" as a second step that immediately follows the history. This example of a small difference is largely a semantic one, however, as each is working to accomplish the same task of recognizing the underlying reason for the patient's presentation to insure a pattern of intervention or referral that is based on facts that span each of the major systems of cardiovascular/pulmonary, integumentary, musculoskeletal, and neuromuscular. A second semantic difference is that the scan examination described here will work to identify a specific pathoanatomical dysfunction, while *The Guide* works within movement-based diagnostic categories known as practice patterns.[6] The pathoanatomical approach is the historical way of addressing neuromuscular and musculoskeletal problems within fields like orthopedics and sports medicine. Within those areas, a pathoanatomical focus and description helps facilitate clear communication. Having made that observation, a well-rounded practitioner will be able to articulate the patient's problem with the language associated with either of these 2 models, depending on the environment. Thus, it could be easily argued that the scan examination to be described below is simply a repackaged version of the *Five Elements of Patient/Client Management Model* ([1] examination,

[2] evaluation, [3] diagnosis, [4] prognosis, and [5] intervention), that also recognizes that each individual will approach patients in his or her own unique way with his or her own individualized system. While making that recognition, the strength of both of these approaches is that they are holistic and use a system to provide quality patient care.

> The redundancy associated with mentioning a "system" multiple times is by design. A key to adult learning is repetition, and as this discussion moves to specifics, it is important to emphasize that a scan exam will only be effective with a sound system that makes sense to the practitioner using it. Individualize the system, but be sure that there is a system in place.

Overview of the Scan Exam

As mentioned previously, 2 of the features needed for an effective scan examination are that the exam needs to be relatively easy to remember and adaptable. Although the labels assigned as memory markers can be anything that makes sense to the examiner, the familiar SOAP (subjective, objective, assessment, and plan), note format will be used here, with 1 modification. Rather than the traditional SOAP format, a SOAGP (with the "g" representing goals), will be used as the framework for the scan examination. Additionally, because the focus of this chapter is on the examination and not on treatment options, the emphasis is on the initial 3 elements of subjective, objective, and assessment, with only minor coverage of the goals and plans. (Although goals and plans are deemphasized here, there is no suggestion that these elements are not important. Other chapters of this book address these sections of the entire exam process in greater detail.

The basic elements of scan examination model used are:

1. *Subjective*—History, systems review, yellow and red flags[36]; the patient's basic information and symptoms
2. *Objective*—Evaluative tests and signs elicited from the patient
3. *Assessment*—Refinement of working hypothesis(es) (normally via deductive thinking), into 1 or more specific problems/dysfunctions, that are supported by collaborative information
4. *Goal*—Based on patient's desires and needs, within the realm of reason; should be stated in terms of both short- and long-term goals
5. *Plan*—Measurable steps designed to accomplish the "goal" listed above

The above provide a framework of labels that describe the basic elements of the examination process. The detail for each section is provided below.

Step 1 of the Scan Exam: Subjective, or the Patient History

An old axiom that "chance (*or luck*) favors the prepared mind"[82] applies strongly to this portion of the examination process. While the patient history might be viewed as a time to ask the patient simply, "Why are you here?", a well-done history is foundational to the scan examination. If ranked in a hierarchy, this may be the most important element of the entire examination process for several reasons. It has been said that approximately 80% of the information needed to determine what is wrong with a patient can be gleaned from a well-organized history.[44,96] Additionally, this is the primary place in the examination where the evaluator has the opportunity to understand the patient's concerns, identify potential yellow and red flags,[36] and most easily accomplish a quick systems review. Thus, the patient history should be approached with the understanding that the time spent is valuable and with a clear purpose to every question asked. An effective patient history will occur only if the evaluator employs a well-organized system and if the evaluator has the didactic background to convert the responses obtained from the patient into working hypotheses based on the body's physiologic response to some form of abnormal anatomy. For example, if a patient with cervical pain that radiates to the shoulder indicates that the pain is largely relieved when resting the involved forearm on their head, they have provided valuable information on a working radiculopathy hypothesis. The abducted position of the shoulder allows the cervical nerve roots to be in a position of relative slack and often decreases the symptoms associated with intervertebral foraminal encroachment. This information can be factored into the findings, if the evaluator is aware of what the patient is telling them with the previous description.

The history typically starts with some of the housekeeping information that is needed to paint a picture of the patient. Factors such as the patient's age, gender, and ethnic background are ascertained. These pieces of information are valuable in that specific problems occur either to a much greater frequency, or exclusively, in individuals of a certain age, gender, or ethnic group. As an example, a slipped capital femoral epiphysis typically occurs in individuals between 10 and 15 years of age, and is twice as common in males as females.[95] Thus, both age and gender are key elements that are factored into the prepared mind when considering the presenting patient. Additionally, while getting slightly ahead of the development of this section, these patients will also report that they have thigh or knee pain, because of the referral pattern of pain from the femoral head.[95] Thus, the anatomic characteristics of referred pain and the high index of suspicion of the joint above and joint below, need to be considered when listening to the patient.

In an effort to keep the subjective portion of the scan examination brief, many if not all of these important background pieces of information can be obtained through a questionnaire that the patient fills out prior to being interviewed. Using a questionnaire has a number of advantages, including the following: the questionnaire (a) provides a built-in system that prevents important information from being overlooked, (b) provides documentation without taking the health care provider's time, (c) utilizes the patient's time while they are waiting to be seen, and (d) is efficient and is a way to accurately collect much more information than typically will be obtained by asking individual questions. It has been shown that in a physical therapy orthopedic setting, the overall percentage of agreement across questionnaire items done as part of a self-administered questionnaire versus a detailed patient-self report by an experienced health care practitioner, was 96%.[13] In light of the time savings and documentation benefits offered by this type of questionnaire, its use in a clinical setting should be seriously considered (Table 3-1 is an example of a questionnaire that could be used with men and women; other excellent questionnaires are provided elsewhere[13,62,81]).

Once the basic information on the patient has been obtained, the history turns to the specific reason that the patient has sought care. This phase of the history typically begins with open-ended questions designed to elicit, in the patient's words, what is wrong. Open-ended questions are those that allow the patient to describe in their own terms what the problem is, how they believed it occurred, and how long they have been living with the symptoms that are present. While providing this time for open-ended questions, the clinician may need to work to keep the patient focused on information relevant to the scan exam. Because time is in short supply, the time spent with open-ended questions should not be a time of idle conversation, but a time that paints a picture of the problem.

Table 3-1 **Preevaluation Questionnaire**

Date:					
Patient's Name	DOB				Age:
Diagnosis	Date of Onset				
Physician	Therapist				
					Precautions:
Medical History			**Do Not Complete: For the Therapist**		
Have you or any immediate family member ever been told you have	**Circle one**		**Relation to Patient**	**Date of Onset**	**Current Status**
Cancer	Yes	No			
Diabetes	Yes	No			
Hypoglycemia	Yes	No			
High blood pressure	Yes	No			
Heart disease	Yes	No			
Angina or chest pain	Yes	No			
Shortness of breath	Yes	No			
Stroke	Yes	No			
Kidney disease/stones	Yes	No			
Urinary tract infection	Yes	No			
Allergies	Yes	No			
Asthma, hay fever	Yes	No			
Rheumatic/scarlet fever	Yes	No			
Hepatitis/jaundice	Yes	No			
Cirrhosis/liver disease	Yes	No			
Polio	Yes	No			
Chronic bronchitis	Yes	No			
Pneumonia	Yes	No			
Emphysema	Yes	No			
Migraine headaches	Yes	No			
Anemia	Yes	No			
Ulcers/stomach problems	Yes	No			
Arthritis/gout	Yes	No			
Other	Yes	No			

(continued)

Table 3-1 Preevaluation Questionnaire *(Continued)*

Medical History		Do Not Complete: For the Therapist		
Have you or any immediate family member ever been told you have	Circle one	Relation to Patient	Date of Onset	Current Status
Medical Testing				
1. Are you taking any prescription or over-the-counter medications?				Yes No
If yes, please list:				
2. Have you had any x-rays or other scans (eg, MRI, etc) done recently?				Yes No
If yes, when and what were the results?				
3. Have you had any laboratory work done recently (eg, urinalysis or blood tests)				Yes No
If yes, when and what were the results?				
4. Please list any operations that you have had and the approximate date of the surgery(ies):				
General Health				
1. Have you had any recent illnesses within the last 3 weeks (eg, colds, influenza, bladder or kidney infection, other?)				Yes No
2. Have you noticed any lumps or thickening of skin or muscle anywhere on your body?				Yes No
3. Do you have any sores that have not healed or any changes in size, shape, or color of a wart or mole?				Yes No
4. Have you had any unexplained weight loss in the past several months?				Yes No
5. Do you smoke or chew tobacco?				Yes No
If yes, how many packs per day?				
For how many months or years?				
6. Do you drink alcohol?				Yes No
If yes, how much do you typically drink in the course of a week?				
7. Do you consume caffeine?				Yes No
If yes, how much in a typical week? (to include coffee, tea, chocolate, and soft drinks)				
8. Are you on any special diet prescribed by a physician?				Yes No
Special Questions for Women				
1. Date of last Pap smear examination:				
2. Date of last breast examination by a physician:				
3. Do you perform monthly self-breast examinations?				Yes No
4. Do you take birth control pills or use an intrauterine device?				Yes No

(continued)

Table 3-1 **Preevaluation Questionnaire** *(Continued)*

Medical History		Do Not Complete: For the Therapist		
Have you or any immediate family member ever been told you have	**Circle one**	**Relation to Patient**	**Date of Onset**	**Current Status**
Special Questions for Men				
1. Do you ever have difficulty with urination? (eg, starting or stopping the flow of urine, or have a very slow flow)	Yes No			
2. Do you every have blood in your urine?	Yes No			
3. Do you every have pain on urination?	Yes No			
Work Environment				
1. Occupation:				
2. Does your job involve:				
a. Prolonged sitting (eg, desk, computer, truck driver)	Yes No			
b. Prolonged standing (eg, equipment operator, sales clerk)	Yes No			
c. Prolonged walking (eg, delivery service, etc)	Yes No			
d. Frequent and repetitive use of large or small equipment	Yes No			
e. Prolonged lifting, bending, twisting, climbing, turning	Yes No			
f. Exposure to chemicals or gases	Yes No			
g. Other: please describe				
3. Do you use any special supports, such as:				
a. Back cushion or neck support	Yes No			
b. Back brace or corset	Yes No			
c. Other kind of brace or support for any body part	Yes No			
For the Physical Therapist:				
Vital signs:				
Resting heart rate:				
Oral temperature:				
Blood pressure:				

Source: Adapted from Goodman C, Snyder T. *Differential Diagnosis in Physical Therapy.* Philadelphia, PA: Saunders; 1990, with permission.[39]

Once that picture has been painted, it is time for the therapist to begin asking specific closed-ended questions that require very brief responses. These questions should all have a specific purpose and potentially reveal something about the patient's underlying problem. For example, asking what makes the pain (typically what brings a patient into the clinic) better or worse addresses a basic truism associated with neuromusculoskeletal pathology: via positioning, range of motion, or pressure a neuromusculoskeletal problem can have the nature of pain changed. If, on the other hand, there is no change in pain in any position or posture, then serious consideration needs to be given to the fact that this problem may lie outside of the scope of a therapist and a referral might be warranted. These probing questions are generally close-ended, they provide the therapist with an opportunity to explore potential yellow or red flags, and they are used to explore a brief systems review (Table 3-2). Effectively performed, this questioning process will be built on a system, permit individualization for each patient seen, and be accomplished and recorded in 5 to 10 minutes.

Prior to providing an example of the subjective (history) portion of the examination, it is important to address several other points including:

1. Recognizing that although the label most frequently used with this section is "subjective," it does not mean that the information provided by a patient is either of less value than that obtained by a physical examination, or that the information is even subjective. Rothstein, in an editorial on subjective and objective measures,[89] eloquently describes measures that are often considered to be entirely subjective, such as pain, can be quantified in a very objective way. Additionally, information that is typically grouped under the heading of "subjective," such as age, race, and gender, are not subjective information at all. In fact, those may be examples of the most objective information obtained in the entire examination. Therefore, the occasional tendency to favor information obtained during the physical exam portion (objective) over that obtained from the patient should be resisted. Both sources of information are vital. Part of the art associated with the interpretation of the information collected is to recognize that while differing elements of the total scan exam may be more reliable than others, it is not as simple as elevating the objective portion of the examination over the subjective portion.[89]
2. Recognizing that pain or lack of function is what typically brings a patient in to be seen, but that the pain is not the problem. There is an underlying cause of the patient's pain or lack of function. A key purpose of the scan examination is to attempt to identify the underlying cause, and then bring forth a plan that is able to address the problem. Therefore, acknowledge that pain is an important symptom, but do not be led by it. Respect it, and then attempt to determine its underlying cause. Acknowledge it for the patient's validation, but do not focus on it as the hallmark of success of failure associated with the intervention. Although more will be said on this later, scenarios can be developed in which a patient would have an increased amount of pain in a follow-up visit, yet the therapist could be pleased with the progress. In the treatment of radicular low back pain with pain radiating down the gluteal region, posterior thigh, to the popliteal fossa, an intervention might be McKenzie style[67] back extension exercises. On a follow-up visit, the pain might be centralized to only the low back region, with pain in that region as great or greater than what was experienced initially. Yet, as a result of the centralization of symptoms, this might be considered a positive development and that treatment plan reinforced and continued. Had the therapist been led only by pain, the increase in pain would have resulted in an abandonment of their approach that was intended to address the underlying cause of the initial pain.
3. Requiring specificity when patient's provide answers to specific questions, such as "Are you experiencing any tingling or decreased sensation?" To a question like the preceding one, many patients will express something like, "I have numbness in my right hand." The follow-up questions that require specificity will focus in on items like: (a) Which side of the hand is affected (palmar aspect, dorsal aspect, or both)? (b) Which finger or fingers is/are affected? (c) Are the fingertips affected? (d) Is the area affected truly numb, or if a pin is stuck in it will you feel it? and (e) Is the altered sensation constant or associated with a given time of day or activity? From this type of follow-up that requires very specific responses, the examiner is able to sort out dermatomes, innervation patterns of specific cutaneous nerves, potential polyneuropathies, potential vascular involvement and positioning or temporal

Table 3-2 **Yellow and Red Flags and an Abridged List of Yellow and Red Flag Items**

Yellow Flags: A yellow flag is metaphorically similar to a yield sign. It indicates a finding that requires some additional attention and follow-up, and *may* warrant a referral to a specialist. (Follow-up questions and the rest of the physical examination will help determine if the finding is manageable in the current environment, or if outside consultation is warranted. Common sense and experience assist greatly in sorting out yellow flags).

***Abridged list* of yellow-flag findings:**

1. Asymmetrical muscle stretch reflexes (old name = DTRs)
2. Present pathologic reflexes (eg, Babinski, Hoffman)
3. Pain of unknown etiology
4. Fatigue
5. Pain that does not fit any dermatomal or cutaneous nerve distribution pattern
6. Pain disproportionate to the findings on physical examination
7. "Give-way weakness" (patient is not able to provide an accurate status of their underlying condition, secondary to pain or some other limitation)
8. Lump or mass in a region like the wrist (need to determine if it is a new problem, if it is gradually resolving over time, the relationship to problem patient is seeking care for, etc)
9. Asymmetrical joint laxity (need to determine time of injury, other treatment, etc)
10. Positive findings on special tests (eg, positive McMurray test implicating a torn meniscus—if definitive diagnosis required over the short-term, then referral would be warranted)
11. Night pain
12. Significant structural scoliosis (needs to be viewed in light of age of patient and past history with this condition)

Red Flags: A red flag is a finding that is clearly outside of the scope of expertise of the therapist, and appropriate care for the patient is dependent on coordination with another health care professional. (While the examination *may* be continued following identifying a "red flag," a course of action at the completion of the examination will be to refer the patient. In some cases, the referral could be immediate, with care directly coordinated between the therapist and the physician referred to. As was the case with yellow flags, common sense and experience assist greatly in identifying findings that require immediate referral.

***Abridged list* of red-flag findings:**

1. Loss of bowel or bladder control
2. Fever or chills
3. Dysphagia of unexplained origin
4. Unexplained weight loss
5. Clear and expected changes in vision (eg, diplopia)
6. Symptoms that are constant and cannot be altered by activity or rest
7. Sudden onset of dizziness or balance problems
8. Sudden weakness or lack of coordination
9. Frequent nausea or vomiting, hemoptysis
10. Night sweats
11. Skin rash of unexplained origin
12. Redness and/or swelling in a joint without any history of injury

events that enhance the symptoms. This will be a level of specificity that the patient is not used to, and will often be met with them having to think about what exactly is involved. Yet, in the hands of an evaluator that has a firm didactic grasp of their anatomy and pathophysiology, this line of specific questioning will permit the formulation of clear hypotheses that can be directly tested.

4. Requiring specificity from the patient when the patient is describing the mechanism of injury. The patient is seeking help and the patient knows prior to making an appointment that the health care provider will want to know "How did this happen?" Because the patient anticipates this, the patient will think back and try to associate any reasonable temporal event with his or her current problem. It might be that the individual presenting with low back pain recalls that a week before the symptoms developed the patient was on an amusement park ride. While no discomfort was noted at the time, in thinking back, that was the only event out of the ordinary and the patient therefore attributes the patient's symptoms to this event. Although intended to help the evaluator, this information could be counterproductive, because apart from timing, there is nothing that really links this event to this episode of low back pain. Specificity in questioning is required to determine if there is a clear mechanism of injury, or if the patient is simply trying to be helpful. A clear mechanism of injury assists the examiner. A possible mechanism of injury needs to be viewed as just that, a possible cause of injury with the equally true possibility that the event and this episode of pain are not related. Because pain of unknown etiology is at least a yellow flag, this second type of response needs to be mentally flagged and viewed in light of the other information obtained over the course of the entire scan examination.
5. Using the information obtained during the subjective portion of the examination to generate a working hypothesis or hypotheses. The danger here is to become too myopic too fast. While the subjective examination may provide up to 80% of the information needed to determine the nature of the patient's problem, it is just part of the scan examination. Use the system developed to stay open-minded, so that less obvious or secondary issues are not missed. A metaphor that illustrates this is the instruction that a radiologist provided to neophyte health care providers in how to read x-rays. He noted that when a radiographic finding is distinct, the eye is drawn to it and unless individual reading the x-ray is disciplined and is using a system, a less obvious (and often more serious) finding will be missed. Therefore, he urged that x-rays should be viewed in a systematic way, to insure that proper attention is paid to all elements visualized. Likewise, when developing a hypothesis or several hypotheses, staying open-minded will best serve the interests of the patient who has entrusted him- or herself to your care. (Table 3-3 provides an abridged list of questions used as part of the subjective examination.)

Example of Questions Typically Found as Part of the Subjective Exam or Patient History—Abridged List

Table 3-1 provides an example of one questionnaire that could be used as part of the examination.

1. *Age:* As mentioned previously with a slipped capital femoral epiphysis, there are certain diseases or injuries that are more prevalent in individuals of a given age. Patients reaching the 35- to 55-year-old age range, for example, are still easily capable of substantial repetitive activity like running the distances associated with marathon training. As a result of the biologic changes associated with the loss of cushioning

Table 3-3 Abridged List of Questions Used as Part of the Subjective Examination

Question	Reason Information Sought	Example	Red or Yellow Flag
What is your age?	Age specificity present with some diseases	Vertebral body epiphyseal aseptic necrosis (Scheuermann disease)	–
Sex? (Typically observed and noted, not asked)	Sex specificity present with some diseases	Juvenile rheumatoid arthritis	–
Current occupation?	Occupation may relate to either the onset of symptoms or serve as a factor in treatment	Heavy industrial worker versus secretary	–
What problem has caused you to seek medical care?	Identifies the patient's perception and location of the current dysfunction	Trauma versus problem of insidious onset	–
Onset of this problem?	Identified the length of time current dysfunction has been present	Acute versus chronic condition	–
Any past medical history of similar or related problem? (If so, how was the condition treated and what was the result?)	Provides insight into past history of dysfunction, rehabilitation status, and effectiveness of prior treatment	Recurring rib dysfunction	–
How is your general health? Have you experienced any unexplained weight loss?	Provides insight into other possible problems that may contribute to the current problem	Rheumatoid arthritis, cancer, cardiac problems, etc	**
Any recent infections, fever, or surgery?	Provides information regarding systemic disease that may be related to this problem	Recent history of bladder infection related to low thoracic or lumbar pain	**
What aggravates your symptoms?	The pathomechanics of provoked pain are identified by the patient	Flexion of the cervical spine reproducing upper thoracic pain	–
What relieves your symptoms?	Provides additional insight into pathomechanics and possible treatment approach	Lying on the affected side decreases pain (this is called autospinting and may suggest pleuropulmonary involvement).[36] Also, beware of nothing relieving symptoms—suggests nonmechanical problem	**
Is there a specific pattern of pain over a 24-hour period?	Mechanical problems tend to become worse throughout the day and are relieved by rest	Muscle strain aggravated by repetitive use	–
Does the pain ever wake you from a sound sleep? If so, are you able to roll over and go back to sleep?	Provides information about the pattern of pain and alerts the examiner to the possibility of nonmechanical problem	Osteoid osteoma (pattern of night pain, typically relieved by aspirin)[40]	**

(continued)

Table 3-3 Abridged List of Questions Used as Part of the Subjective Examination *(Continued)*

Question	Reason Information Sought	Example	Red or Yellow Flag
What hobbies or recreational pursuits do you engage in?	May relate to onset of symptoms or identify factors that will need to be considered in treatment	Serious rugby player versus avid reader	–
Are you aware of strength or sensory changes?	Provides insight into function of the neuromusculoskeletal system	C5 dermatome identified as area of decreased sensation	–
Any episodes of dizziness or vertigo?	Symptoms may be present with vestibular or vertebral artery problems	Vertebral artery problem	**
Current medications?	Relates potentially to both this problem and other medical problems	Steroids—long-term use may be associated with osteoporosis	–
Have x-rays or other special tests been performed? If so, do you know the results?	Provides a more complete picture of what has already been done	X-rays, laboratory work obtained	–
On a scale of 1 to 10, with 10 representing excruciating pain and 1 representing minimal pain, where would you rate your pain over the past 24 hours?	Provides a pseudo-objective level of the patient's current perception of pain, which can be used to gauge progress at a later point in time	Pain currently at 4/10	–

**Potential yellow or red flags that may suggest additional work-up or referral to an appropriate medical specialist.

Source: Adapted from Halle J. Neuromuscular scan examination with selected related topics. In: Flynn T, ed. *The Thoracic Spine and Rib Cage: Musculoskeletal Evaluation and Treatment.* Boston, MA: Butterworth-Heinemann; 1996:121-146, with permission.

in the heel pad and changes in connective tissue, this group of older joggers tend to have an increased prevalence of plantar fasciitis.[65] These are just 2 of literally thousands of conditions where age plays a factor that should be considered in the mix of information collected in the scan exam. Proper understanding of life span issues requires an excellent didactic background in the pathophysiology associated with disease and injury.

One other caveat that should be mentioned with age, is the way that this information is obtained. The standard way of asking a question about age is, "How old are you?" While there are times in our lives when we are looking forward to getting older, for someone beyond the young adult stage, this question may imply that their age is the problem. Two ways of obtaining this information in a more neutral way are to use the questionnaire referred to previously that requests the day, month, and year of birth, or ask the same question without any reference to being old, such as, "What is your age?" Although a very small point, part of your job as a successful evaluator is to make the patient feel comfortable and not at all defensive. If someone is sensitive about their age, one of these minor changes in approach might help facilitate the conversation.

2. *Gender:* Like age, given diseases or injuries are more common in one gender than the other. The aforementioned slipped capital femoral epiphysis is illustrative of a problem that is much more common in males. Other conditions, like rheumatoid arthritis or fibromyalgia, are more common in females.[48,58,93] Additionally, there are conditions that are restricted to one gender or the other that often have symptoms suggestive of a neuromusculoskeletal complaint. A male older than the age of 40 years presenting with low back pain without a clear mechanism of injury, should be questioned about their genitourinary system, specifically about their prostate. This is important because the prostate can refer pain to the low back.[10] Similarly, women of childbearing age, presenting with low back pain should be questioned about their menstrual cycle, as pregnancy and the alteration in hormonal levels can also be responsible for low back pain.[14,94,100] These are but 2 of potentially thousands of conditions that have a predisposition for one gender over the other. An excellent understanding of pathophysiology and the role of gender is needed by the examiner to successfully evaluate the patients they see. Although a full description of this topic is beyond the scope of this chapter, the interested reader is referred to several excellent texts.[37,41]
3. *Ethnic makeup:* The ethnicity of the patient is also a factor that needs to be considered when examining the individual from a holistic perspective. It should be recognized that like age and gender, ethnicity can be a factor in the prevalence of the health problem that the patient is seeking assistance with. It is well recognized that there are ethnic differences in the bone mineral content of various races, with whites experiencing higher fracture rates than either Asians or African Americans.[7] Other injury and disease states, such as hypertension and renal disease, are more prevalent in African American populations than among whites.[27,31] Although these are but 2 examples, they illustrate that the genetics associated with the individual are an important factor to keep in mind when considering various hypotheses and the likelihood of a specific problem in the patient that is presenting for care.

   Closely related to ethnic makeup, is the issue of cultural and socioeconomic factors that can play a role in health and disease. In a recent study examining intimate partner violence in Native American women, it was found that more than half of the women (58.7%) receiving care at a tribally operated clinic in southwest Oklahoma, reported lifetime physical and/or sexual abuse.[63] Almost as striking as the overall lifetime percentage, was the finding that 30.1% of these women reported physical or sexual intimate partner violence in the previous 12 months.[63] These are exceptionally high rates of intimate partner violence and illustrate the need for health care workers to have an understanding of the communities that they serve. This one example serves to drive home the point that the individuals that are served in a health care facility are not simply biologic beings that may have a dysfunction of some type, but they are potentially affected by the totality of their day-to-day existence, including lifestyle, genetics, culture, and the mores of the community in which they live.
4. *Morphology:* The body type of an individual presenting for an examination is also a factor in the likelihood of developing a given injury or dysfunction. The previously described slipped capital femoral epiphysis also has morphology implications, as it tends to occur more in youngsters who are either tall or thin, or short and obese.[95] This is thought to be to the result of a potential hormonal imbalance that may be occurring during a period of growth. Here, again, there are potentially thousands of conditions that are related to body type or structural makeup, such as increased incidence of patellofemoral pain in individuals with alignment or range of motion issues.[3,21,59]

   This is a broad label and includes less-than-perfect biomechanics present in many individuals, such as leg-length discrepancies, range of motion restrictions, muscle imbalances, in addition to the general body type of the individual. The key point here is that the examiner needs to be aware of the potential role of morphology or biomechanics, make a mental note of any characteristics observed, and follow-up with examination procedures that work to either confirm or reject any working hypotheses generated.

5. *Family history:* Family history, like all of the categories discussed above, is a key factor in performing any scan examination. The old adage, "the apple doesn't fall too far from the tree," is applicable to medical conditions as well as personality traits. An individual with a family history of diabetes is more likely to develop a polyneuropathy secondary to diabetes, than an individual without this family history.[20,34] Individuals with parents who have documented Charcot-Marie-Tooth, are at risk for inheriting the gene responsible for this mixed motor and sensory neuropathy, and the examiner needs to consider the patient's complaint in light of this information.[12,53] The role of family history, particularly those conditions with known recessive or dominant gene inheritance patterns, needs to be an important piece of information used to generate working hypotheses. Again, to efficiently use this information, the examiner needs to have excellent didactic preparation and a system where they are able to quickly reference questions that arise. A list of specific conditions associated with family history is beyond the scope of this chapter, and the interested reader is referred to Goodman, Boissonnault, and Fuller.[37]
6. *Past medical history:* The truism of "history tends to repeat itself,"[1] is very applicable when evaluating patients. The past medical history will often provide a piece of information that is directly applicable to why the patient who is being evaluated has a current problem. It may be something as straightforward as a history of carpal tunnel syndrome in the right hand, when the patient is now presenting with left-hand alterations in sensation and strength. Because there is a significantly increased odds ratio of patients with documented carpal tunnel syndrome (distal median neuropathy) having involvement of the contralateral side,[8,24,47] the information provided may give a vital clue. Although the carpal tunnel case is one in which the patient probably also had a high index of suspicion, there are other times when the patient may have not made any linkage between a past medical problem and the patient's current problem. A second example of this is the surgical removal of a lipoma from the dorsal surface of the lower neck. Over time, shoulder pain develops on that side that the patient does not relate to the lipoma resection. An astute examiner will pay particular attention to the manual muscle testing of the upper trunk, as it is not unknown for the spinal accessory nerve to be accidentally resected, resulting in shoulder pain caused by an inability of the trapezius muscle to contribute to normal humeral-scapular rhythm. In addition, the patient may have had this exact problem before, and the patient may also know what helped the patient to recover from the problem previously. Sage questioning may provide a solution to the problem with which the patient presents.
7. *Medications:* Knowledge of the medications that a person is taking is important for a variety of reasons. The medications give you information that the patient may not have thought was important and did not provide to you, even though asked. For example, a person may not mention that they have any cardiovascular problems, but if you find out that they are on a beta blocker, a follow-up question can be asked that clarifies the purpose of this medication. With that example, it is also important to know that the range of the patient's heart rate is limited at the upper extreme, so that any exercise prescription developed for the individual would need to take the medication into account. This one example is compounded by the fact that many individuals today are on multiple medications. Prior to performing an evaluation, it is incumbent upon the examiner to take the time to find out both what the patient is taking and why the

patient is taking those medications. (If the examiner is unsure, the *Physician's Desk Reference* is an excellent source of information on medications.[2])

8. *Mechanism of injury:* In those cases where a patient is able to accurately describe how his or her injury occurred, the patient can provide the examiner with tremendous insight into what is going on. A simple example is an individual who underwent an inversion sprain of the ankle and is able to relate that he or she "rolled over onto the outside of his or her foot, with resulting ankle pain." Knowledge of the anatomy and the pathophysiology of ankle sprains allows the examiner to speculate (hypothesize) as to which lateral ligaments of the ankle have been injured, with the most common pattern being the anterior talofibular ligament first, the calcaneofibular ligament second, and the posterior talofibular ligament third. With a good description of the mechanism of injury, each of these structures can be evaluated and the extent of the injury logically deduced.

   There may be other cases where the mechanism of injury is not particularly clear to the patient, but the patient's description will still aid a great deal. The reason that the mechanism may not be clear is that the injury happened too fast. This is often the case in knee injuries on an athletic field, where there was some sudden event, such as a collision, with resultant knee pain. The fact that the person heard a "pop" at the time of the injury, and that they experienced significant knee joint effusion within an hour of the event, however, is very telling. It has been said that with these two pieces of information, the logical deduction that will be correct the majority of the time is that the individual has sustained an anterior cruciate ligament injury. Therefore, ask questions that will gather all the known information that occurred at or around the time of the injury.

   Be aware, that in the patient's desire to assist you by telling you what happened, the patient may not be truly aware of what occurred. A case that also involves the knee is the individual that sustains a patellar dislocation. It is not unusual for a person who has sustained a dislocation to report that the patella dislocated medially, then relocated in the trochlear groove. Although a medial dislocation is possible, the majority of patellar dislocations occur laterally because the knee is characterized by valgus.[77,98] The patient may report a dislocation to the inside of the knee because that side of the knee hurts as a result of the medial retinaculum that has torn to allow the patella to dislocate. The point that this illustrates is that even though a patient believes he or she knows what happened, the injury may occur so fast that the patient's perception is not entirely accurate. Therefore, listen to what the patient has to say and evaluate the information obtained with a critical mind, factoring in what is known about the most common mechanisms of injury to a particular area.

   A last point is the aforementioned case of the patient desiring to help identify the cause of their problem. When a clear-cut mechanism of injury is not clear, some individuals will think back to all the events that occurred about the same time as the onset of their symptoms. If this is their "best guess," rather than a known mechanism of injury, then this should probably be treated as an idiopathic cause of their problem. At the very least, pain of unknown origin should be treated as a yellow flag, and in many cases, viewed as a red flag. Thus, just because a patient thinks that they know what caused their pain, the evaluator is still required to critically evaluate this information and give it the range of credibility that it warrants.

9. *AM/PM pattern of pain:* The pattern of pain that the patient describes can be very useful in developing a working hypothesis because most neuromusculoskeletal dysfunctions can be relieved by position or rest. It would be expected that pain secondary to somatic dysfunction could be both provoked (see later section on provocative tests), and decreased or eliminated by proper positioning and rest. Somatic dysfunction

can be defined as "impaired or altered function of related components of the somatic (body framework) system; skeletal, arthrodial, and myofascial structures; and related vascular, lymphatic and neural elements.[15] Thus, the pattern of pain that is typically reported for most neuromusculoskeletal disorders is activity or position dependent and relieved by rest or positioning that removes stress from the affected structure. Pain that cannot be influenced by position or rest, or pain that wakes a patient from a sound sleep and keeps them awake, is at a minimum a yellow flag. An example of this type of pain is an osteoid osteoma, which accounts for 10% to 12% of benign bone tumors.[38] Because the pain from this type of a lesion is not directly affected by position and is a consistent irritation at night when rest should be working to relieve pain, the clinician has to factor the pattern of pain into the clinician's thought process. The majority, if not all, of patients with a clear pattern of increased pain at night that is not relieved by position, should be referred for additional work-up.

While the AM/PM pattern of pain should be addressed in an effort to clarify the patient's complaint, there are a couple of other principles that need to be factored into the picture that the patient is telling. First, many conditions have an AM/PM pattern of pain that is not a yellow or red flag, such as early arthritic changes. These patients will often describe that they are stiff (painful) early in the morning, loosen up as they move around, and then tend to stiffen up and become painful again toward the end of the day, when they are tired. This pattern of pain is logical, and if it fits with all of the other collaborative information, then it has provided one more confirmation of the patient's presenting problem. Another example of a logical AM/PM pattern of pain is the patient with carpal tunnel syndrome. These patients often describe "tingling in the hand that interrupts sleep,"[68] and pain that is partially relieved by shaking their hands back and forth. This pattern of pain is explained by the fact that many individuals assume a curled-up position when they sleep, resulting in a flexed-wrist posture that restricts the needed blood flow to an already compromised median nerve that is passing under the transverse carpal ligament. Again, this pattern of pain is logical, can be explained, and even forms the basis for conservative treatment with a resting night splint, and is not a yellow or red flag.

A second consideration is that the brain tends to stay active, even when the patient is attempting to relax. The typical individual is constantly on the go throughout the day, with the eyes providing visual information, the ears hearing all that is going on around the individual, the temperature of the air being constantly assessed, the individual's joints providing feedback regarding position, speed, or some other variable, in addition to the challenges and concerns of the day. When trying to relax and go to sleep at night, vision is eliminated with the eyes closed, the environment is normally quiet, temperature is optimally regulated, and joints are not moving. Therefore, the brain that is still receiving afferent input will have a tendency to focus on the incoming information provided, and the reasonably manageable level of pain may appear more pronounced to the patient in the evening. This is often the case with individuals with a shoulder bursitis or other joint inflammation process. This pattern of pain is also logical and fits with the expected characteristics of a patient with a somatic dysfunction. Focused questioning will identify the pattern of pain as keeping with the collaborative evidence gathered in the examination.

It should also be noted that pain that wakes an individual from a sound sleep is not the key element that elevates the AM/PM pattern of pain to a yellow or red flag. The patient described in the preceding paragraph may wake from a sound sleep if the patient rolls over onto the inflamed shoulder. Although this wakes the patient up, the patient is able to reposition in a way that takes stress off the shoulder, allowing the patient to fall back to sleep. The key point that elevates a patient to a potential yellow or red flag, is when the patient consistently awakens in the middle of the night and once awake, is not able to go back to sleep. This suggests something other than a somatic dysfunction and a work-up by a specialist with the tools to explore systemic conditions or visceral problems should be considered. When this is coupled with a pattern of pain that is not affected by rest or positioning, referral is probably warranted.

10. *Nature of pain:* Pain is important because it is typically what brings the patient into the clinic. Pain can help guide the process, and it needs to be respected when treating a patient. Having said that, a key principle is to not be led by pain (see previous section, point 2, under the subjective examination). Let pain be one piece of information, but do not have the pain experienced by the patient be the focus of either the examination or the treatment plan.

The nature of the pain can often provide a great deal of information that will help identify a potential problem. As a result of the location of receptors in the body and the way that we are physiologically wired, pain caused by a superficial structure tends to be more easily located.[28] Pain caused by visceral structures is often referred.[69] Regions of the body, such as visceral pleura, are insensitive to pain.[72] Some structures, such as nerves, often have pain that radiates.[92] Pain caused by nerve origin may also have descriptive characteristics that help identify a nerve as the structure involved, such as a "bright" or "sharp" pain.[4,46] A full description of the nature of pain is beyond the scope of this chapter, but common characteristics associated with pain have been described elsewhere for the interested reader.[36,40,43,50,62] The key point is that pain can provide valuable clues to what is going on with the patient. Listen to the information provided, know what various descriptions of pain mean, and add this as one piece of the puzzle when assembling the information that will hopefully lead to a collaborative picture of the patient's problem.

11. *Training history:* If the patient is engaged in any athletic, vocational, household repair, or recreational activities that require physical labor, ask about the nature, frequency, duration, and intensity of the activity. Additionally, ask about any changes in the treatment regimen. Individuals presenting for care because of overuse injuries are a significant percentage of the patient population seen. Research shows that errors in training, account for a significant percentage of the injuries that are attributed to overuse problems.[51,54] The most common error associated with the training prescription (activity, frequency, duration, and intensity), is increasing the total volume of the activity too quickly, by ramping up the duration of the activity in too large of increments.

While having unrealistic expectations about how fast mileage or repetitions or sets or some other variable can be added, there are many other training errors that will become evident when listening to a patient's training history. I once had a patient who complained of knee pain. When asked about what he did recreationally, he indicated that he was a jogger. A follow-up question asked about his training mileage, and he indicated that he had run 16 miles yesterday. When questioned further about his typical training week, he indicated that over the past 3 days, he had run 16 miles each day. Although a well-educated individual (a lawyer), he did not see the need to allow his body a chance to recover from training events that were clearly stressful to his body. When a more balanced training program was developed, his symptoms cleared up and his performance improved.

Training errors are numerous and a complete list is beyond the scope of this chapter. One final thought, however, is that the potential errors are not restricted to the training prescription variables listed above. An example with running that should be considered in the questioning process is the type and age of the shoes worn. Many recreational joggers will wear their shoes for much longer periods of time than they were designed to be worn. Thus, the shoe has lost all cushioning properties and additional stress is being directly transferred to the jogger. Also, a jogger may switch shoes to a new brand, and gradually develop symptoms that they do not attribute to the change in shoes. An important point is to recognize that training errors are common and that the patient will often clearly describe what change has brought on a specific problem, not recognizing the connection between their behavior and the injury.

Bottom Line

The above list of 11 items is an abridged list of some of the variables that may be considered in a subjective examination. Each evaluator will build a list over time that suits the evaluator's style and the typical patient population with whom the evaluator is working. Although the exact items may vary from therapist to therapist, there are several truisms that are present with everyone. First, as has been stressed repeatedly, there should be a clear system associated with the subjective evaluation, so that key items are not missed. Second, for every question asked, there should be a specific purpose for the question. Use the information provided to categorize symptoms and other information into a workable hypothesis(es). Third, based on this information, the objective portion of the scan examination is planned. Last, know when the information provided indicates that the problem may be outside of the evaluator's area of expertise. "The mark of a true professional is to know the limits of his/her abilities, and to refer, when appropriate."[42]

Objective/Physical Examination

The objective examination builds on the information provided in the subjective/history portion of the scan exam, with modifications designed in as needed. The objective examination is a fluid process whereby the examiner can begin to test the hypotheses generated from the responses that the patient provided to the therapist. Although a fluid process, it cannot be stressed enough that this evaluation is performed within the context of a system that has key items that should be evaluated with every patient. The system is required to insure that the focus of the examination remains broad (so that some key information is not overlooked), important information is not inadvertently missed, and so that the process of examining the patient is efficient (eg, not having them change positions back and forth numerous times, etc).

Metaphorically, for those familiar with golf, this process is a little like approaching a golf course. A skilled golfer approaches the round with a plan (the system). This individual knows where the hazards are, which side of the fairway is optimal to drive to, what regions are out-of-bounds, and has identified opportunities for either conservative or bold play. While each golf course is different, the basic elements of whatever system used by that individual will be in evidence with every course played. Note that this implies that not all people will utilize the same system when evaluating a golf course, because their unique approach will be based on their particular strengths and weaknesses. This is also true for the objective examination, where the system used by different skilled professionals will not be exactly the same, even though each system will contain virtually all of the same elements. Additionally, as in golf, while the plan (system) reflects that for a par 4, there is a drive, a second shot to the green, and a 2-putt, that plan will be modified as needed as a person progresses through the round. The art and skill of performing at a high level utilizes a well-thought-out plan that can be creatively modified as needed to accomplish the task at hand. In golf, this may mean knowing when to chip back out into the fairway, or when it is appropriate to attempt to blast a shot over trees on a dog-legged fairway. In the examination process, this is knowing when to add on to the framework utilized in the scan examination and follow-up on a lead that will permit a more definitive determination of the patient's problem. The system provides the framework or plan. Based on that information, the evaluator needs to remain flexible and respond to the information provided, both from the subjective (history) and from the physical examination itself. Note that this fluid process is significantly different from following an algorithm that has predetermined sequence of steps that are largely adhered to without a great deal of interpretation. A strong didactic base, coupled with a system and the ability to generate and evaluate multiple hypotheses simultaneously, is needed to perform a competent objective examination.

Although all the information in the preceding paragraph is accurate, it also correctly implies that a skilled evaluator has experience. So, what about the neophyte therapist starting out with the performance of objective examinations? Three suggestions are as follows: (a) Develop a form or series of forms that serve to prompt the evaluation, to insure that no important steps or pieces of information are forgotten. Because each individual approaches the physical examination in his or her own way, individualize this system to fit the style and needs of the person performing the examination. (b) Whenever possible, seek out and develop a relationship with a mentor. Everyone will run into questions or situations that are not clear, where an outside perspective is needed. Develop this type of relationship and ideally have the ability to seek out information on an "as-needed" basis, as well as establish a time where regular exchanges and reviews of patients can take place. (c) Have a preplanned system that permits stepping out of the examination room and going to another location to look up information that is needed to complete a thought or to review information associated with a particular condition. This may be as simple as saying, "Excuse me. I need to follow up on some patient information. I will be back in a minute." If this allows obtaining information as needed, it will result in both learning and improved care provided for the patient being seen.

Record as You Go

Record as you go during the objective examination process. Research shows that no one is able to perform a complex examination that includes modifications on the fly, and remember all of the details associated with that examination.[88] It is not a weakness to pause for a few seconds during the evaluation, and jot down any pertinent findings. My personal preference is to annotate any findings that are not optimal. This includes any subtle limitations of range of motion, any identified areas of less-than-perfect sensation, or any other finding associated with any aspect of the physical examination. The advantage of this is that when evaluating most patients, the majority of their findings will be normal. Therefore, by recording all elements that deviate from normal as you go, you are constructing in your mind a complete picture based on all of the data presented. Then, at some later time, such as the end of the entire evaluation process or after the patient has been treated, the therapist is able to sit down and generate a proper record of the visit, with all data (both normal and less than optimal) incorporated into the note.

In addition to being efficient and assisting with reconstructing an accurate picture of the entire evaluation, this process of generating a cursory annotation followed by a formal note provides the advantage of reviewing the material twice. An important element of a skilled clinician is the insight provided by reflecting on the findings presented. In the first pass, all potential findings are collected in a serial process and tested against the working hypothesis. When then looking at the entirety of the data at the end of the evaluation, it is not unusual for a paradigm shift in thinking to occur, with a new hypothesis leading to a different conclusion and treatment approach. An accurate evaluation is built upon excellent information and reflection. This will only be accomplished by fastidiously recording as you proceed through the examination.

Two last points need to be made associated with recording the information. First, if you did not record it, from a legal standpoint, you did not do it. Annotation is critical to substantiate your findings and treatment plan. Second, annotate in such a way that the information provided is efficient, useful, and indicates that a thorough evaluation was done. In the preface to *The Four-Minute Neurologic Exam,*[35] Stephen Goldberg, MD, makes the observation that "Neuro WNL" ("the neurologic exam is within normal limits") is commonly the last notation on a physical exam report. Regretfully, Dr. Goldberg points out that this often means that virtually no neurologic exam took place. The painful joke in some clinical settings is that the acronym WNL means "We never looked." When providing a summary of the findings, provide enough detail on the tests performed that it is clear what was done and what the findings were. Although this may take an extra minute or two, it shows attention to detail and the fact that the objective examination was taken seriously. Additionally, it provides any other evaluators that follow with an excellent road map, identifying where that patient's problem was on a given date.

Basic Elements of Most Physical Examinations

The following is an abridged list of some of the basic elements that should be included in virtually all scanning examinations. Depending on the types of patients a particular practice sees, this list may not be sufficient and a number of other items should be added. There are several excellent guides that outline many additional examination tests, such as Richard Baxter's *Pocket Guide to Musculoskeletal Assessment*[9] and Mark Dutton's *Orthopaedic Examination, Evaluation, and Intervention.*[25] These references and other pocket guides[45] and texts,[64,101] can be used to effectively build upon the scant framework of a "scan examination." As has been described previously, the scan exam is not intended to be a thorough examination, but rather to provide a system where a quick evaluation can be performed that, at a minimum, identifies that the problem appears to manageable within the neuromusculoskeletal realm, or that the problem is one that requires referral or immediate attention. From the framework provided by the scan examination, other elements can be added to work toward the desired thorough evaluation, as time permits. At a minimum, the following should be incorporated into the scan examination:

1. *Observation:* The observation begins when walking out to the waiting room to meet the patient. Watch how the patient moves from sitting to standing, the contact that the patient makes when shaking hands, and the way that the patient moves back to the examination area. Because everyone responds in a little different way when they know they are being watched, work to carry on a pleasant conversation while surreptitiously paying close attention to the patient's movements. The simple analogy of taking someone's picture when they don't know that you are watching provides a much more realistic view than the "posed" state of saying "cheese" to artificially look relaxed. Similarly, if the clinician asks the patient to walk while watching them, the patient's gait may or may not provide the information that you really want. Do as much as you can while the patient is performing normal activities.

   Observation also includes looking at the individual from a postural perspective, noting any asymmetries in their skeletal frame or musculature. This means that all regions of the body being investigated need to be appropriately exposed, maintaining proper decorum for the patient. Be systematic here also, starting at a location like the malleoli of the ankles, and systematically working up to the head. Look for equal alignment of clear bony landmarks like the fibular heads, greater trochanters, ischial tuberosities, dimples associated with the posterior inferior iliac spines, the iliac crests, etc. Look for folds of the skin that may be present on one side of the trunk but not the other, that could suggest a scoliosis or other issue and are another way to identify a potential structural abnormality. Additionally, look for signs of atrophy, scars, edema, or any other abnormality that provides evidence of a past or current problem. One example of a case where observation can play a key role is the previously mentioned iatrogenic nerve lesion, a transaction of the spinal accessory nerve.[71] During the history, past surgeries may have been asked about, and the patient may relate that nothing has been done to their shoulder, which is the reason they are being seen. By observing a scar over their right upper thorax, a question can be asked about the cause of that scar. The patient relates, "Oh, that really was nothing, just a benign lipoma that was removed from my back." If the therapist recognizes that spinal accessory nerve may have been inadvertently transected through this type of minor surgery and that paralysis of the trapezius can cause shoulder pain, a potential linkage between the scar and the patient's problem needs to be explored. The bottom line is that the therapist is required to take the time to adequately observe the patient, through the use of a system, both statically and actively (Figure 3-2).

2. *Range of motion:* Because this is a scan examination, the key objective is to see if there are any significant limitations and annotate those. The simplest way to assess this is to have a system that incorporates many motions simultaneously and have the patient actively perform that activity or activities. For example, if a patient is able to reach symmetrically behind and up their backs, reaching the mid-scapular region with both hands, then they have demonstrated normal or near normal internal rotation and extension of their shoulders (Figure 3-3). By reaching up over their heads with their arms (normal flexion), then from this position reaching as far down their backs as they can to at least the mid-scapular region, shoulder abduction and external rotation are also assessed. Elbow, wrist and hand motion will be simultaneously assessed during the upcoming strength assessments. If all of the above is normal, then the scan exam can probably proceed to the next element of the evaluator's system.

   In the case where active range of motion is either not symmetrical or if a clear or subtle range limitation is identified, the examiner is obligated to both note it and follow up with a more detailed examination. If weakness happens to the patient's key problem, this may involve an active-assistive approach to ascertain the true range of motion at a given joint. More information may also be obtained by performing passive range of motion, and at the end of the range, providing gentle overpressure. These follow up procedures can be used to assess the true status of the joint and the surrounding inert and contractile structures.[22] The key purpose of the range of motion portion of the scan examination is to determine if the patient moves normally or not. If movement is not normal, identify the limitation. Then, if time permits, follow up the basic assessment with more

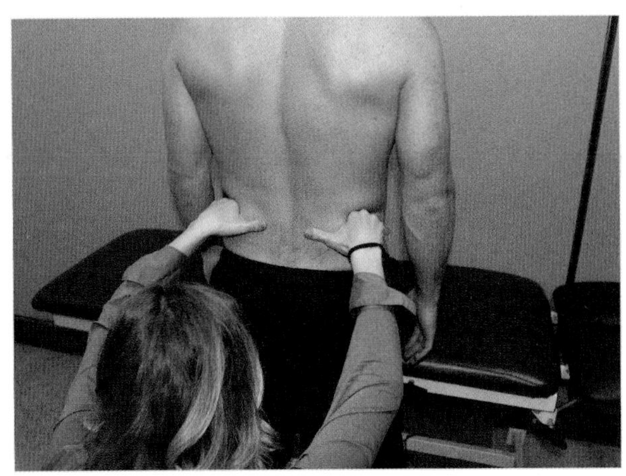

Figure 3-2 Observation of iliac crest height, looking posterior to anterior

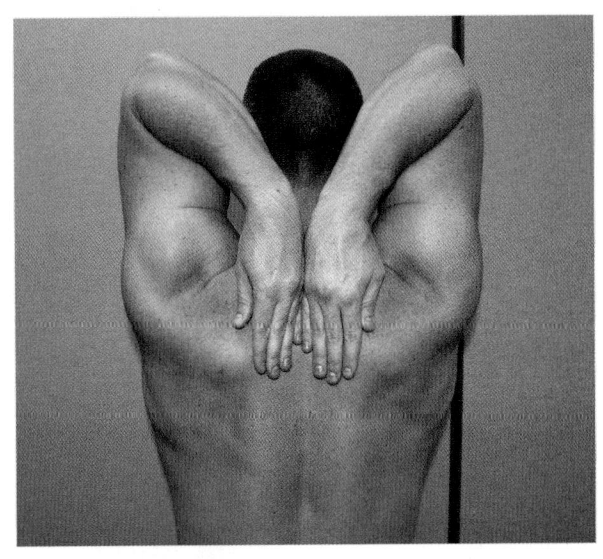

Figure 3-3 Scan exam active-range-of-motion assessment of the upper extremities

detailed manual procedures to determine the true state of the joint and surrounding structures.

In addition to the extent of the range of motion available, the quality of the motion also needs to be assessed. Did the movement flow smoothly without interruption, or did the patient grimace with range of motion that started and slowed in a halting fashion? Assess what the patient is attempting to convey through their movement, and work to factor this into the working hypothesis. Work to identify movement patterns that are limited because of weakness and other patterns that are limited because of pain. Through the quality of the motion, the patient will often tell the examiner as much information as is provided through the history or the actual range-of-motion numbers obtained visually or with a goniometer.

A last point associated with a scan examination is that the range-of-motion assessment is normally done visually, and not assessed in pure planes as is typically done when recording range of motion with a goniometer. The scan exam's purpose is to identify if movement is normal, or if asymmetrical or limited, where this is occurring. Typically, the only time a goniometer would be used during a scan examination is as a type of follow-up, to annotate the previously identified limitation in range of motion.

3. *Strength:* The goal of a scan examination with strength testing is similar to that of range of motion: to identify any clear deficiencies or asymmetries. To that end, the typical scan examination does not involve a manual muscle test of all the muscles in a given region, but rather scans the major muscle groups. For the upper extremities, this may involve the following (all of which can be done in a sitting position):
    a. Resisted shoulder abduction—tests deltoid group and scapular rotators (Figure 3-4).
    b. Resisted shoulder flexion—tests shoulder flexors and scapular stabilizers.
    c. Resisted protraction—to assess the serratus anterior (Figure 3-5).

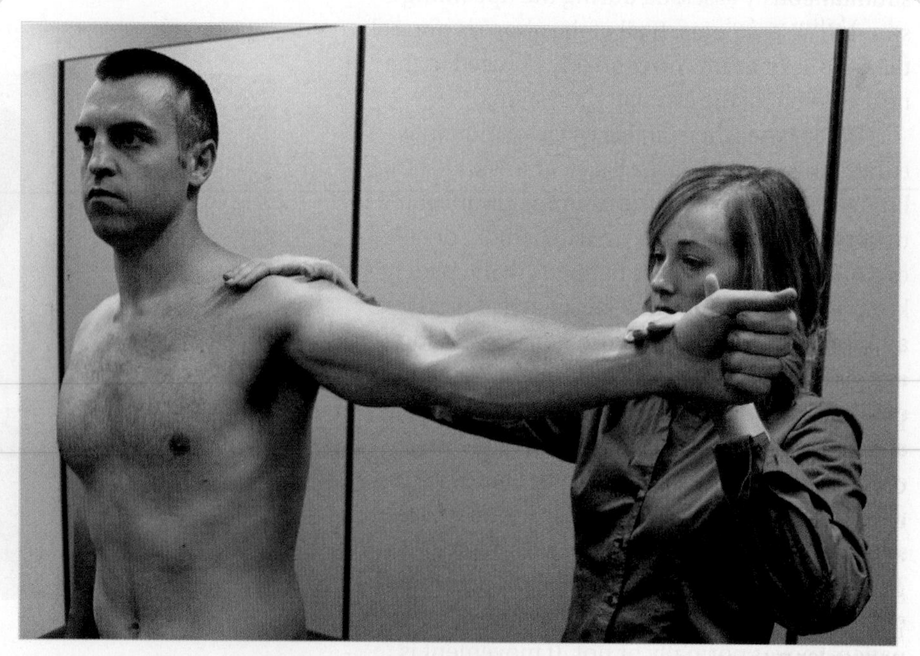

Figure 3-4 **Manual muscle test of the abductors of the shoulder**

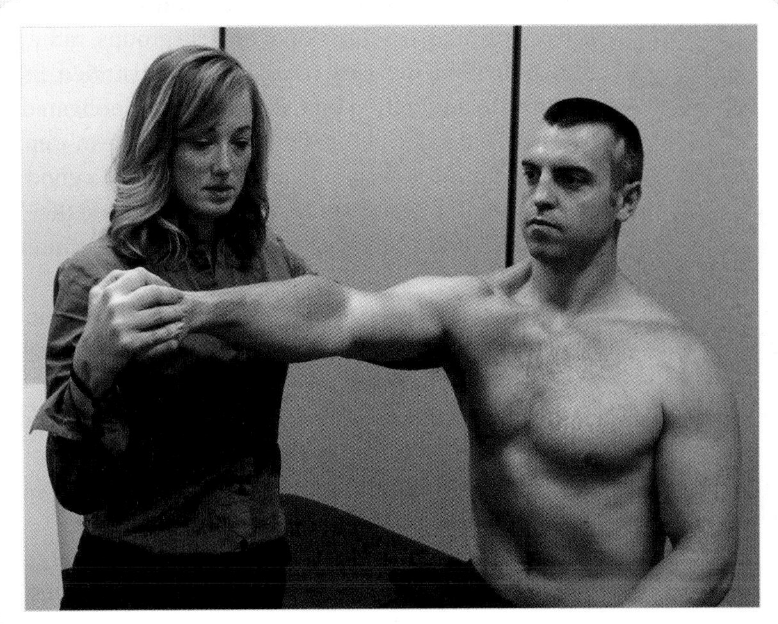

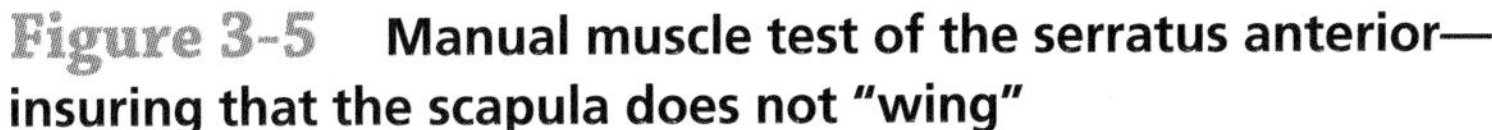

Figure 3-5 Manual muscle test of the serratus anterior—insuring that the scapula does not "wing"

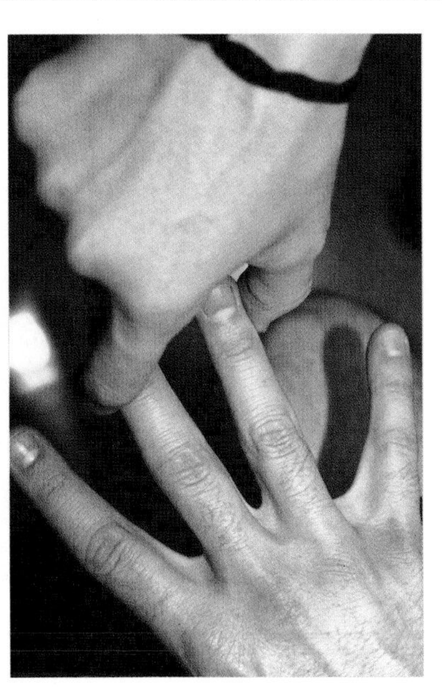

Figure 3-6 Manual muscle test of resisted finger abduction

- **d.** Resisted shoulder internal and external rotation—tests shoulder rotators.
- **e.** Resisted elbow flexion and extension—tests muscles of the arm.
- **f.** Resisted elbow supination and pronation—tests supinators and pronators.
- **g.** Resisted wrist extension and flexion—tests forearm muscles.
- **h.** Grip strength—assesses extrinsic muscles of the anterior forearm.
- **i.** Resisted finger abduction—tests dorsal interossei and abductors of the thumb and little finger (Figure 3-6).
- **j.** Ability to make an "O" with the thumb and index finger, and resist—tests muscles innervated by the anterior interosseous branch of the median nerve (Figure 3-7).
- **k.** Resisted shoulder shrug—assesses the upper trapezius.
- **l.** May also want to assess resisted neck movements (flexion, extension, rotation and side bending), if appropriate—depends on the patient's presentation.

These muscle groups are typically tested in a midrange position because that is where the patient will have near-optimal strength as predicted by the length-tension curve.[29,86] The resisted contractions are typically isometric contractions, as they can be performed quickly and provide a reasonable measure of the amount of resistance that the patient is able to generate. There is not really a need to have the patient demonstrate that he or she can move any particular muscle group through the full range of motion, as this should have already been assessed during the range-of-motion portion of the scan

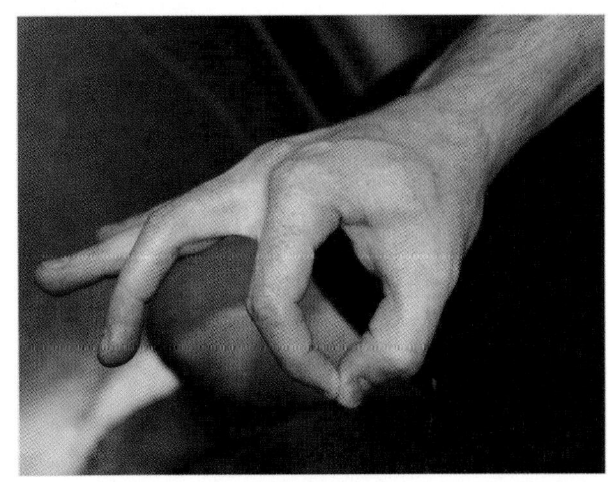

Figure 3-7 The "O" sign—assessing for anterior interosseous nerve integrity

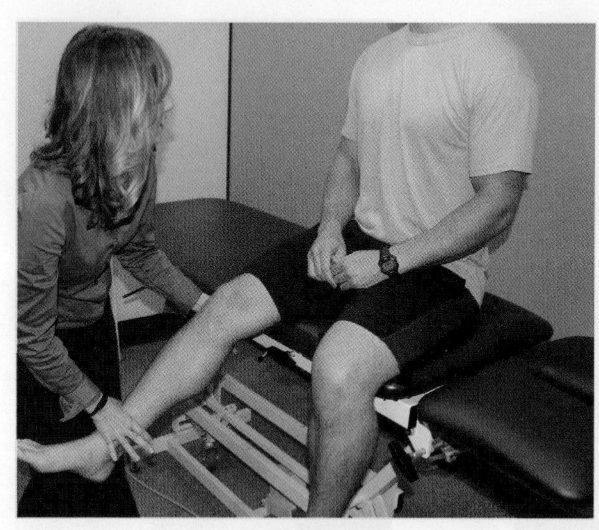

Figure 3-8 **Manual muscle test of the quadriceps—illustrated out of the "closed-packed" position**

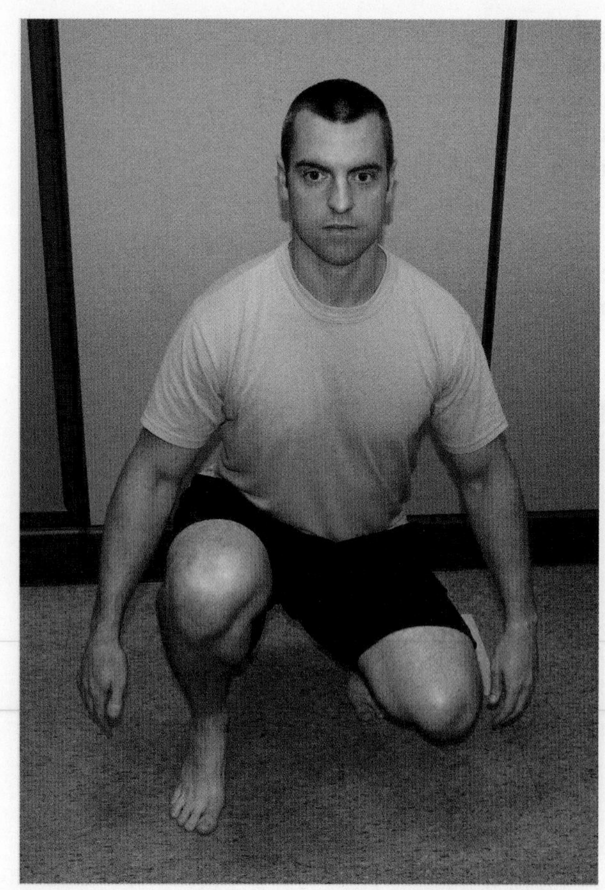

Figure 3-9 **Example of a functional test**

examination. Additionally, note that the above scheme is working to assess functional muscle groups, rather than individual muscles. If weakness is identified, in addition to annotating that, the clinician is obligated to go back at some point and perform a more in-depth examination. The scan examination provides a good overview of the region under investigation, and the framework upon which a more detailed examination can be built.

A similar scheme to the 12 muscle groups outlined above can easily be devised for the lower extremities (Figure 3-8). This may proceed in a manner similar to the muscle groups identified above, working down from the hips, or it may involve a combination of muscle group tests and functional tests. For example, it is probably more meaningful to have a patient walk on his or her toes and then on his or her heels than it is to resist plantarflexion or dorsiflexion. This is because the patient's body weight (particularly with toe walking) will provide more resistance than typically will be provided with a group manual muscle test. If there is any issue with toe walking, quantify the potential weakness with the number of unilateral heel raises that the patient is able to perform, up to a maximum of 25, which is considered normal.[85] One other functional test that can be used is a deep squat, returning to a standing position. For young and flexible patients who can easily perform this maneuver, information is provided about the knee extensors and hip extensors. When this is combined with select group muscle tests, a system can be devised that quickly provides a great deal of information on all of the major muscle groups of the lower extremity. Because this is a scan examination, devise a system that is thorough, but avoids needless redundancy. If a functional test is incorporated into the system used with athletic individuals, then drop out a group muscle test that would be redundant (Figure 3-9). On the other hand, if the patient is an 80-year-old who would typically have difficulty performing a deep squat, have enough flexibility in your system so that age-appropriate tasks are requested, while still examining all desired muscle groups.

As was the case with an upper-quarter scan examination, any identified deficiencies will need to be followed up at some other time with a more detailed evaluation. At the time of the more detailed follow-up, it is both appropriate and expected that individual manual muscle tests will be performed. There are a number of excellent texts that provide great detail on the correct way to perform manual muscle testing.[23,56,85]

In finishing the overview of this element of the scan examination, the role of pain in scanning the strength of major muscle groups should be addressed. If a patient "yields to pain" during a resisted isometric contraction, then nothing can really be said about the status of the contractile unit (muscle, tendon, and tendon-periosteal insertion).[22] This is because the strength could be normal, but the patient is yielding because of discomfort. To record the strength as less than normal would then be inaccurate. All that the clinician can really do is annotate that they could not accurately assess the strength of the muscle group in question, because the patient yielded in response to pain. It may be valuable to state the level of resistance provided prior to yielding (eg, unable to assess patient's true elbow flexion resistance, but patient provided elbow flexion resistance of 4/5 prior to yielding secondary to pain), but that is a personal preference and judgment call. The key point is to recognize that to provide a strength measurement, it needs to be reflective of the patient's best efforts without the overlay of pain or some other factor.

4. *Sensation:* Most of the time if a person has a significant sensory deficit, this typically will be revealed during the history portion of the evaluation. Therefore, insure that the question is asked and listen closely to the patient's response. Additionally, as was outlined previously, require the patient to be precise and identify specific sides of the limb, specific digits, and where any sensory abnormality begins or ends.

   Although the history will provide significant insight into most sensory issues, the clinician remains obligated to perform, at a minimum, a sensory scan examination of the region in question. To do this, the area to be tested should be exposed, the patient should be relaxed and comfortable, and, in keeping with informed consent, should have had the sensory test explained and consented to, prior to the examination. Then, the sensory examination should proceed in a systematic way, usually distal to proximal. The areas assessed should cover all cutaneous peripheral nerves and dermatomes of the region under investigation (see reference 70 for specific cutaneous nerve fields and dermatomes).

   The easiest modality to use for this assessment is light touch, as this can be done with the clinician's fingertips. In the vast majority of cases, because of the initial statement that sensory deficits are usually identified in the history, a scan with light touch is adequate and time efficient. The combination of both a normal history of sensation and normal light touch over a region like the upper extremity in an upper quarter screen, provides a strong foundation to move on to the next element in the overall scan examination. Having stated that, the examiner has to recognize that different modalities are carried by different sensory systems. A patient could have a problem like syringomyelia that affects the anterior white commissures at several levels in the spinal cord, disrupting the anterolateral sensory system. In this patient, light touch should be normal, but the modalities of pain and temperature sensation would be altered. Therefore, for this patient, who is presenting typically with altered sensation in a region like the shoulders bilaterally ("shawl" or "breastplate" sensory deficit),[90] it is imperative that the clinician additionally perform a "sharp-dull" or some other sensory test that evaluates the modalities carried by the anterolateral system.[33] Again, a scan examination is to provide an overview and is used to identify deficits. If a sensory deficiency is identified by either the history or the light touch scan, then the evaluator is obligated to recognize that additional follow-up may need to be done and that sensation involves several systems that are best evaluated by their unique modalities. Additionally, although typically kept in the back of the clinician's mind, there are also other procedures, such as the extinction phenomena,[80] that may need to be utilized in rare cases where central nervous system involvement is suspected (see reference 35 for additional details).

Sensory testing can add a great deal to the testing of a working hypothesis, if the evaluator has a clear picture of the distributions provided by both dermatomes and cutaneous peripheral nerves. Generally, dermatomes are the extension of problems originating at the root or plexus level, and roughly follow the maps outlined in anatomy atlases like Netter's or Grant's atlas of anatomy.[5,76] Dermatomes also overlap, so if only 1 root level is affected, there may be no clear sensory involvement, or the area involved would appear smaller than the anatomy atlases typically convey. For dermatomes, it typically requires that at least 2 levels be affected to have complete sensory loss in a dermatomal distribution. With cutaneous peripheral nerves, however, damage to a given nerve can result in clear sensory loss when only that 1 nerve has been compromised. For example, if a patient sustained a cut or fracture that severed the superficial radial nerve above the wrist, then a sensory loss would occur in a region on the dorsum of the hand between the thumb and index finger.[70] This loss is unique to this peripheral cutaneous nerve and is in keeping with the more distal site of injury. Because this is a sensory nerve at this point (still has some autonomic motor fibers within the nerve, so it is not a pure sensory nerve[70]), there will not be any distal muscles that can be collaboratively tested. Careful sensory testing will provide collaborative information that can be used with the data from the rest of the examination to help identify the underlying problem.

An additional point with sensory testing is that the evaluator needs to clearly ascertain the nature of the sensory dysfunction. For some patients, they have normal sensation but may also complain of tingling. Thus, there really is no deficit, but the patient still is identifying a region that does not feel normal. Some patient's will describe distributions that can only be explained by a vascular dysfunction, so in addition to knowing dermatomes and peripheral cutaneous nerves, the evaluator needs to be aware of vascular regions and the manifestations of a less than optimal vascular system. Finally, there will be some patients with a hypesthesia or allodynia associated with their sensory system. These are typically caused by conditions like complex regional pain syndrome (old name for sympathetic reflex dystrophy) that affect the sensory system by producing an increase in the perceived sensation. Conditions such as complex regional pain syndrome illustrate the need for the evaluator to have an excellent foundational anatomical and physiologic base, understanding the role of autonomic fibers in mixed nerves, in addition to the more frequently considered general sensory afferents. By staying open-minded, collecting the data as it presents, and then working to distill the information within the context of working hypotheses, the evaluating clinician will often be able to use sensation to collaborate the rest of the objective examination.

5. *Palpation:* The history should have provided insight into the region where the patient states the pain is located, if pain is a major factor in the patient's presentation for care. It is the job of the evaluating clinician to know the anatomy of the area well enough that the structures that can be easily palpated are identified and assessed with touch in a systematic way. As has been the case with all elements of the evaluation, the history should have provided the clinician with a set of working hypotheses that need to be distilled down to the one or two most likely involved structures. Additionally, the clinician should have insisted during the history that the patient identify "the bull's-eye" point of pain. In other words, require through questioning that the individual provide a specific location where the patient believes the pain is emanating from, rather than permitting the patient to simply report that "the shoulder hurts." What is the specific location of the center point of pain? With this information, it is much easier to plan the systematic palpation assessment.

Once the focal point of the palpation assessment has been identified, the planned evaluation should begin away from this point. The reasons for beginning away from this centralized point of pain are:

a. It assists in keeping the evaluator from becoming myopic. If the systematic palpation assessment immediately focuses in on the suspected area or structure involved, it is too easy to stop the assessment as soon as the patient expresses that the therapist's palpation causes pain. If this is done, other potentially involved areas or structures are not investigated and potentially important data are missed.

b. By its very nature, palpation is a provocative test that is meant to reproduce the pain that the patient is seeking to stop. Therefore, as part of the process of performing a sound evaluation and establishing maximum rapport with the patient, it makes sense to not immediately reach out and press on an area that the therapist believes will reproduce pain. Start on structures outside of the key area of interest, and systematically work towards what is believed to be the involved structure. The patient then has the knowledge that the therapists is evaluating numerous structures in the area and that the key goal is not to immediately reproduce pain. When a structure is palpated that is painful, this can be compared to the other structures that have been palpated and questions asked about the nature of the pain produced. For example, firm palpation to the coracoid process in the shoulder is uncomfortable for the normal person. If this is reported as painful, the follow-up questions should assess if this reproduces the pain that has caused the patient to present for care, or if this is simply a structure or area that is uncomfortable when palpated. In an ideal world, the goal of palpation is to identify 1 structure or 1 small area that reproduces the same pain that has prompted the patient to seek medical care.

c. Because palpation is expected to be painful, it is probably a good idea to leave the palpation to late in the physical examination. This is closely related to point b above, where a key goal is to establish maximum rapport and not immediately reach out and perform procedures that the therapist expects will hurt the patient. Be gentle, explain what is being done, provide a systematic assessment, and work to design the palpation of a region so that it is towards the end of the overall examination and ideally ends with the palpation of the 1 or 2 structures that are the primary working hypotheses.

Two final caveats are:

a. Palpating an area provides an excellent opportunity for a very close visual inspection of the region. Look for any swelling, potential joint effusion, changes in skin color or texture, atrophy, or evidence of old scars or other sign of injury. If anything out of the ordinary is observed, ask pertinent questions and work those responses into the working hypotheses. Use this time to fully examine the region and make a complete assessment.

b. Understand the potential impact of referred pain and how it may affect the assessment. If pain is referred, there is a good chance that the palpation of a given region will not reproduce the patient's described pain. This is logical, as the real source of the pain is in another region of the body. For example, as a result of the embryologic distribution of root levels associated with the phrenic nerve, an irritation or injury causing pain in the region of the diaphragm may refer pain to the C3 through C5 dermatomes of the neck and shoulder.[69] Although this is where the patient feels pain, this is not the source of the patient's pain, and palpation will not shed any additional light on the matter. It may be that the key finding from this negative result is to prompt the evaluator to think beyond the one region being investigated and consider referred pain as a key source of the problem. If this is the case, and because referred pain if often associated with visceral structures, an additional question that needs to be asked has to do with the nature of the presenting problem. If it is neuromusculoskeletal, then it may still be within the domain of the therapist performing the evaluation. If it is outside of that sphere, then referral to an appropriate specialist may be the ideal course of treatment. Again, a key element associated with anyone performing scanning examinations is to understand the limits of their skills and professional scope of practice, and utilize other members of the health care team when appropriate.

6. *Provocative tests:* Palpation was potentially a provocative test, because by design, the evaluator hopes to be able to put pressure on an involved structure and reproduce the pain that has brought the patient into the clinic. Thus, if the clinician is able to reproduce the patient's exact pain, and if there is an understanding of the structures involved when the pain is reproduced, then the cause of the pain can be understood. In other words, the goal of a provocative test is to reproduce the patient's symptoms, in a controlled environment, where the factors that contribute to the generation of pain can be understood.

   A classic example of a provocative test is the contractile versus inert tissue test described by Cyriax.[22] In a hypothetical case where a clinician is evaluating shoulder pain and has as working hypotheses a potential subdeltoid bursitis versus a supraspinatus tendonitis, a provocative test can be used to potentially distinguish between these 2 clinical problems. The provocative test will really involve 2 elements, one that tests the contractile elements (muscle, tendon, and tenoperiosteal elements), and one that tests the inert structures (a bursa would be an example of an inert structure). For example, with the arm held at the patient's side, the patient is asked to strongly abduct their shoulder while the shoulder is being isometrically stabilized. In the case of supraspinatus tendonitis, this "contractile" structure will be stressed, causing pain that reproduces the patient's symptoms. Because no movement took place (which is the role of the inert bursa), it would not be expected that this isometric contraction would cause any pain, if the involved structure was the subdeltoid bursa. On the basis of this information gained by a pain-producing (provocative) test, the evaluating clinician can make a judgment regarding the structure most likely involved in this patient.

   The flipside of this assessment is to have the patient completely relax her shoulder, putting all of the contractile structures in a state where they are not stressed. Then, the clinician can gently move the shoulder into abduction, through the 50- to 130-degree range of motion where a bursa is often irritated.[73] If this causes pain where the previous isometric contraction did not elicit pain, it suggests that the bursa is the involved anatomical structure.

   Note 5 points in the preceding example.

   - A test was used to intentionally provoke the patient's symptoms, in an effort to understand what is causing the pain. Both of these tests should not result in a finding of pain reproduction, as they are testing different structures. The more specific a given provocative test is, the better the understanding is of the potential cause of pain when it is reproduced.
   - The decision matrix used by the experienced clinician is built upon the collaborative findings of the 2 preceding tests, as well as any other provocative tests that are thought to be appropriate. No one manual test has perfect sensitivity or specificity. Therefore, in an effort to do the best job of identifying the cause of a patient's symptoms, the potential cause of the problem should be looked at

through the use of several tests, and the results from each evaluated against the working hypotheses in a collaborative manner.

- There should be clear communication with the patient that some of the testing done may actually create some discomfort, but this is being intentionally done in an effort to better understand the mechanisms involved in creating the problem. If there is clear communication with the patient, and they know ahead of time that while the evaluator is being as gentle as possible they may still experience pain, it is easier for them to tolerate these tests. As has been stated before, this assists with the development of establishing rapport and aids in the informational exchange.
- The clinician needs to know if the pain caused by a provocative test is the same pain that brought the patient into the clinic. For example, if the patient had been describing a radicular pain from the shoulder, down the lateral aspect of the arm, into the ulnar aspect of the forearm, does the provocative test create this type of pain? If the pain created is limited to the base of the neck with no radicular symptoms, then whatever provocative test was used has not provided a great deal of insight into the patient's primary problem. On the other hand, if the test employed did reproduce these symptoms, then the therapist has an increased understanding of the mechanics involved and is in a much better position to design a treatment program to truly treat the problem.
- Understand that when evaluating the neuromusculoskeletal system, most causes of pain can be mechanically provoked. If at the end of the provocative testing there has not been anything that was able to reproduce the patient's symptoms, the clinician needs to strongly consider that the cause of the pain may not be associated with a neuromusculoskeletal system problem. As was mentioned in the preceding section on pain, this may be a strong indicator that a referral may be warranted.

There are many provocative tests that can be employed, depending on the region evaluated. The classics are procedures like the foraminal encroachment test[60,66] (the Spurling test; see Figure 3-1) for potential cervical radiculopathies, the straight-leg test[84] for lumbar or sacral nerve root problems (Figure 3-10), or the family of

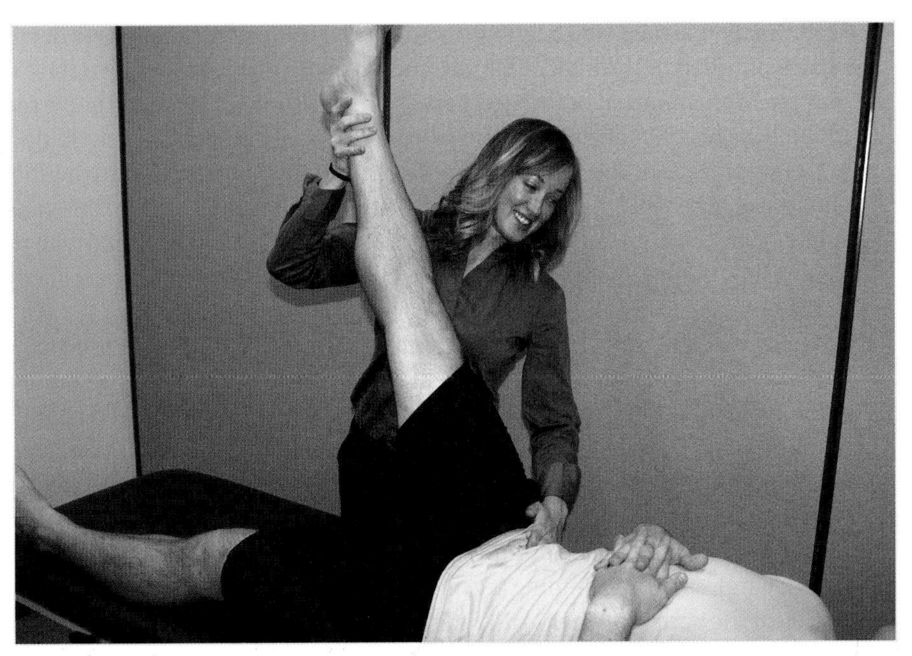

Figure 3-10 Example of a straight-leg raising test

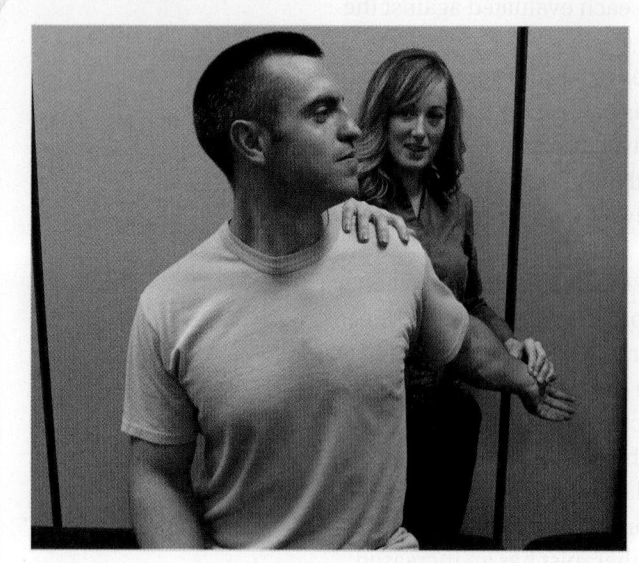

Figure 3-11 Example of a thoracic outlet test

thoracic outlet tests[57,78,83] (Figure 3-11). The purpose of this chapter is not to list all of these tests, but rather to point out their contribution to the evaluation process. A provocative test that is well understood in terms of the structures involved when it is employed, provides a manual testing procedure that gives the clinician tremendous insight into the mechanism of the patient's problem. When combined with other tests in a collaborative fashion, a strongly defendable hypothesis can be generated that can direct a highly effective treatment program. (The interested reader should see the texts by Baxter,[9] Dutton,[25] Flynn,[30] and others that provide a more complete listing of provocative tests and the mechanisms behind them.)

7. *Clearing tests:* A general principle of neuromusculoskeletal assessment is to always evaluate the region (or joint) above and below the primary area of interest. The intent of this principle is to remain broad in the initial evaluation so that areas that often refer pain are not inadvertently missed, and to keep the evaluation from becoming too myopic in its focus. Thus, clearing tests are employed to "clear" a given region as the potential source of the patient's problem, or to "clear" structures that may potentially create a danger for a patient if a particular procedure is employed later in the evaluation or treatment phase.[87] Two examples are provided below to demonstrate these two uses of clearing tests.

In treating an individual with shoulder pain, the neck should always be examined. It is common for a patient to describe pain in the shoulder or arm that is caused by a nerve root or other impingement in the cervical spine. To clear the neck, one of the tests used is the aforementioned foraminal encroachment test (Spurling test). This test, through the combination of neck side bending, rotation, and extension, functions to decrease the space provided by the intervertebral foramen (close down the intervertebral space). In the case of an impinged or irritated nerve root, this should irritate the nerve root, reproduce the patient's symptoms, and serve as a type of provocative test. On the other hand, if this procedure does not elicit any discomfort that radiates toward the shoulder, the findings suggest that the neck can be cleared as an obvious source of this patient's shoulder pain. Thus, the negative finding with the Spurling test, combined with negative findings of any other screening tests used with the cervical spine, work to collectively clear the neck as a likely source of this patient's pain.

Staying with the cervical spine, a second clearing test that is often used in an effort to promote maximum safety for the patient is a vertebral artery test. The combined positioning of the supine patient in an extended, side bent and rotated position for up to 30 seconds,[60] is intended to rule out the vertebral artery as a source of concern should manipulation or other manual procedures be used to treat the cervical spine (Figure 3-12). A positive finding with this test suggests that the patient has a potential restriction of the vertebral artery and should be referred for additional evaluation. On the other hand, a negative finding (eg, no nausea, dizziness, diplopia, etc) is used as a way to clear the vertebral artery and provide the examiner with data that suggests that manipulating the cervical spine should be safe. By employing this vertebral artery test, the therapist is working to promote safety and clear any identifiable potential dangers prior to beginning the treatment program.

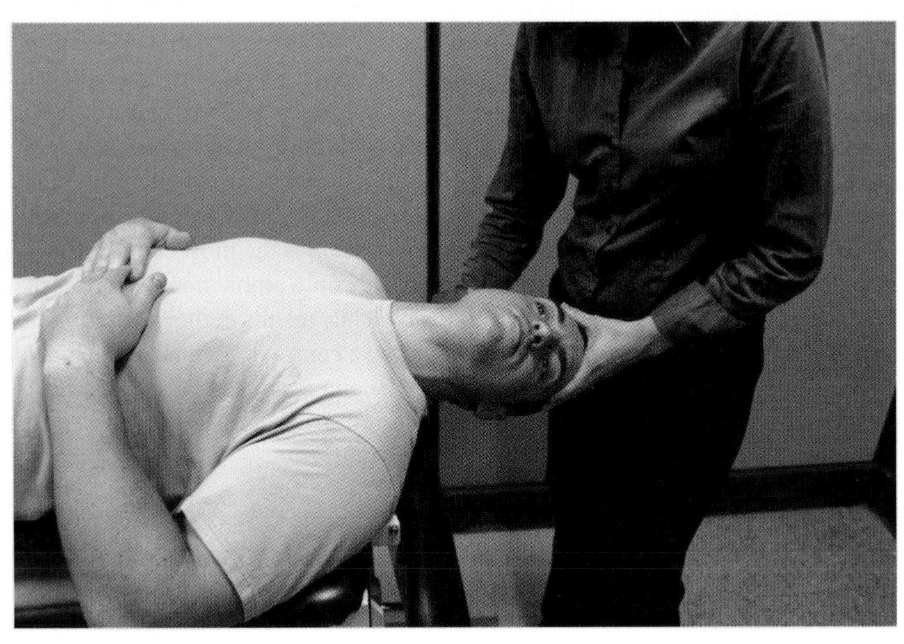

Figure 3-12 **Vertebral artery test position**

Although the goals associated with the clearing tests are admirable, the astute evaluator should understand that negative findings in the 2 commonly used clearing tests do not truly "clear" the neck. An individual can have a cervical radiculopathy in the presence of a negative Spurling test. Additionally, research clearly shows that the vertebral artery test is far from specific when attempting to identify patient's with vertebral artery restrictions, and a negative finding with this test does not necessarily rule out the possibility of a vertebrobasilar insufficiency or provide a safe environment for cervical manipulation.[17,87] These clearing tests are simply one more bit of collaborative information that should be evaluated within the context of the entire examination. In the presence of negative clearing tests, a region like the cervical spine may drop from being the prime hypothesis being investigated, but the cervical spine still needs to be kept in the back of the examiner's mind as a secondary or tertiary hypothesis. Then, as more data are collected, a considered judgment can be made on the best working hypothesis. There should never be a time, however, when the evaluator dismisses a region like the neck as a potential contributor to the problem at hand, simply because the results of 1 or 2 clearing tests were negative.

An additional point that was implied in the section above is that the categorization of tests is not discrete. The Spurling test is both a provocative test and a clearing test. The label designator assigned at any point in time is really the intended use of the test. Regardless of the label assigned, the test remains the same and both types of information (provocative and clearing) are provided when the manual test is employed. The skilled examiner has a well-thought-out system that stays consistent in its key elements and utilizes tests that provide the data upon which defendable judgments can be made. The labeling of a test may assist with description of one of the purposes of a given test to others, or provide a rationale for assigning tests to particular places in an evaluation scheme, but the potentially multiple uses of a given procedure should be clearly recognized by the evaluator performing these tests.

8. *Muscle stretch reflexes:* Muscle stretch reflexes test the integrity of the segmental level reflex arc, as well as provide information on the central nervous system interacting with the reflex arc. In its simplest form, the muscle stretch reflex consists of a sensory receptor (muscle spindle), an afferent neuron, a synapse, an efferent neuron, and the effector organ of skeletal muscle. When a muscle is abruptly stretched, as is the case when a reflex hammer displaces a tendon, the muscle spindles in the homonymous muscle are stretched and generate an action potential that is conveyed to the spinal cord. This signal brought into the central nervous system is the most common example of a monosynaptic reflex, synapsing directly onto alpha motor neurons of the muscle of origin.[55] This excitatory stimulus typically results in the generation of an action potential down the efferent neuron, creating a contraction in all of the muscle fibers innervated by that particular motor unit. The end result, is a visible muscle contraction of the muscle associated with the tendon struck, indicating that the reflex arc is intact (Figure 3-13).

The old term deep tendon reflex *is a misnomer.* For years, the reflex arc described above has been known as a deep tendon reflex. While all clinicians need to be aware of the term because it remains in use today, it should also be understood that a better descriptor is muscle stretch reflex (MSR). The term MSR is more precise, as it accurately conveys that muscle spindles are the sensory organ activated, because the modality that they are most sensitive to is a change in length.[55] This term also conveys the role that muscle spindles have at the muscle of origin, which is to facilitate the muscle and provide the contraction observed. On the other hand, the old term, deep tendon reflex, suggests that the sensory organ of interest resides within the tendon, and the only receptor that would qualify is the Golgi tendon organ. This receptor is not activated by a change in length, but rather by a tension change, which is not significantly affected by a small deflection with a reflex hammer. Additionally, the impact of Golgi tendon activation for the homonymous muscle (muscle of origin) is to inhibit the muscle. This is directly opposite of what is observed when an MSR is evoked. Therefore, in an effort to accurately convey what has been done during the examination, the term MSR should be used, instead of the dated and incorrect term of deep tendon reflex.

Although the preceding paragraph identified the key elements involved with eliciting a segmental level reflex, it failed to convey some of the informational richness that can be obtained from this simple test. In any case where the reflexes are not symmetrical, the findings need to be viewed in light of any other collaborative information available. Additionally, in some cases where the reflex findings are symmetrical but either elevated or depressed, these findings also need to viewed in light of the other collaborative information. Several illustrative examples will be provided in the paragraphs below to assist in the interpretation of findings associated with muscle stretch reflexes (MSRs).

Generally, an asymmetrically depressed or absent reflex is suggestive of pathology that is impacting the reflex arc directly, such as a lower motor neuron problem. The converse is generally true for elevated or "brisk" reflexes, which are commonly viewed as indicating that the central nervous system's normal role of integrating reflexes (serving as a governor) has been disrupted. Thus, an asymmetrical brisk reflex is typically indicative of an upper motor neuron (premotor neuron) problem.[91] In both of the statements made in this paragraph, the term *asymmetrical* has been used because it illustrates the important point that not everyone will have the same response to a reflex hammer tapping a given tendon or muscle belly. Some individuals have bilaterally depressed or even absent reflexes, but these are symmetrical and not

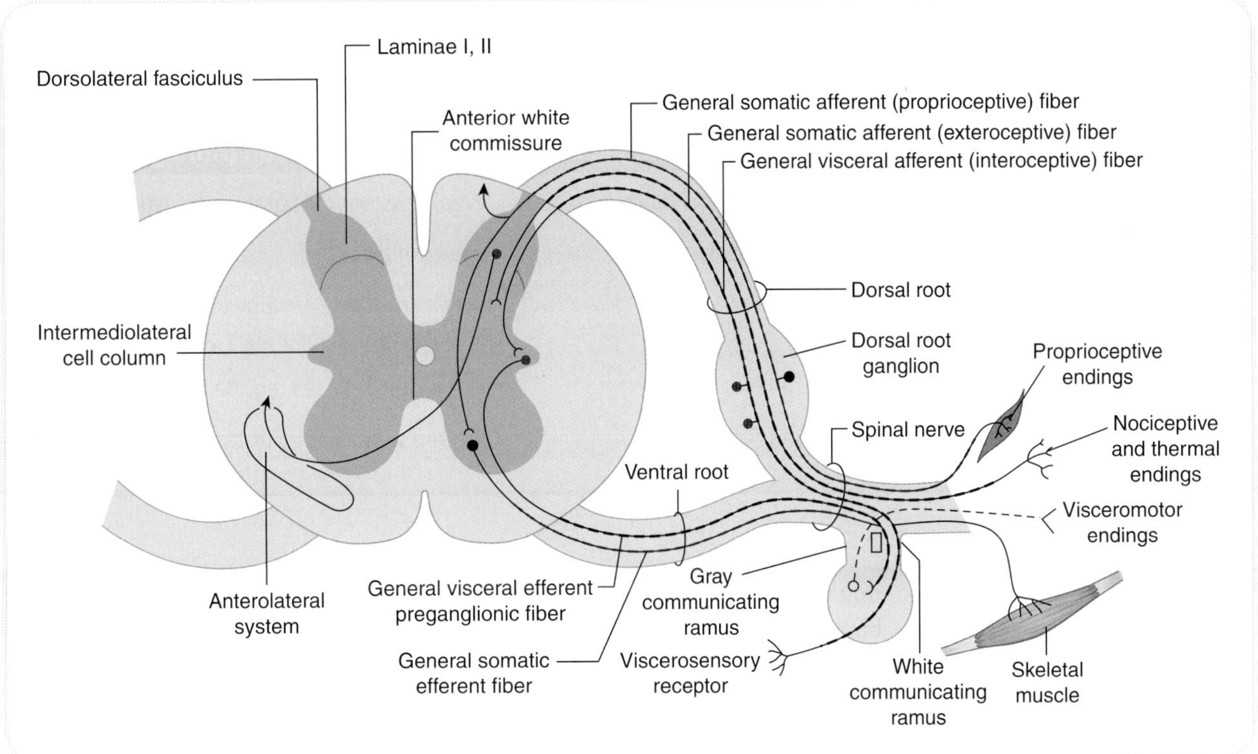

Figure 3-13 **Typical spinal nerve with reflex arc**

(Reproduced with permission from Prentice. *Therapeutic Modalities.* 3rd Ed. New York: McGraw-Hill; 2005.)

restricted to only one of the many MSRs that can be tested. In a similar vein, some individuals have bilaterally brisk reflexes, but this is also relatively uniform throughout all of their reflexes. Therefore, the presence of asymmetrical reflexes, suggests pathology and further investigation. Additionally, while the presence of clearly depressed or clearly elevated reflexes can be a normal finding, the astute clinician must keep this information in the back of their mind and is obligated to investigate further, as this may be a subtle sign of a systemic or symmetrical problem. A few examples are provided below.

Depressed reflexes: In cases where there is complete damage to any element of the reflex arc, such as the afferent or efferent limb, no reflex will be elicited. This would be the case for an individual with a severed peripheral nerve, affecting both the afferent and efferent fibers. Thus, no signal would ever reach the spinal cord, and no efferent signal would consequently be generated. The absence of a reflex, in this case, indicates some type of structural problem that the clinician would need to investigate further. In this simple case, the severed nerve would be accompanied with a host of other findings, such as clear atrophy, sensory loss, and weakness that should make the source of the problem evident (Table 3-4 summarizes upper motor neuron/lower motor neuron signs/symptoms).

A more subtle finding is a depressed, yet intact MSR. This is usually indicative of some type of structural problem that impedes the function of some of the axons within a mixed spinal nerve, with other axons continuing to function normally. A common example of this is the patient with a herniated disk in their lower back. The disk protrusion that compresses the exiting nerve root decrements the function of a percentage of the axons contained within that mixed spinal nerve, so

Table 3-4 Common Upper Motor Neuron/Lower Motor Neuron Signs and Symptoms

Lower Motor Neuron (Abridged List)	Upper Motor Neuron (Abridged List)
Weakness and/or paralysis (flaccid)	Weakness and/or paralysis (spastic)
Hyporeflexia (or areflexia)	Hyperreflexia
Rapid muscle atrophy	No clear muscle atrophy (or slowly developing atrophy that is secondary to disuse)
No pathologic reflexes	Pathologic reflexes (eg, Babinski, Hoffman)
Fasciculations and fibrillations	Altered or loss of voluntary motion

that while the reflex signal is able to be both received via afferents and expressed back to the periphery through efferents, the size of the response is smaller than that found on the unaffected side. In individuals with some type of nerve root compression at the intervertebral foramen, this type of depressed reflex is the expected finding. In severe cases of nerve root impingement, no reflex can be elicited, suggesting that a majority of axons contained within that mixed spinal nerve root are involved.

Note that both the afferent and efferent limb of the reflex arc were included in the discussion of the impact on the reflex arc. Although many clinicians view a depressed reflex as being synonymous with a lower motor neuron problem, it should be recognized that any condition that affects any element of this arc can result in MSR findings that are not normal. While rare, an individual with tabes dorsalis (tertiary syphilis) will have selective destruction of the dorsal columns of the spinal cord and the neurons that project into the dorsal columns.[32] Because these are the same neurons that bring the afferent action potentials into the spinal cord, the death of these neurons means that the afferent limb of the reflex arc is disrupted with minimal or absent MSRs, in the presence of completely healthy lower motor neurons. This "artificial" example is provided to illustrate 2 points. First, any dysfunction within the reflex arc can result in a depressed or absent reflex, so it cannot be considered to be a pure indicator of a lower motor neuron problem. Second, in a case like tabes dorsalis, the depression or absence of MSRs is bilateral and widespread, suggesting that there are other collaborative data available. Thus, the depressed reflex does not stand alone, but is one important piece of the puzzle that is fed into evaluation and compared against the varied working hypotheses that are in play.

Elevated reflexes: In a normally functioning nervous system, the central nervous system (brain and spinal cord), act as a type of "governor" that helps regulate and control the activity generated by the segmental level reflex. If that normal relationship is disrupted by an insult that affects the central nervous system, then the reflex arc is functionally "released" from this governor. This results in an elevated or brisk reflex, when a MSR is elicited.

In the case of a condition, such as a cerebral vascular accident (stroke), affecting one side of the central nervous system, the asymmetrical finding of an elevated MSR on one side would be expected. With a more symmetrical lesion, such as a spinal stenosis narrowing the vertebral foramen (canal) that was affecting the entirety of the spinal cord, bilaterally elevated MSRs would be expected. Both of these cases demonstrate that an altered and elevated MSR provide the clinician with information that the central nervous system is not functioning in the expected way with the segmental level reflex arc, and that the peripheral nervous system is probably not the source of this patient's complaint.

The key issue associated with the MSR testing described above is that it provides the clinician with a direct way of assessing the peripheral nervous system, and an indirect way of examining the central nervous system. This type of testing would not really be needed for the clear-cut example of an individual with a severed nerve; the nature of the problem would be obvious. Similarly, this type of testing is not really necessary for the patient that has clearly experienced a cerebral vascular accident, since again; the nature of the problem would be obvious. However, for the typical patient who is seeking an evaluation for a problem that is not directly obvious, having a tool that is able to simultaneously provide information about both the peripheral and central nervous system is invaluable. And, the information provided can often be the key that helps unlock the puzzle. Two examples illustrate this with relatively obscure cases: (a) A patient presents with symmetrically brisk patellar tendon MSRs and Achilles tendon MSRs, while simultaneously having absent MSRs in the upper extremity. This odd finding could result in additional investigation that unfortunately demonstrates that the patient is suffering from amyotrophic lateral sclerosis (Lou Gering's disease), a mixed upper- and lower-motor-neuron pathology; the MSR findings help direct the rest of the examination and referrals. (b) A second patient, referred for anterior knee pain, is found to have very brisk patellar tendon MSRs bilaterally. Upon further questioning, the patient also discloses that there have been episodes of fluctuating weakness and diplopia (double vision). Appropriate referral and follow-up testing might reveal that this patient is in the early stages of multiple sclerosis and the increase in tone of the lower extremity associated with this condition is responsible for the knee pain.

These 2 rare cases illustrate that a clinician will not find what the clinician is not looking for. The only way to guard against missing examples is to be systematic and know the anatomy and physiology behind the test being employed. MSRs of the region being examined (eg, upper extremity or lower extremity), should be a part of every evaluation done, except perhaps the athletic injury that the clinician personally witnessed. This information should be noted and factored in as part of the working hypotheses being considered.

Commonly tested MSRs and how they are recorded: In the upper extremity, 3 MSRs are commonly tested: biceps brachii (predominantly C5), brachioradialis (predominantly C6), and the triceps brachii (predominantly C7). In the lower extremity, there are 2 commonly tested MSRs and 1 less frequently used MSR. The 2 commonly used reflexes are the quadriceps (predominantly L4) and the gastrocnemius-soleus (predominantly S1). The less commonly employed hamstring reflex is predominantly L5. The hamstring reflex is not used as often because it is much more difficult to elicit and is therefore less reliable and useful. Table 3-5 lists the commonly used reflexes and their grading.

The reflexes are typically graded on a 5-point scale, ranging from 0, indicating an absent reflex, to 4, indicating an extremely brisk reflex.[62] A 2, is considered normal, with anything above or below that value indicative of a finding that is elevated or depressed to some extent. Again, the key finding is not that a reflex deviates from the 2 level. The key findings are that there is asymmetry between limbs, or the symmetrical but unusual MSR is associated with other collaborative findings revealed during the scan examination.

Table 3-5 Commonly Used Muscle Stretch Reflexes[a]

Upper Extremity	Lower Extremity
Biceps brachii reflex (**C5**,6)	Patellar tendon reflex (L2-**4**)
Brachioradialis reflex (C5,**6**)	Hamstring reflex (**L5**, S1-2)
Triceps brachii reflex (C6,**7**,8)	Achilles tendon reflex (L5, **S1**-2)

[a]**Bolding** indicates most prominent root level.

9. *Pathologic reflexes:* Pathologic reflex testing is adjunctive to the MSRs described above. For those patients with an upper-motor-neuron problem, it would be expected that a pathologic reflex could be elicited. The pathologic reflex commonly sought in the lower extremity is the Babinski reflex, which is performed by stroking a blunt object across the sole of the foot, from the lateral side toward the great toe. A "present Babinski" is when this causes the great toe to extend and the other toes to extend and abduct. A response that causes flexion of the great toe and other toes, or withdrawal of the foot is a normal response, and is recorded as a "Babinski not present." The more common elicitation of this reflex that involves stroking the lateral side of the foot progressing to the ball of the foot, is really a combination of 2 pathologic reflexes, the Chaddock and Babinski.[18] For a more complete description of the technique and findings associated with these 2 reflexes and other reflexes of the lower extremity (eg, Oppenheim and Gordon), see Cowan et al.[18]

   The upper limb equivalent to the Babinski is the Hoffman sign (or reflex). This is elicited by having a relaxed and supported hand, and the distal aspect of the middle finger is flipped up in the direction of the fingernail.[18] In an individual who does not have an upper motor neuron lesion, this does not elicit much of a response in the relaxed thumb and index finger of the tested side. In a person with an upper-motor-neuron lesion, the thumb and index finger tend to contract, in a motion that draws these 2 digits toward one another.[18] Because a slight contraction of the thumb and index finger can occur in an individual that has a natural tendency for increased reflexes, it is important to compare one side to the other. If asymmetry is identified, then this present Hoffman reflex needs to be viewed in light of the other collaborative information and prominently figures into the working hypotheses.

   Upper quarter scan examinations should always include testing for the pathologic Hoffman sign, and lower quarter scan examinations should always include testing for the pathologic Babinski reflex. In addition to this minimal level of screening, there are patient conditions in the upper extremity where a Babinski reflex should also be elicited. In the previously mentioned case of an individual with a vertebral foramen spinal stenosis in the cervical region, with symptoms predominantly affecting the upper extremities, a Babinski reflex should be obtained. The demonstration of unilateral or bilaterally present Babinski reflexes provides a great deal of insight into the location of the primary problem (spinal cord compression in the cervical or upper thoracic region with upper motor neuron involvement), and indicates that a referral to a health care provider who can address the base problem is warranted. The bottom line is, pathologic reflexes should always be performed in the region of interest, and a Babinski or other appropriate lower-extremity pathologic reflex should additionally be elicited for those upper-extremity problems where the working hypotheses involve the spinal cord or other elements of the central nervous system (eg, the previously mentioned case of multiple sclerosis).

10. *Special tests:* A scan examination is by definition, a systematic and efficient (implying brief), evaluation of a particular area of interest. Although the 2 most common applications of the scan examination are upper- and lower-quarter screens, the scan examination is adaptable to all regions of the body, such as examining the knee joint or wrist. Recognized within this application to a specific joint or region is the need to always consider the joint or region immediately proximal and distal to that area, as it is common to have referred pain and an initially myopic evaluation does not serve the patient well.

    Recognizing that the standard scan examination is by design brief and efficient, there needs to be adequate flexibility built into the design of the scan examination to permit additional investigation and follow-up of an area of particular interest. This is where special tests come into play. In the case of an individual with knee pain and a history that suggests damage to the ligaments and capsule surrounding the joint, or structures associated with the joint such as bursa, further investigation is warranted. The skilled clinician should employ the appropriate tests to help progress to the next stage of the scan examination, which is the assessment. These tests will assist with the revision or refinement of the working hypotheses into one best hypothesis. The myriad of available special tests is beyond the scope of this chapter, and the interested reader is referred to other sources that provide much more detail on specific tests.[25,37,41,61,64,101]

Final Caveat Prior to the Assessment

The goal of the scan examination to this point has been to collect data. As the clinician proceeds to the assessment, there is a need to be reflective, reexamine mentally each bit of information to determine how it relates to the variety of working hypotheses in play, and, hopefully, distill this data into one best hypothesis that is consistent with the history and objective findings obtained during the examination. This working hypothesis can be expressed as an anatomical or structural problem, the traditional medical diagnosis, or as a listing of physical therapy diagnoses that demonstrate the functional neuromusculoskeletal problems that can be addressed. In either case, the clinician needs to decide what the problem(s) is(are), and begin to formulate a course of action. This leads to the assessment.

Assessment

The assessment typically is the one hypothesis that is most consistent with all the data collected in the preceding scan examination. In most cases, there is a single explanation that has brought a patient in for care. In rare cases, however, there may be several dysfunctions that are occurring simultaneously, and the astute clinician needs to have a flexible enough system to both look for and allow for this possibility. Once all the data have been reviewed, a decision has to be made on what the problem is; identification of one or more issues is necessary to frame an approach on the best way to address the identified problem. The documentation and communication of the assessment may take one of several forms, including the following:

1. One traditional medical diagnosis that provides a pathophysiologic structure that can be addressed by the evaluating clinician (an anatomical or structural diagnosis).
2. Two or more medical diagnoses that provide several pathophysiologic structures that can be addressed by the evaluating clinician (again, an anatomical or structural diagnosis).
3. A physical therapy diagnosis that demonstrates clear biomechanical or neuromusculoskeletal shortcomings that can be addressed and that is consistent with the patient's presenting problem. These issues may range from muscle weakness to range-of-motion limitations, to leg-length discrepancies, to myriad other findings

that become evident during the scan examination with appropriate special tests for follow-up.[6]

4. A decision that a referral to another health care provider is warranted. As has been stressed throughout this chapter, the hallmark of true professionals is knowing the limits of their areas of expertise.[42] A proper referral can be a tremendously valuable service to a patient seeking care.
5. A decision to schedule a follow-up appointment to collect additional data and refine the working hypothesis. A reality of life is that there is not infinite time to perform the most detailed and involved evaluation to investigate every possible dysfunction with each patient. The key purpose of the scan examination is to employ a systematic evaluation so as not to miss potential pathology that requires referral or immediate care. A secondary purpose of the examination is to allow the flexibility for a more in-depth examination at a second or third patient visit. This means that if more information is required, recognize this need and build the collection of the data into a subsequent patient visit. The willingness to admit that not all data can or should be collected during the initial visit permits the time for further reflection, mentorship consultation, and consideration of the potential role of other key systems, such as cardiopulmonary, neurological and integumentary.

The choice of the way to express the assessed findings may be dictated by the environment that the clinician works in, or it may be personal preference. As has been alluded to above, there is a current drive to express physical therapy findings in a form that recognizes that a physical therapy diagnosis (assessment) differs from a medical diagnosis (assessment).[6] Physical therapists cannot typically order tests like x-rays, bones scans, and magnetic resonance imaging, or perform arthroscopic explorations, so they do not have the tools to diagnose fractures, stress reactions of bone, torn menisci, or labral tears. Recognizing that this is absolutely true, it is also true that a patient with a clearly positive Lachman test and pivot shift test to the knee, with a history of hearing "a pop" and experiencing an acute right knee effusion, probably has, at a minimum, a torn anterior cruciate ligament. These collaborative findings can be expressed in the assessment as a list of the physical therapy limitations associated with this condition, such as:

Assessment #1: (1) limited knee joint range of motion of the right knee, (2) knee pain, (3) knee joint effusion, (4) antalgic gait, (5) quadriceps muscle weakness, and (6) altered neuromuscular control; grouped under Preferred Practice Pattern 4D, Impaired joint mobility, motor function, muscle performance, and range of motion associated with connective tissue dysfunction.

This is the nomenclature associated with *The Guide to Physical Therapy Practice*.[6] This assessment would probably also result in a referral to a health care professional, like an orthopedic surgeon, for the additional testing needed to make a definitive diagnosis.

A second way of expressing these findings in the assessment would be to provide a probable anatomical cause of the dysfunction, along with a list of the specific items that physical therapy would work to address. An example of this form of assessment with the same patient described above would be:

Assessment #2: Rule out torn right anterior cruciate ligament

Physical Therapy issues: (1) limited knee joint range of motion, (2) knee pain, (3) knee joint effusion, (4) antalgic gait, (5) quadriceps muscle weakness, and (6) altered neuromuscular control.

Other: Refer to an orthopedic surgeon or other appropriate health care professional for definitive diagnosis.

Neither of these approaches is absolutely correct or incorrect. Assessment #1 follows the basic tenets of *The Guide to Physical Therapy Practice*, which is the profession's definitive document describing the scope of physical therapy practice.[6] In those settings where this type of description works, it should probably be the approach used, as this is in keeping with the recommendations of *The Guide*.[6] Having recognized the key role and importance of *The Guide*, it is also important to recognize that there are limitations associated with using a list of findings to describe the physical therapy diagnosis. Metaphorically, for those entities for which we have established labels recognized by all parties, it is easier to convey information by using the label than by using a list of descriptors. It is easier to say that there is an elephant in the backyard, than to try to describe a big animal that is gray, wrinkled, possessing a tail, with ears bigger than most animals. Although physical therapists cannot examine the genetic code to verify the species of elephant, they are able to identify the basic creature and then convey any specific attributes of that animal that may relate to a specific species. Clearly, great liberty has been taken with the elephant metaphor, but it illustrates that physical therapists do not function in a vacuum, but are part of the traditional medical community. Therefore, the communication tends to be much more straightforward with other health professionals when traditional labels like "rule out anterior cruciate ligament tear" are used. These can be stated in a way that demonstrates that this is not a definitive diagnosis, but rather a strong working hypothesis. When supplemented with the list of attributes that the scan examination has identified that can be addressed by physical therapy, then the communication and, if warranted, referral, are clearer for all involved. Consequently, in those settings where the format of Assessment #2 makes sense, it should be considered.

The bottom line of the assessment is to identify and label the specific items that should be addressed during the next 2 phases of the scan examination: the goal and the plan.

Goal

The "goal" is what the clinician and the patient want to achieve. It is placed in this system in a location that differs from the traditional SOAP (subjective, objective, assessment, and plan) note format. The rationale for this transposition of place in the examination process is that the clinician needs to know where they want to go (the goal), prior to developing a plan to get there. Metaphorically, no one would ever look at a map and plan to head out of town on a specific highway, if they had not first determined where they wanted to end up at the completion of the trip. In a similar vein, the clinician, in consultation with the patient, needs to establish 1 or more goals that meet at least the following minimal list of expectations, if the clinician has determined that the care needed can be provided within the clinician's scope of practice. These 5 expectations are: (a) the goals are realistic, (b) the goals meet the patient's expectations, (c) the goals define what will be achieved in the short term, (d) the goals define what will be achieved in the long term, and (e) the goals are measurable. When the care or additional evaluation needs to be done by another health care professional, the goal may change to linking the patient with the best health care provider for them.

The initial expectation associated with goals is that they are realistic. To a large degree, this is based on the experience and judgment of the clinician, drawing from the information provided during the scan exam evaluation. It is not realistic to assume that the goal(s) associated with care are to have each patient return to an optimal level of function. A patient encountered by the author early in his career was a gentleman in his early to mid-seventies, with longstanding diabetes and bilateral above-knee amputations. He loved to ride trains, and had been referred for transfer training, general conditioning, and household mobility training. He had been in a wheelchair for more than a year, and had new prosthetic limbs. Although the scan exam performed on him utilized the system outlined in this chapter (in terms of history, prepared questions, and a physical examination), the data collected were vital to determining his current physical status, point where a treatment plan should be initiated, and what goals might be sought. While blurring the point of being realistic with the next paragraph on the patient's expectations, this collected data needs to be viewed in light of the wishes of the patient. In this case, back in the late 1970s, the only way to board the steam engine trains that he wanted to ride was to walk up the steps onto the train. Thus, he came to the clinic with an expectation that he would be assisted in learning to walk again, so that he could walk to the train, board it, and ride. Because of his age, level of conditioning, and the extreme energy costs associated with ambulating with the prostheses associated with dual above-knee amputations, this was not a realistic goal. The information obtained from the scan exam provided a starting point to begin formulating what was realistic. This led to the next expectation of the goal(s) established, working to meet the patient's expectations.

Serving the patient and working to meet the patient's needs and expectations is really the fundamental reason that health care is provided. To achieve these elements of care, clinicians need to take the time to find out what the patient wants and expects. The information provided by the patient, coupled with the data obtained during the scan examination, allows a merging of the patient's goals with the clinician's therapeutic goals. When combined in this way, the 2 elements synergistically create a set of goals that are a "force multiplier," in terms of achieving realistic, measurable, results. Referring back to the example in the paragraph above, it was not realistic that the patient would be able to walk to the train, climb a short series of stairs, and ambulate to his seat on the train. Although that goal was out of reach, this individual appeared capable of transfers, short-distance ambulation, and the ability to navigate 2 or 3 steps. Following a frank discussion, a mutually agreed upon set of expectations were outlined and agreed to. These provided the basis for short- and long-term goal development, with measurable/objective landmarks. That these goals took the patient's wants and expectations into account helped to create an environment in which this individual's motivation and drive are still something that I easily recall more than 30 years later.

A more common example of the need to take the patient's wants and expectations into account is when dealing with athletes. Athletic patients who are used to training regularly and are injured with some type of overuse problem typically will not settle for a plan that involves rest. Most of these patients want to continue to train, and while they will be polite to the health care professional who recommends rest, they will often leave the office and start the search for another health care provider who understands their particular needs. The clinician who takes the time to find out what the patient wants and expects should be in a position to educate the patient on what is realistic from the pathophysiologic perspective, while also letting the patient know that the clinician is collaboratively working to achieve the patient's goals. This may mean resting the involved structure or limb while engaging in "active rest" that allows the patient's conditioning to be maintained by some sort of alternate activity. The bottom line here is that the goals established need to be in line with the patient's expectations to enhance compliance and motivation, yet structured within the framework of what the clinician knows is realistic. This creates an environment in which both individuals—the patient and the clinician—are working together as a team for a specific purpose (or outcome).

The mutually established goals should ideally be expressed as both short-term and long-term goals. Metaphorically, no one is comfortable with a global goal like "completing graduate school," or "losing 35 pounds." On the surface, these goals appear so large and unattainable, that it would be extremely easy for the individual working to accomplish the goal to become overwhelmed and discouraged. It makes much more sense to set a series of short-term goals that over time lead to the accomplishment of the global (or long-term) goal. In the case of patient goals, the initial short-term goals set should be something that can be accomplished within a few treatment sessions or a time period of a week or less. The goal should be realistic, measurable, and in the direction of the long-term goal. For the clinician to stay engaged in the patient's progress, the short-term goal should ideally be linked with a recheck of some type, so that there is continuing dialogue between the 2 members of this team. This type of exchange and dialogue also permits the necessary adjustments and reestablishment of new sets of short-term goals, on the way to accomplishing the overall goal.

The long-term goal serves as the finish line. The long-term goal is the destination that the patient and provider are trying to reach. This goal is also established initially, so that it is clear what both the patient and health care provider are striving to achieve. In addition to serving as a roadmap and framework for adjusting the short-term goals on the way to achieving the final goal, this gives both members of this rehabilitation team a feel for where they are on this journey. Achievement of the long-term goal is a logical time to discontinue care.

A point that was alluded to in the preceding paragraphs is that all stated goals must be measurable. This is needed both as a way to objectively track progress and because third-party payers often require it. As the expert in this area, work to identify criteria that are reliable, easily obtained, and directly related to the patient's condition. In addition to being measurable, short-term and long-term goals should have clear timelines associated with them. Although not all the elements of the classic "behavioral objective" will always be in evidence for each goal stated, they should at least be implied, if not explicitly stated. For example, if a short-term goal is to have "10 degrees of additional shoulder flexion in 1 week," the classic elements of who will do what, by when, and to what extent, are all either stated or implied. In this case, the "who" is the patient, so it does not need to be explicitly stated. The "do what," is achieve an additional 10 degrees of shoulder flexion. The "by when," is reflected in the time specification of 1 week, and the "to what extent" implies that the clinician will employ a standard assessment methodology and will require proper form (no substitution). Thus, utilization of an objective system of this type allows progress to be tracked and both members of the rehabilitation team to know where they are at in terms of the final goal.

In those cases where the scan examination reveals that either the patient's or the clinician's goals fall outside of the current health care provider's area of expertise, a referral is indicated. The hallmark of true professionals is knowing their own limitations and referring to other members of the health care team when appropriate.[42] In this case, referral works toward the goal of providing the patient with the best possible care for the patient's particular condition, and it strengthens the entire health care family by having professionals work with each other and draw on specific strengths.

Plan

Once the short-term and long-term goals are identified, it is a relatively straightforward process to determine how to get there. If the metaphor of a trip is considered, once the destination is clear, the map can be looked at and the most efficient trip plotted. Extending this metaphor, if there is a specific sight or person that the budding travelers want to see as part of their trip, that detour can be built into the plan.

From the health care provider's perspective, the basic plan is what should be done, taught, and recommended to the patient. This will be based on a variety of factors, including, but not limited to, the clinician's experience level, equipment available, number of visits allowed by third-party payers, distance that the patient lives from the clinic, and availability of child care for dependents. Within this context, the health care provider is in a position to specify a treatment program, identify where it will be done (eg, in the clinic, at home, or in both locations), identify how often items of this treatment program are performed, and any specifics associated with the program, such as intensity or cautions. The classic exercise prescription should be in evidence here: (a) specificity (what should be done),

(b) frequency (how often the activity should be done, or the number of repetitions and sets expected), (c) duration (how long the activity should be performed), and (d) intensity (what level of performance is expected). When this is provided to the patient in a clear manner and with specific expectations, the likelihood of success of the plan increases dramatically. Other elements that also work toward promoting success are to go through the plan with the patient, having the patient demonstrate any activities that the patient will be doing at home. Instead of simply asking the patient to verbally acknowledge that the patient understands what to do, provide a constructive critique and give the patient an opportunity to ask questions and demonstrate understanding. Then provide the plan in writing, supported with appropriate handouts, videotapes, or other medium that offers a clear reminder for the patient when the patient is trying to do these at home. Additionally, give the patient a specific number or e-mail that the patient can use if questions arise, and ensure that you address them at least once a day.

A home program should be included in almost all treatment programs, because it provides a number of advantages. First, in today's health care environment, no patient will be authorized to come into the clinic for all of the patient's care. It has to be recognized that whether the treatment is elevation of a swollen limb, ambulation instruction, or some form of therapeutic exercise, the patient will do the majority of this care outside of the clinic's walls. Consequently, make use of this reality and have the program performed whenever it is appropriate, within the patient's normal environment. Second, and perhaps more importantly, there is a need to engage the patient in the patient's own care and make the patient responsible for the outcome. There is a tendency today to assume that a patient will seek care and that the health care professional will "fix the patient." This puts all the responsibility on the health care provider and none on the patient. The reality is that the majority of care will take place outside of the clinic, and the patient needs to be both engaged in that care and take responsibility for seeing that it is enacted. A metaphor used earlier described the rehabilitation "team," where the health care provider serves as the coach and the patient functions like the player. Although the coach may be able to recommend the amount of weight that should be lifted, the specific exercises, warm-ups, etc, it is the job of the player to perform the activities to become stronger, faster, more flexible, etc. The patient must assume the bulk of the responsibility for the patient's care, or it should be understood that most treatment interventions will not be successful. While perhaps a poor metaphor, few would argue that even if a patient arranged and kept regular dental checkups every 6 months, if the patient did not brush or floss between those checkups, it would be ludicrous to think that the resulting dental decay and gingivitis was because the dentist had failed the patient. In a similar vein, the patient must be engaged in the patient's own treatment plan, or the chances for optimal success drop logarithmically.

Along with the specific elements of the treatment plan, both within and outside of the clinic, there needs to be a clear recheck system. This should specify when the health care provider and the patient will next meet and assess progress, and when a partial or full reassessment will be performed. This gives the patient a concrete vision of when the patient will have ready access to the patient's health care provider and the patient can prepare questions and concerns for this date. From the health care provider's perspective, this also allows the provider to examine what is possible and make plans for those exchanges with the patient. A useful consideration prior to any recheck appointment is for clinicians to ask themselves 3 basic questions: (a) What should be done if the patient says that they are better? (b) What should be done if the patient says that there has not been a change in their status? (c) What should be done if the patient indicates that the problem has worsened? Over the course of a week, the practicing clinician will hear all of those responses. As "luck (chance) favors the prepared mind,"[82] if these options have been thought through in advance, the clinician will not appear to be stumped in front of the patient. Rather, the clinician will have thought through potential options and be able to appropriately respond to the vast majority of findings at the time of a recheck. This is somewhat analogous to the skilled chess player who is not concerned only with the next move, but has considered all options associated with the next several moves. Anticipating what might occur to the patient, considering options, and being in a position to respond to whatever arises during the recheck, works to increase the knowledge base and skill of the clinician. Ultimately, this leads to improved patient care and, hopefully, the achievement of the majority of mutually stated goals of the patient and clinician.

With a clear plan and recheck system, care is provided, and a regular evaluation of the patient's status is implemented. Judgments are made, and the cycle of reevaluation, assessment of current short-term goals, and plan modification is performed. It is hoped that through the use of a system, such as the one outlined here with the scan examination, that the care provided will be based on objective information, mutually determined goals, and that the plan will successfully address the patient's neuromusculoskeletal problem.

Clinical Pearls

1. **Know sensation patterns extremely well and demand specificity when patients are describing sensory alterations.** This "clinical pearl" revolves around the realization that patients will often present with some pattern of altered sensation, but it will be presented by them in a very general way. For example, patients will present and state that their hand is numb or has some other form of altered sensation. When pressed on this issue and asked to state if the sensory alteration impacts the palm of the hand or the dorsum of the hand, the response is often a bit of confusion and a statement to the effect of "I hadn't really considered that." Further follow-up questions that require additional specificity, such as is the alteration on the thumb side or the little finger side of the hand, may also be met with a lack of clarity. With sensation alterations, requiring the patient to be very specific, while not leading the patient, is critical when working to develop a hypothesis regarding the pathoanatomical reason for the deficiency being described.

   Although different modalities are carried by axons that constitute the dorsal column medial lemniscal system and the anterolateral system (see point 4 under "Basic Elements of Most Physical Examinations" above), the 2 primary sensory distributions that are most useful when sorting out altered sensation patterns are dermatomes and peripheral cutaneous nerves. Dermatomes arise from a single nerve root and their sensory patterns have some overlap, which typically makes a noted deficiency an alteration rather than a loss of sensation.[74] Peripheral cutaneous nerve distributions, on the other hand, represent the region of skin where a traceable nerve provides sensation to a discrete portion of skin.[74] Should a peripheral nerve be completely compromised, it would be expected to not deliver sensation from its distribution. In the more likely case that there is a compromise of some but not all axons, the degree of sensation alteration would be proportional, but the pattern will remain the same. So this pattern is *the key* and is the reason why the examiner needs to know both dermatomes and peripheral cutaneous nerve distributions extremely well. Using the hand and forearm again as an example, if a patient describes altered sensation limited to the palmar surface of the hand, involving the thumb and index finger, and the lateral aspect of the forearm, this is not fully compatible with a potential median nerve problem. The key discrepancy here is that the median nerve cutaneous distribution is limited to the region from the crease of the wrist distally and the lateral forearm should not be involved. In this particular case, with the stated sensory pattern, a more likely cause would be a C6 radiculopathy. If the examiner knows their anatomy and is able to demand that the patient be very specific in identifying the region of any sensory alterations, this can be extremely useful information in determining the nature of the patient's presenting problem.

Two final caveats regarding sensation are that there are other patterns in addition to dermatomes and peripheral cutaneous nerves, and even in the presence of an expected normal side, both sides should be examined. Although dermatomes and peripheral cutaneous nerves are the most common patterns that are being distinguished on a scan examination, other patterns can present, such as the "stocking-glove" pattern of a polyneuropathy. If a patient presents with altered sensation that is symmetrical, particularly of the distal extremities, consider a peripheral neuropathy (polyneuropathy). With the frequency of diabetes in Western societies, this would not be an unexpected complaint when examining patients.[16] These symptoms typically present first in the feet, then the hands, but it is *the pattern* that distinguishes the problem and leads to the working hypothesis. Second, always test both sides. For most patients, this comparison is to provide a compare and contrast between a normal side and a side that is involved with the presenting complaint. If that is the case, this is a useful comparison and it should be documented. But for some conditions, such as the previously referenced potential median neuropathy (eg, carpal tunnel syndrome), research shows that if one side is involved, the likelihood of involvement of the contralateral side may be as high as 90%.[47,79] A careful examination of the contralateral side may identify or suggest the potential of a mild and developing dysfunction that can be addressed early, before it becomes a significant problem.

2. **Use the resources (professionals) within your network to refine your evaluative skills.** The easiest way to summarize this "clinical pearl" is through the analogy of the way evidenced-based information is obtained from libraries. In high school, students learn to use the *Readers Guide to Periodical Literature*. In college, they learn to use *Index Medicus* (PubMed). In graduate school, they learn to use the librarians. While this analogy is a bit tongue-in-cheek, it illustrates that the evolution of seeking information becomes more refined over time and it recognizes the willingness to use professionals to speed up the process. In medicine, there are at least 2 clear realities that have the potential to dramatically increase the accuracy of the examinations performed. First, we are moving into an age of digital records where imaging tests will be available to the health care team. Take the time to review these and work to link the evaluation performed with imaging and other tests that either collaborate or refute the working hypotheses that were developed. Only by testing the hypotheses against defendable standards will any examiner refine their skills. Feedback is required, and this is a good way to obtain it. Second, take the time to develop a network of professionals who can be learned from. To extend the medical imaging example, there are many radiologists who are more than willing to answer questions about what they can deduce from the imaging tests that have been performed. As opportunities present, work to develop a relationship with some of these other members of the health care team so that when questions arise, there is a chance to pose questions and learn from those individuals. This is ideally a two-way exchange, but because most professionals are excited about their specialty area, most are also willing to help mentor other health care professionals who are striving to provide their patient with the best possible care. Although it requires a bit of effort and potentially stepping out of a "comfort zone," obtaining additional information, feedback, and mentoring are all critical in the process of developing increased clinical competence.
3. **Keep an open mind, because some of what we think we know, we do not know.** The easiest example of this is provided by what was a known "truism" at the time of World War II and the Vietnam War. It was then "known" that individuals with flat feet (low-arched feet) were susceptible to an increased injury incidence and this perception negatively impacted their classification status on fitness for active

duty.[11] But when the issue was studied, the finding was that this assumption was not grounded in fact.[19,52] The finding from the Cowan et al article was that "[t]hese findings do not support the hypothesis that low-arched individuals are at increased risk of injury."[19] This interesting historical example demonstrates that it is important to keep an open mind, and continue to look for evidenced-based information upon which decisions are made. Just collect the data and use it to develop the best working hypothesis(es), and base the subsequent treatment approaches on that information.

4. **Don't be intimidated by "cranial nerves" when performing scan examinations.** Although the anatomy and function of cranial nerves initially takes a bit of effort to master, realize that virtually every upper-quarter screen exam will at least examine cranial nerve XI (spinal accessory), as a quick manual muscle test is a shoulder shrug. Additionally, you will be listening to the patient answer questions that will indirectly involve tongue function (cranial nerve XII—hypoglossal), and swallowing (which involves cranial nerves IX and X—glossopharyngeal and vagus). Balance and hearing are assessed with walking and talking, providing information on cranial nerve XIII (vestibulocochlear). If a patient can smile symmetrically, then this finding suggests that the motor portion of cranial nerve VII (facial) is intact. Sensation to the face and muscles of mastication are key roles of cranial nerve V (trigeminal). Tracking of the eyes addresses cranial nerves III, IV, and VI (oculomotor, trochlear, and abducens, respectively). And, the ability to see is a measure that cranial nerve II (optic) is functioning.[75] Although very cursory and most of these tasks are simply observational, some information is provided for 11 of the 12 cranial nerves by performing a shoulder shrug manual muscle test, being a good observer, and knowing what you are looking for. The one nerve that is not assessed in this quick scan is cranial nerve I (olfactory), which assesses the sense of smell. The point of this "clinical pearl" is to illustrate that cranial nerve function can be reasonably monitored during a scan examination, and should any data suggest that a more in-depth follow-up is needed, then a true cranial nerve evaluation can be performed. By keeping an open mind and collecting as much information as possible during a scan examination, it is much less likely that a significant finding will be missed.

Concluding Thoughts

The key element of any scan examination is a systematically applied evaluation to insure that important information is not inadvertently overlooked. This entails approaching the examination with an open mind that is constantly working to assure that if red or yellow flags are identified, they are annotated and appropriately explored. Both of these features are enacted within the context of an evaluation that is time efficient, while remaining flexible, so that data that points to a given working hypothesis can be explored in more detail where there is the opportunity for additional evidence to either collaborate or refute that hypothesis. The data so obtained, provides the framework for the goals and plan to address the patient's presenting condition.

A few concluding thoughts that the novice examiner might find useful are the following:

1. "When hoofbeats are heard, think about horses rather than zebras."[49] What this means is that when data start pointing to several potential hypotheses, the most likely cause is the most commonly occurring hypothesis. If there is another hypothesis that relates to a relatively obscure condition (a zebra), continue to explore the more likely hypothesis first, and in most cases, this will lead to a solution. Having said that, file the

alternative hypothesis away, because on a rare occasion, you will see a zebra and don't want to be so myopic that all that is seen is a horse.

2. Don't approach referring a patient to another health care professional as not being successful. All health care professionals have spheres of expertise and all health care providers should ideally be working to insure that the patient is seen by the most appropriate health care provider. As has been stated previously, the hallmark of true professionals is knowing their own limitations.[42]
3. Although each health care professional will develop his or her own system, a system should always be used. This has been stressed throughout this chapter because it is that important. The only way that data will be systematically collected, joints above and below the region of interest will be explored, and the possibilities of visceral or referred causes of the patient's problem will be kept within the hypotheses explored, is through a system. Use of a system will assist in not missing key elements and in providing higher quality health care.
4. All the evaluative procedures used (basic scan exam and any follow-up special tests) are based on a strong foundational knowledge of anatomy, histology, biomechanics, physiology, neuroscience, and the other foundational elements needed to understand the workings of the human body. Throughout your career, continue to be a student and work to build upon the knowledge base of the profession and the various interrelationships that exist across all of the basic sciences. This type of curiosity will ultimately work to the patient's advantage by having the patient seen by a highly qualified professional.

SUMMARY

1. Use a system to insure that examinations are thorough and reproducible.
2. Listen to the patient and the patient's concerns—the history and the information obtained are vital to the evaluation.
3. Start broad, with an open mind—let the findings guide your hypotheses.
4. Have a rationale for every question asked and every physical exam test performed, so that this information can be translated into usable data.
5. Know your areas of expertise and your limitations—a hallmark of a true professional is knowing when to refer (work within the full health care team).
6. Record as you go throughout the examination to increase accuracy.
7. Understand that while "clearing tests" are important, they do not truly rule out any region of the body.
8. Although most dysfunctions are limited to a single problem, be aware that comorbidities are a real possibility.
9. Develop a plan that meets both the goals of the patient and of the rehabilitation professional.
10. At the time of goal planning, always consider the following options for the follow-up appointment:
    - **a.** What should be the response if the patient is better?
    - **b.** What should be the response if there is no change in the patient?
    - **c.** What should be the response if the patient's problem is worse?

REFERENCES

1. Classic Quotes. Clarence Darrow. 1938. http://answers.yahoo.com/question/index?qid=20080724112054AAVq1tf. Accessed August 7, 2013.
2. *Physician's Desk Reference.* Montvale, NJ: Thomson; 2005.
3. Aglietti P, Rinonapoli E, Stringa G, Taviani A. Tibial osteotomy for the varus osteoarthritic knee. *Clin Orthop Relat Res.* 1983;(176):239-251.
4. Aguggia M. Typical facial neuralgias. *Neurol Sci.* 2005;26:s68-s70.
5. Agur A, Dalley A. *Grant's Atlas of Anatomy.* 12th ed. Philadelphia, PA: Lippincott Williams & Wilkins; 2009.
6. American Physical Therapy Association. Guide to physical therapist practice. *Phys Ther.* 2001;81:9-746.
7. Anderson J, Pollitzer W. Ethnic and genetic differences in susceptibility to osteoporotic fractures. *Adv Nutr Res.* 1994;9:129-149.
8. Bahrami M, Rayegani S, Fereidouni M, Baghbani M. Prevalence and severity of carpal tunnel syndrome (CTS) during pregnancy. *Electromyogr Clin Neurophysiol.* 2005;45:123-125.
9. Baxter R. *Pocket Guide to Musculoskeletal Assessment.* Philadelphia, PA: Saunders; 1998.
10. Benjamin R. Neurologic complications of prostate cancer. *Am Fam Physician.* 2002;65:1834-1840.
11. Bennett J, Stock D. The longstanding problem of flat feet. *J R Army Med Corps.* 1989;135:144-146.
12. Bertorini T, Narayanaswami P, Rashed H. Charcot-Marie-Tooth disease (hereditary motor sensory neuropathies) and hereditary sensory and autonomic neuropathies. *Neurologist.* 2004;10:327-337.
13. Boissonnault W, Badke M. Collecting health history information: the accuracy of a patient self-administered questionnaire in an orthopedic outpatient setting. *Phys Ther.* 2005;85:531-543.
14. Borg-Stein J, Dugan S, Gruber J. Musculoskeletal aspects of pregnancy. *Am J Phys Med Rehabil.* 2005;84:180-192.
15. Bourdillon J, Day E, Bookhout M. Examination, general considerations. In: Bourdillon J, Day E, Bookhout M, eds. *Spinal Manipulation.* 5th ed. Boston, MA: Butterworth-Heinemann; 1992:47-80.
16. Centers for Disease Control and Prevention (CDC). Increasing prevalence of diagnosed diabetes—United States and Puerto Rico, 1995–2010. *MMWR Morb Mortal Wkly Rep.* 2012;61:918-921.
17. Childs JD, Flynn TW, Fritz JM, et al. Screening for vertebrobasilar insufficiency in patients with neck pain: manual therapy decision-making in the presence of uncertainty. *J Orthop Sports Phys Ther.* 2005;35:300-306.
18. Chusid J. Reflexes. In: Chusid J, ed. *Correlative Neuroanatomy & Functional Neurology.* 16th ed. Los Altos, CA: Lange Medical Publications; 1976:206-210.
19. Cowan D, Jones B, Robinson J. Foot morphologic characteristics and risk of exercise-related injury. *Arch Fam Med.* 1993;2:773-777.
20. Crook E, Patel S. Diabetic nephropathy in African-American patients. *Curr Diab Rep.* 2004;4:455-461.
21. Crossley K, Cowan SM, Bennell KL, McConnell J. Patellar taping: is clinical success supported by scientific evidence? *Man Ther.* 2000;5:142-150.
22. Cryrix J. The diagnosis of soft tissue lesions. In: Cyriax J, ed. *Textbook of Orthopaedic Medicine.* 7th ed. London, UK: Spottiswoode Ballantyne; 1978:64-103.
23. Daniels L, Worthingham C. *Muscle Testing: Techniques of Manual Examination.* Philadelphia, PA: W.B. Saunders; 1986.
24. Diaz J. Carpal tunnel syndrome in female nurse anesthetists versus operating room nurses: prevalence, laterality, and impact of handedness. *Anesth Analg.* 2001;93:975-980.
25. Dutton M. *Orthopaedic Examination, Evaluation & Intervention.* New York, NY: McGraw-Hill; 2004.
26. Everwild. "First, do no harm" is not in the Hippocratic oath. 2005.
27. Falkner B. Insulin resistance in African Americans. *Kidney Int Suppl.* 2003;83:S27-S30.
28. Fields H. Pain from deep tissues and referred pain. In: Fields H, ed. *Pain: Mechanisms and Management.* New York, NY: McGraw-Hill; 1987:79-98.
29. Fitts R, McDonald K, Schluter J. The determinants of skeletal muscle force and power: their adaptability with changes in activity pattern. *J Biomech.* 1991;24:111-122.
30. Flynn T. *The Thoracic Spine and Rib Cage.* Newton, MA: Butterworth-Heinemann; 1996.
31. Fogo A. Hypertensive risk factors in kidney disease in African Americans. *Kidney Int Suppl.* 2003;(83):S17-S21.
32. Gardner E, Kandel E. Touch. In: Kandel E, Schwartz J, Jessell T, eds. *Principles of Neural Science.* 4th ed. New York, NY: McGraw-Hill; 2000:451-471.
33. Gardner E, Martin J, Jessell T. The bodily senses. In: Kandel E, Schwartz J, Jessell T, eds. *Principles of Neural Science.* 4th ed. New York, NY: McGraw-Hill; 2000:430-450.
34. Gaylor A, Condren M. Type 2 diabetes mellitus in the pediatric population. *Pharmacotherapy.* 2004;24:871-878.
35. Goldberg S. *The Four Minute Neurologic Exam.* Miami, FL: MedMaster; 1992.
36. Goodman C. Red flags: recognizing signs and symptoms. *Phys Ther Magazine.* 1993;9:55-62.
37. Goodman C, Boissonnault W, Fuller K. *Pathology: Implications for the Physical Therapist.* 2nd ed. Philadelphia, PA: Saunders; 2003.

38. Goodman C, Randall T. Musculoskeletal neoplasms. In: Goodman C, Boissonnault W, Fuller K, eds. *Pathology: Implications for the Physical Therapist*. 2nd ed. Philadelphia, PA: Saunders; 2003:905-928.
39. Goodman C, Snyder T. *Differential Diagnosis in Physical Therapy*. Philadelphia, PA: Saunders; 1990.
40. Goodman C, Snyder T. Systematic origins of musculoskeletal pain: associated signs and symptoms. In: Goodman C, Snyder T, eds. *Differential Diagnosis in Physical Therapy*. Philadelphia, PA: Saunders; 1990:327-345.
41. Goodman C, Snyder T. *Differential Diagnosis in Physical Therapy*. 2nd ed. Philadelphia, PA: Saunders; 1995.
42. Goodman C, Snyder T: Introduction to differential screening in physical therapy. In: Goodman C, Snyder T, eds. *Differential Diagnosis in Physical Therapy*. 2nd ed. Philadelphia, PA: Saunders; 1995:1-23.
43. Goodman C, Snyder T. Oncology. In: Goodman C, Boissonnault W, Fuller K, eds. *Pathology: Implications for the Physical Therapist*. 2nd ed. Philadelphia, PA: Saunders; 2003:236-263.
44. Goodman C, Snyder T. Introduction to the interviewing process. In: Goodman C, Snyder T, eds. *Differential Diagnosis in Physical Therapy*. Philadelphia, PA: Saunders; 1990:7-42.
45. Goodyer P. *Techniques in Musculoskeletal Rehabilitation: Companion Handbook*. New York, NY: McGraw-Hill; 2001.
46. Govind J. Lumbar radicular pain. *Aust Fam Physician*. 2004;33:409-412.
47. Goyal V, Bhatia M, Padma M, Jain S, Maheshwari MC. Electrophysiological evaluation of 140 hands with carpal tunnel syndrome. *J Assoc Physicians India*. 2001;49:1070-1073.
48. Gran J. The epidemiology of chronic generalized musculoskeletal pain. *Best Pract Res Clin Rheumatol*. 2003;17:547-561.
49. Greathouse D, Schreck R, Benson C. The United States Army physical therapy experience: evaluation and treatment of patients with neuromusculoskeletal disorders. *J Orthop Sports Phys Ther*. 1994;19:261-266.
50. Halle J. Neuromuscular scan examination with selected related topics. In: Flynn T, ed. *The Thoracic Spine and Rib Cage: Musculoskeletal Evaluation and Treatment*. Boston, MA: Butterworth-Heinemann; 1996:121-146.
51. Henderson NE, Knapik JJ, Shaffer SW, McKenzie TH, Schneider GM. Injuries and injury risk factors among men and women in U.S. Army Combat Medic Advanced individual training. *Mil Med*. 2000;165:647-652.
52. Hogan M, Staheli L. Arch height and lower limb pain: an adult civilian study. *Foot Ankle Int*. 23:43-47, 200.
53. Houlden H, Blake J, Reilly M. Hereditary sensory neuropathies. *Curr Opin Neurol*. 2004;17:569-577.
54. Jones G, Cowan D, Knapik J. Exercise, training and injuries. *Sports Med*. 1994;18:202-214.
55. Kandel E. Nerve cells and behavior. In: Kandel E, Schwartz J, Jessell T, eds. *Principles of Neural Science*. 4th ed. New York, NY: McGraw-Hill; 2000:19-35.
56. Kendall F, McCreary E, Provance P. Muscles: *Testing and Function*. Baltimore, MD: Williams & Wilkins; 1993.
57. Koknel T. Thoracic outlet syndrome. *Agri*. 2005;17:5-9.
58. Kvien T: Epidemiology and burden of illness of rheumatoid arthritis. *Pharmacoeconomics*. 2004;22: 1-12.
59. Lun V, Meeuwisse WH, Stergiou P, Stefanyshyn D. Relation between running injury and static lower limb alignment in recreational runners. *Br J Sports Med*. 2004;38:576-580.
60. Magee D. Cervical spine. In: Magee D, ed. *Orthopedic Physical Assessment*. 4th ed. Philadelphia, PA: Saunders; 2002:121-182.
61. Magee D. *Orthopedic Physical Assessment*. 4th ed. Philadelphia, PA: Saunders; 2002.
62. Magee D. Principles and concepts. In: Magee D, ed. *Orthopedic Physical Assessment*. 4th ed. Philadelphia, PA: Saunders; 2002:1-66.
63. Malcoe L, Duran B, Montgomery J. Socioeconomic disparities in intimate partner violence against Native American women: a cross-sectional study. *BMC Med*. 2004;2:1-14.
64. Malone T, McPoil T, Nitz A. *Orthopedics and Sports Physical Therapy*. St. Louis, MO: Mosby; 1997.
65. Matheson GO, Macintyre JG, Taunton JE, Clement DB, Lloyd-Smith R. Musculoskeletal injuries associated with physical activity in older adults. *Med Sci Sports Exerc*. 1989;21:379-385.
66. McClure P. The degenerative cervical spine: pathogenesis and rehabilitation concepts. *J Hand Ther*. 2000;13:163-174.
67. McKenzie R. *Treat Your Own Back*. Minneapolis, MN: Orthopedic Physical Therapy Product; 1997.
68. Michlovitz S. Conservative interventions for carpal tunnel syndrome. *J Orthop Sports Phys Ther*. 2004;34: 589-600.
69. Moore K, Dalley A, Agur A. Abdomen. In: Moore K, Dalley A, eds. *Clinically Oriented Anatomy*. 6th ed. Philadelphia, PA: Lippincott Williams & Wilkins; 2010:181-325.
70. Moore K, Dalley A, Agur A. *Clinically Oriented Anatomy*. 6th ed. Philadelphia, PA: Lippincott Williams & Wilkins; 2010.
71. Moore K, Dalley A, Agur A. Neck. In: Moore K, Dalley A, eds. *Clinical Oriented Anatomy*. 6th ed. Philadelphia, PA: Lippincott Williams & Wilkins; 2010:981-1052.
72. Moore K, Dalley A, Agur A. Thorax. In: Moore K, Dalley A, eds. *Clinically Oriented Anatomy*. 6th ed. Philadelphia, PA: Lippincott Williams & Wilkins; 2010:71-180.
73. Moore K, Dalley A, Agur A. Upper limb. In: Moore K, Dalley A, eds. *Clinical Oriented Anatomy*. 6th ed. Philadelphia, PA: Lippincott Williams & Wilkins; 2010:670-819.
74. Moore K, Dalley A, Agur A. Introduction to clinically oriented anatomy. In: Moore K, Dalley A, Agur A, eds. *Clinically Oriented Anatomy*. 6th ed. Philadelphia, PA: Lippincott Williams & Wilkins; 2010:1-79.

75. Moore K, Dalley A, Agur A. Summary of cranial nerves. In: Moore K, Dalley A, Agur A, eds. *Clinically Oriented Anatomy*. 6th ed. Philadelphia, PA: Lippincott Williams & Wilkins; 2010:1053-1082.
76. Netter F. *Atlas of Human Anatomy*. 5th ed. St. Louis, MO: Saunders; 2011.
77. Norkin C, Levangie P. The knee complex. In: Norkin C, Levangie P, eds. *Joint Structure and Function*. 2nd ed. Philadelphia, PA: FA Davis; 1992:337-378.
78. Oates S, Daley R. Thoracic outlet syndrome. *Hand Clin.* 1996;12:705-718.
79. Padua L, Padua R, Nazzaro M, Tonali P. Incidence of bilateral symptoms in carpal tunnel syndrome. *J Hand Surg Br.* 1998;23:603-606.
80. Patten J. The cerebral hemispheres: 1. The lobes of the brain. In: Patten J, ed. *Neurological Differential Diagnosis*. New York, NY: Springer-Verlag; 1977:69-85.
81. Pecoraro RE, Inui TS, Chen MS, Plorde DK, Heller JL. Validity and reliability of a self-administered health history questionnaire. *Public Health Rep.* 1979;94:231-238.
82. QuoteDB. Chance favors the prepared mind. 2005.
83. Rayan G. Thoracic outlet syndrome. *J Shoulder Elbow Surg.* 1998;7:440-451.
84. Rebain R, Baxter G, McDonough S. A systematic review of the passive straight leg raising test as a diagnostic aid for low back pain. *Spine (Phila Pa 1976).* 2002;27:E388-E395.
85. Reese N. Techniques of manual muscle testing: lower extremity. In: Reese N, ed. *Muscle and Sensory Testing*. Philadelphia, PA: Saunders; 1999:234-336.
86. Rhoades R, Tanner G. Skeletal and smooth muscle. In: Rhoades R, Tanner G, eds. *Medical Physiology*. Boston, MA: Little, Brown; 1995:165-192.
87. Richter R, Reinking M. How does evidence on the diagnostic accuracy of the vertebral artery test influence teaching of the test in a professional physical therapy education program. *Phys Ther.* 2005;85:589-599.
88. Rose EA, Deshikachar AM, Schwartz KL, Severson RK. Use of a template to improve documentation and coding. Fam Med 2001;33:516-521.
89. Rothstein J. On defining subjective and objective measurements. *Phys Ther.* 1989;69:577-579.
90. Rowland L. Clinical syndromes of the spinal cord and brain stem. In: Kandel E, Schwartz J, Jessell T, eds. *Principles of Neural Science*. 3rd ed. Norwalk, CT: Appleton & Lange; 1991:711-730.
91. Rowland L. Diseases of the motor unit. In: Kandel E, Schwartz J, Jessell T, eds. *Principles of Neural Science*. 4th ed. New York, NY: McGraw-Hill; 2000:695-712.
92. Saunders D, Daunders R. Evaluation of the spine. In: Saunders D, ed. *Evaluation, Treatment and Prevention of Musculoskeletal Disorders*. 3rd ed. Bloomington, IN: Educational Opportunities; 1993:33-97.
93. Shaver JL. Fibromyalgia syndrome in women. *Nurs Clin North Am.* 2004;39:195-204.
94. Stuge G, Hilde G, Vollestad N. Physical therapy for pregnancy-related low back and pelvic pain: a systematic review. *Acta Obstet Gynecol Scand.* 2003;82:989-990.
95. Tippett S. Considerations with the pediatric patient. In: Prentice W, Voight M, eds. *Techniques in Musculoskeletal Rehabilitation*. New York, NY: McGraw-Hill; 2001: 697-714.
96. Walton L. The symptoms and signs of disease in the nervous system. In: Walton L, ed. *Essentials of Neurology*. New York, NY: Churchill Livingstone, 1989:1-24.
97. Weir CR, Hurdle JF, Felgar MA, Hoffman JM, Roth B, Nebeker JR. Direct text entry in electronic progress notes: an evaluation of input errors. *Methods Inf Med.* 2003;42:61-67.
98. Wilson T, Talwalkar J, Johnson D. Lateral patella dislocation associated with an irreducible posterolateral knee dislocation: literature review. *Orthopedics.* 2005;28:459-461.
99. Wolff A, Bourke J. Reducing medical errors: a practical guide. *Med J Aust.* 2000;173:247-251.
100. Wu WH, Meijer OG, Uegaki K, et al. Pregnancy-related pelvic girdle pain (PPP), I: terminology, clinical presentation, and prevalence. *Eur Spine J.* 2004;13:575-589.
101. Zachazewski J, Magee D, Quillen W. *Athletic Injuries and Rehabilitation*. Philadelphia, PA: Saunders; 1996.

4

Impairments Caused By Pain

Craig R. Denegar and William E. Prentice

OBJECTIVES

After completion of this chapter, the physical therapist should be able to do the following:

- Compare the various types of pain and appraise their positive and negative effects.
- Choose a technique for assessing pain.
- Analyze the characteristics of sensory receptors.
- Examine how the nervous system relays information about painful stimuli.
- Distinguish between the different neurophysiologic mechanisms for pain control for the therapeutic modalities used by clinicians.
- Predict how pain perception can be modified by cognitive factors.

Understanding Pain

The International Association for the Study of Pain defines pain as "an unpleasant sensory and emotional experience associated with actual or potential tissue damage, or described in terms of such damage."[1] Pain is a subjective sensation, with more than 1 dimension and an abundance of descriptors of its qualities and characteristics. In spite of its universality, pain is composed of a variety of human discomforts, rather than being a single entity.[2] The perception of pain can be subjectively modified by past experiences and expectations.[37] Much of what we do to treat patients' pain is to change their perceptions of pain.[3]

Pain does have a purpose. It warns us that something is wrong and can provoke a withdrawal response to avoid further injury. It also results in muscle spasm and guards or protects the injured part. Pain, however, can persist after it is no longer useful. It can become a means of enhancing disability and inhibiting efforts to rehabilitate the patient.[4] Prolonged spasm, which leads to circulatory deficiency, muscle atrophy, disuse habits, and conscious or unconscious guarding, may lead to a severe loss of function.[5] Chronic pain may become a disease state in itself. Often lacking an identifiable cause, chronic pain can totally disable a patient.

Research in recent years has led to a better understanding of pain and pain relief, as well as the psychology of pain, offering new approaches to the treatment of musculoskeletal injury and pain.[6] The evolution of the treatment of pain is, however, incomplete.

The control of pain is an essential aspect of caring for an injured patient. This chapter does not provide a complete explanation of neurophysiology, pain, and pain relief. Several physiology textbooks provide extensive discussions of human neurophysiology and neurobiology to supplement this chapter. Instead, this chapter presents an overview of some theories of pain control, which are intended to provide a stimulus for the clinician to develop his or her own rationale for managing pain.[8]

Types of Pain

Acute Versus Chronic Pain

Traditionally, pain has been categorized as either *acute* or *chronic.* Acute pain is experienced when tissue damage is impending and after injury has occurred. Pain lasting for more than 6 months is generally classified as chronic.[9] More recently, the term *persistent pain* has been used to differentiate chronic pain that defies intervention from conditions in which continuing (persistent) pain is a symptom of a treatable condition.[10,11] More research is devoted to chronic pain and its treatment, but acute and persistent pain confronts the clinician most often.[12]

Referred Pain

Referred pain, which also may be either acute or chronic, is pain that is perceived to be in an area that seems to have little relation to the existing pathology. For example, injury to the spleen often results in pain in the left shoulder. This pattern, known as the Kehr sign, is useful for identifying this serious injury and arranging prompt emergency care. Referred pain can outlast the causative events because of altered reflex patterns, continuing mechanical stress on muscles, learned habits of guarding, or the development of hypersensitive areas, called *trigger points.*

Radiating Pain

Irritation of nerves and nerve roots can cause *radiating pain.* Pressure on the lumbar nerve roots associated with a herniated disc or a contusion of the sciatic nerve can result in pain radiating down the lower extremity to the foot.

Deep Somatic Pain

Deep somatic pain is a type that seems to be **sclerotomic** (associated with a sclerotome, a segment of bone innervated by a spinal segment). There is often a discrepancy between the site of the disorder and the site of the pain.

Pain Assessment

Pain is a complex phenomenon that is difficult to evaluate and quantify because it is subjective and is influenced by attitudes and beliefs of the clinician and the patient. Quantification is hindered by the fact that pain is a very difficult concept to put into words.[13]

Obtaining an accurate and standardized assessment of pain is problematic. Several tools have been developed. These pain profiles identify the type of pain, quantify the intensity of pain, evaluate the effect of the pain experience on the patient's level of function, and/or assess the psychosocial impact of pain.

The pain profiles are useful because they compel the patient to verbalize the pain and thereby provide an outlet for the patient and also provide the clinician with a better understanding of the pain experience. They assess the psychosocial response to pain and injury. The pain profile can assist with the evaluation process by improving communication and directing the clinician toward appropriate diagnostic tests. Finally, these profiles provide a standard measure to monitor treatment progress.[10]

Pain Assessment Scales

The following profiles are used in the evaluation of acute and chronic pain associated with illnesses and injuries.

Visual Analog Scales

Visual analog scales are quick and simple tests to be completed by the patient (Figure 4-1). These scales consist of a line, usually 10 cm in length, the extremes of which are taken to represent the limits of the pain experience.[14] One end is defined as "No Pain" and the other as "Severe Pain." The patient is asked to mark the line at a point corresponding to the severity of the pain. The distance between "No Pain" and the mark represents pain severity. A similar scale can be used to assess treatment effectiveness by placing "No Pain Relief" at one end of the scale and "Complete Pain Relief" at the other. These scales can be completed daily or more often as pretreatment and posttreatment assessments.[15]

Pain Charts

Pain charts can be used to establish spatial properties of pain. These 2-dimensional graphic portrayals are completed by the patient to assess the location of pain and a number of subjective components. Simple line drawings of the body in several postural positions are presented to the patient (Figure 4-2). On these drawings, the patient draws or colors in areas that correspond to the patient's pain experience. Different colors are used for different sensations—for example, blue for aching pain, yellow for numbness or tingling, red for burning pain, and green for cramping pain. Descriptions can be added to the form to enhance the communication value. The form could be completed daily.[16]

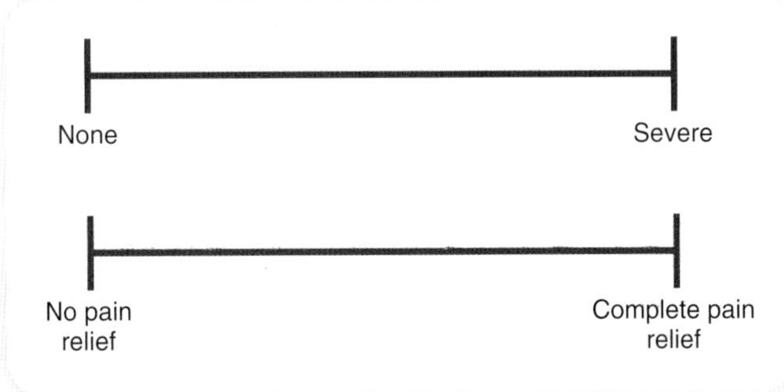

Figure 4-1 Visual analog scales

(Reproduced with permission from Prentice. *Therapeutic Modalities in Rehabilitation*. 4th ed. New York: McGraw-Hill; 2011.)

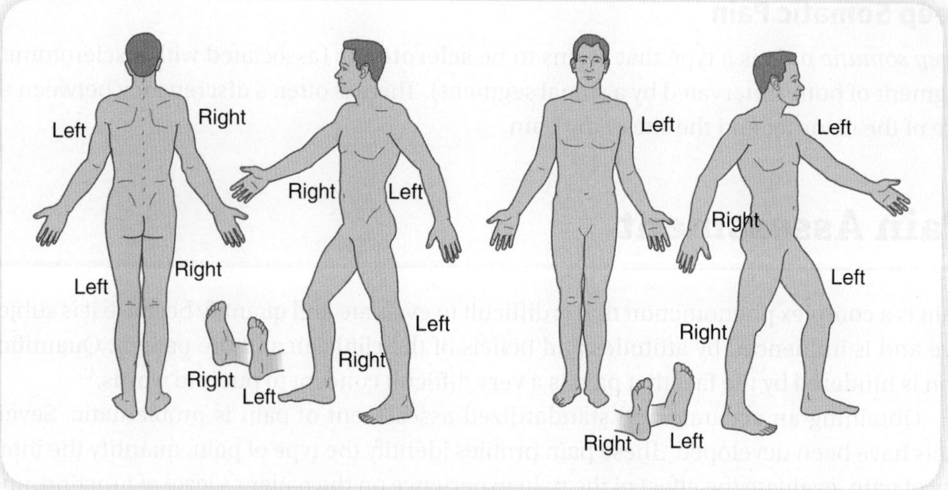

Figure 4-2 **The pain chart**

Use the following instructions: "Please use all of the figures to show me exactly where all your pains are, and where they radiate to. Shade or draw with *blue marker*. Only the patient is to fill out this sheet. Please be as precise and detailed as possible. Use *yellow marker* for numbness and tingling. Use *red marker* for burning or hot areas, and *green marker* for cramping. Please remember: blue = pain, yellow = numbness and tingling, red = burning or hot areas, green = cramping." (Used with permission from Margoles MS. The pain chart: spatial properties of pain. In: Melzack R, ed. *Pain Measurement and Assessment*. New York, NY: Raven Press; 1983.)

McGill Pain Questionnaire

The *McGill Pain Questionnaire* is a tool with 78 words that describe pain (Figure 4-3). These words are grouped into 20 sets that are divided into 4 categories representing dimensions of the pain experience. Although completion of the McGill Pain Questionnaire may take only 20 minutes, it is often frustrating for patients who do not speak English well. The McGill Pain Questionnaire is commonly administered to patients with low back pain. When administered every 2 to 4 weeks, it demonstrates changes in status very clearly.[2]

Activity Pattern Indicators Pain Profile

The *Activity Pattern Indicators Pain Profile* measures patient activity. It is a 64-question, self-report tool that may be used to assess functional impairment associated with pain. The instrument measures the frequency of certain behaviors such as housework, recreation, and social activities.[10]

Numeric Pain Scale

The most common acute pain profile is a *numeric pain scale*. The patient is asked to rate his or her pain on a scale from 1 to 10, with 10 representing the worst pain the patient has experienced or could imagine (Figure 4-4). The question is asked before and after treatment. When treatments provide pain relief, patients are asked about the extent and duration of the relief. In addition, patients may be asked to estimate the portion of the day that they experience pain and about specific activities that increase or decrease their pain. When pain affects sleep, patients may be asked to estimate the amount of sleep they got in the previous 24 hours. In addition, the amount of medication required for pain can be noted. This information helps the clinician assess changes in pain, select appropriate treatments, and communicate more clearly with the patient about the course of recovery from injury or surgery.

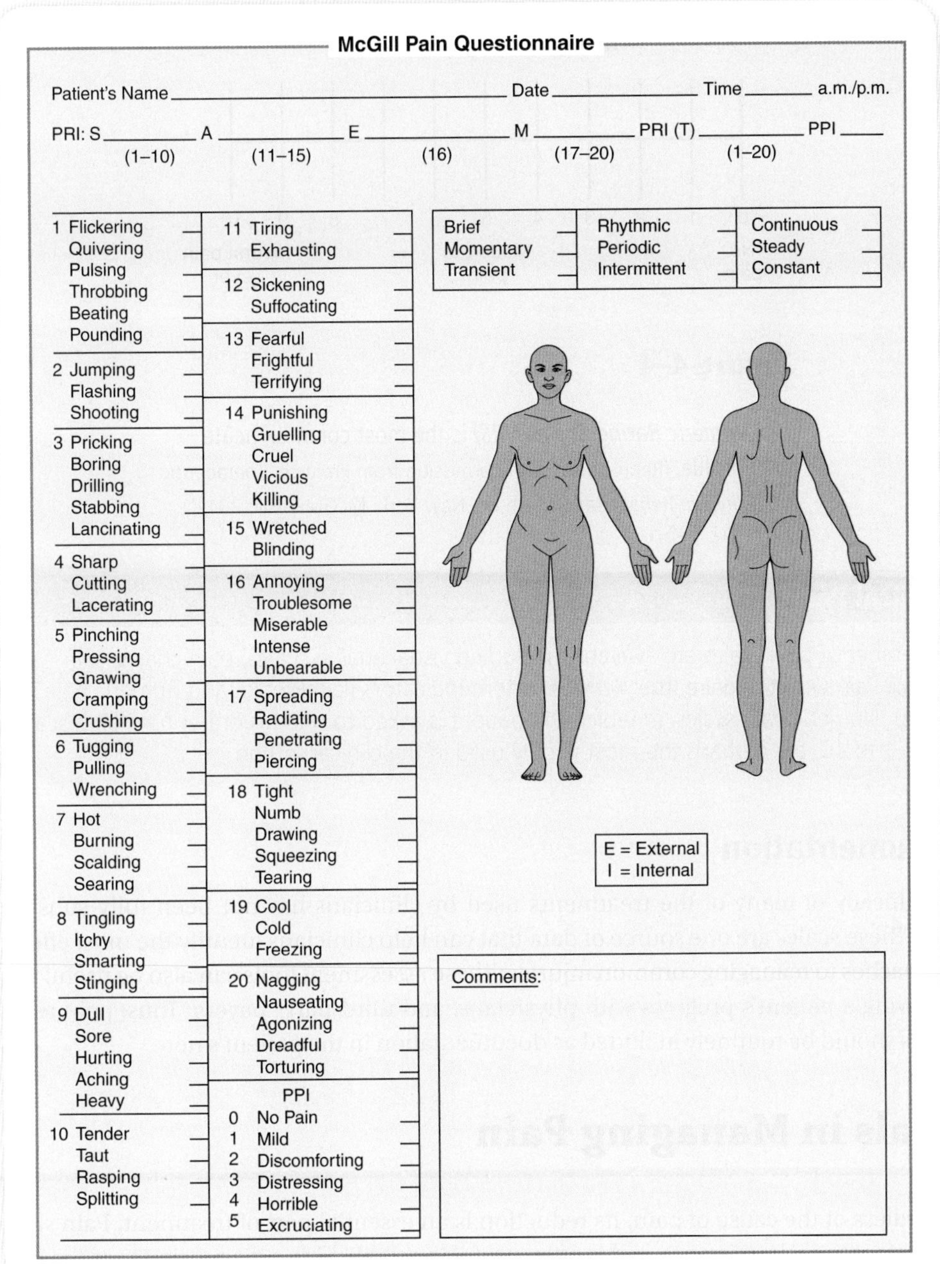

McGill Pain Questionnaire

Patient's Name ______ Date ______ Time ______ a.m./p.m.

PRI: S ______ (1–10) A ______ (11–15) E ______ (16) M ______ (17–20) PRI (T) ______ (1–20) PPI ______

1 Flickering, Quivering, Pulsing, Throbbing, Beating, Pounding

2 Jumping, Flashing, Shooting

3 Pricking, Boring, Drilling, Stabbing, Lancinating

4 Sharp, Cutting, Lacerating

5 Pinching, Pressing, Gnawing, Cramping, Crushing

6 Tugging, Pulling, Wrenching

7 Hot, Burning, Scalding, Searing

8 Tingling, Itchy, Smarting, Stinging

9 Dull, Sore, Hurting, Aching, Heavy

10 Tender, Taut, Rasping, Splitting

11 Tiring, Exhausting

12 Sickening, Suffocating

13 Fearful, Frightful, Terrifying

14 Punishing, Gruelling, Cruel, Vicious, Killing

15 Wretched, Blinding

16 Annoying, Troublesome, Miserable, Intense, Unbearable

17 Spreading, Radiating, Penetrating, Piercing

18 Tight, Numb, Drawing, Squeezing, Tearing

19 Cool, Cold, Freezing

20 Nagging, Nauseating, Agonizing, Dreadful, Torturing

PPI

0 No Pain
1 Mild
2 Discomforting
3 Distressing
4 Horrible
5 Excruciating

Brief	Rhythmic	Continuous
Momentary	Periodic	Steady
Transient	Intermittent	Constant

E = External
I = Internal

Comments:

Figure 4-3 McGill pain questionnaire

The descriptors fall into 4 major groups: sensory, 1 to 10; affective, 11 to 15; evaluative, 16; and miscellaneous, 17 to 20. The rank value for each descriptor is based on its position in the word set. The sum of the rank values is the pain rating index (PRI). The present pain intensity (PPI) is based on a scale of 0 to 5. (Reproduced with permission from Prentice. *Therapeutic Modalities in Rehabilitation*. 4th ed. New York: McGraw-Hill; 2011.)

All of these scales help patients communicate the severity and duration of their pain and appreciate changes that occur. Often in a long recovery, patients lose sight of how much progress has been made in terms of the pain experience and return to functional activities. A review of these pain scales often can serve to reassure the patient; foster a brighter, more positive outlook; and reinforce the commitment to the plan of treatment.

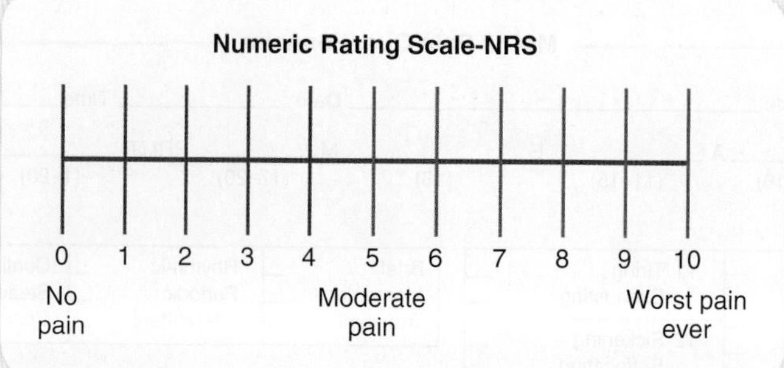

Figure 4-4

The *Numeric Rating Scale (NRS)* is the most common acute pain profile. (Reproduced with permission from Prentice. *Therapeutic Modalities in Rehabilitation*. 4th ed. New York: McGraw-Hill; 2011.)

Clinical Pearl

A number of pain scales are available, including visual analog scales, pain charts, the McGill Pain Questionnaire, the Activity Pattern Indicators Pain Profile, and numeric pain scales. Numeric pain scales, in which the patient is asked to rate his or her pain on a scale from 1 to 10, are perhaps the most widely used in the clinical setting.

Documentation

The efficacy of many of the treatments used by clinicians has not been fully substantiated. These scales are one source of data that can help clinicians identify the most effective approaches to managing common injuries. These assessment tools can also be useful when reviewing a patient's progress with physicians, and third-party payers. Thus, pain assessments should be routinely included as documentation in the patient's note.

Goals in Managing Pain

Regardless of the cause of pain, its reduction is an essential part of treatment. Pain signals the patient to seek assistance and is often useful in establishing a diagnosis. Once the injury or illness is diagnosed, pain serves little purpose. Medical or surgical treatment or immobilization is necessary to treat some conditions, but physical therapy and an early return to activity are appropriate following many injuries.[35] The clinician's objectives are to encourage the body to heal through exercise designed to progressively increase functional capacity and to return the patient to work, recreational, and other activities as swiftly and safely as possible. Pain will inhibit therapeutic exercise. The challenge for the clinician is to control acute pain and protect the patient from further injury while encouraging progressive exercise in a supervised environment.

Pain Perception

The patient's perception of pain can differ markedly from person to person, as can the terminology used to describe the type of pain the patient is experiencing. The clinician commonly asks the patient to describe what the patient's pain feels like during an injury evaluation. The patient often uses terms such as *sharp, dull, aching, throbbing, burning, piercing, localized,* and *generalized.* It is sometimes difficult for the clinician to infer what exactly is causing a particular type of pain. For example, "burning" pain is often associated with some injury to a nerve, but certainly other injuries may produce what the patient is perceiving as "burning" pain. Thus, verbal descriptions of the type of pain should be applied with caution.

Sensory Receptors

A nerve ending is the termination of a nerve fiber in a peripheral structure. It may be a sensory ending (receptor) or a motor ending (effector). Sensory endings can be capsulated (eg, free nerve endings, Merkel corpuscles) or encapsulated (eg, end bulbs of Krause or Meissner corpuscles).

There are several types of sensory receptors in the body, and the clinician should be aware of their existence as well as of the types of stimuli that activate them (Table 4-1). Activation of some of these sense organs with therapeutic agents will decrease the patients perception of pain.

Six different types of receptor nerve endings are commonly described:

1. Meissner corpuscles are activated by light touch.
2. Pacinian corpuscles respond to deep pressure.
3. Merkel corpuscles respond to deep pressure, but more slowly than Pacinian corpuscles, and also are activated by hair follicle deflection.
4. Ruffini corpuscles in the skin are sensitive to touch, tension, and possibly heat; those in the joint capsules and ligaments are sensitive to change in position.

Table 4-1 Some Characteristics of Selected Sensory Receptors

	Stimulus		Receptor	
Type of Sensory Receptors	**General Term**	**Specific Nature**	**Term**	**Location**
Mechanoreceptors	Pressure	Movement of hair in a hair follicle Light pressure Deep pressure Touch	Afferent nerve fiber Meissner corpuscle Pacinian corpuscle Merkel touch corpuscle	Base of hair follicles Skin Skin Skin
Nociceptors	Pain	Distension (stretch)	Free nerve endings	Wall of gastrointestinal tract, pharynx skin
Proprioceptors	Tension	Distension Length changes Tension changes	Corpuscles of Ruffini Muscle spindles Golgi tendon organs	Skin and capsules in joints and ligaments Skeletal muscle Between muscles and tendons
Thermoreceptors	Temperature change	Cold Heat	End bulbs of Krause Corpuscles of Ruffini	Skin Skin and capsules in joints and ligaments

Source: Reproduced with permission from Previte J. *Human Physiology.* New York, NY: McGraw-Hill; 1983.

5. End bulbs of Krause are thermoreceptors that react to a decrease in temperature and touch.[17]
6. Pain receptors, called *nociceptors* or *free nerve endings*, are sensitive to extreme mechanical, thermal, or chemical energy.[3] They respond to noxious stimuli—in other words, to impending or actual tissue damage (eg, cuts, burns, sprains, and so on). The term *nociceptive* is from the Latin *nocere*, to damage, and is used to imply pain information. These organs respond to superficial forms of heat and cold, analgesic balms, and massage.

Proprioceptors found in muscles, joint capsules, ligaments, and tendons provide information regarding joint position and muscle tone. The muscle spindles react to changes in length and tension when the muscle is stretched or contracted. The Golgi tendon organs also react to changes in length and tension within the muscle. See Table 4-1 for a more complete listing.

Some sensory receptors respond to phasic activity and produce an impulse when the stimulus is increasing or decreasing, but not during a sustained stimulus. They adapt to a constant stimulus. Meissner corpuscles and Pacinian corpuscles are examples of such receptors.

Tonic receptors produce impulses as long as the stimulus is present. Examples of tonic receptors are muscle spindles, free nerve endings, and end bulbs of Krause. The initial impulse is at a higher frequency than later impulses that occur during sustained stimulation.

Accommodation is the decline in generator potential and the reduction of frequency that occur with a prolonged stimulus or with frequently repeated stimuli. If some physical agents are used too often or for too long, the receptors may adapt to or accommodate the stimulus and reduce their impulses. The *accommodation* phenomenon can be observed with the use of superficial hot and cold agents, such as ice packs and hydrocollator packs.

As a stimulus becomes stronger, the number of receptors excited increases, and the frequency of the impulses increases. This provides more electrical activity at the spinal cord level, which may facilitate the effects of some physical agents.

Cognitive Influences

Pain perception and the response to a painful experience may be influenced by a variety of cognitive processes, including anxiety, attention, depression, past pain experiences, and cultural influences.[18] These individual aspects of pain expression are mediated by higher centers in the cortex in ways that are not clearly understood.[3] They may influence both the sensory discriminative and motivational affective dimensions of pain.

Many mental processes modulate the perception of pain through descending systems. Behavior modification, the excitement of the moment, happiness, positive feelings, focusing (directed attention toward specific stimuli), hypnosis, and suggestion may modulate pain perception. Past experiences, cultural background, personality, motivation to play, aggression, anger, and fear are all factors that could facilitate or inhibit pain perception. Strong central inhibition may mask severe injury for a period of time.[3] At such times, evaluation of the injury is quite difficult.

Patients with chronic pain may become very depressed and experience a loss of fitness. They tend to be less active and may have altered appetites and sleep habits. They have a decreased will to work and exercise and often develop a reduced sex drive. They may turn to self-abusive patterns of behavior. Tricyclic drugs are often used to inhibit serotonin depletion for the patient with chronic pain.

Just as pain may be inhibited by central modulation, it may also arise from central origins. Phobias, fear, depression, anger, grief, and hostility are all capable of producing pain in the absence of local pathologic processes. In addition, pain memory, which is associated with old injuries, may result in pain perception and pain response that are out of proportion to a new, often minor, injury. Substance abuse can also alter and confound the perception of pain. Substance abuse may cause the chronic pain patient to become more depressed or may lead to depression and psychosomatic pain.

Neural Transmission

Afferent nerve fibers transmit impulses from the sensory receptors toward the brain whereas *efferent* fibers, such as motor neurons, transmit impulses from the brain toward the periphery.[7] First-order or primary afferents transmit the impulses from the sensory receptor to the dorsal horn of the spinal cord (Figure 4-5). There are 4 different types of first-order neurons (Table 4-2). Aα and Aβ are large-diameter afferents that have a *high* (fast) conduction velocity, and Aδ and C fibers are small-diameter fibers with *low* (slow) conduction velocity.

Second-order afferent fibers carry sensory messages up the spinal cord to the brain. They are categorized as wide dynamic range or nociceptive specific. The wide dynamic range second-order afferents receive input from Aβ, Aδ, and C fibers. These second-order afferents serve relatively large, overlapping receptor fields. The nociceptive specific second-order afferents respond exclusively to noxious stimulation. They receive input only from Aδ and C fibers. These afferents serve smaller receptor fields that do not overlap. All of these neurons synapse with third-order neurons, which carry information to various brain centers where the input is integrated, interpreted, and acted upon.

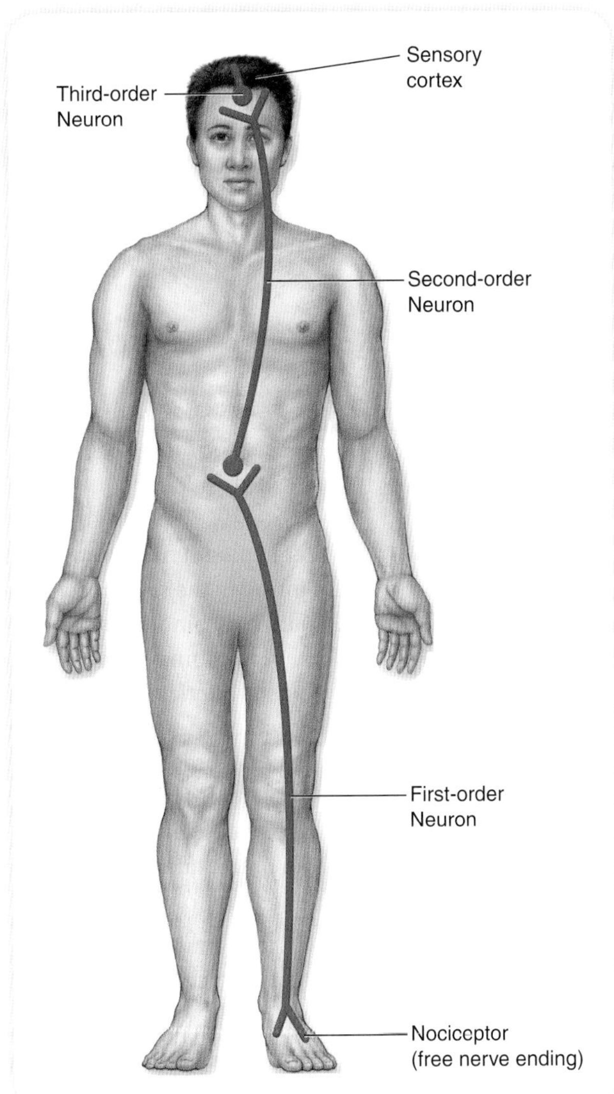

Figure 4-5 Neural afferent transmission

Sensory (pain) information from free nerve endings is transmitted to the sensory cortex in the brain via first-, second-, and third-order neurons. (Reproduced with permission from Prentice. *Therapeutic Modalities in Rehabilitation*. 4th ed. New York: McGraw-Hill; 2011.)

Facilitators and Inhibitors of Synaptic Transmission

For information to pass between neurons, a transmitter substance must be released from the end of one neuron terminal (presynaptic membrane), enter the synaptic cleft, and attach to a receptor site on the next neuron (postsynaptic membrane) (Figure 4-6). In the past, all the activity within the synapse was attributed to *neurotransmitters*, such as acetylcholine. The neurotransmitters, when released in sufficient quantities, are known to cause depolarization of the postsynaptic neuron. In the absence of the neurotransmitter, no depolarization occurs.

It is now apparent that several compounds that are not true neurotransmitters can facilitate or inhibit synaptic activity. *Serotonin, norepinephrine, enkephalin, β-endorphin, dynorphin,* and *substance* P are each important in the body's pain control mechanism.[19]

Enkephalin is an *endogenous* (made by the body) *opioid* that inhibits the depolarization of second-order nociceptive nerve fibers. It is released from *interneurons,*

Table 4-2 Classification of Afferent Neurons

Size	Type	Group	Subgroup	Diameter (μm)	Conduction Velocity (m/s)	Receptor	Stimulus
Large	Aα	I	1a	13 to 22	70 to 120	Proprioceptive mechanoreceptor	Muscle velocity and length change, muscle shortening of rapid speed
	Aα	I	1b			Proprioceptive mechanoreceptor Cutaneous receptors	Muscle length information from touch and pacinian corpuscles
	Aβ	II	Muscle	8 to 13	40 to 70		
	Aβ	II	Skin				
	Aδ	III	Muscle	1 to 4	5 to 15	75% mechanoreceptors and thermoreceptors	Touch, vibration, hair receptors Temperature change
Small	Aδ	III	Skin			25% nociceptors, mechanoreceptors, and thermoreceptors (hot and cold)	Noxious, mechanical, and temperature (>45°C, <10°C)
	C	IV	Muscle	0.2 to 1.0	0.2 to 2.0	50% mechanoreceptors and thermoreceptors	Touch and temperature

enkephalin neurons with short axons. The enkephalins are stored in nerve-ending vesicles found in the *substantia gelatinosa* and in several areas of the brain. When released, enkephalin may bind to presynaptic or postsynaptic membranes.[19]

Norepinephrine is released by the depolarization of some neurons and binds to the postsynaptic membranes. It is found in several areas of the nervous system, including a tract that descends from the pons, which inhibits synaptic transmission between first- and second-order nociceptive fibers, thus decreasing pain sensation.[20]

Other endogenous opioids may be active analgesic agents. These neuroactive peptides are released into the central nervous system and have an action similar to that of morphine, an opiate analgesic. There are specific opiate receptors located at strategic sites, called binding sites, to receive these compounds. β-Endorphin and dynorphin have potent analgesic effects. These are released within the central nervous system by mechanisms that are not fully understood at this time.

Nociception

A nociceptor is a peripheral pain receptor. Its cell body is in the dorsal root ganglion near the spinal cord. Pain is initiated when there is injury to a cell causing a release of 3 chemicals, *substance P*, *prostaglandin*, and *leukotrienes*, that sensitize the nociceptors in and around the area of injury by lowering their depolarization threshold. This is referred to as *primary hyperalgesia,* in which the nerve's threshold to noxious stimuli is lowered, thus enhancing the pain response.[5] Over a period of several hours, *secondary hyperalgesia* occurs, as chemicals spread throughout the surrounding tissues, increasing the size of the painful area and creating hypersensitivity.

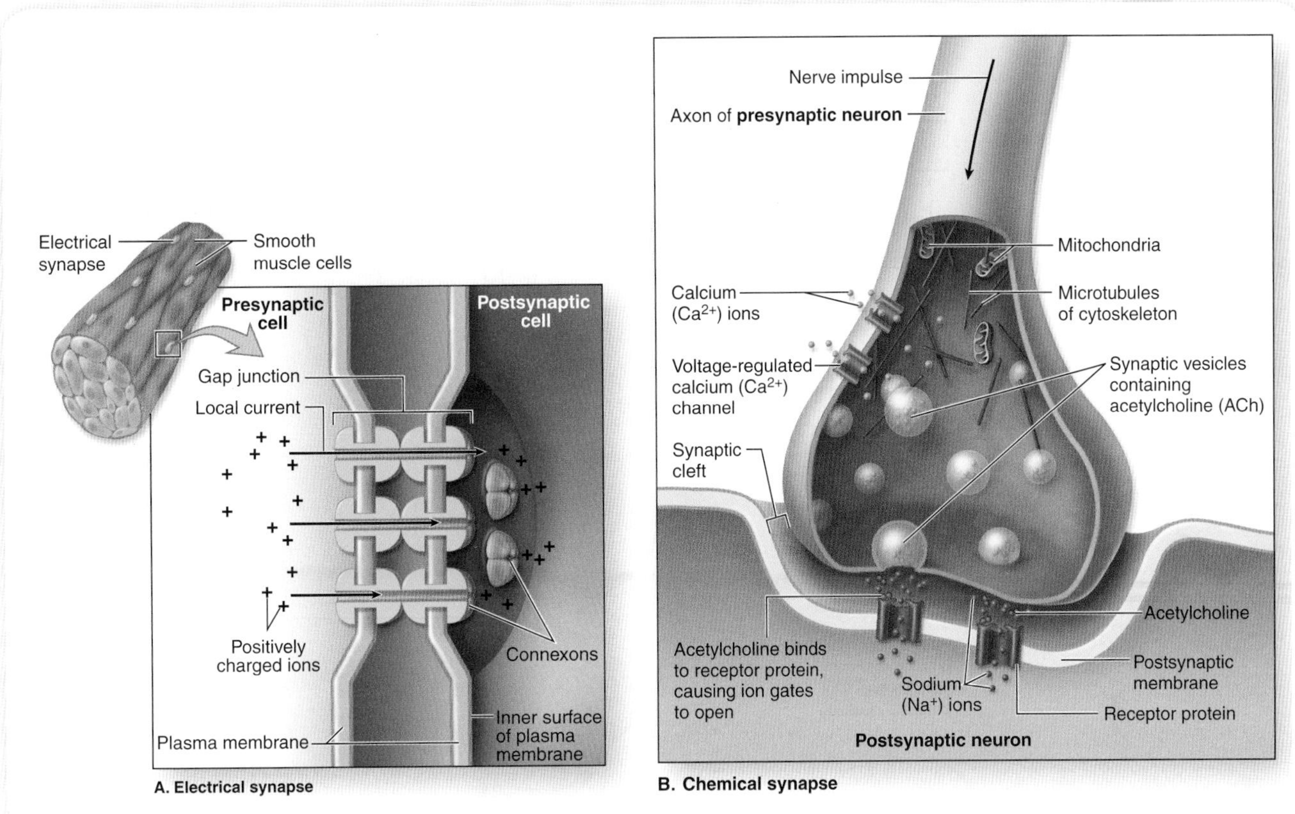

Figure 4-6 **Synaptic transmission**

(Reproduced with permission from McKinley M, O'Loughlin VD. *Human Anatomy.* 2nd ed. New York, NY: McGraw-Hill; 2008.)

Nociceptors initiate the electrical impulses along 2 afferent fibers toward the spinal cord. Aδ and C fibers transmit sensations of pain and temperature from peripheral nociceptors. The majority of the fibers are C fibers. Aδ fibers have larger diameters and faster conduction velocities. This difference results in 2 qualitatively different types of pain, termed *acute* and *chronic.*[19] Acute pain is rapidly transmitted over the larger, faster-conducting Aδ afferent neurons and originates from receptors located in the skin.[19] It is localized and short, lasting only as long as there is a stimulus, such as the initial pain of an unexpected pinprick. Chronic pain is transmitted by the C fiber afferent neurons and originates from both superficial skin tissue and deeper ligament and muscle tissue. This pain is an aching, throbbing, or burning sensation that is poorly localized and less specifically related to the stimulus. There is a delay in the perception of pain following injury, but the pain will continue long after the noxious stimulus is removed.[5]

The various types of afferent fibers follow different courses as they ascend toward the brain. Some Aδ and most C afferent neurons enter the spinal cord through the dorsal horn of the spinal cord and synapse in the substantia gelatinosa with a second-order neuron (Figure 4-7).[20] Most nociceptive second-order neurons ascend to higher centers along 1 of the 3 tracts—the lateral spinothalamic tract, the spinoreticular tract, or the spinoencephalic tract—with the remainder ascending along the spinocervical tract.[20] Approximately 80% of nociceptive second-order neurons ascend to higher centers along the lateral spinothalamic tract.[20] Approximately 90% of the second-order afferents terminate in the thalamus.[20] Third-order neurons project to the sensory cortex and numerous other centers in the central nervous system (see Figure 4-5).

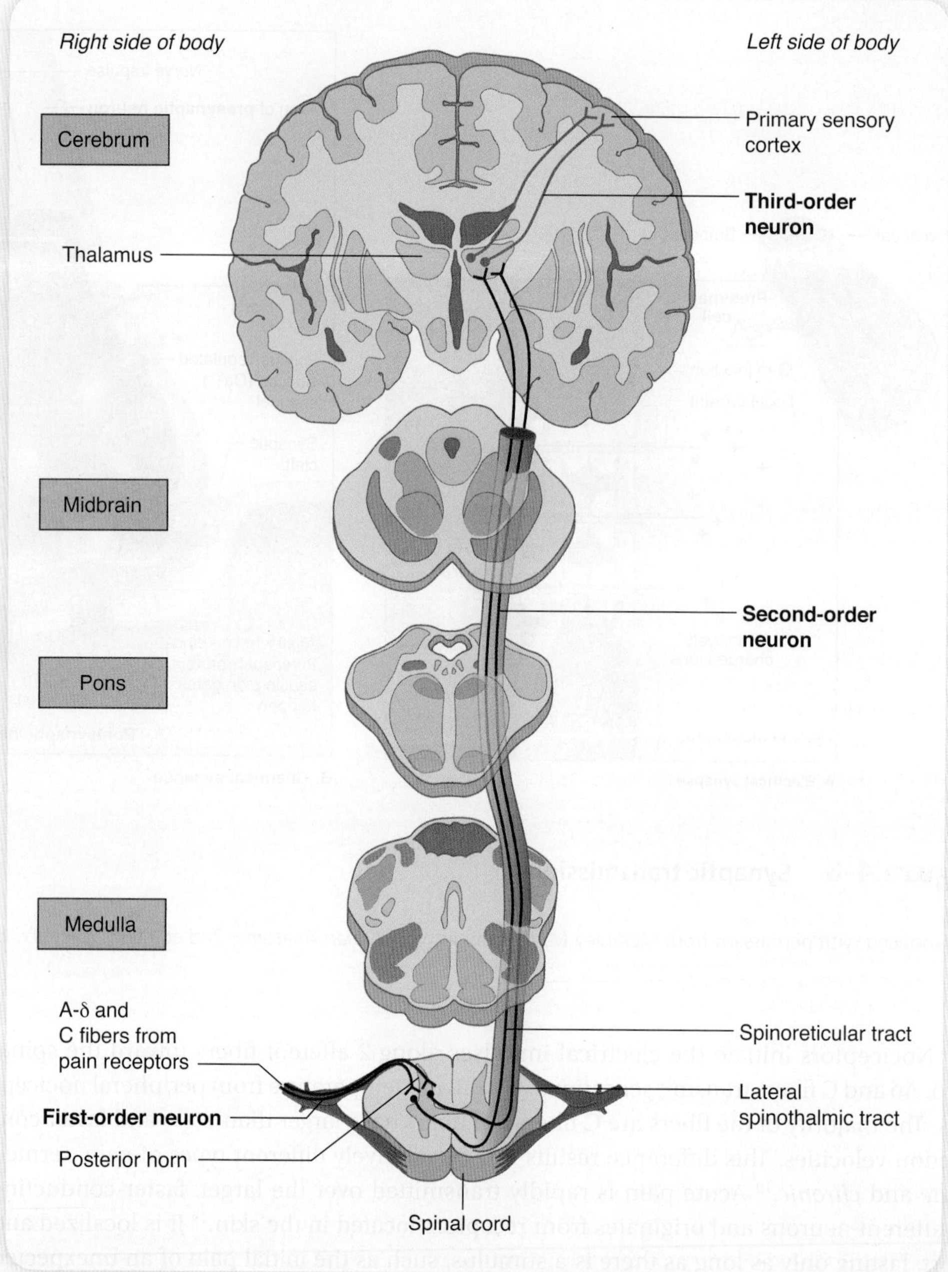

Figure 4-7

The ascending lateral spinothalamic and spinoreticular tract in the spinal cord carries pain information to the cortex. (Reproduced with permission from Prentice. *Therapeutic Modalities in Rehabilitation*. 4th ed. New York: McGraw-Hill; 2011.)

These projections allow us to perceive pain. They also permit the integration of past experiences and emotions that form our response to the pain experience. These connections are also believed to be parts of complex circuits that the clinician may stimulate to manage pain. Most analgesic physical agents are believed to slow or block the impulses ascending along the Aδ and C afferent neuron pathways through direct input into the dorsal horn or through descending mechanisms. These pathways are discussed in more detail in the following section.

Neurophysiologic Explanations of Pain Control

The neurophysiologic mechanisms of pain control through stimulation of cutaneous receptors have not been fully explained.[21] Much of what is known—and current theory—is the result of work involving electroacupuncture and transcutaneous electrical nerve stimulation. However, this information often provides an explanation for the analgesic response to other modalities, such as massage, analgesic balms, and moist heat.

The concepts of the analgesic response to cutaneous receptor stimulation presented here were first proposed by Melzack and Wall[22] and Castel.[23] These models essentially present 3 analgesic mechanisms:

1. Stimulation from ascending Aβ afferents results in blocking impulses at the spinal cord level of pain messages carried along Aδ and C afferent fibers (gate control).
2. Stimulation of descending pathways in the dorsolateral tract of the spinal cord by Aδ and C fiber afferent input results in a blocking of the impulses carried along the Aδ and C afferent fibers.
3. The stimulation of Aδ and C afferent fibers causes the release of endogenous opioids (β-endorphin), resulting in a prolonged activation of descending analgesic pathways.

These theories or models are not necessarily mutually exclusive. Recent evidence suggests that pain relief may result from combinations of dorsal horn and central nervous system activity.[24,25]

The Gate Control Theory of Pain

The gate control theory explains how a stimulus that activates only nonnociceptive nerves can inhibit pain (Figure 4-8).[22] Three peripheral nerve fibers are involved in this mechanism of pain control: Aδ fibers, which transmit noxious impulses associated with intense pain; C fibers, which carry noxious impulses associated with long-term or chronic pain; and Aβ fibers, which carry sensory information from cutaneous receptors but are nonnociceptive and do not transmit pain. Impulses ascending on these fibers stimulate the substantia gelatinosa as they enter the dorsal horn of the spinal cord. Essentially, the nonnociceptive Aβ fibers inhibit the effects of the Aδ and C pain fibers, effectively "closing a gate" to the transmission of their stimuli to the second-order interneurons. Thus, the only information that is transmitted on the second-order neurons through the ascending lateral spinothalamic tract to the cortex is the information from the Aβ fibers. The "pain message" carried along the smaller-diameter Aδ and C fibers is not transmitted to the second-order neurons and never reaches sensory centers.

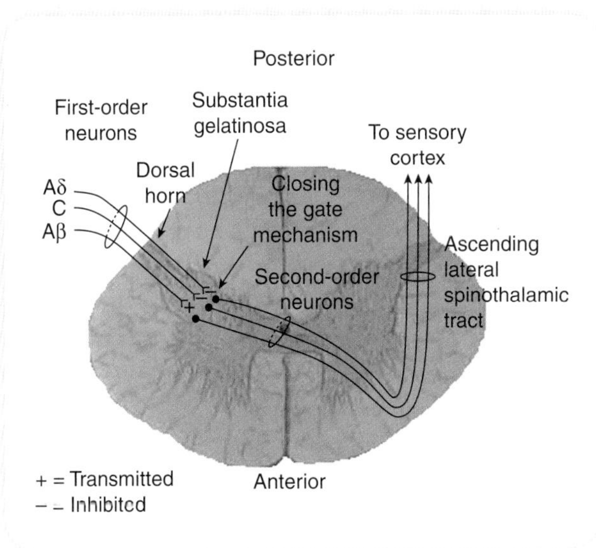

Figure 4-8 Gate control theory

Sensory information carried on Aβ fibers "closes the gate" to pain information carried on Aδ and C fibers in the substantia gelatinosa preventing transmission of pain to sensory centers in the cortex. (Reproduced with permission from Prentice. *Therapeutic Modalities in Rehabilitation*. 4th ed. New York: McGraw-Hill; 2011.)

The discovery and isolation of endogenous opioids in the 1970s led to new theories of pain relief. Castel introduced an endogenous opioid analog to the gate control theory.[23] This theory proposes that increased neural activity in Aβ primary afferent pathways triggers a release of enkephalin from *enkephalin interneurons* found in the dorsal horn.

These neuroactive amines inhibit synaptic transmission in the Aδ and C fiber afferent pathways. The end result, as in the gate control theory, is that the pain message is blocked before it reaches sensory levels.

The concept of sensory stimulation for pain relief, as proposed by the gate control theory, has empirical support. Rubbing a contusion, applying moist heat, or massaging sore muscles decreases the perception of pain. The analgesic response to these treatments is attributed to the increased stimulation of Aβ afferent fibers. A decrease in input along nociceptive Aδ and C afferents also results in pain relief. Cooling afferent fibers decreases the rate at which they conduct impulses. Thus, a 20-minute application of cold is effective in relieving pain because of the decrease in activity, rather than an increase in activity along afferent pathways.

Descending Pain Control

A second mechanism of pain control essentially expands the original gate control theory of pain control and involves input from higher centers in the brain through a descending system (Figure 4-9).[26] Emotions (such as anger, fear, stress), previous experiences, sensory perceptions, and other factors coming from the thalamus in the cerebrum stimulate the *periaqueductal gray* (PAG) matter of the midbrain. The pathway over which this pain reduction takes place is a dorsal lateral projection from cells in the PAG to an area in the medulla of the brainstem called the *raphe nucleus*. When the PAG fires, the raphe nucleus also fires. Serotonergic efferent pathways from the raphe nucleus project to the dorsal horn along the entire length of the spinal cord where they synapse with enkephalin interneurons located in the substantia gelitanosa.[27] The activation of enkephalin interneuron synapses by serotonin suppresses the release of the neurotransmitter substance P from Aδ and C fibers used by the sensory neurons involved in the perception of chronic and/or intense pain. Additionally, enkephalin is released into the synapse between the enkephalin interneuron and the second-order neuron that inhibits synaptic transmission of impulses from incoming Aδ and C fibers to the second-order afferent neurons that transmit the pain signal up the lateral spinothalamic tract to the thalamus (Figure 4-10).[28]

A second descending, noradrenergic pathway projecting from the pons to the dorsal horn has also been identified.[20] The significance of these parallel pathways is not fully understood. It is also not known if these noradrenergic fibers directly inhibit dorsal horn synapses or stimulate the enkephalin interneurons.

This model provides a physiologic explanation for the analgesic response to brief, intense stimulation. The analgesia following acupressure and the use of some transcutaneous electrical nerve stimulators (TENS), such as point stimulators, is attributed to this descending pain control mechanism.[38,39,40]

β-Endorphin and Dynorphin in Pain Control

There is evidence that stimulation of the small-diameter afferents (Aδ and C) can stimulate the release of other endogenous opioids called *endorphins*.[7,17,21,22,25,26,29] β-Endorphin and dynorphin are endogenous opioid peptide neurotransmitters found in the neurons of both the central and peripheral nervous system.[30] The mechanisms regulating the release of β-endorphin and dynorphin have not been fully elucidated. However, it is apparent that these endogenous substances play a role in the analgesic response to some forms of stimuli used in the treatment of patients in pain.

β-Endorphin is released into the blood from the anterior pituitary gland and into the brain and spinal cord from the hypothalamus.[30] In the anterior pituitary gland, it shares a prohormone with adrenocorticotropin. Thus, when β-endorphin is released, so, too, is

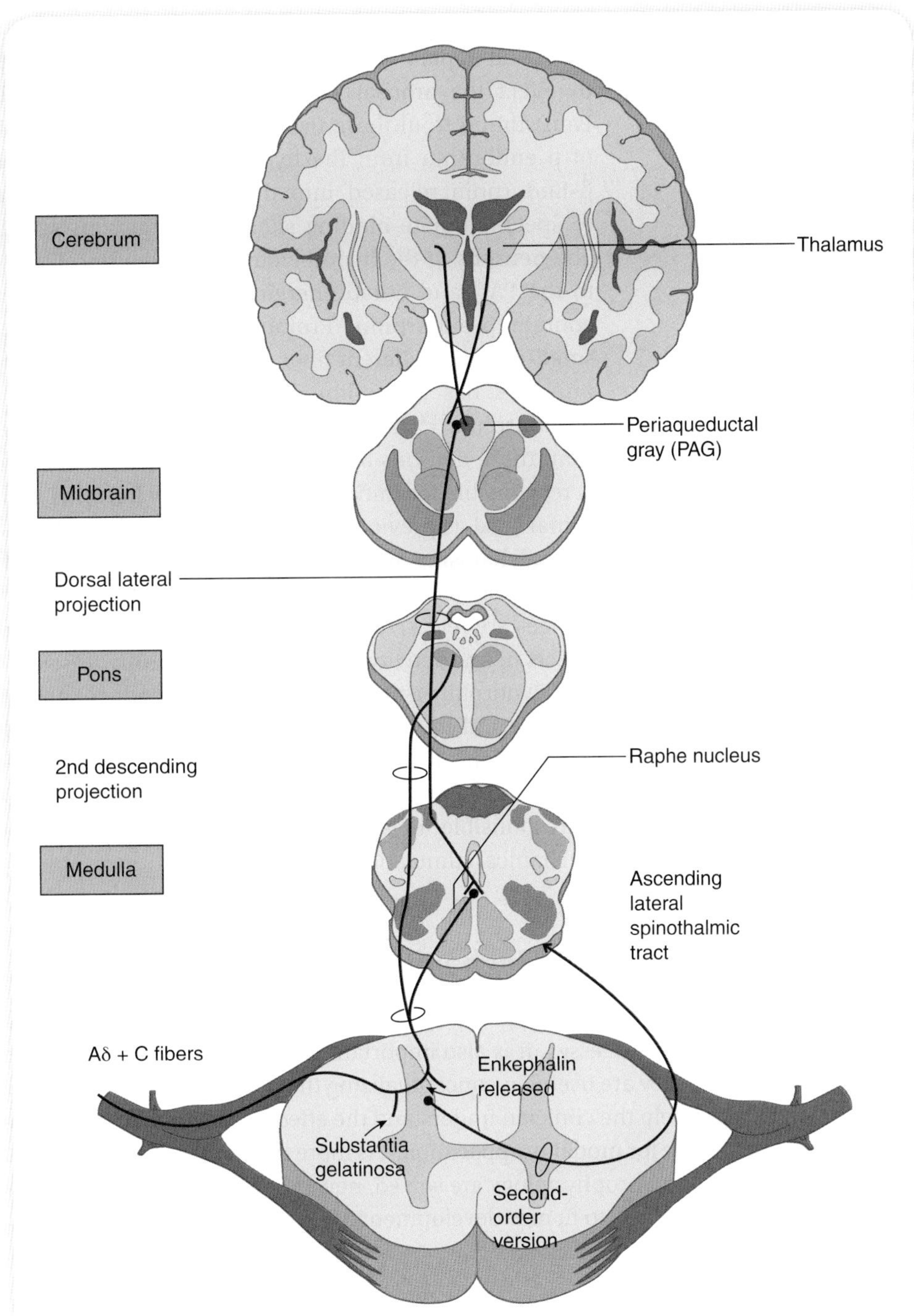

Figure 4-9 Descending pain control

Influence from the thalamus stimulates the periaqueductal gray, the raphe nucleus, and the pons to inhibit the transmission of pain impulses through the ascending tracts. (Reproduced with permission from Prentice. *Therapeutic Modalities in Rehabilitation*. 4th ed. New York: McGraw-Hill; 2011.)

adrenocorticotropin. β-Endorphin does not readily cross the blood-brain barrier,[19] and thus the anterior pituitary gland is not the sole source of β-endorphin.[31,41]

As stated previously, pain information is transmitted to the brainstem and thalamus primarily on 2 different pathways, the spinothalamic and spinoreticular tracts.

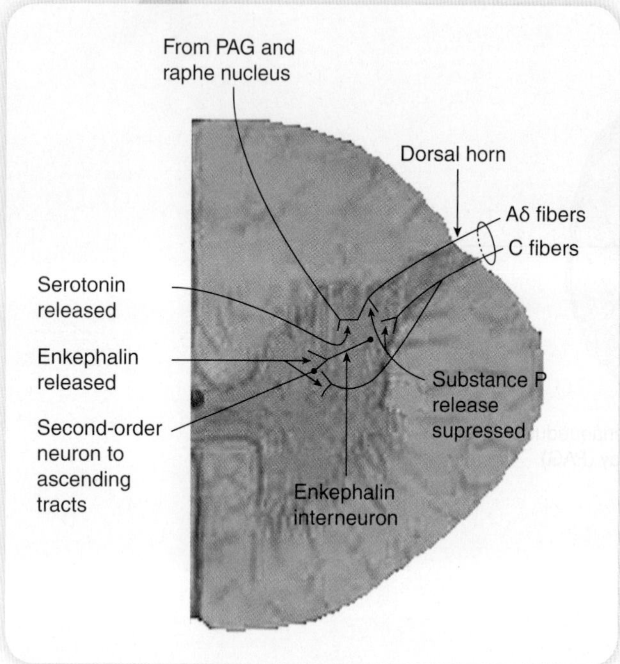

Figure 4-10

The enkephalin interneuron functions to inhibit transmission of pain between the Aδ and C fibers and the second-order neuron to the ascending tracts. (Reproduced with permission from Prentice. *Therapeutic Modalities in Rehabilitation.* 4th ed. New York: McGraw-Hill; 2011.)

Spinothalamic input is thought to effect the conscious sensation of pain, and the spinoreticular tract is thought to effect the arousal and emotional aspects of pain. Pain stimuli from these two tracts stimulate the release of β-endorphin from the hypothalamus (Figure 4-11). β-Endorphin released into the nervous system binds to specific opiate-binding sites in the nervous system. The neurons in the hypothalamus that send projections to the PAG and noradrenergic nuclei in the brainstem contain β-endorphin. Prolonged (20 to 40 minutes) small-diameter afferent fiber stimulation via electroacupuncture has been thought to trigger the release of β-endorphin.[21,41] It is likely that β-endorphin released from these neurons by stimulation of the hypothalamus is responsible for initiating the same mechanisms in the spinal cord as previously described with other descending mechanisms of pain control.[36,43] Once again, further research is needed to clarify where and how these substances are released and how the release of β-endorphin affects neural activity and pain perception.

Dynorphin, a more recently isolated endogenous opioid, is found in the PAG, rostroventral medulla, and the dorsal horn.[20] It has been demonstrated that dynorphin is released during electroacupuncture.[32] Dynorphin may be responsible for suppressing the response to noxious mechanical stimulation.[20]

Summary of Pain Control Mechanisms

The body's pain control mechanisms are probably not mutually exclusive. Rather, analgesia is the result of overlapping processes. It is also important to realize that the theories presented are only models. They are useful in conceptualizing the perception of pain and pain relief. These models will help the clinician understand the effects of therapeutic modalities and form a sound rationale for modality application.[8] As more research is conducted and as the mysteries of pain and neurophysiology are solved, new models will emerge. The clinician should adapt these models to fit new developments.

Pain Management

How should the clinician approach pain? First, the source of the pain must be identified. Unidentified pain may hide a serious disorder, and treatment of such pain may delay the appropriate treatment of the disorder.[33] Once a diagnosis has been made, the clinician must select the therapeutic technique that is most appropriate for each patient, based on their knowledge and professional judgment.[34]

The therapist may choose from a variety of useful pain control strategies including the following:

1. Encourage cognitive processes that influence pain perception, such as motivation, tension diversion, focusing, relaxation techniques, positive thinking, thought stopping, and self-control.

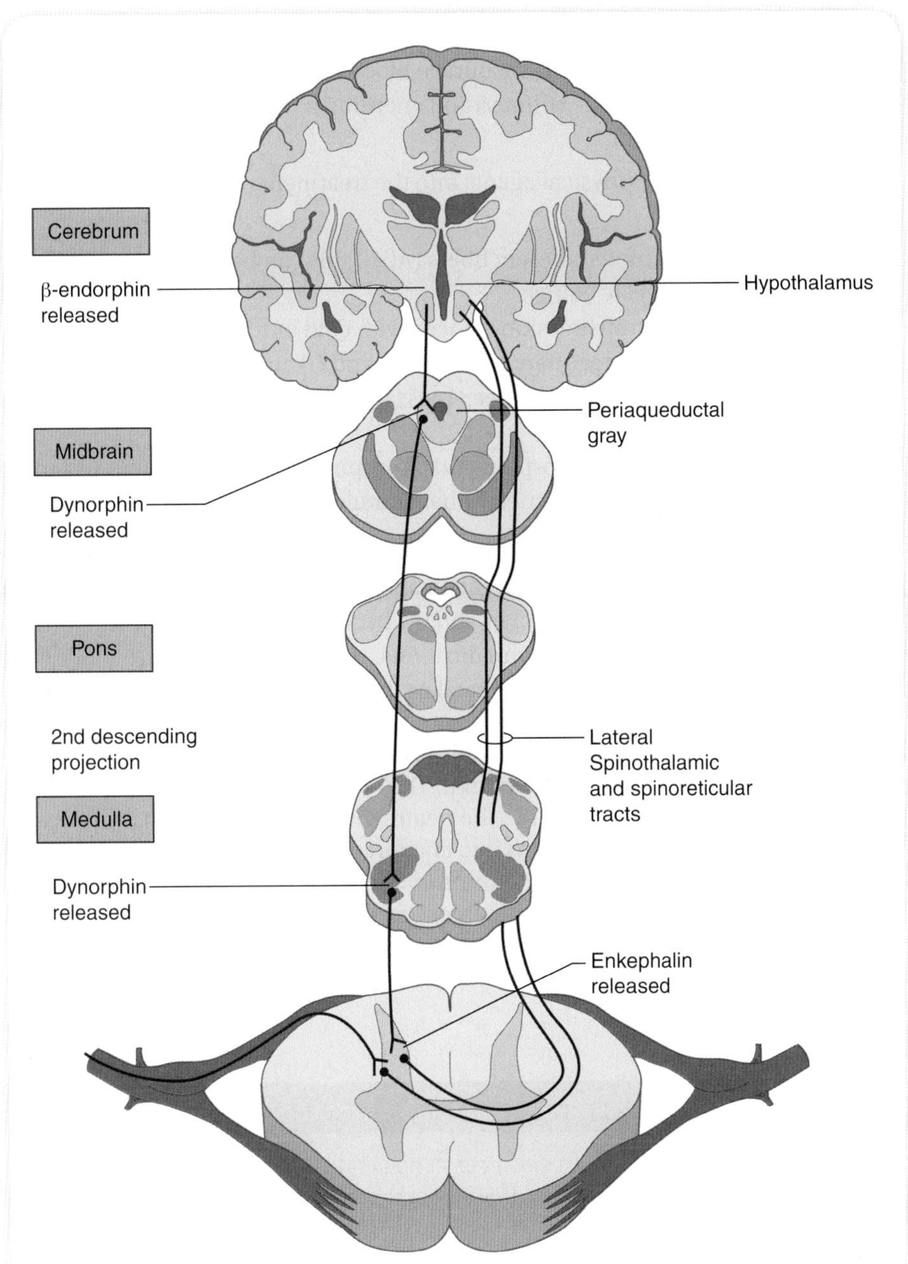

Figure 4-11

β-Endorphin released from the hypothalamus, and dynorphin released from the PAG and the medulla modulate. (Reproduced with permission from Prentice. *Therapeutic Modalities in Rehabilitation*. 4th ed. New York: McGraw-Hill; 2011.)

2. Minimize the tissue damage through the application of proper first aid and immobilization.
3. Maintain a line of communication with the patient. Let the patient know what to expect following an injury. Pain, swelling, dysfunction, and atrophy will occur following injury. The patient's anxiety over these events will increase the patient's perception of pain. Often, a patient who has been told what to expect by someone the patient trusts will be less anxious and suffer less pain.

4. Recognize that all pain, even psychosomatic pain, is very real to the patient.
5. Encourage supervised exercise to encourage blood flow, promote nutrition, increase metabolic activity, and reduce stiffness and guarding if the activity will not cause further harm to the patient.
6. Incorporate appropriate physical agents into the treatment plan. In general, physical agents can be used to:[42]
   a. stimulate large-diameter afferent fibers (Aβ)—this can be done with TENS, massage, and analgesic balms;
   b. decrease pain fiber transmission velocity with cold or ultrasound;
   c. stimulate small-diameter afferent fibers (Aδ and C) and descending pain control mechanisms with acupressure, deep massage, or TENS over acupuncture points or trigger points;
   d. stimulate a release of β-endorphin and dynorphin or other endogenous opioids through prolonged small-diameter fiber stimulation with TENS.[17]

The physician may choose to prescribe oral or injectable medications in the treatment of the patient. The most commonly used medications are classified as analgesics, antiinflammatory agents, or both. The clinician should become familiar with these drugs and note whether the patient is taking any medications. It is also important to work with the referring physician to assure that the patient takes the medications appropriately.

The clinician's approach to the patient has a great impact on the success of the treatment. The patient will not be convinced of the efficacy and importance of the treatment unless the clinician appears confident about it. The clinician must make the patient a participant rather than a passive spectator in the treatment and rehabilitation process.

The goal of most treatment programs is to encourage early pain-free exercise. The physical agents used to control pain do little to promote tissue healing. They should be used to relieve acute pain following injury or surgery or to control pain and other symptoms, such as swelling, to promote progressive exercise. The clinician should not lose sight of the effects of the physical agents or the importance of progressive exercise in restoring the patient's functional ability.

Clinical Pearl

Stimulating the trigger point with an electrical stimulating current will trigger the release of a chemical (β-endorphin) in the brain that will act to modulate pain.

Reducing the perception of pain is as much an art as a science. Selection of the appropriate pain control intervention, proper application, and marketing are all important and will continue to be so even as we increase our understanding of the neurophysiology of pain. There is still the need for a good empirical rationale for the use of a specific pain management approach. The clinician is encouraged to keep abreast of the neurophysiology of pain and the physiology of tissue healing to maintain a current scientific basis for managing the pain experienced by his or her patients.

Clinical Pearl

A modality should provide a significant amount of cutaneous input that would be transmitted to the spinal cord along Aβ fibers. The modalities of choice may include various types of heat or cold, electrical stimulating currents, counterirritants (analgesic balms), or massage.

SUMMARY

1. Pain is a response to a noxious stimulus that is subjectively modified by past experiences and expectations.
2. Pain is classified as either acute or chronic and can exhibit many different patterns.
3. Early reduction of pain in a treatment program will facilitate therapeutic exercise.
4. Stimulation of sensory receptors can modify the patient's perception of pain.
5. There are 3 mechanisms of pain control:
   - **a.** dorsal horn modulation due to the input from large-diameter afferents through a gate control system, the release of enkephalins, or both;
   - **b.** descending efferent fiber activation due to the effects of small-fiber afferent input on higher centers, including the thalamus, raphe nucleus, and PAG region;
   - **c.** the release of endogenous opioids including β-endorphin through prolonged small-diameter afferent stimulation.
6. Pain perception may be influenced by a variety of cognitive processes mediated by the higher brain centers.
7. The selection of a therapeutic modality for controlling pain should be based on current knowledge of neurophysiology and the psychology of pain.
8. The application of specific techniques for the control of pain should not occur until the diagnosis of the injury has been established.
9. The selection of a therapeutic intervention for managing pain should be based on establishing the primary cause of pain.

REFERENCES

1. Merskey H, Albe Fessard D, Bonica J. Pain terms: a list with definitions and notes on usage. *Pain.* 1979;6: 249-252.
2. Melzack R. Concepts of pain measurement. In: Melzack R, ed. *Pain Measurement and Assessment.* New York, NY: Raven Press; 1983.
3. Beissner K, Henderson C, Papaleontiou M. Physical therapists' use of cognitive-behavioral therapy for older adults with chronic pain: a nationwide survey. *Phys Ther.* 2009;89(5):456-469.
4. Deleo J. Basic science of pain. *J Bone Joint Surg Am.* 2006;88(2):58-62.
5. Kahanov L, Kato M, Kaminski T. Therapeutic modalities. Therapeutic effect of joint mobilization: joint mechanoreceptors and nociceptors. *Athl Ther Today.* 2007;12(4):28-31.
6. Fedorczyk J. The role of physical agents in modulating pain. *J Hand Ther.* 1997;10:110-121.
7. Willis W, Grossman R. *Medical Neurobiology.* 3rd ed. St. Louis, MO: Mosby; 1981.
8. Aronson P. Pain theories—a review for application in athletic training and therapy. *Athl Ther Today.* 2002;7(4):8-13.
9. Bowsher D. Central pain mechanisms. In: Wells P, Frampton V, Bowsher D, eds. *Pain Management in Physical Therapy.* Norwalk, CT: Appleton & Lange; 1994.
10. Fishman S, Ballantyne J. *Bonica's Management of Pain.* Philadelphia, PA: Lippincott Williams and Wilkins; 2009.
11. Previte J. *Human Physiology.* New York, NY: McGraw-Hill; 1983.
12. Merskey H, Bogduk N. *Classification of Chronic Pain. Definitions of Chronic Pain Syndromes and Definition of Pain Terms.* 2nd ed. Seattle, WA: International Association for the Study of Pain; 1994.
13. Addison R. Chronic pain syndrome. *Am J Med.* 1985;77:54-58.
14. Mattacola C, Perrin D, Gansneder B. A comparison of visual analog and graphic rating scales for assessing pain following delayed onset muscle soreness. *J Sport Rehabil.* 1997;6:38-46.
15. Huskisson E. Visual analogue scales. Pain measurement and assessment. In: Melzack R, ed. *Pain Measurement and Assessment.* NewYork, NY: Raven Press; 1983.
16. Margoles MS. The pain chart: spatial properties of pain. In: Melzack R, ed. *Pain Measurement and Assessment.* New York, NY: Raven Press; 1983.

17. Saluka K. *Mechanisms and Management of Pain for the Physical Therapist*. Seattle, WA: International Association for the Study of Pain; 2009.

18. Miyazaki T. Pain mechanisms and pain clinic. *Jpn J Clin Sports Med*. 2005;13(2):183.

19. Berne R. *Physiology*. St. Louis, MO: Elsevier Health Sciences; 2004.

20. Jessell T, Kelly D. Pain and analgesia. In: Kandel E, Schwartz J, Jessell T, eds. *Principles of Neural Science*. Norwalk, CT: Appleton & Lange; 1991.

21. Wolf S. Neurophysiologic mechanisms in pain modulation: relevance to TENS. In: Manheimer J, Lampe G, eds. *Sports Medicine Applications of TENS*. Philadelphia, PA: FA Davis; 1984.

22. Melzack R, Wall P. Pain mechanisms: a new theory. *Science*. 1965;150:971-979.

23. Castel J. *Pain Management: Acupuncture and Transcutaneous Electrical Nerve Stimulation Techniques*. Lake Bluff, IL: Pain Control Services; 1979.

24. Allen RJ. Physical agents used in the management of chronic pain by physical therapists. *Phys Med Rehabil Clin N Am*. 2006;17(2):315-345.

25. Clement-Jones V, McLaughlin L, Tomlin S. Increased beta-endorphin but not met-enkephalin levels in human cerebrospinal fluid after electroacupuncture for recurrent pain. *Lancet*. 1980;2:946-948.

26. Chapman C, Benedetti C. Analgesia following electrical stimulation: partial reversal by a narcotic antagonist. *Life Sci*. 1979;26:44-48.

27. Millan MJ. Descending control of pain. *Prog Neurobiol*. 2002;66:355-474.

28. Gebhart G. Descending modulation of pain. *Neurosci Biobehav Rev*. 2004;27:729-737.

29. Sjoland B, Eriksson M. Increased cerebrospinal fluid levels of endorphins after electro-acupuncture. *Acta Physiol Scand*. 1977;100:382-384.

30. Stein C. The control of pain in peripheral tissue by opioids. *N Engl J Med*. 1995;332:1685-1690.

31. Denegar G, Perrin D, Rogol A. Influence of transcutaneous electrical nerve stimulation on pain, range of motion and serum cortisol concentration in females with induced delayed onset muscle soreness. *J Orthop Sports Phys Ther*. 1989;11:101-103.

32. Ho W, Wen H. Opioid-like activity in the cerebrospinal fluid of pain athletes treated by electroacupuncture. *Neuropharmacology*. 1989;28:961-966.

33. Cohen S, Christo P, Moroz L. Pain management in trauma patients. *Am J Phys Med Rehabil*. 2004;83(2):142-161.

34. Curtis N. Understanding and managing pain. *Athl Ther Today*. 2002;7(4):32.

35. Bishop B. Pain: its physiology and rationale for management. *Phys Ther*. 1980;60:13-37.

36. Cheng R, Pomeranz B. Electroacupuncture analgesia could be mediated by at least two pain relieving mechanisms: endorphin and non-endorphin systems. *Life Sci*. 1979;25:1957-1962.

37. Dickerman J. The use of pain profiles in sports medicine practice. *Fam Pract Recertification*. 1992;14(3):35-44.

38. Mayer D, Price D, Rafii A. Antagonism of acupuncture analgesia in man by the narcotic antagonist naloxone. *Brain Res*. 1977;121:368-372.

39. Pomeranz B, Paley D. Brain opiates at work in acupuncture. *New Sci*. 1975;73:12-13.

40. Pomeranz B, Chiu D. Naloxone blockade of acupuncture analgesia: enkephalin implicated. *Life Sci*. 1976;19(10):1757-1762.

41. Pomeranz B, Paley D. Electro-acupuncture hypoalgesia is mediated by afferent impulses: an electrophysiological study in mice. *Exp Neurol*. 1979;66:398-402.

42. Salar G, Job I, Mingringo S. Effects of transcutaneous electrotherapy on CSF beta-endorphin content in athletes without pain problems. *Pain*. 1981;10:169-172.

43. Wen H, Ho W, Ling N. The influence of electroacupuncture on naloxone: induces morphine withdrawal: elevation of immunoassayable beta-endorphin activity in the brain but not in the blood. *Am J Chin Med*. 1979;7:237-240.

5

Impaired Posture and Function

Phil Page

OBJECTIVES

After completion of this chapter, the physical therapist should be able to do the following:

- Describe the interaction of posture and proprioception.
- Articulate the role of posture in functional movement.
- Relate alterations in posture to musculoskeletal pathology.
- Identify key components of a postural assessment.

Introduction and Background

Postural assessment is a mainstay in any evaluation of a patient or client with musculoskeletal pain. The late physical therapist Florence Kendall was a pioneer and clinical guru in postural assessment. Her classic textbook, *Muscle Testing and Function*, serves as the reference for many students and practicing therapists who assess posture. By her definition, posture is the composite alignment of all the joints in the body at any given movement in time.[25] Furthermore, Kendall[25] defined ideal posture as skeletal alignment with minimal stress and strain, conducive to maximal efficiency.

Taking a structural and biomechanical approach, Kendall focused on using a plumb line to identify asymmetries in posture through observations of skeletal alignment. She suggested that a plumb line enabled a therapist to see the postural deviations that occur with respect to the forces of gravity. This static view of the musculoskeletal system is very helpful in observing the relationship between anterior–posterior and medial–lateral force imbalances. For example, a forward head posture indicated by position of the head in front of the frontal plane bisecting the body would create extra work for the posterior spine and muscles to support the head.

Although Kendall's structural approach to postural assessment provides a biomechanical assessment of the musculoskeletal system, the late Vladimir Janda, MD, saw postural assessment as a functional impression of the status of the sensorimotor system. According to Janda, the sensorimotor system is 1 functional unit comprised of the afferent sensory system and the efferent motor system; 2 systems that cannot be considered to function independent of each other.[34] He noted that changes in muscle tension are the first response of the system to nociception. By combining static biomechanical assessment popularized by Kendall with his observation of muscle function, Janda was able to form an early observational description of the possible cause of the patient's musculoskeletal pain from a neurological perspective.[34]

Clinical Pearl

Postural assessment is often a first impression of the status of the sensorimotor system, and should subsequently lead the diagnostic pathway with regard to musculoskeletal dysfunction.

The Role of Proprioception in Posture

Proprioception is vital to maintaining postural alignment, both statically and dynamically. The afferent information from joint mechanoreceptors and muscular receptors provides valuable information needed to maintain postural reflexes and to facilitate normal posture and movement patterns. Dr. Janda proposed 3 key areas of proprioception in the body that provide strong influences on posture: the sole of the foot, sacroiliac joint, and cervical spine. The position of the foot influences posture,[14] while cutaneous and muscle spindle afferents influence upright posture and gait.[9,24,45] The sacroiliac joint[18,51] and cervical spine[1,31] joint capsules are rich in proprioceptors that serve to constantly provide information on joint alignment, which contributes to the maintenance of upright posture. Janda noted the importance of normalizing proprioception from these 3 key areas early in the rehabilitation process because of their role in posture and function.

"Postural stability," sometimes referred to as "balance," can be defined as the ability to maintain one's center of gravity within their base of support. Standing balance results from equilibrium of forces throughout the musculoskeletal system that results in an upright posture in relation to gravity. Postural stability can be further classified into static or dynamic postural stability. Static postures are observed with the body at rest, whereas dynamic postures are observed during movement.

From a structural perspective, faulty postures resulting from segments aligned outside the body's center of gravity may result in postural instability. For example, subjects with increased thoracic kyphosis demonstrate poor postural control[44]; however, inducing a forward head posture in otherwise young healthy subjects does not reduce postural stability.[41]

Postural stability can be considered a "window" into the function of the sensorimotor system. Proper proprioceptive input is critical to maintain postural stability via the somatosensory system.[43] Janda noted that the central nervous system is the primary mediator of chronic musculoskeletal pain.[19] For example, patients with chronic low back pain[39] or neck pain[38] demonstrate poor postural stability; therefore, posture and balance assessments can provide valuable clues to therapists treating patients with chronic musculoskeletal pain.

The Role of Posture in Function

Posture evolves in a predictable manner during the development of a baby, progressing from reflexive mechanisms to integrated mature postural strategies. Postural reflexes such as the asymmetrical tonic neck reflex, symmetrical tonic neck reflex, and the crossed extensor reflexes help provide reflexive movement patterns and alignment during early musculoskeletal development. Posture is highly influenced by neuroflexive mechanisms early in development; however, these mechanisms reduce their influence over time as they become more integrated during maturation. Other postural reflexes, such as righting reactions and automatic postural reactions, are eventually used to maintain upright posture for function, even in adults.

Normal, progressive, human development is essential for proper posture. As it matures, the musculoskeletal system requires appropriate stress and strain for normal development. Maturation of the central nervous system goes hand-in-hand with the development of the musculoskeletal system.[13] Without balanced and adequate forces experienced as a child, postural deviations and faults may present in the adult the musculoskeletal system. This is commonly seen in the posture of a person with a disability where central nervous system maturation has been impaired.

Posture differs between individuals and can change over time. Genetics obviously plays a role in human structure, providing natural variability of "normal" posture. This variability is observable within a population. Posture changes over time as a result of activity or aging. Kuo et al[26] found greater forward head posture (FHP) and increased thoracic kyphosis in healthy older adults, as compared to younger adults.

Athletes, particularly throwers, demonstrate different scapular and shoulder complex postures than nonathletic individuals. For example, overhead athletes exhibit increased scapular internal rotation and anterior tilt in their dominant shoulder as compared to the nondominant shoulder.[33,48] In addition, collegiate baseball players demonstrate different scapular position than high school players.[49] These postural adaptations appear to be a normal progression over sustained participation by these athletes.[40,48]

From a functional perspective, proper posture supports normal joint range of motion, helps place the limbs in appropriate positions for functional activity, and protects the musculoskeletal system from excessive force. For example, a "neutral" position of the lumbar spine and pelvis can help minimize stress on lumbar discs and facets while lifting a heavy object. Similarly, neutral alignment of the scapula is recommended because scapular orientation can influence glenohumeral congruency and may affect shoulder complex muscle activation.[35,47]

Postural alignment also helps explain the concept of "regional interdependence." Movement of one segment of the body may be affected by the positioning of another regional segment either proximally or distally. Some researchers report altered scapular muscle activation with upper extremity tasks in subjects with FHP,[37,47,53] while others[32] report normal shoulder kinematics in healthy subjects despite scapular position asymmetries.

Poor posture can impede range of motion in adjacent joints. For example, FHP is associated with reduced cervical range of motion.[8,11] Quek et al[36] reported that both increased thoracic kyphosis and FHP contribute to decreased cervical range of motion in older adults. Severe kyphotic postures reduce the subacromial space in the shoulder[17]; however, Bullock et al[5] found that an erect sitting posture increased shoulder flexion range of motion by an average of 9 degrees in patients with shoulder impingement. Thus, the role of posture in contribution to, as well as prevention and management of musculoskeletal injuries is an important consideration for clinicians.

The Role of Posture in Pathology

The human body was designed for homeostasis and structural/mechanical balance. All critical systems in the body can function automatically without conscious control. Previously mentioned reflexes, such as the crossed-extensor reflex, facilitate automatic and characteristic responses of the muscular system for protection in response to a painful stimulus. In fact, it is possible that some reflexes are components of longstanding chronic musculoskeletal pain syndromes. Autonomic responses such as "fight or flight" also have subconscious influence on the muscular system. Interestingly, the muscular system receives information from both the central nervous system and the peripheral nervous system, and therefore is influenced both by automatic and voluntary control. Based on these phenomena, Janda noted that muscles have characteristic and predictable responses to pain and pathology which can lead to characteristic postural changes which he described as the "upper crossed"[21] and "lower crossed"[20] muscle imbalance syndromes.

Prolonged muscle imbalance and poor posture can lead to structural changes in muscle. Borstad[3] found a link between pectoralis minor tightness and altered thoracic and scapular postures. Adaptive shortening occurs when muscle that is relatively shorted for a long period of time as a result of poor posture becomes structurally shorter; conversely, adaptive lengthening occurs when a muscle is elongated over a prolonged period of time.[25] Janda noted that both of these posture-related changes in muscle are closely associated with muscle imbalance and result in shifts of the muscle length–tension curve, thus reducing overall muscle strength throughout the full excursion of the muscle, and presenting clinically as "weak" muscles.[22]

Differences in muscular tension on opposite sides of joints can cause muscle imbalance. Muscle imbalances are often propagated by poor posture, creating a vicious cycle. This ultimately can lead to joint dysfunction caused by unbalanced joint stress and pathologic movement (Figure 5-1).

Muscular imbalance may lead to changes in joint orientation that are sometimes reflected in posture. Although muscle imbalance is often seen in arthritic joints, there is little evidence to suggest that muscle imbalance is causative of arthritis, because no prospective studies have been completed. Muscle imbalances are usually associated with postural deviations[19,25]; however, few, if any, prospective cohort studies have established a cause-and-effect relationship between posture and muscle imbalance.

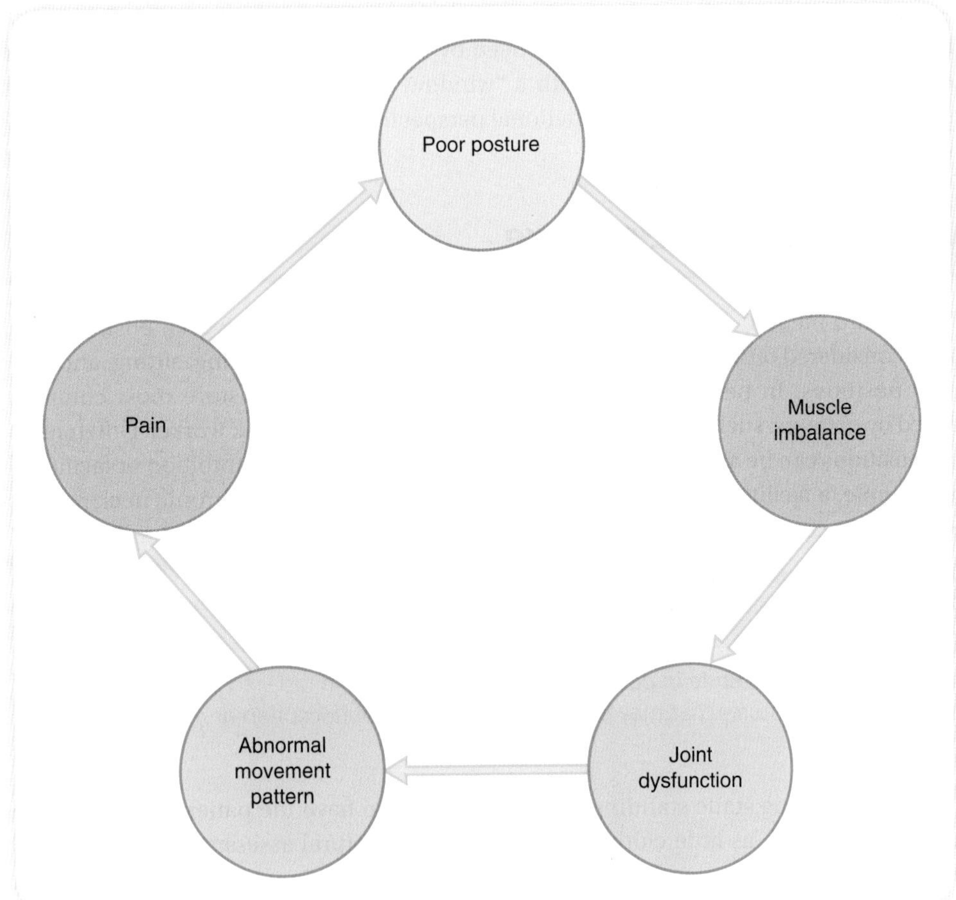

Figure 5-1 Vicious cycle of muscle imbalance

The ability to relate posture to pathology is limited by the ability to quantify postural deviations. Most literature evaluates sagittal plane posture, particularly in the cervicothoracic region by determining the presence of FHP. There appears to be a relationship between cervical pain syndromes and postural deficits. FHP is related to neck pain.[16,23,42,46,55] Lau et al[27] reported that greater thoracic kyphosis was associated with cervical dysfunction and disability.

In addition to neck pain, several researchers have demonstrated a relationship between FHP and headaches of various types.[11,12,16,52] Temporal-mandibular joint dysfunction,[28] craniofacial pain,[4] and even carpal tunnel syndrome[8] are associated with FHP. Despite many studies demonstrating the relationship of poor posture and cervical dysfunction, some researchers have found no such relationship.[10,50,56]

Low back pain is also related to postural deficits, typically involving increased lumbar lordosis or pelvic tilt.[2,6,7,54] Interestingly, Christie et al[7] noted FHP and increased thoracic kyphosis in patients with acute low back pain compared to those with chronic low back pain.

Although there appears to be a relationship between poor posture and spinal dysfunction, shoulder posture and shoulder pain are not as clearly related in the literature. Altered scapular posture, including downward rotation, protraction, and anterior tilt, can decrease the subacromial space.[29] While improving posture in shoulder impingement patients increased active shoulder range of motion,[5,30] postural deficits may not be observed clinically in all patients with shoulder dysfunction.[15]

In summarizing the literature, it is important to recognize that postural deficits may be related to pathology, as well as be influenced by both aging and activity. Postural assessment should provide the clinician with a "window" to the status of the musculoskeletal system from both a structural and functional perspective; however, it should never be diagnostic when used alone.

Assessment of Posture

The standard method of observing posture is in quiet standing. However, posture should not be considered *only* in standing, but also in prone, supine, side-lying, sitting, and quadruped positions. In particular, clinicians should consider the posture most commonly utilized by patients, such as the sitting posture used by an office/desk worker. Different postural positions can be associated with different patterns of muscle inhibition or facilitation. For example, a facilitated upper trapezius muscle in a patient with chronic neck pain may become less activated in a supine position.

Clinical Pearl

Consider assessing posture in positions other than standing in order to incorporate developmental postures that may offer a window into proprioception or motor control.

When assessing static standing posture, it is best to have the patient stand quietly in a well-lit room with as little clothing on as possible. Postural assessment should include both a structural ("alignment") viewpoint and a functional ("muscle tension") viewpoint. Structurally, observe the alignment of structures in relation to gravity; as previously mentioned, Kendall et al[25] advocate for the use of a plumb line for assessing static symmetry in standing posture with relation to a known, static reference system. Functionally, visual skills are the key to postural assessment, as the clinician observes symmetry, contour, and tone of muscles. Dr. Janda suggested that muscles with higher tone (tight muscles) present with a relatively convex appearance, whereas muscles with lower tone (weak muscles) present with a relative concave appearance.[34] Bilateral comparison is a valuable tool in assessing postural muscle function. Subtle visual clues can provide the clinician with valuable information on the presence of possible muscle imbalance syndromes.

Standing posture should be observed from the posterior, anterior, and lateral views; furthermore, the postural assessment should begin from the pelvis with each view and progress to the lower quarter, then the upper quarter, using a standard and reproducible system. If necessary, therapists should consider including a plumb-line structural assessment as described by Kendall. Table 5-1 lists 10 key points for each of the 3 views recommended to focus on muscle imbalances.

Posterior View

Static postural assessment in standing begins by observing the dorsal aspect. Begin by focusing on the position of the pelvis as most dysfunction is first evident at the pelvis. Elevation of the pelvis on one side indicates possible leg-length discrepancy or a tight quadratus lumborum on that side. Note the level of the posterior superior iliac spine for sacroiliac position. A lateral shift of the pelvis may indicate gluteal weakness with a Trendelenburg compensation, or the patient may be compensating for a lumbar disc pathology. Next, examine the gluteus maximus for atrophy, comparing both sides. Generally, smaller muscle size or atrophy specifically of the upper lateral quadrant of the gluteus maximus

Table 5-1 Thirty-Point Postural Assessment: 10 Points in 3 Views

	Posterior	Anterior	Lateral
1. Pelvis and core	Pelvis Gluteals Low Back	Pelvis Abdominals Ribs	Lumbar spine
2. Lower quarter	Adductors Hamstrings Gastroc-soleus Rearfoot	Quads (vastus medialis obliquus) Tibialis anterior Foot	Iliotibial band Knee (hyperextension) Midfoot
3. Upper quarter	Shoulder/deltoid Scapula Head	Face/head Neck Pectorals Arms and hands	Head Cervical lordosis Shoulder Thoracic/scapula Arms and hands

suggests gluteal atrophy and weakness (Figure 5-2). Above the gluteus maximus, examine the lumbar area for asymmetrical atrophy of the region of the multifidus or hypertrophy of the thoracolumbar extensor muscles. Gluteus maximus inhibition is often associated with ipsilateral thoracolumbar hypertrophy as a compensatory mechanism to stabilize the spine and extend the hip during gait.

Next, examine the lower quarter from the posterior view. The inner thigh should be a shallow S-shaped curve. If the upper part of the curve near the groin is more "bulky" creating a deeper S-shaped curve, the one-joint pectineus muscle may be tight (Figure 5-3).

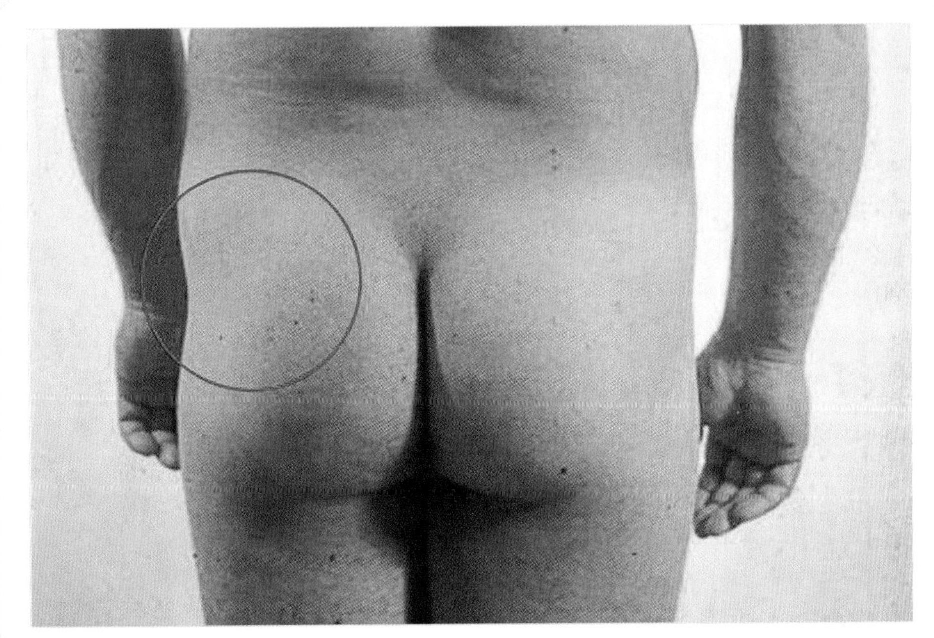

Figure 5-2 **Upper lateral gluteus maximus atrophy suggests gluteal atrophy and weakness**

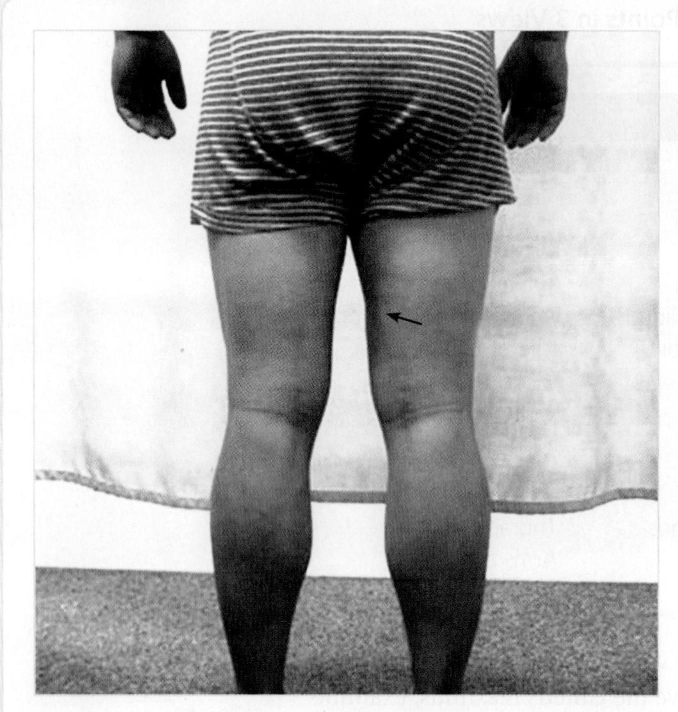

Figure 5-3 One-joint adductor tightness is indicated by a bulky right pectineus and deeper S-shaped curve

Conversely, if there is no S-shaped curve, the 2-joint gracilis muscle may be tight. Next, observe the lower two-thirds of the hamstring above the knee crease; hypertrophy in this region indicates tight hamstrings and is usually associated with weakness of the gluteus maximus on the same side. Moving distally, observe the gastroc-soleus region. If the soleus is tight, it will reduce the demarcation of the gastroc-soleus anastomosis, creating more of a straight line or even a bulge on the medial aspect (Figure 5-4). Finally, observe the rear foot for valgus or varus position, and for navicular drop in the case of over pronation, particularly noting any side-to-side differences.

Move to the upper quarter from a posterior view. Note asymmetrical elevation of the shoulder, indicating tightness of the upper trapezius and weakness of the lower trapezius. Patients with severe bilateral tightness of the upper trapezius may appear to have "gothic" shoulders, reflecting the style of windows on gothic churches. A small "notch" above the insertion of the levator scapula into the superior angle of the scapula indicates tightness. Next, observe the scapulae for their position in 3 dimensions, noting asymmetries

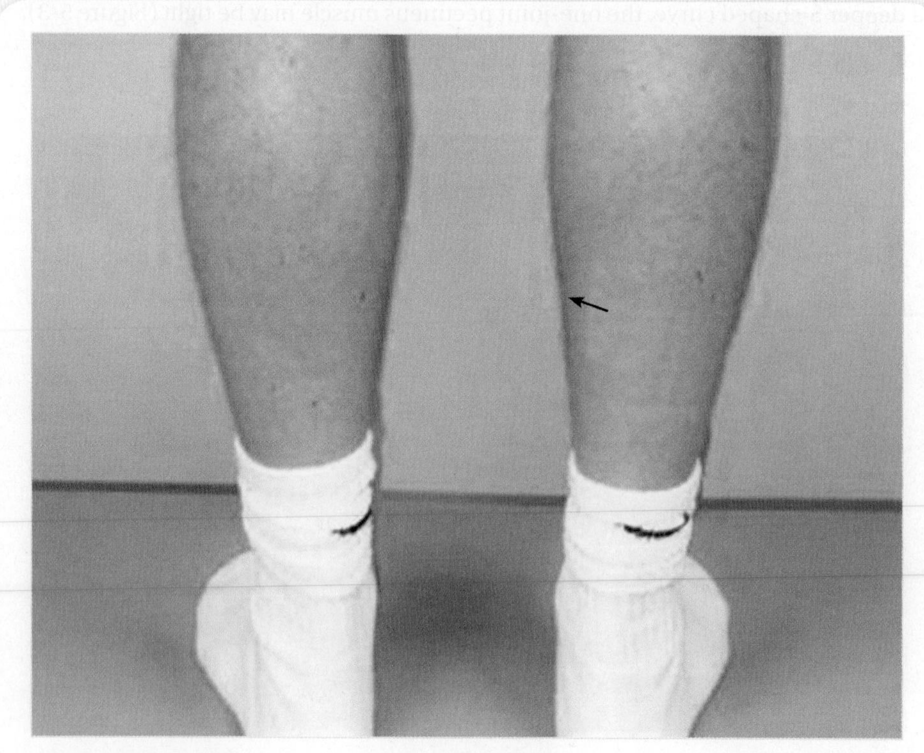

Figure 5-4 From the posterior, right soleus tightness is indicated by a straight line medial to gastrocnemius muscle belly and Achilles region

in protraction/retraction (internal/external rotation), upward/downward rotation, and anterior/posterior tilt. Note any alterations in scapular position or flattening of the mid-scapular area. Scapular position can provide clues about scapular muscle tightness and weakness. Finally, observe any rotation of the head to one side or the other; the trapezius on the side opposite the direction of cervical rotation may be tight.

Anterior View

As with the posterior view, begin the anterior view by observing the pelvis. Look for asymmetry of the anterior superior iliac spines that might indicate a pelvic rotation, upshift, or leg-length discrepancy. Next, examine the abdominal wall for a "lateral line" just to the side of the umbilicus, indicating hypertonicity of the oblique muscles (Figure 5-5).

Janda described a "pseudohernia" where the lateral abdominal wall slightly protrudes above the waist, indicating a possibly inhibited transverse abdominis muscle (see Figure 5-5). Observe the position of the inferior-lateral rib cage for symmetry and position. An inspiratory position of the ribs indicated by protrusion of the ribs signals possible diaphragm dysfunction (Figure 5-6).

Next, observe the vastus medialis muscle above the knee; bulkiness indicates repetitive knee hyperextension. Moving distally, examine the anterior tibialis for atrophy indicated by a groove rather than bulk over the anterior shin. Look for excessive activity of the tibialis anterior or extensor digitorum muscles in front of the ankle and foot, which may indicate a balance dysfunction. Finally, observe the general posture of the feet including pes planus or pes cavus, noting asymmetry.

At the head, examine the face for asymmetries. Janda noted that the middle of the forehead, bridge of the nose, mid-mouth, and mid-jaw should be in a straight line; deviations

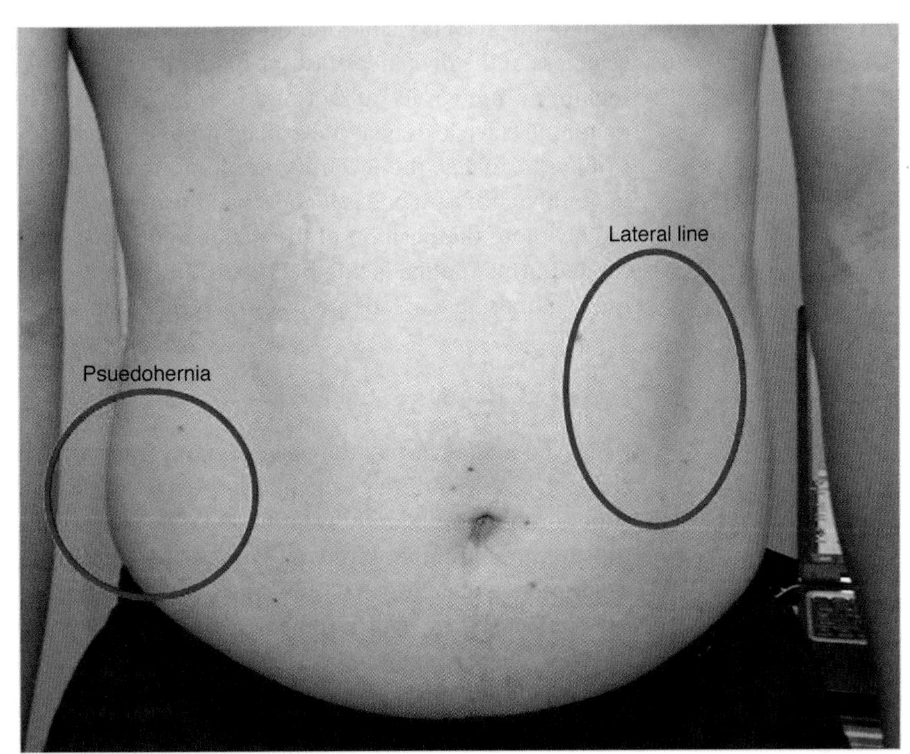

Figure 5-5 **Anterior view of abdomen reveals a lateral line (left oblique tightness) and pseudohernia (right transversus abdominis weakness)**

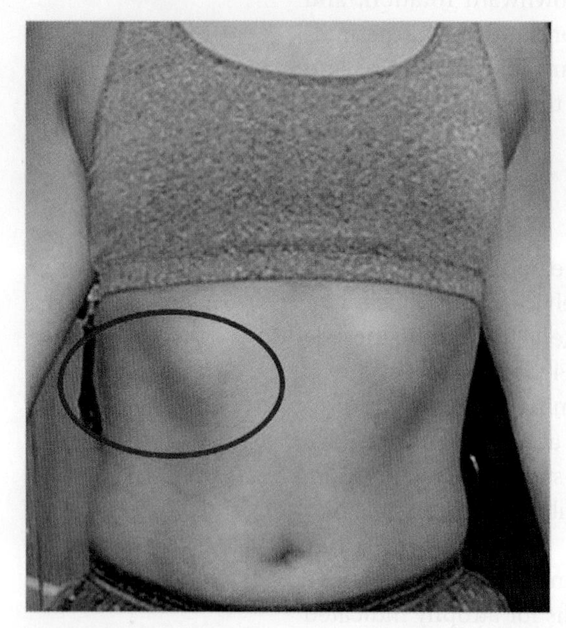

Figure 5-6 Protracted inferior ribs in an inspiratory position suggest diaphragm dysfunction

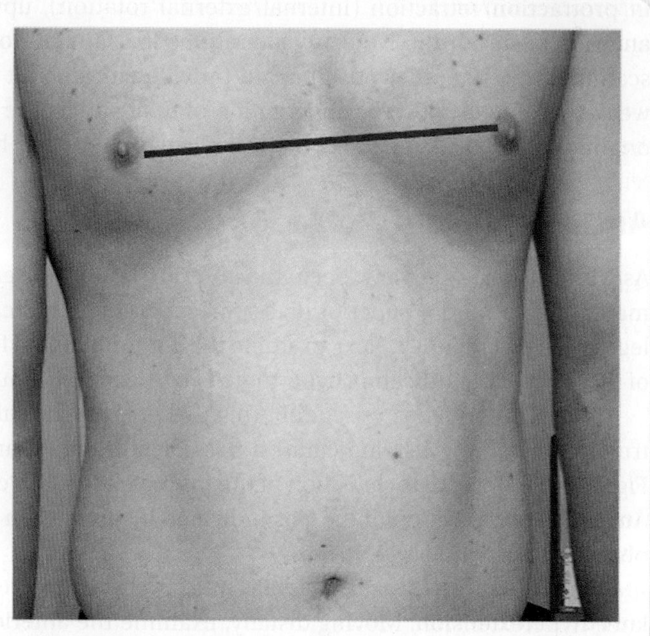

Figure 5-7 Higher nipple level indicates left pectoral tightness

indicate general body asymmetry and subsequent compensations. Note any rotation or abnormal positioning of the head, which may indicate cervical muscle tightness. Observe the anterior neck muscles, particularly noting the sternocleidomastoid (SCM) during respiration. If the clavicular attachment of the SCM is visible, it indicates hypertrophy. A groove medial to the SCM indicates weakness of the deep neck flexors. Next, observe the pectoral region; an increased bulk of one pectoralis muscle underneath the clavicle or near the axillary groove indicates hypertrophy. In males, the level of the nipple line may indicate pectoral tightness if one is higher than the other (Figure 5-7). Finally, note the position of the hands and arms. Internally rotated arms (palms facing backward) indicate tightness of the pectorals and/or latissimus dorsi (Figure 5-8).

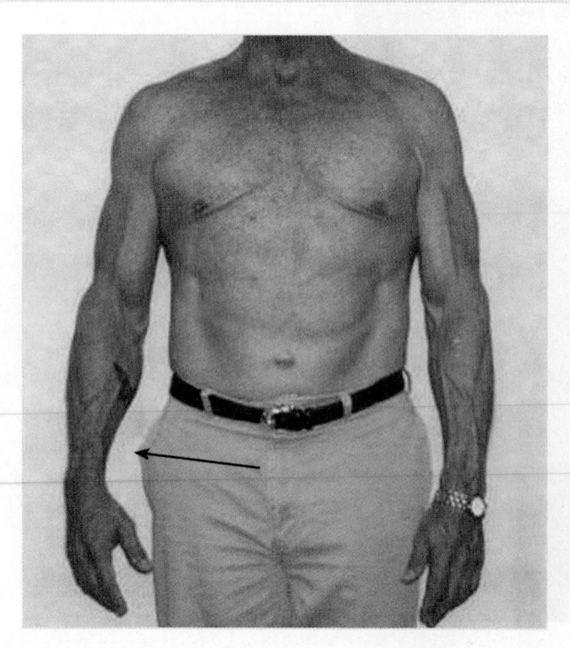

Figure 5-8 Hand rotation and slight abduction suggests right pectoral tightness

Lateral View

Begin the lateral view at the pelvis, noting anterior or posterior pelvic tilt, and pelvic inclination between the anterior superior iliac spines and posterior superior iliac spine. Note the amount of lumbar lordosis (hypo- or hyperlordosis) and the presence of a "swayback" posture. An increased lordosis may be caused by tight hip flexors, and a reduced lordosis may be related to tight hamstrings. Also note the position of the arms and hands. If the arms are positioned anterior to the middle of the body, the pectorals may be tight.

Next, examine the iliotibial tract for flatness or a groove, indicating tightness of the iliotibial band. Janda noted that women tend to present with flatness of the iliotibial band, whereas males present with a groove. Take note any hyperextension of the knee, which may indicate general hypermobility. Observe the foot again for the height of the arch and navicular bone, noting asymmetry.

Finally, observe the position of the head in relation to the body, noting a FHP, which is typically associated with tightness of the SCM and suboccipital extensor muscles. Note the amount of cervical lordosis both in the upper and lower segments; an increased upper cervical lordosis is generally associated with a FHP. Observe the position of the shoulder, more specifically, the relationship of the head of the humerus to the acromion. Normally, one-third of the width of the humerus should be anterior to the acromion; a more anterior humerus indicates tightness of the pectoralis major. Finally, note the amount of thoracic kyphosis, as well as the presence of any scapular malposition.

Conclusion

Good posture is essential for efficient movement and for protecting the musculoskeletal system from excessive stress and strain both at rest and during movement. Although there appears to be a link between posture and cervical dysfunction, the relationship between posture and other musculoskeletal pain remains less clear in the literature. Postural assessment gives clinicians the first clues to the structure and function in musculoskeletal pain. By combining a traditional "plumb-line" assessment of structure with a perspective of muscle balance through patterns of muscle tightness and weakness, clinicians can get a better picture of the status of the sensorimotor system and its influence on musculoskeletal pain syndromes.

SUMMARY

1. Proprioception plays an important role in posture and postural stability.
2. Standing posture gives an impression of the status of the sensorimotor system, but may not be diagnostic when used alone.
3. Consider assessing posture in several postures, including sitting and quadruped.
4. Muscle imbalance syndromes are often associated with postural deficits, but cause and effect between imbalance and posture has not been established.
5. Postural analysis including key points from different views can provide clues to muscle imbalances.

REFERENCES

1. Abrahams VC. The physiology of neck muscles; their role in head movement and maintenance of posture. *Can J Physiol Pharmacol.* 1977;55(3):332-338.
2. Barrey C, Jund J, Noseda O, Roussouly P. Sagittal balance of the pelvis-spine complex and lumbar degenerative diseases. A comparative study about 85 cases. *Eur Spine J.* 2007;16(9):1459-1467.
3. Borstad JD. Resting position variables at the shoulder: evidence to support a posture-impairment association. *Phys Ther.* 2006;86(4):549-557.
4. Braun BL. Postural differences between asymptomatic men and women and craniofacial pain patients. *Arch Phys Med Rehabil.* 1991;72(9):653-656.
5. Bullock MP, Foster NE, Wright CC. Shoulder impingement: the effect of sitting posture on shoulder pain and range of motion. *Man Ther.* 2005;10(1):28-37.
6. Chaleat-Valayer E, Mac-Thiong JM, Paquet J, Berthonnaud E, Siani F, Roussouly P. Sagittal spino-pelvic alignment in chronic low back pain. *Eur Spine J.* 2011;20 Suppl 5: 634-640.

7. Christie HJ, Kumar S, Warren SA. Postural aberrations in low back pain. *Arch Phys Med Rehabil.* 1995;76(3): 218-224.
8. De-la-Llave-Rincon AI, Fernandez-de-las-Penas C, Palacios-Cena D, Cleland JA. Increased forward head posture and restricted cervical range of motion in patients with carpal tunnel syndrome. *J Orthop Sports Phys Ther.* 2009;39(9):658-664.
9. Dorofeev IY, Avelev VD, Shcherbakova NA, Gerasimenko YP. The role of cutaneous afferents in controlling locomotion evoked by epidural stimulation of the spinal cord in decerebrate cats. *Neurosci Behav Physiol.* 2008;38(7):695-701.
10. Edmondston SJ, Chan HY, Ngai GC, et al. Postural neck pain: an investigation of habitual sitting posture, perception of "good" posture and cervicothoracic kinaesthesia. *Man Ther.* 2007;12(4):363-371.
11. Fernandez-de-Las-Penas C, Cuadrado ML, Pareja JA. Myofascial trigger points, neck mobility and forward head posture in unilateral migraine. *Cephalalgia.* 2006;26(9):1061-1070.
12. Fernandez-de-las-Penas C, Perez-de-Heredia M, Molero-Sanchez A, Miangolarra-Page JC. Performance of the craniocervical flexion test, forward head posture, and headache clinical parameters in patients with chronic tension-type headache: a pilot study. *J Orthop Sports Phys Ther.* 2007;37(2):33-39.
13. Frank C, Kobesova A, Kolar P. Dynamic neuromuscular stabilization and sports rehabilitation. *Int J Sports Phys Ther.* 2013;8(1):62-73.
14. Freeman MA, Wyke B. Articular reflexes at the ankle joint: an electromyographic study of normal and abnormal influences of ankle-joint mechanoreceptors upon reflex activity in the leg muscles. *Br J Surg.* 1967;54(12):990-1001.
15. Greenfield B, Catlin PA, Coats PW, Green E, McDonald JJ, North C. Posture in patients with shoulder overuse injuries and healthy individuals. *J Orthop Sports Phys Ther.* 1995;21(5):287-295.
16. Griegel-Morris P, Larson K, Mueller-Klaus K, Oatis CA. Incidence of common postural abnormalities in the cervical, shoulder, and thoracic regions and their association with pain in two age groups of healthy subjects. *Phys Ther.* 1992;72(6):425-431.
17. Gumina S, Di Giorgio G, Postacchini F, Postacchini R. Subacromial space in adult patients with thoracic hyperkyphosis and in healthy volunteers. *Chir Organi Mov.* 2008;91(2):93-96.
18. Hinoki M, Ushio N. Lumbomuscular proprioceptive reflexes in body equilibrium. *Acta Otolaryngol Suppl.* 1975;330:197-210.
19. Janda V. Muscles, central nervous regulation and back problems. In: Korr IM, ed. *Neurobiological Mechanisms in Manipulative Therapy.* New York, NY: Plenum Press; 1978:27-41.
20. Janda V. Muscles and motor control in low back pain: Assessment and management. In: Twomey LT, ed. *Physical Therapy of the Low Back.* New York, NY: Churchill Livingstone; 1987:253-278.
21. Janda V. Muscles and cervicogenic pain syndromes. In: Grand R, ed. *Physical Therapy of the Cervical and Thoracic Spine.* New York, NY: Churchill Livingstone; 1988:153-166.
22. Janda V. Muscle strength in relation to muscle length, pain, and muscle imbalance. In: Harms-Ringdahl K, ed. *Muscle Strength (International Perspectives in Physical Therapy).* Vol 8. Edinburgh, UK: Churchill Livingstone; 1993:83-91.
23. Kapreli E, Vourazanis E, Billis E, Oldham JA, Strimpakos N. Respiratory dysfunction in chronic neck pain patients. A pilot study. *Cephalalgia.* 2009;29(7):701-710.
24. Kavounoudias A, Roll R, Roll JP. Foot sole and ankle muscle inputs contribute jointly to human erect posture regulation. *J Physiol.* 2001;532(Pt 3):869-878.
25. Kendall FP, McCreary EK, Provance PG, Rodgers MM, Romani WA. *Muscles. Testing and Function with Posture and Pain.* 5th ed. Baltimore, MD: Lippincott Williams & Wilkins; 2005.
26. Kuo YL, Tully EA, Galea MP. Video analysis of sagittal spinal posture in healthy young and older adults. *J Manipulative Physiol Ther.* 2009;32(3):210-215.
27. Lau KT, Cheung KY, Chan KB, Chan MH, Lo KY, Chiu TT. Relationships between sagittal postures of thoracic and cervical spine, presence of neck pain, neck pain severity and disability. *Man Ther.* 2010;15(5):457-462.
28. Lee WY, Okeson JP, Lindroth J. The relationship between forward head posture and temporomandibular disorders. *J Orofac Pain.* 1995;9(2):161-167.
29. Lewis JS, Green A, Wright C. Subacromial impingement syndrome: the role of posture and muscle imbalance. *J Shoulder Elbow Surg.* 2005;14(4):385-392.
30. Lewis JS, Wright C, Green A. Subacromial impingement syndrome: the effect of changing posture on shoulder range of movement. *J Orthop Sports Phys Ther.* 2005;35(2):72-87.
31. McLain RF. Mechanoreceptor endings in human cervical facet joints. *Spine (Phila Pa 1976).* 1994;19(5):495-501.
32. Morais NV, Pascoal AG. Scapular positioning assessment: is side-to-side comparison clinically acceptable? *Man Ther.* 2013;18(1):46-53.
33. Oyama S, Myers JB, Wassinger CA, Daniel Ricci R, Lephart SM. Asymmetric resting scapular posture in healthy overhead athletes. *J Athl Train.* 2008;43(6):565-570.
34. Page P, Frank CC, Lardner R. *Assessment and Treatment of Muscle Imbalance: The Janda Approach.* Champaign, IL: Human Kinetics; 2010.
35. Picco BR, Fischer SL, Dickerson CR. Quantifying scapula orientation and its influence on maximal hand force capability and shoulder muscle activity. *Clin Biomech (Bristol, Avon).* 2010;25(1):29-36.
36. Quek J, Pua YH, Clark RA, Bryant AL. Effects of thoracic kyphosis and forward head posture on cervical range of motion in older adults. *Man Ther.* 2013;18(1): 65-71.

37. Raine S, Twomey LT. Head and shoulder posture variations in 160 asymptomatic women and men. *Arch Phys Med Rehabil.* 1997;78(11):1215-1223.
38. Ruhe A, Fejer R, Walker B. Altered postural sway in patients suffering from non-specific neck pain and whiplash associated disorder—a systematic review of the literature. *Chiropr Man Therap.* 2011;19(1):13.
39. Ruhe A, Fejer R, Walker B. Center of pressure excursion as a measure of balance performance in patients with non-specific low back pain compared to healthy controls: a systematic review of the literature. *Eur Spine J.* 2011;20(3):358-368.
40. Seitz AL, Reinold M, Schneider RA, Gill TJ, Thigpen C. Altered 3-dimensional scapular resting posture does not alter scapular motion in the throwing shoulder of healthy professional baseball pitchers. *J Sport Rehabil.* 2011 Nov 16. [Epub ahead of print]
41. Silva AG, Johnson MI. Does forward head posture affect postural control in human healthy volunteers? *Gait Posture.* 2012 Dec 6. [Epub ahead of print]
42. Silva AG, Punt TD, Sharples P, Vilas-Boas JP, Johnson MI. Head posture and neck pain of chronic nontraumatic origin: a comparison between patients and pain-free persons. *Arch Phys Med Rehabil.* 2009;90(4):669-674.
43. Simoneau GG, Ulbrecht JS, Derr JA, Cavanagh PR. Role of somatosensory input in the control of human posture. *Gait Posture.* 1995;3:115-122.
44. Sinaki M, Brey RH, Hughes CA, Larson DR, Kaufman KR. Balance disorder and increased risk of falls in osteoporosis and kyphosis: significance of kyphotic posture and muscle strength. *Osteoporos Int.* 2005;16(8):1004-1010.
45. Sorensen KL, Hollands MA, Patla E. The effects of human ankle muscle vibration on posture and balance during adaptive locomotion. *Exp Brain Res.* 2002;143(1):24-34.
46. Szeto GP, Straker L, Raine S. A field comparison of neck and shoulder postures in symptomatic and asymptomatic office workers. *Appl Ergon.* 2002;33(1):75-84.
47. Thigpen CA, Padua DA, Michener LA, et al. Head and shoulder posture affect scapular mechanics and muscle activity in overhead tasks. *J Electromyogr Kinesiol.* 2010;20(4):701-709.
48. Thomas SJ, Swanik KA, Swanik C, Huxel KC, Kelly JDt. Change in glenohumeral rotation and scapular position after competitive high school baseball. *J Sport Rehabil.* 2010;19(2):125-135.
49. Thomas SJ, Swanik KA, Swanik CB, Kelly JD. Internal rotation and scapular position differences: a comparison of collegiate and high school baseball players. *J Athl Train.* 2010;45(1):44-50.
50. Tsunoda D, Iizuka Y, Iizuka H, et al. Associations between neck and shoulder pain (called katakori in Japanese) and sagittal spinal alignment parameters among the general population. *J Orthop Sci.* 2013;18(2):216-219.
51. Vilensky JA, O'Connor BL, Fortin JD, et al. Histologic analysis of neural elements in the human sacroiliac joint. *Spine (Phila Pa 1976).* 2002;27(11):1202-1207.
52. Watson DH, Trott PH. Cervical headache: an investigation of natural head posture and upper cervical flexor muscle performance. *Cephalalgia.* 1993;13(4):272-284; discussion 232.
53. Weon JH, Oh JS, Cynn HS, Kim YW, Kwon OY, Yi CH. Influence of forward head posture on scapular upward rotators during isometric shoulder flexion. *J Bodyw Mov Ther.* 2010;14(4):367-374.
54. Yahia A, Jribi S, Ghroubi S, Elleuch M, Baklouti S, Habib Elleuch M. Evaluation of the posture and muscular strength of the trunk and inferior members of patients with chronic lumbar pain. *Joint Bone Spine.* 2011;78(3):291-297.
55. Yip CH, Chiu TT, Poon AT. The relationship between head posture and severity and disability of patients with neck pain. *Man Ther.* 2008;13(2):148-154.
56. Zito G, Jull G, Story I. Clinical tests of musculoskeletal dysfunction in the diagnosis of cervicogenic headache. *Man Ther.* 2006;11(2):118-129.

6

Impaired Muscle Performance

Regaining Muscular Strength, Endurance and Power

William E. Prentice

OBJECTIVES

After completion of this chapter, the physical therapist should be able to do the following:

- Define muscular strength, endurance, and power, and discuss their importance in a program of rehabilitation following injury.
- Discuss the anatomy and physiology of skeletal muscle.
- Discuss the physiology of strength development and factors that determine strength.
- Describe specific methods for improving muscular strength.
- Differentiate between muscle strength and muscle endurance.
- Discuss differences between males and females in terms of strength development.

Following all musculoskeletal injuries, there will be some degree of impairment in muscular strength and endurance. For the therapist supervising a rehabilitation program, regaining, and in many instances improving, levels of strength and endurance are critical for discharging and returning the patient to a functional level following injury.

By definition, *muscular strength* is the ability of a muscle to generate force against some resistance. Maintenance of at least a normal level of strength in a given muscle or muscle group is important for normal healthy living. Muscle weakness or imbalance can result in abnormal movement or gait and can impair normal functional movement. Resistance training plays a critical role in injury rehabilitation.

Muscular strength is closely associated with muscular endurance. *Muscular endurance* is the ability to perform repetitive muscular contractions against some resistance for an extended period of time. As we will see later, as muscular strength increases, there tends to be a corresponding increase in endurance. For the average person in the population, developing muscular endurance is likely more important than developing muscular strength because muscular endurance is probably more critical in carrying out the everyday activities of living. This statement becomes increasingly true with age.

Types of Skeletal Muscle Contraction

Skeletal muscle is capable of 3 different types of contraction: *isometric contraction, concentric contraction,* and *eccentric contraction.* An isometric contraction occurs when the muscle contracts to produce tension, but there is no change in muscle length. Considerable force can be generated against some immovable resistance even though no movement occurs. In a concentric contraction, the muscle shortens in length while tension increases to overcome or move some resistance. In an eccentric contraction, the resistance is greater than the muscular force being produced, and the muscle lengthens while producing tension. Concentric and eccentric contractions are considered dynamic movements.[56]

Recently, *econcentric contraction,* which combines both a controlled concentric and a concurrent eccentric contraction of the same muscle over 2 separate joints, has been introduced.[19,30] An econcentric contraction is possible only in muscles that cross at least 2 joints. An example of an econcentric contraction is a prone, open-kinetic-chain hamstring curl. The hamstrings contract concentrically to flex the knee, while the hip tends to flex eccentrically, lengthening the hamstring. Rehabilitation exercises have traditionally concentrated on strengthening isolated single-joint motions, despite the fact that the same muscle is functioning at a second joint simultaneously. Consequently, it has been recommended that the strengthening program includes exercises that strengthen the muscle in the manner in which it contracts functionally. Traditional strength-training programs have been designed to develop strength in individual muscles, in a single plane of motion. However, because all muscles function concentrically, eccentrically, and isometrically in 3 planes of motion, a strengthening program should be multiplanar, concentrating on all 3 types of contraction.[15]

Factors That Determine Levels of Muscular Strength, Endurance, and Power

Size of the Muscle

Muscular strength is proportional to the cross-sectional diameter of the muscle fibers. The greater the cross-sectional diameter or the bigger a particular muscle, the stronger it is, and thus the more force it is capable of generating. The size of a muscle tends to increase in cross-sectional diameter with resistance training. This increase in muscle size is referred to as *hypertrophy*.[42] A decrease in the size of a muscle is referred to as *atrophy*.

Number of Muscle Fibers

Strength is a function of the number and diameter of muscle fibers composing a given muscle. The number of fibers is an inherited characteristic; thus, a person with a large number of muscle fibers to begin with has the potential to hypertrophy to a much greater degree than does someone with relatively few fibers.[38]

Neuromuscular Efficiency

Strength is also directly related to the efficiency of the neuromuscular system and the function of the motor unit in producing muscular force.[46] Initial increases in strength during the first 8 to 10 weeks of a resistance training program can be attributed primarily to increased neuromuscular efficiency.[59] Resistance training will increase neuromuscular efficiency in 3 ways: there is an increase in the number of motor units being recruited, in the firing rate of each motor unit, and in the synchronization of motor unit firing.[7]

Biomechanical Considerations

Strength in a given muscle is determined not only by the physical properties of the muscle but also by biomechanical factors that dictate how much force can be generated through a system of levers to an external object.[31,38,63]

Position of Tendon Attachment

If we think of the elbow joint as one of these lever systems, we would have the biceps muscle producing flexion of this joint (Figure 6-1). The position of attachment of the biceps muscle on the forearm will largely determine how much force this muscle is capable of

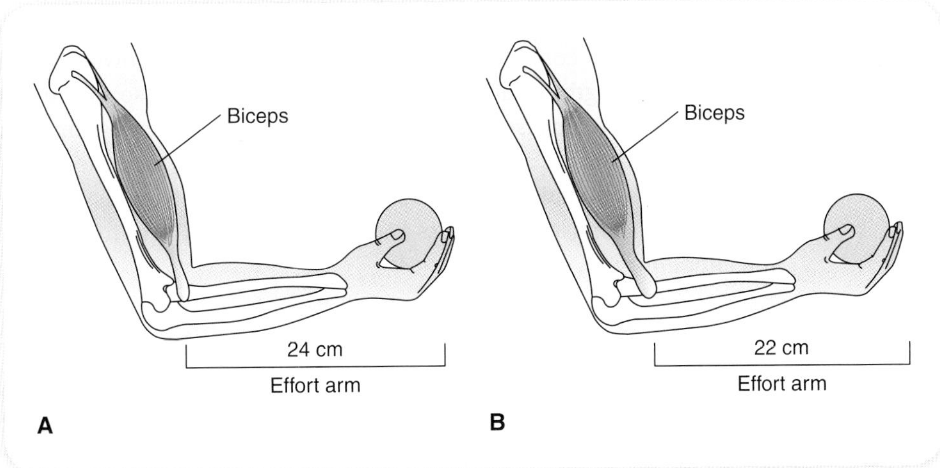

Figure 6-1

The position of attachment of the muscle tendon on the lever arm can affect the ability of that muscle to generate force. **B** should be able to generate greater force than **A** because the tendon attachment on the lever arm is closer to the resistance. (Reproduced with permission from Prentice. *Principles of Athletic Training*. 14th ed. New York: McGraw-Hill; 2011.)

generating. If there are 2 individuals, A and B, and A has a biceps attachment that is closer to the fulcrum (the elbow joint) than does B, then A must produce a greater effort with the biceps muscle to hold the weight at a right angle, because the length of the effort arm will be greater than that for B.

Length–Tension Relationship

The length of a muscle determines the tension that can be generated. By varying the length of a muscle, different tensions can be produced.[31] Figure 6-2 illustrates this length–tension relationship. At position *B* in the curve, the interaction of the crossbridges between the actin and myosin myofilaments within the sarcomere is at maximum. Setting a muscle at this particular length will produce the greatest amount of tension. At position *A*, the muscle is shortened, and at position *C*, the muscle is lengthened. In either case, the interaction between the actin and myosin myofilaments through the crossbridges is greatly reduced, thus the muscle is not capable of generating significant tension.

Clinical Pearl

The patient who is able to move more weight has a mechanical advantage. For example, if the tendinous insertion of the hamstrings is more distal, a longer lever arm is created and thus less force is required to move the same resistance.

Age

The ability to generate muscular force is also related to age.[4] Both men and women seem to be able to increase strength throughout puberty and adolescence, reaching a peak around 20 to 25 years of age, at which time, this ability begins to level off, and in some cases decline. After about age 25, a person generally loses an average of 1% of his or her maximal remaining strength each year. Thus, at age 65 years, a person would have only approximately 60% of the strength he or she had at age 25 years.[45] This loss in muscle strength is definitely related to individual levels of physical activity. People who are more active, or perhaps continue to strength-train, considerably decrease this tendency toward declining muscle strength. In addition to retarding this decrease in muscular strength, exercise can also have an effect in slowing the decrease in cardiorespiratory endurance and flexibility, as well as slowing increases in body fat. Thus, strength maintenance is important for all individuals regardless of age for achieving total wellness and good health as well as in rehabilitation after injury.[62]

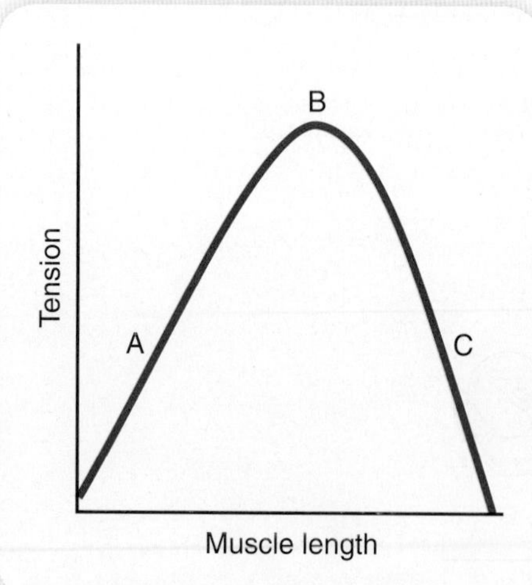

Figure 6-2 The length–tension relation of the muscle

Greatest tension is developed at point *B*, with less tension developed at points *A* and *C*. (Reproduced with permission from Prentice. *Principles of Athletic Training*. 14th ed. New York: McGraw-Hill; 2011.)

Overtraining

Overtraining in a physically active patient can have a negative effect on the development of muscular strength. Overtraining is an imbalance between exercise and recovery in which the training program exceeds the body's physiologic and psychological limits. Overtraining can result in psychological breakdown (staleness) or physiologic breakdown that can involve musculoskeletal injury, fatigue, or sickness. Engaging in proper and efficient resistance training, eating a proper diet, and getting appropriate rest can all minimize the potential negative effects of overtraining.

Fast-Twitch Versus Slow-Twitch Fibers

All fibers in a particular motor unit are either *slow-twitch fibers* or *fast-twitch fibers*. Each kind has distinctive metabolic and contractile capabilities.

Slow-Twitch Fibers

Slow-twitch fibers are also referred to as *type I* or *slow-oxidative* fibers. They are more resistant to fatigue than fast-twitch fibers; however, the time required to generate force is much greater in slow-twitch fibers.[29] Because they are relatively fatigue resistant, slow-twitch fibers are associated primarily with long-duration, aerobic-type activities.

Fast-Twitch Fibers

Fast-twitch fibers are capable of producing quick, forceful contractions but have a tendency to fatigue more rapidly than slow-twitch fibers. Fast-twitch fibers are useful in short-term, high-intensity activities, which mainly involve the anaerobic system. Fast-twitch fibers are capable of producing powerful contractions, whereas slow-twitch fibers produce a long-endurance force. There are 2 subdivisions of fast-twitch fibers. Although both types of fast-twitch fibers are capable of rapid contraction, *type IIa fibers* or *fast-oxidative-glycolytic* fibers are moderately resistant to fatigue, whereas *type IIb fibers* or *fast-glycolytic* fibers fatigue rapidly and are considered the "true" fast-twitch fibers. Recently, a third group of fast-twitch fibers, *type IIx,* has been identified in animal models. Type IIx fibers are fatigue resistant and are thought to have a maximum power capacity less than that of type IIb but greater than that of type IIa fibers.[45]

Ratio in Muscle

Within a particular muscle are both types of fibers, and the ratio of the 2 types in an individual muscle varies with each person.[32] Muscles whose primary function is to maintain posture against gravity require more endurance and have a higher percentage of slow-twitch fibers. Muscles that produce powerful, rapid, explosive strength movements tend to have a much higher percentage of fast-twitch fibers.

Because this ratio is genetically determined, it can play a large role in determining ability for a given sport activity. Sprinters and weightlifters, for example, have a large percentage of fast-twitch fibers in relation to slow-twitch fibers.[16] Conversely, marathon runners generally have a higher percentage of slow-twitch fibers. The question of whether fiber types can change as a result of training has to date not been conclusively resolved.[10] However, both types of fibers can improve their metabolic capabilities through specific strength and endurance training.[7]

The Physiology of Strength Development

Muscle Hypertrophy

There is no question that resistance training to improve muscular strength results in an increased size, or hypertrophy, of a muscle. What causes a muscle to hypertrophy? A number of theories have been proposed to explain this increase in muscle size.[22]

First, some evidence exists that there is an *increase in the number of muscle fibers (hyperplasia)* as a result of fibers splitting in response to training.[39] However, this research has been conducted in animals and should not be generalized to humans. It is generally accepted that the number of fibers is genetically determined and does not seem to increase with training.

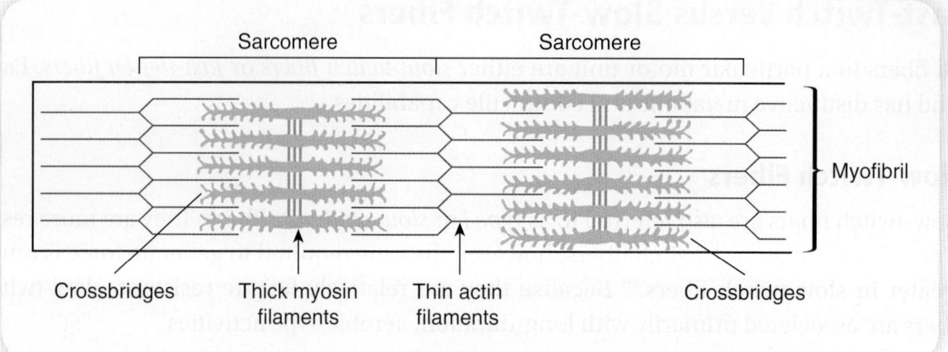

Figure 6-3

Muscles contract when an electrical impulse from the central nervous system causes the myofilaments in a muscle fiber to move closer together.

Second, it has been hypothesized that because the muscle is working harder in resistance training, more blood is required to supply that muscle with oxygen and other nutrients. Thus, it is thought that *the number of capillaries is increased.* This hypothesis is only partially correct; no *new* capillaries are formed during resistance training; however, a number of dormant capillaries might become filled with blood to meet this increased demand for blood supply.[45]

A third theory to explain this increase in muscle size seems the most credible. Muscle fibers are composed primarily of small protein filaments, called *myofilaments,* which are contractile elements in muscle. Myofilaments are small contractile elements of protein within the sarcomere. There are 2 distinct types of myofilaments: thin *actin* myofilaments and thicker *myosin* myofilaments. Fingerlike projections, or crossbridges, connect the actin and myosin myofilaments. When a muscle is stimulated to contract, the crossbridges pull the myofilaments closer together, thus shortening the muscle and producing movement at the joint that the muscle crosses (Figure 6-3).[5]

Clinical Pearl

Individuals have a particular ratio of fast-twitch to slow-twitch muscle fibers. Those who have a higher ratio of slow-twitch to fast-twitch fibers are better at endurance activities. Because this ratio is genetically determined, it would be surprising if someone who is good at endurance activity could also be good at sprint-type activities.

These *myofilaments increase in size and number* as a result of resistance training, causing the individual muscle fibers to increase in cross-sectional diameter.[58] This increase is particularly present in men, although women will also see some increase in muscle size. More research is needed to further clarify and determine the specific reasons for muscle hypertrophy.

Reversibility

If resistance training is discontinued or interrupted, the muscle will atrophy, decreasing in both strength and mass. Adaptations in skeletal muscle that occur in response to resistance training can begin to reverse in as little as 48 hours. It does appear that consistent exercise of a muscle is essential to prevent reversal of the hypertrophy that occurs from strength training.

Other Physiologic Adaptations to Resistance Exercise

In addition to muscle hypertrophy, there are a number of other physiologic adaptations to resistance training.[40] The strength of noncontractile structures, including tendons and ligaments, is increased. The mineral content of bone is increased, thus making the bone stronger and more resistant to fracture. Maximal oxygen uptake is improved when resistance training is of sufficient intensity to elicit heart rates at or above training levels. However, it must be emphasized that these increases are minimal and that if increased maximal oxygen uptake is the goal, aerobic exercise rather than resistance training is recommended. There is also an increase in several enzymes important in aerobic and anaerobic metabolism.[3,25,26] All of these adaptations contribute to strength and endurance.

Techniques of Resistance Training

There are a number of different techniques of resistance training for strength improvement, including functional strength training, isometric exercise, progressive resistive exercise, isokinetic training, circuit training, plyometric exercise, and calisthenic exercise. Regardless of the specific strength-training technique used, the therapist should integrate functional strengthening activities that involve multiplanar, eccentric, concentric, and isometric contractions.

The Overload Principle

Regardless of which of these techniques is used, one basic principle of reconditioning is extremely important. For a muscle to improve in strength, it must be forced to work at a higher level than it is accustomed to. In other words, the muscle must be overloaded. Without overload, the muscle will be able to maintain strength as long as training is continued against a resistance to which the muscle is accustomed, but no additional strength gains will be realized. This maintenance of existing levels of muscular strength may be more important in resistance programs that emphasize muscular endurance rather than strength gains. Many individuals can benefit more in terms of overall health by concentrating on improving muscular endurance. However, to most effectively build muscular strength, resistance training requires a consistent, increasing effort against progressively increasing resistance.[38,56]

Resistive exercise is based primarily on the principles of overload and progression. If these principles are applied, all of the following resistance training techniques will produce improvement of muscular strength over time.

In a rehabilitation setting, progressive overload is limited to some degree by the healing process. If the therapist takes an aggressive approach to rehabilitation, the rate of progression is perhaps best determined by the injured patient's response to a specific exercise. Exacerbation of pain or increased swelling should alert the therapist that their rate of progression is too aggressive.

Functional Strength Training

For many years, the strength-training techniques in conditioning or rehabilitation programs have focused on isolated, single-plane exercises used to elicit muscle hypertrophy in a specific muscle. These exercises have a very low neuromuscular demand because they are performed primarily with the rest of the body artificially stabilized on stable pieces of equipment.[15] The central nervous system controls the ability to integrate the proprioceptive function of a number of individual muscles that must act collectively to produce a specific movement pattern that occurs in three planes of motion. If the body is designed to move in 3 planes of motion, then isolated training does little to improve functional ability. When strength training using isolated, single-plane, artificially stabilized exercises, the entire body is not being prepared to deal with the imposed demands of normal daily activities (walking up or down stairs, getting groceries out of the trunk, etc).[26] Functional strength training provides a unique approach that may revolutionize the way the sports medicine community thinks about strength training. To understand the approach to functional strength training, the athletic trainer must understand the concept of the *kinetic chain* and must realize that the entire kinetic chain is an integrated functional unit. The kinetic chain is composed of not only muscle, tendons, fasciae, and ligaments but also the articular system and the neural system.

All of these systems function simultaneously as an integrated unit to allow for structural and functional efficiency. If any system within the kinetic chain is not working efficiently, the other systems are forced to adapt and compensate; this can lead to tissue overload, decreased performance, and predictable patterns of injury. The functional integration of the systems allows for optimal neuromuscular efficiency during functional activities.[15] During functional movements, some muscles contract concentrically (shorten) to produce movement, others contract eccentrically (lengthen) to allow movement to occur, and still other muscles contract isometrically to create a stable base on which the functional movement occurs. These functional movements occur in 3 planes. Functional strength training uses integrated exercises designed to improve functional movement patterns in terms of not only increased strength and improved neuromuscular control but also high levels of stabilization strength and dynamic flexibility.[15]

Unlike traditional strength-training techniques, which use barbells, dumbbells, or exercise machines and single-plane exercises day after day, a primary principle of functional strength training is to make use of training variations to force constant neural adaptations instead of concentrating solely on morphologic changes. Exercise variables that can be changed include the plane of motion, body position, base of support, upper- or lower-extremity symmetry, the type of balance modality, and the type of external resistance.[15] Table 6-1 lists these exercise training variables. Figure 6-4 provides examples of functional strengthening exercises.

Table 6-1 Exercise Training Variables

Plane of Motion	Body Position	Base of Support	Upper-Extremity Symmetry	Lower-Extremity Symmetry	Balance Modality	External Resistance
Sagittal	Supine	Exercise bench	2 arms	2 legs	Floor	Barbell
Frontal	Prone	Stability ball	Alternate arms	Staggered stance	Sport beam	Dumbbell
Transverse	Sidelying	Balance modality	1 arm	1 leg	½ foam roll	Cable machines
Combination	Sitting	Other	1 arm w/rotation	2-leg unstable	Airex pad	Tubing
	Kneeling			Staggered stance unstable	Dyna disc	Medicine balls
	Half kneeling			1-leg unstable	BOSU	Power balls
	Standing				Proprio shoes	Bodyblade
					Sand	Other

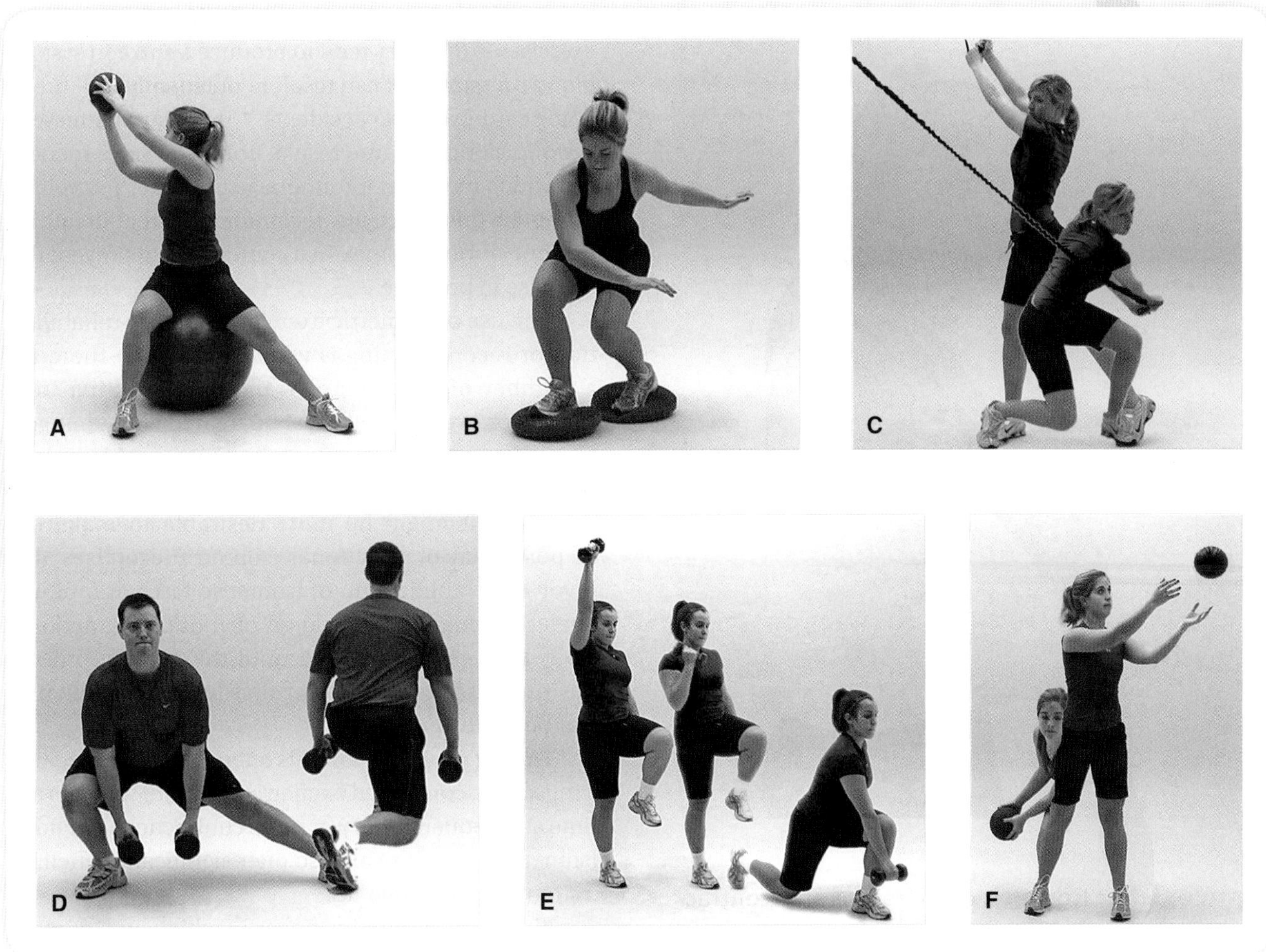

Figure 6-4 Functional strengthening exercises use simultaneous movements (concentric, eccentric, and isometric contractions) in 3 planes on either stable or unstable surfaces

A. Stability ball diagonal rotations with weighted ball. **B.** Tandem stance on DynaDisc with trunk rotation. **C.** Standing diagonal rotations with cable or tubing resistance. **D.** Weight-resisted multiplanar lunges. **E.** Front lunge balance to one-arm press. **F.** Weighted-ball double arm rotation toss from squat.

Isometric Exercise

An *isometric exercise* involves a muscle contraction in which the length of the muscle remains constant while tension develops toward a maximal force against an immovable resistance (Figure 6-5).[6] An isometric contraction provides stabilization strength that helps maintain normal length-tension and force-couple relationships that are critical for normal joint arthrokinematics. Isometric exercises are capable of increasing muscular strength.[54] However, strength gains are relatively specific, with as much as a 20% overflow to the joint angle at which training is performed. At other angles, the strength curve drops off dramatically because of a lack of motor activity at that angle. Thus, strength is increased at the specific angle of exertion, but there is no corresponding increase in strength at other positions in the range of motion.

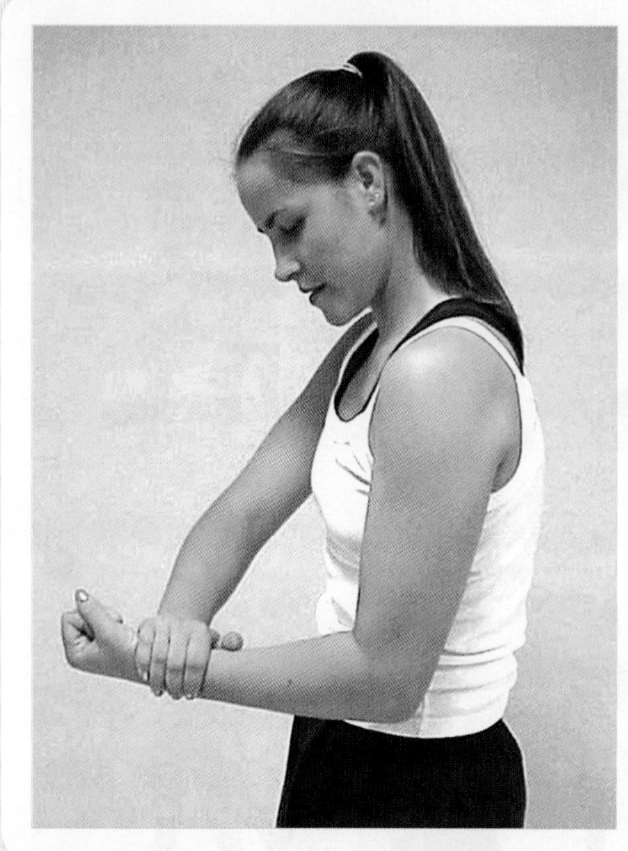

Figure 6-5 **Isometric exercises involve contraction against some immovable resistance**

Another major disadvantage of these isometric exercises is that they tend to produce a spike in systolic blood pressure that can result in potentially life-threatening cardiovascular accidents.[29] This sharp increase in systolic blood pressure results from a Valsalva maneuver, which increases intrathoracic pressure. To avoid or minimize this effect, it is recommended that breathing be done during the maximal contraction to prevent this increase in pressure.

The use of isometric exercises in injury rehabilitation or reconditioning is widely practiced. There are a number of conditions or ailments resulting from trauma or overuse that must be treated with strengthening exercises. Unfortunately, these problems can be exacerbated with full range-of-motion resistance exercises. It might be more desirable to make use of positional or functional isometric exercises that involve the application of isometric force at multiple angles throughout the range of motion. Functional isometrics should be used until the healing process has progressed to the point that full-range activities can be performed.

During rehabilitation, it is often recommended that a muscle be contracted isometrically for 10 seconds at a time at a frequency of 10 or more contractions per hour. Isometric exercises can also offer significant benefit in a strengthening program.[64]

There are certain instances in which an isometric contraction can greatly enhance a particular movement. For example, one of the exercises in power weight lifting is a squat. A squat is an exercise in which the weight is supported on the shoulders in a standing position. The knees are then flexed, and the weight is lowered to a three-quarter squat position, from which the lifter must stand completely straight once again.

It is not uncommon for there to be one particular angle in the range of motion at which smooth movement is difficult because of insufficient strength. This joint angle is referred to as a sticking point. A power lifter will typically use an isometric contraction against some immovable resistance to increase strength at this sticking point. If strength can be improved at this joint angle, then a smooth, coordinated power lift can be performed through a full range of movement.

Clinical Pearl

Doing isometric exercise will help a patient gain strength for that specific tension point.

Progressive Resistive Exercise

A second technique of resistance training is perhaps the most commonly used and most popular technique for improving muscular strength in a rehabilitation program. *Progressive resistive exercise* uses exercises that strengthen muscles through a contraction that overcomes some fixed resistance such as with dumbbells, barbells, various exercise machines, or resistive elastic tubing. Progressive resistive exercise uses isotonic, or *isodynamic,* contractions in which force is generated while the muscle is changing in length.

Concentric Versus Eccentric Contractions

Isotonic contractions can be concentric or eccentric. In performing a bicep curl, to lift the weight from the starting position the biceps muscle must contract and shorten in length. This shortening contraction is referred to as a concentric or positive contraction. If the biceps muscle does not remain contracted when the weight is being lowered, gravity would cause this weight to simply fall back to the starting position. Thus, to control the weight as it is being lowered, the biceps muscle must continue to contract while at the same time gradually lengthening. A contraction in which the muscle is lengthening while still applying force is called an eccentric or negative contraction.

It is possible to generate greater amounts of force against resistance with an eccentric contraction than with a concentric contraction, because eccentric contractions require a much lower level of motor unit activity to achieve a certain force than do concentric contractions. Because fewer motor units are firing to produce a specific force, additional motor units can be recruited to generate increased force. In addition, oxygen use is much lower during eccentric exercise than in comparable concentric exercise. Thus, eccentric contractions are less resistant to fatigue than concentric contractions. The mechanical efficiency of eccentric exercise can be several times higher than that of concentric exercise.[56]

Traditionally, progressive resistive exercise has concentrated primarily on the concentric component without paying much attention to the importance of the eccentric component.[56] The use of eccentric contractions, particularly in rehabilitation of various sport-related injuries, has received considerable emphasis in recent years. Eccentric contractions are critical for deceleration of limb motion, especially during high-velocity dynamic activities.[35] For example, a baseball pitcher relies on an eccentric contraction of the external rotators of the glenohumeral joint to decelerate the humerus, which might be internally rotating at speeds as high as 8000 degrees per second. Certainly, strength deficits or an inability of a muscle to tolerate these eccentric forces can predispose an injury. Thus, in a rehabilitation program, the therapist should incorporate eccentric strengthening exercises. Eccentric contractions are possible with all free weights, with the majority of isotonic exercise machines, and with most isokinetic devices. Eccentric contractions are used with plyometric exercise discussed in Chapter 10 and can also be incorporated with functional proprioceptive neuromuscular facilitation strengthening patterns discussed in Chapter 12.

In progressive resistive exercise, it is essential to incorporate both concentric and eccentric contractions.[33] Research has clearly demonstrated that the muscle should be overloaded and fatigued both concentrically and eccentrically for the greatest strength improvement to occur.[4,22,45] When training specifically for the development of muscular strength, the concentric portion of the exercise should require 1 to 2 seconds, while the eccentric portion of the lift should require 2 to 4 seconds. The ratio of the concentric component to the eccentric component should be approximately 1:2. Physiologically, the muscle will fatigue much more rapidly concentrically than eccentrically.

Free Weights Versus Exercise Machines

Various types of exercise equipment can be used with progressive resistive exercise, including free weights (barbells and dumbbells) and exercise machines such as Cybex, Universal, Paramount, Tough Stuff, Icarian Fitness, King Fitness, Body Solid, Pro-Elite, Life Fitness,

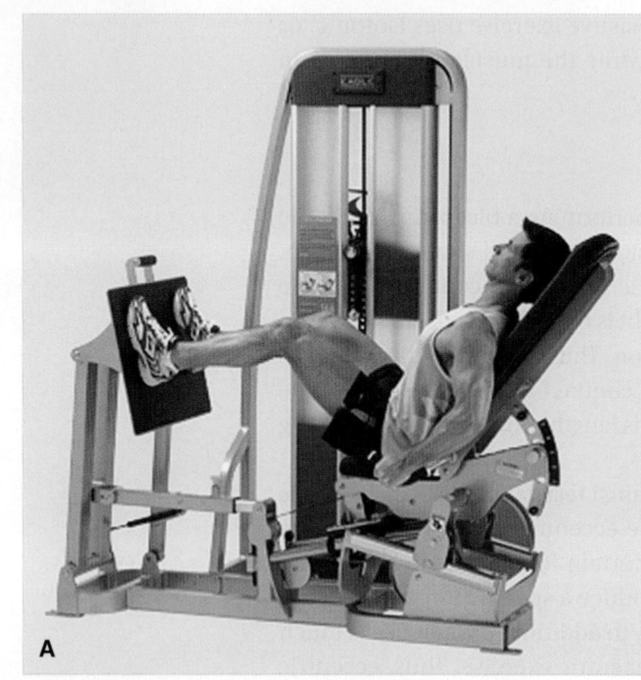

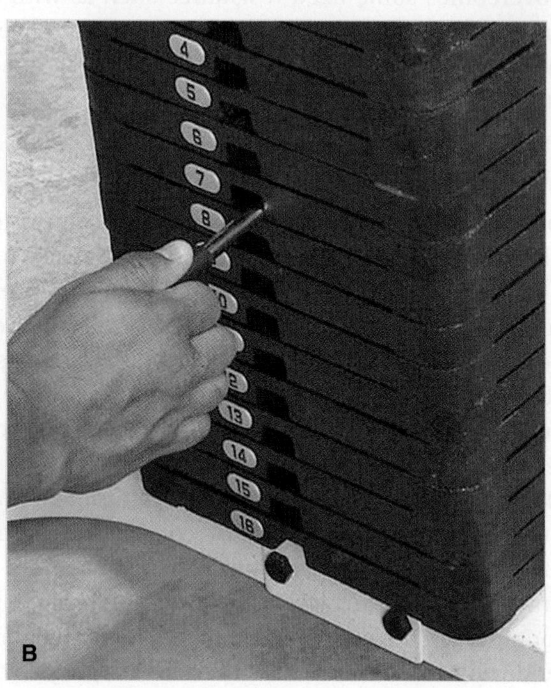

Figure 6-6 Isotonic equipment

A. Most exercise machines are isotonic. **B.** Resistance can be easily changed by changing the key in the stack of weights.

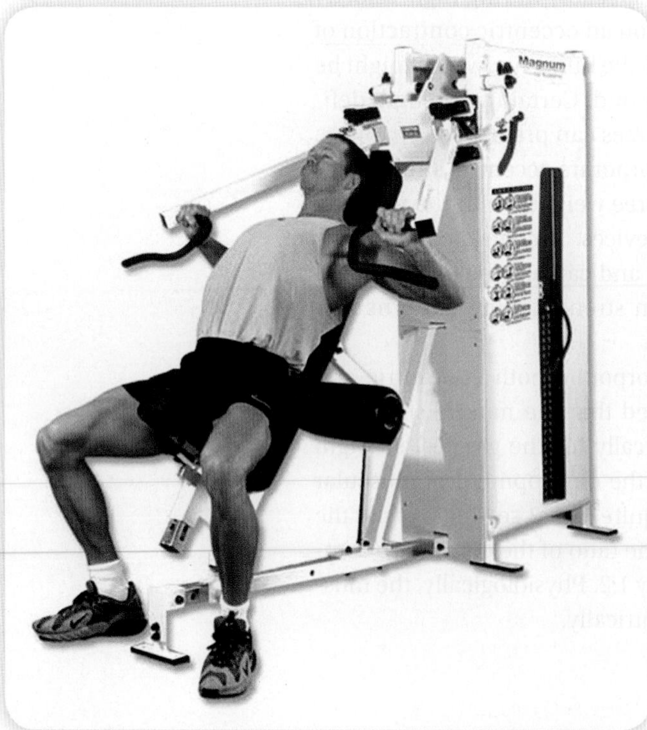

Figure 6-7 Bench press exercise machine with a stack of weights

Nautilus, BodyCraft, Yukon, Flex, CamBar, GymPros, Nugym, BodyWorks, DP, Soloflex, and Body Master (Figure 6-6). Dumbbells and barbells require the use of iron plates of varying weights that can be easily changed by adding or subtracting equal amounts of weight to both sides of the bar. The exercise machines for the most part have stacks of weights that are lifted through a series of levers or pulleys. The stack of weights slides up and down on a pair of bars that restrict the movement to only one plane. Weight can be increased or decreased simply by changing the position of a weight key.

There are advantages and disadvantages to free weights and machines. The exercise machines are relatively safe to use in comparison with free weights. For example, a bench press with free weights requires a partner to help lift the weight back onto the support racks if the lifter does not have enough strength to complete the lift; otherwise the weight might be dropped on the chest. With the machines the weight can be easily and safely dropped without fear of injury (Figure 6-7).

It is also a simple process to increase or decrease the weight by moving a single weight key with the exercise machines, although changes can generally be made only in increments of 10 or 15 pounds. With free weights, iron plates must be added or removed from each side of the barbell.

The biggest disadvantage in using exercise machines is that with few exceptions the design constraints of the machine allow only single-plane motion, limiting or controlling more functional movements that occur in multiple planes simultaneously.

Anyone who has strength-trained using free weights and exercise machines realizes the difference in the amount of weight that can be lifted. Unlike the machines, free weights have no restricted motion and can thus move in many different directions, depending on the forces applied. With free weights, an element of neuromuscular control on the part of the lifter to stabilize the weight and prevent it from moving in any other direction than vertical will usually decrease the amount of weight that can be lifted.[66]

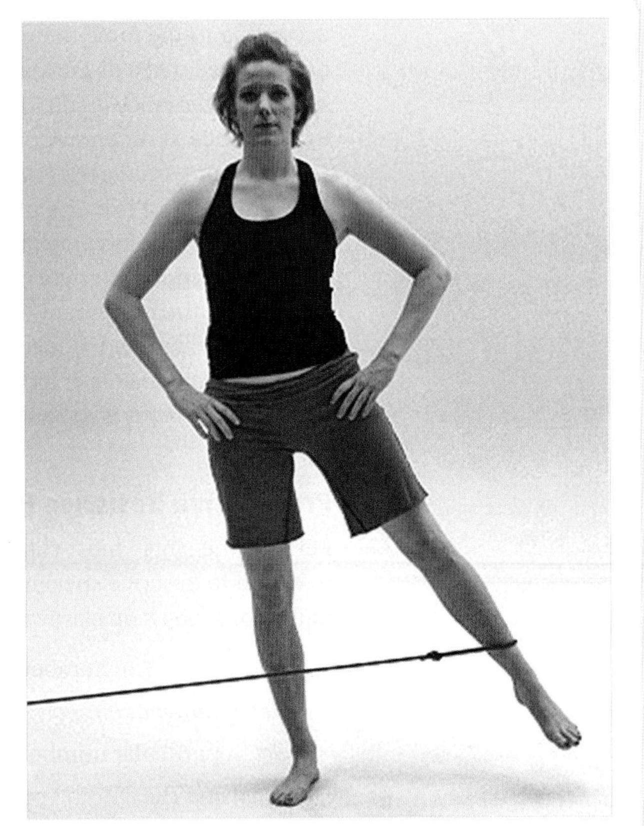

Figure 6-8 Strengthening exercises using surgical tubing are widely used in rehabilitation

Surgical Tubing or Thera-Band

Surgical tubing or Thera-Band, as a means of providing resistance, has been widely used in rehabilitation (Figure 6-8). The advantage of exercising with surgical tubing or Thera-Band is that movement can occur in multiple planes simultaneously. Thus, exercise can be done against resistance in more functional movement planes. Chapters 10 and 12 discuss the use of surgical tubing exercise in plyometrics and proprioceptive neuromuscular facilitation strengthening techniques. Surgical tubing can be used to provide resistance with the majority of the strengthening exercises shown in Chapters 25-32.

Regardless of which type of equipment is used, the same principles of progressive resistive exercise may be applied.

Clinical Pearl

Exercise machines typically are safer and more comfortable than free weights. It is easier to change the resistance, and the weight increments are small for easy progressions. Many of the machines utilize some type of cam for accommodating resistance. However, they are expensive and can be used only for one specific joint movement. Dumbbells or free weights are more versatile as well as cheaper. They also implement an additional aspect of training, as it requires neuromuscular control to balance the weight throughout the full range of motion.

Variable Resistance

One problem often mentioned in relation to progressive resistive exercise reconditioning is that the amount of force necessary to move a weight through a range of motion changes according to the angle of pull of the contracting muscle. It is greatest when the angle of pull is approximately 90 degrees. In addition, once the inertia of the weight has been overcome and momentum has been established, the force required to move the resistance varies according to the force the muscle can produce through the range of motion. Thus, it has been argued that a disadvantage of any type of isotonic exercise is that the force required to move the resistance is constantly changing throughout the range of movement. This change in resistance at different points in the range of motion has been labeled *accommodating resistance* or *variable resistance.*

A number of exercise machine manufacturers have attempted to alleviate this problem of changing force capabilities by using a cam in the machine's pulley system. The cam is individually designed for each piece of equipment so that the resistance is variable throughout the movement. The cam is intended to alter resistance so that the muscle can handle a greater load, but at the points where the joint angle or muscle length is mechanically disadvantageous, it reduces the resistance to muscle movement. Whether this design does what it claims is debatable.

Progressive Resistive Exercise Techniques

Perhaps the single most confusing aspect of progressive resistive exercise is the terminology used to describe specific programs.[32] The following list of terms with their operational definitions may help clarify the confusion:

Repetitions: The number of times a specific movement is repeated

Repetition maximum (RM): The maximum number of repetitions at a given weight

Set: A particular number of repetitions

Intensity: The amount of weight or resistance lifted

Recovery period: The rest interval between sets

Frequency: The number of times an exercise is done in a week's period

Recommended Techniques of Resistance Training

Specific recommendations for techniques of improving muscular strength are controversial among therapists. A considerable amount of research has been done in the area of resistance training relative to (a) the amount of weight to be used; (b) the number of repetitions; (c) the number of sets; and (d) the frequency of training.

A variety of specific programs have been proposed that recommend the optimal amount of weight, number of sets, number of repetitions, and frequency for producing maximal gains in levels of muscular strength. However, regardless of the techniques used, the healing process must dictate the specifics of any strength-training program. Certainly, to improve strength, the muscle must be progressively overloaded. The amount of weight used and the number of repetitions must be sufficient to make the muscle work at higher intensity than it is accustomed to. This factor is the most critical in any resistance training program. The resistance training program must also be designed to ultimately meet the specific competitive needs of the patient.

Resistance training programs were initially designed by power lifters and bodybuilders. Programs or routines commonly used in training and conditioning include the following:

Single set: One set of 8 to 12 repetitions of a particular exercise performed at a slow speed.

Tri-sets: A group of 3 exercises for the same muscle group performed using 2 to 4 sets of each exercise with no rest between sets.

Multiple sets: Two or 3 warm-up sets with progressively increasing resistance followed by several sets at the same resistance.

Supersets: Either 1 set of 8 to 10 repetitions of several exercises for the same muscle group performed one after another, or several sets of 8 to 10 repetitions of 2 exercises for the same muscle group with no rest between sets.

Pyramids: One set of 8 to 12 repetitions with light resistance, then an increase in resistance over 4 to 6 sets until only 1 or 2 repetitions can be performed. The pyramid can also be reversed going from heavy to light resistance.

Split routine: Workouts exercise different muscle groups on successive days. For example, Monday, Wednesday, and Friday might be used for upper-body muscles, and Tuesday, Thursday, and Saturday for lower-body muscles.

Circuit training: This technique may be useful to the therapist for maintaining or perhaps improving levels of muscular strength or endurance in other parts of the body while the patient allows for healing and reconditioning of an injured body part. Circuit training uses a series of exercise stations, each of which involves weight training, flexibility, calisthenics, or brief aerobic exercises. Circuits can be designed to accomplish many different training goals. With circuit training the patient moves rapidly from one station to the next, performing whatever exercise is to be done at that station within a specified time period. A typical circuit would consist of 8 to 12 stations, and the entire circuit would be repeated three times.

Circuit training is most definitely an effective technique for improving strength and flexibility. Certainly, if the pace or time interval between stations is rapid and if workload is maintained at a high level of intensity with heart rates at or above target training levels, the cardiorespiratory system may benefit from this circuit. However, there is little research evidence that circuit training is very effective in improving cardiorespiratory endurance. It should be, and is most often, used as a technique for developing and improving muscular strength and endurance.[27]

Techniques of Resistance Training Used in Rehabilitation

One of the first widely accepted strength-development programs to be used in a rehabilitation program was developed by DeLorme and was based on a repetition maximum (RM) of 10.[18] The amount of weight used is what can be lifted exactly 10 times (Table 6-2).

Zinovieff proposed the Oxford technique, which, like the DeLorme program, was designed to be used in beginning, intermediate, and advanced levels of rehabilitation.[68] The only difference is that the percentage of maximum was reversed in the 3 sets (Table 6-3). The McQueen technique[48] differentiates between beginning to intermediate and advanced levels, as in shown in Table 6-4.

The Sanders program (Table 6-5) was designed to be used in the advanced stages of rehabilitation and was based on a formula

Table 6-2 The DeLorme Program

Set	Amount of Weight	Repetitions
1	50% of 10 RM	10
2	75% of 10 RM	10
3	100% of 10 RM	10

Table 6-3 The Oxford Technique

Set	Amount of Weight	Repetitions
1	100% of 10 RM	10
2	75% of 10 RM	10
3	50% of 10 RM	10

Table 6-4 The McQueen Technique

Set	Amount of Weight	Repetitions
3 (Beginning/ intermediate)	100% of 10 RM	10
4 to 5 (Advanced)	100% of 2 to 3 RM	2 to 3

Table 6-5 The Sanders Program

Sets	Amount of Weight	Repetitions
Total of 4 sets (3 times per week)	100% of 5 RM	5
Day 1, 4 sets	100% of 5 RM	5
Day 2, 4 sets	100% of 3 RM	5
Day 3, 1 set	100% of 5 RM	5
2 sets	100% of 3 RM	5
2 sets	100% of 2 RM	5

Table 6-6 Knight's DAPRE Program

Sets	Amount of Weight	Repetitions
1	50% of RM	10
2	75% of RM	6
3	100% of RM	Maximum
4	Adjusted working weight[a]	Maximum

[a]See Table 6-7.

Table 6-7 DAPRE Adjusted Working Weight

Number of Repetitions Performed During Third Set	Adjusted Working Weight During Fourth Set	Next Exercise Session
0 to 2	–5 to 10 lb	–5 to 10 lb
3 to 4	–0 to 5 lb	Same weight
5 to 6	Same weight	±0 to 10 lb
7 to 10	±5 to 10 lb	±5 to 15 lb
11	±10 to 15 lb	±10 to 20 lb

Table 6-8 The Berger Adjustment Technique

Sets	Amount of Weight	Repetitions
3	100% of 10 RM	6 to 8

that used a percentage of body weight to determine starting weights.[56] The following percentages represent median starting points for different exercises:

Barbell squat—45% of body weight
Barbell bench press—30% of body weight
Leg extension—20% of body weight
Universal bench press—30% of body weight
Universal leg extension—20% of body weight
Universal leg curl—10% to 15% of body weight
Universal leg press—50% of body weight
Upright rowing—20% of body weight

Knight applied the concept of progressive resistive exercise in rehabilitation. His Daily Adjusted Progressive Resistive Exercise (DAPRE) program (Tables 6-6 and 6-7) allows for individual differences in the rates at which patients progress in their rehabilitation programs.[37]

Berger proposed a technique that is adjustable within individual limitations (Table 6-8). For any given exercise, the amount of weight selected should be sufficient to allow 6 to 8 RM in each of the 3 sets, with a recovery period of 60 to 90 seconds between sets. Initial selection of a starting weight might require some trial and error to achieve this 6 to 8 RM range. If at least 3 sets of 6 RM cannot be completed, the weight is too heavy and should be reduced. If it is possible to do more than 3 sets of 8 RM, the weight is too light and should be increased.[8] Progression to heavier weights is then determined by the ability to perform at least 8 RM in each of 3 sets. When progressing weight, an increase of approximately 10% of the current weight being lifted should still allow at least 6 RM in each of 3 sets.[9]

For rehabilitation purposes, strengthening exercises should be performed on a daily basis initially, with the amount of weight, number of sets, and number of repetitions governed by the injured patient's response to the exercise. As the healing process progresses and pain or swelling is no longer an issue, a particular muscle or muscle group should be exercised consistently every other day. At that point, the frequency of weight training should be at least 3 times per week but no more than 4 times per week. It is common for serious weightlifters to lift every day; however, they exercise different muscle groups on successive days.

It has been suggested that if training is done properly, using both concentric and eccentric contractions, resistance training is necessary only twice each week. However, this schedule has not been sufficiently documented.

Isokinetic Exercise

An *isokinetic exercise* involves a muscle contraction in which the length of the muscle is changing while the contraction is performed at a constant velocity.[11] In theory, maximal resistance is provided throughout the range of motion by the machine. The resistance provided by the machine will move only at some preset speed, regardless of the torque applied to it by the individual. Thus, the key to isokinetic exercise is not the resistance but the speed at which resistance can be moved.

Few isokinetic devices are still available commercially (Figure 6-9). In general, they rely on hydraulic, pneumatic, and mechanical pressure systems to produce this constant velocity of motion. Most isokinetic devices are capable of resisting concentric and eccentric contractions at a fixed speed to exercise a muscle.

Isokinetics as a Conditioning Tool

Isokinetic devices are designed so that regardless of the amount of force applied against a resistance, it can only be moved at a certain speed. That speed will be the same whether maximal force or only half the maximal force is applied. Consequently, in isokinetic training, it is absolutely necessary to exert as much force against the resistance as possible (maximal effort) for maximal strength gains to occur.[11] Maximal effort is one of the major problems with an isokinetic strength-training program.

Anyone who has been involved in a resistance training program knows that on some days it is difficult to find the motivation to work out. Because isokinetic training requires a maximal effort, it is very easy to "cheat" and not go through the workout at a high level of intensity. In a progressive resistive exercise program, the patient knows how much weight has to be lifted for how many repetitions. Thus, isokinetic training is often more effective if

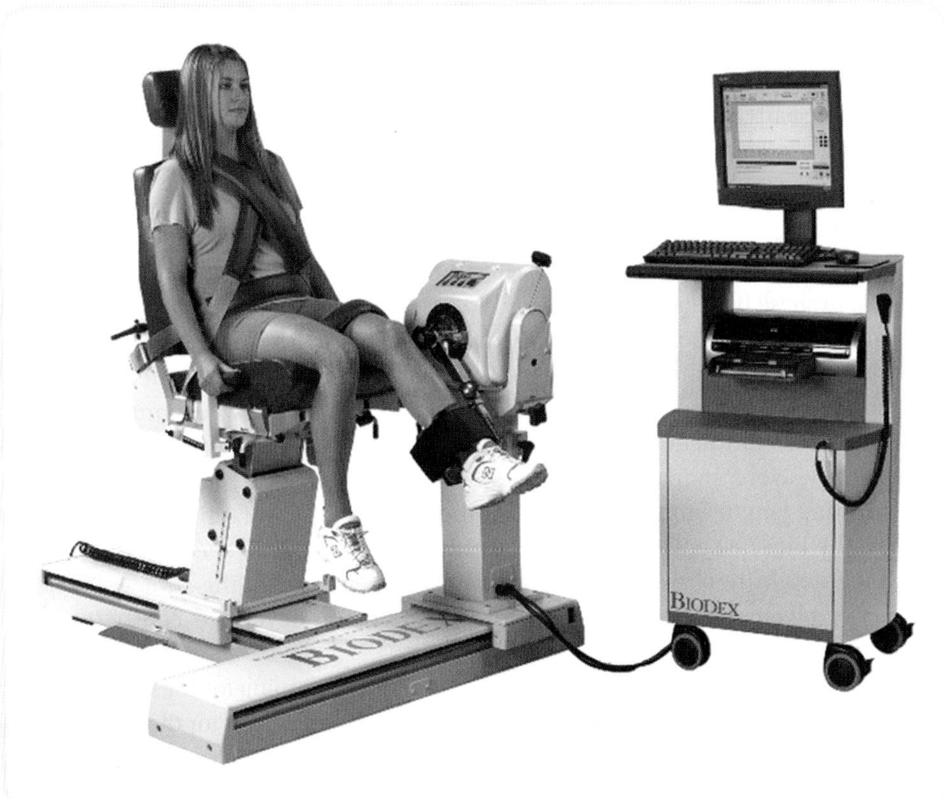

Figure 6-9 The Biodex is an isokinetic device that provides resistance at a constant velocity

a partner system is used, primarily as a means of motivation toward a maximal effort. When isokinetic training is done properly with a maximal effort, it is theoretically possible that maximal strength gains are best achieved through the isokinetic training method in which the velocity and force of the resistance are equal throughout the range of motion. However, there is no conclusive research to support this theory.

Whether this changing force capability is a deterrent to improving the ability to generate force against some resistance is debatable. In real life, it does not matter whether the resistance is changing; what is important is that an individual develops enough strength to move objects from one place to another.

Another major disadvantage of using isokinetic devices as a conditioning tool is their cost. With initial purchase costs ranging between $50,000 and $80,000 and the necessity of regular maintenance and software upgrades, the use of an isokinetic device for general conditioning or resistance training is, for the most part, unrealistic. Thus, isokinetic exercises are primarily used as a diagnostic and rehabilitative tool.

Isokinetics in Rehabilitation

Isokinetic strength testing gained a great deal of popularity throughout the 1980s in rehabilitation settings. This trend stems from its providing an objective means of quantifying existing levels of muscular strength and thus becoming useful as a diagnostic tool.[49]

Because the capability exists for training at specific speeds, comparisons have been made regarding the relative advantages of training at fast or slow speeds in a rehabilitation program. The research literature seems to indicate that strength increases from slow-speed training are relatively specific to the velocity used in training. Conversely, training at faster speeds seems to produce a more generalized increase in torque values at all velocities. Minimal hypertrophy was observed only while training at fast speeds, affecting only type II or fast-twitch fibers.[17,52] An increase in neuromuscular efficiency caused by more effective motor unit firing patterns has been demonstrated with slow-speed training.[45]

During the early 1990s, the value of isokinetic devices for quantifying torque values at functional speeds was questioned.

Plyometric Exercise

Plyometric exercise has also been referred to in the literature as reactive neuromuscular training. It is a technique that is being increasingly incorporated into later stages of the rehabilitation program by therapists. Plyometric training includes specific exercises that encompass a rapid stretch of a muscle eccentrically, followed immediately by a rapid concentric contraction of that muscle to facilitate and develop a forceful explosive movement over a short period of time.[13,20] The greater the stretch put on the muscle from its resting length immediately before the concentric contraction, the greater the resistance the muscle can overcome. Plyometrics emphasize the speed of the eccentric phase. The rate of stretch is more critical than the magnitude of the stretch. An advantage to using plyometric exercises is that they can help to develop eccentric control in dynamic movements.[43]

Plyometric exercises involve hops, bounds, and depth jumping for the lower extremity and the use of medicine balls and other types of weighted equipment for the upper extremity.[12,14] Depth jumping is an example of a plyometric exercise in which an individual jumps to the ground from a specified height and then quickly jumps again as soon as ground contact is made (Figure 6-10).[53]

Plyometrics tend to place a great deal of stress on the musculoskeletal system. The learning and perfection of specific jumping skills and other plyometric exercises must be

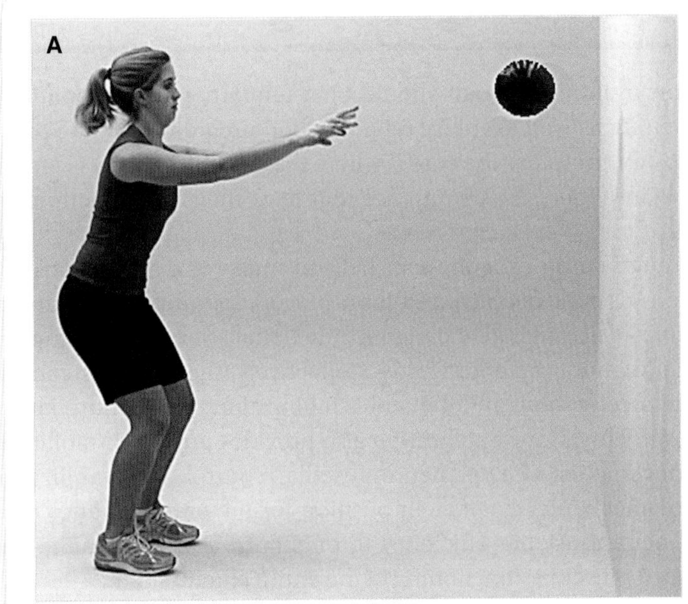

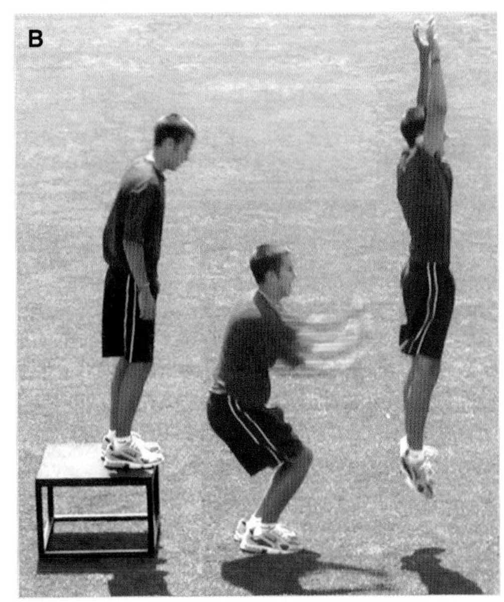

Figure 6-10 **Plyometric exercises**

A. Upper extremity plyometric exercise using a medicine ball. **B.** Depth jumping lower extremity plyometric exercise.

technically correct and specific to one's age, activity, physical, and skill development. Chapter 10 discusses plyometric exercise in detail.

Calisthenic Strengthening Exercises

Calisthenics, or free exercise, is one of the more easily available means of developing strength. Isotonic movement exercises can be graded according to intensity by using gravity as an aid, by ruling gravity out, by moving against gravity, or by using the body or a body part as a resistance against gravity. Most calisthenics require the individual to support the body or move the total body against the force of gravity. Pushups are a good example of a vigorous antigravity exercise (Figure 6-11*A*). Calisthenic-like exercises are used in functional strength training, which was discussed earlier. To be considered maximally effective, the isotonic calisthenic exercise, like all types of exercise, must be performed in an exacting manner and in full range of motion. In most cases, 10 or more repetitions are performed for each exercise and are repeated in sets of 2 or 3. Some free exercises use an isometric, or holding, phase instead of a full range of motion. Examples of these exercises are back extensions and situps (Figure 6-11*B*). When the exercise produces maximum muscle tension, it is held between 6 and 10 seconds and then repeated 1 to 3 times.

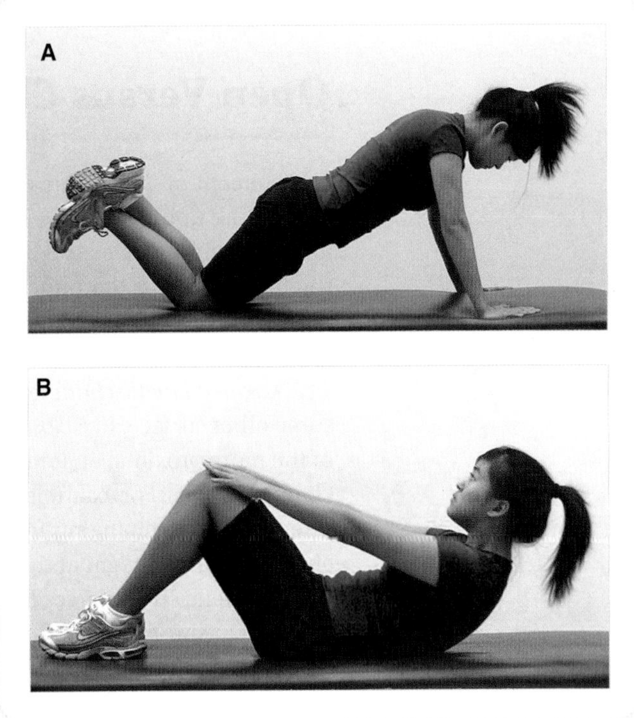

Figure 6-11 **Calisthenic exercises use body weight as resistance**

A. Pushups. **B.** Situps.

Core Stabilization Strengthening

A dynamic core stabilization training program should be a fundamental component of all comprehensive strengthening as well as injury rehabilitation programs.[34,36] The *core* is defined as the lumbo-pelvic-hip complex. The core is where the center of gravity is located and where all movement begins. There are 29 muscles that have their attachment to the lumbo-pelvic-hip complex.

A core stabilization strengthening program can help to improve dynamic postural control; ensure appropriate muscular balance and joint movement around the lumbo-pelvic-hip complex; allow for the expression of dynamic functional strength; and improve neuromuscular efficiency throughout the entire body. Collectively, these factors contribute to optimal acceleration, deceleration, and dynamic stabilization of the entire kinetic chain during functional movements. Core stabilization also provides proximal stability for efficient lower-extremity movements. Greater neuromuscular control and stabilization strength will offer a more biomechanically efficient position for the entire kinetic chain, therefore allowing optimal neuromuscular efficiency throughout the kinetic chain. This approach facilitates a balanced muscular functioning of the entire kinetic chain.[15]

Many patients develop the functional strength, power, neuromuscular control, and muscular endurance in specific muscles to perform functional activities. However, relatively few patients have developed the muscles required for stabilization. The body's stabilization system has to be functioning optimally to effectively utilize the strength, power, neuromuscular control, and muscular endurance that they have developed in their prime movers. If the extremity muscles are strong and the core is weak, then there will not be enough force created to produce efficient movements. A weak core is a fundamental problem of inefficient movements that leads to injury.[15] Chapter 15 discusses core stabilization techniques in detail.

Open Versus Closed Kinetic Chain Exercises

The concept of the kinetic chain deals with the anatomical functional relationships that exist in the upper and lower extremities. In a weightbearing position, the lower extremity kinetic chain involves the transmission of forces among the foot, ankle, lower leg, knee, thigh, and hip. In the upper extremity, when the hand is in contact with a weightbearing surface, forces are transmitted to the wrist, forearm, elbow, upper arm, and shoulder girdle.

An *open kinetic chain* exists when the foot or hand is not in contact with the ground or some other surface. In a *closed kinetic chain,* the foot or hand is weight bearing. Movements of the more proximal anatomical segments are affected by these open versus closed kinetic chain positions. For example, the rotational components of the ankle, knee, and hip reverse direction when changing from open to closed kinetic chain activity. In a closed kinetic chain, the forces begin at the ground and work their way up through each joint. Also, in a closed kinetic chain, forces must be absorbed by various tissues and anatomical structures, rather than simply dissipating as would occur in an open chain.

In rehabilitation, the use of closed-chain strengthening techniques has become a treatment of choice for many therapist. Most functional activities involve some aspect of weight bearing with the foot in contact with the ground or the hand in a weightbearing position, so closed kinetic chain strengthening activities are more functional than open-chain activities. Consequently, rehabilitative exercises should be incorporated that emphasize strengthening of the entire kinetic chain rather than an isolated body segment. Chapter 11 discusses closed-kinetic-chain activities in detail.

Training for Muscular Strength Versus Muscular Endurance

Muscular endurance was defined as the ability to perform repeated muscle contractions against resistance for an extended period of time. Most resistance-training experts believe that muscular strength and muscular endurance are closely related.[21,50,57] As one improves, there is a tendency for the other to also improve.

It is generally accepted that when resistance training for strength, heavier weights with a lower number of repetitions should be used.[65] Conversely, endurance training uses relatively lighter weights with a greater number of repetitions.

It has been suggested that endurance training should consist of 3 sets of 10 to 15 repetitions,[9] using the same criteria for weight-selection progression and frequency as recommended for progressive resistive exercise. Thus, suggested training regimens for muscular strength and endurance are similar in terms of sets and numbers of repetitions.[55] Persons who possess great levels of strength tend to also exhibit greater muscular endurance when asked to perform repeated contractions against resistance.[48]

Resistance Training Differences Between Males and Females

The approach to strength training is no different for females than for males. However, some obvious physiologic differences exist between the genders.

The average female will not build significant muscle bulk through resistance training. Significant muscle hypertrophy is dependent on the presence of the steroidal hormone *testosterone.* Testosterone is considered a male hormone, although all females possess some level of testosterone in their systems. Women with higher testosterone levels tend to have more masculine characteristics, such as increased facial and body hair, a deeper voice, and the potential to develop a little more muscle bulk.[23,50] For the average female, developing large, bulky muscles through strength training is unlikely, although muscle tone can be improved. Muscle tone basically refers to the firmness of tension of the muscle during a resting state.

The initial stages of a resistance training program are likely to rapidly produce dramatic increases in levels of strength.[1] For a muscle to contract, an impulse must be transmitted from the nervous system to the muscle. Each muscle fiber is innervated by a specific motor unit. By overloading a particular muscle, as in weight training, the muscle is forced to work more efficiently. Efficiency is achieved by getting more motor units to fire, thus causing more muscle fibers to contract, which results in a stronger contraction of the muscle. Consequently, both women and men often see extremely rapid gains in strength when a weight-training program is first begun.[28] In females, these initial strength gains, which can be attributed to improved neuromuscular efficiency, tend to plateau, and minimal improvement in muscular strength is realized during a continuing resistance training program. These initial neuromuscular strength gains are also seen in males, although their strength continues to increase with appropriate training.[1] Again, females who possess higher testosterone levels have the potential to increase their strength further because they are able to develop greater muscle bulk.

Differences in strength levels between males and females are best illustrated when strength is expressed in relation to body weight minus fat. The reduced *strength-to-bodyweight ratio* in women is the result of their percentage of body fat. The strength-to-bodyweight ratio can be significantly improved through resistance training by decreasing the body fat percentage while increasing lean weight.[45]

The absolute strength differences are considerably reduced when body size and composition are considered. Leg strength can actually be stronger in females than in males, although upper extremity strength is much greater in males.[45]

Resistance Training in the Adolescent

The principles of resistance training discussed previously may be applied to adolescents. There are certainly a number of sociologic questions regarding the advantages and disadvantages of younger, in particular prepubescent, individuals engaging in rigorous strength-training programs. From a physiologic perspective, experts have for years debated the value of strength training in adolescents. Recently, a number of studies have indicated that if properly supervised, adolescents can improve strength, power, endurance, balance, and proprioception; develop a positive body image; improve sport performance; and prevent injuries.[41] A prepubescent child can experience gains in levels of muscle strength without muscle hypertrophy.[51]

A therapist supervising a rehabilitation program for an injured adolescent should certainly incorporate resistive exercise into the program. However, close supervision, proper instruction, and appropriate modification of progression and intensity based on the extent of physical maturation of the individual is critical to the effectiveness of the resistive exercises.[41]

Specific Resistive Exercises Used in Rehabilitation

Because muscle contractions results in joint movement, the goal of resistance training in a rehabilitation program should be either to regain and perhaps increase the strength of a specific muscle that has been injured or to increase the efficiency of movement about a given joint.[45]

The exercises included throughout Chapters 25-32 show exercises for all motions about a particular joint rather than for each specific muscle. These exercises are demonstrated using free weights (dumbbells or bar weights) and some exercise machines. Other strengthening techniques widely used for injury rehabilitation involving isokinetic exercise, plyometrics, core stability training, closed kinetic chain exercises, and proprioceptive neuromuscular facilitation strengthening techniques are discussed in greater detail in subsequent chapters.

SUMMARY

1. Muscular strength may be defined as the maximal force that can be generated against resistance by a muscle during a single maximal contraction.
2. Muscular endurance is the ability to perform repeated isotonic or isokinetic muscle contractions or to sustain an isometric contraction without undue fatigue.
3. Muscular endurance tends to improve with muscular strength, thus training techniques for these 2 components are similar.
4. Muscular strength and endurance are essential components of any rehabilitation program.

5. Muscular power involves the speed with which a forceful muscle contraction is performed.
6. The ability to generate force is dependent on the physical properties of the muscle, neuromuscular efficiency, as well as the mechanical factors that dictate how much force can be generated through the lever system to an external object.
7. Hypertrophy of a muscle is caused by increases in the size and perhaps the number of actin and myosin protein myofilaments, which result in an increased cross-sectional diameter of the muscle.
8. The key to improving strength through resistance training is using the principle of overload within the constraints of the healing process.
9. Five resistance training techniques that can improve muscular strength are isometric exercise, progressive resistive exercise, isokinetic training, circuit training, and plyometric training.
10. Improvements in strength with isometric exercise occur at specific joint angles.
11. Progressive resistive exercise is the most common strengthening technique used by the therapist for rehabilitation after injury.
12. Circuit training involves a series of exercise stations consisting of resistance training, flexibility, and calisthenic exercises that can be designed to maintain fitness while reconditioning an injured body part.
13. Isokinetic training provides resistance to a muscle at a fixed speed.
14. Plyometric exercise uses a quick eccentric stretch to facilitate a concentric contraction.
15. Closed kinetic chain exercises might provide a more functional technique for strengthening of injured muscles and joints in the athletic population.
16. Females can significantly increase their strength levels but generally will not build muscle bulk as a result of strength training because of their relative lack of the hormone testosterone.

REFERENCES

1. Akima H, Takahashi H, Kuno SY. Early phase adaptations of muscle use and strength to isokinetic training. *Med Sci Sports Exerc.* 1999;31(4):588-594.
2. Allerheiligen W. Speed development and plyometric training. In: Baechle T, ed. *Essentials of Strength Training.* Champaign, IL: Human Kinetics; 1994.
3. Alway SE, MacDougall JD, Sale DG, Sutton JR, McComas AJ. Functional and structural adaptations in skeletal muscle of trained athletes. *J Appl Physiol.* 1988;64:1114-1120.
4. Astrand PO, Rodahl K. *Textbook of Work Physiology: Physiological Bases of Exercise.* Champaign, IL: Human Kinetics; 2003.
5. Baechle T, ed. *Essentials of Strength Training and Conditioning.* Champaign, IL: Human Kinetics; 2008.
6. Baker D, Wilson G, Carlyon B. Generality vs. specificity: a comparison of dynamic and isometric measures of strength and speed-strength. *Eur J Appl Physiol.* 1994;68:350-355.
7. Bandy W, Lovelace-Chandler V, McKitrick-Bandy B. Adaptation of skeletal muscle to resistance training. *J Orthop Sports Phys Ther.* 1990;12(6):248-255.
8. Berger R. *Conditioning for Men.* Boston: Allyn & Bacon; 1973.
9. Berger R. Effect of varied weight training programs on strength. *Res Q Exerc Sport.* 1962;33:168.
10. Booth F, Thomason D. Molecular and cellular adaptation of muscle in response to exercise: Perspectives of various models. *Physiol Rev.* 1999;71:541-585.
11. Brown LE. *Isokinetics in Human Performance.* Champaign, IL: Human Kinetics; 2000.
12. Bruce-Low S, Smith D. Explosive exercises in sports training: a critical review. *J Exerc Physiol Online.* 2007;10(1):21.
13. Chu D. *Jumping into Plyometrics.* Champaign, IL: Human Kinetics; 1998.
14. Chu D. Plyometrics in sports injury rehabilitation and training. *Athl Ther Today.* 1999;4(3):7.

15. Clark M. *Integrated Training for the New Millennium.* Calabasas, CA: National Academy of Sports Medicine; 2001.
16. Costill D, Daniels J, Evan W, Fink W, Krahenbuhl G, Saltin B. Skeletal muscle enzymes and fiber compositions in male and female track athletes. *J Appl Physiol.* 1976;40:149-154.
17. Coyle E, Feiring D, Rotkis T, et al. Specificity of power improvements through slow and fast speed isokinetic training. *J Appl Physiol.* 1981;51:1437-1442.
18. DeLorme T, Wilkins A. *Progressive Resistance Exercise.* New York: Appleton-Century-Crofts; 1951.
19. Deudsinger RH. Biomechanics in clinical practice. *Phys Ther.* 1984;64:1860-1868.
20. Duda M. Plyometrics: a legitimate form of power training. *Phys Sportsmed.* 1988;16:213.
21. Dudley GA, Fleck SJ. Strength and endurance training: are they mutually exclusive? *Sports Med.* 1987;4(2):79-85.
22. Etheridge G, Thomas T. Physiological and bio-medical changes of human skeletal muscle induced by different strength training programs. *Med Sci Sports Exerc.* 1982;14:141.
23. Fahey T. Weight Training Basics. St. Louis, MO: McGraw-Hill; 2005.
24. Faulkner J, Green H, White T. Response and adaptation of skeletal muscle to changes in physical activity. In: Bouchard C, Shepard R, Stephens J, eds. *Physical Activity, Fitness, and Health.* Champaign, IL: Human Kinetics; 1994.
25. Fleck SJ, Kramer WJ. *Designing Resistance Training Programs.* Champaign, IL: Human Kinetics; 2004.
26. Gabriel D, Kamen G. Neural adaptation to resistive exercise: mechanisms and recommendations for training practices. *Sports Med.* 2006;26(2):133-149.
27. Gettman L. Circuit weight training: a critical review of its physiological benefits. *Phys Sportsmed.* 1981;9(1):44.
28. Gravelle BL, Blessing DL. Physiological adaptation in women concurrently training for strength and endurance. *J Strength Cond Res.* 2000;14(1):5.
29. Graves JE, Pollack M, Jones A, Colvin AB, Leggett SH. Specificity of limited range of motion variable resistance training. *Med Sci Sports Exerc.* 1989;21:84-89.
30. Hakkinen K. Neuromuscular adaptations during concurrent strength and endurance training versus strength training. *Eur J Appl Physiol.* 2002;89:42-52.
31. Harmen E. The biomechanics of resistance training. In: Baechle T, ed. *Essentials of Strength Training.* Champaign, IL: Human Kinetics; 1994.
32. Hickson R, Hidaka C, Foster C. Skeletal muscle fiber type, resistance training and strength-related performance. *Med Sci Sports Exerc.* 1994;26:593-598.
33. Horobagyi T, Katch FI. Role of concentric force in limiting improvement in muscular strength. *J Appl Physiol.* 1990;68:650-658.
34. Jones M, Trowbridge C. Four ways to a safe, effective strength training program. *Athl Ther Today.* 1998;3(2):4.
35. Kaminski TW, CWabbersen V, Murphy RM. Concentric versus enhanced eccentric hamstring strength training: Clinical implications. *J Athl Train.* 1998;33(3):216-221.
36. King MA. Core stability: creating a foundation for functional rehabilitation. *Athl Ther Today.* 2000;5(2): 6-13.
37. Knight K, Ingersoll C. Isotonic contractions may be more effective than isometric contractions in developing muscular strength. *J Sport Rehabil.* 2001;10(2):124.
38. Komi P. Endocrine responses to resistance exercises. In: *Strength and Power in Sport.* London, UK: Blackwell Scientific; 2003.
39. Kraemer W. General adaptation to resistance and endurance training programs. In: Baechle T, ed. *Essentials of Strength Training.* Champaign, IL: Human Kinetics; 1994.
40. Kraemer WJ, Ratamess N. Fundamentals of resistance training: progression and exercise prescription. *Med Sci Sports Exerc.* 2004;36(4):674-688.
41. Kraemer WJ, Fleck SJ. *Strength Training for Young Athletes.* Champaign, IL: Human Kinetics; 2004.
42. Kraemer WJ. ACSM Position stand. Progression models in resistance training for healthy adults. *Med Sci Sports Exerc.* 2002;34(2):364-380.
43. Kramer J, Morrow A, Leger A. Changes in rowing ergometer, weight lifting, vertical jump and isokinetic performance in response to standard and standard plus plyometric training programs. *Int J Sports Med.* 1993;14(8):440-454.
44. Mastropaolo J. A test of maximum power theory for strength. *Eur J Appl Physiol.* 1992;65:415-420.
45. McArdle W, Katch F, Katch V. *Exercise Physiology, Energy, Nutrition, and Human Performance.* Philadelphia, PA: Lea & Febiger; 2006.
46. McComas A. Human neuromuscular adaptations that accompany changes in activity. *Med Sci Sports Exerc.* 1994;26(12):1498-1509.
47. McGlynn GH. A reevaluation of isometric training. *J Sports Med Phys Fitness.* 1972;12:258-260.
48. McQueen I. Recent advance in the techniques of progressive resistance. *Br Med J.* 1954;11:11993.
49. Nicholas JJ. Isokinetic testing in young nonathletic able-bodied subjects. *Arch Phys Med Rehabil.* 1989;70(3):210-213.
50. Nygard CH, Luophaarui T, Suurnakki T, Ilmarinen J. Muscle strength and muscle endurance of middle-aged women and men associated to type, duration and intensity of muscular load at work. *Int Arch Occup Environ Health.* 1998;60(4):291-297.
51. Ozmun J, Mikesky A, Surburg P. Neuromuscular adaptations following prepubescent strength training. *Med Sci Sports Exerc.* 1994;26:510-514.
52. Pipes T, Wilmore J. Isokinetic vs. isotonic strength training in adult men. *Med Sci Sports Exerc.* 1975;7:262-274.
53. Radcliffe JC, Farentinos RC. *High-Powered Plyometrics.* Champaign, IL: Human Kinetics; 1999.

54. Rehfeldt H, Caffiber G, Kramer H, Küchler G. Force, endurance time, and cardiovascular responses in voluntary isometric contractions of different muscle groups. *Biomed Biochim Acta.* 1989;48(5-6):S509-S514.

55. Sale D, MacDougall D. Specificity in strength training: a review for the coach and athlete. *Can J Appl Sport Sci.* 1986;6:87-92.

56. Sanders M. Weight training and conditioning. In: Sanders B, ed. *Sports Physical Therapy.* Norwalk, CT: Appleton & Lange; 1997:239-250.

57. Sandler D. Speed and strength through plyometrics. In: *Sports Power.* Champaign, IL: Human Kinetics; 2005:107-144.

58. Soest A, Bobbert M. The role of muscle properties in control of explosive movements. *Biol Cybern.* 1993;69:195-204.

59. Staron RS, Karapondo DL, Kreamer WJ. Skeletal muscle and adaptations during early phase of heavy resistance training in men and women. *J Appl Physiol.* 1994;76:1247-1255.

60. Stone J. Rehabilitation—speed of movement/muscular power. *Athl Ther Today.* 1998;3(5):10.

61. Stone J. Rehabilitation—muscular endurance. *Athl Ther Today.* 1998;3(4):21.

62. Stone M, Sands W. Maximum strength and strength training—a relationship to endurance? *Strength Cond J.* 2006;28(3):44.

63. Strauss RH, ed. *Sports Medicine.* Philadelphia, PA: WB Saunders; 1991.

64. Ulmer HV, Knieriemen W, Warlo T, Zech B. Interindividual variability of isometric endurance with regard to the endurance performance limit for static work. *Biomed Biochim Acta.* 1989;48(5-6):S504-S508.

65. Van Etten L, Verstappen E, Westerterp K. Effect of body building on weight training induced adaptations in body composition and muscular strength. *Med Sci Sports Exerc.* 1994;6:515-521.

66. Weltman A, Stamford B. Strength training: free weights vs. machines. *Phys Sportsmed.* 1982;10:197.

67. Yates JW. Recovery of dynamic muscular endurance. *Eur J Appl Physiol.* 1987;56(6):662.

68. Zinovieff A. Heavy resistance exercise: the Oxford technique. *Br J Physiol Med.* 1951;14:129.

7

Impaired Endurance

Maintaining Aerobic Capacity and Endurance

Patrick D. Sells and William E. Prentice

OBJECTIVES **After completion of this chapter, the physical therapist should be able to do the following:**

- Explain the relationships between heart rate, stroke volume, cardiac output, and rate of oxygen use.
- Describe the function of the heart, blood vessels, and lungs in oxygen transport.
- Describe the oxygen transport system and the concept of maximal rate of oxygen use.
- Describe the principles of continuous and interval training and the potential of each technique for improving aerobic activity.
- Describe the difference between aerobic and anaerobic activity.
- Describe the principles of reversibility and detraining.
- Describe caloric threshold goals associated with various stages of exercise programming.

Although strength and flexibility are commonly regarded as essential components in any injury rehabilitation program, often relatively little consideration is given toward maintaining aerobic capacity and cardiorespiratory endurance. When musculoskeletal injury occurs, the patient is forced to decrease physical activity and levels of cardiorespiratory endurance may decrease rapidly. Thus, the therapist must design or substitute alternative activities that allow the individual to maintain existing levels of aerobic capacity during the rehabilitation period. Furthermore, the importance of maintaining and improving functional capacity is becoming increasingly evident regardless of musculoskeletal injury. Recent research demonstrates a reduction in risk for cardiovascular disease is associated with improved levels of aerobic capacity. Sandvik et al[46] reported mortality rates according to fitness quartiles over 16 years of follow-up. The number of deaths in the least-fit portion of the study outnumbered the deaths of the most fit by a margin of 61 to 11 deaths from cardiovascular causes.[46] Myers et al studied 6213 subjects referred for treadmill testing and concluded that exercise capacity is a more powerful predictor of mortality among men than other established risk factors for cardiovascular disease.[41]

By definition, *cardiorespiratory endurance* is the ability to perform whole-body activities for extended periods of time without undue fatigue.[11,16] The cardiorespiratory system provides a means by which oxygen is supplied to the various tissues of the body. Without oxygen, the cells within the human body cannot possibly function and ultimately cell death will occur. Thus, the cardiorespiratory system is the basic life-support system of the body.[2,11]

Training Effects on the Cardiorespiratory System

Basically, transport of oxygen throughout the body involves the coordinated function of 4 components: heart, blood vessels, blood, and lungs. The improvement of cardiorespiratory endurance through training occurs because of increased capability of each of these 4 elements in providing necessary oxygen to the working tissues.[56] A basic discussion of the training effects and response to exercise that occur in the heart, blood vessels, blood, and lungs should make it easier to understand why the training techniques discussed later are effective in improving cardiorespiratory endurance.

Adaptation of the Heart to Exercise

The heart is the main pumping mechanism and circulates oxygenated blood throughout the body to the working tissues. The heart receives deoxygenated blood from the venous system and then pumps the blood through the pulmonary vessels to the lungs, where carbon dioxide is exchanged for oxygen. The oxygenated blood then returns to the left atrium of the heart, into the left ventricle, from which it exits through the aorta to the arterial system and is circulated throughout the body, supplying oxygen to the tissues.

Heart Rate

As the body begins to exercise, the working tissues require an increased supply of oxygen (via transport on red blood cells) to meet the increased metabolic demand (cardiac output). The working tissues use the decreasing concentration of oxygen as a signal to vasodilate the blood vessels in the tissue. This decreases the resistance to blood flow and allows for a decrease velocity of flow, and thereby increasing O_2 extraction.[49] Increases in heart rate occur as one response to meet the demand. The heart is capable of adapting to this increased demand through several mechanisms. *Heart rate* shows a gradual adaptation to an increased workload by increasing proportionally to the intensity of the exercise and will plateau at a given level after approximately 2 to 3 minutes (Figure 7-1).[12] Increases in heart rate produced by exercise are met by a decrease in diastolic filling time. Heart rate parameters change with age, body position, type of exercise, cardiovascular disease, heat and humidity, medications, and blood volume. Conditions that exist in any patient should be taken into consideration when prescribing exercise to improve aerobic endurance. The commonly used equation to predict maximal heart rate (MHR) is 220 – age for healthy men and women. However, the formula has limitations to persons who fall outside the "apparently healthy" classification and should be used with caution. Monitoring heart rate is an indirect method of estimating oxygen consumption.[16] Additionally, any medications should be considered prior to assessment or evaluation of heart rate response. For example, patients taking beta blockers will have an attenuated heart rate response to exercise. In general, heart rate and oxygen consumption have a linear relationship with exercise intensity. The greater the intensity of the exercise, the higher the heart rate. This relationship is least consistent at very-low and very-high intensities of exercise (Figure 7-2). During higher-intensity activities, MHR may be achieved before maximum oxygen consumption, which can continue to rise despite reaching an age predicted heart rate.[38] Because of these existing relationships, it should be apparent that the rate of oxygen consumption can be estimated by monitoring the heart rate.[13]

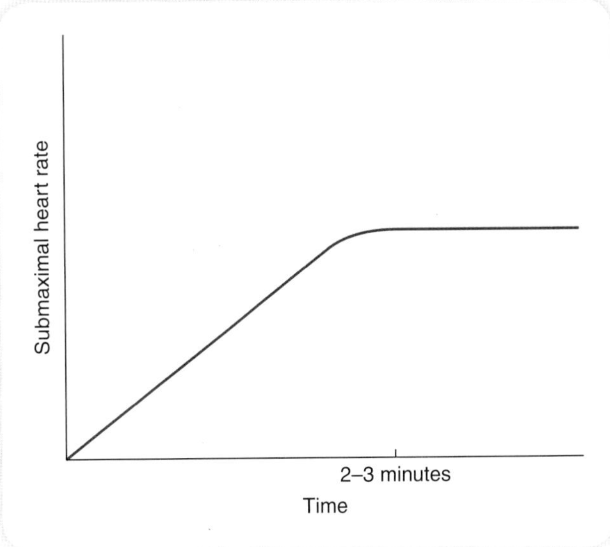

Figure 7-1 Plateau heart rate

For the heart rate to plateau at a given level, 2 to 3 minutes are required.

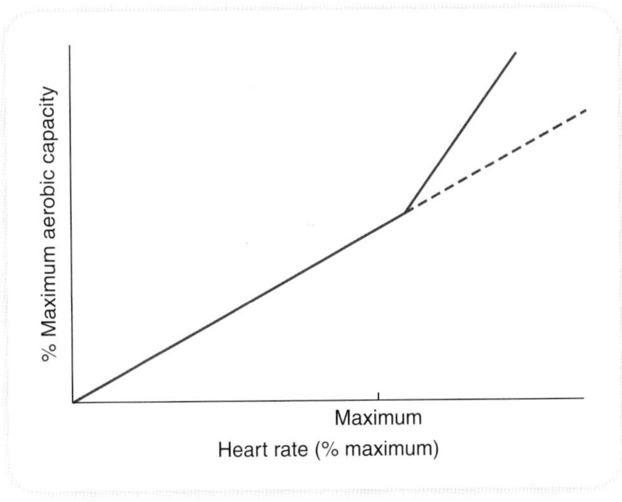

Figure 7-2 Maximum heart rate

Maximum heart rate is achieved at about the same time as maximal aerobic capacity.

Stroke Volume

A second mechanism by which the cardiovascular system is able to adapt to increased demands of cardiac output during exercise is to increase *stroke volume* (the volume of blood being pumped out with each beat).[12] Stroke volume is equal to the difference between end diastolic volume and end systolic volume. Tyical values for stroke volume range from 60 to 100 mL per beat at rest and 100 to 120 mL per beat at maximum.[18] Stroke volume will continue to increase only to the point at which diastolic filling time is simply too short to allow adequate filling. This occurs at approximately 40% to 50% of maximal aerobic capacity, or at a heart rate of 110 to 120 beats per minute; above this level, increases in the cadiac output are accounted for by increases in heart rate (Figure 7-3).[18]

Cardiac Output

Stroke volume and heart rate collectively determine the volume of blood being pumped through the heart in a given unit of time. Approximately 5 L of blood are pumped through

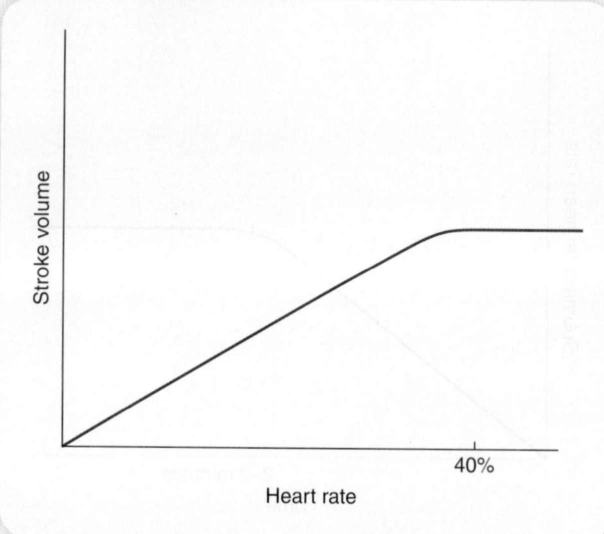

Figure 7-3 Stroke volume plateaus

Stroke volume plateaus at approximately 40% of maximal heart rate.

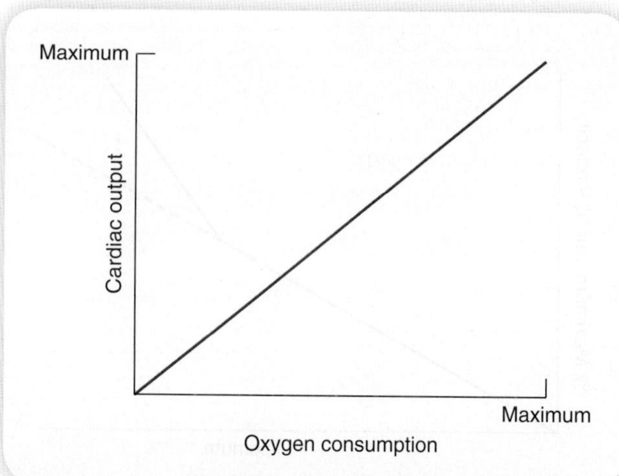

Figure 7-4 Cardiac output limits maximal aerobic capacity

the heart during each minute at rest. This is referred to as the *cardiac output*, which indicates how much blood the heart is capable of pumping in exactly 1 minute. Thus cardiac output is the primary determinant of the maximal rate of oxygen consumption possible (Figure 7-4). During exercise, cardiac output increases to approximately 4 times that experienced during rest (to approximately 20 L) in the normal individual, and may increase as much as 6 times in the elite endurance athlete (to approximately 31 L).

Cardiac output = stroke volume × heart rate

The above equation illustrates that any factor that will impact heart rate or stroke volume can either increase or decrease cardiac output. For example, an increase in venous return of blood from working muscle will increase the end diastolic volume. This increased volume will increase stroke volume via the Frank Starling mechanism[49] and, therefore, cardiac output.[57] Heart rate is regulated by the autonomic nervous system as well as circulating levels of Epinephrine secreted from the adrenal medulla. Conversely, conditions that resist ventricular outflow (high blood pressure or an increase in afterload) will result in a decrease in cardiac output. Conversely, a condition that would decrease venous return (peripheral artery disease) would decrease stroke volume and attenuate cardiac output. Figure 7-5 outlines the factors that regulate both stroke volume and heart rate.

A commonly reported benefit of aerobic conditioning is a reduced resting heart rate and a reduced heart rate at a standard exercise load. This reduction in heart rate is explained by an increase in stroke volume brought about by increased venous return and to increased contractile conditions in the myocardium. The heart becomes more efficient because it is capable of pumping more blood with each stroke. Because the heart is a muscle, it can hypertrophy, or increase in size and strength as a result of aerobic exercise, to some extent, but this is in no way a negative effect of training.

Training Effect

Increased stroke volume × decreased heart rate = cardiac output

During exercise, females tend to have a 5% to 10% higher cardiac output than males at all intensities. This is likely the result of a lower concentration of hemoglobin in the female, which is compensated for during exercise by an increased cardiac output.[59]

Adaptation in Blood Flow

The amount of blood flowing to the various organs increases during exercise. However, there is a change in overall distribution of cardiac output: the percentage of total cardiac output to the nonessential organs is decreased, whereas it is increased to active skeletal muscle.

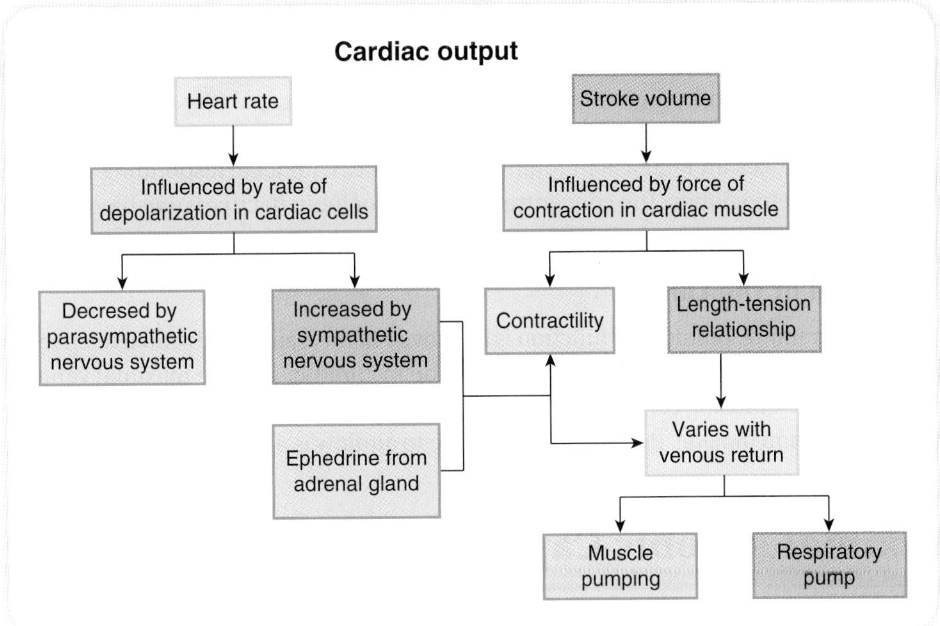

Figure 7-5 **The factors effecting cardiac output**

Volume of blood flow to the heart muscle or myocardium increases substantially during exercise, even though the percentage of total cardiac output supplying the heart muscle remains unchanged. The increase in flow to skeletal muscle is brought about by withdrawal of sympathetic stimulation to arterioles, and vasodilation is maintained by intrinsic metabolic control.[40] Trained persons have a higher capillary density than their untrained counterparts to better accommodate the increased supply and demand. In skeletal muscle, there is increased formation of blood vessels or capillaries, although it is not clear whether new ones form or dormant ones simply open up and fill with blood.[49]

The total peripheral resistance (TPR) is the sum of all forces that resist blood flow within the vascular system. TPR decreases during exercise primarily because of vessel vasodilation in the active skeletal muscles.

Blood Pressure

Blood pressure in the arterial system is determined by the cardiac output in relation to TPR to blood flow as follows:

$$BP = CO \times TPR$$

where BP = blood pressure, CO = cardiac output, and TPR = total peripheral resistance.

Blood pressure is created by contraction of the myocardium. Contraction of the ventricles of the heart creates systolic pressure, and relaxation of the heart creates diastolic pressure. Blood pressure is regulated centrally by neural activity on peripheral arterioles and locally by metabolites produced during exercise. During exercise, there is a decrease in TPR (via decreased vasoconstriction) and an increase in cardiac output. Systolic pressure increases in proportion to oxygen consumption and cardiac output, whereas diastolic pressure shows little or no increase.[6] Failure of systolic pressure to increase with increased exercise intensity is considered an abnormal response to exercise and is a general indication to stop an exercise test or session.[1] Blood pressure falls below preexercise levels after exercise and may stay low for several hours. There is general agreement that engaging in consistent aerobic exercise will produce modest reductions in both systolic and diastolic blood pressure at rest as well as during submaximal exercise.[10,15]

Adaptations in the Blood

Oxygen is transported throughout the system bound to *hemoglobin.* Found in red blood cells, hemoglobin is an iron-containing protein that has the capability of easily accepting or giving up molecules of oxygen as needed. Training for improvement of cardiorespiratory endurance produces an increase in total blood volume, with a corresponding increase in the amount of hemoglobin. The concentration of hemoglobin in circulating blood does not change with training; it may actually decrease slightly.

Adaptation of the Lungs

As a result of training, pulmonary function is improved in the trained individual relative to the untrained individual. The volume of air that can be inspired in a single maximal ventilation is increased. The diffusing capacity of the lungs is also increased, facilitating the exchange of oxygen and carbon dioxide. Pulmonary resistance to air flow is also decreased.[35]

Maximal Aerobic Capacity

The maximal amount of oxygen that can be used during exercise is referred to as *maximal aerobic capacity* (exercise physiologists refer to this as $\dot{V}O_{2max}$). It is considered to be the best indicator of the level of cardiorespiratory endurance. Maximal aerobic capacity is most often presented in terms of the volume of oxygen used relative to body weight per unit of time ($mL \times kg^{-1} \times min^{-1}$).[3]

It is common to see aerobic capacity expressed in metabolic equivalents (METs). Resting oxygen consumption is generally considered to be 3.5 $mL \times kg^{-1} \times min^{-1}$ or 1 MET. Therefore, an exercise intensity of 10 METs is equivalent to a $\dot{V}O_2$ of 35 $mL \times kg^{-1} \times min^{-1}$. A normal maximal aerobic capacity for most collegiate men and women would fall in the range of 35 to 50 $mL \times kg^{-1} \times min^{-1}$.[35]

Rate of Oxygen Consumption

The performance of any activity requires a certain rate of oxygen consumption, which is about the same for all persons, depending on their present level of fitness. Generally, the greater the rate or intensity of the performance of an activity, the greater will be the oxygen consumption. Each person has his or her own maximal rate of oxygen consumption. The person's ability to perform an activity is closely related to the amount of oxygen required by that activity. This ability is limited by the maximal amount of oxygen the person is capable of delivering into the lungs. Fatigue occurs when insufficient oxygen is supplied to muscles. It should be apparent that the greater the percentage of maximal aerobic capacity required during an activity, the less time the activity may be performed (see Figure 7-6).

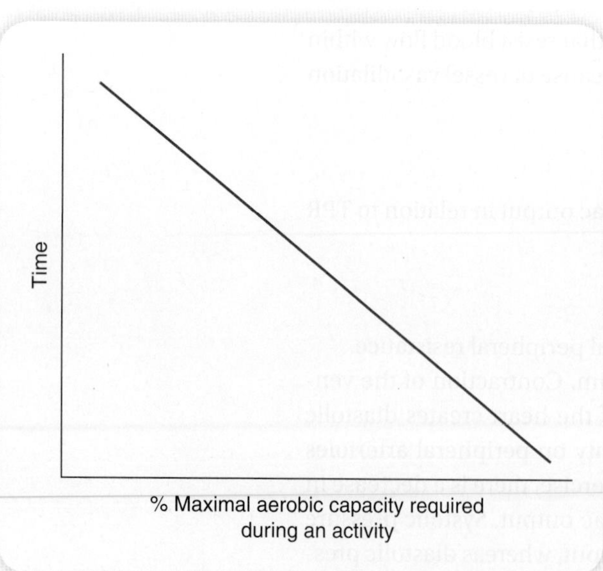

Figure 7-6 Maximal aerobic capacity required during activity

The greater the percentage of maximal aerobic capacity required during an activity, the less time that activity can be performed.

Three factors determine the maximal rate at which oxygen can be used: (a) external respiration, involving the ventilatory process or pulmonary function; (b) gas transport, which is accomplished by the cardiovascular system (that is, the heart, blood vessels, and blood); and (c) internal (cellular) respiration, which involves the use of oxygen by the cells to produce energy. Exercise physiologists generally discuss the limiting factors of maximal aerobic capacity based on healthy human subjects in a controlled environment.[4,27,28] Under these conditions, research presents agreement that the ability to transport oxygen through the heart, lungs, and blood is the limiting factor to the overall rate of oxygen consumption. This indicates that this is not the ability of the mitochondria to consume oxygen that limits $\dot{V}O_{2max}$. A high maximal aerobic capacity within a person's range indicates that all 3 systems are working well.

Maximal Aerobic Capacity: An Inherited Characteristic

The maximal rate at which oxygen can be used is a genetically determined characteristic; we inherit a certain range of maximal aerobic capacity, and the more active we are, the higher the existing maximal aerobic capacity will be within that range.[47,58] Therefore, a training program is capable of increasing maximal aerobic capacity to its highest limit within our range.[43,50,58]

Fast-Twitch Versus Slow-Twitch Muscle Fibers

The range of maximal aerobic capacity inherited is in a large part determined by the metabolic and functional properties of skeletal muscle fibers. As discussed in detail in Chapter 6, there are 3 distinct types of muscle fibers, *slow-twitch* and 2 variations of *fast-twitch* fibers, each of which has distinctive metabolic and contractile capabilities. Because they are relatively fatigue resistant, slow-twitch fibers are associated primarily with long-duration, aerobic-type activities. The slow-twitch fibers depend on oxidative phosphorylation to generate adenosine triphosphate (ATP) to provide the energy needed for muscle contraction. Fast-twitch fibers are useful in short-term, high-intensity activities, which mainly involve the anaerobic system. Intermediated fast-twitch fibers demonstrate a reliance on glycolysis to produce ATP. These intermediate fibers also have the ability to adapt based on specific training regimens.[49] In general, if a patient has a high ratio of slow-twitch to fast-twitch muscle fibers, the patient will be able to use oxygen more efficiently and thus will have a higher maximal aerobic capacity.

Cardiorespiratory Endurance and Work Ability

Cardiorespiratory endurance plays a critical role in our ability to carry out normal daily activities.[40] Fatigue is closely related to the percentage of maximal aerobic capacity that a particular workload demands.[49] For example, Figure 7-7 presents 2 people, A and B. A has maximal aerobic capacity of 50 mL/kg per minute, whereas B has a maximal aerobic capacity of only 40 mL/kg per minute. If both A and B are exercising at the same intensity, then A will be working at a much lower percentage of maximal aerobic capacity than B. Consequently, A should be able to sustain his or her activity over a much longer period of time. Everyday activities may be adversely affected if the ability to use oxygen efficiently is impaired. Thus, improvement of cardiorespiratory endurance should be an essential component of any conditioning program and must be included as part of the rehabilitation program for the injured patient.[9]

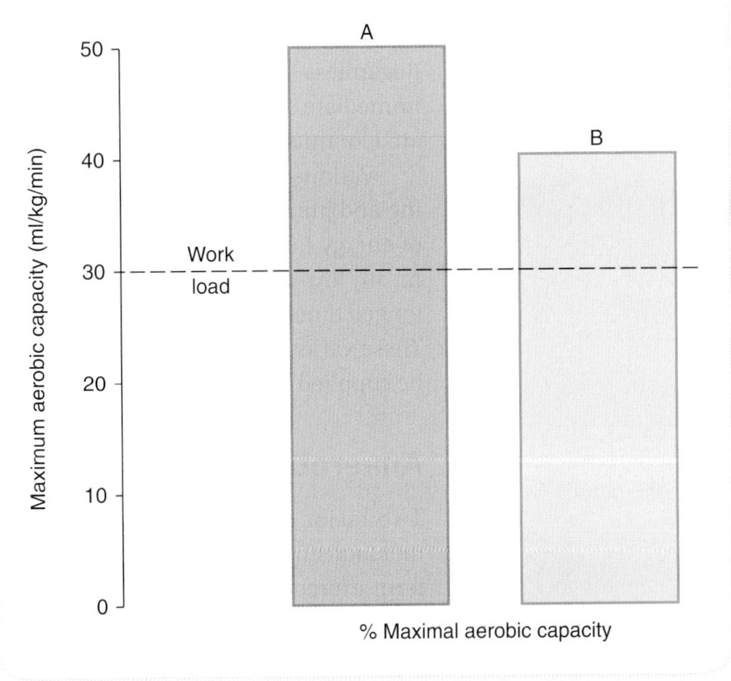

Figure 7-7

Patient A should be able to work longer than patient B as a result of a lower percentage use of maximal aerobic capacity.

Regardless of the training technique used for the improvement of cardiorespiratory endurance, one principal goal remains the same: *to increase the ability of the cardiorespiratory system to supply a sufficient amount of oxygen to working muscles.* Without oxygen, the body is incapable of producing energy for an extended period of time.

Producing Energy for Exercise

All living systems need to perform a variety of activities, such as growing, generating energy, repairing damaged tissues, and eliminating wastes. All of these activities are referred to as being metabolic or as cellular *metabolism*.

Muscles are metabolically active and must generate energy to move. Energy is produced from the breakdown of certain nutrients from foodstuffs. This energy is stored in a compound called ATP, which is the ultimate usable form of energy for muscular activity. ATP is produced in the muscle tissue from blood glucose or glycogen. Fats and proteins can also be metabolized to generate ATP. Glucose not needed immediately can be stored as glycogen in the resting muscle and liver. Stored glycogen in the liver can later be converted back to glucose and transferred to the blood to meet the body's energy needs.[7]

It is important to understand that the intensity and duration of exercise selected as an intervention will have implications on the source of "fuel" to engage in the activity. The "fuel" is the ATP needed for muscular contraction. Exercise intensity and duration effect the source or pathway that is used to supply the ATP; that is, does the ATP come from the breakdown of circulating blood glucose (glycolysis) or from the Krebs cycle and the electron transport chain (oxidative phosphorlization)?

If the combination of duration and intensity is low (40% to 50% of $\dot{V}o_{2max}$), the body relies more heavily on fats stored in adipose tissue to meet its energy needs. The longer the duration of an activity, the greater the amount of fat used, especially during the later stages of endurance events. During rest and submaximal exertion, both fat and carbohydrates are used to provide energy in approximately a 60%-to-40% ratio. Carbohydrate must be available to use fat. If glycogen is totally depleted, fat cannot be completely metabolized. Regardless of the nutrient source that produces ATP, it is always available in the cell as an immediate energy source. When all available sources of ATP are used, more must be generated for muscular contraction to continue.[8,29]

Various sports activities involve specific demands for energy. For example, sprinting and jumping are high-energy-output activities, requiring a relatively large production of energy for a short time. Long-distance running and swimming, on the other hand, are mostly low-energy-output activities per unit of time, requiring energy production for a prolonged time. Other physical activities demand a blend of both high- and low-energy output. These various energy demands can be met by the different processes in which energy can be supplied to the skeletal muscles.[17]

Anaerobic Versus Aerobic Metabolism

Two major energy-generating systems function in muscle tissue: anaerobic and aerobic metabolism. Each of these systems produces ATP.[21] Activities that demand intensive, short-term exercise need ATP that is rapidly available and metabolized to meet energy needs. The primary source for ATP production in short-term high-intensity exercise is phosphocreatine system. Tissues only store enough phosphocreatine to generate ATP for events lasting approximately 10 seconds or less. After a few seconds of intensive exercise, however, the small stores of ATP are used up. The body then utilizes stored glycogen as an energy source. Glycogen can be broken down to supply glucose, which is then metabolized within the muscle cells to generate ATP for muscle contractions.[38]

Glucose can be metabolized to generate small amounts of ATP energy without the need for oxygen. This energy system is referred to as *anaerobic metabolism* (occurring in the absence of oxygen). As exercise continues, the body has to rely on a more complex form of carbohydrate and fat metabolism to generate ATP. This second energy system requires oxygen and is therefore referred to as *aerobic metabolism* (occurring in the presence of oxygen). The aerobic system of producing energy generates considerably more ATP than the anaerobic one.

In most activities, both aerobic and anaerobic systems function simultaneously. The degree to which the 2 major energy systems are involved is determined by the intensity and duration of the activity.[55] If the intensity of the activity is such that sufficient oxygen can be supplied to meet the demands of working tissues, the activity is considered to be *aerobic*. Conversely, if the activity is of high-enough intensity, or the duration is such that there is insufficient oxygen available to meet energy demands, the activity becomes *anaerobic*.[51]

Excess Postexercise Oxygen Consumption

As the intensity of the exercise increases and insufficient amounts of oxygen are available to the tissues, an oxygen deficit is incurred. Oxygen deficit occurs in the beginning of exercise (within the first 2 to 3 minutes) when the oxygen demand is greater than the oxygen supplied. It was been hypothesized that this oxygen debt was caused by lactic acid produced during anaerobic activity, and this debt must be "paid back" during the postexercise period. However, there is presently a different rationale for this oxygen deficit, which is currently referred to as "excess postexercise oxygen consumption." It is theoretically caused by disturbances in mitochondrial function from an increase in temperature.[38] Additional explanations include evidence of both a "fast" and a "slow" component. The fast components include the restoration of phosphocreatine levels depleted in the earliest seconds of exercise, and replacing stored muscle and blood oxygen content. The slow portion is accounted for by providing the energy for the elevated respiratory rate and heart rate, elevated levels of catecholamines and gluconeogenesis, the conversion of lactic acid to glucose.[44]

Techniques for Maintaining Cardiorespiratory Endurance

Several different training techniques may be incorporated into a rehabilitation program through which cardiorespiratory endurance can be maintained. Certainly, a primary consideration for the therapist is whether the injury involves the upper or lower extremity. With injuries that involve the upper extremity, weightbearing activities can be used, such as walking, running, stair climbing, and modified aerobics. However, if the injury is to the lower extremity, alternative non-weightbearing activities, such as swimming or stationary cycling, may be necessary. The goal of the therapist is to try to maintain cardiorespiratory endurance throughout the rehabilitation process.

The principles of the training techniques discussed next can be applied to running, cycling, swimming, stair climbing, or any other activity designed to maintain levels of cardiorespiratory fitness.

Continuous Training

Continuous training involves the following considerations:

- The frequency of the activity
- The intensity of the activity
- The type of activity
- The time (duration) of the activity

Frequency of Training

The American College of Sports Medicine (ACSM) recommends that most adults engage in moderate-intensity cardiorespiratory exercise training for ≥30 min•day^{-1} on ≥5 days•wk^{-1} for a total of ≥150 min•wk^{-1}, vigorous-intensity cardiorespiratory exercise training for ≥20 min•day^{-1} on ≥3 days•wk^{-1} (≥75 min•wk^{-1}), or a combination of moderate- and vigorous-intensity exercise to achieve a total energy expenditure of ≥500 to 1000 MET•min•wk^{-1}.[1] A competitive athlete should be prepared to train as often as 6 times per week. Everyone should take off at least 1 day per week to give damaged tissues a chance to repair themselves.

Intensity of Training

The intensity of exercise is also a critical factor, although recommendations regarding training intensities vary.[25] This statement is particularly true in the early stages of training, when the body is forced to make a magnitude of adjustments to increased workload demands. The ACSM guidelines regarding intensity of exercise recommend the following: 55%/65% to 90% of MHR, or 40%/50% to 85% of maximum oxygen uptake reserve ($\dot{V}O_2R$) or MHR reserve (hear rate reserve [HRR]). HRR and $\dot{V}O_2R$ are calculated from the difference between resting and maximum heart rate and resting and maximum $\dot{V}O_2$, respectively. To estimate training intensity, a percentage of this value is added to the resting heart rate and/or resting $\dot{V}O_2$ and is expressed as a percentage of HRR or $\dot{V}O_2R$. The lower-intensity values, that is, 40% to 49% of $\dot{V}O_2R$ or HRR and 55% to 64% of MHR, are most applicable to individuals who are quite unfit. These intensities require the therapist to either know the person's maximal values or use a prediction equation to estimate these intensities. A great rule of thumb is to always go with actual data over prediction data when available. There are many limitations to prediction equations. Because of the linear relationship between heart rate, oxygen consumption, and exercise intensity, it becomes a relatively simple process to identify a specific workload (pace) that will make the heart rate plateau at the desired level.[52] By monitoring heart rate, we know whether the pace is too fast or too slow to achieve the desired range of intensity.[33] Prior to selecting an exercise intensity, the therapist should consider several factors, including current level of fitness, medications, cardiovascular risk profile, an individual's likes and dislikes, and patient's goals and objectives.[1]

Monitoring Heart Rate There are several methods for measuring heart rate response during exercise. These include, but are not limited to, palpation of the heart rate at the radial or carotid artery, pulse oximetry, telemetry (heart rate monitors), and electrocardiography. One of the easiest methods is to palpate the radial artery. This assessment can be done by the patient or the therapist. The carotid artery is simple to find, especially during exercise. However, there are pressure (baro) receptors located in the carotid artery that, if subjected to hard pressure from the 2 fingers, will slow down the heart rate, giving a false indication of exactly what the heart rate is. Thus, the pulse at the radial artery proves the most accurate measure of heart rate. Regardless of where the heart rate is taken, it should be recorded prior to exercise, during exercise to ensure target intensities, and monitored following exercise to ensure recovery. Another factor must be considered when measuring heart rate during exercise. The patient is trying to elevate heart rate to a specific target rate and maintain it at that level during the entire workout.[22] Heart rate can be increased or decreased by speeding up or slowing down the pace. Based on the fact that heart rates will attain a steady state or plateau to a prescribed work rate in 2 to 3 minutes, the therapist should allow sufficient time prior to assessment of heart rate. Thus, the patient should be actively engaged in the workout for 2 to 3 minutes before measuring pulse.[61]

There are several formulas that will easily allow the therapist to identify a target training heart rate.[42] Exact determination of MHR involves exercising a patient at a maximal level and monitoring the heart rate using an electrocardiography. This process is difficult outside of a laboratory. However, an approximate estimate of MHR for both males and females in the population is thought to be 220 beats per minute.[45] MHR is related to age. With aging,

MHR decreases.[34] Thus, a relatively simple estimate of MHR would be MHR = 220 – age. For a 40-year-old patient, MHR would be approximately 180 beats per minute (220 – 40 = 180). If you are interested in working at 70% of your MHR, the target heart rate can be calculated by multiplying 0.7 × (220 – age). The intensity range of 70% to 85% of MHR approximates 55% to 75% of $\dot{V}O_{2max}$. Again using a 40-year-old person as an example, a target heart rate would be 126 beats per minute (0.7 × [220 – 40] = 126).

Another commonly used formula that takes into account your current level of fitness is the Karvonen equation, sometimes referred to as the *HRR* method.[26,30]

Target training HR = Resting HR + (0.6[Maximum HR – Resting HR])

Resting heart rate generally falls between 60 and 80 beats per minute. A 40-year-old patient with a resting pulse of 70 beats per minute, according to the Karvonen equation, would have a target training heart rate of 136 beats per minute (70 + 0.6[180 – 70] = 136).

Regardless of the formula used, to see minimal improvement in cardiorespiratory endurance, the patient must train with the heart rate elevated to at least 60% of its maximal rate.[1,23,31] Exercising at a 70% level is considered moderate, because activity can be continued for a long period of time with little discomfort and still produce a training effect.[39] In a trained individual, it is not difficult to sustain a heart rate at the 85% level.[14]

Clinical Pearl

In the event that the physical therapist has data indicating that the heart rate is at the ventilatory threshold, that rate can be used to prescribe exercise. The risk of a cardiac event increases, the closer the heart rate is to the ventilatory threshold; therefore, prescribing exercise 10 beats per minute below that level will keep the risk low.

Rating of Perceived Exertion Rating of perceived exertion can be used in addition to monitoring heart rate to indicate exercise intensity.[5] During exercise, individuals are asked to rate subjectively on a numerical scale from 6 to 20 exactly how they feel relative to their level of exertion (Table 7-1). More intense exercise that requires a higher level of oxygen consumption and energy expenditure is directly related to higher subjective ratings of perceived exertion. The use of a rating-of-perceived-exertion scale is the preferred method of monitoring the exercise intensity of individuals who are taking medications, beta blockers for example, that attenuate the normal heart rate response to exercise. Over a period of time, patients can be taught to exercise at a specific rating of perceived exertion that relates directly to more objective measures of exercise intensity.[20,40]

Table 7-1 Rating of Perceived Exertion

Scale	Verbal Rating
6	
7	Very, very light
8	
9	Very light
10	
11	Fairly light
12	
13	Somewhat hard
14	
15	Hard
16	
17	Very hard
18	
19	Very, very hard
20	

Source: Borg GA. Psychophysical basis of perceived exertion. *Med Sci Sports Exerc* 1982;14:377.

Type of Exercise

The type of activity used in continuous training must be aerobic. Aerobic activities are activities that generally involve repetitive, whole-body, large-muscle movements that are rhythmical in nature and use large amounts of oxygen, elevate the heart rate, and maintain it at that level for an extended period of time. Examples of aerobic activities are walking, running, jogging, cycling, swimming, rope skipping, stepping, aerobic dance exercise, rollerblading, and cross-country skiing.

The advantage of these aerobic activities as opposed to more intermittent activities, such as racquetball, squash, basketball, or tennis, is that aerobic activities are easy to regulate in intensity by either speeding up or slowing down the pace.[37] Because we already know that a given intensity of the workload elicits a given heart rate, these aerobic activities allow us to maintain heart rate at a specified or target level. Intermittent activities involve variable speeds and intensities that cause the heart rate to fluctuate considerably. Although these intermittent activities will improve cardiorespiratory endurance, they are much more difficult to monitor in terms of intensity. It is important to point out that any type of activity, from gardening to aerobic exercise, can improve fitness.[42]

Time (Duration)

For minimal improvement to occur, the patient must participate in at least 20 minutes of continuous activity with the heart rate elevated to its working level. The ACSM recommends duration of training to be 20 to 60 minutes of continuous or intermittent (minimum of 10-minute bouts accumulated throughout the day) aerobic activity. Duration varies with the intensity of the activity. Lower-intensity activity should be conducted over a longer period of time (30 minutes or more). Patients training at higher levels of intensity should train at least 20 minutes or longer "because of the importance of 'total fitness' and that it is more readily attained with exercise sessions of longer duration and because of the potential hazards and adherence problems associated with high-intensity activity, moderate-intensity activity of longer duration is recommended for adults not training for athletic competition" (see the Appendix).

Generally, the greater the duration of the workout, the greater the improvement in cardiorespiratory endurance.

Interval Training

Unlike continuous training, *interval training* involves activities that are more intermittent. Interval training consists of alternating periods of relatively intense work and active recovery. It allows for performance of much more work at a more intense workload over a longer period of time than if working continuously. It is most desirable in continuous training to work at an intensity of approximately 60% to 80% of MHR. Obviously, sustaining activity at a relatively high intensity over a 20-minute period is extremely difficult. The advantage of interval training is that it allows work at this 80% or higher level for a short period of time followed by an active period of recovery during which you may be working at only 30% to 45% of MHR. Thus, the intensity of the workout and its duration can be greater than with continuous training.

There are several important considerations in interval training. The training period is the amount of time in which continuous activity is actually being performed, and the recovery period is the time between training periods. A set is a group of combined training and recovery periods, and a repetition is the number of training/recovery periods per set. Training time or distance refers to the rate or distance of the training period. The training/recovery ratio indicates a time ratio for training versus recovery.

An example of interval training is a patient exercising on a stationary bike. An interval workout involves 10 repetitions of pedaling at a maximum speed for 20 seconds followed by pedaling at 40% of maximum speed for 90 seconds. During this interval training session, heart rate will probably increase to 85% to 95% of maximal level while pedaling at maximum speed and will probably fall to the 35% to 45% level during the recovery period.

Older adults should exercise some caution when using interval training as a method for improving cardiorespiratory endurance. The intensity levels attained during the active periods may be too high and create undue risk for the older adult.

Caloric Thresholds and Targets

The interplay between the duration, intensity, and frequency of exercise creates a caloric expenditure from exercise sessions. The amount of caloric expenditure is important to a wide range of patients, including those interested in weight loss, as well as those under very strenuous training regimens. General acceptance exists such that the health benefits and training changes associated with exercise programs are related to the total amount of work (indicated by caloric expenditure) completed during training.[1] These caloric thresholds may be different to elicit improvements in $\dot{V}O_{2max}$, weight loss, or risk of premature chronic disease. The ACSM recommends a range of 150 to 400 calories of energy expenditure per day in exercise or physical activity. Expenditure of 1000 kcal per week should be the initial goal for those not previously engaged in regular activity. Patients should be moved toward the upper end of the recommendation (300 to 400 kcal per day) to obtain optimal fitness. The estimation of caloric expenditure is easily accomplished using the METs associated with a given activity and the formula[1]:

$$(MET \times 3.5 \times \text{body weight in kg})/200 = \text{kcal/min}$$

Numerous charts and tables exist that estimate activities in terms of intensity requirements expressed in METs. If a weekly goal of 1000 kcal is established for a 70-kg person at an intensity of 6 METs, the caloric expenditure would be calculated as follows:

$$(6 \times 3.5 \times 70 \text{ kg})/200 = \text{kcal/min}$$

At an exercise intensity of 6 METs, the patient would need to exercise 136 minutes to achieve the 1000 kcal goal. If the patient wants to exercise 4 days each week, 34 minutes of exercise each of the 4 days will be required.

The primary goal of weight loss is to consume or burn more calories than are taken in (eaten). The calories used during exercise can be added to the calories cut from the diet to calculate total caloric deficit needed to create weight loss. The aforementioned patient could reduce his or her caloric intake by 400 kcal each day. This will total 2800 kcal that have been restricted from the diet. These calories are then added to the 1000 kcal used for exercise. A pound of fat is equivalent to 3500 kcal. The combination of reduced caloric intake and increased used of kcal for exercise in the example is 3800 kcal, or slightly more than 1 pound of weight loss in 1 week.

Combining Continuous and Interval Training

As indicated previously, most physical activities involve some combination of aerobic and anaerobic metabolism.[60] Continuous training is generally done at an intensity level that primarily uses the aerobic system. In interval training, the intensity is sufficient to necessitate a greater percentage of anaerobic metabolism.[19] Therefore, for the physically active patient, the therapist should incorporate both training techniques into a rehabilitation program to maximize cardiorespiratory fitness.

Detraining

Physical training promotes a wide range of physiologic training. These include increased size and number of mitochondria, increased capillary bed density, changes in resting and exercise heart rate, blood pressure, myocardial oxygen consumption, and improved

$\dot{V}O_{2max}$ to mention a few. It would seem logical that if the stimulus (exercise) is removed, these changes will dissipate. Long periods of inactivity are associated with the reversal of the aforementioned changes. Improvements may be lost in as little as 12 days to as long as several months to see a complete reversal of changes.

SUMMARY

1. The therapist should routinely incorporate activities that will help maintain levels of cardiorespiratory endurance into the rehabilitation program.
2. Cardiorespiratory endurance involves the coordinated function of the heart, lungs, blood, and blood vessels to supply sufficient amounts of oxygen to the working tissues.
3. The best indicator of how efficiently the cardiorespiratory system functions is the maximal rate at which oxygen can be used by the tissues.
4. Heart rate is directly related to the rate of oxygen consumption. It is therefore possible to predict the intensity of the work in terms of a rate of oxygen use by monitoring heart rate.
5. Aerobic exercise involves an activity in which the level of intensity and duration is low enough to provide a sufficient amount of oxygen to supply the demands of the working tissues.
6. In anaerobic exercise, the intensity of the activity is so high that oxygen is being used more quickly than it can be supplied; thus, an oxygen debt is incurred that must be repaid before working tissue can return to its normal resting state.
7. Continuous or sustained training for maintenance of cardiorespiratory endurance involves selecting an activity that is aerobic in nature and training at least 3 times per week for a time period of no less than 20 minutes with the heart rate elevated to at least 60% of maximal rate.
8. Interval training involves alternating periods of relatively intense work followed by active recovery periods. Interval training allows performance of more work at a relatively higher workload than continuous training.
9. Aerobic exercise is a very powerful tool when considering the decreased mortality and morbidity associated with improvements in functional capacity. The therapist with a working knowledge of the principles of exercise prescription and testing are best capable of ensuring the safety and effectiveness of interventions.

REFERENCES

1. American College of Sports Medicine. *ACSM's Guidelines for Exercise Testing and Prescription*. 8th ed. Philadelphia, PA: Lippincott Williams & Wilkins; 2010:366.
2. Åstrand PO, Rodahl K. *Textbook of Work Physiology*. New York, NY: McGraw-Hill; 1986.
3. Åstrand PO. Åstrand-rhyming nomogram for calculation of aerobic capacity from pulse rate during submaximal work. *J Appl Physiol.* 1954;7:218.
4. Bassett D, Howley E. Limiting factors for maximal oxygen uptake and determinants of endurance performance. *Med Sci Sports Exerc.* 2000;32:70-84.
5. Borg GA. Psychophysical basis of perceived exertion. *Med Sci Sports Exerc.* 1982;14:377.
6. Brooks G, Fahey T, White T. *Exercise Physiology: Human Bioenergetics and Its Applications*. New York, NY: McGraw-Hill; 2004.

7. Brooks G, Mercier J. The balance of carbohydrate and lipid utilization during exercise: The crossover concept. *J Appl Physiol.* 1994;76:2253-2261.
8. Cerretelli P. Energy sources for muscle contraction. *Sports Med.* 1992;13:S106-S110.
9. Chillag SA. Endurance patients: physiologic changes and nonorthopedic problems. *South Med J.* 1986; 79:1264.
10. Convertino VA. Aerobic fitness, endurance training, and orthostatic intolerance. *Exerc Sport Sci Rev.* 1987;15:223.
11. Cooper KH. *The Aerobics Program for Total Well-Being.* New York, NY: Bantam Books; 1982.
12. Cox M. Exercise training programs and cardiorespiratory adaptation. *Clin Sports Med.* 1991;10:19-32.
13. deVries H. *Physiology of Exercise for Physical Education and Athletics.* Dubuque, IA: William C. Brown; 1986.
14. Dicarlo L, Sparling P, Millard-Stafford M. Peak heart rates during maximal running and swimming: implications for exercise prescription. *Int J Sports Med.* 1991;12: 309-312.
15. Durstein L, Pate R, Branch D. Cardiorespiratory responses to acute exercise. In: American College of Sports Medicine. *Resource Manual for Guidelines for Exercise Testing and Prescription.* Philadelphia, PA: Lea & Febiger; 1993.
16. Fahey T, ed. *Encyclopedia of Sports Medicine and Exercise Physiology.* New York, NY: Garland; 1995.
17. Fox E, Bowers R, Foss M. *The Physiological Basis of Physical Education and Athletics.* Philadelphia, PA: Saunders; 1981.
18. Franklin B. Cardiorespiratory responses to acute exercise. In: American College of Sports Medicine. *Resource Manual for Guidelines for Exercise Testing and Prescription,* 4th ed. Philadelphia, PA: Lippincott Williams & Wilkins; 2010:164.
19. Gaesser GA, Wilson LA. Effects of continuous and interval training on the parameters of the power-endurance time relationship for high-intensity exercise. *Int J Sports Med.* 1988;9:417.
20. Glass S, Whaley M, Wegner M. A comparison between ratings of perceived exertion among standard protocols and steady state running. *Int J Sports Med.* 1991;12:77-82.
21. Green J, Patla A. Maximal aerobic power: neuromuscular and metabolic considerations. *Med Sci Sports Exerc.* 1992;24:38-46.
22. Greer N, Katch F. Validity of palpation recovery pulse rate to estimate exercise heart rate following four intensities of bench step exercise. *Res Q Exerc Sport.* 1982;53:340.
23. Hage P. Exercise guidelines: Which to believe? *Phys Sportsmed.* 1982;10:23.
24. Haskell WL, Lee IM, Pate RR, et al. Physical activity and public health: updated recommendation for adults from the American College of Sports Medicine and the American Heart Association. *Med Sci Sports Exerc.* 2007;39(8):1423-1434.
25. Hawley J, Myburgh K, Noakes T. Maximal oxygen consumption: a contemporary perspective. In: Fahey T, ed. *Encyclopedia of Sports Medicine and Exercise Physiology.* New York, NY: Garland; 1995.
26. Hickson RC, Foster C, Pollac M, et al. Reduced training intensities and loss of aerobic power, endurance, and cardiac growth. *J Appl Physiol.* 1985;58:492.
27. Hill A, Long C, Lupton H. Muscular exercise, Lactic acid and the supply and utilization of oxygen. Parts VII-VIII. *Proc R Soc Lond B Biol Sci.* 1924;97:155-176.
28. Hill A, Lupton H. Muscular exercise, Lactic acid and the supply and utilization of oxygen. *Q J Med.* 1923;16: 135-171.
29. Honig C, Connett R, Gayeski T. O_2 transport and its interaction with metabolism. *Med Sci Sports Exerc.* 1992;24:47-53.
30. Karvonen MJ, Kentala E, Mustala O. The effects of training on heart rate: a longitudinal study. *Ann Med Exp Biol Fenn.* 1957;35:305.
31. Koyanagi A, Yamamoto K, Nishijima K. Recommendation for an exercise prescription to prevent coronary heart disease. *J Med Syst.* 1993;17:213-217.
32. Lee IM, Rexrode KM, Cook NR, Manson JE, Buring JE. Physical activity and coronary heart disease in women: is "no pain, no gain" passe? *JAMA.* 2001;285(11):1447-1454.
33. Levine G, Balady G. The benefits and risks of exercise testing: the exercise prescription. *Adv Intern Med.* 1993;38:57-79.
34. Londeree B, Moeschberger M. Effect of age and other factors on maximal heart rate. *Res Q Exerc Sport.* 1982;53:297.
35. MacDougall D, Sale D. Continuous vs. interval training: a review for the patient and coach. *Can J Appl Sport Sci.* 1981;6:93.
36. Manson JE, Greenland P, LaCroix AZ, et al. Walking compared with vigorous exercise for the prevention of cardiovascular events in women. *N Engl J Med.* 2002;347:716-725.
37. Marcinik EJ, Hogden K, Mittleman K, et al. Aerobic/calisthenic and aerobic/circuit weight training programs for Navy men: a comparative study. *Med Sci Sports Exerc.* 1985;17:482.
38. McArdle W, Katch F, Katch V. *Exercise Physiology, Energy, Nutrition, and Human Performance.* Philadelphia, PA: Lippincott Williams & Wilkins; 2001.
39. Mead W, Hartwig R. Fitness evaluation and exercise prescription. *Fam Pract.* 1981;13:1039.
40. Monahan T. Perceived exertion: an old exercise tool finds new applications. *Phys Sportsmed.* 1988; 16:174.
41. Myers J, Praksah M, Froelicher V, Do D, Partington S, Atwood J. Exercise capacity and mortality among men referred for exercise testing. *N Engl J Med.* 346 (11): 793-8041, 2002.
42. Pate R, Pratt M, Blair S. Physical activity and public health: a recommendation from the CDC and ACSM. *JAMA.* 1995;273:402-407.
43. Powers S. Fundamentals of exercise metabolism. In: American College of Sports Medicine. *Resource Manual for Guidelines for Exercise Testing and Prescription.* Philadelphia, PA: Lea & Febiger; 1993:133.

44. Powers S, Howley E. *Exercise Physiology: Theory and Application to Fitness and Performance.* New York, NY: McGraw Hill; 2009.

45. Rowland TW, Green GM. Anaerobic threshold and the determination of training target heart rates in premenarcheal girls. *Pediatr Cardiol.* 1989; 10:75.

46. Sandvik L, Erikssen J, Thaulow E, Erikssen G, Mundal R, Rodahl K. Physical fitness as a predictor of mortality among healthy, middle-aged Norwegian men. *N Engl J Med.* 1993;328:533-537.

47. Saltin B, Strange S. Maximal oxygen uptake: old and new arguments for a cardiovascular limitation. *Med Sci Sports Exerc.* 1992;24:30-37.

48. Sesso HD, Paffenbarger RS Jr, Lee IM. Physical activity and coronary heart disease in men: the Harvard Alumni Health Study. *Circulation.* 2000;102(9):975-980.

49. Silverthorn, D. *Human Physiology. An Integrated Approach.* Boston, MA: Pearson; 2012.

50. Smith M, Mitchell J. Cardiorespiratory adaptations to exercise training. In: American College of Sports Medicine. *Resource Manual for Guidelines for Exercise Testing and Prescription.* Philadelphia, PA: Lea & Febiger; 1993.

51. Stachenfeld N, Eskenazi M, Gleim G. Predictive accuracy of criteria used to assess maximal oxygen consumption. *Am Heart J.* 1992;123:922-925.

52. Swain D, Abernathy K, Smith C. Target heart rates for the development of cardiorespiratory fitness. *Med Sci Sports Exerc.* 1994;26:112-116.

53. Tanaka H, Monahan KD, Seals DR. Age-predicted maximal heart rate revisited. *J Am Coll Cardiol.* 2001;37(1):153-156.

54. Tanasescu M, Leitzmann MF, Rimm EB, Willett WC, Stampfer MJ, Hu FB. Exercise type and intensity in relation to coronary heart disease in men. *JAMA.* 2002;288(16):1994-2000.

55. Vago P, Mercier M, Ramonatxo M, et al. Is ventilatory anaerobic threshold a good index of endurance capacity? *Int J Sports Med.* 1987;8:190.

56. Wagner P. Central and peripheral aspects of oxygen transport and adaptations with exercise. *Sports Med.* 1991;11:133-142.

57. Weltman A, Weltman J, Ruh R, et al. Percentage of maximal heart rate reserve, and $\dot{V}O_2$ peak for determining endurance training intensity in sedentary women. *Int J Sports Med.* 1989;10:212. Review.

58. Weymans M, Reybrouck T. Habitual level of physical activity and cardiorespiratory endurance capacity in children. *Eur J Appl Physiol.* 1989;58:803.

59. Williford HN, Scharff-Olson M, Blessing DL. Exercise prescription for women: Special considerations. *Sports Med.* 1993;15:299-311.

60. Wilmore J, Costill D. *Physiology of Sport and Exercise.* Champaign, IL: Human Kinetics; 1994.

61. Zhang Y, Johnson M, Chow N. Effect of exercise testing protocol on parameters of aerobic function. *Med Sci Sports Exerc.* 1991;23:625-630.

62. U.S. Department of Health and Human Services. *Physical Activity Guidelines Advisory Committee Report,* 2008. Publication No. U0049. Washington, DC: ODPHP; 2008.

Appendix

Med Sci Sports Exerc. 2011;43(7):1334-1359.

American College of Sports Medicine Position Stand

Quantity and Quality of Exercise for Developing and Maintaining Cardiorespiratory, Musculoskeletal, and Neuromotor Fitness in Apparently Healthy Adults: Guidance for Prescribing Exercise

Carol Ewing Garber, PhD, FACSM, (Chair); Bryan Blissmer, PhD; Michael R. Deschenes, PhD, FACSM; Barry A. Franklin, PhD, FACSM; Michael J. Lamonte, PhD, FACSM; I-Min Lee, MD, ScD, FACSM; David C. Nieman, PhD, FACSM; David P. Swain, PhD, FACSM

Summary

The purpose of this Position Stand is to provide guidance to professionals who counsel and prescribe *individualized* exercise to apparently healthy adults of all ages. These recommendations also may apply to adults with certain chronic diseases or disabilities, when appropriately evaluated and advised by a health professional. This document supersedes the 1998 American College of Sports Medicine (ACSM) Position Stand, "The Recommended Quantity and Quality of Exercise for Developing and Maintaining Cardiorespiratory and Muscular Fitness, and Flexibility in Healthy Adults." The scientific evidence demonstrating the beneficial effects of exercise is indisputable, and the benefits of exercise far outweigh the risks in most adults. A program of regular exercise that includes cardiorespiratory, resistance, flexibility, and neuromotor exercise training *beyond* activities of daily living to improve and maintain physical fitness and health is *essential* for most adults. The ACSM recommends that most adults engage in moderate-intensity cardiorespiratory exercise training for ≥30 min•day^{-1} on ≥5 days•wk^{-1} for a total of ≥150 min•wk^{-1}, vigorous-intensity cardiorespiratory exercise training for ≥20 min•day^{-1} on ≥3 days•wk^{-1} (≥75 min•wk^{-1}), or a combination of moderate- and vigorous-intensity exercise to achieve a total energy expenditure of ≥500 to 1000 MET•min•wk^{-1}. On 2 to 3 days•wk^{-1}, adults should also perform resistance exercises for each of the major muscle groups, and neuromotor exercise involving balance, agility, and coordination. Crucial to maintaining joint range of movement, completing a series of flexibility exercises for each the major muscle-tendon groups (a total of 60 s per exercise) on ≥2 days•wk^{-1} is recommended. The exercise program should be modified according to an individual's habitual physical activity, physical function, health status, exercise responses, and stated goals. Adults who are unable or unwilling to meet the exercise targets outlined here still can benefit from engaging in amounts of exercise *less than* recommended. In addition to exercising regularly, there are health benefits in concurrently reducing total time engaged in sedentary pursuits and also by interspersing frequent, short bouts of standing and physical activity between periods of sedentary activity, even in physically active adults. Behaviorally based exercise interventions, the use of behavior change strategies, supervision by an experienced fitness instructor, and exercise that is pleasant and enjoyable can improve adoption and adherence to prescribed exercise programs. Educating adults about and screening for signs and symptoms of CHD (coronary heart disease) and gradual progression of exercise intensity and volume may reduce the risks of exercise.[54] Consultations with a medical professional and diagnostic exercise testing for CHD are useful when clinically indicated but are not recommended for universal screening to enhance the safety of exercise.

Many people are currently involved in cardiorespiratory fitness and resistance training programs, and efforts to promote participation in all forms of physical activity are being developed and implemented. Thus, the need for guidelines for exercise prescription is apparent. Based on the existing evidence concerning exercise prescription for healthy adults and the need for guidelines, the ACSM makes few recommendations for the quantity and quality of training for developing and maintaining cardiorespiratory fitness, body composition, muscular strength and endurance, and flexibility in the healthy adult.

How Much Physical Activity is Needed to Improve Health and Cardiorespiratory Fitness?

Several studies have supported a dose–response relationship between chronic physical activity levels and health outcomes,[24,62] such that greater benefit is associated with higher amounts of physical activity. Data regarding the specific quantity and quality of physical activity for the attainment of the health benefits are less clear. Epidemiologic studies have estimated the *volume* of physical activity needed to achieve specific health benefits, typically expressed as kilocalories per week (kcal•wk^{-1}), MET-minutes per week (MET•min•wk^{-1}), or MET-hours per week (MET•h•wk^{-1}). Large prospective cohort studies of diverse populations[32,36,48,53] clearly show that an energy expenditure of approximately 1000 kcal•wk^{-1} of moderate-intensity physical activity (or about 150 min•wk^{-1}) is associated with lower rates of CVD (cardiovascular disease) and premature mortality. This is equivalent to an intensity of about 3 to 5.9 METs (for people weighing ~68 to 91 kg) and 10 MET•h•wk^{-1}. Ten MET-hours per week can also be achieved with ≥20 min•day^{-1} of vigorous-intensity (≥~6 METs) physical activity performed ≥3 days•wk^{-1} or for a total of ~75 min•wk^{-1}. Previous investigations have suggested that there may be a dose–response relationship between energy expenditure and depression, but additional study is needed to confirm this possibility.[25]

Muscular Strength and Endurance, Body Composition, and Flexibility

1. **Resistance training.** Resistance training should be an integral part of an adult fitness program and of a sufficient intensity to enhance strength, muscular endurance, and maintain fat-free mass. Resistance training should be progressive in nature, individualized, and provide a stimulus to all the major muscle groups. One set of 8 to 10 exercises that conditions the major muscle groups 2 to 3 days per week is recommended. Multiple-set regimens may provide greater benefits if time allows. Most persons should complete 8 to 12 repetitions of each exercise; however, for older and more frail persons (aged approximately 50 to 60 years and above), 10 to 15 repetitions may be more appropriate.

2. **Flexibility training.** Flexibility exercises should be incorporated into the overall fitness program sufficient to develop and maintain range of motion. These exercises should stretch the major muscle groups and be performed a minimum of 2 to 3 days per week. Stretching should include appropriate static and/or dynamic techniques.

8

Impaired Mobility

Restoring Range of Motion and Improving Flexibility

William E. Prentice

OBJECTIVES

After completion of this chapter, the physical therapist should be able to do the following:

- Define flexibility and describe its importance in injury rehabilitation.
- Identify factors that limit flexibility.
- Differentiate between active and passive range of motion.
- Explain the difference between dynamic, static, and proprioceptive neuromuscular facilitation stretching.
- Discuss the neurophysiologic principles of stretching.
- Describe stretching exercises that may be used to improve flexibility at specific joints throughout the body.
- Compare and contrast the various manual therapy techniques including myofascial release, strain/counterstrain, positional release, soft tissue mobilization, and massage that can be used to improve mobility and range of motion.

When injury occurs, there is almost always some associated loss of the ability to move normally. Loss of motion may be a result of pain, swelling, muscle guarding, or spasm; inactivity resulting in shortening of connective tissue and muscle; loss of neuromuscular control; or some combination of these factors. Restoring normal range of motion following injury is one of the primary goals in any rehabilitation program.[90] Thus the therapist must routinely include exercise designed to restore normal range of motion to regain normal function.

Flexibility has been defined as the ability to move a joint or series of joints through a full, nonrestricted, pain-free range of motion.[2,3,28,40,46,72,88] Flexibility is dependent on a combination of (a) joint range of motion, which may be limited by the shape of the articulating surfaces and by capsular and ligamentous structures surrounding that joint; and (b) muscle flexibility, or the ability of the musculotendinous unit to lengthen.[102] Flexibility involves the ability of the neuromuscular system to allow for efficient movement of a joint through a range of motion.[3,31,48,52,83,105]

Flexibility can be discussed in relation to movement involving only 1 joint, such as the knees, or movement involving a whole series of joints, such as the spinal vertebral joints, that must all move together to allow smooth bending or rotation of the trunk. Lack of flexibility in 1 joint or movement can affect the entire kinetic chain. A person might have good range of motion in the ankles, knees, hips, back, and one shoulder joint but lack normal movement in the other shoulder joint; this is a problem that needs to be corrected before the person can function normally.[11,20]

This chapter concentrates primarily on rehabilitative techniques used to increase the length of the musculotendinous unit and its associated fascia, as well as restricted neural tissue. In addition, a discussion of a variety of manual therapy techniques including myofascial release, strain/counterstrain, positional release therapy, soft-tissue mobilization, and massage as they relate to improving mobility will be included. Joint mobilization and traction techniques used to address tightness in the joint capsule and surrounding ligaments are discussed in Chapter 13. Loss of the ability to control movement as a result of impairment in neuromuscular control was discussed in Chapter 9.

Importance of Flexibility to the Patient

Maintaining a full, nonrestricted range of motion has long been recognized as essential to normal daily living. Lack of flexibility can also create uncoordinated or awkward movement patterns resulting from lost neuromuscular control. In most patients, functional activities require relatively "normal" amounts of flexibility.[77] However some sport activities, such as gymnastics, ballet, diving, karate, and especially dance require increased flexibility for superior performance[23] (Figure 8-1).

It has also been generally accepted that flexibility is essential for improving performance in physical activities.[25] However, a review of the evidence-based information in the literature looking at the relationship between flexibility and improved performance is, at best, conflicting and inconclusive.[43,59,104] Although many studies done over the years have suggested that stretching improves performance,[11,59,76,111] several recent studies have found that stretching causes decreases in performance parameters such as strength, endurance, power, joint position sense, and reaction times.[9,13,30,42,43,61,65,70,78,83,85,93,106,110]

The same can be said when examining the relationship between flexibility and reducing the incidence of injury. While it is generally accepted that good flexibility reduces the likelihood of injury, a true cause-and-effect relationship has not been clearly established in the literature.[4,5,19,76,107,110]

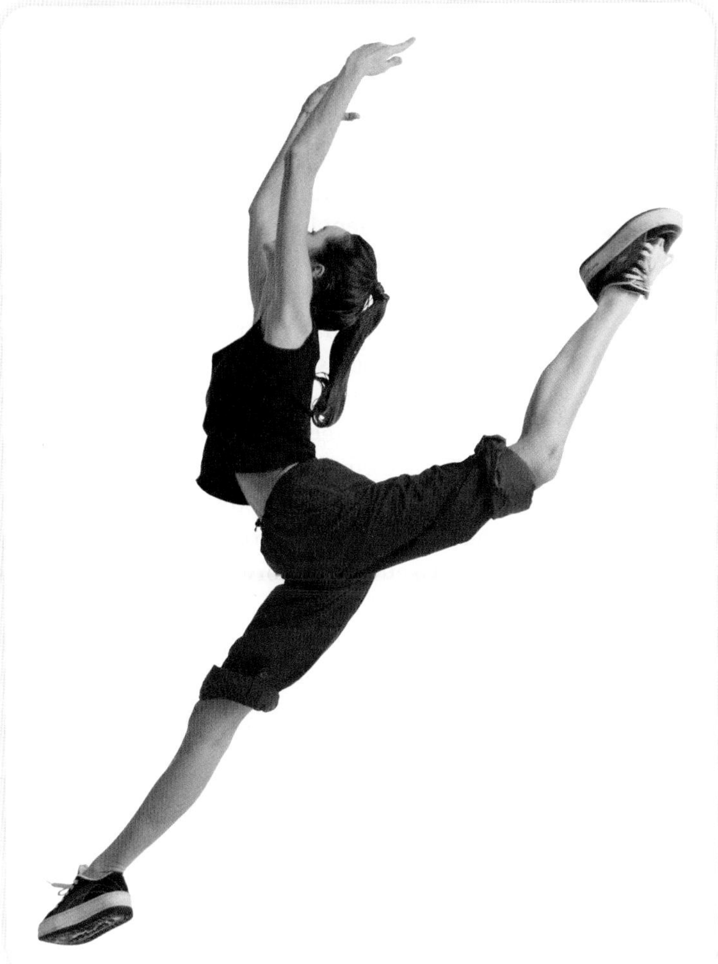

Figure 8-1 Extreme flexibility

Certain dance and athletic activities require extreme flexibility for successful performance.

Anatomic Factors That Limit Flexibility

A number of anatomic factors can limit the ability of a joint to move through a full, unrestricted range of motion.[84] *Muscles* and their tendons, along with their surrounding fascial sheaths, are most often responsible for limiting range of motion. When performing stretching exercises to improve flexibility about a particular joint, you are attempting to take advantage of the highly elastic properties of a muscle. Over time it is possible to increase the elasticity, or the length that a given muscle can be stretched. Persons who have a good deal of movement at a particular joint tend to have highly elastic and flexible muscles.

Connective tissue surrounding the joint, such as ligaments on the joint capsule, can be subject to contractures. Ligaments and joint capsules have some elasticity; however, if a joint is immobilized for a period of time, these structures tend to lose some elasticity and actually shorten. This condition is most commonly seen after surgical repair of an unstable joint, but it can also result from long periods of inactivity.

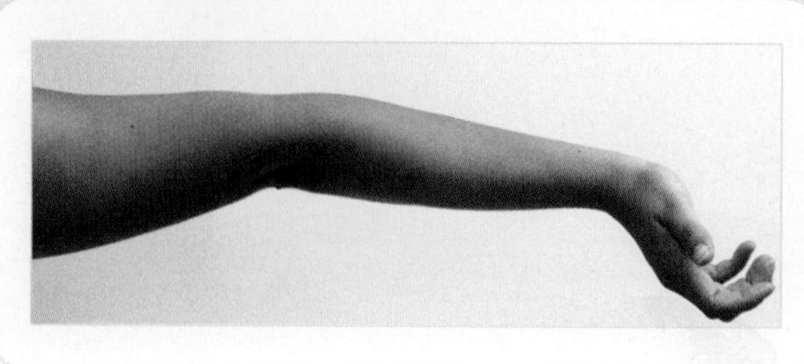

Figure 8-2

Excessive joint motion, such as the hyperextended elbow, can predispose a joint to injury.

It is also possible for a person to have relatively slack ligaments and joint capsules. These people are generally referred to as being loose-jointed. Examples of this trait would be an elbow or knee that hyperextends beyond 180 degrees (Figure 8-2). Frequently, there is instability associated with loose-jointedness that can present as great a problem in movement as ligamentous or capsular contractures.

Bony structure can restrict the end point in the range. An elbow that has been fractured through the joint might lay down excess calcium in the joint space, causing the joint to lose its ability to fully extend. However, in many instances we rely on bony prominences to stop movements at normal end points in the range.

Fat can also limit the ability to move through a full range of motion. A person who has a large amount of fat on the abdomen might have severely restricted trunk flexion when asked to bend forward and touch the toes. The fat can act as a wedge between 2 lever arms, restricting movement wherever it is found.

Skin might also be responsible for limiting movement. For example, a person who has had some type of injury or surgery involving a tearing incision or laceration of the skin, particularly over a joint, will have inelastic scar tissue formed at that site. This scar tissue is incapable of stretching with joint movement.

Over time, skin contractures caused by scarring of ligaments, joint capsules, and musculotendinous units are capable of improving elasticity to varying degrees through stretching. With the exception of bone structure, age, and gender, all the other factors that limit flexibility can be altered to increase range of joint motion.

Neural tissue tightness resulting from acute compression, chronic repetitive microtrauma, muscle imbalances, joint dysfunction, or poor posture can create morphologic changes in neural tissues. These changes might include intraneural edema, tissue hypoxia, chemical irritation, or microvascular stasis—all of which could stimulate nociceptors, creating pain. Pain causes muscle guarding and spasm to protect the inflamed neural structures, and this alters normal movement patterns. Eventually neural fibrosis results, which decreases the elasticity of neural tissue and prevents normal movement within surrounding tissues.[21]

Active and Passive Range of Motion

Active range of motion, also called *dynamic flexibility,* refers to the degree to which a joint can be moved by a muscle contraction, usually through the midrange of movement. Dynamic flexibility is not necessarily a good indicator of the stiffness or looseness of a joint because it applies to the ability to move a joint efficiently, with little resistance to motion.[48]

Passive range of motion, sometimes called *static flexibility,* refers to the degree to which a joint can be passively moved to the end points in the range of motion. No muscle contraction is involved to move a joint through a passive range.

When a muscle actively contracts, it produces a joint movement through a specific range of motion.[83,100] However, if passive pressure is applied to an extremity, it is capable of moving farther in the range of motion. It is essential in sports activities that an extremity be capable of moving through a nonrestricted range of motion.[87]

Passive range of motion is important for injury prevention. There are many situations in physical activity in which a muscle is forced to stretch beyond its normal active limits. If the

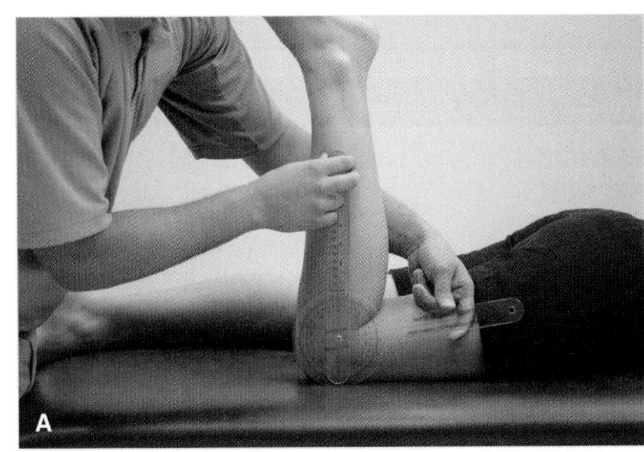

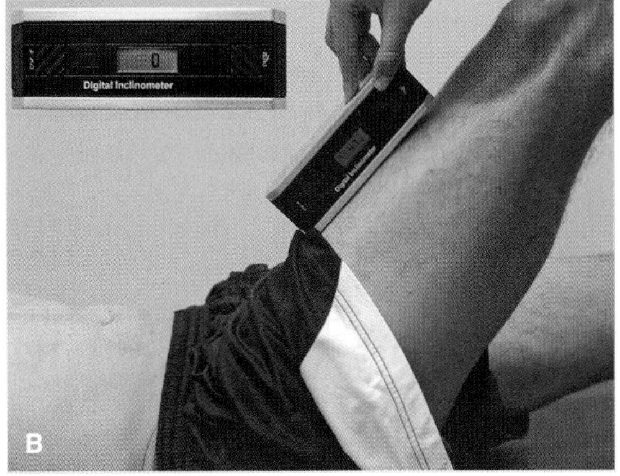

Figure 8-3

Measurement of active knee joint flexion using (**A**) a universal goniometer, or (**B**) a digital goniometer.

muscle does not have enough elasticity to compensate for this additional stretch, it is likely that the musculotendinous unit will be injured.

Assessment of Active and Passive Range of Motion

Accurate measurement of active and passive range of joint motion is difficult.[50] Various devices have been designed to accommodate variations in the size of the joints, as well as the complexity of movements in articulations that involve more than 1 joint.[50] Of these devices, the simplest and most widely used is the *goniometer* (Figure 8-3).

A goniometer is a large protractor with measurements in degrees. By aligning the individual arms of the goniometer parallel to the longitudinal axis of the 2 segments involved in motion about a specific joint, it is possible to obtain reasonably accurate measurement of range of movement. To enhance reliability, standardization of measurement techniques and methods of recording active and passive ranges of motion are critical in individual clinics where successive measurements might be taken by different therapists to assess progress.[49] Table 8-1 provides a list of what would be considered normal active ranges for movements at various joints.

The goniometer has an important place in a rehabilitation setting, where it is essential to assess improvement in joint flexibility to modify injury rehabilitation programs.

In some clinics a digital inclinometer is used instead of a goniometer. An inclinometer is a more precise measuring instrument with high reliability that has most often been used in research settings. Digital inclinometers are affordable and can easily be used to accurately measure range of motion of all joints of the body from complex movements of the spine and large joints of the extremities to the small joints of fingers and toes.

Stretching to Improve Mobility

The goal of any effective stretching program should be to improve the range of motion at a given articulation by altering the extensibility of the neuromusculotendinous units that produce movement at that joint. It is well documented that exercises that stretch these

Table 8-1 Active Ranges of Joint Motions

Joint	Action	Degrees of Motion
Shoulder	Flexion	0 to 180
	Extension	0 to 50
	Abduction	0 to 180
	Medial rotation	0 to 90
	Lateral rotation	0 to 90
	Flexion	0 to 90
Elbow	Flexion	0 to 160
Forearm	Pronation	0 to 90
	Supination	0 to 90
Wrist	Flexion	0 to 90
	Extension	0 to 70
	Abduction	0 to 25
	Adduction	0 to 65
Hip	Flexion	0 to 125
	Extension	0 to 15
	Abduction	0 to 45
	Adduction	0 to 15
	Medial rotation	0 to 45
	Lateral rotation	0 to 45
Knee	Flexion	0 to 140
Ankle	Plantarflexion	0 to 45
	Dorsiflexion	0 to 20
Foot	Inversion	0 to 30
	Eversion	0 to 10

neuromusculotendinous units and their fascia over time will increase the range of movement possible about a given joint.[41,80]

For many years the efficacy of stretching in improving range of motion has been theoretically attributed to neurophysiologic phenomena involving the stretch reflex. However, a recent study that extensively reviewed the existing literature suggested that improvements in range of motion resulting from stretching must be explained by mechanisms other than the stretch reflex.[19] Studies reviewed indicate that changes in the ability to tolerate stretch and/or the viscoelastic properties of the stretched muscle are possible mechanisms.

Clinical Pearl

A goniometer can be used to measure the angle between the femur and the fibula, giving you degrees of flexion and extension. To maximize consistency in measurement, it is helpful if the same person takes sequential goniometric measurement.

Neurophysiologic Basis of Stretching

Every muscle in the body contains various types of mechanoreceptors that, when stimulated, inform the central nervous system of what is happening with that muscle.[22] Two of these mechanoreceptors are important in the stretch reflex: the *muscle spindle* and the *Golgi tendon organ.* Both types of receptors are sensitive to changes in muscle length. The Golgi tendon organs are also affected by changes in muscle tension.[15]

When a muscle is stretched, both the muscle spindles and the Golgi tendon organs immediately begin sending a volley of sensory impulses to the spinal cord. Initially impulses coming from the muscle spindles inform the central nervous system that the muscle is being stretched. Impulses return to the muscle from the spinal cord, causing the muscle to reflexively contract, thus resisting the stretch.[68] The Golgi tendon organs respond to the change in length and the increase in tension by firing off sensory impulses of their own to the spinal cord. If the stretch of the muscle continues for an extended period of time (at least 6 seconds), impulses from the Golgi tendon organs begin to override muscle spindle impulses. The impulses from the Golgi tendon organs, unlike the signals from the muscle spindle, cause a reflex relaxation of the antagonist muscle. This reflex relaxation serves as a protective mechanism that will allow the muscle to stretch through relaxation without exceeding the extensibility limits, which could damage the muscle fibers.[12] This relaxation of the antagonist muscle during contractions is referred to as *autogenic inhibition.*

In any synergistic muscle group, a contraction of the agonist causes a reflex relaxation in the antagonist muscle, allowing it to stretch and protecting it from injury. This phenomenon is referred to as reciprocal inhibition[92] (see Figure 12-32).

Effects of Stretching on the Physical and Mechanical Properties of Muscle

The neurophysiologic mechanisms of both autogenic and reciprocal inhibition result in reflex relaxation with subsequent lengthening of a muscle. Thus the mechanical properties of that muscle that physically allow lengthening to occur are dictated via neural input.

Both muscle and tendon are composed largely of noncontractile collagen and elastin fibers. Collagen enables a tissue to resist mechanical forces and deformation, whereas elastin composes highly elastic tissues that assist in recovery from deformation.[62]

Collagen has several mechanical and physical properties that allow it to respond to loading and deformation, permitting it to withstand high tensile stress.[103] The mechanical properties of collagen include (a) *elasticity,* which is the capability to recover normal length after elongation; (b) *viscoelasticity,* which allows for a slow return to normal length and shape after deformation; and (c) *plasticity,* which allows for permanent change or deformation. The physical properties include (a) *force-relaxation,* which indicates the decrease in the amount of force needed to maintain a tissue at a set amount of displacement or deformation over time; (b) the *creep response,* which is the ability of a tissue to deform over time while a constant load is imposed; and (c) *hysteresis,* which is the amount of relaxation a tissue has undergone during deformation and displacement. If the mechanical and physical limitations of connective tissue are exceeded, injury results.

Unlike tendon, muscle also has active contractile components that are the actin and myosin myofilaments. Collectively the contractile and noncontractile elements determine the muscle's capability of deforming and recovering from deformation.[112]

Both the contractile and the noncontractile components appear to resist deformation when a muscle is stretched or lengthened. The percentage of their individual contribution to resisting deformation depends on the degree to which the muscle is stretched or deformed and on the velocity of deformation. The noncontractile elements are primarily resistant to the degree of lengthening, while the contractile elements limit high-velocity deformation. The greater the stretch, the more the noncontractile components contribute.[103]

Lengthening of a muscle via stretching allows for viscoelastic and plastic changes to occur in the collagen and elastin fibers. The viscoelastic changes that allow slow deformation with imperfect recovery are not permanent. However, plastic changes, although difficult to achieve, result in residual or permanent change in length due to deformation created by long periods of stretching.

The greater the velocity of deformation, the greater the chance for exceeding that tissue's capability to undergo viscoelastic and plastic change.[112]

Effects of Stretching on the Kinetic Chain

Joint hypomobility is one of the most frequently treated causes of pain. However, the etiology can usually be traced to faulty posture, muscular imbalances, and abnormal neuromuscular control. Once a particular joint has lost its normal arthrokinematics, the muscles around that joint attempt to minimize the stress at that involved segment. Certain muscles become tight and hypertonic to prevent additional joint translation. If one muscle becomes tight or changes its degree of activation, then synergists, stabilizers, and neutralizers have to compensate, leading to the formation of complex neuromusculoskeletal dysfunctions.

Muscle tightness and hypertonicity have a significant impact on neuromuscular control. Muscle tightness affects the normal length–tension relationships. When one muscle in a force-couple becomes tight or hypertonic, it alters the normal arthrokinematics of the involved joint. This affects the synergistic function of the entire kinetic chain, leading to abnormal joint stress, soft-tissue dysfunction, neural compromise, and vascular/lymphatic stasis. These result in alterations in recruitment strategies and stabilization strength. Such compensations and adaptations affect neuromuscular efficiency throughout the kinetic chain. Decreased neuromuscular control alters the activation sequence or firing order of different muscles involved, and a specific movement is disturbed. Prime movers may be slow to activate, while synergists, stabilizers, and neutralizers substitute and become overactive. When this is the case, new joint stresses will be encountered.[21] For example, if the psoas is tight or hyperactive, then the gluteus maximus will have decreased neural drive. If the gluteus maximus (prime mover during hip extension) has decreased neural drive, then synergists (hamstrings), stabilizers (erector spinae), and neutralizers (piriformis) substitute and become overactive (synergistic dominance). This creates abnormal joint stress and decreased neuromuscular control during functional movements.

Muscle tightness also causes reciprocal inhibition. Increased muscle spindle activity in a specific muscle will cause decreased neural drive to that muscle's functional antagonist. This alters the normal force-couple activity, which, in turn, affects the normal arthrokinematics of the involved segment. For example, if a patient has tightness or hypertonicity in the psoas, then the functional antagonist (gluteus maximus) can be inhibited (decreased neural drive), causing decreased neuromuscular control. This, in turn, leads to *synergistic dominance*—the neuromuscular phenomenon that occurs when synergists compensate for a weak and/or inhibited muscle to maintain force production capabilities.[21] This process alters the normal force-couple relationships, which, in turn, creates a chain reaction.

Importance of Increasing Muscle Temperature Prior to Stretching

To most effectively stretch a muscle during a program of rehabilitation, intramuscular temperature should be increased prior to stretching.[75] Increasing the temperature has a positive effect on the ability of the collagen and elastin components within the musculotendinous unit to deform. Also, the capability of the Golgi tendon organs to reflexively relax the muscle through autogenic inhibition is enhanced when the muscle is heated. It appears that the optimal temperature of muscle to achieve these beneficial effects is 39°C (103°F). This increase in intramuscular temperature can be achieved either through low-intensity warm-up–type exercise or through the use of various therapeutic modalities.[27,44,91] It is recommended that exercise be used as the primary means for increasing intramuscular temperature.

The use of cold prior to stretching also has been recommended.[26] Cold appears to be most useful when there is some muscle guarding associated with delayed-onset muscle soreness.[82]

Clinical Pearl

Applying certain therapeutic modalities, such as ice and/or electrical stimulating currents, can decrease pain and discourage muscle guarding to increase range of motion. Delayed-onset muscle soreness will usually begin to subside at about 48 hours following a workout.

Stretching Techniques

Stretching techniques for improving flexibility have evolved over the years.[57] The oldest technique for stretching is *dynamic stretching* (ballistic), which makes use of repetitive bouncing motions. A second technique, known as *static stretching,* involves stretching a muscle to the point of discomfort and then holding it at that point for an extended time. This technique has been used for many years. Another group of stretching techniques known collectively as *proprioceptive neuromuscular facilitation* (PNF) techniques, involving alternating contractions and stretches, also has been recommended (Figure 8-4).[58,108] Most recently, emphasis has been on the contribution of *stretching myofascial tissue,* as well as *stretching tight neural tissue,* in enhancing the ability of the neuromuscular system to efficiently control movement through a full range of motion. Researchers have had considerable discussion about which of these techniques is most effective for improving range of motion, and no clear-cut consensus currently exists.[11,32,41,66,80,86]

Agonist Versus Antagonist Muscles

Before discussing the different stretching techniques, it is essential to define the terms *agonist muscle* and *antagonist muscle.* Most joints in the body are capable of more than 1 movement. The knee joint, for example, is capable of flexion and extension. Contraction of the quadriceps group of muscles on the front of the thigh causes knee extension, whereas contraction of the hamstring muscles on the back of the thigh produces knee flexion.

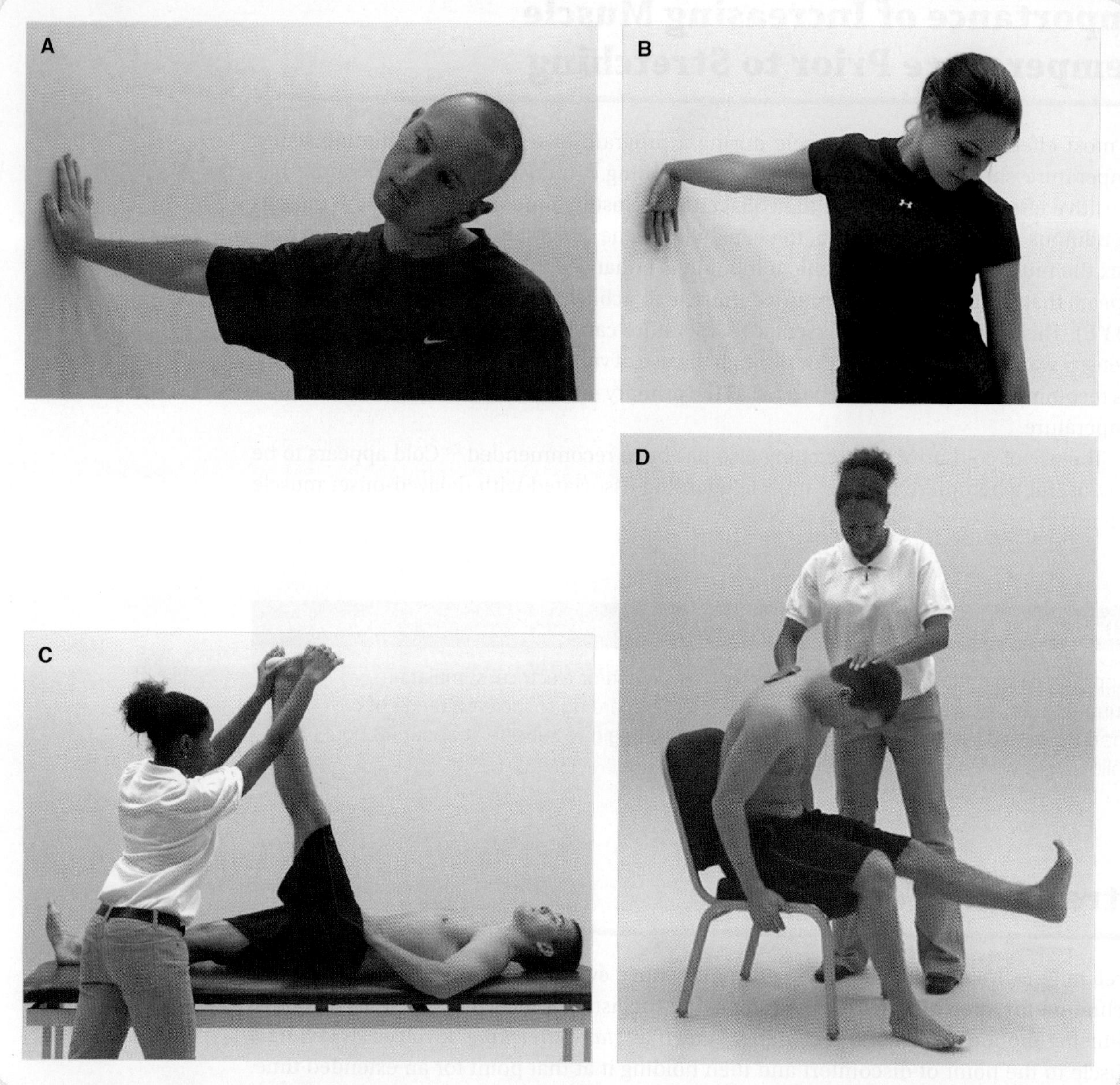

Figure 8-4 Neural tension stretches

A. Median nerve. B. Radial nerve. C. Sciatic nerve. D. Slump position.

To achieve knee extension, the quadriceps group contracts while the hamstring muscles relax and stretch. Muscles that work in concert with one another in this manner are called *synergistic muscle groups*.[8] The muscle that contracts to produce a movement, in this case the quadriceps, is referred to as the *agonist muscle*. The muscle being stretched in response to contraction of the agonist muscle is called the *antagonist muscle*.[40] In this example of knee extension, the antagonist muscle would be the hamstring group. Some degree of balance in strength must exist between agonist and antagonist muscle groups. This balance is necessary for normal, smooth, coordinated movement, as well as for reducing the likelihood of muscle strain caused by muscular imbalance. Comprehension of this synergistic muscle action is essential to understanding the various techniques of stretching.

Dynamic Stretching

In dynamic stretching, repetitive contractions of the agonist muscle are used to produce quick stretches of the antagonist muscle.

Over the years, many fitness experts have questioned the safety of the dynamic stretching technique.[47,68] Their concerns have been primarily based on the idea that dynamic stretching creates somewhat uncontrolled forces within the muscle that can exceed the extensibility limits of the muscle fiber, thus producing small microtears within the musculotendinous unit.[35,39,74,112] Certainly this might be true in sedentary individuals or perhaps in individuals who have sustained muscle injuries.

However, many physical activities are dynamic and require a repeated dynamic contraction of the agonist muscle. The antagonist contracting eccentrically to decelerate the dynamic stretching of the antagonist muscle before engaging in this type of activity should allow the muscle to gradually adapt to the imposed demands and reduce the likelihood of injury. Because dynamic stretching is more functional, it should be integrated into a reconditioning program during the later stages of healing when appropriate.

A progressive velocity flexibility program has been proposed that takes the patient through a series of stretching exercises where the velocity of the stretch and the range of lengthening are progressively controlled.[81] The stretching exercises progress from slow static stretching to slow, short, end-range stretching, to slow, full-range stretching, to fast, short, end-range stretching, and to fast, full-range stretching. This program allows the patient to control both the range and the speed with no assistance from a therapist.

Clinical Pearl

Ballistic stretching is dynamic stretching that is useful prior to activity because it is a functional stretch. It mimics activity that will be performed during competition. However, there is some speculation that because it is an uncontrolled stretch, it may lead to injury, especially in sedentary individuals. Static stretching is convenient because it can be done on any muscle and it doesn't require a partner. It is not very functional. PNF stretching will most likely provide the greatest increase in range of motion, but it is a little more time-consuming and requires a partner.

Static Stretching

The static stretching technique is another extremely effective and widely used technique of stretching.[52] This technique involves stretching a given antagonist muscle passively by placing it in a maximal position of stretch and holding it there for an extended time. Recommendations for the optimal time for holding this stretched position vary, ranging from as short as 3 seconds to as long as 60 seconds.[48] Several studies indicate that holding a stretch for 15 to 30 seconds is the most effective for increasing muscle flexibility.[6,64,67] Stretches lasting longer than 30 seconds seem to be uncomfortable. A static stretch of each muscle should be repeated 3 or 4 times. A static stretch can be accomplished by using a contraction of the agonist muscle to place the antagonist muscle in a position of stretch. A passive static stretch requires the use of body weight, assistance from a therapist or partner, or use of a T-bar, primarily for stretching the upper extremity.

> **Clinical Pearl**
>
> A static stretch should be held for approximately 30 seconds. This allows time for the Golgi tendon organs to override the muscle spindles and produce a reflex muscle relaxation. The patient should stretch to the point where tightness or resistance to stretch is felt but it should not be painful. The stretch should be repeated 3 to 5 times.

Proprioceptive Neuromuscular Facilitation Stretching Techniques

Proprioceptive neuromuscular facilitation techniques were first used by therapists for treating patients who had various neuromuscular disorders.[58] More recently, PNF stretching exercises have increasingly been used as a stretching technique for improving flexibility.[15,24,64,71,73]

There are 3 different PNF techniques used for stretching: contract-relax, hold-relax techniques, and slow reversal-hold-relax.[102] All 3 techniques involve some combination of alternating isometric or isotonic contractions and relaxation of both agonist and antagonist muscles (a 10-second pushing phase followed by a 10-second relaxing phase).

Contract-relax is a stretching technique that moves the body part passively into the agonist pattern. The patient is instructed to push by contracting the antagonist (the muscle that will be stretched) isotonically against the resistance of the therapist. The patient then relaxes the antagonist while the therapist moves the part passively through as much range as possible to the point where limitation is again felt. This contract-relax technique is beneficial when range of motion is limited by muscle tightness.

Hold-relax is very similar to the contract-relax technique. It begins with an isometric contraction of the antagonist (the muscle that will be stretched) against resistance, combined with light pressure from the therapist to produce maximal stretch of the antagonist. This technique is appropriate when there is muscle tension on one side of a joint and may be used with either the agonist or the antagonist. This techniques is also referred to as a *muscle energy* technique and will be discussed in Chapter 12.[16]

Slow reversal-hold-relax, also occasionally referred to as the *contract-relax-agonist-contraction* technique, begins with an isotonic contraction of the agonist, which often limits range of motion in the agonist pattern, followed by an isometric contraction of the antagonist (the muscle that will be stretched) during the push phase. During the relax phase, the antagonists are relaxed while the agonists are contracting, causing movement in the direction of the agonist pattern and thus stretching the antagonist. This technique, like the contract-relax and hold-relax, is useful for increasing range of motion when the primary limiting factor is the antagonistic muscle group.

PNF stretching techniques can be used to stretch any muscle in the body.[11,28,29,34,71,74,79,82,86,102] PNF stretching techniques are perhaps best performed with a partner, although they may also be done using a wall as resistance.

Comparing Stretching Techniques

Although all 3 stretching techniques discussed to this point have been demonstrated to effectively improve flexibility, there is still considerable debate as to which technique produces the greatest increases in range of movement.[7] The dynamic technique is recommended for anyone who is involved in dynamic activity, despite its potential for causing muscle soreness in the sedentary individual. In physically active individuals, it is unlikely that dynamic stretching will result in muscle soreness.

Static stretching is perhaps the most widely used technique. It is a simple technique and does not require a partner. A fully nonrestricted range of motion can be attained through static stretching over time.

Much research has been done comparing dynamic and static stretching techniques for the improvement of flexibility. Static and dynamic stretching appear to be equally effective in increasing flexibility, and there is no significant difference between the two.[36] However, much of the literature states that with static stretching there is less danger of exceeding the extensibility limits of the involved joints because the stretch is more controlled. Most of the literature indicates that dynamic stretching is apt to cause muscular soreness, especially in sedentary individuals, whereas static stretching generally does not cause soreness and is commonly used in injury rehabilitation of sore or strained muscles.[35,109] Static stretching is likely a much safer stretching technique, especially for sedentary individuals. However, because many physical activities involve dynamic movement, stretching in a warm-up should begin with static stretching followed by dynamic stretching, which more closely resembles the dynamic activity. PNF stretching techniques are capable of producing dramatic increases in range of motion during one stretching session.[14] Studies comparing static and PNF stretching suggest that PNF stretching is capable of producing greater improvement in flexibility over an extended training period.[45,46,82] The major disadvantage of PNF stretching is that a partner is usually required to assist with the stretch, although stretching with a therapist or partner can have some motivational advantages.

How long increases in muscle flexibility can be sustained once stretching stops is debatable.[38,94,113] One study indicated that a significant loss of flexibility was evident after only 2 weeks.[113] It was recommended that flexibility can be maintained by engaging in stretching activities at least once a week. However, to see improvement in flexibility, stretching must be done 3 to 5 times per week.[37]

Stretching Neural Structures

The therapist should be able to differentiate between tightness in the musculotendinous unit and abnormal neural tension. The patient should perform both active and passive multiplanar movements that create tension in the neural structures that are exacerbating pain, limiting range of motion, and increasing neural symptoms, including numbness and tingling.[21] For example, the straight-leg raising test not only applies pressure to the sacroiliac joint cell but also may indicate a problem in the sciatic nerve (Figure 8-4*C*). Internally rotating and adducting the hip increases the tension on the neural structures in both the greater sciatic notch and the intervertebral foramen. An exacerbation of pain from 30 degrees to 60 degrees indicates some sciatic nerve involvement. If dorsiflexing the ankle with maximum straight leg raising increases the pain, then the pain is likely caused by some nerve root (L3-4, S1-3) or sciatic nerve irritation. Figure 8-4 shows the assessment and stretching positions for neural tension in the median, radial, and sciatic nerves as well as the vertebral nerve roots in the spine.

Specific Stretching Exercises

Chapters 25 to 32 include various stretching exercises that may be used to improve flexibility at specific joints or in specific muscle groups throughout the body. The stretching exercises shown in Figure 8-5 are examples that may be done statically; they may also be done with a partner using a PNF technique. There are many possible variations to each of these exercises.[54] The patient may also perform static stretching exercises using a stability ball (Figure 8-6). The exercises selected are those that seem to be the most effective for stretching of various muscle groups. Table 8-2 provides a list of guidelines and precautions for stretching.

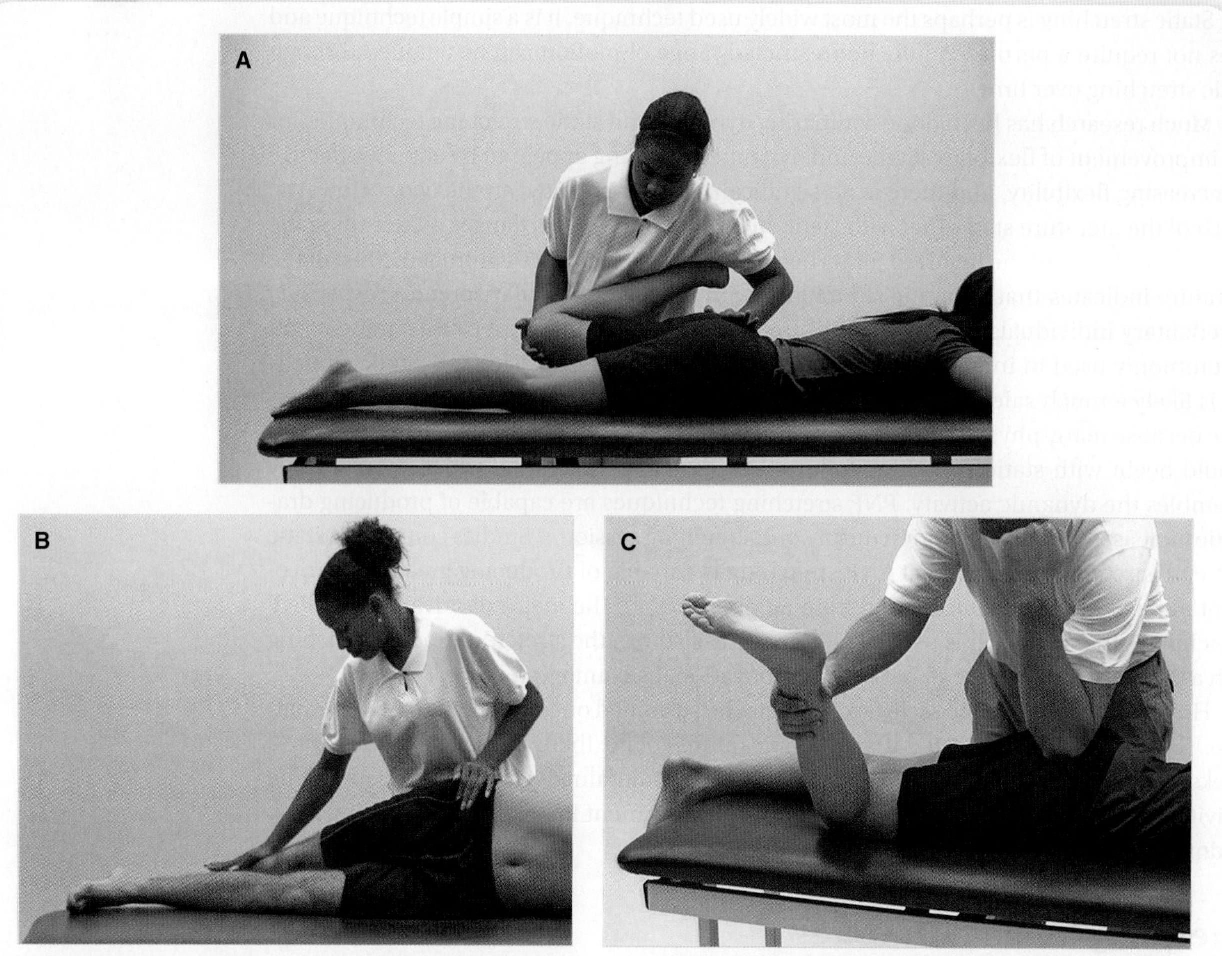

Figure 8-5

Examples of stretching exercises that may be done statically or using a PNF technique. **A.** Quadriceps. **B.** Hip abductors. **C.** Piriformis.

Alternative Stretching Techniques

The Pilates Method of Stretching

The Pilates method is a somewhat different approach to stretching for improving flexibility. This method has become extremely popular and widely used among personal fitness trainers, physical therapists, and some therapists. Pilates is an exercise technique devised by German-born Joseph Pilates, who established the first Pilates studio in the United States before World War II. The Pilates method is a conditioning program that improves muscle control, flexibility, coordination, strength, and tone.[10] The basic principles of Pilates exercise are to make patients more aware of their bodies as single integrated units, to improve body alignment and breathing, and to increase efficiency of movement. Unlike other exercise programs, the Pilates method does not require the repetition of exercises but instead consists of a sequence of carefully performed movements, some of which are carried out on specially designed equipment (Figure 8-7). However,

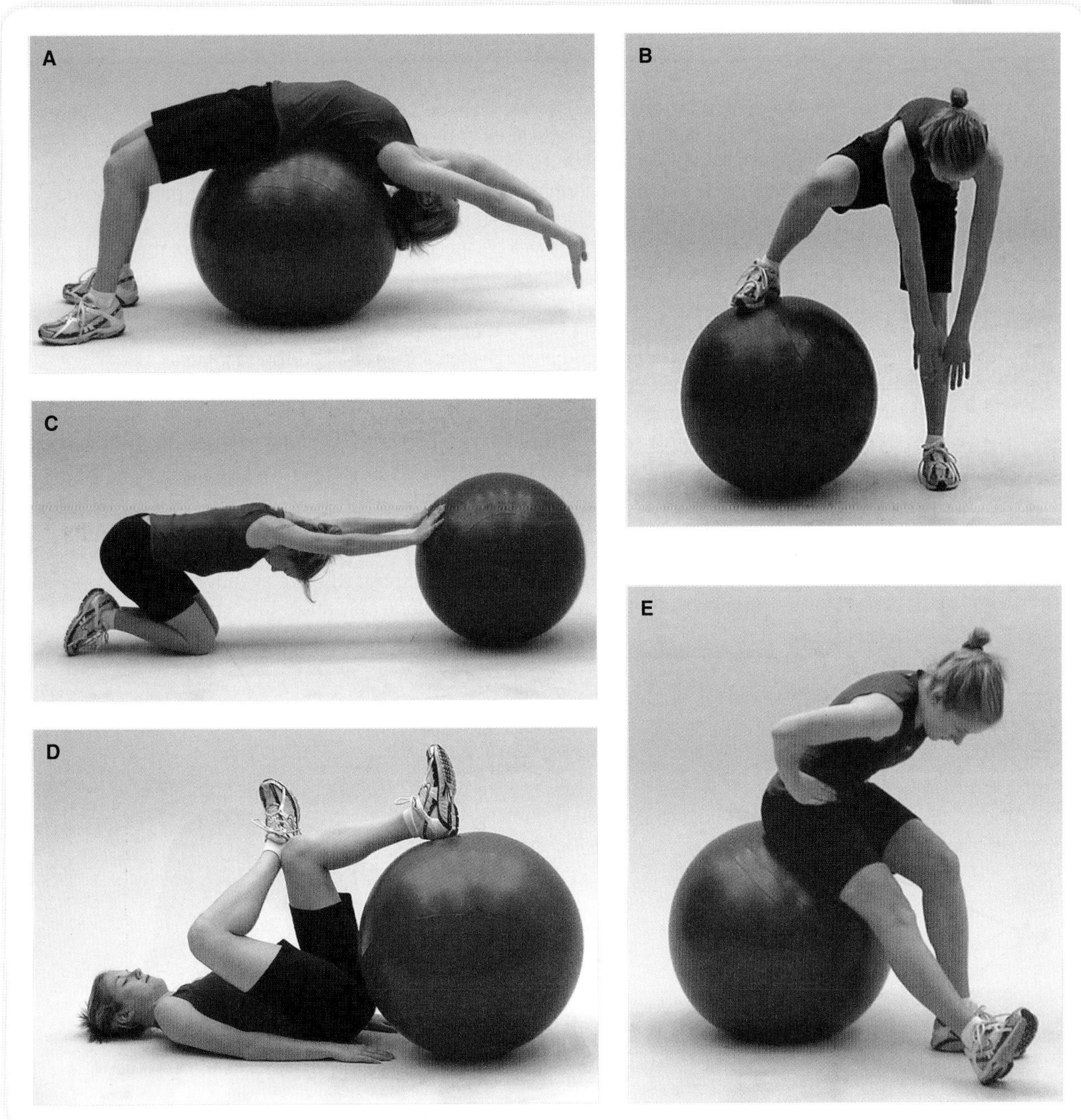

Figure 8-6 **Static stretching using a stability ball**

A. Back extension. **B**. Standing abductor stretch. **C**. Latissimus dorsi stretch. **D**. Piriformis stretch. **E**. Seated hamstring stretch.

the majority of Pilates exercises are performed on a mat or floor without equipment (Figure 8-8). Each exercise is designed to stretch and strengthen the muscles involved. There is a specific breathing pattern for each exercise to help direct energy to the areas being worked, while relaxing the rest of the body. The Pilates method works many of the deeper muscles together, improving coordination and balance, to achieve efficient and graceful movement. The goal for the patient is to develop a healthy self-image through the attainment of better posture, proper coordination, and improved flexibility. This

Table 8-2 Guidelines and Precautions for a Sound Stretching Program[60,96,97,101]

- Warm up using a slow jog or fast walk before stretching vigorously.
- To increase flexibility, the muscle must be stretched within pain tolerances and tissue healing limitations to attain functional or normal range of motion.
- Stretch only to the point where tightness or resistance to stretch, or perhaps some discomfort, is felt. Stretching should not be painful.[1]
- Increases in range of motion will be specific to whatever muscle or joint is being stretched.
- Exercise caution when stretching muscles that surround painful joints. Pain is an indication that something is wrong and should not be ignored.
- Avoid overstretching the ligaments and capsules that surround joints.
- Exercise caution when stretching the low back and neck. Exercises that compress the vertebrae and their discs can cause damage.
- Stretching from a seated rather than a standing position takes stress off the low back and decreases the chances of back injury.
- Be sure to continue normal breathing during a stretch. Do not hold your breath.
- Static and PNF techniques are most often recommended for individuals who want to improve their range of motion.
- Dynamic stretching should be done only by those who are already flexible or accustomed to stretching, and should be done only after static stretching.

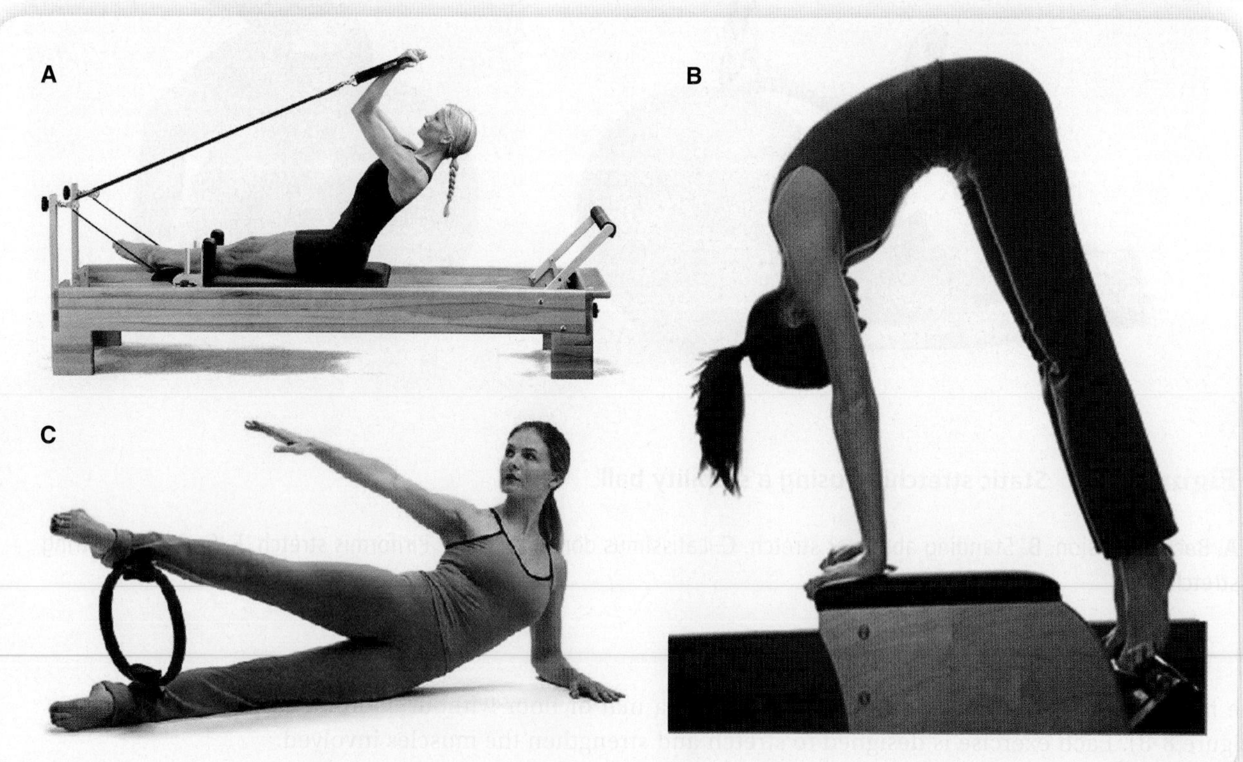

Figure 8-7 Pilates techniques using equipment

A. Reformer. B. Wunda chair. C. Magic ring.

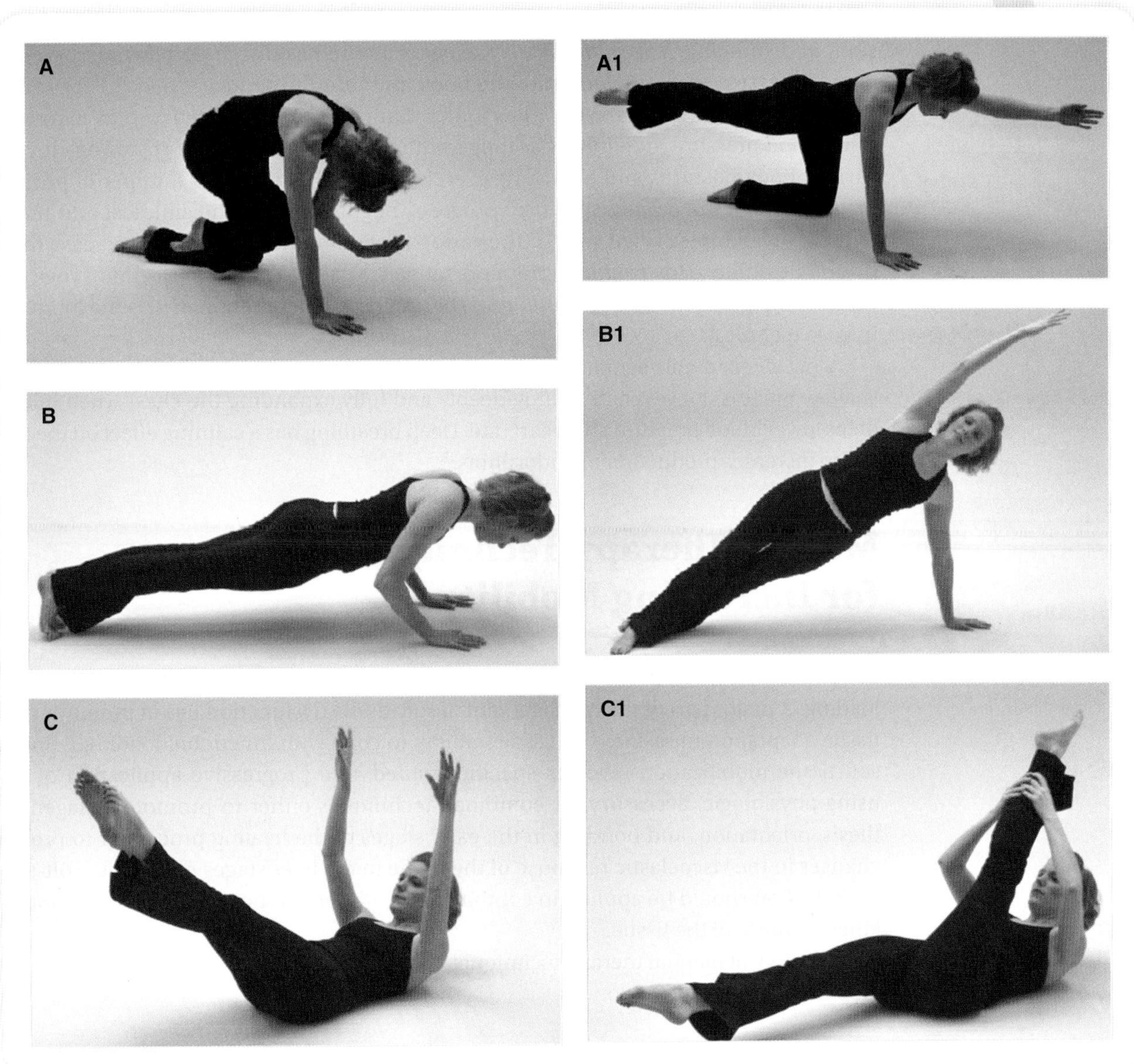

Figure 8-8 **Pilates floor exercises**

A. Alternating arm, opposite-leg extensions. **B**. Push-up to a side plank. **C**. Alternating leg scissors.

method concentrates on body alignment, lengthening all the muscles of the body into a balanced whole, and building endurance and strength without putting undue stress on the lungs and heart. Pilates instructors believe that problems such as soft-tissue injuries can cause bad posture, which can lead to pain and discomfort. Pilates exercises aim to correct this.

Yoga

Yoga originated in India approximately 6000 years ago. Its basic philosophy is that most illness is related to poor mental attitudes, posture, and diet. Practitioners of yoga maintain that stress can be reduced through combined mental and physical approaches. Yoga can help an individual cope with stress-induced behaviors like overeating, hypertension, and smoking. Yoga's meditative aspects are believed to help alleviate psychosomatic illnesses. Yoga aims to unite the body and mind to reduce stress.[56] For example, Dr. Chandra Patel, a yoga expert, has found that persons who practice yoga can reduce their blood pressure indefinitely as long as they continue to practice yoga. Yoga involves various body postures and breathing exercises. Hatha yoga uses a number of positions through which the practitioner may progress, beginning with the simplest and moving to the more complex (Figure 8-9). The various positions are intended to increase mobility and flexibility. However, practitioners must use caution when performing yoga positions. Some positions can be dangerous, particularly for someone who is inexperienced in yoga technique.

Slow, deep, diaphragmatic breathing is an important part of yoga. Many people take shallow breaths; however, breathing deeply and fully expanding the chest when inhaling helps lower blood pressure and heart rate. Deep breathing has a calming effect on the body. It also increases production of endorphins.[56]

Manual Therapy Techniques for Increasing Mobility

Following injury, soft tissue loses some of its ability to tolerate the demands of functional loading. A major part of the management of soft-tissue dysfunction lies in promoting soft-tissue adaptation to restore the tissue's ability to cope with functional loading.[53] Specific soft-tissue mobilization involves specific, graded, and progressive application of force using physiologic, accessory, or combined techniques either to promote collagen synthesis, orientation, and bonding in the early stages of the healing process or to promote changes in the viscoelastic response of the tissue in the later stages of healing. Soft-tissue mobilization should be applied in combination with rehabilitation regimes to restore the kinetic control of the tissue.[53]

A variety of manual therapy techniques can be used in injury rehabilitation to improve mobility and range of motion.

Myofascial Release Stretching

Myofascial release is a term that refers to a group of techniques used for the purpose of relieving soft tissue from the abnormal grip of tight fascia.[57] It is essentially a form of stretching that has been reported to have significant impact in treating a variety of conditions.[73] Some specialized training is necessary for the therapist to understand specific techniques of myofascial release.[89] It is also essential to have an in-depth understanding of the fascial system.

Fascia is a type of connective tissue that surrounds muscles, tendons, nerves, bones, and organs. It is essentially continuous from head to toe and is interconnected in various sheaths or planes. Fascia is composed primarily of collagen along with some elastic fibers. During movement the fascia must stretch and move freely. If there is damage to the fascia owing to injury, disease, or inflammation, it will not only affect local adjacent structures but may also affect areas far removed from the site of the injury.[69] Thus it may be necessary to release tightness both in the area of injury and in distant areas. It will tend to soften and release in response to gentle pressure over a relatively long period of time.

Myofascial release has also been referred to as soft-tissue mobilization. Soft-tissue mobilization should not be confused with joint mobilization, although it must be

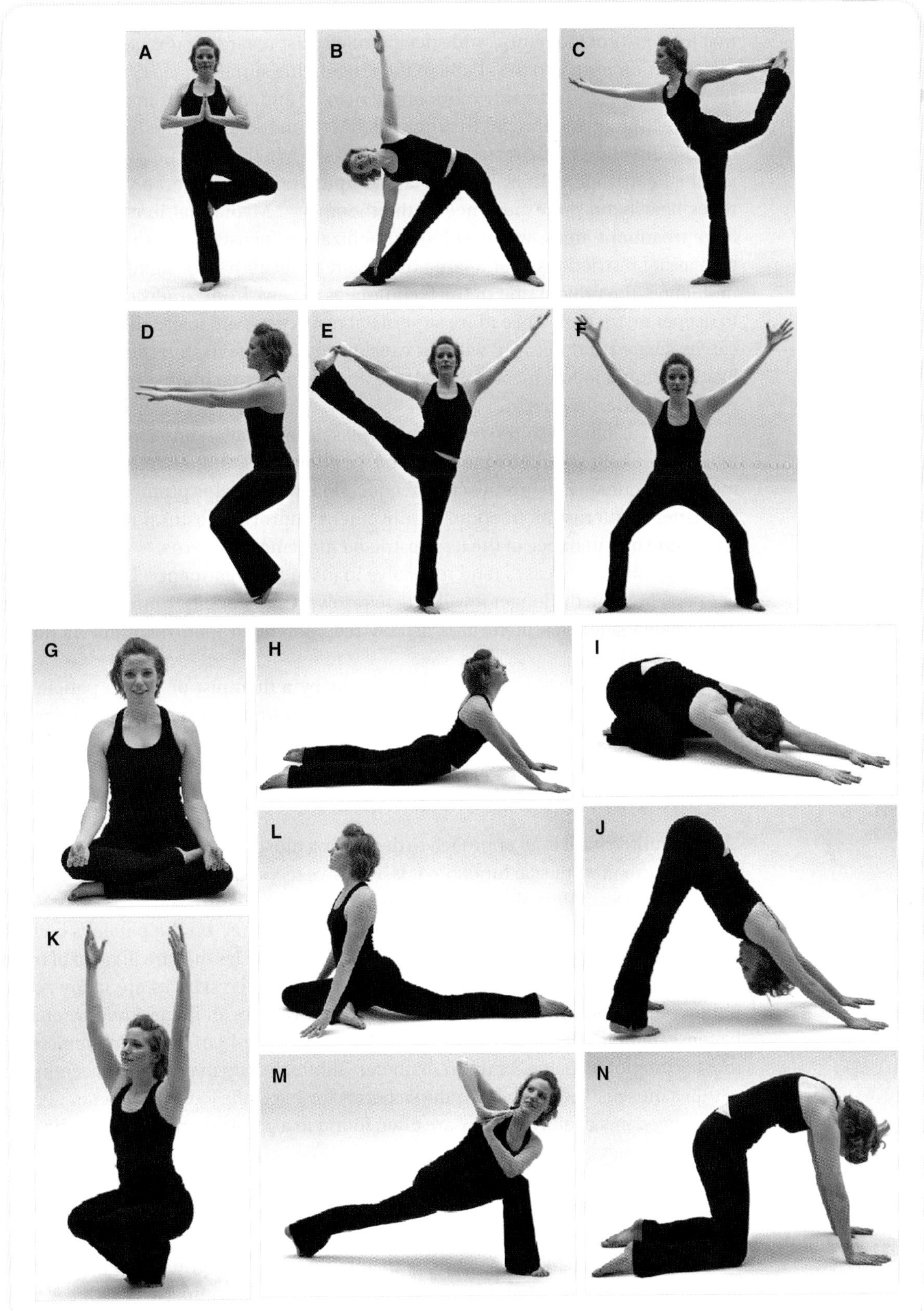

Figure 8-9 Yoga positions

A. Tree. **B**. Triangle. **C**. Dancer. **D**. Chair. **E**. Extended hand to big toe. **F**. Big mountain. **G**. Lotus. **H**. Cobra. **I**. Downward facing dog. **J**. Static squat. **K**. Pigeon. **L**. Child. **M**. Runner's lunge with twist. **N**. Cat.

emphasized that the two are closely related.[57] Joint mobilization is used to restore normal joint arthrokinematics, and specific rules exist regarding direction of movement and joint position based on the shape of the articulating surfaces (see Chapter 13). Myofascial restrictions are considerably more unpredictable and may occur in many different planes and directions.[98] Myofascial treatment is based on localizing the restriction and moving into the direction of the restriction, regardless of whether that follows the arthrokinematics of a nearby joint. Thus, myofascial manipulation is considerably more subjective and relies heavily on the experience of the therapist.[69] Myofascial manipulation focuses on large treatment areas, whereas joint mobilization focuses on a specific joint. Releasing myofascial restrictions over a large treatment area can have a significant impact on joint mobility.[73] The progression of the technique is to work from superficial fascial restrictions to deeper restriction. Once more superficial restrictions are released, the deep restrictions can be located and released without causing any damage to superficial tissue. Joint mobilization should follow myofascial release and will likely be more effective once soft-tissue restrictions are eliminated.

As extensibility is improved in the myofascia, elongation and stretching of the musculotendinous unit should be incorporated. In addition, strengthening exercises are recommended to enhance neuromuscular reeducation, which helps promote new, more efficient movement patterns. As freedom of movement improves, postural reeducation may help ensure the maintenance of the less-restricted movement patterns.

Generally, acute cases tend to resolve in just a few treatments. The longer a condition has been present, the longer it will take to resolve. Occasionally, dramatic results will occur immediately after treatment. It is usually recommended that treatment be done at least 3 times per week.

Myofascial release can be done manually by a therapist or by the patient stretching using a foam roller.[89] Figure 8-10 shows examples of stretching using the foam roller.

Strain-Counterstrain Technique

Strain-counterstrain is an approach to decreasing muscle tension and guarding that may be used to normalize muscle function. It is a passive technique that places the body in a position of greatest comfort, thereby relieving pain.[1,55]

In this technique, the therapist locates "tender points" on the patient's body that correspond to areas of dysfunction in specific joints or muscles that are in need of treatment.[99] These tender points are not located in or just beneath the skin, as are many acupuncture points, but instead are deeper in muscle, tendon, ligament, or fascia. They are characterized by tense, tender, edematous spots on the body. They are 1 cm or less in diameter, with the most acute points being 3 mm in diameter, although they may be a few centimeters long within a muscle. There can be multiple points for 1 specific joint dysfunction. Points might be arranged in a chain, and they are often found in a painless area opposite the site of pain and/or weakness.[55]

The therapist monitors the tension and level of pain elicited by the tender point while moving the patient into a position of ease or comfort. This is accomplished by markedly shortening the muscle.[99] When this position of ease is found, the tender point is no longer tense or tender. When this position is maintained for a minimum of 90 seconds, the tension in the tender point and in the corresponding joint or muscle is reduced or cleared. By slowly returning to a neutral position, the tender point and the corresponding joint or muscle remains pain-free with normal tension. For example, with neck pain and/or tension headaches, the tender point may be found on either the front or back of the patient's neck and shoulders. The therapist will have the patient lie on the patient's back and will gently

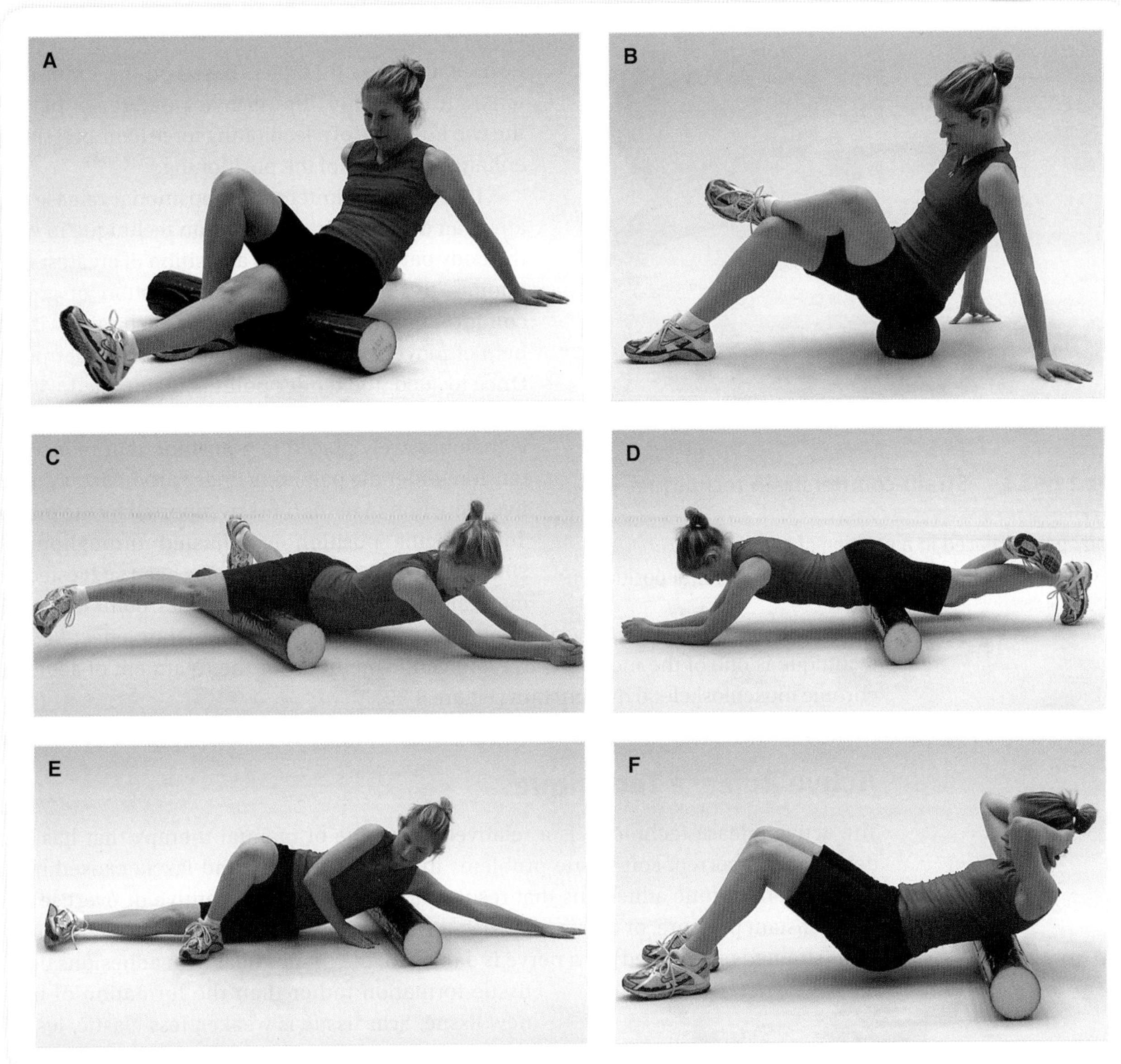

Figure 8-10 Myofascial release stretching using a foam roller or firm ball

A. Hamstrings. **B**. Piriformis. **C**. Adductors. **D**. Quadriceps. **E**. Latissimus dorsi. **F**. Rhomboids.

and slowly bend the patient's neck until that tender point is no longer tender. After holding that position for 90 seconds, the therapist gently and slowly returns the neck to its resting position. When that tender point is pressed again, the patient should notice a significant decrease in pain there (Figure 8-11).[99]

The physiologic rationale for the effectiveness of the strain-counterstrain technique can be explained by the stretch reflex.[2] When a muscle is placed in a stretched position, impulses from the muscle spindles create a reflex contraction of the muscle in response to stretch. With strain-counterstrain, the joint or muscle is placed not in a position of stretch but instead in a slack position. Thus, muscle spindle input is reduced and the muscle is relaxed, allowing for a decrease in tension and pain.[2]

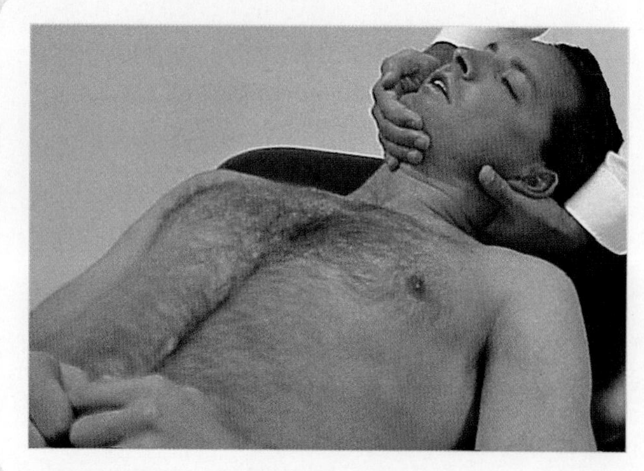

Figure 8-11 **Strain-counterstrain technique**

The body part is placed in a position of comfort for 90 seconds and then slowly moved back to a neutral position.

Positional Release Therapy

Positional release therapy is based on the strain-counterstrain technique. The primary difference between the two is the use of a facilitating force (compression) to enhance the effect of the positioning.[17,18,90,95]

Like strain-counterstrain, positional release therapy is an osteopathic mobilization technique in which the body part is moved into a position of greatest relaxation.[33] The therapist finds the position of greatest comfort and muscle relaxation for each joint with the help of movement tests and diagnostic tender points. Once located, the tender point is maintained with the palpating finger at a subthreshold pressure. The patient is then passively placed in a position that reduces the tension under the palpating finger producing a subjective reduction in tenderness as reported by the patient. This specific position is adjusted throughout the 90-second treatment period. It has been suggested that maintaining contact with the tender point during the treatment period exerts a therapeutic effect.[17,18] This technique is one of the most effective and gentle methods for the treatment of acute and chronic musculoskeletal dysfunction (Figure 8-12).[90]

Active Release Technique

The active release technique is a relatively new type of manual therapy that has been developed to correct soft-tissue problems in muscle, tendon, and fascia caused by the formation of fibrotic adhesions that result from acute injury, repetitive or overuse injuries, constant pressure, or tension injuries.[63] When a muscle, tendon, fascia, or ligament is torn (strained or sprained) or a nerve is damaged, the tissues heal with adhesions or scar tissue formation rather than the formation of brand new tissue. Scar tissue is weaker, less elastic, less pliable, and more pain-sensitive than healthy tissue.

These fibrotic adhesions disrupt the normal muscle function, which, in turn, affects the biomechanics of the joint complex and can lead to pain and dysfunction. Soft-tissue mobilization provides a way to diagnose and treat the underlying causes of cumulative trauma disorders that, left uncorrected, can lead to inflammation, adhesions, fibrosis, and muscle imbalances. All of these can result in weak and tense tissues, decreased circulation, hypoxia, and symptoms of peripheral nerve entrapment, including numbness, tingling, burning, and aching.[63] Soft-tissue mobilization is a deep-tissue technique used for breaking down scar tissue/adhesions and restoring function and movement.[63] In soft-tissue mobilization, the therapist first locates through palpation those adhesions in the muscle, tendon, or fascia that are causing the problem. Once these are located, the therapist traps the affected muscle by applying pressure or tension with the thumb or finger over these lesions

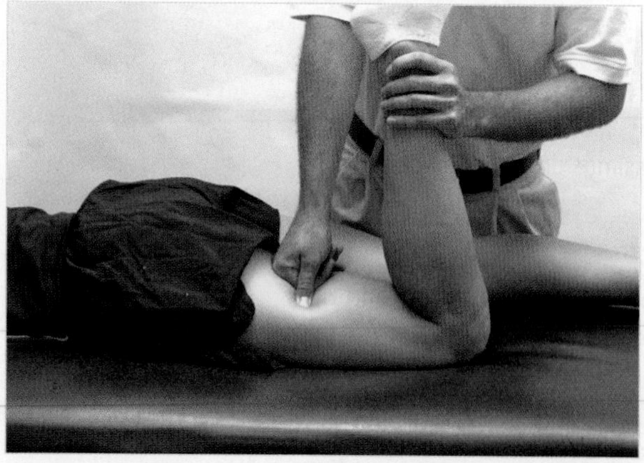

Figure 8-12

The positional release technique places the muscle in a position of comfort with the finger or thumb exerting submaximal pressure on a myofascial trigger point.

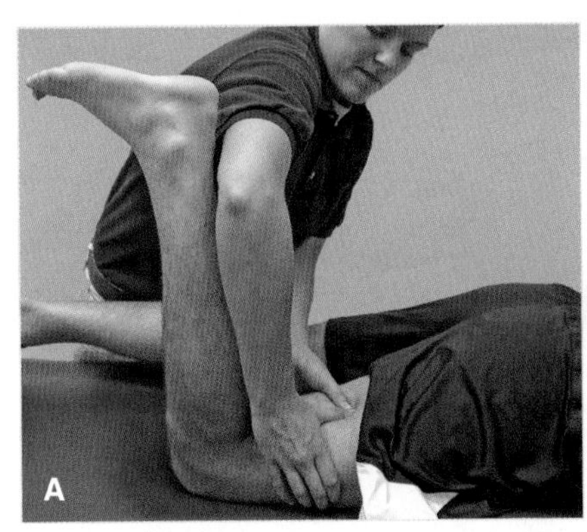

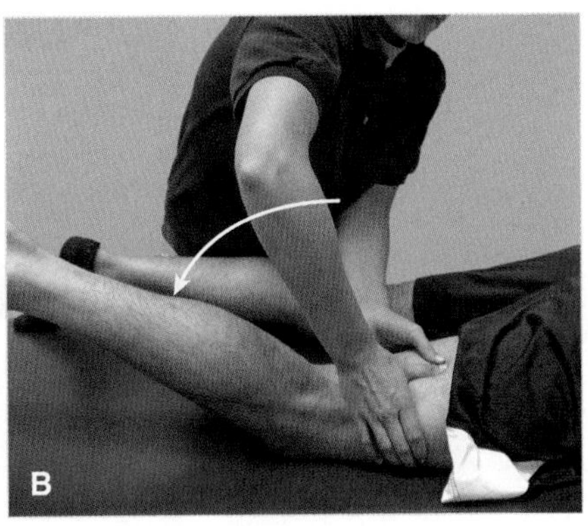

Figure 8-13 Soft-tissue mobilization technique

The muscle is elongated from a shortened position while static pressure is applied to the tender point.

in the direction of the fibers. Then the patient is asked to actively move the body part such that the musculature is elongated from a shortened position while the therapist continues to apply tension to the lesion (Figure 8-13). This should be repeated 3 to 5 times per treatment session. By breaking up the adhesions, the technique improves the patient's condition by softening and stretching the scar tissue, resulting in increased range of motion, increased strength, and improved circulation, optimizing healing. Treatments tend to be uncomfortable during the movement phases as the scar tissue or adhesions tear apart.[63] This is temporary and subsides almost immediately after the treatment. An important part of soft-tissue mobilization is for the patient to heed the therapist's recommendations regarding activity modification, stretching, and exercise.

Graston Technique

The Graston Technique is an instrument-assisted soft-tissue mobilization that enables clinicians to effectively break down scar tissue and fascial restrictions as well as stretch connective tissue and muscle fibers (Figure 8-14).[36,51] The technique utilizes 6 hand-held specially designed stainless steel instruments shaped to fit the contour of the body, to scan an area, locate, and then treat the injured tissue that is causing pain and restricting motion.[51] A clinician normally will palpate a painful area looking for usual nodules, restrictive barriers or tissue tensions. The instruments help to magnify existing restrictions and the clinician can feel these through the instruments.[36] Then the clinician can utilize the instruments to supply precise pressure to break up scar tissue, relieving the discomfort and helping to restore normal function. The instruments, with a narrow surface area at their edge, have the ability to separate fibers.

A specially designed lubricant is applied to the skin prior to using the instrument, allowing the instrument to glide over the skin without causing irritation. Using a cross-friction massage in multiple directions, which involves using the instruments to stroke or rub against the grain of the scar tissue, the clinician creates small amounts of trauma to the affected area.[36] This temporarily causes inflammation in the area, increasing the rate and amount of blood flow in and around the area. The theory is that this process helps initiate and promote the healing process of the affected soft tissues. It is common for the patient to experience some discomfort during the procedure and possibly some bruising.

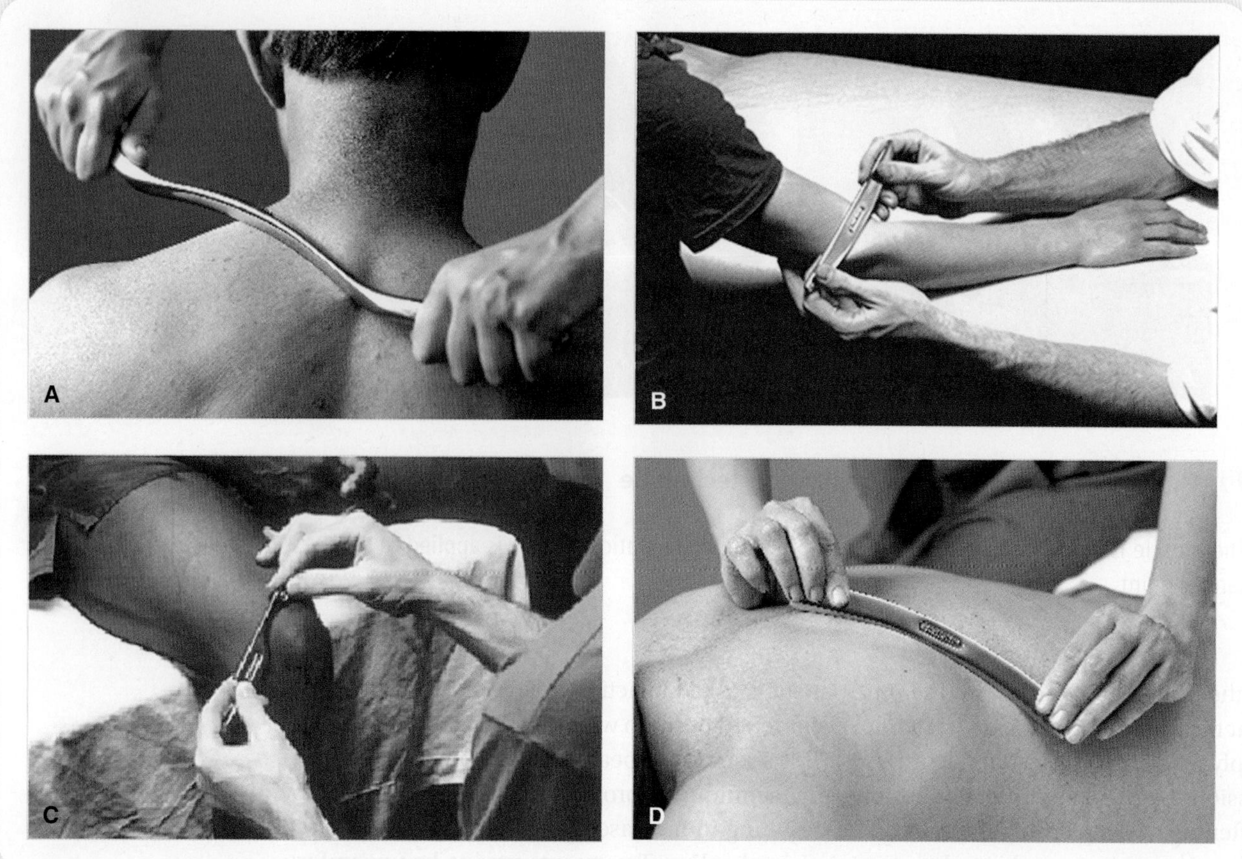

Figure 8-14

The Graston Technique uses handheld stainless steel instruments to locate and then separate existing restrictions within a muscle. (Courtesy of The Graston Technique.)

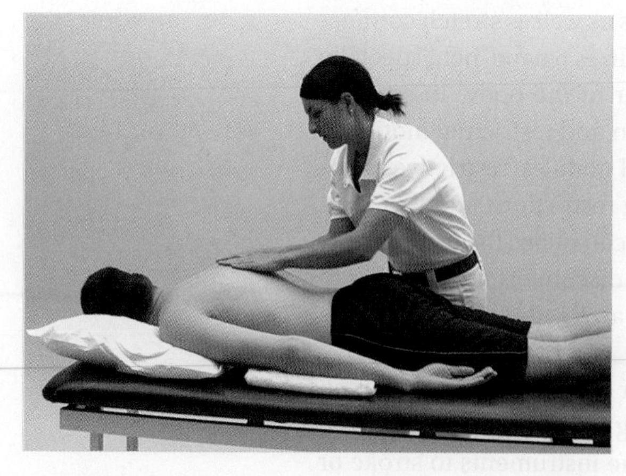

Figure 8-15

Massage can be an extremely effective technique for improving mobility and range of motion.

Ice application following the treatment may ease the discomfort. It is recommended that an exercise, stretching, and strengthening program be used in conjunction with the technique to help the injured tissues heal.

Massage

Massage is a mechanical stimulation of the tissues by means of rhythmically applied pressure and stretching (Figure 8-15).[83] Over the years, many claims have been made relative to the therapeutic benefits of massage, but few are based on well-controlled, well-designed studies. Therapists have used massage to increase flexibility and coordination as well as to increase pain threshold; to decrease neuromuscular excitability in the muscle being massaged; to stimulate circulation, thus improving energy transport to the muscle; to facilitate healing and restore joint mobility; and to remove lactic acid, thus alleviating muscle cramps.[83]

How these effects can be accomplished is determined by the specific approaches used with massage techniques and how they are applied. Generally, the effects of massage are either *reflexive* or *mechanical.* The effect of massage on the nervous system differs greatly according to the method employed, the pressure exerted, and the duration of applications. Through the reflex mechanism, sedation is induced. Slow, gentle, rhythmical, and superficial *effleurage* may relieve tension and soothe, rendering the muscles more relaxed. This indicates an effect on sensory and motor nerves locally and some central nervous system response. The mechanical approach seeks to make mechanical or histologic changes in myofascial structures through direct force applied superficially.[83]

Among the massage techniques used by therapists are the following[83]:

1. *Hoffa massage*—the classic form of massage, strokes include effleurage, petrissage, percussion or tapotement, and vibration.
2. *Friction massage*—used to increase the inflammatory response, particularly in case of chronic tendinitis or tenosynovitis.
3. *Acupressure*—massage of acupuncture and trigger points, used to reduce pain and irritation in anatomical areas known to be associated with specific points.
4. *Connective tissue massage*—a stroking technique used on layers of connective tissue, a relatively new form of treatment in this country, primarily affecting circulatory pathologies.
5. *Myofascial release*—used for the purpose of relieving soft tissue from the abnormal grip of tight fascia.
6. *Rolfing*—a system devised to correct inefficient structure by balancing the body within a gravitational field through a technique involving manual soft-tissue manipulation.
7. *Trager*—attempts to establish neuromuscular control so that more normal movement patterns can be routinely performed.

SUMMARY

1. Flexibility is the ability of the neuromuscular system to allow for efficient movement of a joint or a series of joints smoothly through a full range of motion.
2. Flexibility is specific to a given joint, and the term *good flexibility* implies that there are no joint abnormalities restricting movement.
3. Flexibility can be limited by muscles and tendons and their fascia, joint capsules or ligaments, fat, bone structure, skin, or neural tissue.
4. *Passive range of motion* refers to the degree to which a joint can be passively moved to the end points in the range of motion. *Active range of motion* refers to movement through the midrange of motion resulting from active contraction.
5. Measurement of joint flexibility is accomplished through the use of a goniometer or an inclinometer.
6. An agonist muscle is one that contracts to produce joint motion, while the antagonist muscle is stretched with contraction of the agonist.
7. Increases in flexibility can be attributed to neurophysiologic adaptations involving the stretch reflex and associated muscle spindles and Golgi tendon organs, changes in the viscoelastic and plastic properties of muscle, adaptations and changes in the kinetic chain, and alterations in intramuscular temperature.
8. Dynamic, static, and PNF techniques have all been used as stretching techniques for improving flexibility.

9. Stretching of tight neural structures and myofascial release stretching are also used to reestablish a full range of motion.
10. Strain-counterstrain is a passive technique that places a body part in a position of greatest comfort to decrease muscle tension and guarding, and to relieve pain.
11. Positional release therapy is similar to strain-counterstrain. Pressure is maintained on a tender point with the body part in a position of comfort for 90 seconds.
12. The active release technique is a deep-tissue technique used for breaking down scar tissue and adhesions and restoring function and movement.
13. Massage is the mechanical stimulation of tissue by means of rhythmically applied pressure and stretching. It allows the therapist, as a health care provider, to help a patient overcome pain and relax through the application of the therapeutic massage techniques.

REFERENCES

1. Alexander KM. Use of strain-counterstrain as an adjunct for treatment of chronic lower abdominal pain. *Phy Ther Case Rep.* 1999;2(5):205-208.
2. Allerheiliger W. Stretching and warm-up. In: Baechle T, ed. *Essentials of Strength Training.* Champaign, IL: Human Kinetics; 1994.
3. Alter M. *The science of flexibility.* Champaign, IL: Human Kinetics; 2004.
4. Andersen JC. Stretching before and after exercise: effect on muscle soreness and injury risk. *J Athl Train.* 2005;40(3):218-220.
5. Armiger P. Preventing musculotendinous injuries: a focus on flexibility. *Athl Ther Today.* 2000;5(4):20.
6. Bandy WD, Irion JM. The effect of time of static stretch on the flexibility of the hamstring muscles. *Phys Ther.* 1994;74:845-852.
7. Bandy WD, Irion JM, Briggler M. The effect of static stretch and dynamic range of motion training on the flexibility of the hamstring muscles. *J Orthop Sports Phys Ther.* 1998;27(4):295.
8. Basmajian J. *Therapeutic Exercise.* 4th ed. Baltimore, MD: Lippincott Williams & Wilkins; 1984.
9. Behm DG, Bambury A, Cahill F, Power K. Effect of acute static stretching on force, balance, reaction time, and movement time. *Med Sci Sports Exerc.* 2004;36(8):1397-1402.
10. Bernardo L. The effectiveness of Pilates training in healthy adults: an appraisal of the research literature. *J Bodyw Mov Ther.* 2007;11(2):106-110.
11. Blahnik J. *Full Body Flexibility.* Champaign, IL: Human Kinetics; 2004.
12. Blanke D. Flexibility. In: Mellion M, ed. *Sports Medicine Secrets.* Philadelphia, PA: Hanley & Belfus; 2002.
13. Boyle P. The effect of static and dynamic stretching on muscle force production. *J Sports Sci.* 2004;22(3): 273-274.
14. Burke DG, Culligan CJ, Holt LE. The theoretical basis of proprioceptive neuromuscular facilitation. *J Strength Cond Res.* 2000;14(4):496-500.
15. Carter AM, Kinzey SJ, Chitwood LF, Cole JL. Proprioceptive neuromuscular facilitation decreases muscle activity during the stretch reflex in selected posterior thigh muscles. *J Sport Rehabil.* 2000;9(4):269-278.
16. Chaitlow L. *Muscle Energy Techniques.* Philadelphia, PA: Churchill Livingstone; 2006.
17. Chaitlow L. *Positional Release Techniques (Advanced Soft Tissue Techniques).* Philadelphia, PA: Churchill Livingstone; 2002.
18. Chaitlow L. Positional release techniques in the treatment of muscle and joint dysfunction. *Clin Bull Myofascial Ther.* 1998;3(1):25-35.
19. Chalmers G. Re-examination of the possible role of golgi tendon organ and muscle spindle reflexes in proprioceptive neuromuscular facilitation muscle stretching. *Sports Biomech.* 2004;3(1):159-183.
20. Chapman EA, deVries HA, Swezey R. Joint stiffness: Effect of exercise on young and old men. *J Gerontol.* 1972;27:218.
21. Clark M. *Integrated Training for the New Millennium.* Calabasas, CA: National Academy of Sports Medicine; 2001.
22. Condon SA, Hutton RS. Soleus muscle EMG activity and ankle dorsiflexion range of motion from stretching procedures. *Phys Ther.* 1987;67:24-30.
23. Corbin C, Fox K. Flexibility: the forgotten part of fitness. *J Phys Educ.* 1985;16(6):191.
24. Corbin C, Noble L. Flexibility. *J Phys Educ Rec Dance.* 1980;51:23.
25. Corbin C, Noble L. Flexibility: a major component of physical fitness. In: Cundiff DE, ed. *Implementation of Health Fitness Exercise Programs.* Reston, VA: American

Alliance for Health, Physical Education, Recreation and Dance; 1985.

26. Cornelius W, Jackson A. The effects of cryotherapy and PNF on hip extensor flexibility. *J Athl Train.* 1984;19:183-184.
27. Cornelius WL, Hagemann RW Jr, Jackson AW. A study on placement of stretching within a workout. *J Sports Med Phys Fitness.* 1988;28(3):234.
28. Cornelius WL. *PNF and Other Flexibility Techniques.* Arlington, VA: Computer Microfilm International; 1986.
29. Cornelius WL. Two effective flexibility methods. *Athlet Train.* 1981;16(1):23.
30. Cornwell A. The acute effects of passive stretching on active musculotendinous stiffness. *Med Sci Sports Exerc.* 1997;29(5):281.
31. Couch J. *Runners World Yoga Book.* Mountain View, CA: World; 1982.
32. Cross KM, Worrell TW. Effects of a static stretching program on the incidence of lower extremity musculotendinous strains. *J Athl Train.* 1999;34(1):11.
33. D'Ambrogio K, Roth G. *Positional Release Therapy: Assessment and Treatment of Musculoskeletal Dysfunction.* St. Louis, MO: Mosby-Year Book; 1996.
34. Decoster L, Cleland J, Altieri C. The effects of hamstring stretching on range of motion: a systematic literature review. *J Orthop Sports Phys Ther.* 2005;3(6):377-387.
35. DeLuccio J. Instrument assisted soft tissue mobilization utilizing Graston technique: a physical therapist's perspective. *Orthop Phys Ther Pract.* 2006;18(3):32-34.
36. deVries HA. Evaluation of static stretching procedures for improvement of flexibility. *Res Q.* 1962;3:222-229.
37. De Deyne PG. Application of passive stretch and its implications for muscle fibers. *Phys Ther.* 2001;81(2):819-827.
38. DePino GM, Webright WG, Arnold BL. Duration of maintained hamstring flexibility after cessation of an acute static stretching protocol. *J Athl Train.* 2000;35(1):56.
39. Entyre BR, Abraham LD. Ache-reflex changes during static stretching and two variations of proprioceptive neuromuscular facilitation techniques. *Electroencephalogr Clin Neurophysiol.* 1986;63: 174-179.
40. Entyre BR, Abraham LD. Antagonist muscle activity during stretching: a paradox reassessed. *Med Sci Sports Exerc.* 1988;20:285-289.
41. Entyre BR, Lee EJ. Chronic and acute flexibility of men and women using three different stretching techniques. *Res Q Exerc Sport.* 1988;59:222-228.
42. Fowles JR, Sale DG, MacDougall JD. Reduced strength after passive stretch of the human plantar flexors. *J Appl Physiol.* 2000;89(3):1179-1188.
43. Ferreira G, Nunes T, Teixeira I. Gains in flexibility related to measures of muscular performance: Impact of flexibility on muscular performance. *Clin J Sport Med.* 2007;17(4):276-281.
44. Funk D, Swank AM, Adams KJ, Treolo D. Efficacy of moist heat pack application over static stretching on hamstring flexibility. *J Strength Cond Res.* 2001;15(1):123-126.
45. Godges JJ, MacRae H, Longdon C, et al. The effects of two stretching procedures on hip range of motion and joint economy. *J Orthop Sports Phys Ther.* 1989;11:350-357.
46. Gribble P, Prentice W. Effects of static and hold-relax stretching on hamstring range of motion using the Flex-Ability LE 1000. *J Sport Rehabil.* 1999;8(3):195.
47. Hedrick A. Dynamic flexibility training. *Strength Cond J.* 2000;22(5):33-38.
48. Herling J. It's time to add strength training to our fitness programs. *J Phys Educ Program.* 1981;79:17.
49. Heyward VH. Assessing flexibility and designing stretching programs. In: Heyward VH, ed. *Advanced Fitness Assessment and Exercise Prescription.* 6th ed. Champaign, IL: Human Kinetics; 2010:265–282.
50. Holt LE TW. Pelham, Burke DG. Modifications to the standard sit-and-reach flexibility protocol. *J Athl Train.* 1999;34(1):43.
51. Howitt S. The conservative treatment of trigger thumb using Graston techniques and active release techniques. *J Can Chiropr Assoc.* 2006;50(4):249-254.
52. Humphrey LD. Flexibility. *J Phys Educ Rec Dance.* 1981;52:41.
53. Hunter G. Specific soft tissue mobilization in the management of soft tissue dysfunction. *Man Ther.* 1998;3(1):2-11.
54. Ishii DK. Flexibility strexercises for co-ed groups. *Scholastic Coach.* 1976;45:31.
55. Jones L. *Strain-Counterstrain.* Boise, ID: Jones; 1995.
56. Kaplan B, Pierce M. *Yoga for Your Life: A practice Manual of Breath and Movement for Everybody.* New York, NY: Sterling Publishing; 2008.
57. Keirns M, ed. *Myofascial Release in Sports Medicine.* Champaign, IL: Human Kinetics; 2000.
58. Knott M, Voss P. *Proprioceptive Neuromuscular Facilitation.* 3rd ed. New York, NY: Harper & Row; 1985.
59. Kokkonen J, Nelson A. Chronic static stretching improves exercise performance. *Med Sci Sports Exerc.* 2007;39(10):1825-1831.
60. Kokkonen JE, Nelson C, Arnold G. Chronic stretching improves sport specific skills. *Med Sci Sports Exerc.* 1997;29(5):67.
61. Kokkonen JN, Nelson AG, Arnall DA. Acute stretching inhibits strength endurance. *Med Sci Sports Exerc.* 2001;35(5):s11.
62. Kubo K, Kanehisa H, Fukunaga T. Effect of stretching training on the viscoelastic properties of human tendon structures in vivo. *J Appl Physiol.* 2002;92(2):595-601.
63. Leahy M. Improved treatments for carpal tunnel and related syndromes. *Chiropr Sports Med.* 1995;9(1):6.
64. Lentell G, Hetherington T, Eagan J, et al. The use of thermal agents to influence the effectiveness of a low-load prolonged stretch. *J Orthop Sports Phys Ther.* 1992;5:200-207.

65. Liemohn W. Flexibility and muscular strength. *J Phys Educ Rec Dance.* 1988;59(7):37.
66. Louden KL, Bolier CE, Allison AK, et al. Effects of two stretching methods on the flexibility and retention of flexibility at the ankle joint in runners. *Phys Ther.* 1985;65:698.
67. Madding SW JG. Wong, Hallum A. Effects of duration of passive stretching on hip abduction range of motion. *J Orthop Sports Phys Ther.* 1987;8:409-416.
68. Mann D, Whedon C. Functional stretching: implementing a dynamic stretching program. *Athl Ther Today.* 2001;6(3):10-13.
69. Manheim C. *Myofascial Release Manual.* Thorofare, NJ: Slack; 2001.
70. Marek S, Cramer J, Fincher L. Acute effects of static and proprioceptive neuromuscular facilitation stretching on muscle strength and power output. *J Athl Train.* 2005;40(2):94-103.
71. Markos PD. Ipsilateral and contralateral effects of proprioceptive neuromuscular facilitation techniques on hip motion and electromyographic activity. *Phys Ther.* 1979;59:1366-1373.
72. McAtee R. *Facilitated Stretching.* Champaign, IL: Human Kinetics; 2007.
73. McClellan E, Padua D, Prentice W. Effects of myofascial release and static stretching on active range of motion and muscle activity. *J Athl Train.* 2000;35(3):329.
74. Moore M, Hutton R. Electromyographic investigation of muscle stretching techniques. *Med Sci Sports Exerc.* 1980;12:322-329.
75. Murphy P. Warming up before stretching advised. *Phys Sportsmed.* 1986;14(3):45.
76. Nelson R. An update on flexibility. *Natl Strength Cond Assoc.* 2005;27(1):10-16.
77. Norris C. *Flexibility Principles and Practices.* London, UK: A&C Black; 1995.
78. Power K, Behm D, Cahill F, Carroll M, Young W. An acute bout of static stretching: effects on force and jumping performance. *Med Sci Sports Exerc.* 2004;36(8): 1389-1396.
79. Prentice WE, Kooima E. The use of PNF techniques in rehabilitation of sport-related injury. *Athlet Train..* 1986;21(1):26-31.
80. Prentice WE. A comparison of static stretching and PNF stretching for improving hip joint flexibility. *J Athl Train.* 1983;18:56-59.
81. Prentice WE. A review of PNF techniques—implications for athletic rehabilitation and performance. *Forum Medicum.* 1989;51:1-13.
82. Prentice WE. An electromyographic analysis of heat or cold and stretching for inducing muscular relaxation. *J Orthop Sports Phys Ther.* 1982;3:133-140.
83. Prentice W. Sports massage. In: Prentice W, ed. *Therapeutic Modalities in Sports Medicine and Athletic Training.* New York, NY: McGraw-Hill; 2009:349-372.
84. Rasch P. *Kinesiology and Applied Anatomy.* Philadelphia, PA: Lea & Febiger; 1989.
85. Rubini E, Costa A. The effects of stretching on strength performance. *Sports Med.* 2007;37(3):213.
86. Sady SP, Wortman M, Blanke D. Flexibility training: ballistic, static, or proprioceptive neuromuscular facilitation? *Arch Phys Med Rehabil.* 1982;63: 261-263.
87. Sapega AA, Quedenfeld T, Moyer R, et al. Biophysical factors in range-of-motion exercise. *Phys Sportsmed.* 1981;9(12):57.
88. Schilling BK, Stone MH. Stretching: acute effects on strength and power performance. *Strength Cond J.* 2000;22(1):44.
89. Sefton J. Myofascial release for athletic trainers, part 1. *Athl Ther Today.* 2004;9(1):40.
90. Schiowitz S. Facilitated positional release. *J Am Osteopath Assoc.* 1990;90(2):145-146, 151-155.
91. Shellock F, Prentice WE. Warm-up and stretching for improved physical performance and prevention of sport related injury. *Sports Med.* 1985;2:267-278.
92. Shindo M, Harayama H, Kondo K, et al. Changes in reciprocal Ia inhibition during voluntary contraction in man. *Exp Brain Res.* 1984;53:400-408.
93. Siatras T, Papadopoulos G, Maeletzi D, Gerodimos V, Kellis P. Static and dynamic acute stretching effect on gymnasts' speed in vaulting. *Ped Ex Sci.* 2003;15: 383-391.
94. Spernoga SG, Uhl TL, Arnold BL, Gansneder BM. Duration of maintained hamstring flexibility after a one time, modified hold-relax stretching protocol. *J Athl Train.* 2001;36(1):44-48.
95. Speicher T. Top 10 positional release therapy techniques to break the chain of pain, part 1. *Athl Ther Today.* 2006;11(5):60.
96. St. George F. *The Stretching Handbook: Ten Steps to Muscle Fitness.* Roseville, IL: Simon & Schuster; 1997.
97. Stamford B. A stretching primer. *Phys Sportsmed.* 1994;22(9):85-86.
98. Stone J. Myofascial release. *Athl Ther Today.* 2000;5(4):34-35.
99. Stone J. Strain-counterstrain. *Athl Ther Today.* 2000;5(6):30.
100. Surburg P. Flexibility/range of motion. In: Winnick JP, ed. *The Brockport Physical Fitness Training Guide.* Champaign, IL: Human Kinetics; 1999.
101. Surburg P. Flexibility training program design. In: Miller P, ed. *Fitness Programming and Physical Disability.* Champaign, IL: Human Kinetics; 1995.
102. Tanigawa MC. Comparison of the hold relax procedure and passive mobilization on increasing muscle length. *Phys Ther.* 1972;52:725.
103. Taylor DC, Brooks DE, Ryan JB. Viscoelastic characteristics of muscle: passive stretching versus muscular contractions. *Med Sci Sports Exerc.* 1997;29(12):1619-1624.

104. Thacker S, Gilchrist J, Stroup D. The impact of stretching on sports injury risk: a systematic review of the literature. *Med Sci Sports Exerc.* 2004;36(3):371-378.
105. Tobias M, Sullivan JP. *Complete Stretching.* New York, NY: Knopf; 1992.
106. Van Hatten B. Passive versus active stretching. *Phys Ther.* 2005;85(1):80.
107. Van Mechelen P. Prevention of running injuries by warm-up, cool-down, and stretching. *Am J Sports Med.* 1993;21(5):711-719.
108. Voss DE, Lonta MK, Myers GJ. *Proprioceptive Neuro-Muscular Facilitation: Patterns and Techniques.* 3rd ed. Philadelphia, PA: Lippincott Williams & Wilkins; 1985.
109. Wessel J, Wan A. Effect of stretching on intensity of delayed-onset muscle soreness. *J Sports Med.* 1984;2:83-87.
110. Winters MV, Blake GC, Trost J. Passive versus active stretching of hip flexor muscles in subjects with limited hip extension: A randomized clinical trial. *Phys Ther.* 2004;84(9):800-807.
111. Worrell T, Smith T, Winegardner J. Effect of hamstring stretching on hamstring muscle performance. *J Orthop Sports Phys Ther.* 1994;20(3):154-159.
112. Zachewski J. Flexibility for sports. In: Sanders B, ed. *Sports Physical Therapy.* Norwalk, CT: Appleton & Lange; 1990:201-238.
113. Zebas CJ, Rivera ML. Retention of flexibility in selected joints after cessation of a stretching exercise program. In: Dotson CO, Humphrey HJ, eds. *Exercise Physiology: Current Selected Research Topics.* New York, NY: AMS Press; 1985.

9

Impaired Neuromuscular Control

Reactive Neuromuscular Training

Michael L. Voight and Gray Cook

OBJECTIVES **After completion of this chapter, the physical therapist should be able to do the following:**

- Explain why neuromuscular control is important in the rehabilitation process.
- Define and discuss the importance of proprioception in the neuromuscular control process.
- Define and discuss the different levels of central nervous system motor control and the neural pathways responsible for the transmission of afferent and efferent information at each level.
- Define and discuss the 2 motor mechanisms involved with interpreting afferent information and coordinating an efferent response.
- Develop a rehabilitation program that uses various techniques of neuromuscular control exercises.

What Is Neuromuscular Control and Why Is It Important?

The basic goal in rehabilitation is to enhance one's ability to function within the environment and to perform the specific activities of daily living (ADL). The entire rehabilitation process should be focused on improving the functional status of the patient. The concept of functional training is not new. In fact, functional training has been around for many years. It is widely accepted that to get better at a specific activity, or to get stronger for an activity, one must practice that specific activity. Therefore, the functional progression for return to ADL can be defined as breaking the specific activities down into a hierarchy and then performing them in a sequence that allows for the acquisition or reacquisition of that skill.

From a historical perspective, the rehabilitation process following injury has focused upon the restoration of muscular strength, endurance, and joint flexibility without any consideration of the role of the neuromuscular mechanism. This is a common error in the rehabilitation process. We cannot assume that clinical programs alone using traditional methods will lead to a safe return to function. Limiting the rehabilitation program to these traditional programs alone often results in an incomplete restoration of ability and quite possibly leads to an increased risk of reinjury.

The overall objective of the functional exercise program is to return the patient to the preinjury level as quickly and as safely as possible. Specific training activities should be designed to restore both dynamic stability about the joint and specific ADL skills. To accomplish this objective, a basic tenet of exercise physiology is employed. The SAID (specific adaptations to imposed demands) principle states that the body will adapt to the stress and strain placed upon it.[130] Patients cannot succeed in ADL if they have not been prepared to meet all of the demands of their specific activity.[130] Reactive neuromuscular training (RNT) is not intended to replace traditional rehabilitation, but rather to help bridge the gap left by traditional rehabilitation in a complementary fashion via proprioceptive and balance training in order to promote a more functional return to activity.[130] The main objective of the RNT program is to facilitate the unconscious process of interpreting and integrating the peripheral sensations received by the central nervous system (CNS) into appropriate motor responses.

Terminology: What Do We Really Need to Know?

Success in skilled performance depends upon how effectively the individual detects, perceives, and uses relevant sensory information. Knowing exactly where our limbs are in space and how much muscular effort is required to perform a particular action is critical for the successful performance in all activities requiring intricate coordination of the various body parts. Fortunately, information about the position and movement of various body parts is available from the peripheral receptors located in and around the articular structures.

About the normal healthy joint, both static and dynamic stabilizers serve to provide support. The role of the capsule-ligamentous tissues in the dynamic restraint of the joint has been well established in the literature.[2,3,19,33,45-50,110] Although the primary role of these structures is mechanical in nature by providing structural support and stabilization to the joint, the capsuloligamentous tissues also play an important sensory role by detecting joint position and motion.[33,34,105] Sensory afferent feedback from the receptors in the capsuloligamentous structures projects directly to the reflex and cortical pathways, thereby mediating reactive muscle activity for dynamic restraint.[2,3,33,34,67] The efferent motor response that ensues from the sensory information is called neuromuscular control. Sensory information is sent to the CNS to be processed, and appropriate motor activities are executed.

Physiology of Proprioception

Although there has been no definitive definition of proprioception, Beard et al described proprioception as consisting of 3 similar components: (a) a static awareness of joint position, (b) kinesthetic awareness, and (c) a closed-loop efferent reflex response required for the regulation of muscle tone and activity.[7] From a physiologic perspective, proprioception is a specialized variation of the sensory modality of touch. Specifically defined, proprioception is the cumulative neural input to the CNS from mechanoreceptors in the joint capsules, ligaments, muscles, tendons, and skin.

A rehabilitation program that addresses the need for restoring normal joint stability and proprioception cannot be constructed until one has a total appreciation of both the mechanical and sensory functions of the articular structures.[12] Knowledge of the basic physiology of how these muscular and joint mechanoreceptors work together in the production of smooth controlled coordinated motion is critical in developing a rehabilitation training program. This is because the role of the joint musculature extends beyond absolute strength and the capacity to resist fatigue. Simply restoring mechanical restraints or strengthening the associated muscles neglects the smooth coordinated neuromuscular controlling mechanisms required for joint stability.[12] The complexity of joint motion necessitates synergy and synchrony of muscle firing patterns, thereby permitting proper joint stabilization, especially during sudden changes in joint position, which is common in functional activities. Understanding these relationships and functional implications will allow the clinician greater variability and success in returning patients safely back to their playing environment.

Sherrington first described the term proprioception in the early 1900s when he noted the presence of receptors in the joint capsular structures that were primarily reflexive in nature.[77,105] Since that time, mechanoreceptors have been morphohistologically identified about the articular structures in both animal and human models. Mechanoreceptors are specialized end organs that function as biologic transducers that can convert the mechanical energy of physical deformation (elongation, compression, and pressure) into action nerve potentials yielding proprioceptive information.[45] Although receptor discharge varies according to the intensity of the distortion, mechanoreceptors can also be based upon their discharge rates. Quickly adapting receptors cease discharging shortly after the onset of a stimulus, while slowly adapting receptors continue to discharge while the stimulus is present.[21,33,45] About the healthy joint, quickly adapting receptors are responsible for providing conscious and unconscious kinesthetic sensations in response to joint movement or acceleration, while slowly adapting mechanoreceptors provide continuous feedback and thus proprioceptive information relative to joint position.[21,45,71]

Once stimulated, mechanoreceptors are able to adapt. With constant stimulation, the frequency of the neural impulses decreases. The functional implication is that mechanoreceptors detect change and rates of change, as opposed to steady-state conditions.[104] This input is then analyzed in the CNS for joint position and movement.[139] The status of the articular structures is sent to the CNS so that information regarding static versus dynamic conditions, equilibrium versus disequilibrium, or biomechanical stress and strain relations can be evaluated.[129,130] Once processed and evaluated, this proprioceptive information becomes capable of influencing muscle tone, motor execution programs, and cognitive somatic perceptions or kinesthetic awareness.[92] Proprioceptive information also protects the joint from damage caused by movement exceeding the normal physiologic range of motion and helps to determine the appropriate balance of synergistic and antagonistic forces. All of this information helps to generate a somatosensory image within the CNS. Therefore, the soft tissues surrounding a joint serve a double purpose: they provide biomechanical support to the bony partners making up the joint, keeping them in relative anatomic alignment, and through an extensive afferent neurologic network, they provide valuable proprioceptive information.

Before the 1970s, articular receptors in the joint capsule were held primarily responsible for joint proprioception.[104] Since then there has been considerable debate as to whether muscular and articular mechanoreceptors interact. As originally described, the articular mechanoreceptors were located primarily on the parts of the joint capsule that are stretched the most when the joint is moved. This led investigators to believe that these receptors were primarily responsible for perception of joint motion. Skoglund found individual receptors that were active at very specific locations in the range of limb movement (eg, from 150 to 180 degrees of joint angle for a particular cell).[113] Another cell would fire at a different set of joint angles. By integrating the information, the CNS could "know" where the limb was in space by detecting which receptors were active. The problem with this theory is that several studies have shown that the majority of the capsular receptors only respond at the extremes of the range of motion or during other situations when a strong stimulus is imparted onto the structures such as distraction or compression.[21,43,48,49] Furthermore, other studies found that the nature of the firing pattern is dependent on whether the movement is active or passive.[14] In addition, the mechanoreceptor firing is dependent on the direction of motion from the joint.[115] The fact that the firing pattern of the joint receptors is dependent on factors other than simple position sense has seriously challenged the thought that the articular mechanoreceptors alone are the means by which the system determines joint position.

A more contemporary viewpoint is that muscle receptors play a more important role in signaling joint position.[25,42] There are 2 main types of muscle receptors that provide complementary information about the state of the muscles. The muscle spindle is located within the muscle fibers and is most active when the muscle is stretched. The Golgi tendon organ (GTO) is located in the junction between the muscle and the tendon, and is most active when the muscle contracts.

Muscle Spindle

The muscle spindle consists of 3 main components: small muscle fibers called *intrafusal fibers* that are innervated by the gamma efferent motor neurons, and types Ia and II afferent neurons (Figure 9-1). The intrafusal fibers are made up of 2 types—bag and chain fibers—the polar ends of which provide a tension on the central region of the spindle, called the *equatorial region.* The sensory receptors located here are sensitive to the length of the equatorial region when the spindle is stretched. The major neurologic connection to this sensory region is the Ia afferent fiber, whose output is related to the length of the equatorial region (position information) as well as to the rate of change in length of this region (velocity information). The spindle connects to the alpha motor neurons for the same muscle, providing excitation to the muscle when it is stretched.

There has been a great deal of controversy about what the spindle actually signals to the CNS.[36] A major conceptual problem in the past was that the output of the Ia afferent that presumably signals stretch or velocity is related to 2 separate factors.[102] First, Ia output is increased by the elongation of the overall muscle via elongation of the spindle as a whole. However, the Ia output is also related to the stretch placed on the equatorial region by the intrafusal fibers by the gamma motor neurons. Therefore, the CNS would have difficulty in interpreting changes in the Ia output as being caused by changes in the overall muscle length with a constant gamma motor neuron activity, changes in gamma motor neuron activity with a constant muscle length, or perhaps changes in both.[102] Another problem was

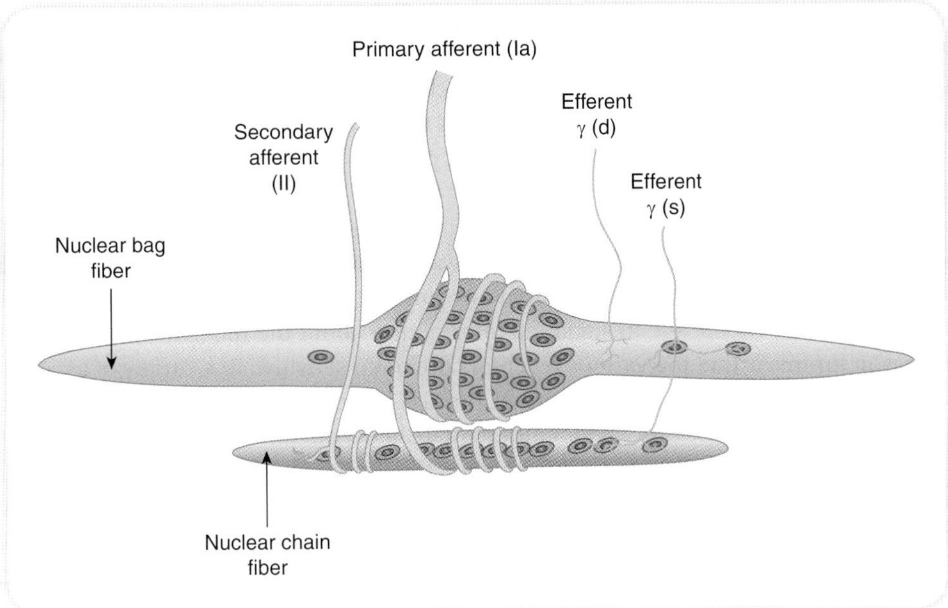

Figure 9-1 The anatomy of muscle receptors

Muscle spindle and GTO. (Reproduced, with permission, from Shumway-Cook A, Woollacott M. Physiology of motor control. In: Shumway-Cook A, Woollacott M, eds. *Motor Control: Theory and Practical Applications*. Baltimore, MD: Williams & Wilkins; 1995:53.)

presented by Gelfan and Carter, who suggested that there was no strong evidence that the Ia afferent fibers actually sent their information to the primary sensory cortex.[39] Because of these factors, it was widely held that the muscle spindle was not important for the conscious perception of movement or position.

Goodwin et al were the first to refute this viewpoint.[43] They found as much as 40 degrees of misalignment of arm that had vibration applied to the biceps tendon.[43] The vibration of the tendon produces a small, rapid, alternating stretch and release of the tendon, which affects the muscle spindle and distorts the output of the Ia afferents from the spindles located in the vibrated muscle. The interpretation was that the vibration distorted the Ia information coming from the same muscle, which led to a misperception of the limb's position. Others have found the same results when applying vibration to a muscle tendon.[97,108,109] This information supports the idea that the muscle spindle is important in providing information to the CNS about limb position and velocity of movement.

Golgi Tendon Organ

The GTOs are tiny receptors located in the junction where the muscle "blends into" the tendon. They are ideally located to provide information about the tension within the muscles because they lie in series with the muscle force-producing contractile elements. The GTO has been shown to produce an inhibition of the muscle in which it is located when a stretch to the active muscle is produced. The fact that a stretch force near the physiologic limit of the muscle was required to induce the tendon organ to fire led to the speculation that this receptor was primarily a protective receptor that would prevent the muscle from contracting so forcibly that it would rupture the tendon. Houk and Henneman[62] and Stuart et al[119] have provided a more precise understanding of the sensitivity of the GTOs. Anatomic evidence reveals that each organ is connected to only a small group (3 to 25) of muscle fibers, not to the entire muscle as had been previously suspected. Therefore, the GTO appears to be in a good position to sense the tensions produced in a limited number of individual motor units, not in the whole muscle. Houk and Henneman determined that the tendon organs could respond to forces of less than 0.1 G.[62] Therefore, the GTOs are very sensitive detectors for active tension in localized portions of a muscle, in addition to having a protective function.

It is most likely that the muscle and joint receptors work complementarily to one another in this complex afferent system, with each modifying the function of the other.[15,46,52,61] An important concept is that any one of the receptors in isolation from the others is generally ineffective in signaling information about the movements of the body. The reason for this is that the various receptors are often sensitive to a variety of aspects of body motion at the same time. For example, the GTOs probably cannot signal information about movement, because they cannot differentiate between the forces produced in a static contraction and the same forces produced when the limb is moving.[102] Although the spindle is sensitive to muscle length, it is also sensitive to the rate of change in length (velocity) and to the activity in the intrafusal fibers that are known to be active during contractions. Therefore, the spindle confounds information about the position of the limb and the level of contraction of the muscle. The joint receptors are sensitive to joint position, but their output can be affected by the tensions applied and by the direction of movement.

Because both the articular and muscle receptors have well-described cortical connections to substantiate a central role in proprioception, some have suggested that the CNS combines and integrates the information in some way to resolve the ambiguity in the signals produced by any one of the receptors.[102,138] Producing an ensemble of information by combining the various separate sources could enable the generation of less ambiguous information about movement.[36] Therefore, the sensory mechanoreceptors may represent a continuum rather than separate distinct classes of receptor.[105] This concept is further illustrated by research that demonstrated a relationship between the muscle spindle sensory afferent and joint mechanoreceptors.[18] McCloskey has also demonstrated a relationship between the cutaneous afferent and joint mechanoreceptors.[78] These studies suggest a complex role for the joint mechanoreceptors in smooth, coordinated, and controlled movement.

Neural Pathways

Information generated and encoded by the mechanoreceptors in the muscle tendon units is projected upward via specialized pathways toward the cortex, where it is further analyzed and integrated with other sensory inputs.[99] Proprioceptive information is relayed to the cerebral cortex via 1 of 2 major ascending systems: the dorsal column and the spinothalamic tract. Both of these pathways involve 3 orders of neurons and 3 synapses in transmitting sensory input from the periphery to the cortex. The primary afferent, which is connected to the peripheral receptor, synapses with a second neuron in the spinal cord or lower brain, depending upon the type of sensation. Before reaching the cerebral cortex, all sensory information passes through an important group of nuclei located in the area of the brain called the *diencephalon*. It is within this group of more than 30 nuclei, collectively called the *thalamus*, that neurophysiologists consider the initial stages of sensory integration and perceptual awareness to begin. Therefore, the second neuron then conveys the information to the thalamus where it synapses with the third and final neuron in the area of the thalamus called the *ventroposterolateral* area. The thalamus achieves these functions by "gating out" irrelevant sensory inputs and directing those that are relevant to an impending or ongoing action toward primary sensory areas within the cortex. The sensory pathways finally terminate in the primary sensory areas located in different regions of the cortex. It is at this point that we become consciously aware of the sensations.

The final perception of what is occurring in the environment around us is achieved after all of these sensations are integrated and then interpreted by the association areas that lie adjacent to the various primary sensory areas associated with the different types of sensory input. With the assistance of memory, objects seen or felt can be interpreted in a meaningful way. The dorsal column plays an important role in motor control because of its speed in transmission. For proprioception to play a protective role through reflex muscle splinting, the information must be transmitted and processed rapidly. The heavily myelinated and wide-diameter axons within this system transmit at speeds of 80 to 100 m/s. This characteristic facilitates rapid sampling of the environment, which enhances the accuracy of motor actions about to be executed and of those already in progress. By comparison, nociceptor transmission occurs at a rate of approximately 1 m/s. Thus proprioceptive information may play a more significant role than pain in the prevention of injuries.

In contrast to the transmission properties associated with the dorsal column system, neurons that make up the spinothalamic tract are small in diameter (some of which are unmyelinated) and conduct slowly (1 to 40 m/s). The 4 spinocerebellar tracts also convey important proprioceptive information from the neuromuscular receptors to the cerebellum. Unlike the dorsal column, these pathways do not synapse in either the thalamus or cerebral cortex. As a result, the proprioceptive information conveyed by the spinocerebellar tracts does not lead to conscious perceptions of limb position. The afferent sources are believed to contribute to kinesthesia.

Assessment of Joint Proprioception

Assessment of proprioception is valuable for identifying proprioceptive deficits. If deficiencies in proprioception can be clinically diagnosed in a reliable manner, a clinician would know when and if a problem exists and when the problem has been corrected.[130] There are several ways to measure or assess proprioception about a joint. From an anatomic perspective, histologic studies can be conducted to identify mechanoreceptors within the specific joint structures. Neurophysiologic testing can assess sensory thresholds and nerve conduction velocities.[6,20,31] From a clinical perspective, proprioception can be assessed by measuring the components that make up the proprioceptive mechanism: kinesthesia (perception of motion) and joint position sensibility (perception of joint position).[17]

Measuring either the angle or time threshold to detection of passive motion can assess kinesthetic sensibility.[112] With the subject seated, the patient's limb is mechanically rotated at a slow constant angular velocity (2 degrees per second). With passive motion, the capsuloligamentous structures come under tension and deform the mechanoreceptors located within. The mechanoreceptor deformation is converted into an electrical impulse, which is then processed within the CNS. Patients are instructed to stop the lever arm movement as soon as they perceive motion. Depending on which measurement is used, either the time to detection or degrees of angular displacement is recorded.

Joint position sense is assessed through the reproduction of both active and passive joint repositioning. The examiner places the limb at a preset target angle and holds it there for a minimum of 10 seconds to allow the patient to mentally process the target angle. Following this, the limb is returned to the starting position. The patient is asked to either actively reproduce or stop the device when passive repositioning of the angle has been achieved (Figure 9-2). The examiner measures the ability of an individual to accurately reproduce the preset target angle position. The angular displacement is recorded as the error in degrees from the preset target angle. Active angle reproduction measures the ability of both the muscle and capsular receptors while passive repositioning primarily measures the capsular receptors. With both tests of proprioception, the patient is blindfolded during

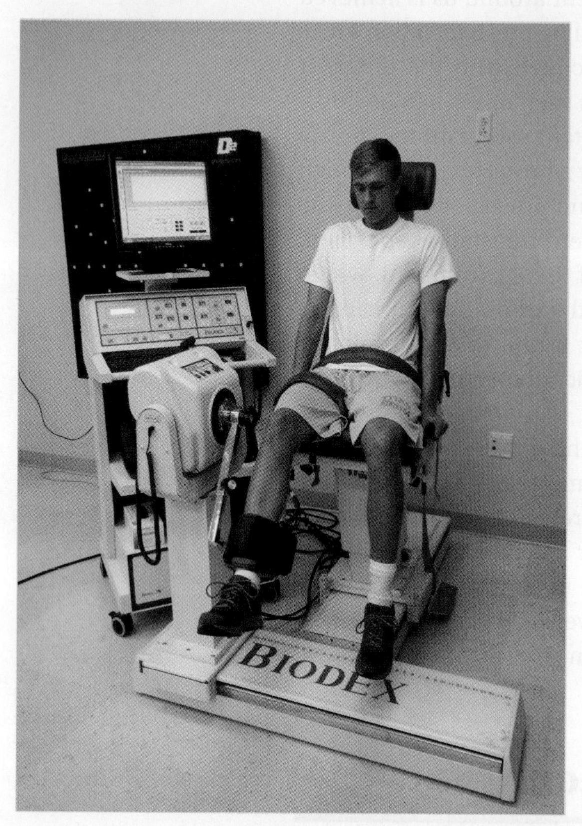

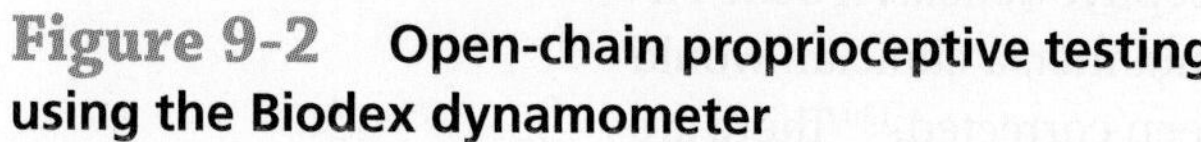
Figure 9-2 Open-chain proprioceptive testing using the Biodex dynamometer

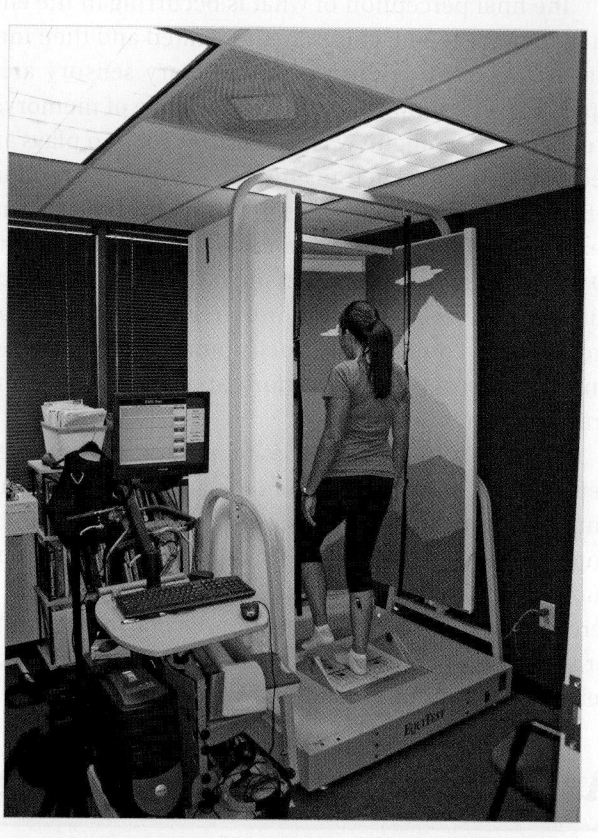

Figure 9-3 EMG assessment of reflex muscle firing as a result of perturbation on the NeuroCom EquiTest

testing to eliminate all visual cueing. In patients with unilateral involvement, the contralateral uninjured limb can serve as an external control for comparison.

The main limitation to current proprioceptive testing is that neither time/angle threshold to detection of passive motion provides an assessment of the unconscious reflex arc believed to provide dynamic joint stability. The assessment of reflex capabilities is usually performed by measuring the latency of muscular activation to involuntary perturbation through electromyogram (EMG) interpretation of firing patterns of those muscles crossing the respective joint (Figure 9-3).[132] The ability to quantify the sequence of muscle firing can provide a valuable tool for the assessment of asynchronous neuromuscular activation patterns following injury.[74,140] A delay or lag in the firing time of the dynamic stabilizers about the joint can result in recurrent joint subluxation and joint deterioration.

Proprioception and Motor Control

The efferent response that is produced as the result of the proprioceptive afferent input is termed *neuromuscular control*. In general, there are 2 motor control mechanisms involved in the interpretation of afferent information and coordinating an efferent response.[54] One of the ways in which motor control is achieved relies heavily on the concept that sensory feedback information is used to regulate our movements. This is a more traditional viewpoint of motor control. The closed-loop system of motor control emphasizes the essential role of the reactive or sensory feedback in the planning, execution, and modification of action. The closed-loop systems involve the processing of feedback against a reference of correctness, the determination of error, and a subsequent correction.[102] The feedback mechanism of motor control relies on the numerous reflex pathways in an attempt to continuously adjust ongoing muscle activation.[29,102] The receptors for the feedback supplied to closed-loop systems are the eyes, vestibular apparatus, joint receptors, and muscle receptors. One important point to note about the closed-loop system of feedback motor control is that this loop requires a great deal of time for a stimulus to be processed and yield a response. Rapid actions do not provide sufficient time for the system to (a) generate an error, (b) detect the error, (c) determine the correction, (d) initiate the correction, and (e) correct the movement before a rapid movement is completed.[102] The best example of this concept is demonstrated by the left jab of former boxing champion Muhammad Ali. The movement itself was approximately 40 milliseconds, yet visually detecting an aiming error and correcting it during the same movement should require approximately 200 milliseconds.[102] The movement is finished before any correction can begin. Therefore, closed-loop feedback control models seem to have their greatest strength in explaining movements that are very slow in time or that have very high movement accuracy requirements.[102]

In contrast, a more contemporary theory emphasizes the open-loop system, which focuses upon the a priori generation of action plans in anticipation of movement produced by a central executor somewhere in the cerebral cortex.[102] The ability to prepare the muscles prior to movement is called *pretuning* or *feed-forward motor control*. The springlike qualities of a muscle can be exploited (through preactivation) by the CNS in anticipation of movements and joint loads. This concept has been termed feed-forward motor control, in which prior sensory feedback (experience) concerning a task is fed forward to preprogram muscle activation patterns.[62] Vision serves an important feed-forward function by preparing the motor system in advance of the actual movement. Preactivated muscles can provide quick compensation for external loads and are critical for dynamic joint stability. Researchers have shown that corrections for rapid changes in body position can occur far more rapidly (30 to 80 milliseconds) than the closed-loop latencies of 200 milliseconds that were previously reported.[27,63,69] Therefore, the motor control system operates with a feed-forward mode in order to send some signals "ahead of" the movement that (a) readies the system for the upcoming motor command and/or (b) readies the system for the receipt of some particular kind of feedback information.

Anticipatory muscle activity contributes to the dynamic restraint system in several capacities. By increasing muscle activation levels in anticipation of an external load, the stiffness properties of the entire muscular unit can be increased.[84] Stiffness is one of the measures used to describe the characteristics of elastic materials. It is defined in terms of the amount of tension increase required to increase the length of the object by a certain amount. From a mechanical perspective, muscle stiffness can be defined as the ratio of the change of force to the change in length. If a spring is very stiff, a great deal of tension is needed to increase its length by a given amount; for a less-stiff spring, much less tension is required. When a muscle is stretched, the change in tension is instantaneous, just as the change in length of a spring. An increase in tension would offset the perturbation or deforming force and bring the system back to its original position. Research demonstrates that the muscle spindle is responsible for the maintenance of the muscle stiffness when the muscle is stretched, so that it can still act as a spring in the control of an unexpected perturbation.[60,63,86] Therefore, stiff muscles can resist stretching episodes more effectively, have greater tone, and provide a more effective dynamic restraint to joint displacement. Increased muscle stiffness can improve the stretch sensitivity of the muscle spindle system while at the same time reduce the electromechanical delay required to develop muscle tension.[28,60,80,84] Heightening the stretch sensitivity can improve the reactive capabilities of the muscle by providing additional sensory feedback.[28]

Central Nervous System Motor Control Integration

It has already been established that the CNS input provided by the peripheral mechanoreceptors and the visual and vestibular receptors is integrated by the CNS to generate a motor response.[26] In addition to the many conscious modifications that can be made while movement is in progress, certain neural connections within the CNS contribute to the modification of movements in progress by providing sensory information at a subconscious level. The influence of some of these reflexive loops is limited to local control of muscle force, but others are capable of influencing force levels in muscle groups quite distant from those originally stimulated. These longer reflex loops are therefore capable of modifying movements to a much larger extent than the shorter reflex loops that are confined to single segments within the spinal cord.

In general, the CNS response falls under 3 categories or levels of motor control: spinal reflexes, brainstem processing, and cognitive cerebral cortex program planning. The goal of the rehabilitation process is to retrain the altered afferent pathways so as to enhance the neuromuscular control system. To accomplish this goal, the objective of the rehabilitation program should be to hyperstimulate the joint and muscle receptors so as to encourage maximal afferent discharge to the respective CNS levels.[12,71,122,126,127]

First Level of Integration: The M1 Reflex

When faced with an unexpected load, the first reflexive muscle response is a burst of EMG activity that occurs after between 30 and 50 milliseconds. The afferent fibers of the mechanoreceptors synapse with the spinal interneurons and produce a reflexive facilitation or inhibition of the motor neurons.[122,126,131] The monosynaptic stretch reflex or M1 reflex is one of the most rapid reflexes underlying limb control (Figure 9-4). The latency or time of this response is very short because it involves only 1 synapse and the information has a relatively short distance to travel. Unfortunately, the muscle response is brief, which does not result in much added contraction of the muscle. The M1 short reflex loop is most often called into play when minute adjustments in muscle length are needed. The stimulus of small muscular stretches occurs during postural sways or when our limbs are subjected to unanticipated loads. Therefore, this mechanism is responsible for regulating motor control of the antagonistic and synergistic patterns of muscle contraction.[99] These adjustments are necessary when misalignment exists between intended muscle length and actual muscle length. This misalignment is most likely to occur in situations where unexpected forces are applied to the limb or the muscle begins to fatigue. In the situation of involuntary and undesirable lengthening of muscles about a joint during conditions of abnormal stress, the short M1 loop must provide for reflex muscle splinting in order to prevent injury from occurring. The M1 reflex occurs at an unconscious level and is not affected by outside factors. These responses can occur simultaneously to control limb position and posture. Because they can occur at the same time, are in parallel, are subconscious, and are without cortical interference, they do not require attention and are thus automatic.

There are 2 important short reflex loops acting in the body: the stretch reflex and the gamma reflex loop. The stretch reflex (Figure 9-5) is triggered when the length of an extrafusal muscle fiber is altered, causing the sensory endings within the muscle spindle to be mechanically deformed. Once deformed, these sensory endings fire, sending nerve impulses into the spinal cord via an afferent sensory neuron located just outside the spinal cord. The information from the Ia afferent is sent essentially to 2 places: to the alpha motor

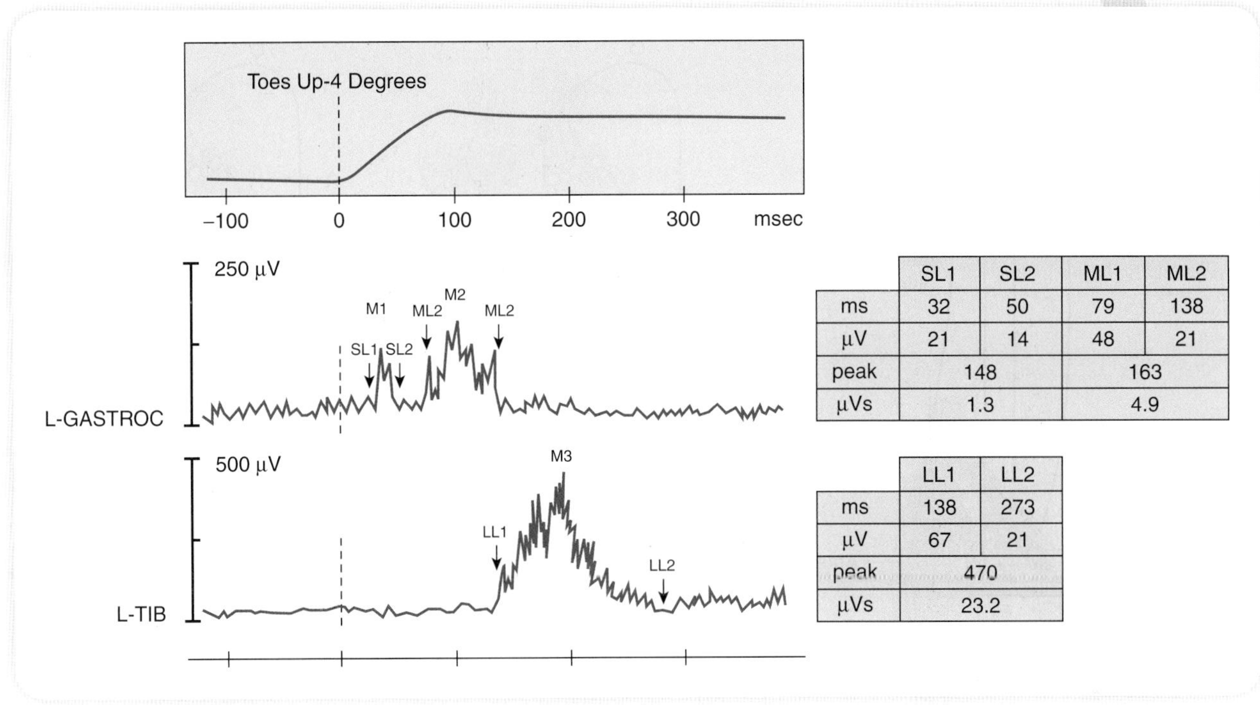

	SL1	SL2	ML1	ML2
ms	32	50	79	138
µV	21	14	48	21
peak	148		163	
µVs	1.3		4.9	

	LL1	LL2
ms	138	273
µV	67	21
peak	470	
µVs	23.2	

Figure 9-4 CNS levels of integration: short- and long-loop postural reflexes

The components of the evoked postural assessment: (M1) myotatic reflex (SL1, SL2), (M2) segmental (polysynaptic) response (ML1, ML2), and (M3) long-loop response (LL1, LL2) involving the brainstem, cortex, and ascending and descending spinal pathways (LL, long loop; ML, mediam loop; SL, short loop). (Reproduced, with permission, from NeuroCom International, Clackamas, OR.)

neurons in the same muscle and upward to the various sensory regions in the cerebral cortex. As soon as these impulses reach the spinal cord, they are transferred to alpha motor neurons that innervate the very same muscle that houses the activated muscle spindles. The loop time, or the time from the initial stretch until the extrafusal fibers are increased in their innervation, is approximately 30 to 40 milliseconds in humans.[102] Stimulation of the muscle spindle ceases when the muscle contracts, because the spindle fibers, which lie parallel to the extrafusal fibers, return to their original length. It is through the operation of this reflex that we are able to continuously alter muscle tone and/or make subtle adjustments in muscle length during movement. These latter adjustments may be in response to external factors producing unexpected loads or forces on the moving limbs.

Consider, for example, what happens when an additional load is applied to an already loaded limb being held in a given position in space.[27] The muscles of the limb are set at a given length, and alpha motor neurons are firing so as to maintain the desired limb position in spite of the load and gravity. Now an additional load is added to the end of the limb, causing the muscles to lengthen as the limb drops. This stretching of the extrafusal muscle fibers results in almost simultaneous stretching of the muscle spindle, which then fires and sends signals to the spinal cord and alpha motor neurons that serve the same muscle. The firing rate of these alpha motor neurons is subsequently increased, causing the muscles in the dropping limb to be further contracted, and the limb is restored to its previous position. Visual information to the stimulus of loading would also lead to increased contraction in the falling limb, but initiating the corrective response consciously would involve considerably longer delays because of additional processing at the cortical level.[27] The short-loop M1 stretch reflex response times

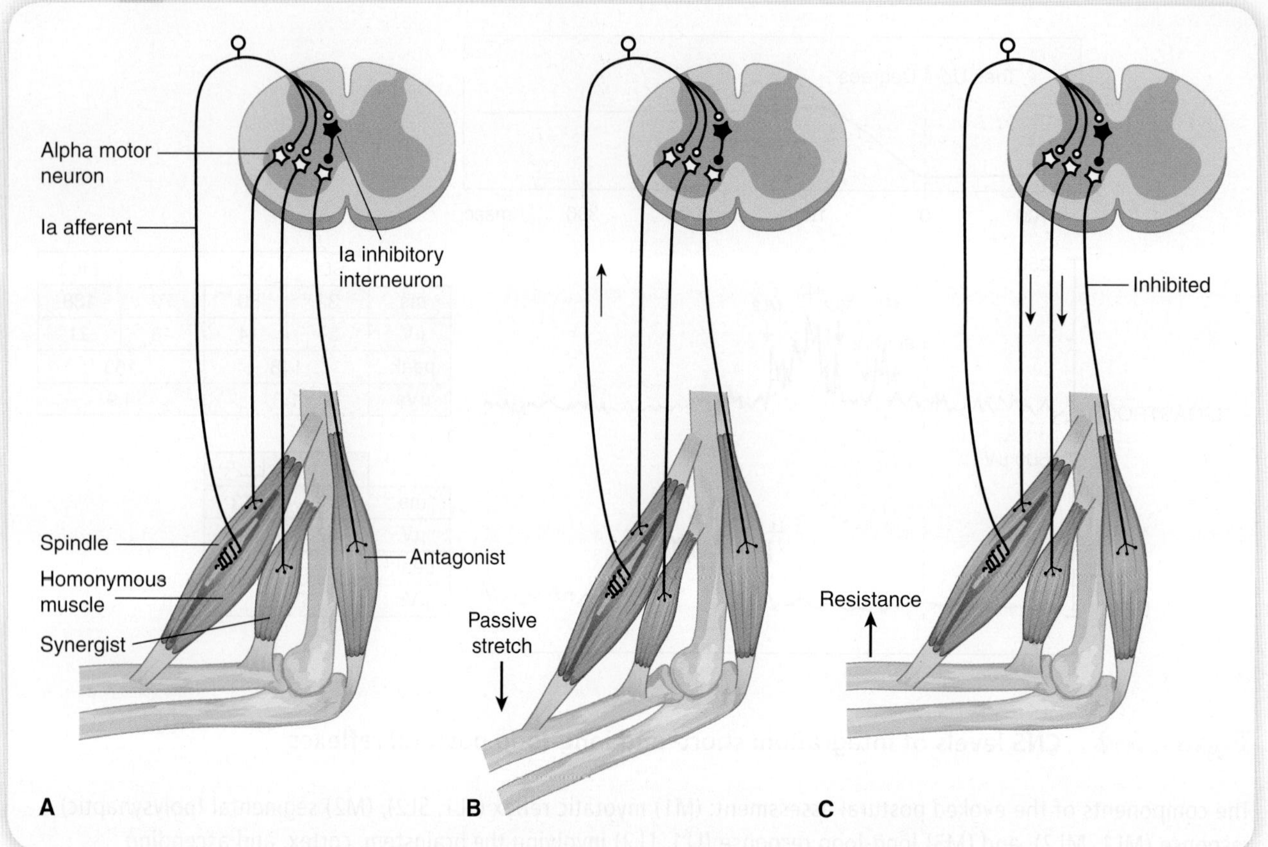

Figure 9-5 Excitation of the muscle spindle is responsible for the stretch reflex

A. Ia afferent fibers making monosynaptic excitatory connections to alpha motor neurons innervating the same muscle from which they arise and motor neurons innervating synergist muscles. They also inhibit motor neurons to antagonist muscles through an inhibitory interneuron. **B.** When a muscle is stretched, the Ia afferents increase their firing rate. **C.** This leads to contraction of the same muscle and its synergists and relaxation of the antagonist. The reflex therefore tends to counteract the stretch, enhancing the springlike properties of the muscle. (Reproduced, with permission, from Gordon J, Ghez C. Muscle receptors and stretch reflexes. In: Kandel E, et al, eds. *Principles of Neural Science*. 3rd ed. East Norwalk, CT, Appleton & Lange; 1991:576.)

are possible within 30 to 50 milliseconds.[58] Visual-based corrections involved corrective delays on the order of 150 to 200 milliseconds.[58] Given that the rapid correction is required for injury prevention, it is important that these short-loop reflex pathways are available for use.

Muscle spindles also play an important role in the ongoing control and modification of movement by virtue of their involvement in a spinal reflex loop known as the gamma reflex loop. The afferent information from the muscle spindle synapses with both the alpha and gamma motor neurons. The alpha motor neuron sends the information it receives to the muscles involved in the movements. The gamma motor neuron sends the same information back to the muscle spindle, which can be stimulated to begin firing at its polar ends. The independent innervation of the muscle spindle by the gamma motor neuron is thought to be important during muscle contractions when the intrafusal fibers of the spindle would normally be slack. Gamma activation of the spindle results in stretching of the intrafusal fibers even though the extrafusal fibers are contracting. In essence, the gamma system takes up the slack in the spindle caused by muscle contraction, thereby making corrections in minute changes in length of the muscle more quickly.

In the short-loop system of spinal control, the activity of the Ia afferent fibers is determined by 2 things: (a) the length and the rate of the stretch of the extrafusal muscle fibers, and (b) the amount of tension in the intrafusal fibers, which is determined by the firing of the gamma efferent fibers. Both alpha and gamma motor neurons can be controlled by higher motor centers, and are thought to be "coordinated" in their action by a process termed *alpha-gamma coactivation*.[44,98] Therefore, the output to the main body of the muscle is determined by (a) the level of innervation provided directly from higher centers and (b) the amount of added innervation provided indirectly from the Ia afferent.[102] This helps to explain how an individual can respond quickly to an unexpected event without conscious involvement of the CNS. When an unexpected event or perturbation causes a muscle to stretch, the spindle's sensory receptors are stimulated. The resulting Ia afferent firing causes a stretch reflex that will increase the activity in the main muscle, all within 40 milliseconds. All of this activity occurs at the same level of the spinal cord as did the innervation of the muscle in the first place. Consequently, no high centers are involved in this 40-millisecond loop.

At this level of motor control, activities to encourage short-loop reflex joint stabilization should dominate.[12,71,110,126] These activities are characterized by sudden alterations in joint position that require reflex muscle stabilization. With sudden alterations or perturbations, both the articular and muscular mechanoreceptors are stimulated for the production of reflex stabilization. Rhythmic stabilization exercises encourage monosynaptic cocontraction of the musculature, thereby producing a dynamic neuromuscular stabilization.[114] These exercises serve to build a foundation for dynamic stability.

Second Level of Integration: The M2 Reflex

For larger adjustments in limb and overall body position, it is necessary to involve the longer reflex loops that extend beyond single segments within the spinal cord. When the muscle spindle is stretched and the Ia afferent fibers are activated, the information is relayed to the spinal cord, where it synapses with the alpha motor neuron. Additionally, information is sent to higher levels of control, where the Ia information is integrated with other information in the sensory and motor centers in the cerebral cortex to produce a more complete response to the imposed stretch. Approximately 50 to 80 milliseconds after an unexpected stimulus, there is a second burst of EMG activity (see Figure 9-4). Because the pathways involved in these neural circuits travel to the more distant subcortical and cortical levels of the CNS to connect with structures such as the motor cortex and cerebellum within the larger projection system, the reflex requires more time or has a longer latency.[51] Therefore, the 80-millisecond loop time for this activity corresponds not only to the additional distance that the impulses have to travel, but also to the multiple synapses that must take place to close the circuit. Both the M1 and M2 responses are responsible for the reflex response that occurs when a tendon is tapped. An example of this occurs when the patellar tendon is tapped with a reflex hammer. The quadriceps muscle is stretched, initiating a reflex response that contracts the quadriceps and produces an involuntary extension of the lower leg.

Even though there is a time lapse for the longer-loop reflexes to take place, there are 2 important advantages for these reflexes. First, the EMG activity from the long-loop reflex is far stronger than that involved in the monosynaptic stretch reflex. The early short-loop monosynaptic reflex system does not result in much actual increase in force. The long-loop reflex can, however, produce enough force to move the limb/joint back into a more neutral position. Second, because the long-loop reflexes are organized in a higher center, they are more flexible than the monosynaptic reflex. By allowing for the involvement of a few other sources of sensory information during the response, an individual can voluntarily adjust the size or amplitude of the M2 response for a given input to generate a powerful response when the goal is to hold the joint as firmly as possible, or to produce no response if the goal is to release under the increasing load. The ability to regulate this response allows an individual to prepare the limb to conform to different environmental demands.

The second level of motor control interaction is at the level of the brainstem.[11,122,130] At this level, afferent mechanoreceptors interact with the vestibular system and visual input from the eyes to control or facilitate postural stability and equilibrium of the body.[12,71,122,127,130] Afferent mechanoreceptor input also works in concert with the muscle spindle complex by inhibiting antagonistic muscle activity under conditions of rapid lengthening and periarticular distortion, both of which accompany postural disruption.[92,126] In conditions of disequilibrium where simultaneous neural input exists, a neural pattern is generated that affects the muscular stabilizers, thereby returning equilibrium to the body's center of gravity.[122] Therefore, balance is influenced by the same peripheral afferent mechanism that mediates joint proprioception and is at least partially dependent upon the individual's inherent ability to integrate joint position sense with neuromuscular control.[120]

Integration of Balance Training: The Second Level of Motor Control

Both proprioception and balance training have been advocated to restore motor control to the lower extremity. In the clinic, the term "balance" is often used without a clear definition.[30] It is important to remember that proprioception and balance are not the same. Proprioception is a precursor of good balance and adequate function. Balance is the process by which we control the body's center of mass with respect to the base of support, whether it is stationary or moving.

Berg attempted to define balance in 3 ways: the ability to maintain a position, the ability to voluntarily move, and the ability to react to a perturbation.[9] All 3 of these components of balance are important in the maintenance of upright posture. Static balance refers to an individual's ability to maintain a stable antigravity position while at rest by maintaining the center of mass within the available base of support. Dynamic balance involves automatic postural responses to the disruption of the center of mass position. Reactive postural responses are activated to recapture stability when an unexpected force displaces the center of mass.[85]

Postural sway is a commonly used indicator of the integrity of the postural control system. Horak defined postural control as the ability to maintain equilibrium and orientation in the presence of gravity.[57,142] Researchers measure postural sway as either the maximum or the total excursion of center of pressure while standing on a forceplate. Little change is noted in healthy adults in quiet standing, but the frequency, amplitude, and total area of sway increase with advancing age or when vision or proprioceptive inputs are altered.[32,59,89,91]

To maintain balance, the body must make continual adjustments. Most of what is currently known about postural control is based upon stereotypical postural strategies activated in response to anteroposterior perturbation.[57,58,85] Horak and Nashner described several different strategies used to maintain balance.[58] These strategies include the ankle, hip, and stepping strategies. These strategies adjust the body's center of gravity so that the body is maintained within the base of support to prevent the loss of balance or falling. There are several factors that determine which strategy would be the most effective response to postural challenge: speed and intensity of the displacing forces, characteristics of the support surface, and magnitude of the displacement of the center of mass. The automatic postural responses can be categorized as a class of functionally organized long-loop responses that produce muscle activation that brings the body's center of mass into a state of equilibrium.[85] Each of the strategies has reflex, automatic, and volitional components that interact to match the response to the challenge.

Small disturbances in the center of gravity can be compensated by motion at the ankle. The ankle strategy repositions the center of mass after small displacements caused by slow-speed perturbations, which usually occur on a large, firm, supporting surface. The oscillations around the ankle joint with normal postural sway are an example of the ankle strategy. Anterior sway of the body is counteracted by gastrocnemius activity, which pulls the body posterior. Conversely, posterior sway of the body is counteracted by contraction of the anterior tibial muscles. If the disturbance in the center of gravity is too great to be counteracted by motion at the ankle, the patient will use a hip or stepping strategy to maintain the center of gravity within the base of support.[82] The hip strategy uses rapid compensatory hip flexion or extension to redistribute the body weight within the available base of support when the center of mass is near the edge of the sway envelope. The hip strategy is usually in response to a moderate or large postural disturbance, especially on an uneven, narrow, or moving surface. The hip strategy is often employed while standing on a bus that is rapidly accelerating. When sudden, large-amplitude forces displace the center of mass beyond the limits of control, a step is used to enlarge the base of support and redefine a new sway envelope. New postural control can then be reestablished. An example of the stepping strategy is the uncoordinated step that often follows a stumble on an unexpected or uneven sidewalk.

The maintenance of balance requires the integration of sensory information from a number of different systems: vision, vestibular, and proprioception. For most healthy adults, the preferred sense for postural control comes from proprioceptive information. Therefore, if proprioception is altered or diminished, balance will also be altered. The functional assessment of the combined peripheral, visual, and vestibular contributions to neuromuscular control can be measured with computerized balance measures of postural stability.[23] The sensory organization test protocol is used to evaluate the relative contribution of vision, vestibular, and proprioceptive input to the control of postural stability when conflicting sensory input occurs.[85] Postural sway is assessed (NeuroCom Smart System) under 6 increasingly challenging conditions (Figure 9-6). Baseline sway is recorded in quiet standing with the eyes open. The reliance on vision is evaluated by asking the patient to close the eyes. A significant increase in sway or loss of balance suggests an overreliance on visual input.[85,107,143] Sensory integration is evaluated when the visual surround moves in concert with sway (sway-referenced vision), creating inaccurate visual input.[103] The patient is then retested on a support surface that moves with sway (sway-referenced support), thereby reducing the quality and availability of proprioceptive input for sensory integration. With the eyes open, vision and vestibular input contribute to the postural responses. With the eyes closed, vestibular input is the primary source of information, because proprioceptive input is altered. The most challenging condition includes sway-referenced vision and sway-referenced support surface.[57,85,107]

Balance activities, both with and without visual input, will enhance motor function at the brainstem level.[11,122] It is important that these activities remain specific to the types of activities or skills that will be required of the athlete upon return to sport.[96] Static balance activities should be used as a precursor to more dynamic skill activity.[96] Static balance skills can be initiated once the individual is able to bear weight on the lower extremity. The general progression of static balance activities is to progress from bilateral to unilateral and from eyes open to eyes closed.[71,96,122,133,134] With balance training, it is important to remember that sensory systems respond to environmental manipulation. To stimulate or facilitate the proprioceptive system, vision must be disadvantaged. This can be accomplished in several ways: remove vision with either the eyes closed or blindfolded, destabilize vision by demanding hand and eye movements (ball toss) or moving the visual surround, or confuse vision with unstable visual cues that disagree with the proprioceptive and vestibular inputs (sway referencing).

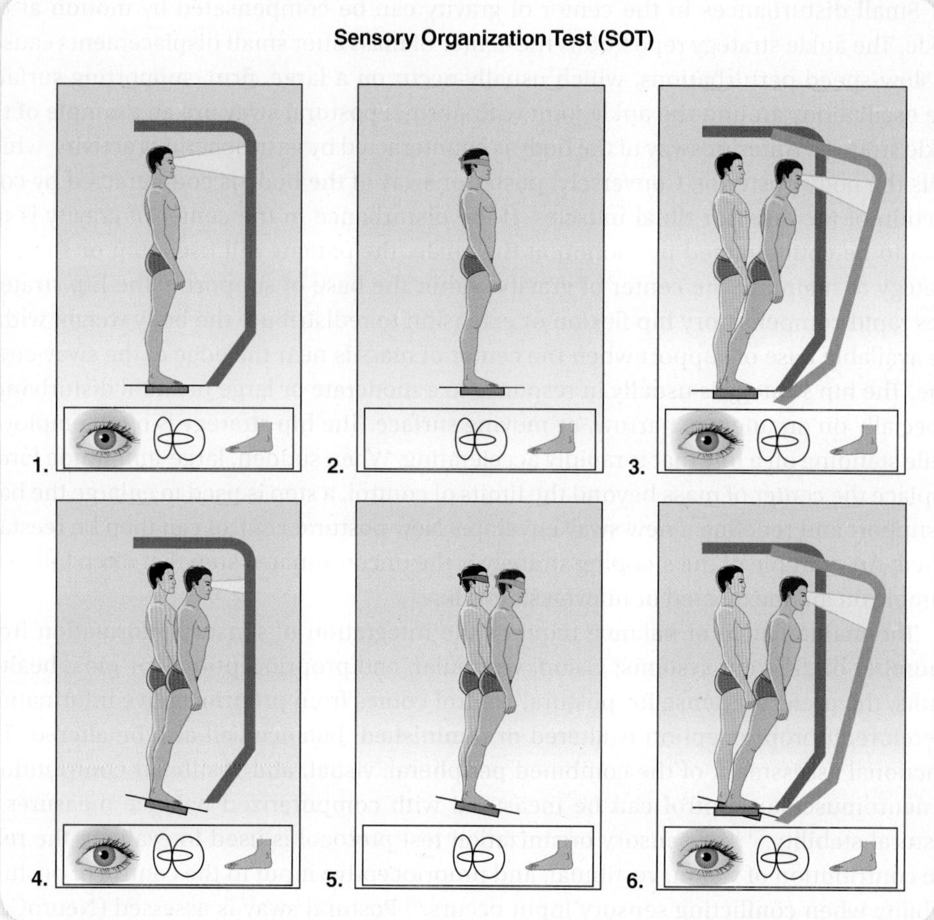

Figure 9-6

The sensory organization conditions integrating vestibular, visual, and somatosensory contributions to balance. (Reproduced, with permission, from NeuroCom International, Clackamas, OR.)

To stimulate vision, proprioception must be either destabilized or confused. The logical progression to destabilize proprioception is to progress the balance training from a stable surface to an unstable surface such as a minitramp, balance board, or dynamic stabilization trainer.[71,122,130] As joint position changes, dynamic stabilization must occur for the patient to control the unstable surface (Figure 9-7). Vision can be confused during balance training by having the patient stand on a compliant surface such as a foam mat or using a sway-referenced moving forceplate. Disadvantaging both vision and proprioceptive information can stimulate the vestibular system. This can be accomplished by several different methods. Absent vision with an unstable or compliant surface is achieved with eyes-closed training on an unstable surface. Demanding hand and eye movements while on a floor mat or foam pad will destabilize both vision and proprioception. A moving surround with a moving forceplate will confuse both vision and proprioceptive input.

The patients should initially perform the static balance activities while concentrating on the specific task (position sense and neuromuscular control) to facilitate and maximize sensory output. As the task becomes easier, activities to distract the athlete's concentration (catching a ball or performing mental exercises) should be incorporated into the training program. This will help to facilitate the conversion of conscious to unconscious motor programming.[122,130] Balance training exercises should induce joint perturbations in order to facilitate reflex muscle activation.

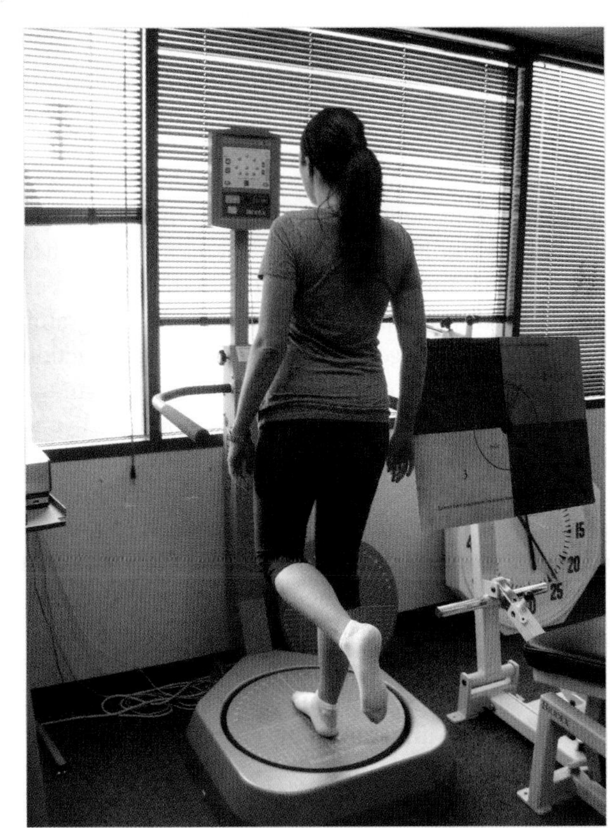

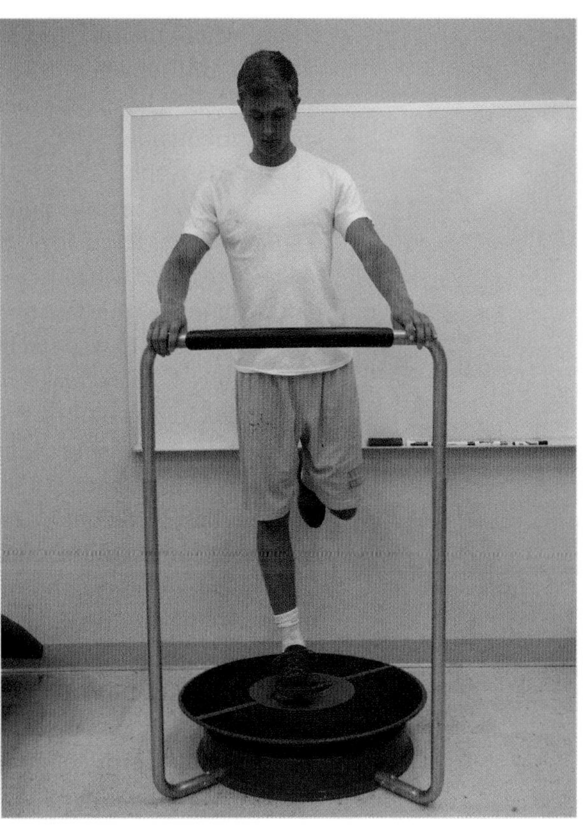

Figure 9-7

Unstable surface training on the Biodex Stability Trainer.

Several studies have assessed the effect of lower-quarter injury on standing balance. Usually the balance characteristics of the injured extremity are compared to those of the uninjured extremity. Mizuta et al measured postural sway in 2 groups: a functionally stable group and a functionally unstable group, both of which had unilateral anterior cruciate ligament (ACL)-deficient knees.[83] An additional group of individuals was also studied to serve as a control group. When compared to the control group, impairment in standing balance was found in the functionally unstable group, but not in the functionally stable group. These results suggest that stabiliometry was a useful tool in the assessment of functional knee stability. Both Friden et al and Gauffin et al demonstrated impaired standing balance during unilateral stance in individuals with chronic ACL-deficient knees.[35,38] Following injury to the lower quarter, impaired standing balance may be caused by the loss of muscular coordination, which could have resulted from the loss of normal proprioceptive feedback.[4,67]

Third Level of Integration: The Voluntary Reaction—Time Response (M3)

The final response that occurs when an unexpected load is applied to the limb is the voluntary long-loop reaction or M3 response (see Figure 9-4). Seen as the third burst of EMG activity, it is a powerful and sustained response that brings the limb back into the desired position. The latency of the M3 response is approximately 120 to 180 milliseconds, depending upon the task and the circumstances. Information is processed at the cerebral cortex, where the mechanoreceptors interact and influence cognitive awareness of body position and movement in which motor commands are initiated for voluntary movements.[12,92,99,122] It is in this region of the primary sensory cortex that there is a high degree of spatial orientation.

The M3 response is very flexible and can be modified by a host of factors such as verbal instructions or anticipation of the incoming sensory information. The delay in the M3 response makes it sensitive to a number of stimulus alternatives. Therefore, the individual's ability to respond will require some conscious attention. Training at this level of the cerebral cortex stimulates the conversion of conscious programming to unconscious programming. These responses have often been referred to as *triggered reactions*. Triggered reactions are prestructured, coordinated reactions in the same or closely related musculature that are "triggered" into action by the mechanoreceptors. The triggered reaction may bypass the information-processing centers because the reaction is stereotyped, predictable, and well practiced. These reactions have latencies from 80 to 180 milliseconds and are far more variable than the latencies of the faster reflexes.[102] The triggered reactions can be learned and can become a more or less automatic response. The individual does not have to spend time processing a response reaction and programming; the reaction is just "triggered off" almost as if it were automatic.[101] Thus, with training, the speed of the M3 response could be increased so as to produce a more automatic reflex response.

The appreciation of joint position at the highest or cognitive level needs to be included in the RNT program. These types of activities are initiated on the cognitive level and include programming motor commands for voluntary movement. The repetitions of these movements will maximally stimulate the conversion of conscious programming to unconscious programming.[12,71,122,126,127,130] The term for this type of training is the *forced-use paradigm*. By making a task significantly more difficult or asking for multiple tasks, we bombard the CNS with input. The CNS attempts to sort and process this overload information by opening additional neural pathways. When the individual goes back to a basic task of ADL, the task becomes easier. This information can then be stored as a central command and ultimately performed without continuous reference to the conscious mind as a "triggered response."[12,71,122,126,127] As with all training, the single greatest obstacle to motor learning is the conscious mind. We must get the conscious mind out of the act!

Coordinating the Muscle Response with Unexpected Loads

The relative roles of these 3 muscle responses depend upon the duration of the movement. As previously discussed, the quickest action occurring in the body has a movement time of approximately 40 milliseconds. When this type or action occurs, the M2 response is incapable of completing or modifying the activity once it is initiated. Even the M1 response has only enough time to begin influencing the muscles near the end of the movement. As the movement time increases, there is a greater potential for the M1 and M2 responses to contribute to the intended action. Movements that take a longer time to be completed (>100 milliseconds) allow both the M1 and M2 responses sufficient time to contribute to all levels of the action. Only when the duration of the movement is 300 milliseconds or longer is there potential for the M3 long-loop response to be involved in amending the movement. Therefore, for movements that take longer than 300 milliseconds for individuals to complete, closed-loop control is possible at several levels of integration at the same time.

Why Is Response Time Important?

When an unexpected load is placed upon a joint, ligamentous damage occurs after the passing of between 70 and 90 milliseconds unless an appropriate response ensues.[7,94,140] Therefore, reactive muscle activity must occur with sufficient magnitude in the 40- to 80-millisecond time frame after loading begins, in order to protect the capsuloligamentous structures. The closed-loop system of CNS integration may not be fast enough to produce a response to increase muscle stiffness. Simply, there is no time for the system to process the information and process the feedback about the condition. Failure of the dynamic restraint system to control these abnormal forces will expose the static structures to excessive forces. In this case, the open-loop system of anticipation becomes more important in producing the desired response. Preparatory muscle activity in anticipation of joint loading can influence the reactive muscle activation patterns. Anticipatory activation increases the sensitivity of the muscle spindles, thereby allowing the unexpected perturbations to be detected more quickly.[29]

Very quick movements are completed before feedback can be used to produce an action to alter the course of movement.[61] Therefore, if the movement is fast enough, a mechanism like a motor program would have to be used to control the entire action, with the movement being carried out without any feedback. Fortunately, the open-loop control system allows the motor control system to organize an entire action ahead of time. For this to occur, previous knowledge of the following needs to be preprogrammed into the primary sensory cortex:

- The particular muscles that are needed to produce an action.
- The order in which these muscles need to be activated.
- The relative forces of the various muscle contractions.
- The relative timing and sequencing of these actions.
- The duration of the respective contractions.

In the open-loop system, movement is organized in advance by a program that sets up some kind of neural mechanism or network that is preprogrammed. A classic example of this occurs in the body as postural adjustments are made before the intended movement. When an individual raises the arm up into forward flexion, the first muscle groups to fire are not even in the shoulder girdle region. The first muscles to contract are those in the lower back and legs (approximately 80 milliseconds before noticeable activity in the shoulder).[8] Because the shoulder muscles are linked to the rest of the body, their contraction affects posture. If no preparatory compensations in posture were made, raising the arm would shift the center of gravity forward, causing a slight loss of balance. The feed-forward motor control system takes care of this potential problem by preprogramming the appropriate postural modification first, rather than requiring the body to make adjustments after the arm begins to move.

Lee has demonstrated that these preparatory postural adjustments are not independent of the arm movement, but rather a part of the total motor pattern.[70] When the arm movements are organized, the motor instructions are preprogrammed to adjust posture first and then move the arm. Therefore, arm movement and postural control are not separate events, but rather different parts of an integrated action that raises the arm while maintaining balance. Lee showed that these EMG preparatory postural adjustments disappear when the individual leans against some type of support prior to raising the arm. The motor control system recognizes that advance preparation of postural control is not needed when the body is supported against the wall.

It is important to remember that most motor tasks are a complex blend of both open- and closed-loop operations. Therefore, both types of control are often at work simultaneously. Both feed-forward and feedback neuromuscular control can enhance dynamic stability if the sensory and motor pathways are frequently stimulated.[71] Each time a signal passes through a sequence of synapses, the synapses become more capable of transmitting the same signal.[50,56] When these pathways are "facilitated" regularly, memory of that signal is created and can be recalled to program future movements.[50,102]

Reestablishing Proprioception and Neuromuscular Control

Although the concept and value of proprioceptive mechanoreceptors have been documented in the literature, treatment techniques directed at improving their function generally have not been incorporated into the overall rehabilitation program. The neurosensory function of the capsuloligamentous structures has taken a backseat to the mechanical structural role. This is mainly a result of the lack of information about how mechanoreceptors contribute to the specific functional activities and how they can be specifically activated.[37,42] Following injury to the capsuloligamentous structures, it is thought that a partial deafferentation of the joint occurs as the mechanoreceptors become disrupted. This partial deafferentation, which is secondary to injury, may be related to either direct or indirect injury. Direct trauma effects include disruption of the joint capsule or ligaments, whereas posttraumatic joint effusion or hemarthrosis[67] can illustrate indirect effects.

Whether a direct or indirect cause, the resultant partial deafferentation alters the afferent information into the CNS and, therefore, the resulting reflex pathways to the dynamic stabilizing structures. These pathways are required by both the feed-forward and feedback motor control systems to dynamically stabilize the joint. A disruption in the proprioceptive pathway will result in an alteration of position and kinesthesia.[4,111] Barrack et al showed an increase in the threshold to detect passive motion in a majority of patients with ACL rupture and functional instability.[4] Corrigan et al, who also found diminished proprioception after ACL rupture, confirmed this finding.[24] Diminished proprioceptive sensitivity also has been shown to cause giving way or episodes of instability in the ACL-deficient knee.[13] Injury to the capsuloligamentous structures not only reduces the joint's mechanical stability but also diminishes the capability of the dynamic neuromuscular restraint system. Consequently, any aberration in joint motion and position sense will impact both the feed-forward and feedback neuromuscular control systems. Without adequate anticipatory muscle activity, the static structures may be exposed to insult unless the reactive muscle activity can be initiated to contribute to dynamic restraint.

Deficits in the neuromuscular reflex pathways may have a detrimental effect on the motor control system as a protective mechanism. Diminished sensory feedback can alter the reflex stabilization pathways, thereby causing a latent motor response when faced with unexpected forces or trauma. Beard et al demonstrated disruption of the protective reflex arc in subjects with ACL deficiency.[7] A significant deficit in reflex activation of the hamstring muscles after a 100-newton anterior shear force in a single-legged closed-chain position was identified, as compared to the contralateral uninjured limb.[7] Beard demonstrated that the latency was directly related to the degree of knee instability; the greater the instability, the greater the latency. Other researchers found similar alterations in the muscle-firing patterns in the ACL-deficient patient.[65,116,140] Solomonow et al found that a direct stress applied to the ACL resulted in reflex hamstring activity, thereby contributing to the maintenance of joint stability.[116] Although this response was also present in ACL-deficient knees, the reflex was significantly slower.

Although it has been demonstrated that a proprioceptive deficit occurs following knee injury, both kinesthetic awareness and reposition sense can be at least partially restored with surgery and rehabilitation. A number of studies have examined proprioception following ACL reconstruction. Barrett measured proprioception after autogenous graft repair and found that the proprioception was better than that of the average ACL-deficient patient, but still significantly worse than the proprioception in the normal knee.[5] Barrett further noted that the patient's satisfaction was more closely correlated with the patient's proprioception than with the patient's clinical score.[5] Harter et al could not demonstrate a significant difference in the reproduction of passive positioning between the operative and nonoperative knee at an average of 3 years after ACL reconstruction.[53] Kinesthesia has been reported to be restored after surgery as detected by the threshold to the detection of passive motion in the midrange of motion.[4] A longer threshold to the detection of passive motion was observed in the ACL-reconstructed knee compared with the contralateral uninvolved knee when tested at the end range of motion.[4] Lephart et al found similar results in patients after either arthroscopically assisted patellar tendon autograft or allograft ACL reconstruction.[74] The importance of incorporating a proprioceptive element in any comprehensive rehabilitation program is justified based upon the results of these studies.

The effects of how surgical and nonsurgical interventions may facilitate the restoration of the neurosensory roles is unclear; however, it has been shown that ligamentous retensioning coupled with rehabilitation can restore proprioceptive sensitivity.[72] As afferent input is altered after joint injury, proprioceptive rehabilitation must focus on restoring proprioceptive sensitivity to retrain these altered afferent pathways and enhance the sensation of joint movement. Restoration may be facilitated by (a) enhancing mechanoreceptor sensitivity, (b) increasing the number of mechanoreceptors stimulated, and (c) enhancing the compensatory sensation from the secondary receptor sites. Research should be directed toward developing new techniques to improve proprioceptive sensitivity.

Methods to improve proprioception after injury or surgery could improve function and decrease the risk for reinjury. Ihara and Nakayama demonstrated a reduction in the neuromuscular lag time with dynamic joint control following a 3-week training period on an unstable board.[65] The maintenance of equilibrium and improvement in reaction to sudden perturbations on the unstable board served to improve the neuromuscular coordination. This phenomenon was first reported by Freeman and Wyke in 1967, when they found that proprioceptive deficits could be reduced with training on an unstable surface.[33] They found that proprioceptive training through stabiliometry, or training on an unstable surface, significantly reduced the episodes of giving way following ankle sprains. Tropp et al confirmed the work of Freeman by demonstrating that the results of stabiliometry could be improved with coordination training on an unstable board.[124] Hocherman et al also showed an improvement in the movement amplitude on an unstable board and the weight distribution on the feet found in hemiplegic patients who received training on an unstable board.[55]

Barrett[5] has demonstrated the relationship between proprioception and function. Barrett's study suggests that limb function relies more on proprioceptive input than on strength during activity. Borsa et al also found a high correlation between diminished kinesthesia with the single-leg hop test.[12] The single-leg hop test was chosen for its integrative measure of neuromuscular control, because a high degree of proprioceptive sensibility and functional ability is required to successfully propel the body forward and land safely on the limb. Giove et al reported a higher success rate in returning athletes to competitive sports through adequate hamstring rehabilitation.[40] Tibone et al and Ihara and Nakayama found that simple hamstring strengthening alone was not adequate; it was necessary to obtain voluntary or reflex-level control on knee instability in order to return to functional activities.[65,121] Walla et al found that 95% of patients were able to successfully avoid surgery after ACL injury when they were able to achieve "reflex-level" hamstring control.[136] Ihara and Nakayama found that the reflex arc between stressing the ACL and hamstring contraction could be shortened with training.[65] With the use of unstable boards, the researchers were able to successfully decrease the reaction time. Because afferent input is altered after joint injury, proprioceptive sensitivity to retrain these altered afferent pathways is critical to shorten the time lag of muscular reaction so as to counteract the excessive strain on the passive structures and to guard against injury.

What About Muscle Fatigue?

It has been well established in the literature that muscle fatigue can play a major role in destabilizing a joint.[100,111,117,129] With fatigue, an increase in knee joint laxity has been noted in both males and females.[100,117,118] More importantly, the body's ability to receive and accurately process proprioceptive information is affected by muscular fatigue. There is evidence that exercise to the point of clinical fatigue does have an effect on proprioception.[111,129] Research demonstrates that the ability to learn or make improvement in joint position sense is severely impaired with muscle fatigue.[75,100] Likewise, muscle fatigue alters both kinesthesia and joint position sense.[2,111,129] Skinner et al showed that the reproduction of passive positioning was significantly diminished following a fatigue protocol.[111] Voight et al also demonstrated a significant proprioceptive deficit following a fatigue protocol.[129] This suggests that patients who are fatigued may have a change in their proprioceptive abilities and are more prone to injury. Following a lower-quarter isokinetic fatigue protocol, postural sway as measured with EMG and forceplates is also increased following muscular fatigue.[66,129] This suggests that muscular fatigue results in a possible motor control deficit. In addition to disruption balance or postural sway, Nyland et al also demonstrated on EMG that muscular fatigue affects muscle activity by extending the latency of the muscle firing.[87]

Modifying Afferent/Efferent Characteristics: How Do We Do It?

The mechanoreceptors in and around the respective joints offer information about the change of position, motion, and loading of the joint to the CNS, which, in turn, stimulates the muscles around the joint to function.[65] If a time lag exists in the neuromuscular reaction, injury may occur. The shorter the time lag, the less stress to the ligaments and other soft-tissue structures about the joint. Therefore, the foundation of neuromuscular control is to facilitate the integration of peripheral sensations relative to joint position and then process this information into an effective efferent motor response. The main objective of the rehabilitation program for neuromuscular control is to develop or reestablish the afferent and efferent characteristics about the joint that are essential for dynamic restraint.[71]

There are several different afferent and efferent characteristics that contribute to the efficient regulation of motor control. As discussed previously, these characteristics include the sensitivity of the mechanoreceptors and facilitation of the afferent neural pathways, enhancing muscle stiffness, and the production of reflex muscle activation. The specific rehabilitation techniques must also take into consideration the levels of CNS integration. For the rehabilitation program to be complete, each of the 3 levels must be addressed in order to produce dynamic stability. The plasticity of the neuromuscular system permits rapid adaptations during the rehabilitation program that enhance preparatory and reactive activity.[7,56,65,71,74,141] Specific rehabilitation techniques that produce adaptations that enhance the efficiency of these neuromuscular techniques include balance training, biofeedback training, reflex facilitation through reactive training, and eccentric and high-repetition/low-load exercises.[41,71]

Objectives of Neuromuscular Control: Reactive Neuromuscular Training

RNT activities are designed to restore functional stability about the joint and to enhance motor control skills. The RNT program centers around the stimulation of both the peripheral and central reflex pathways to the skeletal muscles. The first objective that should be addressed in the RNT program is the restoration of dynamic stability. Reliable kinesthetic and proprioceptive information provides the foundation on which dynamic stability and motor control are based. It has already been established that altered afferent information into the CNS can alter the feed-forward and feedback motor control systems. Therefore, the first objective of the RNT program is to restore the neurosensory properties of the damaged structures while at the same time enhancing the sensitivity of the secondary peripheral afferents.[74] The restoration of dynamic stability allows for the control of abnormal joint translation during functional activities. For this to occur, the reestablishment of dynamic stability is dependent upon the CNS receiving appropriate information from the peripheral receptors. If the information into the system is altered or inappropriate for the stimulus, a bad motor response will ensue.

To facilitate appropriate kinesthetic and proprioceptive information to the CNS, joint reposition exercises should be used to provide a maximal stimulation of the peripheral mechanoreceptors.[135] The use of closed kinetic chain activities creates axial loads that maximally stimulate the articular mechanoreceptors via the increase in compressive forces.[22,45] The use of closed-chain exercises not only enhances joint congruency and neurosensory feedback but also minimizes the shearing stresses about the joint.[128] At the same time, the muscle receptors are facilitated by both the change in length and tension.[22,45] The objective is to induce unanticipated perturbations, thereby stimulating reflex stabilization. The persistent use of these pathways will decrease the response time when faced with an unanticipated joint load.[88] In addition to weightbearing exercises, joint repositioning exercises can be used to enhance the conscious appreciation of proprioception. Rhythmic stabilization exercises can be included early in the RNT program to enhance neuromuscular coordination in response to unexpected joint translation. The intensity of the exercises can be manipulated by increasing either the weight loaded across the joint or the size of the perturbation. The addition of a compressive sleeve, wrap, or taping about the joint can also provide additional proprioceptive information by stimulating the cutaneous mechanoreceptors.[5,71,76,90] Following the restoration of range of motion and strength, dynamic stability can be enhanced with reflex stabilization and basic motor learning exercises.

The second objective of the RNT program is to encourage preparatory agonist-antagonist cocontraction. Efficient coactivation of the musculature restores the normal force couples that are necessary to balance joint forces and increase joint congruency, thereby reducing the loads imparted onto the static structures.[71] The cornerstone of rehabilitation during this phase is postural stability training. Environmental conditions are manipulated to produce a sensory response. Specifically, the 3 variables of balance that are manipulated include bilateral to unilateral stance, eyes open to eyes closed, and stable to unstable surfaces. The use of unstable surfaces allows the clinician to use positions of compromise in order to produce maximal afferent input into the spinal cord, thereby producing a reflex response. Dynamic coactivation of the muscles about the joint to produce a stabilizing force requires both the feed-forward and feedback motor control systems. In order to facilitate these pathways, the joint must be placed into positions of compromise in order for the patient to develop reactive stabilizing strategies. Although it was once believed that the speed of the stretch reflexes could not be directly enhanced, efforts to do so have been successful in human and animal studies. This has significant implications for reestablishing the reactive capability of the dynamic restraint system. Reducing the electromechanical delay between joint loading and the protective muscle activation can increase dynamic stability. In the controlled clinical environment, positions of vulnerability can be used safely.

Proprioceptive training for functionally unstable joints following injury has been documented in the literature.[65,106,123,125,135] Tropp et al[124] and Wester et al[137] reported that ankle disk training significantly reduced the incidence of ankle sprain. Concerning the mechanism of effects, Tropp et al suggested that unstable surface training reduced the proprioceptive deficit.[124] Sheth et al demonstrated changes with healthy adults in the patterns of contractions on the inversion and eversion musculature before and after training on an unstable surface.[106] They concluded that the changes would be supported by the concept of reciprocal Ia inhibition via the mechanoreceptors in the muscles. Konradsen and Ravin also suggested that the afferent input from the calf musculature was responsible for dynamic protection against sudden ankle inversion stress.[68] Pinstaar et al reported that postural sway was restored after 8 weeks of ankle disk training when carried out 3 to 5 times a week.[93] Tropp and Odenrick also showed that postural control improved after 6 weeks of training when performed 15 minutes per day.[125] Bernier and Perrin, whose program consisted of balance exercises progressing from simple to complex sessions (3 times a week for 10 minutes), also found that postural sway was improved after 6 weeks of training.[10] Although there were some differences in each of these training programs, the postural control improved after 6 to 8 weeks of proprioceptive training for participants with functional instability of the ankle.

Once dynamic stability has been achieved, the focus of the RNT program is to restore ADL and sport-specific skills. Exercise and training drills should be incorporated into the program that will refine the physiologic parameters that are required for the return to preinjury levels of function. Emphasis in the RNT program must be placed upon a progression from simple to complex neuromotor patterns that are specific to the demands placed upon the patient during function. The training program should begin with simple activities, such as walking/running, and then progress to highly complex motor skills requiring refined neuromuscular mechanisms including proprioceptive and kinesthetic awareness that provide reflex joint stabilization.

Exercise Program/Progression

Dynamic reactive neuromuscular control activities should be initiated into the overall rehabilitation program once adequate healing has occurred. The progression to these activities is predicated on the athlete satisfactorily completing the activities that are considered prerequisites for the activity being considered. Keeping this in mind, the progression of activities must be goal-oriented and specific to the tasks that will be expected of the athlete.

The general progression for activities to develop dynamic reactive neuromuscular control is from slow-speed to fast-speed activities, from low-force to high-force activities, and from controlled to uncontrolled activities. Initially, these exercises should evoke a balance reaction or weight shift in the lower extremities and ultimately progress to a movement pattern. These reactions can be as simple as a static control with little or no visible movement or as complex as a dynamic plyometric response requiring explosive acceleration, deceleration, or change in direction. The exercises will allow the clinician to challenge the patient using visual and/or proprioceptive input via tubing and other devices (medicine balls, foam rolls, visual obstacles). Although these exercises will improve physiologic parameters, they are specifically designed to facilitate neuromuscular reactions. Therefore, the clinician must be concerned with the kinesthetic input and quality of the movement patterns rather than the particular number of sets and repetitions. Once fatigue occurs, motor control becomes poor and all training effects are lost. Therefore, during the exercise progression, all aspects of normal motor control/movement should be observed. These should include isometric, concentric, and eccentric muscle control; articular loading and unloading; balance control during weight shifting and direction changes; controlled acceleration and deceleration; and demonstration of both conscious and unconscious control.

Phase I: Static Stabilization (Closed-Chain Loading/Unloading)

Phase I involves minimal joint motion and should always follow a complete open-chain exercise program that restores near-full active range of motion. The patient should stand bearing full weight with equal distribution on the affected and unaffected lower extremity. The feet should be positioned approximately shoulder-width apart. Greater emphasis can be placed on the affected lower extremity by having the patient put the unaffected lower extremity on a 6- to 8-inch stool or step bench. This flexes the hip and knee and forces a greater weight shift to the affected side, yet allows the unaffected extremity to assist with balance reactions (Figure 9-8). The weightbearing status then progresses to having the unaffected extremity suspended in front or behind the body, forcing a single-leg stance on the affected side (Figure 9-9). The patient is then asked to continue the single-leg stance while shifting weight to the forefoot and toes by lifting the heel and plantarflexing the ankle. This places the complete responsibility for weightbearing and balance reactions on the affected lower extremity. This position will also require slight flexion of the hip and knee. Support devices are often helpful and can minimize confusion. When the patient is first

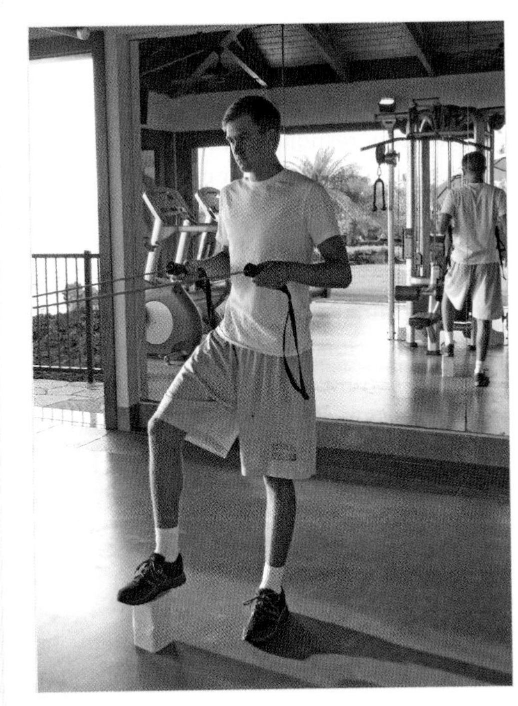

Figure 9-8 **Static stabilization**

Weight shifting technique to enhance transfer onto the left leg.

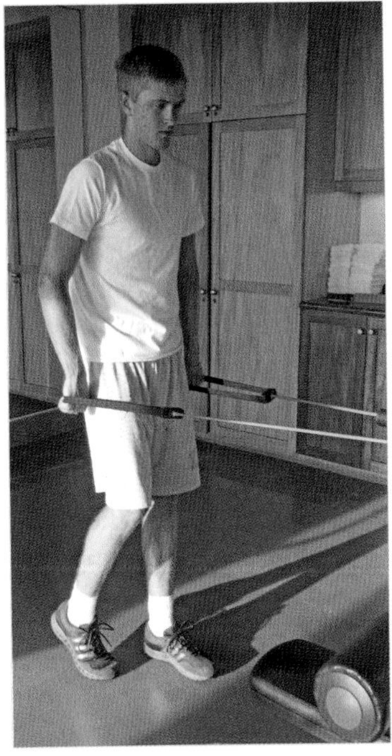

Figure 9-9

Static stabilization: Uniplanar anterior weight shift.

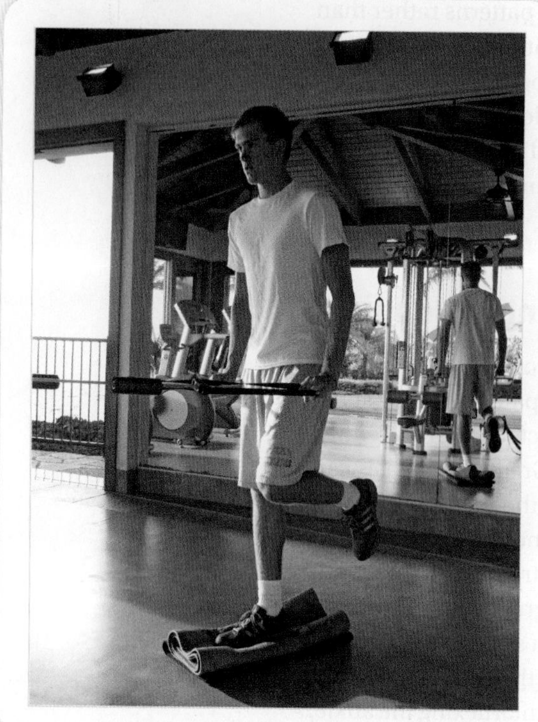

Figure 9-10

Static stabilization: Single-leg stance/unstable surface.

asked to progress weight bearing to the forefoot and toes, a heel lift device can be used. A support device can also be used to place the ankle in dorsiflexion, inversion, or eversion to increase kinesthetic input or decrease biomechanical stresses on the hip, knee, and ankle.

At each progression, the clinician may ask that the patient train with eyes closed to decrease the visual input and increase kinesthetic awareness. The clinician may also use an unstable surface with training in this phase to increase the demands on the mechanoreceptor system. The unstable surface will facilitate the reflex pathways mediated by the peripheral efferent receptors. Single or multidirectional rocker devices will assist the progression to the next phase (Figure 9-10).

The physiologic rationale for this phase of RNT is the use of static compression of the articular structures to produce maximal output of the mechanoreceptors, thereby facilitating isometric contractions of the musculature and providing a dynamic reflex stabilization. The self-generated oscillations will help increase the interplay between visual, mechanoreceptor, and equilibrium reaction. Changes in the isometric muscle tension will assist in the sensitization of the muscle spindle (gamma bias).

The exercise tubing technique used in this phase is called *oscillating technique for isometric stabilization* (OTIS). The technique can be used to stimulate muscle spindle and mechanoreceptor activity. The exercises involve continuously loaded short-arc movements of 1 body part, which, in turn, causes an isometric stabilization reaction of the involved body part. This is accomplished by pulling 2 pieces of tubing toward the body and returning the tubing to a start position in a smooth rhythmical fashion with increasing speeds. Resistance builds as the tubing is stretched. This forces a transfer of weight in the direction of the tubing. Because the involved body part is only required to react or respond to a simple stimulus, the oscillating stimulus will produce an isometric contraction in the lower extremity that must produce a stabilizing force in the direction opposite to the tubing pull. The purpose of this technique is to quickly involve the proprioceptive system with minimal verbal and visual cueing. Ognibene et al demonstrated a significant improvement in both single-leg postural stability and reaction time with a 4-week training program using OTIS techniques.[88]

Change in direction—according to anterior, posterior, medial, and lateral weight shifting—will create specific planar demands. Each technique is given a name, which is related to the weight shift produced by the applied tension. The body will then react with an equal and opposite stabilization response. Consequently, the exercise is named for the cause and not the effect. The goal during this phase is static stabilization. Numerous successful repetitions demonstrating stability are required to achieve motor learning and control.

Uniplanar Exercise

Anterior Weight Shift The patient faces the tubing and pulls the tubing toward the body using a smooth, comfortable motion. This causes forward weight shift that is stabilized with an isometric counterforce consisting of hip extension, knee extension, and ankle plantarflexion. There should be little or no movement noted in the lower extremity. If movement is noted, resistance should be decreased to achieve the desired stability (see Figure 9-9).

Lateral Weight Shift The patient stands with the affected side facing the tubing. The tubing is pulled by 1 hand in front of the body and by the other hand behind the body to equalize the force and minimize the rotation. This causes a lateral weight shift (LWS), which is stabilized with an isometric counterforce consisting of hip abduction, knee cocontraction, and ankle eversion.

Medial Weight Shift The patient stands with the unaffected side facing the tubing. The tubing is pulled in the same fashion as above. This causes a medial weight shift (MWS), which is stabilized with an isometric counterforce consisting of hip adduction, knee cocontraction, and ankle inversion.

Posterior Weight Shift The patient stands with his/her back to the tubing in the frontal plane. The tubing is pulled to the body from behind, causing a posterior weight shift (PWS), which is stabilized by an isometric counterforce consisting of hip flexion, knee flexion, and ankle dorsiflexion.

Multiplanar Exercise

The basic exercise program can be progressed to multiplanar activity by combining the proprioceptive neuromuscular facilitation chop and lift patterns of the upper extremities. The chop patterns from the affected and unaffected side will cause a multiplanar stress requiring isometric stabilization. The patient will now be forced to automatically integrate the isometric responses that were developed in the previous uniplanar exercises. The force will be representative of the proprioceptive neuromuscular facilitation diagonals of the lower extremities (Figure 9-11). The lift patterns from the affected to the unaffected side will add multiplanar stress in the opposite direction (Figure 9-12). Changing the resistance, speed of movement, or spatial orientation relative to the resistance can make modifications to the multiplanar exercise. If resistance is increased, the movement speed should be decreased to allow for a strong stabilizing counterforce. If the speed of movement is increased, then

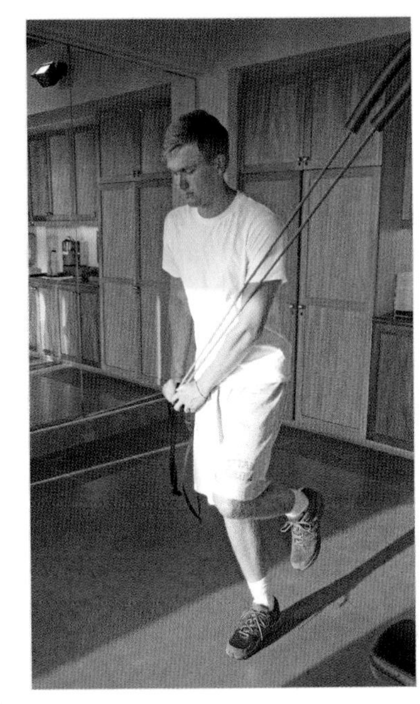

Figure 9-11

Static stabilization: Multiplanar PNF chop technique to provide rotational stress.

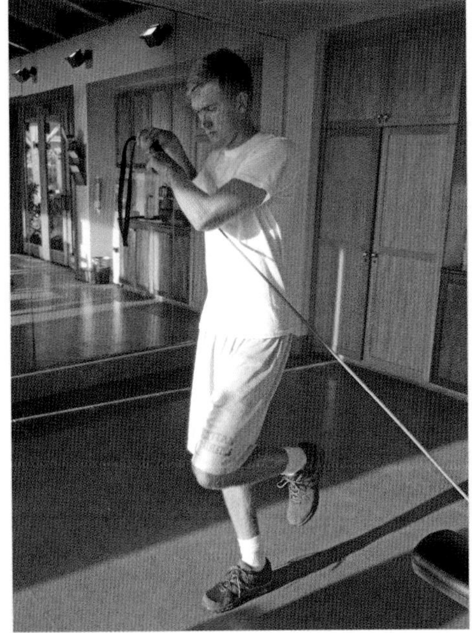

Figure 9-12

Static stabilization: Multiplanar PNF lift technique to provide rotation stress.

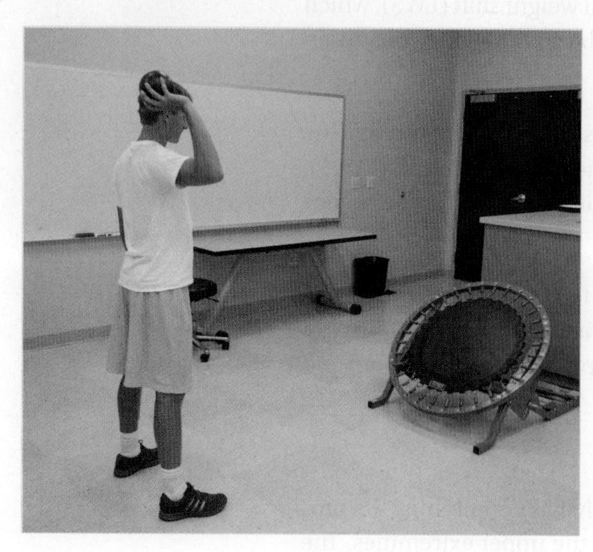

Figure 9-13 **Static stabilization**

ITIS technique in unilateral stance using a Plyoball and plyoback for an impulse stimulus.

resistance should be decreased to allow for a quick counterforce response. By altering the angle of the body in relation to the resistance, the quality of the movement is changed. A greater emphasis can be placed on one component while reducing the emphasis on another component.

Technique Modification

These techniques can also be used with medicine ball exercises. The posture and position are nearly the same, but the medicine ball does not allow for the oscillations provided by the tubing. The medicine ball provides impulse activity and a more complex gradient of loading and unloading (Figure 9-13). This is referred to as impulse technique for isometric stabilization (ITIS). As described, the patient is positioned to achieve the desired stress. The medicine ball is then used with a rebounding device or thrown by the clinician. Progression to ball toss while stabilizing on an unstable surface will disrupt concentration, thereby facilitating the conversion to unconscious reflex adaptation.

The elastic tubing and medicine ball techniques are similar in position but differ somewhat in physiologic demands. Therefore, they should be used to complement each other and not replace or substitute the other at random. When performing an ITIS activity with a medicine ball, the force exerted by the exercise device names the weight shift. The tubing will exert a pull and the ball will exert a push; therefore, they will be performed from the opposite sides to achieve the same weight shift.

Phase II: Transitional Stabilization (Conscious Controlled Motion Without Impact)

Phase II replaces isometric activity with controlled concentric and eccentric activity progressing through a full range of functional motion. The forces of gravity are coupled with tubing to simulate stress in both the vertical and horizontal planes. In phase I, gravitational forces statically load the neuromuscular system. Varying degrees of imposed lateral stress via the tubing are used to stimulate isometric stabilization. Phase II requires that the movement occur in the presence of varying degrees of imposed lateral stress. The movement stimulates the mechanoreceptors in 2 ways: (a) articular movement causes capsular stretch in a given direction at a given speed and (b) the changes in the body position cause loading and unloading of the articular structures and pressure changes in the intracapsular fluid. The exercises in this phase use simple movements such as the squat and lunge. The addition of tubing adds a horizontal stress. Other simple movements such as walking, sidestepping, and the lateral slide board can also be emphasized to stimulate a more efficient and controlled movement.

The physiologic rationales for activities in this phase are the stimulation of dynamic postural responses and facilitation of concentric and eccentric contractions via the compression and translation of the articular structures. This, in turn, helps to increase muscle stiffness, which has a significant role in producing dynamic stabilization about the joint by resisting and absorbing joint loads.[80,81] Research has established that eccentric loading increases both muscle stiffness and tone.[16,95] Chronic overloading of the musculotendinous unit via eccentric contractions will result in not only connective tissue proliferation but also a desensitization of the GTO and increased muscle spindle activity.[64]

The self-generated movements require dynamic control in the midrange and static control at the end range of motion. Because a change in direction is required at the end ranges of motion, the interplay between visual, mechanoreceptor, and equilibrium reactions continues to increase. The "gamma bias" now responds to changes in both length and tension of the involved musculature.

Assisted techniques can also be used in this phase to progress patients who may find phase II exercise fatiguing or difficult. Assisted exercise is used to reduce the effect of gravity on the body or an extremity to allow for an increase in the quality or quantity of a desired movement. The assisted technique will offset the weight of the body or extremity by a percentage of the total weight. This will allow improved range of motion, a reduction in substitution, minimal eccentric stress, and a reduction in fatigue. The closed-chain tubing program can also benefit from assisted techniques, which allow for a reduction in vertical forces by decreasing relative body weight on one or both lower extremities.

The need for assisted exercise is only transitional in nature. The goal is to progress from unweighted to weight with overloading. The tubing, if used effectively, can also provide an overloading effect by causing exaggerated weight shifting. This overloading will be referred to as resisted techniques for all closed-chain applications. The 2 basic exercises used are the squat and the lunge.

Squat

The squat is used first because it employs symmetrical movement of the lower extremities. This allows the affected lower extremity to benefit from the visual and proprioceptive feedback from the unaffected lower extremity. The clinician should observe the patient's posture and look for weight shifting, which almost always occurs away from the affected limb. Each joint can be compared to its unaffected counterpart. In performing the squat, a weight shift may be provided in 1 of 4 different directions. The tubing is used to assist, resist, and modify movement patterns. The PWS works to identify closed-chain ankle dorsiflexion. A chair or bench can be used as a range-of-motion block (range-limiting device) when necessary. This minimizes fear and increases safety. The anterior weight shift (AWS) provides an anterior pull that helps facilitate the hip flexion mobility during the descent. Medial and lateral changes may be provided with resistance in order to promote weight bearing on the involved side or decrease weight bearing on the involved side as progression is made (Figure 9-14). The varying weight shifts may be used to intentionally increase the load or resistance on a particular side for means of strengthening or to facilitate a neuromuscular response on the opposite side. For example, an individual who is reluctant to weight bear on the involved side may be helped in doing so by causing increased weight shift to the uninvolved side. This will create the need to shift weight to the involved side, thus encouraging a joint response to the required stimulus.

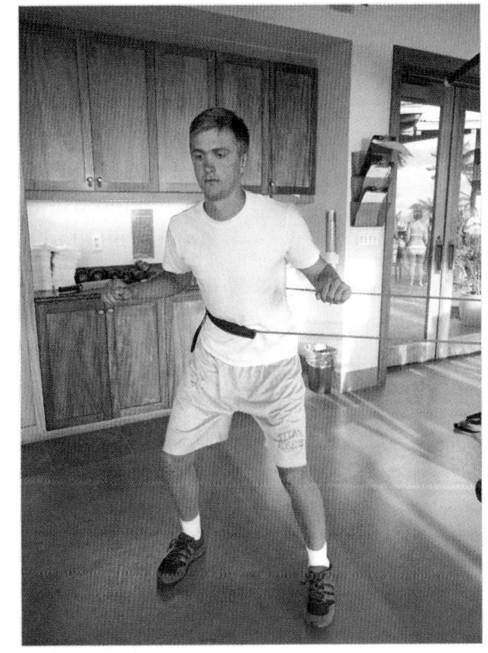

Figure 9-14 **Transitional stabilization**

Resisted squat with an LWS in the home health setting.

Assisted Technique The patient faces the tubing, which is placed at a descending angle and is attached to a belt. The belt is placed under the buttocks to simulate a swing. A bench is used to allow a proper stopping point. The elastic tension of the tubing is at its greatest when the patient is in the seated position and decreases as the mechanical advantage increases. Therefore, the tension curve of the tubing complements the needs of the patient. The next 4 exercises follow the assisted squat in difficulty. The tubing is now used to cause weight shifting and demands a small amount of dynamic stability.

Anterior Weight Shift The patient faces the tubing, which comes from a level halfway between the hips and the knees and attaches to a belt. The belt is worn around the waist and causes an AWS. During the squat movement, the ankles plantarflex as the knees extend.

Posterior Weight Shift The patient faces away from the tubing at the same level as above and attaches to a belt. The belt is worn around the waist and causes a PWS. This places a greater emphasis on the hip extensors and less emphasis on the knee extensors and plantar flexors.

Medial Weight Shift The patient stands with the unaffected side toward the tubing at the same level as above. The belt is around the waist and causes an MWS. This places less stress on the affected lower extremity and allows the patient to lean onto the affected lower extremity without incurring excessive stress or loading.

Lateral Weight Shift The patient stands with the affected side toward the tubing that is at the same level as above. The belt is worn around the waist, which causes a weight shift onto the affected lower extremity. This exercise will place a greater stress on the affected lower extremity, thereby demanding increased balance and control. The exercise simulates a single-leg squat but adds balance and safety by allowing the unaffected extremity to remain on the ground.

Lunge

The lunge is more specific in that it simulates sports and normal activity. The exercise decreases the base while at the same time producing the need for independent disassociation. The range of motion can be stressed to a slightly higher degree. If the patient is asked to alternate the lunge from the right to the left leg, the clinician can easily compare the quality of the movement between the limbs. When performing the lunge, the patient may often use exaggerated extension movements of the lumbar region to assist weak or uncoordinated hip extension. This substitution is not produced during the squat exercise. Therefore, the lunge must be used not only as an exercise but also as a part of the functional assessment. The substitution must be addressed by asking the patient to maintain a vertical torso (note that the assisted technique will assist the clinician in minimizing this substitution).

Assisted Technique—Forward Lunge The patient faces away from the tubing, which descends at a sharp angle (approximately 60 degrees). This angle parallels the patient's center of gravity, which moves forward and down (Figure 9-15). This places a stretch on the tubing and assists the patient up from the low point of the lunge position. The ability to perform a lunge with correct technique is often negated as a result of the inability to support one's body weight. The assisted lunge corrects this by modifying the load required of the patient, thus improving the quality of the movement. The assistance also minimizes eccentric demands for deceleration when lowering and provides balance assistance by helping the patient focus on the center of gravity (anatomically located within the hip and pelvic region). The patient is asked to first alternate the activity to provide kinesthetic feedback. The clinician can then use variations of full and partial motion to stimulate the appropriate control before moving on to the next exercise.

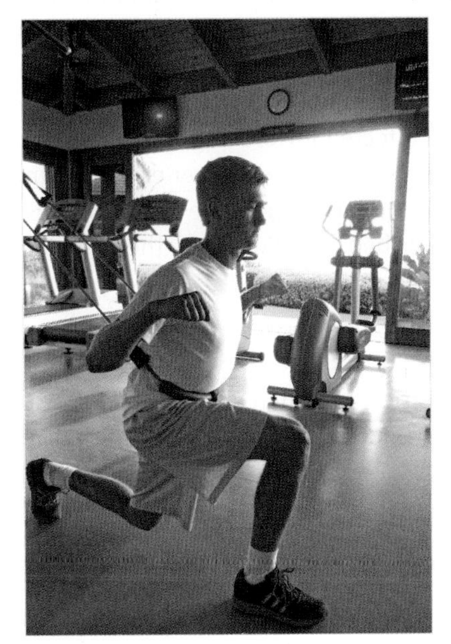

Figure 9-15

Transitional stabilization: Assisted lunge technique.

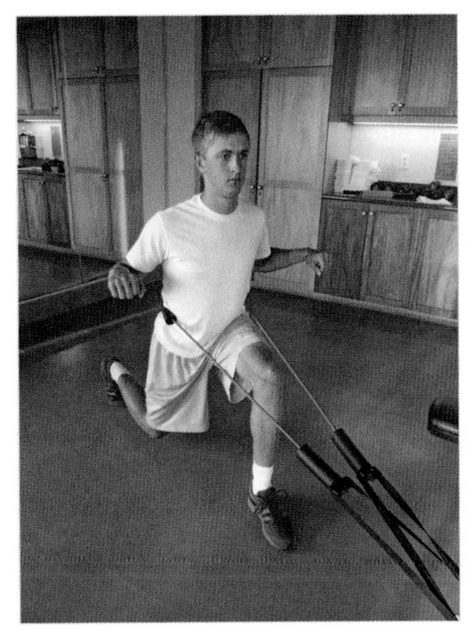

Figure 9-16 **Transitional stabilization**

Resisted forward lunge to facilitate deceleration stress.

Resisted Technique—Forward Lunge The patient faces the tubing, which is at an ascending angle from the floor to the level of the waist (Figure 9-16). The tubing will now increase the eccentric loading on the quadriceps with the deceleration or the downward movement. For the upward movement, the patient is asked to focus on hip extension and not knee extension. The patient must learn to initiate movement from the hip and not from lumbar hyperextension or excessive knee extension. Initiation of hip extension should automatically stimulate isometric lumbar stabilization along with the appropriate amounts of knee extension and ankle plantarflexion. A foam block is often used to protect the rear knee from flexing beyond 90 degrees and touching the floor. The block can also be made larger to limit range of motion at any point in the lunge.

Resisted Technique—Lateral and Medial Weight Shift Forward lunges can be performed to stimulate static lateral and medial stabilization during dynamic flexion and extension movements of the lower extremities. The LWS lunge is performed by positioning the patient with the affected lower extremity toward the direction of resistance. The tubing is placed at a level halfway between the waist and the ankle. The patient is then asked to perform a lunge with minimal lateral movement. This movement stimulates static lateral stabilization of the hip, knee, ankle, and foot during dynamic flexion (unloading) and extension (loading). The MWS lunge is performed by positioning the patient with the affected extremity opposite to the resistance. The tubing is attached as described in the LWS. The movement stimulates static medial stabilization of the affected lower extremity in the presence of dynamic flexion and extension.

The lunge techniques teach weight shifting onto the affected lower extremity during lateral body movements. The assisted technique lateral lunge complements the assisted technique forward lunge, because it also reduces relative body weight while allowing closed-chain function. The prime mover is the unaffected lower extremity that moves the center of gravity over the affected lower extremity for the sole purpose of visual and proprioceptive input prior to excessive loading. The resisted technique lateral lunge complements the resisted technique forward lunge, because it also provides an overloading effect on the affected lower extremity. In this exercise, the affected lower extremity is the prime mover, as well as the primary weightbearing extremity. The affected lower extremity must not only produce the weight shift but also react, respond, and repeat the movement. Sets, repetitions, and resistance for all of the exercises described are selected by the clinician to produce the appropriate reaction without pain or fatigue.

Technique Modification

As in phase I, the medicine ball can be used to add variety and increase stimulation. However, it is used to stimulate control in the beginning, middle, and end ranges of the squat and lunges. The tubing can also be used to create ITIS and OTIS applications to reinforce stability throughout the range of motion.

Functional Testing

Functional testing provides objective criteria and can help the clinician to justify a progression to phase III or an indication that the patient should continue working in phase II. A single-leg body weight squat or lunge can be performed. The quality and quantity of the repetitions are compared to the unaffected lower extremity and a deficit can be calculated. An isotonic leg press machine can also be used in this manner by setting the weight at the patient's body weight and comparing the repetitions. Open-chain isotonic and isokinetic testing can also be helpful in identifying problem areas when specificity is needed. Regardless of the mode of testing, it is recommended that the affected lower extremity display 70% to 80% of the capacity demonstrated by the unaffected lower extremity, or no more than a 20% to 30% strength deficit. When the patient has met these criteria, the patient can move safely into phase III.

Phase III: Dynamic Stabilization (Unconscious Control/Loading)

Phase III introduces impact and ballistic exercise to the patient. This movement will produce a stretch-shortening cycle that has been described in plyometric exercises. Plyometric function is not a result of the magnitude of the prestretch, but rather relies on the rate of stretch to produce a more forceful contraction. This is done in 2 ways.

1. The stretch reflex is a neuromuscular response to tension produced in the muscle passively. The muscle responds with an immediate contraction to reorient itself to the new position, protect it, and maintain posture. If a voluntary contraction is added in conjunction with this reflex, a more forceful contraction can be produced.
2. The elastic properties of the tendon allow it to temporarily store energy and release it. When a quick prestretch is followed by a voluntary contraction, the tendon will add to the strength of the contraction by providing force in the direction opposite to the prestretch.

Dynamic training at this level can increase the descending cortical drive to the large motor nerves of the skeletal muscles as well as the small efferent nerves of the muscle spindle.[79] If both the muscle tension and efferent output to the muscle spindles are increased, the stretch sensitivity of the muscle spindle will also be increased, thereby reducing the reflex latency.[64] Both feed-forward and feedback loops are used concurrently to superimpose stretch reflexes on preprogrammed motor activity.

As has been previously discussed, there have been previous studies that were directed toward reducing muscle reaction times.[7,65,141] Ihara and Nakayama significantly reduced the latency of muscle reaction times with a 3-week training period of unanticipated perturbations via the use of unstable wobble boards.[65] Both Beard et al and Wojtys et al found similar results when comparing agility training with traditional strength training.[7,141] Reducing the muscle reaction time in order to produce a protective response following an abnormal joint load will enhance dynamic stability about the joint.

Before the patient is asked to learn any new techniques, the patient is instructed to demonstrate unconscious control by performing various phase II activities while throwing and catching the medicine ball. The squat and lunge exercises are performed with various applications of tubing at the waist level. This activity removes the attention from the lower extremity exercise, thereby stimulating unconscious control. The forces added by throwing and catching the medicine ball stimulate balance reactions needed for the progression to plyometric activities. Simple rope jumping is another transitional exercise that can be used to provide early plyometric information. The double-leg rope jumping is done first. The patient is then asked to perform alternating leg jumping. Rope jumping is effective in building confidence and restoring a plyometric rhythm to movement. Four-way resisted stationary running is an exercise technique used to orient the patient to light plyometric activity.

Resisted Walking

Resisted walking uses the same primary components as in gait training. The applied resistance of the tubing, however, allows for a reactive response unavailable in nonresisted activities. For example, a patient may present with a slight Trendelenburg gait associated with a weak gluteus medius. By initiating a program that would incorporate a progression such as that used with the squat, the patient should be able to progress to resisted walking. The addition of resistance permits for increased loading and also brings about the need for improved balance and weight shift.

Resisted Hopping

Bilateral hopping should be introduced following adequate training with the jump rope, then followed by increased unilateral training. The use of resistance in the hopping technique is to promote increased resistance in 1 of 4 directions. This increased resistance is used to simulate those forces normally seen on the field or court in the return to activity. Introduction of the program should begin with bilateral training and then progress to a unilateral format, which may be accommodated with box drills or diagonal training. At higher levels, implementing cones, hurdles, and/or foam rolls may be used in order to increase the plyometric demands during the hopping drills.

Resisted Running

Resisted running simply involves jogging or running in place with tubing attached to a belt around the waist. The clinician can analyze the jogging or running activity because it is a stationary drill. The tubing resistance is applied in 4 different directions, providing simulation of the different forces that the patient will experience as the patient returns to full activity.

1. The PWS run causes a balance reaction that results in an AWS (opposite direction) and simulates the acceleration phase of jogging or running (Figure 9-17). The patient faces opposite the direction of the tubing resistance and should be encouraged to stay on the toes (for all running exercises). The initial light stepping activity can be progressed to jogging and then running. The most advanced form of the PWS run involves the exaggeration of the hip flexion called "high knees." Exaggeration of hip

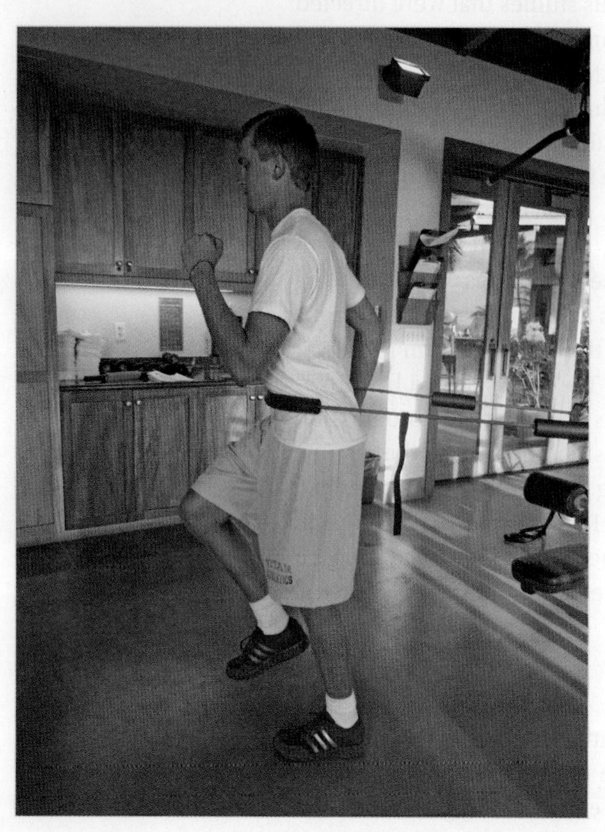

Figure 9-17

Dynamic stabilization—stationary run with a posterior weight shift.

flexion helps to stimulate a plyometric action in the hip extensors, thus facilitating acceleration. This form of exercise lends itself to slow, controlled endurance conditioning (greater than 3 minutes), or interval training, which depends greatly on the intensity of the resistance, cadence, and rest periods. The interval-training program is most effective and shows the greatest short-term gains. Intervals can be 10 seconds to 1 minute; however, the most common drills are 15 to 30 seconds in length. The patient is usually allowed a 1- to 2-minute rest and is required to perform 3 to 5 sets. To make sure that the patient is delivering maximum intensity, the clinician should count the number of foot touches (repetitions) that occur during the interval. The clinician needs to only count the touches of the affected lower extremity. The patient is then asked to equal or exceed the amount of foot touches on the next interval (set). This is also extremely effective as a functional test for acceleration. The interval time/repetitions can be recorded and compared to future tests. The clinician should note that the PWS places particular emphasis on the hip flexors and extensors, as well as the plantar flexors of the ankle.

2. The MWS run follows the same progression as the PWS run (from light jogging to high knees) with the resistance now applied medial to the affected lower extremity (which causes an automatic weight shift laterally). Endurance training, interval training, and testing should also be performed for this technique. This technique simulates the forces that the patient will experience when cutting or turning quickly away from the affected side. This drill is the same as in phase I MWS. Although the phase I MWS is static, the same muscles are responsible for dynamic stability. This exercise represents the forces that the patient will encounter when sprinting into a turn on the affected side.
3. The LWS run should follow the same progression as above except that the resistance is now lateral to the affected lower extremity (which causes an automatic MWS). This technique simulates the forces that the patient will experience when cutting or turning quickly toward the affected side.

   When performing the MWS and LWS runs, high knees should be used when working on acceleration. Instructing the patient to perform exaggerated knee flexion or "butt kicks" can emphasize deceleration. The exaggeration of knee flexion places greater plyometric stress on the knee, which has a large amount of eccentric responsibility during deceleration. This exercise represents the forces that the patient will encounter when sprinting into a turn on the unaffected side.
4. The AWS run is probably the most difficult technique to perform correctly and is therefore taught last. The tubing that is set to pull the patient forward stimulates a PWS. This technique simulates deceleration and eccentric loading of the knee extensors. The patient should start with light jogging on the toes and progress to butt kicks. This is a plyometric exercise that incorporates exaggerated knee flexion and extension. This exercise serves to assist the patient in developing the

eccentric/concentric reactions that are required in function. The clinician should note that injuries occur more frequently during deceleration and direction changes than on acceleration or straightforward running. Therefore, AWS training is extremely important to the athlete returning to the court or field.

Resisted Bounding

The bounding exercise is a progression taken from both the hopping and running exercise to increase demands placed on the horizontal component. Therefore, bounding is an exercise technique that places greater emphasis on the lateral movements. The progression of the bounding exercises follows the same weight-shifting sequence as the previous running exercise. Side-to-side bounding in a lateral resisted exercise promotes symmetrical balance and endurance required for progression to higher-level strength and power applications. Distraction activities also may be included in the bounding and/or running exercises in order to promote increased upper extremity demands and to detract from visual and/or verbal reference needed on the lower extremity.

It is suggested that the patient be taught how to perform the bounding exercise without the tubing first. A foam roll, cone, or other obstacle can be used to simulate jump height and/or distance. The tubing can then be added to provide the secondary forces to cause anterior, lateral, medial, or posterior weight shifting. Bounding should be taught as a jump from one foot to another. A single lateral bound can be used as a supplementary functional test. Measurements can be taken for a left and right lateral bound. Bounding is only considered valid if the patient can maintain his or her balance when landing. To standardize the bounding exercise, the body height is used for the bound stride and markers can be placed for the left and right foot landings.

1. The AWS lateral combines lateral motion with an automatic PWS or deceleration reaction. It is slightly more demanding than the stationary running exercises because the body weight is driven to a greater distance.
2. The LWS bound causes an excessive lateral plyometric force and will help to develop lateral acceleration and deceleration in the affected lower extremity. This is the most strenuous of the lateral bounding activities because it actually accelerates the body weight onto the affected lower extremity. This is, however, necessary so that the clinician can observe the ability of the affected limb to perform a quick direction change and controlled acceleration/deceleration.
3. The MWS bound is used as an assisted plyometric exercise. The patient works with the total body weight but impact is greatly lowered by reducing both acceleration and deceleration forces. This exercise is an excellent transitional exercise at the end of phase II as well as at the beginning of phase III. It also serves as a warm-up drill providing submaximal stimulation of the proprioceptive system prior to a phase III exercise session.
4. The PWS bound facilitates an anterior lateral push-off of each leg and stimulates an AWS. This exercise assists in teaching acceleration and lateral cutting movements.

Multidirectional Drills

Multidirectional drills include jumping (2-foot takeoff followed by a 2-foot landing), hopping (1-foot takeoff followed by a landing on the same foot), and bounding (1-foot takeoff followed by an opposite-foot landing). A series of floor markers can be placed in various patterns to simulate functional movements. A weight shift can be produced in any direction by the orientation of the tubing. Obstacles can also be used to make the exercise more complicated.

The jumping exercise can be developed to simulate downhill skiing, while the hopping exercise can be designed to stress single-leg push-off for vertical jumping sports such as basketball and volleyball.

SUMMARY

1. There has been increased attention to the development of balance and proprioception in the rehabilitation and reconditioning of athletes following injury. It is believed that injury results in altered somatosensory input that influences neuromuscular control.
2. If static and dynamic balance and neuromuscular control are not reestablished following injury, then the patient will be susceptible to recurrent injury and the patient's performance may decline.
3. The following rules should be employed when designing the RNT program:
   - Make sure that the exercise program is specific to the patient's needs. The most important thing to consider during the rehabilitation of patients is that they should be performing functional activities that simulate their ADL requirements. This rule applies to not only the specific joints involved but also the speed and amplitude of movement required in ADL.
   - Practice does appear to be task specific in both athletes and people who have motor-control deficits.[73] As retraining of balance continues, it is best to practice complex skills in their entirety rather than in isolation, because the skills will transfer more effectively.[1]
   - Make sure to include a significant amount of "controlled chaos" in the program. Unexpected activities with the ADL are by nature unstable. The more the patient rehearses in this type of environment, the better the patient will react under unrehearsed conditions.
   - Progress from straight-plane to multiplane movement patterns. In ADL, movement does not occur along a single joint or plane of movement. Therefore, exercise for the kinetic chain must involve all 3 planes simultaneously.
   - Begin your loading from the inside out. Load the system first with body weight and then progress to external resistance. The core of the body must be developed before the extremities.
   - Have causative cures as a part of the rehabilitation process. The cause of the injury must eventually become a part of the cure. If rotation and deceleration were the cause of the injury, then use this as a part of the rehabilitation program in preparation for return to activity.
   - Be progressive in nature. Remember to progress from simple to complex. The function progression breaks an activity down into its component parts and then performs them in a sequence that allows for the acquisition or reacquisition of the activity. Basic conditioning and skill acquisition must be acquired before advanced conditioning and skill acquisition.
   - Always ask: Does the program make sense? If it does not make sense, chances are that it is not functional and therefore not optimally effective.
   - Make the rehabilitation program fun. The first 3 letters of functional are FUN. If it is not fun, then compliance will suffer and so will the results.
   - An organized progression is the key to success. Failing to plan is planning to fail.

REFERENCES

1. Barnett M, Ross D, Schmidt R, Todd B. Motor skills learning and the specificity of training principle. *Res Q Exerc Sport.* 1973;44:440-447.
2. Barrack RL, Lund PJ, Skinner HB. Knee joint proprioception revisited. *J Sport Rehabil.* 1994;3:18-42.
3. Barrack RL, Skinner HB. The sensory function of knee ligaments. In: Daniel D, ed. *Knee Ligaments: Structure, Function, Injury, and Repair*. New York, NY: Raven Press; 1990.
4. Barrack RL, Skinner HB, Buckley SL. Proprioception in the anterior cruciate deficient knee. *Am J Sports Med.* 1989;17:1-6.
5. Barrett DS. Proprioception and function after anterior cruciate reconstruction. *J Bone Joint Surg Br.* 1991;73:833-837.
6. Basmajian JV, ed. *Biofeedback: Principles and Practice for Clinicians*. Baltimore, MD: Williams and Wilkins; 1979.
7. Beard DJ, Dodd CF, Trundle HR, et al. Proprioception after rupture of the ACL: an objective indication of the need for surgery? *J Bone Joint Surg Br.* 1993;75:311.
8. Bernier JN, Perrin DH. Effect of coordination training on proprioception of the functionally unstable ankle. *J Orthop Sports Phys Ther.* 1998;27:264-275.
9. Belen'kii VY, Gurfinkle VS, Pal'tsev YI. Elements of control of voluntary movements. *Biofizika.* 1967;12:135-141.
10. Berg K. Balance and its measure in the elderly: a review. *Physiother Can.* 1989;41:240-246.
11. Blackburn TA, Voight ML. Single leg stance: development of a reliable testing procedure. In: *Proceedings of the 12th International Congress of the World Confederation for Physical Therapy*. Alexandria, VA: APTA; 1995.
12. Borsa PA, Lephart SM, Kocher MS, Lephart SP. Functional assessment and rehabilitation of shoulder proprioception for glenohumeral instability. *J Sport Rehabil.* 1994;3:84-104.
13. Borsa PA, Lephart SM, Irrgang JJ, Safran MR, Fu F. The effects of joint position and direction of joint motion on proprioceptive sensibility in anterior cruciate ligament deficient athletes. *Am J Sports Med.* 1997;25:336-340.
14. Boyd IA, Roberts TDM. Proprioceptive discharges from stretch-receptors in the knee joint of the cat. *J Physiol.* 1953;122:38-59.
15. Braxendale RA, Ferrel WR, Wood L. Responses of quadriceps motor units to mechanical stimulation of knee joint receptors in decerebrate cat. *Brain Res.* 1988;453:150-156.
16. Bulbulian R, Bowles DK. The effect of downhill running on motor neuron pool excitability. *J Appl Physiol.* 1992;73(3): 968-973.
17. Burgess PR. Signal of kinesthetic information by peripheral sensory receptors. *Annu Rev Neurosci.* 1982;5:171.
18. Cafarelli E, Bigland B. Sensation of static force in muscles of different length. *Exp Neurol.* 1979;65:511-525.
19. Ciccotti MR, Kerlan R, Perry J, Pink M. An electromyographic analysis of the knee during functional activities: I. The normal profile. *Am J Sports Med.* 1994;22:645-650.
20. Ciccotti MR, Kerlan R, Perry J, Pink M. An electromyographic analysis of the knee during functional activities: II. The anterior cruciate ligament—deficient knee and reconstructed profiles. *Am J Sports Med.* 1994;22:651-658.
21. Clark FJ, Burgess PR. Slowly adapting receptors in cat knee joint: can they signal joint angle? *J Neurophysiol.* 1975;38:1448-1463.
22. Clark FJ, Burgess RC, Chapin JW, Lipscomb WT. Role of intramuscular receptors in the awareness of limb position. *J Neurophysiol.* 1985;54:1529-1540.
23. Cohen H, Keshner E. Current concepts of the vestibular system reviewed: Visual/vestibular interaction and spatial orientation. *Am J Occup Ther.* 1989;43:331-338.
24. Corrigan JP, Cashman WF, Brady MP. Proprioception in the cruciate deficient knee. *J Bone Joint Surg Br.* 1992;74:247-250.
25. Cross MJ, McCloskey DI. Position sense following surgical removal of joints in man. *Brain Res.* 1973;55:443-445.
26. Crutchfield A, Barnes M. *Motor Control and Motor Learning in Rehabilitation*. Atlanta, GA: Stokesville; 1993.
27. Dewhurst DJ. Neuromuscular control system. *IEEE Trans Biomed Eng.* 1965;14:167-171.
28. Dietz VJ, Schmidtbleicher D. Interaction between preactivity and stretch reflex in human triceps brachii during landing from forward falls. *J Physiol.* 1981;311:113-125.
29. Dunn TG, Gillig SE, Ponser ES, Weil N. The learning process in biofeedback: is it feed-forward or feedback? *Biofeedback Self Regul.* 1986;11:143-155.
30. Ekdhl C, Jarnlo G, Anderson S. Standing balance in healthy subjects. *Scand J Rehabil Med.* 1989;21:187-195.
31. Eklund J. Position sense and state of contraction: the effects of vibration. *J Neurol Neurosurg Psychiatry.* 1972;35:606.
32. Era P, Heikkinen E. Postural sway during standing and unexpected disturbances of balance in random samples of men of different ages. *J Gerontol.* 1985;40:287-295.
33. Freeman MAR, Wyke B. Articular reflexes of the ankle joint. An electromyographic study of normal and abnormal influences of ankle-joint mechanoreceptors upon reflex activity in leg muscles. *Br J Surg.* 1967;54:990-1001.
34. Freeman MAR, Wyke B. Articular contributions to limb reflexes. *Br J Surg.* 1966;53:61-69.
35. Friden T, Zatterstrom R, Lindstand A, Moritz U. Disability in anterior cruciate ligament insufficiency: An analysis of 19 untreated patients. *Acta Orthop Scand.* 1990;61:131-135.

36. Gandevia SC, Burke D. Does the nervous system depend on kinesthetic information to control natural limb movements? *Behav Brain Sci.* 1992;15:614-632.
37. Gandevia SC, McCloskey DI. Joint sense, muscle sense and their contribution as position sense, measured at the distal interphalangeal joint of the middle finger. *J Physiol.* 1976;260:387-407.
38. Gauffin H, Pettersson G, Tegner Y, Tropp H. Function testing in patients with old rupture of the anterior cruciate ligament. *Int J Sports Med.* 1990;11:73-77.
39. Gelfan S, Carter S. Muscle sense in man. *Exp Neurol.* 1967;18:469-473.
40. Giove TP, Miller SJ, Kent BE, Sanford TL, Garrick JG. Non-operative treatment of the torn anterior cruciate ligament. *J Bone Joint Surg Am.* 1983;65:184-192.
41. Glaros AG, Hanson K. EMG biofeedback and discriminative muscle control. *Biofeedback Self Regul.* 1990;15:135-143.
42. Glenncross D, Thornton E. Position sense following joint injury. *Am J Sports Med.* 1981;21:23-27.
43. Goodwin GM, McCloskey DI, Matthews PC. The contribution of muscle afferents to kinesthesia shown by vibration induced illusions of movement and by effects of paralyzing joint afferents. *Brain.* 1972;95:705-748.
44. Granit R. *The Basis of Motor Control.* New York, NY: Academic Press; 1970.
45. Grigg P. Peripheral neural mechanisms in proprioception. *J Sport Rehabil.* 1994;3:1-17.
46. Grigg P. Response of joint afferent neurons in cat medial articular nerve to active and passive movements of the knee. *Brain Res.* 1976;118:482-485.
47. Grigg P, Finerman GA, Riley LH. Joint position sense after total hip replacement. *J Bone Joint Surg Am.* 1973;55:1016-1025.
48. Grigg P, Hoffman AH. Ruffini mechanoreceptors in isolated joint capsule. Reflexes correlated with strain energy density. *Somatosens Mot Res.* 1984;2:149-162.
49. Grigg P, Hoffman AH. Properties of Ruffini afferents revealed by stress analysis of isolated sections of cats knee capsule. *J Neurophysiol.* 1982;47:41-54.
50. Guyton AC. *Textbook of Medical Physiology.* 6th ed. Philadelphia, PA: WB Saunders; 1991.
51. Haddad B. Protection of afferent fibers from the knee joint to the cerebellum of the cat. *Am J Physiol.* 1953;172:511-514.
52. Hagood SM, Solomonow R, Baratta BH, et al. The effect of joint velocity on the contribution of the antagonist musculature to knee stiffness and laxity. *Am J Sports Med.* 1990;18:182-187.
53. Harter RA, Osternig LR, Singer SL, Larsen RL, Jones DC. Long-term evaluation of knee stability and function following surgical reconstruction for anterior cruciate ligament insufficiency. *Am J Sports Med.* 1988;16:434-442.
54. Hellenbrant FA. Motor learning reconsidered: a study of change. In: *Neurophysiologic Approaches to Therapeutic Exercise.* Philadelphia, PA: FA Davis; 1978.
55. Hocherman S, Dickstein R, Pillar T. Platform training and postural stability in hemiplegia. *Arch Phys Med Rehabil.* 1984;65:588-592.
56. Hodgson JA, Roy RR, DeLeon R, et al. Can the mammalian lumbar spinal cord learn a motor task? *Med Sci Sports.* 1994;26:1491-1497.
57. Horak FB. Clinical measurement of postural control in adults. *Phys Ther.* 1989;67:1881-1885.
58. Horak FB, Nashner LM. Central programming of postural movements. Adaptation to altered support surface configurations. *J Neurophysiol.* 1986;55:1369-1381.
59. Horak FB, Shupert CL, Mirka A. Components of postural dyscontrol in the elderly. *Neurobiol Aging.* 1989;10:727-738.
60. Houk JC. Regulation of stiffness by skeletomotor reflexes. *Annu Rev Physiol.* 1979;41:99-114.
61. Houk JC, Crago PE, Rymer WZ. Function of the dynamic response in stiffness regulation: A predictive mechanism provided by non-linear feedback. In: Taylor A, Prochazka A, eds. *Muscle Receptors and Feedback.* London, UK: Macmillan; 1981.
62. Houk JC, Henneman E. Responses of Golgi tendon organs to active contractions of the soleus muscle in the cat. *J Neurophysiol.* 1967;30:466-481.
63. Houk JC, Rymer WZ. Neural controls of muscle length and tension. In: Brooks VB, ed. *Handbook of Physiology: Section 1: The Nervous System, Vol. 2: Motor Control.* Bethesda, MD: American Physiological Society; 1981.
64. Hutton RS, Atwater SW. Acute and chronic adaptations of muscle proprioceptors in response to increased use. *Sports Med.* 1992;14:406-421.
65. Ihara H, Nakayama A. Dynamic joint control training for knee ligament injuries. *Am J Sports Med.* 1986;14:309-315.
66. Johnson RB, Howard ME, Cawley PW, Losse GM. Effect of lower extremity muscular fatigue on motor control performance. *Med Sci Sports.* 1998;30:1703-1707.
67. Kennedy JC, Alexander IJ, Hayes KC. Nerve supply to the human knee and its functional importance. *Am J Sports Med.* 1982;10:329-335.
68. Konradsen L, Ravin JB. Prolonged peroneal reaction time in ankle instability. *Int J Sports Med.* 1991;12:290-292.
69. Lee RG, Murphy JT, Tatton WG. Long latency myotatic reflexes in man: Mechanisms, functional significance, and changes in patients with Parkinson's disease or hemiplegia. In: Desmedt J, ed. *Advances in Neurology.* Basel, Switzerland: Karger; 1983.
70. Lee WA. Anticipatory control of postural and task muscles during rapid arm flexion. *J Mot Behav.* 1980;12:185-196.
71. Lephart SM. Reestablishing proprioception, kinesthesia, joint position sense and neuromuscular control in rehabilitation. In: Prentice WE, ed. *Rehabilitation Techniques in Sports Medicine.* 2nd ed. St. Louis, MO: Mosby; 1994.

72. Lephart SM, Henry TJ. Functional rehabilitation for the upper and lower extremity. *Orthop Clin North Am.* 1995;26:579-592.

73. Lephart SM, Kocher MS, Fu FH, et al. Proprioception following ACL reconstruction. *J Sport Rehabil.* 1992;1:188-196.

74. Lephart SM, Pincivero DM, Giraldo JL, Fu F. The role of proprioception in the management and rehabilitation of athletic injuries. *Am J Sports Med.* 1997;25:130-137.

75. Marks R, Quinney HA. Effect of fatiguing maximal isokinetic quadriceps contractions on the ability to estimate knee position. *Percept Mot Skills.* 1993;77:1195-1202.

76. Matsusaka N, Yokoyama S, Tsurusaki T, et al. Effect of ankle disk training combined with tactile stimulation to the leg and foot in functional instability of the ankle. *Am J Sports Med.* 2001;29(1):25-30.

77. Matthews PC. Where does Sherrington's "muscular sense" originate? Muscle, joints, corollary discharges? *Annu Rev Neurosci.* 1982;5:189.

78. McCloskey DI. Kinesthetic sensitivity. *Physiol Rev.* 1978;58:763-820.

79. McComas AJ. Human neuromuscular adaptations that accompany changes in activity. *Med Sci Sports.* 1994;26:1498-1509.

80. McNair PJ, Marshall RN. Landing characteristics in subjects with normal and anterior cruciate ligament deficient knee joints. *Arch Phys Med Rehabil.* 1994;75:584-589.

81. McNair PJ, Wood GA, Marshall RN. Stiffness of the hamstring muscles and its relationship to function in anterior cruciate deficient individuals. *Clin Biomech (Bristol, Avon).* 1992;7:131-173.

82. Melville-Jones GM, Watt GD. Observations of the control stepping and hopping in man. *J Physiol.* 1971;219:709-727.

83. Mizuta H, Shiraishi M, Kubota K, Kai K, Takagi K. A stabiliometric technique for the evaluation of functional instability in the anterior cruciate ligament-deficient knee. *Clin J Sport Med.* 1992;2:235-239.

84. Morgan DL. Separation of active and passive components of short-range stiffness of muscle. *Am J Physiol.* 1977;32:45-49.

85. Nashner LM. Sensory, neuromuscular, and biomechanical contributions to human balance. In: Duncan PW, ed. *Balance: Proceedings of the APTA Forum.* Alexandria, VA: APTA; 1986:550.

86. Nichols TR, Houk JC. Improvement of linearity and regulation of stiffness that results from actions of stretch reflex. *J Neurophysiol.* 1976;39:119-142.

87. Nyland JA, Shapiro R, Stine RL, et al. Relationship of fatigued run and rapid stop to ground reaction forces, lower extremity kinematics, and muscle activation. *J Orthop Sports Phys Ther.* 1994;20:132-137.

88. Ognibene J, McMahan K, Harris M, Dutton S, Voight M. Effects of unilateral proprioceptive perturbation training on postural sway and joint reaction times of healthy subjects. In: *Proceedings of National Athletic Training Association Annual Meeting.* Champaign, IL: Human Kinetics; 2000.

89. Palta AE, Winter DA, Frank JS. Identification of age-related changes in the balance control system. In: Duncan PW, ed. *Balance: Proceedings of the APTA Forum.* Alexandria, VA: APTA; 1986.

90. Perlau RC, Frank C, Fick G. The effects of elastic bandages on human knee proprioception in the uninjured population. *Am J Sports Med.* 1995;23:251-255.

91. Peterka RJ, Black OF. Age related changes in human postural control: sensory organization tests. *J Vestib Res.* 1990;1:73-85.

92. Phillips CG, Powell TS, Wiesendanger M. Protection from low threshold muscle afferents of hand and forearm area 3A of Babson's cortex. *J Physiol.* 1971;217:419-446.

93. Pinstaar A, Brynhildsen J, Tropp H. Postural corrections after standardized perturbations of single limb stance: Effect of training and orthotic devices in patients with ankle instability. *Br J Sports Med.* 1996;30:151-155.

94. Pope MH, Johnson DW, Brown DW, Tighe C. The role of the musculature in injuries to the medial collateral ligament. *J Bone Joint Surg Am.* 1972;61:398-402.

95. Pousson M, Hoecke JV, Goubel F. Changes in elastic characteristics of human muscle and induced by eccentric exercise. *J Biomech.* 1990;23:343-348.

96. Rine RM, Voight ML, Laporta L, Mancini R. A paradigm to evaluate ankle instability using postural sway measures. *Phys Ther.* 1994;74:S72.

97. Rogers DK, Bendrups AP, Lewis MM. Disturbed proprioception following a period of muscle vibration in humans. *Neurosci Lett.* 1985;57:147-152.

98. Rothwell J. *Control of Human Voluntary Movement.* 2nd ed. London, UK: Chapman & Hall; 1994.

99. Rowinski, MJ. Afferent neurobiology of the joint. In: The role of eccentric exercise. In: *ProClinics.* Shirley, NY: Biodex; 1988.

100. Sakai H, Tanaka S, Kurosawa H, Masujima A. The effect of exercise on anterior knee laxity in female basketball players. *Int J Sports Med.* 1992;13:552-554.

101. Schmidt RA. The acquisition of skill: some modifications to the perception-action relationship through practice. In: Heuer H, Sanders AF, eds. *Perspectives on Perception and Action.* Hillsdale, NJ: Erlbaum; 1987.

102. Schmidt RA. *Motor Control and Learning.* Champaign, IL: Human Kinetics; 1988.

103. Schulmann D, Godfrey B, Fisher A. Effect of eye movements on dynamic equilibrium. *Phys Ther.* 1987;67:1054-1057.

104. Schulte MJ, Happel LT. Joint innervation in injury. *Clin Sports Med.* 1990;9:511-517.

105. Sherrington CS. *The Interactive Action of the Nervous System.* New Haven, CT: Yale University Press; 1911.

106. Sheth P, Yu B, Laskowski ER, et al. Ankle disk training influences reaction times of selected muscles in a simulated ankle sprain. *Am J Sports Med.* 1997;25:538-543.

107. Shumway-Cook A, Horak FB. Assessing the influence of sensory interaction on balance. *Phys Ther.* 1986;66:1548-1550.

108. Sittig AC, Denier van der Gon JJ, Gielen CM. Different control mechanisms for slow and fast human arm movements. *Neurosci Lett.* 1985;22:S128.

109. Sittig AC, Denier van der Gon JJ, Gielen CM. Separate control of arm position and velocity demonstrated by vibration of muscle tendon in man. *Exp Brain Res.* 1985;60:445-453.

110. Skinner HB, Barrack RL, Cook SD, Haddad RJ. Joint position sense in total knee arthroplasty. *J Orthop Res.* 1984;1:276-283.

111. Skinner HB, Wyatt MP, Hodgdon JA, Conrad DW, Barrack RI. Effect of fatigue on joint position sense of the knee. *J Orthop Res.* 1986;4:112-118.

112. Skoglund CT. Joint receptors and kinesthesia. In: Iggo A, ed. *Handbook of Sensory Physiology.* Berlin, Germany: Springer-Verlag; 1973.

113. Skoglund S. Anatomical and physiological studies of the knee joint innervation in the cat. *Acta Physiol Scand Suppl.* 1956;36(Suppl 124):1-101.

114. Small C, Waters CL, Voight ML. Comparison of two methods for measuring hamstring reaction time using the Kin-Com Isokinetic Dynamometer. *J Orthop Sports Phys Ther.* 1994;19.

115. Smith JL. Sensorimotor integration during motor programming. In: Stelmach GE, ed. *Information Processing in Motor Control and Learning.* New York, NY: Academic Press; 1978.

116. Solomonow M, Baratta R, Zhou BH, et al. The synergistic action of the anterior cruciate ligament and thigh muscles in maintaining joint stability. *Am J Sports Med.* 1987;15:207-213.

117. Steiner ME, Brown C, Zarins B, et al. Measurements of anterior–posterior displacement of the knee: A comparison of results with instrumented devices and with clinical examination. *J Bone Joint Surg Am.* 1990;72:1307-1315.

118. Stoller DW, Markoff KL, Zager SA, Shoemaker SC. The effect of exercise, ice, and ultrasonography on torsional laxity of the knee. *Clin Orthop.* 1983;174:172-180.

119. Stuart DG, Mosher CG, Gerlack RL, Reinking RM. Mechanical arrangement and transducing properties of Golgi tendon organs. *Exp Brain Res.* 1972;14:274-292.

120. Swanik CB, Lephart SM, Giannantonio FP, Fu F. Reestablishing proprioception and neuromuscular control in the ACL-injured athlete. *J Sport Rehabil.* 1997;6:183-206.

121. Tibone JE, Antich TJ, Funton GS, Moynes DR, Perry J. Functional analysis of anterior cruciate ligament instability. *Am J Sports Med.* 1986;14:276-284.

122. Tippett S, Voight ML. *Functional Progressions for Sports Rehabilitation.* Champaign, IL: Human Kinetics; 1995.

123. Tropp H, Askling C, Gillquist J. Prevention of ankle sprains. *Am J Sports Med.* 1985;13:259-262.

124. Tropp H, Ekstrand J, Gillquist J. Factors affecting stabiliometry recordings of single leg stance. *Am J Sports Med.* 1984;12:185-188.

125. Tropp H, Odenrick P. Postural control in single limb stance. *J Orthop Res.* 1988;6:833-839.

126. Voight ML. Proprioceptive concerns in rehabilitation. In: *Proceedings of the 25th FIMS World Congress of Sports Medicine.* Athens, Greece: International Sports Medicine Federation; 1994.

127. Voight ML. *Functional Exercise Training.* Presented at the 1990 National Athletic Training Association Annual Conference, Indianapolis, IN; 1990.

128. Voight ML, Bell S, Rhodes D. Instrumented testing of tibial translation during a positive Lachman's test and selected closed-chain activities in anterior cruciate deficient knees. *J Orthop Sports Phys Ther.* 1992;15:49.

129. Voight ML, Blackburn TA, Hardin JA. Effects of muscle fatigue on shoulder proprioception. *J Orthop Sports Phys Ther.* 1996;21:348-352.

130. Voight ML, Cook G, Blackburn TA. Functional lower quarter exercises through RNT. In: Bandy WD, ed. *Current Trends for the Rehabilitation of the Athlete.* Lacrosse, WI: Sports Physical Therapy Section Home Study Course; 1997.

131. Voight ML, Draovitch P. Plyometric training. In: Albert M, ed. *Muscle Training in Sports and Orthopaedics.* New York, NY: Churchill Livingstone; 1991.

132. Voight ML, Nashner LM, Blackburn TA. Neuromuscular function changes with ACL functional brace use: a measure of reflex latencies and lower quarter EMG responses [abstract]. In: *Conference Proceedings.* American Orthopedic Society for Sports Medicine; 1998.

133. Voight ML, Rine RM, Apfel P, et al. The effects of leg dominance and AFO on static and dynamic balance abilities. *Phys Ther.* 1993;73(6):S51.

134. Voight ML, Rine RM, Briese K, Powell C. Comparison of sway in double versus single leg stance in unimpaired adults. *Phys Ther.* 1993;73(6):S51.

135. Voss DE, Ionta MK, Myers BJ. *Proprioceptive Neuromuscular Facilitation: Patterns and Techniques.* Philadelphia, PA: Harper & Row; 1985.

136. Walla DJ, Albright JP, McAuley E, Martin V, Eldridge V, El-Khoury G. Hamstring control and the unstable anterior cruciate ligament-deficient knee. *Am J Sports Med.* 1985;13:34-39.

137. Wester JU, Jespersen SM, Nielsen KD, et al. Wobble board training after partial sprains of the lateral ligaments of the ankle: A prospective randomized study. *J Orthop Sports Phys Ther.* 1996;23:332-336.

138. Wetzel MC, Stuart DC. Ensemble characteristics of cat locomotion and its neural control. *Prog Neurobiol.* 1976;7:1-98.

139. Willis WD, Grossman RG. *Medical Neurobiology*. 3rd ed. St Louis, MO: Mosby; 1981.

140. Wojtys E, Huston L. Neuromuscular performance in normal and anterior cruciate ligament-deficient lower extremities. *Am J Sports Med.* 1994;22:89-104.

141. Wojtys E, Huston L, Taylor PD, Bastian SD. Neuromuscular adaptations in isokinetic, isotonic, and agility training programs. *Am J Sports Med.* 1996;24(2):187-192.

142. Woollacott MH. Postural control mechanisms in the young and the old. In: Duncan PW, ed. *Balance: Proceedings of the APTA Forum*. Alexandria, VA: APTA; 1990.

143. Woollacott MH, Shumway-Cook A, Nashner LM. Aging and posture control: changes in sensory organs and muscular coordination. *Int J Aging Hum Dev.* 1986;23:97-114.

10

Plyometric Exercise in Rehabilitation

Michael L. Voight and Steven R. Tippett

OBJECTIVES **After completion of this chapter, the physical therapist should be able to do the following:**

- Define plyometric exercise and identify its function in a rehabilitation program.
- Describe the mechanical, neurophysiologic, and neuromuscular control mechanisms involved in plyometric training.
- Discuss how biomechanical evaluation, stability, dynamic movement, and flexibility should be assessed before beginning a plyometric program.
- Explain how a plyometric program can be modified by changing intensity, volume, frequency, and recovery.
- Discuss how plyometrics can be integrated into a rehabilitation program.
- Recognize the value of different plyometric exercises in rehabilitation.

What Is Plyometric Exercise?

In sports training and rehabilitation of athletic injuries, the concept of specificity has emerged as an important parameter in determining the proper choice and sequence of exercise in a training program. The jumping movement is inherent in numerous sport activities such as basketball, volleyball, gymnastics, and aerobic dancing. Even running is a repeated series of jump-landing cycles. Consequently, jump training should be used in the design and implementation of the overall training program.

Peak performance in sport requires technical skill and power. Skill in most activities combines natural athletic ability and learned specialized proficiency in an activity. Success in most activities is dependent upon the speed at which muscular force or power can be generated. Strength and conditioning programs throughout the years have attempted to augment the force production system to maximize the power generation. Because power combines strength and speed, it can be increased by increasing the amount of work or force that is produced by the muscles or by decreasing the amount of time required to produce the force. Although weight training can produce increased gains in strength, the speed of movement is limited. The amount of time required to produce muscular force is an important variable for increasing the power output. Plyometrics is a form of training that attempts to combine speed of movement with strength.

The roots of plyometric training can be traced to Eastern Europe, where it was known simply as jump training.[19,20,39–41] The term *plyometrics* was coined by an American track and field coach, Fred Wilt.[46] The development of the term is confusing. *Plyo-* comes from the Greek word *plythein*, which means "to increase." *Plio* is the Greek word for "ore," and metric literally means "to measure." Practically, plyometrics is defined as a quick, powerful movement involving prestretching the muscle and activating the stretch-shortening cycle to produce a subsequently stronger concentric contraction. It takes advantage of the length-shortening cycle to increase muscular power.[12]

In the late 1960s and early 1970s, when the Eastern Bloc countries began to dominate sports requiring power, their training methods became the focus of attention. After the 1972 Olympics, articles began to appear in coaching magazines outlining a strange new system of jumps and bounds that had been used by the Soviets to increase speed. Valery Borzov, the 100-meter gold medalist, credited plyometric exercise for his success. As it turns out, the Eastern Bloc countries were not the originators of plyometrics, just the organizers. This system of hops and jumps has been used by American coaches for years as a method of conditioning. Both rope jumping and bench hops have been used to improve quickness and reaction times. The organization of this training method has been credited to the legendary Soviet jump coach Yuri Verhoshanski, who, during the late 1960s, began to tie this method of miscellaneous hops and jumps into an organized training plan.[39–41] The main purpose of plyometric training is to heighten the excitability of the nervous system for improved reactive ability of the neuromuscular system.[43] Therefore, any type of exercise that uses the myotatic stretch reflex to produce a more powerful response of the contracting muscle is plyometric in nature. All movement patterns in both athletes and activities of daily living involve repeated stretch-shortening cycles. Picture a jumping athlete preparing to transfer forward energy to upward energy. As the final step is taken before jumping, the loaded leg must stop the forward momentum and change it into an upward direction. As this happens, the muscle undergoes a lengthening eccentric contraction to decelerate the movement and prestretch the muscle. This prestretch energy is then immediately released in an equal and opposite reaction, thereby producing kinetic energy. The neuromuscular system must react quickly to produce the concentric shortening contraction to prevent falling and produce the upward change in direction. Most elite athletes will naturally exhibit with great ease this ability to use stored kinetic energy. Less-gifted athletes can train this ability and enhance their production of power. Consequently, specific functional exercise to emphasize this rapid change of direction must be used to prepare patients and athletes for return to activity.[17] Because plyometric exercises train specific movements in a biomechanically accurate manner, the muscles, tendons, and ligaments are all strengthened in a functional manner.

Most of the literature to date on plyometric training has focused on the lower quarter.[1] Because all movements in athletics involve a repeated series of stretch-shortening cycles, adaptation of the plyometric principles can be used to enhance the specificity of training in other sports or activities that require a maximum amount of muscular force in a minimal amount of time. Whether the athlete is jumping or throwing, the musculature around the involved joints must first stretch and then contract to produce the explosive movement. Because of the muscular demands during the overhead throw, plyometrics have been advocated as a form of conditioning for the overhead throwing athlete.[42,45] Although the principles are similar, different forms of plyometric exercises should be applied to the upper extremity to train the stretch-shortening cycle. Additionally, the intensity of the upper extremity plyometric program is usually less than that of the lower extremity, as a result of the smaller muscle mass and type of muscle function of the upper extremity compared to the lower extremity.

The role of the core muscles of the abdominal region and the lumbar spine in providing a vital link for stability and power cannot be overlooked. Plyometric training for these muscles can be incorporated in isolated drills as well as functional activities.

Biomechanical and Physiologic Principles of Plyometric Training

The goal of plyometric training is to decrease the amount of time required between the yielding eccentric muscle contraction and the initiation of the overcoming concentric contraction. Normal physiologic movement rarely begins from a static starting position, but rather is preceded by an eccentric prestretch that loads the muscle and prepares it for the ensuing concentric contraction.[11] The coupling of this eccentric-concentric muscle contraction is known as the stretch-shortening cycle. The physiology of this stretch-shortening cycle can be broken down into 2 components: proprioceptive reflexes and the elastic properties of muscle fibers.[43] These components work together to produce a response, but they are discussed separately to aid understanding.

Mechanical Characteristics

The mechanical characteristics of a muscle can best be represented by a 3-component model (Figure 10-1). A contractile component, a series elastic component (SEC), and a parallel elastic component all interact to produce a force output. Although the contractile component is usually the focal point of motor control, the SEC and parallel elastic component also play an important role in providing stability and integrity to the individual fibers when a muscle is lengthened.[43] During this lengthening process, energy is stored within the musculature in the form of kinetic energy.

When a muscle contracts in a concentric fashion, most of the force that is produced comes from the muscle fiber filaments sliding past one another. Force is registered

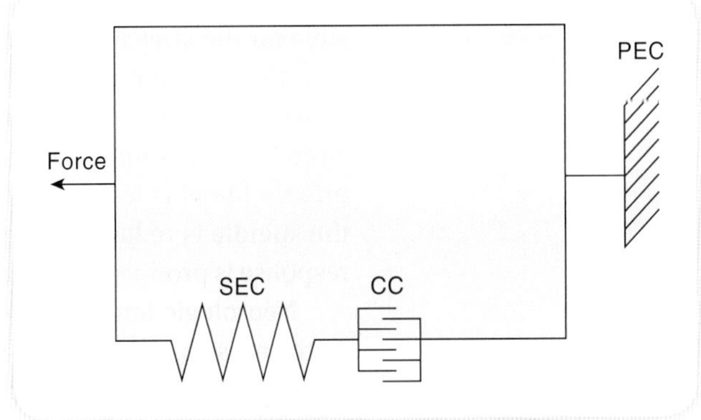

Figure 10-1 Three-component model

externally by being transferred through the SEC. When eccentric contraction occurs, the muscle lengthens like a spring. With this lengthening, the SEC is also stretched and allowed to contribute to the overall force production. Therefore, the total force production is the sum of the force produced by the contractile component and the stretching of the SEC. An analogy would be the stretching of a rubber band. When a stretch is applied, potential energy is stored and applied as it returns to its original length when the stretch is released. Significant increases in concentric muscle force production have been documented when immediately preceded by an eccentric contraction.[2,4,9] This increase might be partly a result of the storage of elastic energy, because the muscles are able to use the force produced by the SEC. When the muscle contracts in a concentric manner, the elastic energy that is stored in the SEC can be recovered and used to augment the shortening contraction. The ability to use this stored elastic energy is affected by 3 variables: time, magnitude of stretch, and velocity of stretch.[23] The concentric contraction can be magnified only if the preceding eccentric contraction is of short range and performed quickly without delay.[2,4,9] Bosco and Komi proved this concept experimentally when they compared damped versus undamped jumps.[4] Undamped jumps produced minimal knee flexion upon landing and were followed by an immediate rebound jump. With damped jumps, the knee flexion angle increased significantly. The power output was much higher with the undamped jumps. The increased knee flexion seen in the damped jumps decreased elastic behavior of the muscle, and the potential elastic energy stored in the SEC was lost as heat. Similar investigations produced greater vertical jump height when the movement was preceded by a countermovement as opposed to a static jump.[2,5,6,29]

The type of muscle fiber involved in the contraction can also affect storage of elastic energy. Bosco et al noted a difference in the recoil of elastic energy in slow-twitch versus fast-twitch muscle fibers.[7] This study indicates that fast-twitch muscle fibers respond to a high-speed, small-amplitude prestretch. The amount of elastic energy used was proportional to the amount stored. When a long, slow stretch is applied to muscle, slow- and fast-twitch fibers exhibit a similar amount of stored elastic energy; however, this stored energy is used to a greater extent with the slow-twitch fibers. This trend would suggest that slow-twitch muscle fibers might be able to use elastic energy more efficiently in ballistic movement characterized by long and slow prestretching in the stretch-shortening cycle.

Neurophysiologic Mechanisms

The proprioceptive stretch reflex is the other mechanism by which force can be produced during the stretch-shortening cycle.[10] Mechanoreceptors located within the muscle provide information about the degree of muscular stretch. This information is transmitted to the central nervous system and becomes capable of influencing muscle tone, motor execution programs, and kinesthetic awareness.[43] The mechanoreceptors that are primarily responsible for the stretch reflex are the Golgi tendon organs and muscle spindles.[31] The muscle spindle is a complex stretch receptor that is located in parallel within the muscle fibers. Sensory information regarding the length of the muscle spindle and the rate of the applied stretch is transmitted to the central nervous system. If the length of the surrounding muscle fibers is less than that of the spindle, the frequency of the nerve impulses from the spindle is reduced. When the muscle spindle becomes stretched, an afferent sensory response is produced and transmitted to the central nervous system.

Neurologic impulses are, in turn, sent back to the muscle, causing a motor response. As the muscle contracts, the stretch on the muscle spindle is relieved, thereby removing the original stimulus. The strength of the muscle spindle response is determined by the rate of stretch.[31] The more rapidly the load is applied to the muscle, the greater the firing frequency of the spindle and resultant reflexive muscle contraction.

The Golgi tendon organ lies within the muscle tendon near the point of attachment of the muscle fiber to the tendon. Unlike the facilitatory action of the muscle spindle, the Golgi tendon organ has an inhibitory effect on the muscle by contributing to a tension-limiting reflex. Because the Golgi tendon organs are in series alignment with the contracting muscle fibers, they become activated with tension or stretch within the muscle. Upon activation, sensory impulses are transmitted to the central nervous system. These sensory impulses cause an inhibition of the alpha motor neurons of the contracting muscle and its synergists, thereby limiting the amount of force produced. With a concentric muscle contraction, the activity of the muscle spindle is reduced because the surrounding muscle fibers are shortening. During an eccentric muscle contraction, the muscle stretch reflex generates more tension in the lengthening muscle. When the tension within the muscle reaches a potentially harmful level, the Golgi tendon organ fires, thereby reducing the excitation of the muscle. The muscle spindle and Golgi tendon organ systems oppose each other, and increasing force is produced. The descending neural pathways from the brain help to balance these forces and ultimately control which reflex will dominate.[34]

The degree of muscle fiber elongation is dependent upon 3 physiologic factors. Fiber length is proportional to the amount of stretching force applied to the muscle. The ultimate elongation or deformation is also dependent upon the absolute strength of the individual muscle fibers. The stronger the tensile strength, the less elongation that will occur. The last factor for elongation is the ability of the muscle spindle to produce a neurophysiologic response. A muscle spindle with a low sensitivity level will result in a difficulty in overcoming the rapid elongation and therefore produce a less powerful response. Plyometric training will assist in enhancing muscular control within the neurologic system.[10]

The increased force production seen during the stretch-shortening cycle is a result of the combined effects of the storage of elastic energy and the myotatic reflex activation of the muscle.[2,4,5,8,9,30,36] The percentage of contribution from each component is unknown.[5] The increased amount of force production is dependent upon the time frame between the eccentric and concentric contractions.[9] This time frame can be defined as the amortization phase.[15] The amortization phase is the electromechanical delay between eccentric and concentric contraction during which time the muscle must switch from overcoming work to acceleration in the opposite direction. Komi found that the greatest amount of tension developed within the muscle during the stretch-shortening cycle occurred during the phase of muscle lengthening just before the concentric contraction.[28] The conclusion from this study was that an increased time in the amortization phase would lead to a decrease in force production.

Physiologic performance can be improved by several mechanisms with plyometric training. Although there has been documented evidence of increased speed of the stretch reflex, the increased intensity of the subsequent muscle contraction might be best attributed to better recruitment of additional motor units.[13,21] The force-velocity relationship states that the faster a muscle is loaded or lengthened eccentrically, the greater the resultant force output. Eccentric lengthening will also place a load on the elastic components of the muscle fibers. The stretch reflex might also increase the stiffness of the muscular spring by recruiting additional muscle fibers.[13,21] This additional stiffness might allow the muscular system to use more external stress in the form of elastic recoil.[13]

Another possible mechanism by which plyometric training can increase the force or power output involves the inhibitory effect of the Golgi tendon organs on force production. Because the Golgi tendon organ serves as a tension-limiting reflex, restricting the amount of force that can be produced, the stimulation threshold for the Golgi tendon organ becomes a limiting factor. Bosco and Komi have suggested that plyometric training can desensitize the Golgi tendon organ, thereby raising the level of inhibition.[4] If the level of inhibition is raised, a greater amount of force production and load can be applied to the musculoskeletal system.

Neuromuscular Coordination

The last mechanism in which plyometric training might improve muscular performance centers around neuromuscular coordination. The speed of muscular contraction can be limited by neuromuscular coordination. In other words, the body can move only within a set speed range, no matter how strong the muscles are. Training with an explosive prestretch of the muscle can improve the neural efficiency, thereby increasing neuromuscular performance. Plyometric training can promote changes within the neuromuscular system that allow the individual to have better control of the contracting muscle and its synergists, yielding a greater net force even in the absence of morphologic adaptation of the muscle. This neural adaptation can increase performance by enhancing the nervous system to become more automatic.

In summary, effective plyometric training relies more on the rate of stretch than on the length of stretch. Emphasis should center on the reduction of the amortization phase. If the amortization phase is slow, the elastic energy is lost as heat and the stretch reflex is not activated. Conversely, the quicker the individual is able to switch from yielding eccentric work to overcoming concentric work, the more powerful the response.

Program Development

Specificity is the key concept in any training program. Sport-specific activities should be analyzed and broken down into basic movement patterns. These specific movement patterns should then be stressed in a gradual fashion, based upon individual tolerance to these activities. Development of a plyometric program should begin by establishing an adequate strength base that will allow the body to withstand the large stress that will be placed upon it. A greater strength base will allow for greater force production because of increased muscular cross-sectional area. Additionally, a larger cross-sectional area can contribute to the SEC and subsequently store a greater amount of elastic energy.

Plyometric exercises can be characterized as rapid eccentric loading of the musculoskeletal complex.[13] This type of exercise trains the neuromuscular system by teaching it to more readily accept the increased strength loads.[3] Also, the nervous system is more readily able to react with maximal speed to the lengthening muscle by exploiting the stretch reflex. Plyometric training attempts to fine tune the neuromuscular system, so all training programs should be designed with specificity in mind.[33] This goal will help to ensure that the body is prepared to accept the stress that will be placed upon it during return to function.

Plyometric Prerequisites

Biomechanical Examination

Before beginning a plyometric training program, a cursory biomechanical examination and a battery of functional tests should be performed to identify potential contraindications or precautions. Lower-quarter biomechanics should be sound to help ensure a stable base of support and normal force transmission. Biomechanical abnormalities of the lower quarter are not contraindications for plyometrics but can contribute to stress failure-overuse injury if not addressed. Before initiating plyometric training, an adequate strength base of the stabilizing musculature must be present. Functional tests are very effective to screen for an adequate strength base before initiating plyometrics. Poor strength in the lower extremities will result in a loss of stability when landing and also increase the amount of stress that is absorbed by the weightbearing tissues with high-impact forces, which will reduce performance and increase the risk of injury. The Eastern Bloc countries arbitrarily placed a 1-repetition maximum in the squat at 1.5 to 2 times the individual's body weight before initiating lower-quarter plyometrics.[3] If this were to hold true, a 200-pound individual would have to squat 300–400 pounds before beginning plyometrics. Unfortunately, not many individuals would meet this minimal criteria. Clinical and practical experience has demonstrated that plyometrics can be started without that kind of leg strength.[13] A simple functional parameter to use in determining whether an individual is strong enough to initiate a plyometric training program has been advocated by Chu.[14] Power squat testing with a weight equal to 60% of the individual's body weight is used. The individual is asked to perform 5 squat repetitions in 5 seconds. If the individual cannot perform this task, emphasis in the training program should again center on the strength-training program to develop an adequate base.

Because eccentric muscle strength is an important component to plyometric training, it is especially important to ensure an adequate eccentric strength base is present. Before an individual is allowed to begin a plyometric regimen, a program of closed-chain stability training that focuses on eccentric lower-quarter strength should be initiated. In addition to strengthening in a functional manner, closed-chain weightbearing exercises also allow the individual to use functional movement patterns. The same holds true for adequate upper-extremity strength prior to initiating an upper-extremity plyometric program. Closed-chain activities, such as wall pushups, traditional pushups, and their modification, as well as functional tests, can be utilized to ascertain readiness for upper-extremity plyometrics.[24,37,38] Once cleared to participate in the plyometric program, precautionary safety tips should be adhered to.

PLYOMETRIC STATIC STABILITY TESTING

Single-leg stance—30 seconds
- Eyes open
- Eyes closed

Single-leg 25% squat—30 seconds
- Eyes open
- Eyes closed

Single-leg 50% squat—30 seconds
- Eyes open
- Eyes closed

Stability Testing

Stability testing before initiating plyometric training can be divided into 2 subcategories: static stability and dynamic movement testing. Static stability testing determines the individual's ability to stabilize and control the body. The muscles of postural support must be strong enough to withstand the stress of explosive training. Static stability testing should begin with simple movements of low motor complexity and progress to more difficult high motor skills. The basis for lower-quarter stability centers around single-leg strength. Difficulty can be increased by having the individual close his or her eyes. The basic static tests are one-leg standing and single-leg quarter squats that are held for 30 seconds. An individual should be able to perform one-leg standing for 30 seconds with eyes open and closed before the initiation of plyometric training. The individual should be observed for shaking or wobbling of the extremity joints. If there is more movement of a weightbearing joint in one direction than the other, the musculature producing the movement in the opposite direction needs to be assessed for specific weakness. If weakness is determined, the individual's program should be limited and emphasis placed on isolated strengthening of the weak muscles. For dynamic jump exercises to be initiated, there should be no wobbling of the support leg during the quarter knee squats.

After an individual has satisfactorily demonstrated both single-leg static stance and a single-leg quarter squat, more dynamic tests of eccentric capabilities can be initiated.

Once an individual has stabilization strength, the concern shifts toward developing and evaluating eccentric strength. The limiting factor in high-intensity, high-volume plyometrics is eccentric capabilities. Eccentric strength can be assessed with stabilization jump tests. If an individual has an excessively long amortization phase or a slow switching from eccentric to concentric contractions, the eccentric strength levels are insufficient.

Dynamic Movement Testing

Dynamic movement testing assesses the individual's ability to produce explosive, coordinated movement. Vertical or single-leg jumping for distance can be used for the lower quarter. Researchers have investigated the use of single-leg hop for distance and a determinant for return to play after knee injury. A passing score on their test is 85% in regard to symmetry. The involved leg is tested twice, and the average between the two trials is recorded. The noninvolved leg is tested in the same fashion, and then the scores of the noninvolved leg are divided by the scores of the involved leg and multiplied by 100. This provides the symmetry index score. Another functional test that can be used to determine whether an individual is ready for plyometric training is the ability to long jump a distance equal to the individual's height.

In the upper quarter, the medicine ball toss is used as a functional assessment. The seated chest press is used as a measure of upper body power. To perform this test, the patient sits tall with their back against the back rest of a chair. While holding onto a medicine ball (4 kg for men and 2 kg for women and juniors), the patient tries to chest pass the ball as far as possible keeping their back in contact with the chair. This should be repeated until the longest pass has been measured. Use the distance from where the ball bounces to the patient's chest as the distance. As can be seen in Table 10-1, under 17 feet for men and 15 feet for women is an indicator of power weakness.

The situp-and-throw test is a great test to assess abdominal and lat power. The situp evaluates core power, while the overhead throw evaluates the lat and trunk power. To perform this test, the patient lies supine with the patient's knees bent and feet flat on the ground, while holding onto a medicine ball with both hands (4 kg for men and 2 kg for women and juniors) with the ball directly over the patient's head like a soccer throw-in. Next, have the patient try to sit up and throw the ball as far as possible. This should be repeated until the longest pass has been measured. Use the distance from where the ball bounces to the patient's chest as the distance (Table 10-2).

Table 10-1 Seated Chest Pass Test

	Distance in Feet			
	Excellent	Good	Average	Needs Work
Female				
Adult	>21	17 to 21	15 to 17	<15
Junior (<16)	>19	16 to 19	14 to 16	<14
Male				
Adult	>24	20 to 24	17 to 20	<17
Junior (<16 years)	>20	18 to 20	15 to 18	<15

Table 10-2 Situp-and-Throw Test

	Distance in Feet			
	Excellent	Good	Average	Needs Work
Female				
Adult	>21	17 to 21	15 to 17	<15
Junior (<16)	>19	16 to 19	14 to 16	<14
Male				
Adult	>24	20 to 24	17 to 20	<17
Junior (<16)	>20	18 to 20	15 to 18	<15

Flexibility

Another important prerequisite for plyometric training is general and specific flexibility, because a high amount of stress is applied to the musculoskeletal system. Consequently, all plyometric training sessions should begin with a general warm-up and flexibility exercise program. The warm-up should produce mild sweating.[26] The flexibility exercise program should address muscle groups involved in the plyometric program and should include static and short dynamic stretching techniques.[25]

Plyometric Prerequisites Summary When the individual can demonstrate static and dynamic control of their body weight with single-leg squats or adequate medicine ball throws for the upper extremity and core, low-intensity in-place plyometrics can be initiated. Plyometric training should consist of low-intensity drills and progress slowly in deliberate fashion. As skill and strength foundation increase, moderate-intensity plyometrics can be introduced. Mature patients with strong weight-training backgrounds can be introduced to ballistic-reactive plyometric exercises of high intensity.[14] Once the individual has been classified as beginner, intermediate, or advanced, the plyometric program can be designed and initiated.

Plyometric Program Design

As with any conditioning program, the plyometric training program can be manipulated through training variables: direction of body movement, weight of the individual, speed of the execution, external load, intensity, volume, frequency, training age, and recovery (Table 10-3).

Direction of Body Movement

Horizontal body movement is less stressful than vertical movement. This is dependent upon the weight of the patient and the technical proficiency demonstrated during the jumps.

Weight of the Patient

The heavier the patient, the greater the training demand placed on the patient. What might be a low-demand in-place jump for a lightweight patient might be a high-demand activity for a heavyweight patient.

Table 10-3 Chu's Plyometric Categories

In-place jumping
Standing jumps
Multiple-response jumps and hops
In-depth jumping and box drills
Bounding
High-stress sport-specific drills

Speed of Execution of the Exercise

Increased speed of execution on exercises like single-leg hops or alternate-leg bounding raises the training demand on the individual.

External Load

Adding an external load can significantly raise the training demand. Do not raise the external load to a level that will significantly slow the speed of movement.

Intensity

Intensity can be defined as the amount of effort exerted. With traditional weight lifting, intensity can be modified by changing the amount of weight that is lifted. With plyometric training, intensity can be controlled by the type of exercise that is performed. Double-leg jumping is less stressful than single-leg jumping. As with all functional exercise, the plyometric exercise program should progress from simple to complex activities. Intensity can be further increased by altering the specific exercises. The addition of external weight or raising the height of the step or box will also increase the exercise intensity.[22]

Volume

Volume is the total amount of work that is performed in a single workout session. With weight training, volume would be recorded as the total amount of weight that was lifted (weight times repetitions). Volume of plyometric training is measured by counting the total number of foot contacts. The recommended volume of foot contacts in any one session will vary inversely with the intensity of the exercise. A beginner should start with low-intensity exercise with a volume of approximately 75- to 100-foot contacts. As ability is increased, the volume is increased to 200- to 250-foot contacts of low-to-moderate intensity.

Frequency

Frequency is the number of times an exercise session is performed during a training cycle. With weight training, the frequency of exercise has typically been 3 times weekly. Unfortunately, research on the frequency of plyometric exercise has not been conducted. Therefore, the optimum frequency for increased performance is not known. It has been suggested that 48 to 72 hours of rest are necessary for full recovery before the next training stimulus.[14] Intensity, however, plays a major role in determining the frequency of training. If an adequate recovery period does not occur, muscle fatigue will result with a corresponding increase in neuromuscular reaction times. The beginner should allow at least 48 hours between training sessions.

Training Age

Training age is the number of years an individual has been in a formal training program. At younger training ages, the overall training demand should be kept low. Prepubescent and pubescent individuals of both genders are engaged in more intense physical training programs. Many of these programs contain plyometric drills. Because youth sports involve plyometric movements, training for these sports should also involve plyometric activities. The literature does not have long-term data looking at the effects of plyometric activities on human articular cartilage and long bone growth. Research demonstrates that plyometric training does indeed result in strength gains in prepubescent individuals, and that plyometric training may in fact contribute to increased bone mineral content in young females.[18,47]

Recovery

Recovery is the rest time used between exercise sets. Manipulation of this variable will depend on whether the goal is to increase power or muscular endurance. Because plyometric training is anaerobic in nature, a longer recovery period should be used to allow restoration of metabolic stores. With power training, a work rest ratio of 1:3 or 1:4 should be used. This time frame will allow maximal recovery between sets. For endurance training, this work-to-rest ratio can be shortened to 1:1 or 1:2. Endurance training typically uses circuit training, where the individual moves from one exercise set to another with minimal rest in between.

The beginning plyometric program should emphasize the importance of eccentric versus concentric muscle contractions. The relevance of the stretch-shortening cycle with decreased amortization time should be stressed. Initiation of lower-quarter plyometric training begins with low-intensity in-place and multiple-response jumps. The individual should be instructed in proper exercise technique. The feet should be nearly flat in all landings, and the individual should be encouraged to "touch and go." An analogy would be landing on a hot bed of coals. The goal is to reverse the landing as quickly as possible, spending only a minimal amount of time on the ground.

Success of the plyometric program will depend on how well the training variables are controlled, modified, and manipulated. In general, as the intensity of the exercise is increased, the volume is decreased. The corollary to this is that as volume increases, the intensity is decreased. The overall key to successfully controlling these variables is to be flexible and listen to what the individual's body is telling you. The body's response to the program will dictate the speed of progression. Whenever in doubt as to the exercise intensity or volume, it is better to underestimate to prevent injury.

Before implementing a plyometric program, the athletic trainer should assess the type of patient that is being rehabilitated and whether plyometrics are suitable for that individual. In most cases, plyometrics should be used in the latter phases of rehabilitation, starting in the advanced strengthening phase once the patient has obtained an appropriate strength base.[36,38] When utilizing plyometric training in the uninjured population, the application of plyometric exercise should follow the concept of periodization.[43] The concept of periodization refers to the year-round sequence and progression of strength training, conditioning, and sport-specific skills.[45] There are 4 specific phases in the year-round periodization model: the competitive season, postseason training, the preparation phase, and the transitional phase.[43] Plyometric exercises should be performed in the latter stages of the preparation phase and during the transitional phase for optimal results and safety. To obtain the benefits of a plyometric program, the individual should (a) be well conditioned with sufficient strength and endurance, (b) exhibit athletic abilities, (c) exhibit coordination and proprioceptive abilities, and (d) be free of pain from any physical injury or condition.

It should be remembered that the plyometric program is not designed to be an exclusive training program for the individual. Rather, it should be one part of a well-structured

Table 10-4 Upper-Extremity Plyometric Drills

I. Warm-up drills	Plyoball trunk rotation Plyoball side bends Plyoball wood chops External rotation (ER)/internal rotation (IR) with tubing Proprioceptive neuromuscular feedback (PNF) D2 pattern with tubing
II. Throwing movements—standing position	Two-hand chest pass Two-hand overhead soccer throw Two-hand side throw overhead Tubing ER/IR (Both at side and 90-degree abduction) Tubing PNF D2 pattern One-hand baseball throw One-hand IR side throw One-hand ER side throw Plyo pushup (against wall)
III. Throwing movements—seated position	Two-hand overhead soccer throw Two-hand side-to-side throw Two-hand chest pass One-hand baseball throw
IV. Trunk drills	Plyoball sit-ups Plyoball sit-up and throw Plyoball back extension Plyoball long sitting side throws
V. Partner drills	Overhead soccer throw Plyoball back-to-back twists Overhead pullover throw Kneeling side throw Backward throw Chest pass throw
VI. Wall drills	Two-hand chest throw Two-hand overhead soccer throw Two-hand underhand side-to-side throw One-hand baseball throw One-hand wall dribble
VII. Endurance drills	One-hand wall dribble Around-the-back circles Figure 8 through the legs Single-arm ball flips

training program that includes strength training, flexibility training, cardiovascular fitness, and sport-specific training for skill enhancement and coordination. By combining the plyometric program with other training techniques, the effects of training are greatly enhanced.

Tables 10-4 and 10-5 suggest upper-extremity and lower-extremity plyometric drills.

Table 10-5 **Lower-Extremity Plyometric Drills**

I. Warm-up drills	Double-leg squats Double-leg leg press Double-leg squat-jumps Jumping jacks
II. Entry-level drills—two-legged	Two-legged drills Side to side (floor/line) Diagonal jumps (floor/4 corners) Diagonal jumps (4 spots) Diagonal zig-zag (6 spots) Plyo leg press Plyo leg press (four corners)
III. Intermediate-level drills	Two-legged box jumps One-box side jump Two box side jumps Two-box side jumps with foam Four-box diagonal jumps Two-box with rotation One-/2-box with catch One-/two-box with catch (foam) Single-leg movements Single-leg plyo leg press Single-leg side jumps (floor) Single-leg side-to-side jumps (floor/4 corners) Single-leg diagonal jumps (floor/4 corners)
IV. Advanced-level drills	Single-leg box jumps One-box side jumps Two-box side jumps Single-leg plyo leg press (4 corners) Two-box side jumps with foam Four-box diagonal jumps One-box side jumps with rotation Two-box side jumps with rotation One-box side jump with catch One-box side jump rotation with catch Two-box side jump with catch Two-box side jump rotation with catch
V. Endurance/agility plyometrics	Side-to-side bounding (20 ft) Side jump lunges (cone) Side jump lunges (cone with foam) Altering rapid step-up (forward) Lateral step-overs High stepping (forward) High stepping (backward) Depth jump with rebound jump Depth jump with catch Jump and catch (Plyoball)

Guidelines for Plyometric Programs

The proper execution of the plyometric exercise program must continually be stressed. A sound technical foundation from which higher-intensity work can build should be established. It must be remembered that jumping is a continuous interchange between force reduction and force production. This interchange takes place throughout the entire body: ankle, knee, hip, trunk, and arms. The timing and coordination of these body segments yields a positive ground reaction that will result in a high rate of force production.[16]

As the plyometric program is initiated, the individual must be made aware of several guidelines.[43] Any deviation from these guidelines will result in minimal improvement and increased risk for injury. These guidelines include the following:

1. Plyometric training should be specific to the individual goals. Activity-specific movement patterns should be trained. These sport-specific skills should be broken down and trained in their smaller components and then rebuilt into a coordinated activity-specific movement pattern.
2. The quality of work is more important than the quantity of work. The intensity of the exercise should be kept at a maximal level.
3. The greater the exercise intensity level, the greater the recovery time.
4. Plyometric training can have its greatest benefit at the conclusion of the normal workout. This pattern will best replicate exercise under a partial to total fatigue environment that is specific to activity. Only low- to medium-stress plyometrics should be used at the conclusion of a workout, because of the increased potential of injury with high-stress drills.
5. When proper technique can no longer be demonstrated, maximum volume has been achieved and the exercise must be stopped. Training improperly or with fatigue can lead to injury.
6. The plyometric training program should be progressive in nature. The volume and intensity can be modified in several ways:
   a. Increase the number of exercises.
   b. Increase the number of repetitions and sets.
   c. Decrease the rest period between sets of exercise.
7. Plyometric training sessions should be conducted no more than 3 times weekly in the preseason phase of training. During this phase, volume should prevail. During the competitive season, the frequency of plyometric training should be reduced to twice weekly, with the intensity of the exercise becoming more important.
8. Dynamic testing of the individual on a regular basis will provide important progression and motivational feedback.
9. In addition to proper technique and exercise dosage, proper equipment is also required. Equipment should allow for the safe performance of the activity, landing surfaces should be even and allow for as much shock absorption as possible, and footwear should provide adequate shock absorption and forefoot support.

The key element in the execution of proper technique is the eccentric or landing phase. The shock of landing from a jump is not absorbed exclusively by the foot but rather is a combination of the ankle, knee, and hip joints all working together to absorb the shock of landing and then transferring the force.

Integrating Plyometrics into the Rehabilitation Program: Clinical Concerns

When used judiciously, plyometrics are a valuable asset in the sports rehabilitation program.[35] Clinical plyometrics should involve loading of the healing tissue. These activities may include (a) medial/lateral loading, (b) rotational loading, and (c) shock absorption/deceleration loading. In addition, plyometric drills will be divided into (a) in-place activities (activities that can be performed in essentially the same or small amount of space), (b) dynamic distance drills (activities that occur across a given distance), and (c) depth jumping (jumping down from a predetermined height and performing a variety of activities upon landing). Simple jumping drills (bilateral activities) can be progressed to hopping (unilateral activities).

Medial-Lateral Loading

Virtually all sporting activities involve cutting maneuvers. Inherent to cutting activities is adequate function in the medial and lateral directions. A plyometric program designed to stress the individual's ability to accept weight on the involved lower extremity and then perform cutting activities off that leg is imperative. Individuals who have suffered sprains to the medial or lateral capsular and ligamentous complex of the ankle and knee, as well as the hip abductor/adductor and ankle invertor/evertor muscle strains, are candidates for medial-lateral plyometric loading. Medial-lateral loading drills should be implemented following injury to the medial soft tissue around the knee after a valgus stress. By gradually imparting progressive valgus loads, tissue tensile strength is augmented.[48] In the rehabilitation setting, bilateral support drills can be progressed to unilateral valgus loading efforts. Specifically, lateral jumping drills are progressed to lateral hopping activities. However, the medial structures must also be trained to accept greater valgus loads sustained during cutting activities. As a prerequisite to full-speed cutting, lateral bounding drills should be performed. These efforts are progressed to activities that add acceleration, deceleration, and momentum. Lateral sliding activities that require the individual to cover a greater distance can be performed on a slide board. If a slide board is not available, the same movement pattern can be stressed with plyometrics (Figure 10-2).

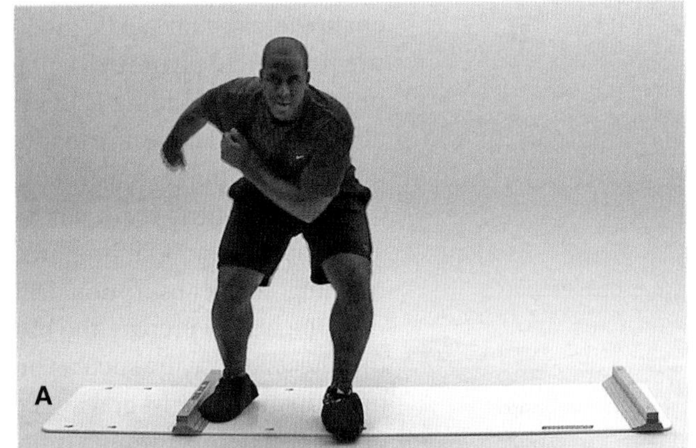

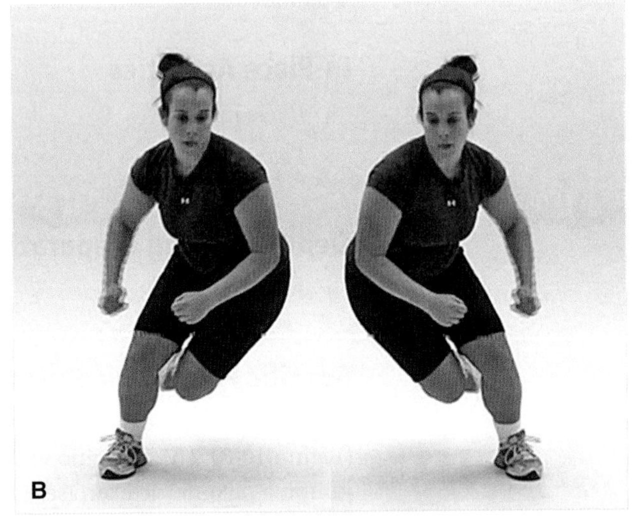

Figure 10-2

A. Slideboard ice skater glides. **B.** Ice skaters.

In-Place Activities

- Lateral bounding (quick step valgus loading)
- Slide bounds

Dynamic Distance Drills

- Crossovers

Rotational Loading

Because rotation in the knee is controlled by the cruciate ligaments, menisci, and capsule, plyometric activities with a rotational component are instrumental in the rehabilitation program after injury to any of these structures. As previously discussed, care must be taken not to exceed healing time constraints when using plyometric training.

In-Place Activities

- Spin jumps

Dynamic Distance Drills

- Lateral hopping

Shock Absorption (Deceleration Loading)

Perhaps some of the most physically demanding plyometric activities are shock absorption activities, which place a tremendous amount of stress upon muscle, tendon, and articular cartilage. As previously stated, the majority of lower-quarter sport function occurs in the closed kinetic chain. Lower-extremity plyometrics are an effective functional closed-chain exercise that can be incorporated into the rehabilitation program. Through the eccentric prestretch, plyometrics place added stress on the tendinous portion of the contractile unit. Eccentric loading is beneficial in the management of tendinitis.[44] Through a gradually progressed eccentric loading program, healing tendinous tissue is stressed, yielding an increase in ultimate tensile strength.

This eccentric load can be applied through jump-down exercises (see Figure 10-6) Therefore, in the final preparation for a return to sports involving repetitive jumping and hopping, shock absorption drills should be included in the rehabilitation program.[27]

One way to prepare the individual for shock absorption drills is to gradually maximize the effects of gravity, such as beginning in a gravity-minimized position and progressing to performance against gravity. Popular activities to minimize gravity include water activities or assisted efforts through unloading jumps and hops in the supine position on a leg press or similar device.

In-Place Activities

- Cycle jumps
- Five-dot drill

Depth Jumping Preparation

- Jump-downs

Specific Plyometric Exercises

Plyometric drills can be categorized into (a) weighted ball toss plyometric exercises (Figure 10-3); (b) dynamic weighted ball plyometric exercises (Figure 10-4); (c) in-place jumping plyometric exercises (Figure 10-5), which involve activities that can be performed in essentially the same or small amount of space; and (d) depth jumping and bounding plyometric exercises (Figure 10-6) that may involve jumping down from a predetermined height and performing a variety of activities upon landing or activities that occur across a given distance. In-place jumping drills (bilateral activities) can be progressed to hopping (unilateral activities).

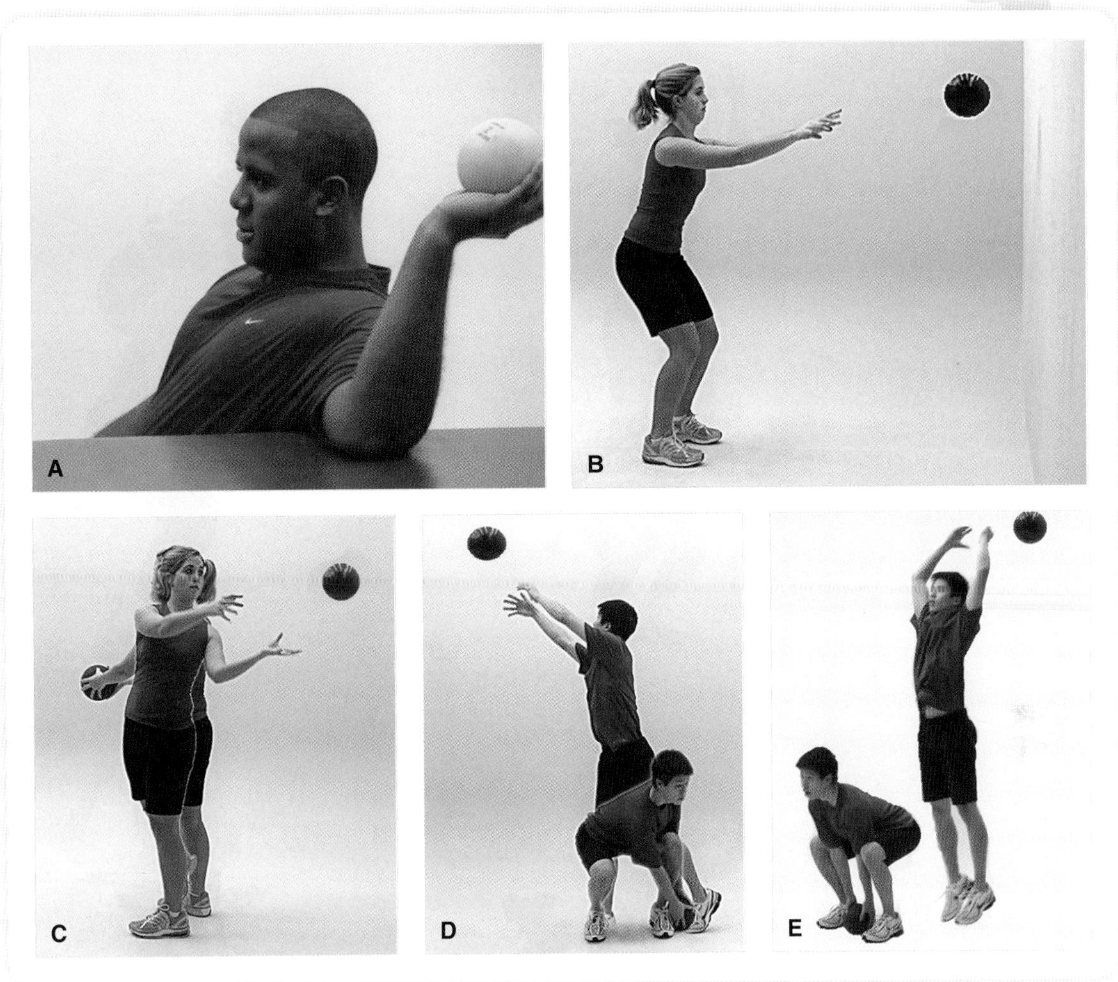

Figure 10-3

A. Single-arm weight ball throw. **B.** Weighted ball two-arm chest pass. **C.** Weighted ball reverse toss with rotation. **D.** Back extension-rotation weighted ball throw. **E.** Overhead weighted ball throw.

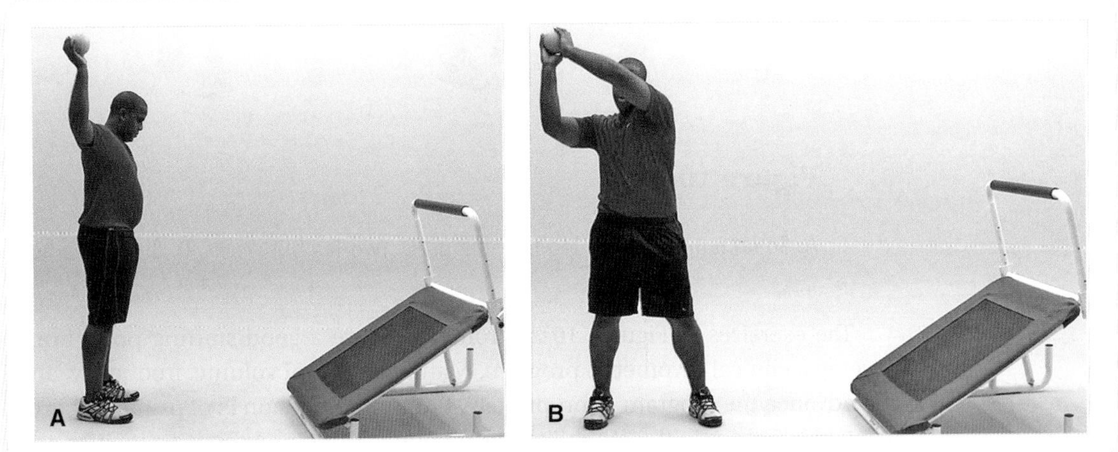

Figure 10-4

A. Plyoback standing single-arm ball toss. **B.** Plyoback two-arm toss with rotation.

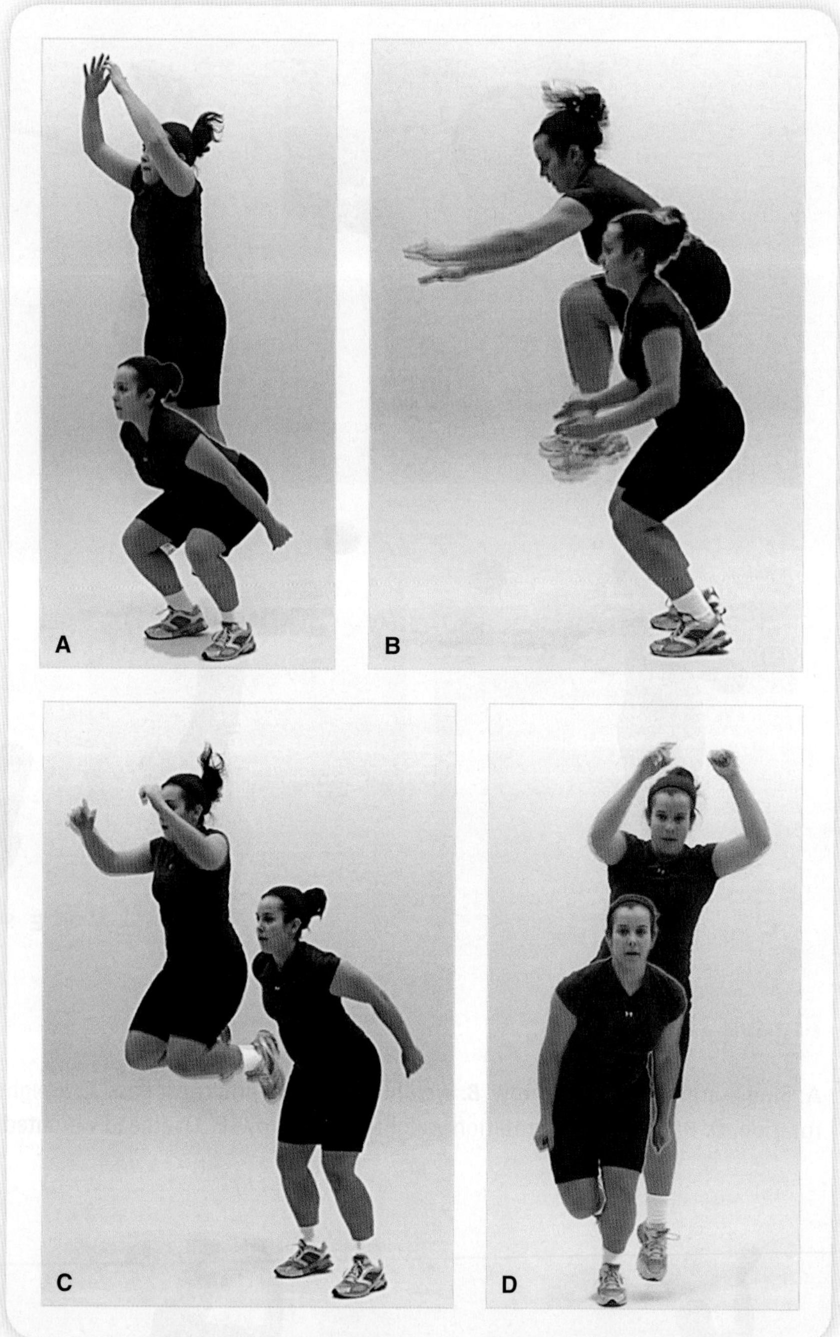

Figure 10-5

A. Squat jumps. **B.** Two-leg tuck jumps. **C.** Two-leg butt kicks. **D.** Single-leg hops.

The exercises in Figures 10-3 through 10-6 are a good starting point from which to develop a clinical plyometric program. Manipulations of volume, frequency, and intensity can advance the program appropriately. Proper progression is of prime importance when using plyometrics in the rehabilitation program. These progressive activities are reinjuries waiting to happen if the progression does not allow for adequate healing or development of an adequate strength base.[32] A close working relationship fostering open communication and acute observation skills is vital in helping ensure that the program is not overly aggressive.

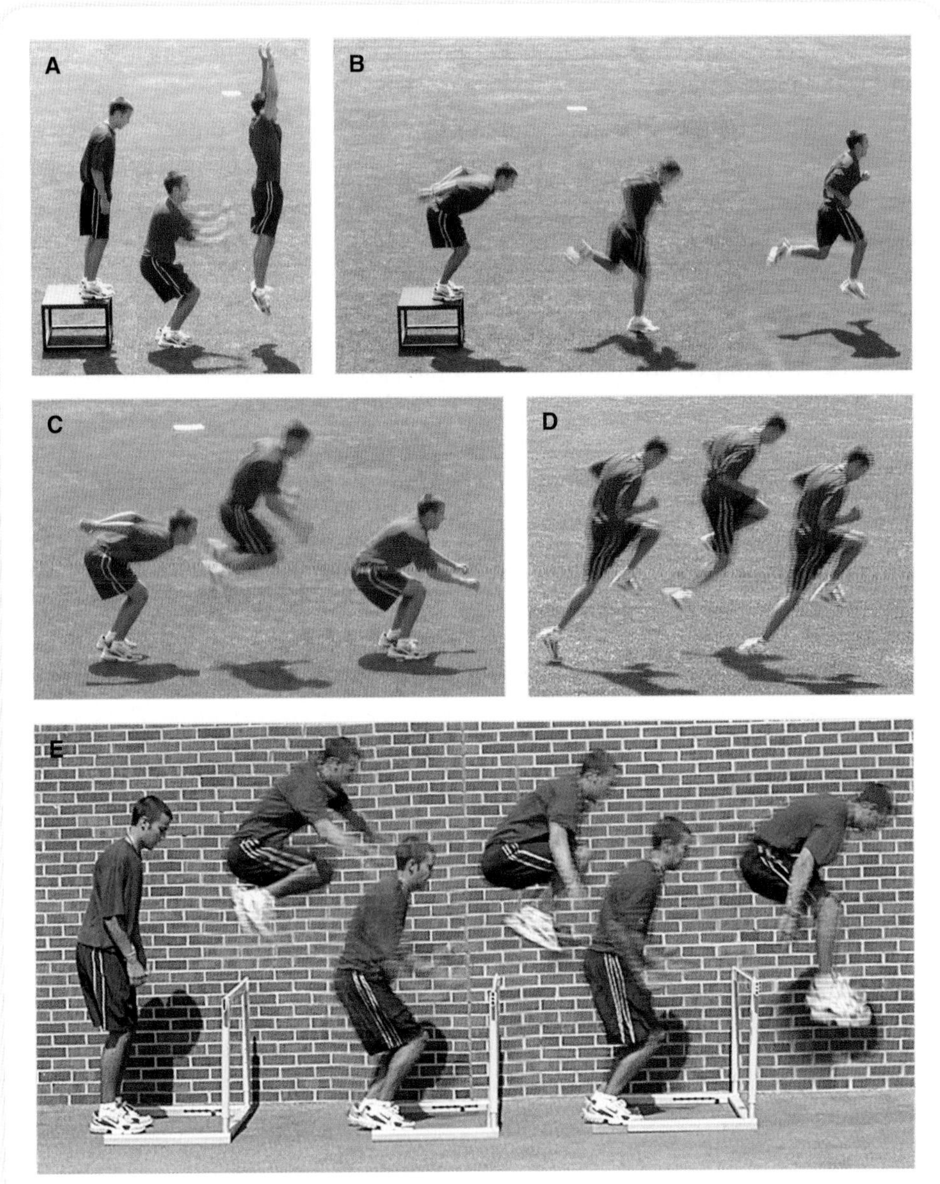

Figure 10-6

A. Depth jump to vertical jump. **B.** Depth jump to bounding. **C.** Repeat two-leg standing long jumps. **D.** Single-leg hops for distance. **E.** Three-hurdle jumps.

SUMMARY

1. Although the effects of plyometric training are not yet fully understood, it still remains a widely used form of combining strength with speed training to functionally increase power. Although the research is somewhat contradictory, the neurophysiologic concept of plyometric training is based on a sound foundation.
2. A successful plyometric training program should be carefully designed and implemented after establishing an adequate strength base.

3. The effects of this type of high-intensity training can be achieved safely if the individual is supervised by a knowledgeable person who uses common sense and follows the prescribed training regimen.
4. The plyometric training program should use a large variety of different exercises, because year-round training often results in boredom and a lack of motivation.
5. Program variety can be manipulated with different types of equipment or kinds of movement performed.
6. Continued motivation and an organized progression are the keys to successful training.
7. Plyometrics are also a valuable asset in the rehabilitation program after a sport injury.
8. Used after both upper- and lower-quarter injury, plyometrics are effective in facilitating joint awareness, strengthening tissue during the healing process, and increasing sport-specific strength and power.
9. The most important considerations in the plyometric program are common sense and experience.

REFERENCES

1. Adams T. An investigation of selected plyometric training exercises on muscular leg strength and power. *Track Field Q Rev.* 1984;84(1):36-40.
2. Asmussen E, Bonde-Peterson F. Storage of elastic energy in skeletal muscles in man. *Acta Physiol Scand.* 1974;91:385.
3. Bielik E, Chu D, Costello F, et al. Roundtable: 1. Practical considerations for utilizing plyometrics. *Strength Cond J.* 1986;8:14.
4. Bosco C, Komi PV. Potentiation of the mechanical behavior of the human skeletal muscle through prestretching. *Acta Physiol Scand.* 1979;106:467.
5. Bosco C, Komi PV. Muscle elasticity in athletes. In: Komi PV, ed. *Exercise and Sports Biology.* Champaign, IL: Human Kinetics; 1982;191-197.
6. Bosco C, Tarkka J, Komi PV. Effect of elastic energy and myoelectric potentiation of triceps surae during stretch-shortening cycle exercise. *Int J Sports Med.* 1982;2:137.
7. Bosco C, Tihanyia J, Komi PV, et al. Store and recoil of elastic energy in slow and fast types of human skeletal muscles. *Acta Physiol Scand.* 1987;16:343.
8. Cavagna GA, Dusman B, Margaria R. Positive work done by a previously stretched muscle. *J Appl Physiol.* 1968;24:21.
9. Cavagna G, Saibene F, Margaria R. Effect of negative work on the amount of positive work performed by an isolated muscle. *J Appl Physiol.* 1965;20:157.
10. Chimera, N, Swanik, K, Swanik C. Effects of plyometric training on muscle-activation strategies and performance in female athletes. *J Athl Train.* 2004;39(1): 24-31.
11. Chmielewski T, Myer G, Kauffman D. Plyometric exercise in the rehabilitation of athletes: physiological responses and clinical application. *J Orthop Sports Phys Ther.* 2006;36(5):308-319.
12. Chu D. Plyometric exercise. *Strength Cond J.* 1984;6:56.
13. Chu D. *Conditioning/Plyometrics.* Paper presented at 10th Annual Sports Medicine Team Concept Conference, San Francisco, CA; December, 1989.
14. Chu D. *Jumping into Plyometrics.* Champaign, IL: Leisure Press; 1992.
15. Chu D, Plummer L. The language of plyometrics. *Strength Cond J.* 1984;6:30.
16. Cissik J. Plyometric fundamentals. *NSCA Perform Train J.* 2004;3(2):9-13.
17. Curwin S, Stannish WD. *Tendinitis: Its Etiology and Treatment.* Lexington, MA: Collamore Press; 1984.
18. Diallo O, Dore E, Duchercise P, et al. Effects of plyometric training followed by a reduced training programme on physical performance in prepubescent soccer players. *J Sports Med Phys Fitness.* 2001;41:342-48.
19. Dunsenev CI. Strength training for jumpers. *Soviet Sports Rev.* 1979;14:2.
20. Dunsenev CI. Strength training of jumpers. *Track Field Q.* 1982;82:4.
21. Ebben W, Simenz C, Jensen R. Evaluation of plyometric intensity using electromyography. *J Strength Cond Res.* 2008;22(3):861.
22. Ebben W. Practical guidelines for plyometric intensity. *NSCA Perform Train J.* 2007;6(5):12.
23. Enoka RM. *Neuromechanical Basis of Kinesiology.* Champaign, IL: Human Kinetics; 1989.
24. Goldbeck T, Davies G. Test-retest reliability of the closed chain upper extremity stability test: a clinical field test. *J Sport Rehabil.* 2000;9:35-45.
25. Javorek I. Plyometrics. *Strength Cond J.* 1989;11:52.
26. Jensen C. Pertinent facts about warming. *Athl J.* 1975;56:72.
27. Katchajov S, Gomberaze K, Revson A. Rebound jumps. *Mod Athl Coach.* 1976;14(4):23.

28. Komi PV. Physiological and biomechanical correlates of muscle function: effects of muscle structure and stretch shortening cycle on force and speed. In: Terjung R, ed. *Exercise and Sports Sciences Review*. Lexington, MA: Collamore Press; 1984;81-122.
29. Komi PV, Bosco C. Utilization of stored elastic energy in leg extensor muscles by men and women. *Med Sci Sports Exerc.* 1978;10(4):261.
30. Komi PV, Buskirk E. Effects of eccentric and concentric muscle conditioning on tension and electrical activity of human muscle. *Ergonomics.* 1972;15:417.
31. Lundon P. A review of plyometric training. *Strength Cond J.* 1985;7:69.
32. Pretz, R. Plyometric exercises for overhead-throwing athletes. *Strength Cond J.* 2006;28(1):36.
33. Rach PJ, Grabiner DM, Gregor JR, et al. *Kinesiology and Applied Anatomy*. 7th ed. Philadelphia, PA: Lea & Febiger; 1989.
34. Rowinski M. *The Role of Eccentric Exercise*. Shirley, NY: Biodex Corp, Pro Clinica; 1988.
35. Shiner J, Bishop T, Cosgarea A. Integrating low-intensity plyometrics into strength and conditioning programs. *Strength Cond J.* 2005;27(6):10.
36. Thomas DW. Plyometrics—more than the stretch reflex. *Strength Cond J*. 1988;10:49.
37. Tippett S. Closed chain exercise. *Orthop Phys Ther Clin N Am.* 1992;1:253-267.
38. Tippett S, Voight M. *Functional Progressions for Sport Rehabilitation*. Champaign, IL: Human Kinetics; 1995.
39. Verhoshanski Y. Are depth jumps useful? *Yesis Rev Soviet Phys Educ Sport* 1969;4:74-79.
40. Verhoshanski Y, Chornonson G. Jump exercises in sprint training. *Track Field Q* 1967;9:1909.
41. Verkhoshanski Y. Perspectives in the improvement of speed-strength preparation of jumpers. *Yesis Rev Soviet Phys Educ Sport* 1969;28-29.
42. Voight M, Bradley D. Plyometrics. In: Davies GJ, ed. *A Compendium of Isokinetics in Clinical Usage and Rehabilitation Techniques*. 4th ed. Onalaska, WI: S & S; 1994;225-244.
43. Voight M, Draovitch P. Plyometrics. In: Albert M, ed. *Eccentric Muscle Training in Sports and Orthopedics.* New York, NY: Churchill Livingstone; 1991:45-73.
44. Von Arx F. Power development in the high jump. *Track Techn.* 1984;88:2818-19.
45. Wilk KE, Voight LM, Keirns AM, Gambetta V, Andrews J, Dillman CJ. Stretch-shortening drills for the upper extremities: theory and clinical application. *J Orthop Sports Phys Ther.* 1993;17:225-39.
46. Wilt F. Plyometrics—what it is and how it works. *Athl J.* 1975;55b:76.
47. Witzke K, Snow C. Effects of plyometric jump training on bone mass in adolescent girls. *Med Sci Sports Exerc.* 2000;32:1051-57.
48. Woo SL, Inoue M, McGurk-Burleson E, et al. Treatment of the medial collateral ligament injury: Structure and function of canine knees in response to differing treatment regimens. *Am J Sports Med.* 1987;15(1):22-29.

11

Open- versus Closed-Kinetic-Chain Exercise in Rehabilitation

William E. Prentice

OBJECTIVES

After completion of this chapter, the physical therapist should be able to do the following:

- Differentiate between the concepts of an open kinetic chain and a closed kinetic chain.
- Contrast the advantages and disadvantages of using open- versus closed-kinetic-chain exercise.
- Recognize how closed-kinetic-chain exercises can be used to regain neuromuscular control.
- Analyze the biomechanics of closed-kinetic-chain exercise in the lower extremity.
- Compare how both open- and closed-kinetic-chain exercises should be used in rehabilitation of the lower extremity.
- Identify the various closed-kinetic-chain exercises for the lower extremity.
- Examine the biomechanics of closed-kinetic-chain exercises in the upper extremity.
- Explain how closed-kinetic-chain exercises are used in rehabilitation of the upper extremity.
- Recognize the various types of closed-kinetic-chain exercises for the upper extremity.

Over the years, the concept of *closed-kinetic-chain exercise* has received considerable attention as a useful and effective technique of rehabilitation, particularly for injuries involving the lower extremity.[81] The ankle, knee, and hip joints constitute the kinetic chain for the lower extremity. When the distal segment of the lower extremity is stabilized or fixed, as is the case when the foot is weight bearing on the ground, the kinetic chain is said to be closed. Conversely, in an *open kinetic chain*, the distal segment is mobile and not fixed. Traditionally, rehabilitation strengthening protocols have used open-kinetic-chain exercises such as knee flexion and extension on a knee machine.[71]

Closed-kinetic-chain exercises are used more often in rehabilitation of injuries to the lower extremity, but they are also useful in rehabilitation protocols for certain upper-extremity activities. For the most part, the upper extremity functions in an open kinetic chain with the hand moving freely. But there are a number of activities in which the upper extremity functions in a closed kinetic chain.[80]

Despite the recent popularity of closed-kinetic-chain exercises, it must be stressed that both open- and closed-kinetic-chain exercises have their place in the rehabilitative process.[21] This chapter clarifies the role of both open- and closed-kinetic-chain exercises in that process.

Concept of the Kinetic Chain

The concept of the kinetic chain was first proposed in the 1970s and initially referred to as the *link system* by mechanical engineers.[69] In this link system, pin joints connect a series of overlapping, rigid segments (Figure 11-1). If both ends of this system are connected to an immovable frame, there is no movement of either the proximal or the distal end. In this closed link system, each moving body segment receives forces from, and transfers forces to, adjacent body segments and thus either affects or is affected by the motion of those components.[29] In a closed link system, movement at one joint produces predictable movement at all other joints.[69] In reality, this type of closed link system does not exist in either the upper or the lower extremity. However, when the distal segment in an extremity (that is, the foot or hand) meets resistance or is fixed, muscle recruitment patterns and joint movements are different than when the distal segment moves freely.[69] Thus, 2 systems—a closed system and an open system—have been proposed.

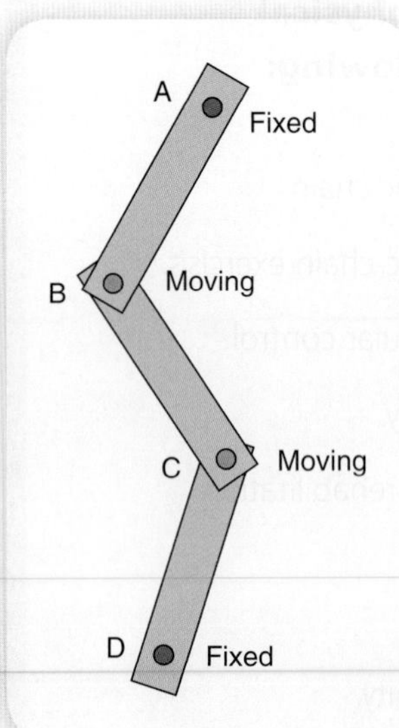

Figure 11-1

If both ends of a link system are fixed, movement at one joint produces predictable movement at all other joints.

Whenever the foot or the hand meets resistance or is fixed, as is the case in a closed kinetic chain, movement of the more proximal segments occurs in a predictable pattern. If the foot or hand moves freely in space as in an open kinetic chain, movements occurring in other segments within the chain are not necessarily predictable.[13]

To a large extent, the term *closed-kinetic-chain exercise* has come to mean "weightbearing exercise." However, although all weightbearing exercises involve some elements of closed-kinetic-chain activities, not all closed-kinetic-chain activities are weight bearing.[67]

Muscle Actions in the Kinetic Chain

Muscle actions that occur during open-kinetic-chain activities are usually reversed during closed-kinetic-chain activities. In open-kinetic-chain exercise, the origin is fixed and muscle contraction produces movement at the insertion. In closed-kinetic-chain exercise, the insertion is fixed and the muscle acts to move the origin. Although this may be important biomechanically, physiologically the muscle can lengthen, shorten, or remain the same length, and thus it makes little difference whether the origin or insertion is moving in terms of the way the muscle contracts.

Concurrent Shift in a Kinetic Chain

The concept of the *concurrent shift* applies to biarticular muscles that have distinctive muscle actions within the kinetic chain during weightbearing activities.[39] For example, in a closed kinetic chain simultaneous hip and knee extension occur when a person stands from a seated position. To produce this movement, the rectus femoris shortens across the knee while it lengthens across the hip. Conversely, the hamstrings shorten across the hip and simultaneously lengthen across the knee. The resulting concentric and eccentric contractions at opposite ends of the muscle produce the concurrent shift. This type of contraction occurs during functional activities including walking, stair climbing, and jumping and cannot be reproduced by isolated open-kinetic-chain knee flexion and extension exercises.[39]

The concepts of the reversibility of muscle actions and the concurrent shift are hallmarks of closed-kinetic-chain exercises.[67]

Advantages and Disadvantages of Open- versus Closed-Kinetic-Chain Exercises

Open- and closed-kinetic-chain exercises offer distinct advantages and disadvantages in the rehabilitation process. The choice to use one or the other depends on the desired treatment goal. Characteristics of closed-kinetic-chain exercises include increased joint compressive forces, increased joint congruency (and thus stability) decreased shear forces, decreased acceleration forces, large resistance forces, stimulation of proprioceptors, and enhanced dynamic stability—all of which are associated with weight bearing. Characteristics of open-kinetic-chain exercises include increased acceleration forces, decreased resistance forces, increased distraction and rotational forces, increased deformation of joint and muscle mechanoreceptors, concentric acceleration and eccentric deceleration forces, and promotion of functional activity. These are typical of non-weightbearing activities.[46]

From a biomechanical perspective, it has been suggested that closed-kinetic-chain exercises are safer and produce stresses and forces that are potentially less of a threat to healing structures than open-kinetic-chain exercises.[62] Coactivation or cocontraction of agonist and antagonist muscles must occur during normal movements to provide joint stabilization. Cocontraction, which occurs during closed-kinetic-chain exercise, decreases the shear forces acting on the joint, thus protecting healing soft-tissue structures that might otherwise be damaged by open-chain exercises.[29] Additionally, weightbearing activity increases joint compressive forces, further enhancing joint stability.

It has also been suggested that closed-kinetic-chain exercises, particularly those involving the lower extremity, tend to be more functional than open-kinetic-chain exercises because they involve weightbearing activities.[79] The majority of activities performed in daily living, such as walking, climbing, and rising to a standing position, as well as in most sport activities, involve a closed-kinetic-chain system. Because the foot is usually in contact with the ground, activities that make use of this closed system are said to be more functional. With the exception of a kicking movement, there is no question that closed-kinetic-chain exercises are more activity specific, involving exercise that more closely approximates the desired activity. For example, knee extensor muscle strength in a closed kinetic chain is more closely related to jumping ability than knee extensor strength in a closed kinetic chain.[8] In a clinical setting, specificity of training must be emphasized to maximize carry-over to functional activities.[67]

With open-kinetic-chain exercises, motion is usually isolated to a single joint. Open-kinetic-chain activities may include exercises to improve strength or range of motion.[34] They may be applied to a single joint manually, as in proprioceptive neuromuscular facilitation or joint mobilization techniques, or through some external resistance using an exercise machine. Isolation-type exercises typically use a contraction of a specific muscle or group of muscles that produces usually single plane and occasionally multiplanar movement.[32] Isokinetic exercise and testing is usually done in an open kinetic chain and can provide important information relative to the torque production capability of that isolated joint.[4]

When there is some dysfunction associated with injury, the predictable pattern of movement that occurs during closed-kinetic-chain activity might not be possible because of pain, swelling, muscle weakness, or limited range of motion. Thus, movement compensations result that interfere with normal motion and muscle activity. If only closed-kinetic-chain exercise is used, the joints proximal or distal to the injury might not show an existing deficit. Without using open-kinetic-chain exercises that isolate specific joint movements, the deficit might go uncorrected, thus interfering with total rehabilitation.[19] The therapist should use the most appropriate open- or closed-kinetic-chain exercise for the given situation.

Closed-kinetic-chain exercises use varying combinations of isometric, concentric, and eccentric contractions that must occur simultaneously in different muscle groups, creating multiplanar motion at each of the joints within the kinetic chain. Closed-kinetic-chain activities require synchronicity of more complex agonist and antagonist muscle actions.[27]

Clinical Pearl

An exercise bike is a good tool when rehabilitating lower-extremity injuries. The patient can work through a full range of motion without bearing weight. The seat height can be adjusted to target a specific range of motion. And most muscles of the leg are utilized. Most bikes have an option of upper-body activity as well. A stair-climber or elliptical machine provides weightbearing exercise that is nonimpact. Later in closed-chain progression, lateral step-ups can be used for neuromuscular control and increased quadriceps firing.

Using Closed-Kinetic-Chain Exercises to Regain Neuromuscular Control

Chapter 9 stressed that proprioception, joint position sense, and kinesthesia are critical to the neuromuscular control of body segments within the kinetic chain. To perform a motor skill, muscular forces, occurring at the correct moment and magnitude, interact to move body parts in a coordinated manner.[56] Coordinated movement is controlled by the central nervous system that integrates input from joint and muscle mechanoreceptors acting within the kinetic chain. Smooth coordinated movement requires constant integration of receptor, feedback, and control center information.[56]

In the lower extremity, a functional weightbearing activity requires muscles and joints to work in synchrony and in synergy with one another. For example, taking a single step requires concentric, eccentric, and isometric muscle contractions to produce supination and pronation in the foot; ankle dorsiflexion and plantarflexion; knee flexion, extension, and rotation; and hip flexion, extension, and rotation. Lack of normal motion secondary to injury in one joint will affect the way another joint or segment moves.[56]

To perform this single step in a coordinated manner, all of the joints and muscles must work together. Thus, exercises that act to integrate, rather than isolate, all of these functioning elements would seem to be the most appropriate. Closed-kinetic-chain exercises, which recruit foot, ankle, knee, and hip muscles in a manner that reproduces normal loading and movement forces in all of the joints within the kinetic chain, are similar to functional mechanics and would appear to be most useful.[56]

Quite often, open-kinetic-chain exercises are used primarily to develop muscular strength while little attention is given to the importance of including exercises that reestablish proprioception and joint position sense.[1] Closed-kinetic-chain activities facilitate the integration of proprioceptive feedback coming from Pacinian corpuscles, Ruffini endings, Golgi-Mazzoni corpuscles, Golgi-tendon organs, and Golgi-ligament endings through the functional use of multijoint and multiplanar movements.[13]

Biomechanics of Open- versus Closed-Kinetic-Chain Activities in the Lower Extremity

Open- and closed-kinetic-chain exercises have different biomechanical effects on the joints of the lower extremity.[18] Walking along with the ability to change direction requires coordinated joint motion and a complex series of well-timed muscle activations. Biomechanically, shock absorption, foot flexibility, foot stabilization, acceleration and deceleration, multiplanar motion, and joint stabilization must occur in each of the joints in the lower extremity for normal function.[33,56] Some understanding of how these biomechanical events occur during both open- and closed-kinetic-chain activities is essential for the therapist.

Foot and Ankle

The foot's function in the support phase of weight bearing during gait is twofold. At heel strike, the foot must act as a shock absorber to the impact or ground reaction forces and then adapt to the uneven surfaces. Subsequently, at push-off, the foot functions as a rigid lever to transmit the explosive force from the lower extremity to the ground.[77]

As the foot becomes weight bearing at heel strike, creating a closed kinetic chain, the subtalar joint moves into a pronated position in which the talus adducts and the plantar flexes while the calcaneus everts. Pronation of the foot unlocks the midtarsal joint and allows the foot to assist in shock absorption. It is important during initial impact to reduce the ground reaction forces and distribute the load evenly on many different anatomical structures throughout the lower-extremity kinetic chain. As pronation occurs at the subtalar joint, there is obligatory internal rotation of the tibia and slight flexion at the knee. The dorsiflexors contract eccentrically to decelerate plantarflexion. In an open kinetic chain, when the foot pronates, the talus is stationary while the foot everts, abducts, and dorsiflexes. The muscles that evert the foot appear to be most active.[77]

The foot changes its function from being a shock absorber to being a rigid lever system as the foot begins to push off the ground. In weight bearing in a closed kinetic chain, supination consists of the talus abducting and dorsiflexing on the calcaneus while the calcaneus inverts on the talus. The tibia externally rotates and produces knee extension. During supination the plantarflexors stabilize the foot, decelerate the tibia, and flex the knee. In an open kinetic chain, supination consists of the calcaneus inverting as the talus adducts and plantarflexes. The foot moves into adduction and plantarflexion, around the stabilized talus.[77] Changes in foot position (ie, pronation or supination) appear to have little or no effect on the electromyogram (EMG) activity of the vastus medialis or the vastus lateralis.[37]

Knee Joint

It is essential for the therapist to understand forces that occur around the knee joint. Palmitier et al proposed a biomechanical model of the lower extremity that quantifies 2 critical

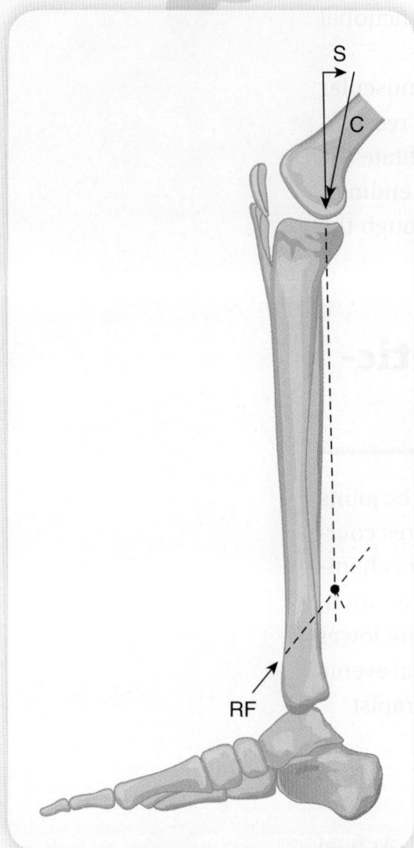

Figure 11-2

Mathematical model showing shear and compressive force vectors. C, compressive; S, shear.

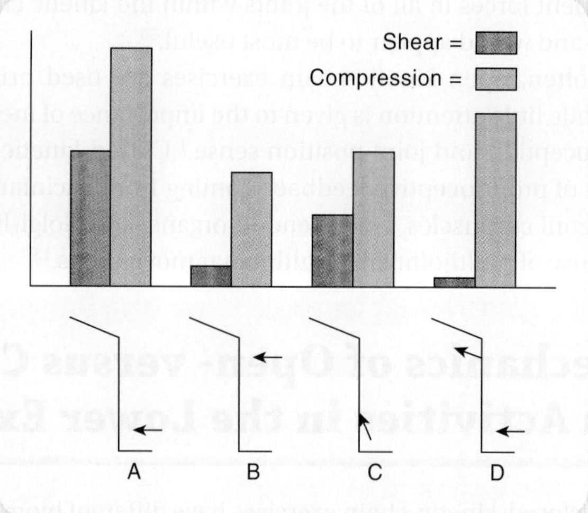

Figure 11-3 Resistive forces applied in different positions alter the magnitude of the shear and compressive forces

A. Resistive force applied distally. **B.** Resistive force applied proximally. **C.** Resistive force applied axially. **D.** Resistive force applied distally with hamstring cocontraction.

forces at the knee joint (Figure 11-2).[53] A *shear force* occurs in a posterior direction that would cause the tibia to translate anteriorly if not checked by soft-tissue constraints, primarily the anterior cruciate ligament (ACL).[14] The second force is a *compressive force* directed along a longitudinal axis of the tibia. Weightbearing exercises increase joint compression, which enhances joint stability.

In an open-kinetic-chain seated knee-joint exercise, as a resistive force is applied to the distal tibia, the shear and compressive forces would be maximized (Figure 11-3*A*). When a resistive force is applied more proximally, shear force is significantly reduced, as is the compressive force (Figure 11-3*B*).[30] If the resistive force is applied in a more axial direction, the shear force is also smaller (Figure 11-3*C*). If a hamstring cocontraction occurs, the shear force is minimized (Figure 11-3*D*).

Closed-kinetic-chain exercises induce hamstring contraction by creating a flexion moment at both the hip and the knee, with the contracting hamstrings stabilizing the hip and the quadriceps stabilizing the knee.[74] A *moment* is the product of force and distance from the axis of rotation. Also referred to as torque, it describes the turning effect produced when a force is exerted on the body that is pivoted about some fixed point (Figure 11-4). Cocontraction of the hamstring muscles helps to counteract the tendency of the quadriceps to cause anterior tibial translation.[73] Cocontraction of the hamstrings is most efficient in reducing shear force when the resistive force is directed in an axial orientation relative to the tibia, as is the case in a weightbearing exercise.[53] Several studies have shown that cocontraction is useful in stabilizing the knee joint and decreasing shear forces.[36,41,54,68]

The tension in the hamstrings can be further enhanced with slight anterior flexion of the trunk.[50] Trunk flexion moves the center of gravity anteriorly, decreasing the knee flexion moment and thus reducing knee shear force and decreasing patellofemoral compression forces.[52] Closed-kinetic-chain exercises try to minimize the flexion moment at the knee while increasing the flexion moment at the hip.

A flexion moment is also created at the ankle when the resistive force is applied to the bottom of the foot. The soleus stabilizes ankle flexion and creates a knee extension moment, which again helps to neutralize anterior shear force (see Figure 11-4). Thus the entire lower-extremity kinetic chain is recruited by applying an axial force at the distal segment.

In an open-kinetic-chain exercise involving seated leg extensions, the resistive force is applied to the distal tibia, creating a flexion moment at the knee only.[70] This negates the effects of a hamstring cocontraction and produces maximal shear force at the knee joint. Shear forces created by isometric open-kinetic-chain knee flexion and extension at 30 and 60 degrees of knee flexion are greater than those with closed-kinetic-chain exercises.[47] Decreased anterior tibial displacement during isometric closed-kinetic-chain knee flexion at 30 degrees when measured by knee arthrometry has also been demonstrated.[78]

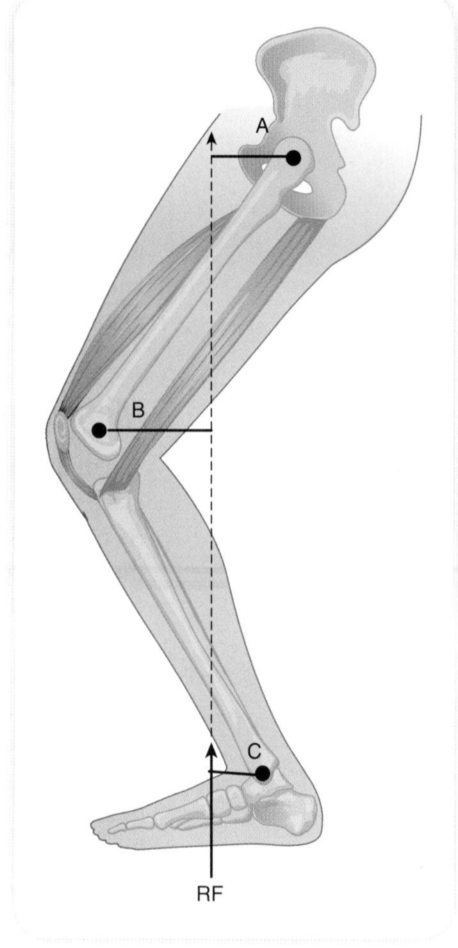

Figure 11-4

Closed-kinetic-chain exercises induce hamstring contraction by creating a flexion moment at (**A**) hip, (**B**) knee, and (**C**) ankle.

Patellofemoral Joint

The effects of open- versus closed-kinetic-chain exercises on the patellofemoral joint must also be considered. In open-kinetic-chain knee extension exercise, the flexion moment increases as the knee extends from 90 degrees of flexion to full extension, increasing tension in the quadriceps and patellar tendon.[6] Thus the patellofemoral joint reaction forces are increased, with peak force occurring at 36 degrees of joint flexion.[25] As the knee moves toward full extension, the patellofemoral contact area decreases, causing increased contact stress per unit area.[7,38]

In closed-kinetic-chain exercise, the flexion moment increases as the knee flexes, once again causing increased quadriceps and patellar tendon tension and thus an increase in patellofemoral joint reaction forces.[61] However, the patella has a much larger surface contact area with the femur, and contact stress is minimized.[7,25,38] Closed-kinetic-chain exercises might be better tolerated in the patellofemoral joint because contact stress is minimized.[6]

Closed-Kinetic-Chain Exercises for Rehabilitation of Lower-Extremity Injuries

For many years, therapists have made use of open-kinetic-chain exercises for lower-extremity strengthening. This practice has been partly a result of design constraints of existing resistive exercise machines. However, the current popularity of closed-kinetic-chain exercises can be attributed primarily to a better understanding of the kinesiology and biomechanics, along with the neuromuscular control factors, involved in rehabilitation of lower-extremity injuries.

For example, the course of rehabilitation after injury to the anterior ACL has changed drastically over the years. (Specific rehabilitation protocols are discussed in detail in Chapter 29.) Technologic advances have created significant improvement in surgical techniques, and this has allowed therapists to change their philosophy of rehabilitation. The current literature provides a great deal of support for accelerated rehabilitation programs that recommend the extensive use of closed-kinetic-chain exercises.[9,15,20,25,48,62,75,82]

Because of the biomechanical and functional advantages of closed-kinetic-chain exercises described earlier, these activities are perhaps best suited to rehabilitation of the ACL.[35] The majority of these studies also indicate that closed-kinetic-chain exercises can be safely incorporated into the rehabilitation protocols very early.[57] Some therapists recommend beginning within the first few days after surgery.

Several different closed-kinetic-chain exercises have gained popularity and have been incorporated into rehabilitation protocols.[43] Among those exercises commonly used are the minisquat, wall slides, lunges, leg press, stair-climbing machines, lateral step-up, terminal knee extension using tubing, and stationary bicycling, slide boards, biomechanical ankle platform system (BAPS) boards, and the Fitter.

Minisquats, Wall Slides, and Lunges

The minisquat (Figure 11-5) or wall slide (Figure 11-6) involves simultaneous hip and knee extension and is performed in a 0- to 40-degree range.[82] As the hip extends, the rectus femoris contracts eccentrically while the hamstrings contract concentrically. Concurrently, as the knee extends, the hamstrings contract eccentrically while the rectus femoris contracts concentrically. Both concentric and eccentric contractions occur simultaneously at either end of both muscles, producing a concurrent shift contraction. This type of contraction is necessary during weightbearing activities.[63] It will be elicited with all closed-kinetic-chain exercises and is impossible with isolation exercises.[69]

These concurrent shift contractions minimize the flexion moment at the knee. The eccentric contraction of the hamstrings helps to neutralize the effects of a concentric quadriceps contraction in producing anterior translation of the tibia.[22] Henning et al found that the half squat produced significantly less anterior shear at the knee than did an open-chain exercise in full extension.[31] A full squat markedly increases the flexion

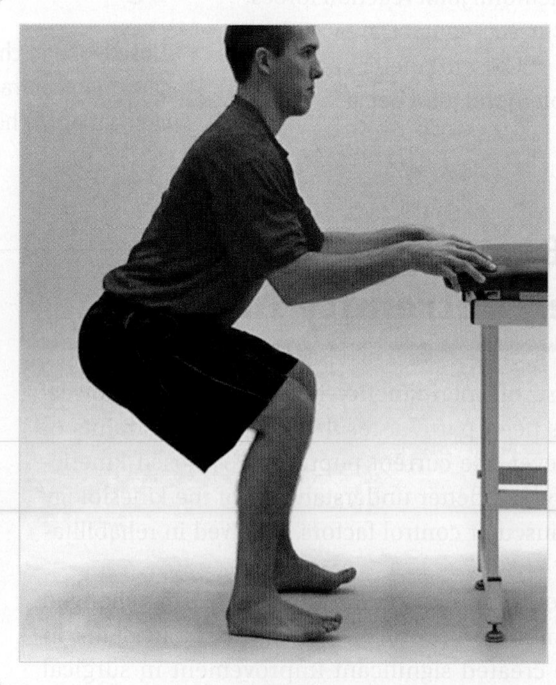

Figure 11-5 Minisquat performed in 0- to 40-degree range

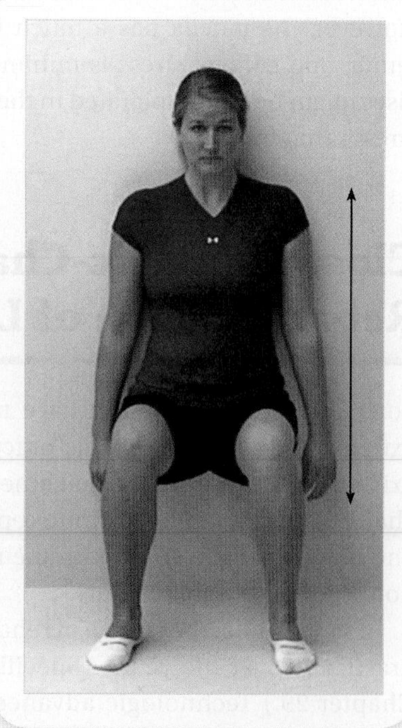

Figure 11-6 Standing wall slide

moment at the knee and thus increases anterior shear of the tibia. As mentioned previously, slightly flexing the trunk anteriorly will also increase the hip flexion moment and decrease the knee moment. It appears that increasing the width of the stance in a wall squat has no effect on EMG activity in the quadriceps.[2] However, moving the feet forward does seem to increase activity in the quadriceps as well as the plantarflexors.[11]

Lunges should be used later in a rehabilitation program to facilitate eccentric strengthening of the quadriceps to act as a decelerator (Figure 11-7).[24,81] Like the minisquat and wall slide, it facilitates cocontraction of the hamstring muscles.[23]

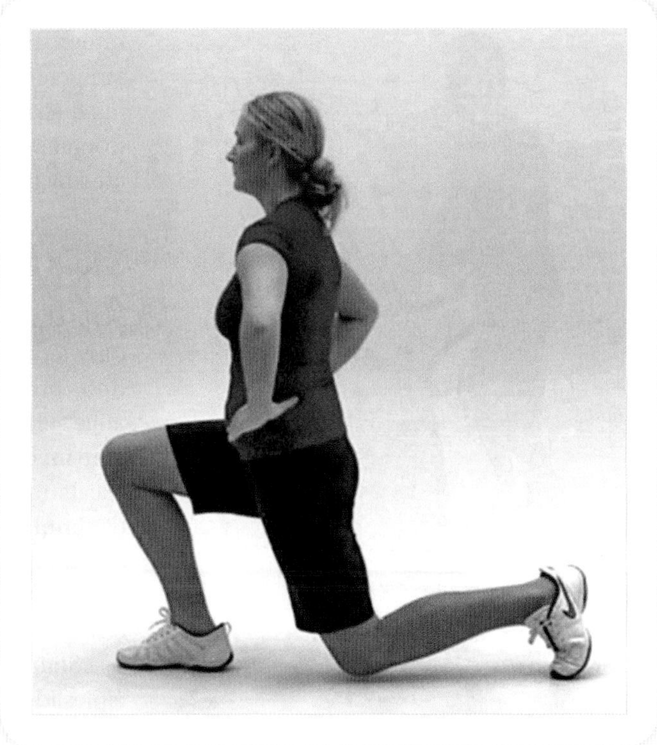

Figure 11-7 Lunges are done to strengthen quadriceps eccentrically

Leg Press

Theoretically, the leg press takes full advantage of the kinetic chain and at the same time provides stability, which decreases strain on the lower back.[45] It also allows exercise with resistance lower than body weight and the capability of exercising each leg independently (Figure 11-8).[53] It has been recommended that leg-press exercises be performed in a 0- to 60-degree range of knee flexion.[82]

It has also been recommended that leg-press machines allow full hip extension to take maximum advantage of the kinetic chain.[5] Full hip extension can only be achieved in a supine position. In this position, full hip and knee flexion and extension can occur, thus reproducing the concurrent shift and ensuring appropriate hamstring recruitment.[53]

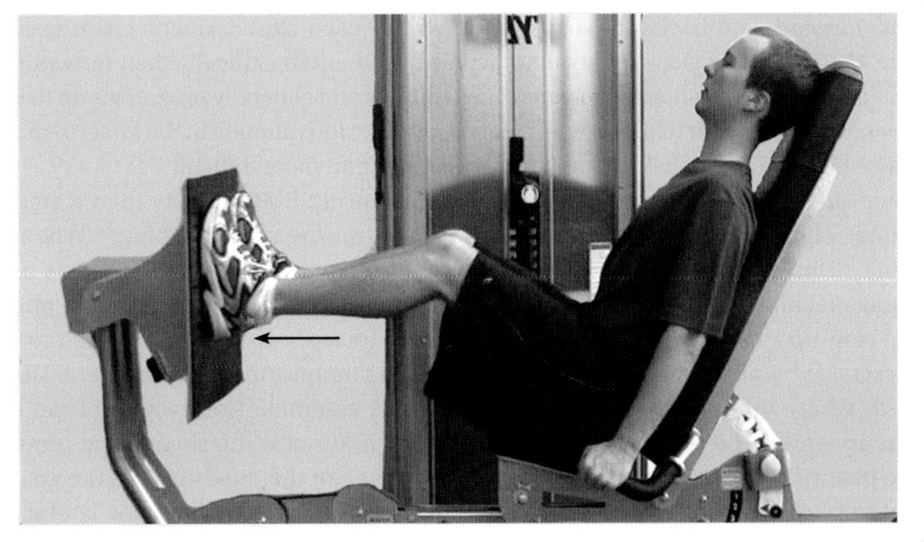

Figure 11-8 Leg-press

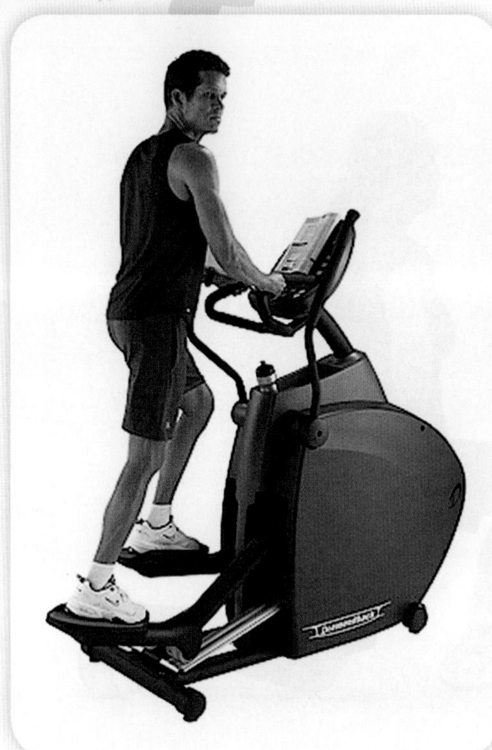

Figure 11-9 Stepping machine

(Courtesy Diamandback Fitness.)

The footplates should also be designed to move in an arc of motion rather than in a straight line. This movement would facilitate hamstring recruitment by increasing the hip flexion moment and decreasing the knee moment. Footplates should be fixed perpendicular to the frontal plane of the hip to maximize the knee extension moment created by the soleus.

Stair Climbing

Stair-climbing machines have gained a great deal of popularity, not only as a closed-kinetic-chain exercise device useful in rehabilitation, but also as a means of improving cardiorespiratory endurance (Figure 11-9). Stair-climbing machines have two basic designs. One involves a series of rotating steps similar to a department store escalator, while the other uses 2 footplates that move up and down to simulate a stepping-type movement. With the latter type of stair climber, also sometimes referred to as a stepping machine, the foot never leaves the footplate, making it a true closed-kinetic-chain exercise device.

Stair climbing involves many of the same biomechanical principles identified with the leg-press exercise.[51] When exercising on the stair climber, the body should be held erect with only slight trunk flexion, thus maximizing hamstring recruitment through concurrent shift contractions while increasing the hip flexion moment and decreasing the knee flexion moment.

Exercise on a stepping machine produces increased EMG activity in the gastrocnemius.[84] Because the gastrocnemius attaches to the posterior aspect of the femoral condyles, increased activity of this muscle could produce a flexion moment of the femur on the tibia. This motion would cause posterior translation of the femur on the tibia, increasing strain on the ACL. Peak firing of the quadriceps might offset the effects of increased EMG activity in the gastronemius.[17]

Step-ups

Lateral, forward, and backward step-ups are widely used closed-kinetic-chain exercises (Figure 11-10). Lateral step-ups seem to be used more often clinically than forward step-ups. Step height can be adjusted to patient capabilities and generally progresses up to about 8 inches. Heights greater than 8 inches create a large flexion moment at the knee, increasing anterior shear force and making hamstring cocontraction more difficult.[12,17]

Step-ups elicit significantly greater mean hamstring EMG activity than a stepping machine, whereas the quadriceps are more active during stair climbing.[85] When performing a step-up, the entire body weight must be raised and lowered, whereas on the stepping machine the center of gravity is maintained at a relatively constant height. The lateral step-up can produce increased muscle and joint shear forces compared to stepping exercise.[17] Caution should be exercised by the therapist in using the lateral step-up in cases where minimizing anterior shear forces is essential. Contraction of the hamstrings appears to be of insufficient magnitude to neutralize the shear force produced by the quadriceps.[12] In situations where strengthening of the quadriceps is the goal, the lateral step-up has been recommended as a beneficial exercise.[86] However, lateral stepping exercises have failed to increase isokinetic strength of the quadriceps muscle. It also appears that concentric quadriceps contractions produce more EMG activity than eccentric contractions in a lateral step-up.[60]

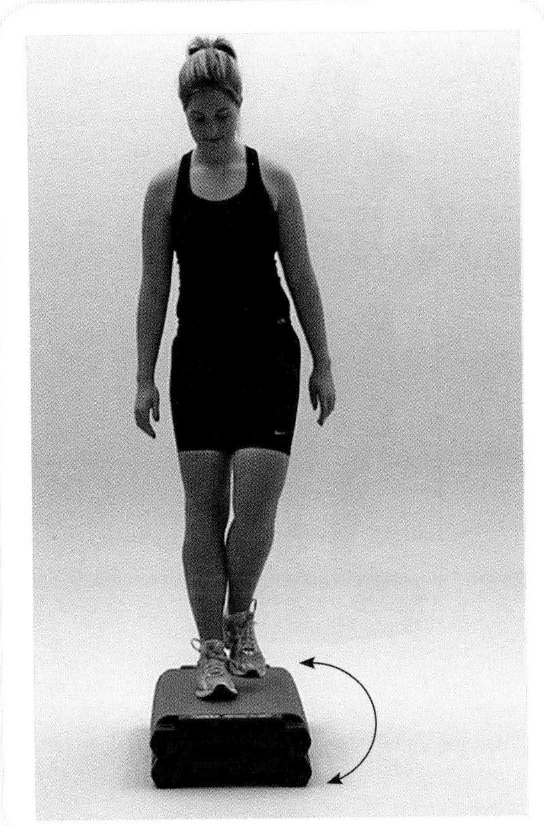

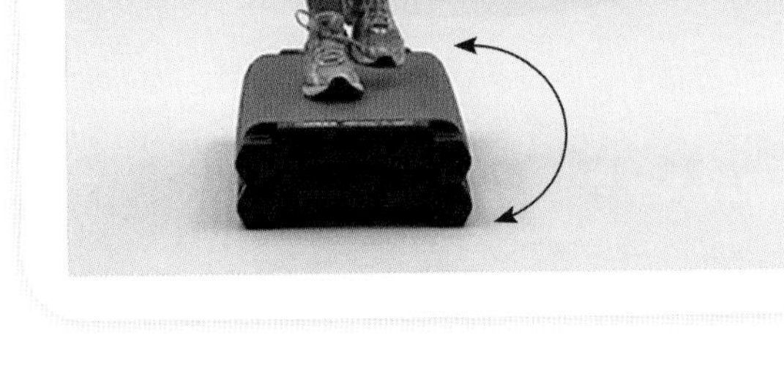

Figure 11-10 **Lateral step-ups**

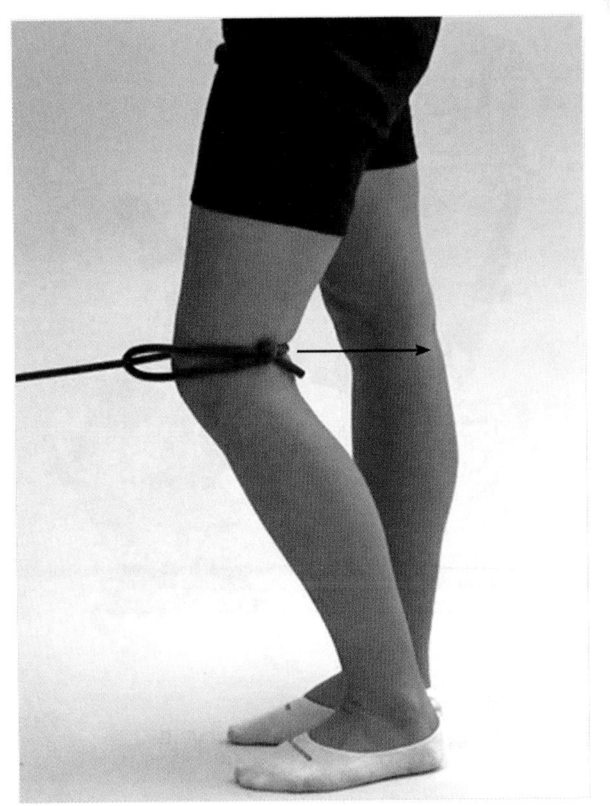

Figure 11-11 **Terminal knee extensions using surgical tubing resistance**

Terminal Knee Extensions Using Surgical Tubing

It has been reported in numerous studies that the greatest amount of anterior tibial translation occurs between 0 and 30 degrees of flexion during open-kinetic-chain exercise.[26,28,40,51,54,55,82] At one time, therapists avoided open-kinetic-chain terminal knee extension after surgery. Unfortunately, this practice led to quadriceps weakness, flexion contracture, and patellofemoral pain.[58]

Closed-kinetic-chain terminal knee extensions using surgical tubing resistance have created a means of safely strengthening terminal knee extension (Figure 11-11).[59] Application of resistance anteriorly at the femur produces anterior shear of the femur, which eliminates any anterior translation of the tibia. This type of exercise performed in the 0- to 30-degree range also minimizes the knee flexion moment, further reducing anterior shear of the tibia. The use of rubber tubing produces an eccentric contraction of the quadriceps when moving into knee flexion. Weightbearing terminal knee extensions with tubing increase the EMG activity in the quadriceps.[85]

Stationary Bicycling

The stationary bicycle can be of significant value as a closed-kinetic-chain exercise device (Figure 11-12).

The advantage of stationary bicycling over other closed-kinetic-chain exercises for rehabilitation is that the amount of the weightbearing force exerted by the injured lower

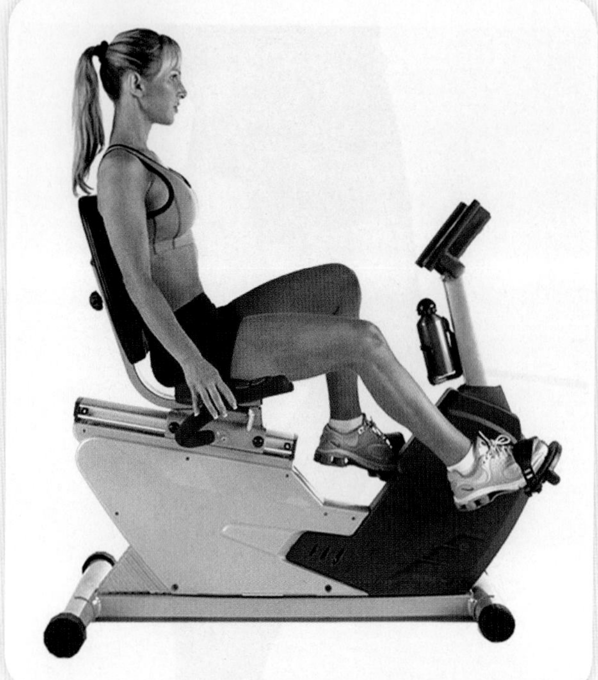

Figure 11-12 Stationary bicycle

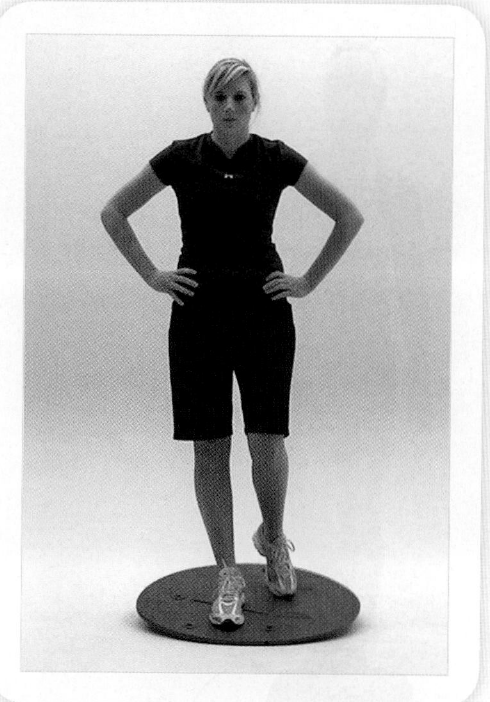

Figure 11-13 BAPS board exercise

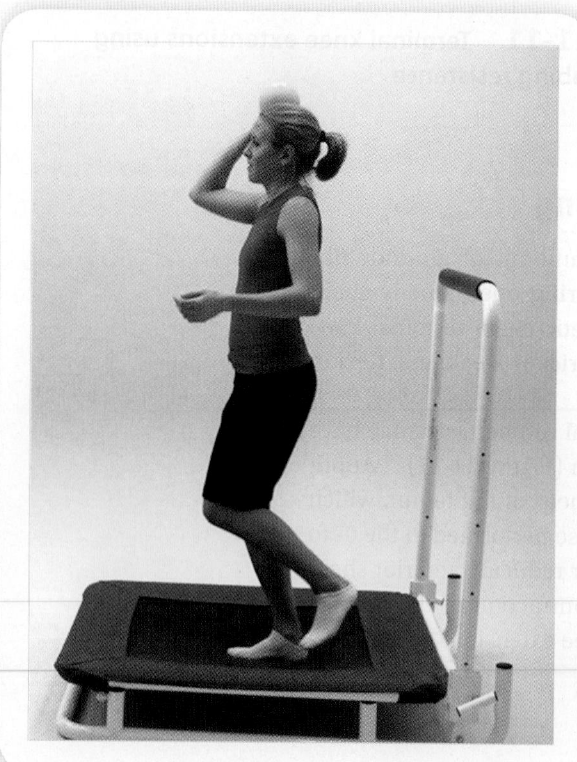

Figure 11-14

Minitramp provides an unstable base of support to which other functional plyometric activities may be added.

extremity can be adapted within patient limitations. The seat height should be carefully adjusted to minimize the knee flexion moment on the downstroke. However, if the stationary bike is being used to regain range of motion in flexion, the seat height should be adjusted to a lower position that uses passive motion of the injured extremity. Toe clips will facilitate hamstring contractions on the upstroke.

BAPS Board and Minitramp

The BAPS board (Figure 11-13) and minitramp (Figure 11-14) both provide an unstable base of support that helps to facilitate reestablishing proprioception and joint position sense in addition to strengthening. Working on the BAPS board allows the therapist to provide stress to the lower extremity in a progressive and controlled manner.[13] It allows the patient to work simultaneously on strengthening and range of motion, while trying to regain neuromuscular control and balance. The minitramp may be used to accomplish the same goals, but it can also be used for more advanced plyometric training.

Slide Boards and Fitter

Shifting the body weight from side to side during a more functional activity on either a slide board (Figure 11-15) or a Fitter (Figure 11-16) helps to reestablish dynamic control

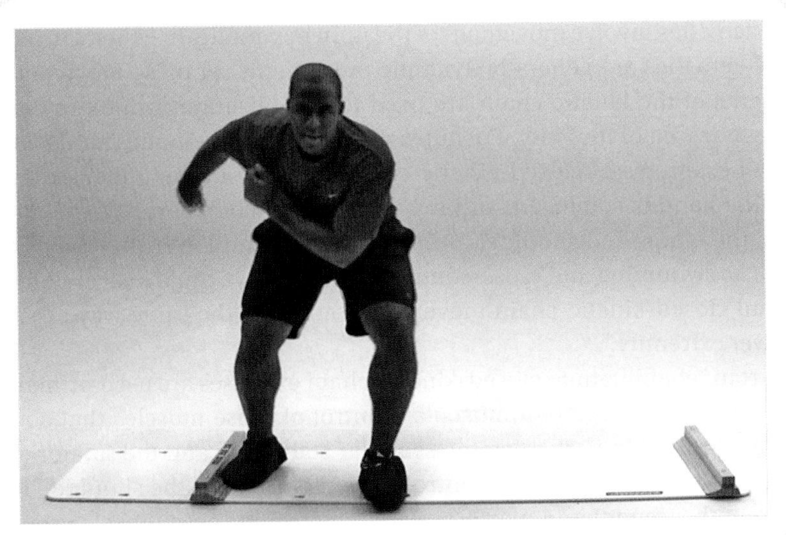

Figure 11-15 Slide board training

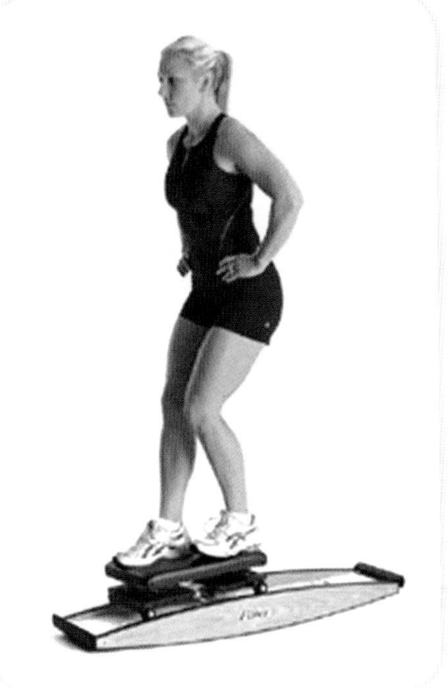

Figure 11-16 The fitter is useful for weight shifting

(Courtesy Fitter International, Inc.)

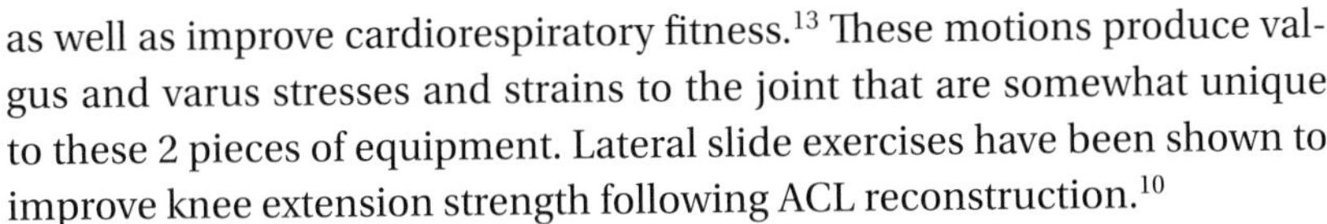

as well as improve cardiorespiratory fitness.[13] These motions produce valgus and varus stresses and strains to the joint that are somewhat unique to these 2 pieces of equipment. Lateral slide exercises have been shown to improve knee extension strength following ACL reconstruction.[10]

Clinical Pearl

Neuromuscular control and balance are crucial to performance. The BAPS board and minitramp provide unstable surfaces on which the patient is required to stand. Such controlled systems are ideal because they challenge proprioception more than the stable ground. The patient who has mastered balance on an apparatus such as the minitramp can be progressed to functional activity such as catching a ball while balancing on an unstable surface.

Clinical Pearl

Unique to the slide board are the valgus and varus strains elicited by the movement. Too much valgus stress while the ligament and musculature are still weak could exacerbate the injury.

Biomechanics of Open- versus Closed-Kinetic-Chain Activities in the Upper Extremity

Although it is true that closed-kinetic-chain exercises are most often used in rehabilitation of lower-extremity injuries, there are many injury situations where closed-kinetic-chain exercises should be incorporated into upper-extremity rehabilitation protocols.[64]

Unlike the lower extremity, the upper extremity is most functional as an open-kinetic-chain system. Most activities involve movement of the upper extremity in which the hand moves freely. These activities are generally dynamic movements. In these movements, the proximal segments of the kinetic chain are used for stabilization, while the distal segments have a high degree of mobility. Pushups, chinning exercises, and handstands in gymnastics are all examples of closed-kinetic-chain activities in the upper extremity. In these cases, the hand is stabilized, and muscular contractions around the more proximal segments, the elbow and shoulder, function to raise and lower the body. Still other activities such as swimming and cross-country skiing involve rapid successions of alternating open-and closed-kinetic-chain movements, much in the same way as running does in the lower extremity.[83]

For the most part in rehabilitation, closed-kinetic-chain exercises are used primarily for strengthening and establishing neuromuscular control of those muscles that act to stabilize the shoulder girdle.[76] In particular, the scapular stabilizers and the rotator cuff muscles function at one time or another to control movements about the shoulder. It is essential to develop both strength and neuromuscular control in these muscle groups, thus allowing them to provide a stable base for more mobile and dynamic movements that occur in the distal segments.[76]

It must also be emphasized that although traditional upper-extremity rehabilitation programs have concentrated on treating and identifying the involved structures, the body does not operate in isolated segments but instead works as a dynamic unit.[49] More recently, rehabilitation programs have integrated closed-kinetic-chain exercises with core stabilization exercises and more functional movement programs.[65] Therapists should recognize the need to address the importance of the legs and trunk as contributors to upper-extremity function and routinely incorporate therapeutic exercises that address the entire kinetic chain.[49]

Clinical Pearl

Closed-chain exercises in which the arm is fixed and the shoulder joint is perturbed cause contraction of the scapular stabilizers and the rotator cuff. This encourages overall stability of the joint.

Shoulder Complex Joint

Closed-kinetic-chain weightbearing activities can be used to both promote and enhance dynamic joint stability. Most often closed-kinetic-chain exercises are used with the hand fixed and thus with no motion occurring. The resistance is then applied either axially or rotationally. These exercises produce both joint compression and approximation, which act to enhance muscular cocontraction about the joint producing dynamic stability.[83]

Two essential force couples must be reestablished around the glenohumeral joint: the anterior deltoid along with the infraspinatus and teres minor in the frontal plane, and the subscapularis counterbalanced by the infraspinatus and teres minor in the transverse plane. These opposing muscles act to stabilize the glenohumeral joint by compressing the humeral head within the glenoid via muscular cocontraction.

The scapular muscles function to dynamically position the glenoid relative to the position of the moving humerus, resulting in a normal scapulohumeral rhythm of movement. However, they must also provide a stable base on which the highly mobile humerus can function. If the scapula is hypermobile, the function of the entire upper extremity will be impaired. Thus force couples between the inferior trapezius counterbalanced by the upper trapezius and levator scapula—and the rhomboids and middle trapezius counterbalanced by the serratus anterior—are critical in maintaining scapular stability. Again, closed-kinetic-chain activities done with the hand fixed should be used to enhance scapular stability.[44]

Elbow

The elbow is a hinged joint that is capable of 145 degrees of flexion from a fully extended position. In some cases of joint hyperelasticity, the joint can hyperextend a few degrees beyond neutral. The elbow consists of the humeroulnar, humeroradial, and radioulnar articulations. The concave radial head articulates with the convex surface of the capitellum of the distal humerus and is connected to the proximal ulna via the annular ligament. The proximal radioulnar joint constitutes the forearm that permits approximately 90 degrees of pronation and 80 degrees of supination when working in conjunction with the elbow joint.

In some activities, the elbow functions in an open kinetic chain. In other activities, the elbow must possess static stability and adequate dynamic strength to be able to transfer force to a hitting implement.[42]

Open- and Closed-Kinetic-Chain Exercises for Rehabilitation of Upper-Extremity Injuries

Most typically, closed-kinetic-chain glenohumeral joint exercises are used during the early phases of a rehabilitation program, particularly in the case of an unstable shoulder to promote cocontraction and muscle recruitment, in addition to preventing shutdown of the rotator cuff secondary to pain and/or inflammation.[3,66] Likewise, closed-kinetic-chain exercise should be used during the late phases of a rehabilitation program to promote muscular endurance of muscles surrounding the glenohumeral and scapulothoracic joints. They may also be used during the later stages of rehabilitation in conjunction with open-kinetic-chain activities to enhance some degree of stability, on which highly dynamic and ballistic motions may be superimposed. At some point during the middle stages of the rehabilitation program, traditional open-kinetic-chain strengthening exercises for the rotator cuff, deltoid, and other glenohumeral and scapular muscles must be incorporated.[34,83]

In the elbow, exercises should also be designed to enhance muscular balance and neuromuscular control of the surrounding agonists and antagonists. Closed-kinetic-chain exercise should be used to improve dynamic stability of the more proximal muscles surrounding the elbow in those activities where the elbow must provide some degree of proximal stability. Open-kinetic-chain exercises for strengthening flexion, extension, pronation, and supination are essential to regain high-velocity dynamic movements of the elbow that are necessary in throwing-type activities.

Clinical Pearl

Open-chain exercises will allow you to apply significant resistance and isolate the muscle. With side-lying exercises it is easy to teach the patient to isolate the muscle. Once that is accomplished, more functional closed-chain exercises can be implemented. Closed-chain exercises will encourage neuromuscular control, as the patient is expected to balance in addition to targeting the particular muscle.

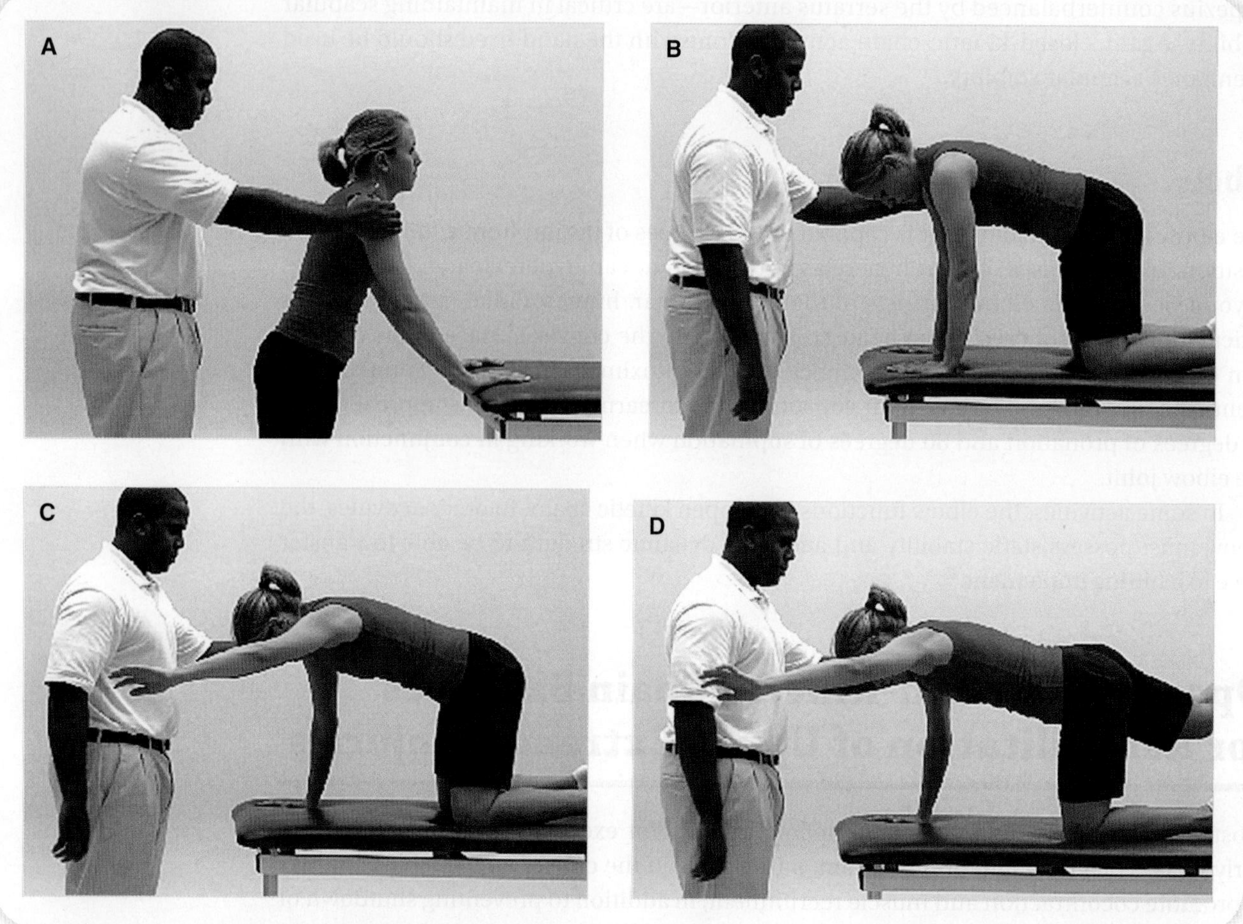

Figure 11-17 Weight shifting

A. Standing. B. Quadruped. C. Tripod. D. Opposite knee and arm.

Weight Shifting

A variety of weight-shifting exercises can be done to assist in facilitating glenohumeral and scapulothoracic dynamic stability through the use of axial compression.[16] Weight shifting can be done in standing, quadruped, tripod, or biped (opposite leg and arm), with weight supported on a stable surface such as the wall or a treatment table (Figure 11-17), or on a movable, unstable surface such as a BAPS board, a wobble board, stability ball, or a Plyoball (Figure 11-18). Shifting may be done side to side, forward and backwards, or on a diagonal. Hand position may be adjusted from a wide base of support to one hand placed on top of the other to increase difficulty. The patient can adjust the amount of weight being supported as tolerated. The therapist can provide manual force of resistance in a random manner to which the patient must rhythmically stabilize and adapt. A diagonal 2 (D2) proprioceptive neuromuscular facilitation pattern may be used in a tripod to force the contralateral support limb to produce a co-contraction and thus stabilization (Figure 11-19).[83] Rhythmic stabilization can also be used regain neuromuscular control of the scapular muscles with the hand in a closed kinetic chain and random pressure applied to the scapular borders (Figure 11-20).

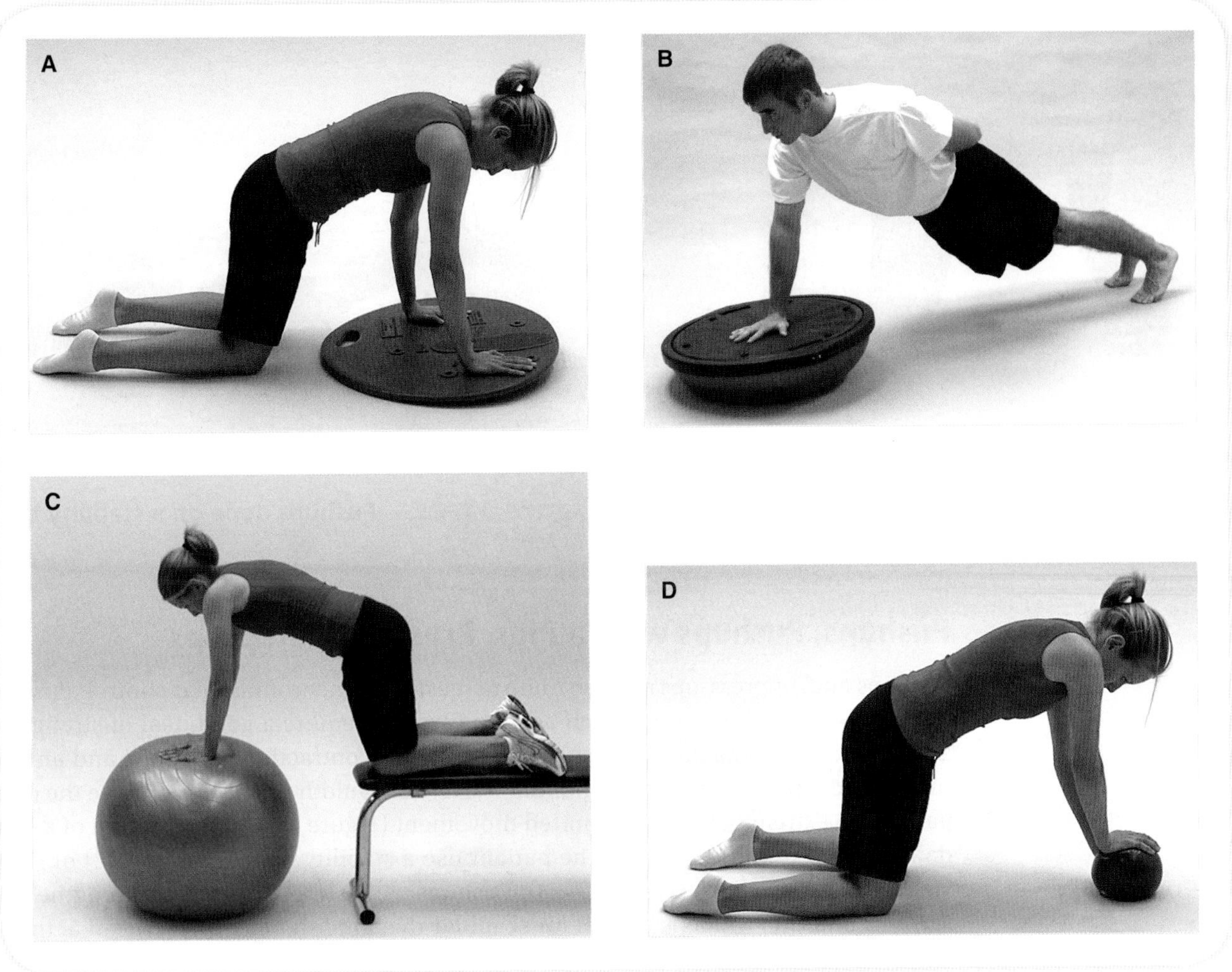

Figure 11-18 **Weight shifting**

A. On a BAPS board. **B**. On a Bosu Balance Trainer. **C**. On a stability ball. **D**. On a Plyoball.

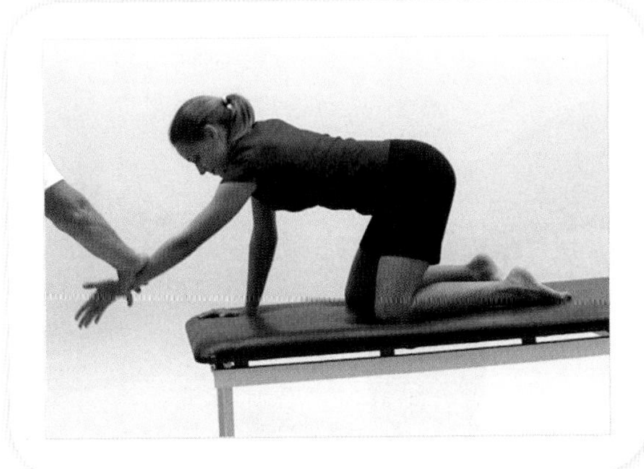

Figure 11-19

D2 proprioceptive neuromuscular facilitation pattern in a tripod to produce stabilization in the contralateral support limb.

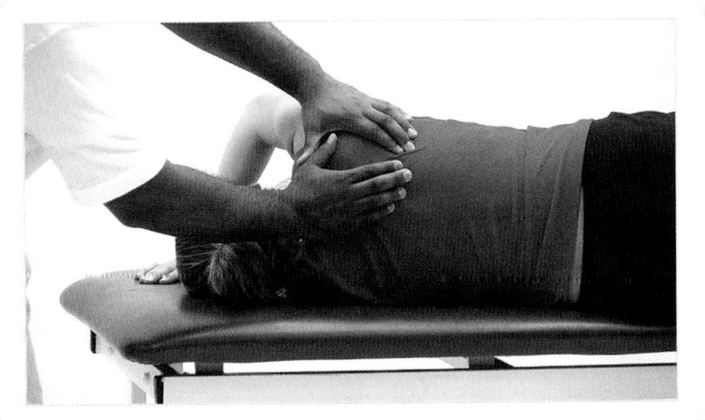

Figure 11-20 **Rhythmic stabilization for the scapular muscles**

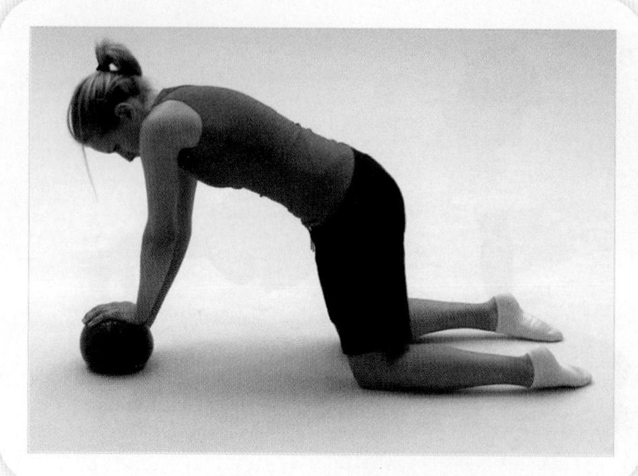

Figure 11-21 Pushups done on a Plyoball

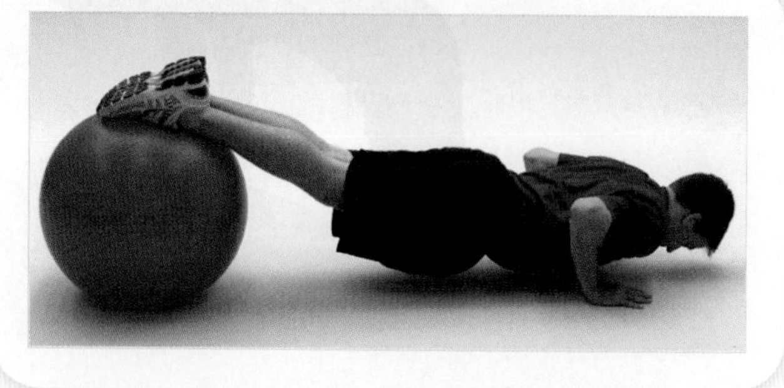

Figure 11-22 Pushups done on a stability ball

Pushups, Pushups with a Plus, Press-ups, Step-ups

Pushups and/or press-ups are also done to reestablish neuromuscular control. Pushups done on an unstable surface such as on a Plyoball require a good deal of strength in addition to providing an axial load that requires cocontraction of agonist and antagonist force couples around the glenohumeral and scapulothoracic joints, while the distal part of the extremity has some limited movement (Figure 11-21). A variation of a standard pushup would be to have the patient use a stability ball (Figure 11-22) or doing wall or corner pushups (Figure 11-23). Pushups with a plus are done to strengthen the serratus anterior, which is critical for scapular dynamic stability in overhead activities (Figure 11-24). Press-ups involve an isometric contraction of the glenohumeral stabilizers (Figure 11-25).

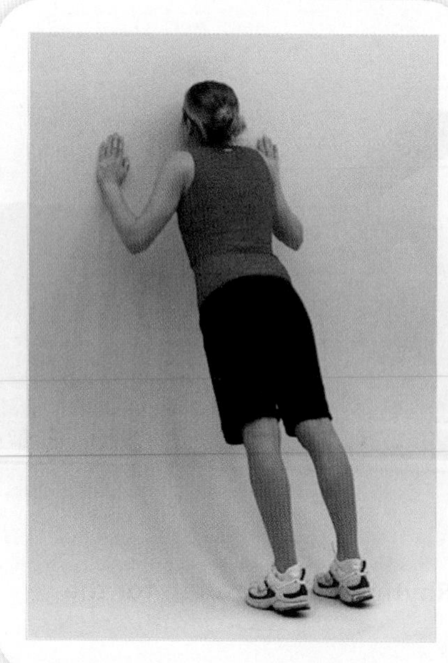

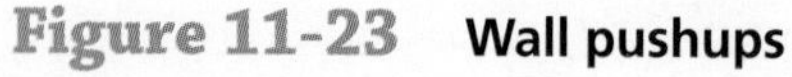

Figure 11-23 Wall pushups

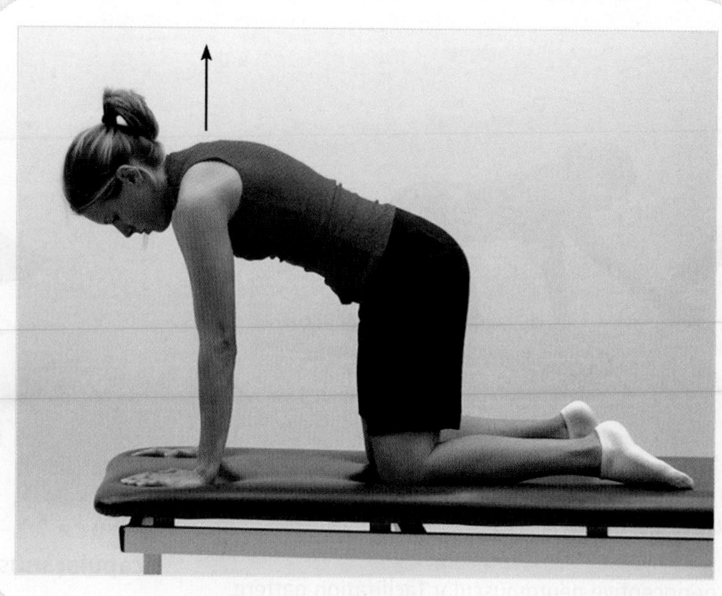

Figure 11-24 Pushups with a plus

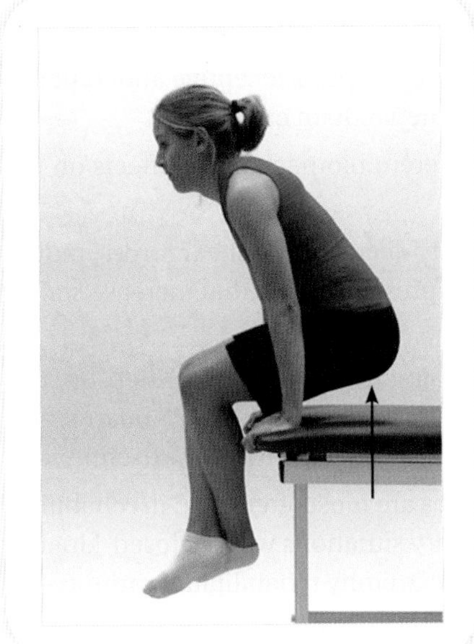

Figure 11-25 Press-ups

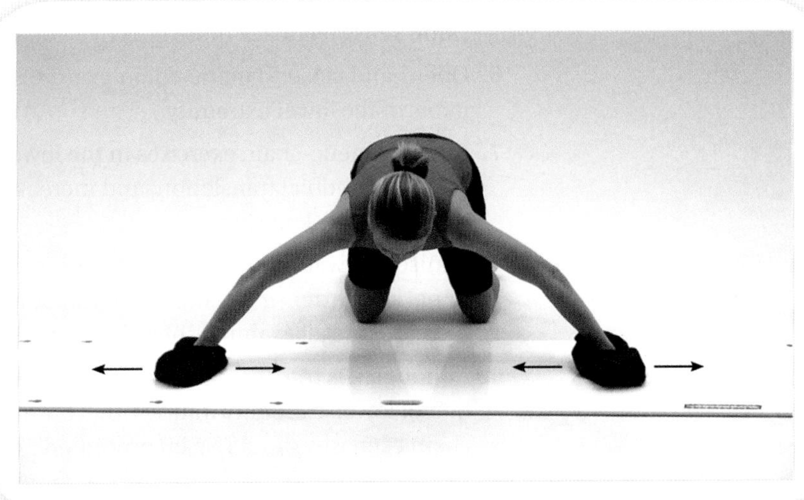

Figure 11-26 Slide board strengthening exercise

> **Clinical Pearl**
>
> Any exercise that perturbs the shoulder complex will cause the scapular stabilizers to fire. Pushups with a plus are done to strengthen the serratus anterior. Pushups performed on a BAPS board or on a Plyoball also promote stability and neuromuscular control of the shoulder complex.

Slide Board

Upper-extremity closed-kinetic-chain exercises performed on a slide board are useful not only for promoting strength and stability but also for improving muscular endurance.[72,83] In a kneeling position, the patient uses a reciprocating motion, sliding the hands forward and backward, side to side, in a "wax on-wax off" circular pattern, or both hands laterally (Figure 11-26). It is also possible to do wall slides in a standing position.

SUMMARY

1. A closed-kinetic-chain exercise is one in which the distal segment of the extremity is fixed or stabilized. In an open kinetic chain, the distal segment is mobile and not fixed.
2. Both open- and closed-kinetic-chain exercises have their place in the rehabilitative process.
3. The concepts of the reversibility of muscle actions and the concurrent shift are hallmarks of closed-kinetic-chain exercises.
4. Open- and closed-kinetic-chain exercises offer distinct advantages and disadvantages in the rehabilitation process. The choice to use one or the other depends on the desired treatment goal.

5. It has been suggested that closed-kinetic-chain exercises are safer because of muscle cocontraction and joint compression; that closed-kinetic-chain exercises tend to be more functional; and that they facilitate the integration of proprioceptive and joint position sense feedback more effectively than open-kinetic-chain exercises.
6. Open- and closed-kinetic-chain exercises have different biomechanical effects on the joints of the lower extremity.
7. Closed-kinetic-chain exercises in the lower extremity decrease the shear forces, reducing anterior tibial translation, and increase the compressive forces that increase stability around the knee joint.
8. Minisquat, wall slides, lunges, leg press, stair-climbing machines, lateral step-up, terminal knee extension using tubing, stationary bicycling, slide boards, BAPS boards, and the Fitter are all examples of closed-kinetic-chain activities for the lower extremity.
9. Although it is true that closed-kinetic-chain exercises are most often used in rehabilitation of lower-extremity injuries, there are many injury situations where closed-kinetic-chain exercises should be incorporated into upper-extremity rehabilitation protocols.
10. Closed-kinetic-chain exercises in the upper extremity are used primarily for strengthening and establishing neuromuscular control of those muscles that act to stabilize the shoulder girdle.
11. Closed-kinetic-chain activities, such as pushups, press-ups, weight shifting, and slide board exercises, are strengthening exercises used primarily for improving shoulder stabilization in the upper extremity.

REFERENCES

1. Andersen S, Terwilliger D, Denegar C. Comparison of open- versus closed-kinetic-chain test positions for measuring joint position sense. *J Sport Rehabil.* 1995;4(3):165-171.
2. Anderson R, Courtney C, Carmeli E. EMG analysis of the vastus medialis/vastus lateralis muscles utilizing the unloading narrow and wide-stance squats. *J Sport Rehabil.* 1998;7(4):236.
3. Andrews J, Dennison J, Wilk K. The significance of closed-chain kinetics in upper extremity injuries from a physician's perspective. *J Sport Rehabil.* 1995;5(1): 64-70.
4. Augustsson J, Esko A, Thornee R, Karlsson J. Weight training of the thigh muscles using closed vs. open kinetic chain exercises: a comparison of performance enhancement. *J Orthop Sports Phys Ther.* 1998;27(1):3.
5. Azegami M, Yanagihashi R. Effects of multi-joint angle changes on EMG activity and force of lower extremity muscles during maximum isometric leg press exercises. *J Phys Ther Sci.* 2007;19(1):65.
6. Bakhtiary A, Fatemi E. Open versus closed kinetic chain exercises for patellar chondromalacia. *Br J Sports Med.* 2008;42(2):99.
7. Baratta R, Solomonow M, Zhou B. Muscular coactivation: the role of the antagonist musculature in maintaining knee stability. *Am J Sports Med.* 1988;16(2):113-122.
8. Blackburn JR, Morrissey CM. The relationship between open and closed kinetic chain strength of the lower limb and jumping performance. *J Orthop Sports Phys Ther.* 1988;27(6):431.
9. Blair D, Willis R. Rapid rehabilitation following anterior cruciate ligament reconstruction. *Athl Train.* 1991;26(1):32-43.
10. Blanpied P, Carroll R, Douglas T, Lyons M. Effectiveness of lateral slide exercise in an anterior cruciate ligament reconstruction rehabilitation home exercise program. *J Orthop Sports Phys Ther.* 2000;30(10):602.
11. Blanpied P. Changes in muscle activation during wall slides and squat-machine exercise. *J Sport Rehabil.* 1999;8(2):123.
12. Brask B, Lueke R, Soderberg G. Electromyographic analysis of selected muscles during the lateral step-up. *Phys Ther.* 1984;64(3):324-329.
13. Bunton E, Pitney W, Kane A. The role of limb torque, muscle action and proprioception during closed-kinetic-chain rehabilitation of the lower extremity. *J Athl Train.* 1993;28(1):10-20.
14. Butler D, Noyes F, Grood E. Ligamentous restraints to anterior-posterior drawer in the human knee: A biomechanical study. *J Bone Joint Surg Am.* 1980;62:259-270.

15. Case J, DePalma B, Zelko R. Knee rehabilitation following anterior cruciate ligament repair/reconstruction: an update. *Athl Train*. 1991;26(1):22-31.
16. Cipriani D, Escamilla R. Open- and closed-chain rehabilitation for the shoulder complex. In: Andrews J, Wilk K, eds. *The Athlete's Shoulder*. New York, NY: Churchill Livingstone; 2008:603-626.
17. Cook T, Zimmerman C, Lux K, et al. EMG comparison of lateral step-up and stepping machine exercise. *J Orthop Sports Phys Ther*. 1992;16(3):108-113.
18. Cordova ML. Considerations in lower extremity closed kinetic chain exercise: a clinical perspective. *Athl Ther Today*. 2001;6(2):46-50.
19. Davies G. The need for critical thinking in rehabilitation. *J Sport Rehabil*. 1995;4(1):1-22.
20. Decarlo MS, Shelbourne KD, McCarroll JR, Rettig AC. A traditional versus accelerated rehabilitation following ACL reconstruction: a one-year follow-up. *J Orthop Sports Phys Ther*. 1992;15(6):309-316.
21. Ellenbecker TS, Davies JG. *Closed Kinetic Chain Exercise: a Comprehensive Guide to Multiple-Joint Exercise*. Champaign, IL: Human Kinetics; 2001.
22. Escamilla RF. Knee biomechanics of the dynamic squat exercise. *Med Sci Sports Exerc*. 2001;33(1):127-141.
23. Escamilla R, Zheng N. Patellofemoral compressive force and stress during the forward and side lunges with and without a stride. *Clin Biomech (Bristol, Avon)*. 2008;23(8):1026.
24. Farrokhi S, Pollard C. Trunk position influences the kinematics, kinetics, and muscle activity of the lead lower extremity during the forward lunge exercise. *J Orthop Sports Phys Ther*. 2008;38(7):403.
25. Fu F, Woo S, Irrgang J. Current concepts for rehabilitation following anterior cruciate ligament reconstruction. *J Orthop Sports Phys Ther*. 1992;15(6):270-278.
26. Fukubayashi T, Torzilli P, Sherman M. An in-vitro biomechanical evaluation of anterior/posterior motion of the knee: tibial displacement, rotation, and torque. *J Bone Joint Surg Br*. 1982;64:258-264.
27. Grahm V, Gehlsen G, Edwards J. Electromyographic evaluation of closed- and open-kinetic-chain knee rehabilitation exercises. *J Athl Train*. 1993;28(1):23-33.
28. Grood E, Suntag W, Noyes F, et al. Biomechanics of knee extension exercise. *J Bone Joint Surg Am*. 1984;66:725-733.
29. Harter R. Clinical rationale for closed-kinetic-chain activities in functional testing and rehabilitation of ankle pathologies. *J Sport Rehabil*. 1995;5(1):13-24.
30. Heijne A, Fleming B. Strain on the anterior cruciate ligament during closed kinetic chain exercises. *Med Sci Sports Exerc*. 2004;36(6):935-941.
31. Henning S, Lench M, Glick K. An in-vivo strain gauge study of elongation of the anterior cruciate ligament. *Am J Sports Med*. 1985;13:22-26.
32. Herrington L, Al-Sherhi A. Comparison of single and multiple joint quadriceps exercise in anterior knee pain rehabilitation. *J Orthop Sports Phys Ther*. 2007;37(4):155.
33. Herrington L. Knee-joint position sense: the relationship between open and closed kinetic chain tests. *J Sport Rehabil*. 2005;14(4):356.
34. Hillman S. Principles and techniques of open-kinetic-chain rehabilitation: the upper extremity. *J Sport Rehabil*. 1994;3(4):319-330.
35. Hooper DM, Morrissey MC, Drechsler W. Open and closed kinetic chain exercises in the early period after anterior cruciate ligament reconstruction: Improvements in level walking, stair ascent, and stair descent. *Am J Sports Med*. 2001;29(2):167-174.
36. Hopkins JT, Ingersoll CD, Sandrey AM. An electromyographic comparison of 4 closed chain exercises. *J Athl Train*. 1999;34(4):353.
37. Hung YJ, Gross TM. Effect of foot position on electromyographic activity of the vastus medialis oblique and vastus lateralis during lower-extremity weight bearing activities. *J Orthop Sports Phys Ther*. 1999;29(2):93-105.
38. Hungerford D, Barry M. Biomechanics of the patellofemoral joint. *Clin Orthop*. 1979;144:9-15.
39. Irrgang J, Safran M, Fu F. The knee: Ligamentous and meniscal injuries. In: Zachazewski J, McGee D, Quillen W, eds. *Athletic Injuries and Rehabilitation*. Philadelphia, PA: WB Saunders; 1995:623-692.
40. Jurist K, Otis V. Anteroposterior tibiofemoral displacements during isometric extension efforts. The roles of external load and knee flexion angle. *Am J Sports Med*. 1985;13:254-258.
41. Kaland S, Sinkjaer T, Arendt-Neilsen L, et al. Altered timing of hamstring muscle action in anterior cruciate ligament deficient patients. *Am J Sports Med*. 1990;18(3):245-248.
42. Ben Kibler W, Sciascia A. Kinetic chain contributions to elbow function and dysfunction in sports. *Clin Sports Med*. 2004;23(4):545-552.
43. Kleiner D, Drudge T, Ricard M. An electromyographic comparison of popular open- and closed-kinetic-chain knee rehabilitation exercises. *J Athl Train*. 1994;29(2):156-157.
44. Kovaleski JE, Heitman R, Gurchiek L, Tyundle T. Reliability and effects of arm dominance on upper extremity isokinetic force, work, and power using the closed chain rider system. *J Athl Train*. 1990;34(4):358.
45. LaFree J, Mozingo A, Worrell T. Comparison of open-kinetic-chain knee and hip extension to closed-kinetic-chain leg press performance. *J Sport Rehabil*. 1995;3(2):99-107.
46. Lepart S, Henry T. The physiological basis for open- and closed-kinetic-chain rehabilitation for the upper extremity. *J Sport Rehabil*. 1995;5(1):71-87.
47. Lutz G, Stuart M, Franklin H. Rehabilitative techniques for athletes after reconstruction of the anterior cruciate ligament. *Mayo Clin Proc*. 1990;65:1322-1329.

48. Malone T, Garrett W. Commentary and historical perspective of anterior cruciate ligament rehabilitation. *J Orthop Sports Phys Ther.* 1992;15(6):265-269.
49. McMullen J, Uhl TL. A kinetic chain approach for shoulder rehabilitation. *J Athl Train.* 2000;35(3):329.
50. Mesfar W, Shirazi-Adl A. Knee joint biomechanics in open-kinetic-chain flexion exercises. *Clin Biomech (Bristol, Avon).* 2008;23(4):477.
51. Nisell R, Ericson MO, Németh G, Ekholm J. Tibiofemoral joint forces during isokinetic knee extension. *Am J Sports Med.* 1989;17:49-54.
52. Ohkoshi Y, Yasuda K, Kaneda K, Wada T, Yamanaka M. Biomechanical analysis of rehabilitation in the standing position. *Am J Sports Med.* 1991;19(6):605-611.
53. Palmitier RA, An KN, Scott SG, Chao EY. Kinetic-chain exercise in knee rehabilitation. *Sports Med.* 1991;11(6):402-413.
54. Renström P, Arms SW, Stanwyck TS, Johnson RJ, Pope MH. Strain within the anterior cruciate ligament during hamstring and quadriceps activity. *Am J Sports Med.* 1986;14:83-87.
55. Reynolds N, Worrell T, Perrin D. Effect of lateral step-up exercise protocol on quadriceps isokinetic peak torque values and thigh girth. *J Orthop Sports Phys Ther.* 1992;15(3):151-156.
56. Rivera J. Open- versus closed-kinetic-chain rehabilitation of the lower extremity: a functional and biomechanical analysis. *J Sport Rehabil.* 1994;3(2):154-167.
57. Ross MD, Denegar CR, Winzenried AJ. Implementation of open and closed kinetic chain quadriceps strengthening exercises after anterior cruciate ligament reconstruction. *J Strength Cond Res.* 2001;15(4):466-473.
58. Sachs RA, Daniel DM, Stone ML, Garfein RF. Patellofemoral problems after anterior cruciate ligament reconstruction. *Am J Sports Med.* 1989;17:760-765.
59. Schulthies SS, Ricard MD, Alexander KJ, Myrer WJ. An electromyographic investigation of 4 elastic-tubing closed kinetic chain exercises after anterior cruciate ligament reconstruction. *J Athl Train.* 1998;33(4):328-335.
60. Selseth A, Dayton M, Cardova M, Ingersoll C, Merrick M. Quadriceps concentric EMG activity is greater than eccentric EMG activity during the lateral step-up exercise. *J Sport Rehabil.* 2000;9(2):124.
61. Sheehy P, Burdett RC, Irrgang JJ, VanSwearingen J. An electromyographic study of vastus medialis oblique and vastus lateralis activity while ascending and descending stairs. *J Orthop Sports Phys Ther.* 1998;27(6):423-429.
62. Shellbourne D, Nitz P. Accelerated rehabilitation after anterior cruciate ligament reconstruction. *Am J Sports Med.* 1990;18:292-299.
63. Shields, Madhavan S. Neuromuscular control of the knee during a resisted single-limb squat exercise. *Am J Sports Med.* 2005;33(10):1520-1526.
64. Smith D. Incorporating kinetic-chain integration, part 1: concepts of functional shoulder movement. *Athl Ther Today.* 2006;11(4):63.
65. Smith D. Incorporating kinetic-chain integration, part 2: functional shoulder rehabilitation. *Athl Ther Today.* 2006;11(5):63.
66. Smith J, Dahm D, Kotajarvi B. Electromyographic activity in the immobilized shoulder girdle musculature during ipsilateral kinetic chain exercises. *Arch Phys Med Rehabil.* 2007;88(11):1377-1383.
67. Snyder-Mackler L. Scientific rationale and physiological basis for the use of closed-kinetic-chain exercise in the lower extremity. *J Sport Rehabil.* 1995;5(1):2-12.
68. Solomonow M, Baratta R, Zhou BH, et al. The synergistic action of the anterior cruciate ligament and thigh muscles in maintaining joint stability. *Am J Sports Med.* 1987;15:207-213.
69. Steindler A. *Kinesiology of the Human Body Under Normal and Pathological Conditions.* Springfield, IL: Charles C. Thomas; 1977.
70. Stensdotter A, Hodges P, Mellor R. Quadriceps activation in closed and in open kinetic chain exercise. *Med Sci Sports Exerc.* 2003;35(12):2043-2047.
71. Stiene H, Brosky T, Reinking M. A comparison of closed-kinetic-chain and isokinetic joint isolation exercise in patients with patellofemoral dysfunction. *J Orthop Sports Phys Ther.* 1996;24(3):136-141.
72. Stone J, Lueken J, Partin N. Closed-kinetic-chain rehabilitation of the glenohumeral joint. *J Athl Train.* 1993;28(1):34-37.
73. Tagesson S, Öberg B, Good L. A comprehensive rehabilitation program with quadriceps strengthening in closed versus open kinetic chain exercise in patients with anterior cruciate ligament deficiency. *Am J Sports Med.* 2008;36(2):298.
74. Tang SFT, Chen CK, Hsu R, Chou SW, Hong WH, Lew LH. Vastus medialis obliquus and vastus lateralis activity in open and closed kinetic chain exercises in patients with patellofemoral pain syndrome: an electromyographic study. *Arch Phys Med Rehabil.* 2001;82(10):1441-1445.
75. Tovin B, Tovin T, Tovin M. Surgical and biomechanical considerations in rehabilitation of patients with intra-articular ACL reconstructions. *J Orthop Sports Phys Ther.* 1992;15(6):317-322.
76. Ubinger ME, Prentice WE, Guskiewicz MK. Effect of closed kinetic chain training on neuromuscular control in the upper extremity. *J Sport Rehabil.* 1999;8(3):184-194.
77. Valmassey R. *Clinical Biomechanics of the Lower Extremities.* St. Louis, MO: Mosby; 1996.
78. Voight M, Bell S, Rhodes D. Instrumented testing of tibial translation during a positive Lachman's test and selected closed-chain activities in anterior cruciate deficient knees. *J Orthop Sports Phys Ther.* 1992;15:49.
79. Voight M, Cook G. Clinical application of closed-chain exercise. *J Sport Rehabil.* 1995;5(1):25-44.
80. Voight M, Tippett S. *Closed Kinetic Chain.* Paper presented at 41st Annual Clinical Symposium of the National Athletic Trainers Association, Indianapolis, June 12, 1990.

81. Wawrzyniak J, Tracy J, Catizone P. Effect of closed-chain exercise on quadriceps femoris peak torque and functional performance. *J Athl Train.* 1996;31(4): 335-345.
82. Wilk K, Andrew J. Current concepts in the treatment of anterior cruciate ligament disruption. *J Orthop Sports Phys Ther.* 1992;15(6):279-293.
83. Wilk K, Arrigo C, Andrews J. Closed- and open-kinetic-chain exercise for the upper extremity. *J Sport Rehabil.* 1995;5(1):88-102.
84. Willett G, Karst G, Canney E, Gallant D, Wees J. Lower limb EMG activity during selected stepping exercises. *J Sport Rehabil.* 1998;7(2):102.
85. Willett G, Paladino J, Barr K, Korta J, Karst G. Medial and lateral quadriceps muscle activity during weight-bearing knee extension exercise. *J Sport Rehabil.* 1998;7(4):248.
86. Worrell TW, Crisp E, LaRosa C. Electromyographic reliability and analysis of selected lower extremity muscles during lateral step-up conditions. *J Athl Train.* 1998;33(2):156.

12

Proprioceptive Neuromuscular Facilitation Techniques in Rehabilitation

William E. Prentice

OBJECTIVES **After completion of this chapter, the physical therapist should be able to do the following:**

- Explain the neurophysiologic basis of proprioceptive neuromuscular facilitation (PNF) techniques.
- Discuss the rationale for use of PNF techniques.
- Identify the basic principles of using PNF in rehabilitation.
- Demonstrate the various PNF strengthening and stretching techniques.
- Describe PNF patterns for the upper and lower extremity, for the upper and lower trunk, and for the neck.
- Discuss the concept of muscle energy technique and explain how it is similar to PNF.

Proprioceptive neuromuscular facilitation (PNF) is an approach to therapeutic exercise based on the principles of functional human anatomy and neurophysiology.[10] It uses proprioceptive, cutaneous, and auditory input to produce functional improvement in motor output and can be a vital element in the rehabilitation process of many conditions and injuries.

The therapeutic techniques of PNF were first used in the treatment of patients with paralysis and various neuromuscular disorders in the 1950s. Originally the PNF techniques were used for strengthening and enhancing neuromuscular control. Since the early 1970s, the PNF techniques have also been used extensively as a technique for increasing flexibility and range of motion.[8,9,16,17,18,30,34,36,45,54,67,71]

This discussion should guide the therapist in using the principles and techniques of PNF as a component of a rehabilitation program.

Proprioceptive Neuromuscular Facilitation as a Technique for Improving Strength and Enhancing Neuromuscular Control

Original Concepts of Facilitation and Inhibition

Most of the principles underlying modern therapeutic exercise techniques can be attributed to the work of Sherrington,[63] who first defined the concepts of facilitation and inhibition.

According to Sherrington, an impulse traveling down the corticospinal tract or an afferent impulse traveling up from peripheral receptors in the muscle causes an impulse volley that results in the discharge of a limited number of specific motor neurons, as well as the discharge of additional surrounding (anatomically close) motor neurons in the subliminal fringe area. An impulse causing the recruitment and discharge of additional motor neurons within the subliminal fringe is said to be facilitatory. Any stimulus that causes motor neurons to drop out of the discharge zone and away from the subliminal fringe is said to be inhibitory.[40] Facilitation results in increased excitability, and inhibition results in decreased excitability of motor neurons.[75] Thus, the function of weak muscles would be aided by facilitation, and muscle spasticity would be decreased by inhibition.[26]

Sherrington attributed the impulses transmitted from the peripheral stretch receptors via the afferent system as being the strongest influence on the alpha motor neurons.[63] Therefore, the therapist should be able to modify the input from the peripheral receptors and thus influence the excitability of the alpha motor neurons. The discharge of motor neurons can be facilitated by peripheral stimulation, which causes afferent impulses to make contact with excitatory neurons and results in increased muscle tone or strength of voluntary contraction. Motor neurons can also be inhibited by peripheral stimulation, which causes afferent impulses to make contact with inhibitory neurons, resulting in muscle relaxation and allowing for stretching of the muscle.[63] PNF should be used to indicate any technique in which input from peripheral receptors is used to facilitate or inhibit.[26]

Several different approaches to therapeutic exercise based on the principles of facilitation and inhibition have been proposed. Among these are the Bobath method,[5,6] Brunnstrom method,[60] Rood method,[58] and Knott and Voss method,[37] which they called PNF. Although each of these techniques is important and useful, the PNF approach of Knott and Voss probably makes the most explicit use of proprioceptive stimulation.[37]

Rationale for Use

As a positive approach to injury rehabilitation, PNF is aimed at what the patient can do physically within the limitations of the injury. It is perhaps best used to decrease deficiencies in strength, flexibility, and neuromuscular coordination in response to demands that are placed on the neuromuscular system.[39] The emphasis is on selective reeducation of individual motor elements through development of neuromuscular control, joint stability, and coordinated mobility. Each movement is learned and then reinforced through repetition in an appropriately demanding and intense rehabilitative program.[59]

The body tends to respond to the demands placed on it. The principles of PNF attempt to provide a maximal response for increasing strength and neuromuscular control.[69,70] These principles should be applied with consideration of their appropriateness in achieving a particular goal. It is well accepted that the continued activity during a rehabilitation program is essential for maintaining or improving strength. Therefore, an intense program should offer the greatest potential for recovery.[53]

The PNF approach is holistic, integrating sensory, motor, and psychological aspects of a rehabilitation program. It incorporates reflex activities from the spinal levels and upward, either inhibiting or facilitating them as appropriate.

The brain recognizes only gross joint movement and not individual muscle action. Moreover, the strength of a muscle contraction is directly proportional to the activated motor units. Therefore, to increase the strength of a muscle, the maximum number of motor units must be stimulated to strengthen the remaining muscle fibers.[30,37] This "irradiation," or overflow effect, can occur when the stronger muscle groups help the weaker groups in completing a particular movement. This cooperation leads to the rehabilitation goal of return to optimal function. [4,37] The principles of PNF, as discussed in the next section, should be applied to reach that ultimate goal.

Clinical Pearl

PNF is used to strengthen gross motor patterns instead of specific muscle actions.

Basic Principles of Proprioceptive Neuromuscular Facilitation

Margret Knott, in her text on PNF,[37] emphasized the importance of the principles rather than specific techniques in a rehabilitation program. These principles are the basis of PNF that must be superimposed on any specific technique. The principles of PNF are based on sound neurophysiologic and kinesiologic principles and clinical experience.[59] Application of the following principles can help promote a desired response in the patient being treated.

1. The patient must be taught the PNF patterns regarding the sequential movements from starting position to terminal position. The therapist has to keep instructions brief and simple. It is sometimes helpful for the therapist to passively move the patient through the desired movement pattern to demonstrate precisely what is to be done. The patterns should be used along with the techniques to increase the effects of the treatment.
2. When learning the patterns, the patient is often helped by looking at the moving limb. This visual stimulus offers the patient feedback for directional and positional control.
3. Verbal cues are used to coordinate voluntary effort with reflex responses. Commands should be firm and simple. Commands most commonly used with PNF techniques are "push" and "pull," which ask for an isotonic contraction; "hold," which asks for an isometric or stabilizing contraction; and "relax."
4. Manual contact with appropriate pressure is essential for influencing direction of motion and facilitating a maximal response because reflex responses are greatly

affected by pressure receptors. Manual contact should be firm and confident to give the patient a feeling of security. The manner in which the therapist touches the patient influences their confidence as well as the appropriateness of the motor response or relaxation.[59] A movement response may be facilitated by the hand over the muscle being contracted to facilitate a movement or a stabilizing contraction.

5. Proper mechanics and body positioning of the therapist are essential in applying pressure and resistance. The therapist should stand in a position that is in line with the direction of movement in the diagonal movement pattern. The knees should be bent and close to the patient such that the direction of resistance can easily be applied or altered appropriately throughout the range.
6. The amount of resistance given should facilitate a maximal response that allows smooth, coordinated motion. The appropriate resistance depends to a large extent on the capabilities of the patient. It may also change at different points throughout the range of motion. Maximal resistance may be applied with techniques that use isometric contractions to restrict motion to a specific point; it may also be used in isotonic contractions throughout a full range of movement.
7. Rotational movement is a critical component in all of the PNF patterns because maximal contraction is impossible without it.
8. Normal timing is the sequence of muscle contraction that occurs in any normal motor activity resulting in coordinated movement.[37] The distal movements of the patterns should occur first. The distal movement components should be completed no later than halfway through the total PNF pattern. To accomplish this, appropriate verbal commands should be timed with manual commands. Normal timing may be used with maximal resistance or without resistance from the therapist.
9. Timing for emphasis is used primarily with isotonic contractions. This principle superimposes maximal resistance, at specific points in the range, upon the patterns of facilitation, allowing overflow or irradiation to the weaker components of a movement pattern. The stronger components are emphasized to facilitate the weaker components of a movement pattern.
10. Specific joints may be facilitated by using traction or approximation. Traction spreads apart the joint articulations, and approximation presses them together. Both techniques stimulate the joint proprioceptors. Traction increases the muscular response, promotes movement, assists isotonic contractions, and is used with most flexion antigravity movements. Traction must be maintained throughout the pattern. Approximation increases the muscular response, promotes stability, assists isometric contractions, and is used most with extension (gravity-assisted) movements. Approximation may be quick or gradual and repeated during a pattern.
11. Giving a quick stretch to the muscle before muscle contraction facilitates a muscle to respond with greater force through the mechanisms of the stretch reflex. It is most effective if all the components of a movement are stretched simultaneously. However, this quick stretch can be contraindicated in many orthopedic conditions because the extensibility limits of a damaged musculotendinous unit or joint structure might be exceeded, exacerbating the injury.

Basic Strengthening Techniques

Each of the principles described in the previous section should be applied to the specific techniques of PNF. These techniques may be used in a rehabilitation program to strengthen or facilitate a particular agonistic muscle group.[29,43,44] The choice of a specific technique depends on the deficits of a particular patient.[56] Specific techniques or combinations of techniques should be selected on the basis of the patient's problem.[3]

Clinical Pearl

The rhythmic initiation technique promotes strength by first introducing the movement pattern passively. The patient will slowly progress to active assistive and then resistive exercises through the movement pattern.

The following techniques are most appropriately used for the development of muscular strength and endurance, as well as for reestablishing neuromuscular control.

Rhythmic Initiation

The rhythmic initiation technique involves a progression of initial passive, then active-assistive, followed by active movement against resistance through the agonist pattern. Movement is slow, goes through the available range of motion, and avoids activation of a quick stretch. It is used for patients who are unable to initiate movement and who have a limited range of motion because of increased tone. It may also be used to teach the patient a movement pattern.

Repeated Contraction

Repeated contraction is useful when a patient has weakness either at a specific point or throughout the entire range. It is used to correct imbalances that occur within the range by repeating the weakest portion of the total range. The patient moves isotonically against maximal resistance repeatedly until fatigue is evidenced in the weaker components of the motion. When fatigue of the weak components becomes apparent, a stretch at that point in the range should facilitate the weaker muscles and result in a smoother, more coordinated motion. Again, quick stretch may be contraindicated with some musculoskeletal injuries. The amount of resistance to motion given by the therapist should be modified to accommodate the strength of the muscle group. The patient is commanded to push by using the agonist concentrically and eccentrically throughout the range.

Slow Reversal

Slow reversal involves an isotonic contraction of the agonist followed immediately by an isotonic contraction of the antagonist. The initial contraction of the agonist muscle group facilitates the succeeding contraction of the antagonist muscles. The slow-reversal technique can be used for developing active range of motion of the agonists and normal reciprocal timing between the antagonists and agonists, which is critical for normal coordinated motion.[55] The patient should be commanded to push against maximal resistance by using the antagonist and then to pull by using the agonist. The initial agonistic push facilitates the succeeding antagonist contraction.

Slow-Reversal-Hold

Slow-reversal-hold is an isotonic contraction of the agonist followed immediately by an isometric contraction, with a hold command given at the end of each active movement. The direction of the pattern is reversed by using the same sequence of contraction with no relaxation before shifting to the antagonistic pattern. This technique can be especially useful in developing strength at a specific point in the range of motion.

Rhythmic Stabilization

Rhythmic stabilization uses an isometric contraction of the agonist, followed by an isometric contraction of the antagonist to produce cocontraction and stability of the 2 opposing muscle groups. The command given is always "hold," and movement is resisted in each direction. Rhythmic stabilization results in an increase in the holding power to a point where the position cannot be broken. Holding should emphasize cocontraction of agonists and antagonists.

Clinical Pearl

Rhythmic stabilization can be used to facilitate strength and stability at a joint by stimulating cocontraction of the opposing muscles that support the joint. PNF strengthening using the D1 and D2 patterns will encourage control in overhead activities.

Clinical Pearl

The movements required for sport are multiplanar movements. PNF strengthening is more functional and is not limited by the design constraints of an exercise machine. Also, PNF technique allows the therapist to adjust the amount of manual resistance throughout the range of motion according to the patient's capabilities.

Treating Specific Problems with Proprioceptive Neuromuscular Facilitation Techniques

PNF-strengthening techniques can be useful in a variety of different conditions. To some extent the choice of the most effective technique for a given situation is dictated by the state of the existing condition and the capabilities and limitations of the individual patient.[72] There are some advantages to using PNF techniques in general.

Relative to strengthening, the PNF techniques are not encumbered by the design constraints of commercial exercise machines, although some of the newer exercise machines have been designed to accommodate triplanar motion and thus will allow for PNF patterned motion.[9] With the PNF patterns, movement can occur in 3 planes simultaneously, thus more closely resembling a functional movement pattern. The amount of resistance applied by the therapist can be easily adjusted and altered at different points through the range of motion to meet patient capabilities.[38] The therapist can choose to concentrate on the strengthening through the entire range of motion or through a very specific range. Combinations of several strengthening techniques can be used concurrently within the same PNF pattern.[51] Rhythmic initiation is useful in the early stages of rehabilitation when the patient is having difficulty moving actively through a pain-free arc. Passive movement can allow the patient to maintain a full range while using an active contraction to move through the available pain-free range. Slow reversal should be used to help improve muscular endurance. Slow-reversal-hold is used to correct existing weakness at specific points in the range of motion through isometric strengthening.

Rhythmic stabilization is used to achieve stability and neuromuscular control about a joint.[11,21] This technique requires cocontraction of opposing muscle groups and is useful in creating a balance in the existing force couples.

Clinical Pearl

Proper body and hand positioning will maximize the therapist ability to provide sufficient resistance. The therapist should stand in a position that is in line with the direction of movement in the diagonal movement pattern. The knees should be bent and the stance close to the patient, so that the direction and amount of resistance can easily be applied or altered appropriately throughout the range of movement.

Proprioceptive Neuromuscular Facilitation Patterns

The PNF patterns are concerned with gross movement as opposed to specific muscle actions. The techniques identified previously can be superimposed on any of the PNF patterns. The techniques of PNF are composed of both rotational and diagonal exercise patterns that are similar to the motions required in most sports and normal daily activities.

The exercise patterns have 3 component movements: flexion-extension, abduction-adduction, and internal-external rotation. Human movement is patterned and rarely involves straight motion because all muscles are spiral in nature and lie in diagonal directions.

The PNF patterns described by Knott and Voss[37] involve distinct diagonal and rotational movements of the upper extremity, lower extremity, upper trunk, lower trunk, and neck. The exercise pattern is initiated with the muscle groups in the lengthened or stretched position. The muscle group is then contracted, moving the body part through the range of motion to a shortened position.

The upper and lower extremities all have 2 separate patterns of diagonal movement for each part of the body, which are referred to as the diagonal 1 (D1) and diagonal 2 (D2) patterns. These diagonal patterns are subdivided into D1 moving into flexion, D1 moving into extension, D2 moving into flexion, and D2 moving into extension. Figures 12-1 and 12-2 illustrate the PNF patterns for the upper and lower extremities, respectively. The patterns are named according to the proximal pivots at either the shoulder or the hip (for example, the glenohumeral joint or femoroacetabular joint).

Tables 12-1 and 12-2 describe specific movements in the D1 and D2 patterns for the upper extremities. Figures 12-3 through 12-10 show starting and terminal positions for each of the diagonal patterns in the upper extremity.

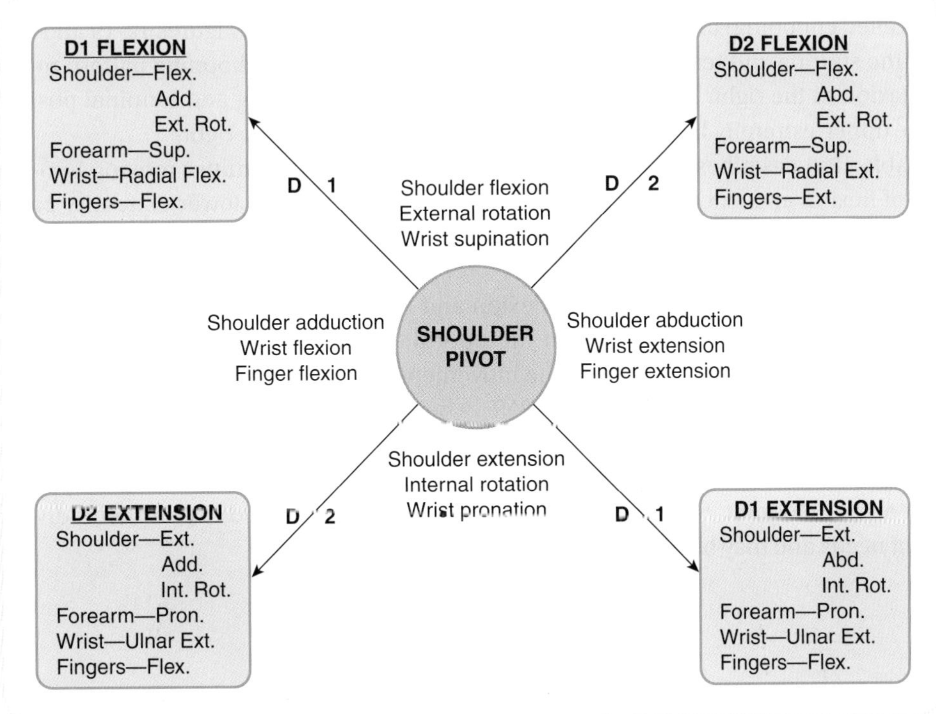

Figure 12-1 PNF patterns of the upper extremity

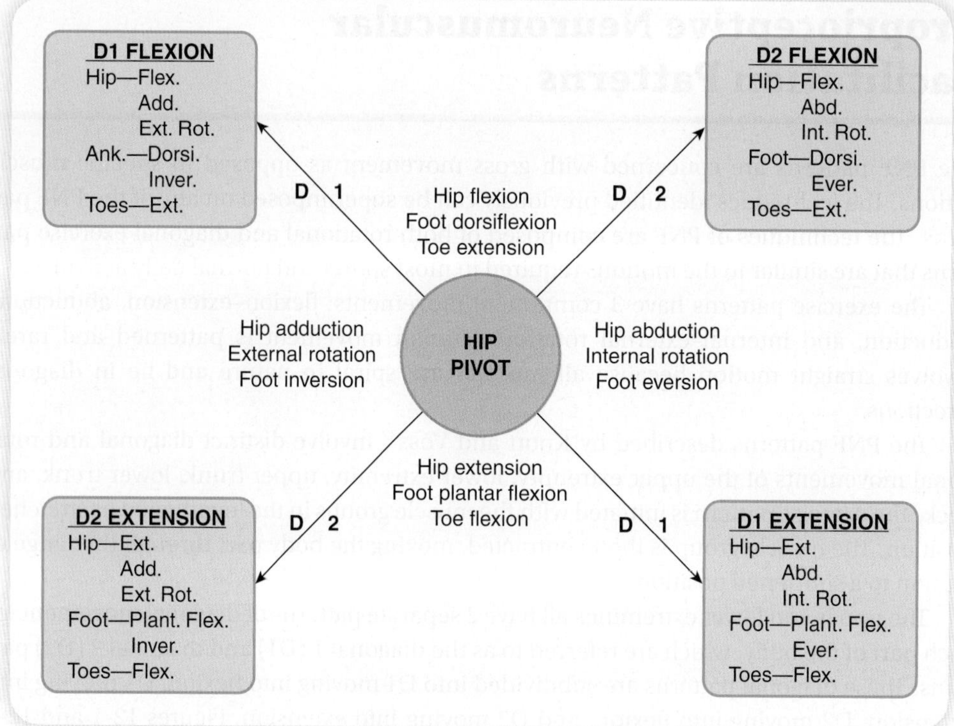

Figure 12-2 PNF patterns of the lower extremity

Tables 12-3 and 12-4 describe specific movements in the D1 and D2 patterns for the lower extremities. Figures 12-11 through 12-18 show the starting and terminal positions for each of the diagonal patterns in the lower extremity.

Table 12-5 describes the rotational movement of the upper trunk moving into extension (also called chopping) and moving into flexion (also called lifting). Figures 12-19 and 12-20 show the starting and terminal positions of the upper-extremity chopping pattern moving into flexion to the right. Figures 12-21 and 12-22 show the starting and terminal positions for the upper-extremity lifting pattern moving into extension to the right.

Table 12-6 describes rotational movement of the lower extremities moving into positions of flexion and extension. Figures 12-23 and 12-24 show the lower-extremity pattern moving into flexion to the left. Figures 12-25 and 12-26 show the lower-extremity pattern moving into extension to the left.

The neck patterns involve simply flexion and rotation to one side (Figures 12-27 and 12-28) with extension and rotation to the opposite side (Figures 12-29 and 12-30). The patient should follow the direction of the movement with their eyes.

The principles and techniques of PNF, when used appropriately with specific patterns, can be an extremely effective tool for rehabilitation of injuries.[65] They can be used to strengthen weak muscles or muscle groups and to improve the neuromuscular control about an injured joint. Specific techniques selected for use should depend on individual patient needs and may be modified accordingly.[14,15]

Table 12-1 D1 Upper-Extremity Movement Patterns

Body Part	Moving into Flexion		Moving into Extension	
	Starting Position (Figure 12-3)	Terminal Position (Figure 12-4)	Starting Position (Figure 12-5)	Terminal Position (Figure 12-6)
Shoulder	Extended Abducted Internally rotated	Flexed Adducted Externally rotated	Flexed Adducted Externally rotated	Extended Adducted Internally rotated
Scapula	Depressed Retracted Downwardly rotated	Flexed Protracted Upwardly rotated	Elevated Protracted Upwardly rotated	Depressed Retracted Downwardly rotated
Forearm	Pronated	Supinated	Supinated	Pronated
Wrist	Ulnar extended	Radially flexed	Radially flexed	Ulnar extended
Finger and thumb	Extended Abducted	Flexed Adducted	Flexed Adducted	Extended Abducted
Hand position for therapist[a]	Left and inside of volar surface of hand Right hand underneath arm in cubital fossa of elbow		Left hand on back of elbow on humerus Right hand on dorsum of hand	
Verbal command	Pull		Push	

[a]For patient's right arm.

Table 12-2 D2 Upper-Extremity Movement Patterns

Body Part	Moving into Flexion		Moving into Extension	
	Starting Position (Figure 12-7)	Terminal Position (Figure 12-8)	Starting Position (Figure 12-9)	Terminal Position (Figure 12-10)
Shoulder	Extended Abducted Internally rotated	Flexed Adducted Externally rotated	Flexed Adducted Externally rotated	Extended Adducted Internally rotated
Scapula	Depressed Retracted Downwardly rotated	Flexed Protracted Upwardly rotated	Elevated Protracted Upwardly rotated	Depressed Retracted Downwardly rotated
Forearm	Pronated	Supinated	Supinated	Pronated
Wrist	Ulnar extended	Radially flexed	Radially flexed	Ulnar extended
Finger and thumb	Flexed Abducted	Extended Adducted	Extended Adducted	Flexed Abducted
Hand position for therapist[a]	Left and on back of humerus Right hand on dorsum of hand		Left hand on volar surface of humerus Right hand on cubital fossa of elbow	
Verbal command	Push		Pull	

[a]For patient's right arm.

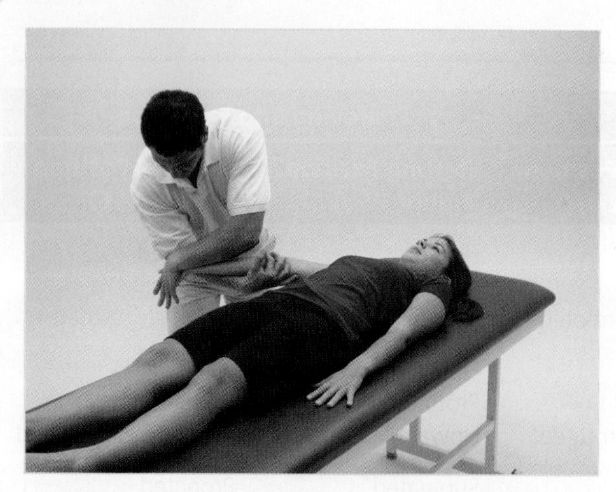

Figure 12-3

D1 upper-extremity movement pattern moving into flexion. Starting position.

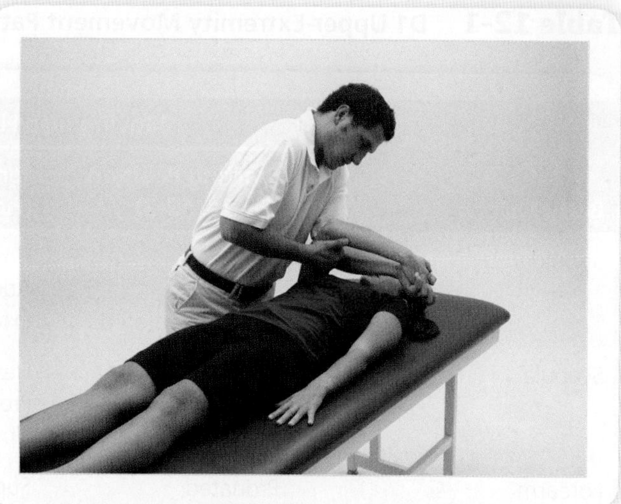

Figure 12-4

D1 upper-extremity movement pattern moving into flexion. Terminal position.

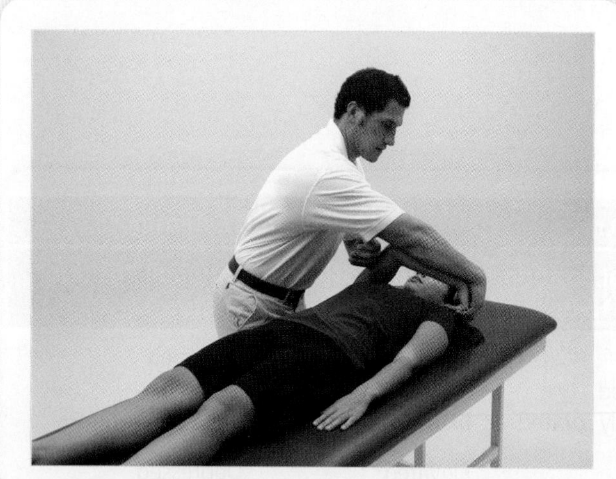

Figure 12-5

D1 upper-extremity movement pattern moving into extension. Starting position.

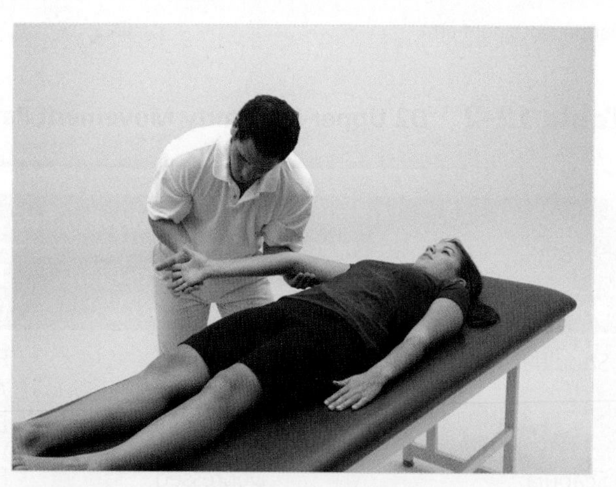

Figure 12-6

D1 upper-extremity movement pattern moving into extension. Terminal position.

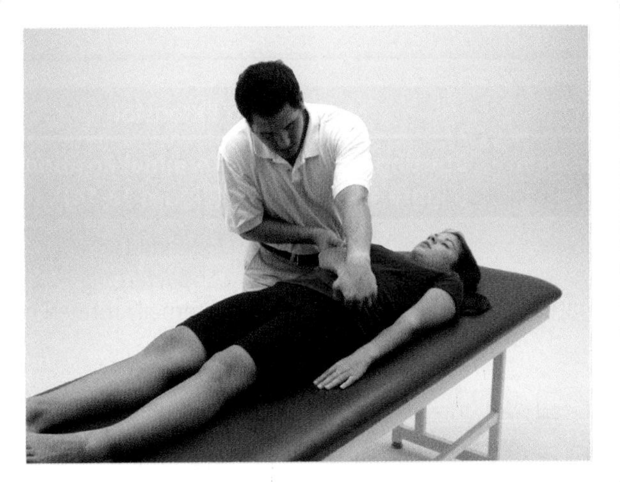

Figure 12-7

D2 upper-extremity movement pattern moving into flexion. Starting position.

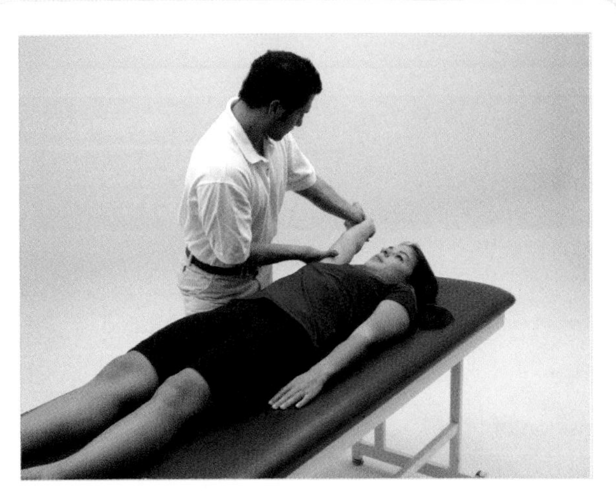

Figure 12-8

D2 upper-extremity movement pattern moving into flexion. Terminal position.

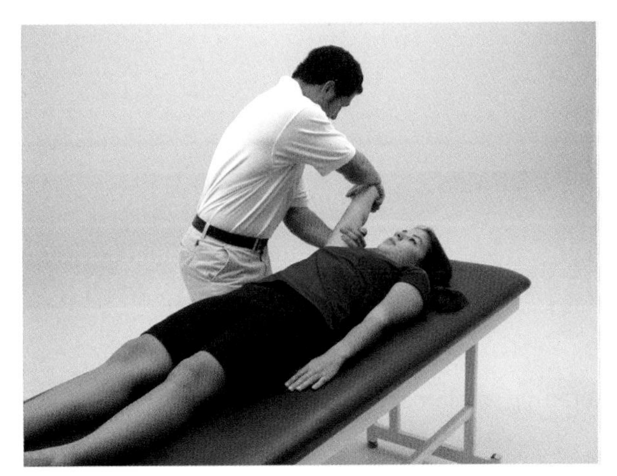

Figure 12-9

D2 upper-extremity movement pattern moving into extension. Starting position.

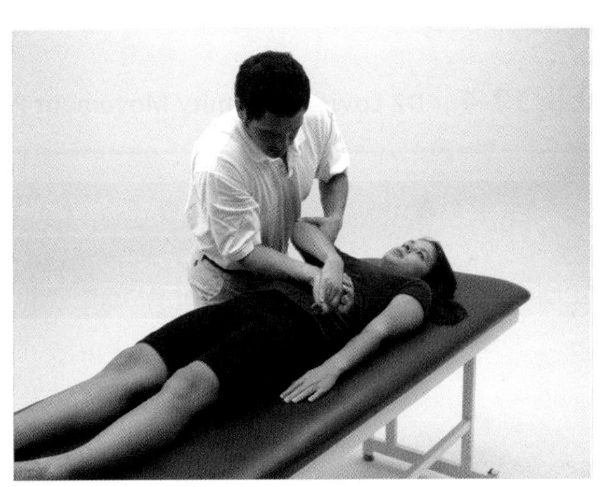

Figure 12-10

D2 upper-extremity movement pattern moving into extension. Terminal position.

Table 12-3 D1 Lower-Extremity Movement Patterns

	Moving into Flexion		Moving into Extension	
Body Part	Starting Position (Figure 12-11)	Terminal Position (Figure 12-12)	Starting Position (Figure 12-13)	Terminal Position (Figure 12-14)
Hip	Extended Abducted Internally rotated	Flexed Adducted Externally rotated	Flexed Adducted Externally rotated	Extended Abducted Internally rotated
Knee	Extended	Flexed	Flexed	Extended
Position of tibia	Externally rotated	Internally rotated	Internally rotated	Externally rotated
Ankle and foot	Plantarflexed Everted	Dorsiflexed Inverted	Dorsiflexed Inverted	Plantarflexed Everted
Toes	Flexed	Extended	Extended	Flexed
Hand position for therapist[a]	Right hand on dorsomedial surface of foot Left hand on anteromedial thigh near patella		Right hand on lateral plantar surface of foot Left hand on posterolateral thigh near popliteal crease	
Verbal command	Pull		Push	

[a]For patient's right leg.

Table 12-4 D2 Lower-Extremity Movement Patterns

	Moving into Flexion		Moving into Extension	
Body Part	Starting Position (Figure 12-15)	Terminal Position (Figure 12-16)	Starting Position (Figure 12-17)	Terminal Position (Figure 12-18)
Hip	Extended Adducted Externally rotated	Flexed Abducted Internally rotated	Flexed Abducted Internally rotated	Extended Adducted Externally rotated
Knee	Extended	Flexed	Flexed	Extended
Position of tibia	Externally rotated	Internally rotated	Internally rotated	Externally rotated
Ankle and foot	Plantarflexed Inverted	Dorsiflexed Everted	Dorsiflexed Everted	Plantarflexed Inverted
Toes	Flexed	Extended	Extended	Flexed
Hand position for therapist[a]	Right hand on dorsolateral surface of foot Left hand on anterolateral thigh near patella		Right hand on medial plantar surface of foot Left hand on posteromedial thigh near popliteal crease	
Verbal command	Pull		Push	

[a]For patient's right leg.

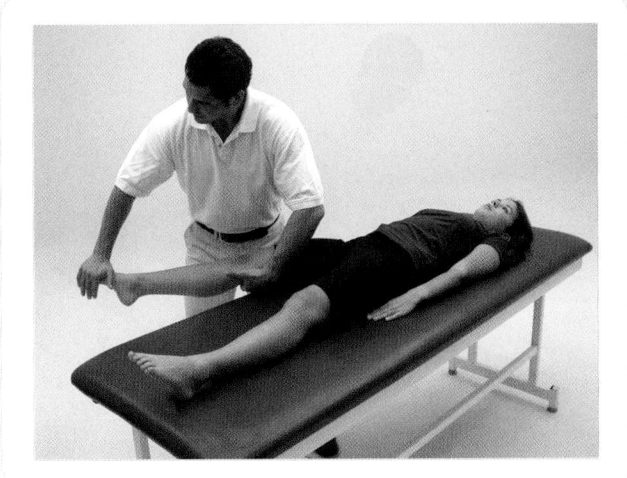

Figure 12-11

D1 lower-extremity movement pattern moving into flexion. Starting position.

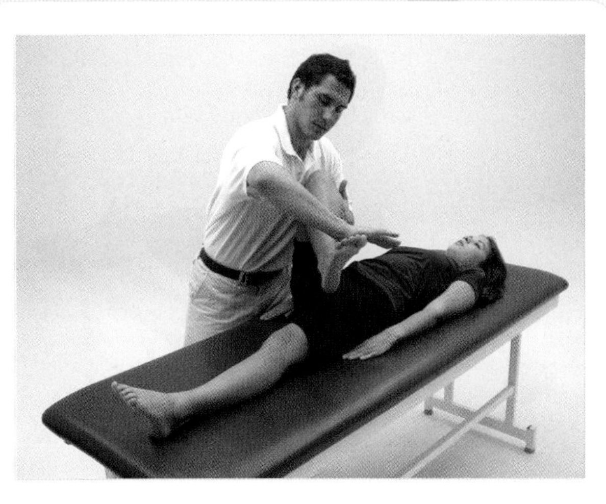

Figure 12-12

D1 lower-extremity movement pattern moving into flexion. Terminal position.

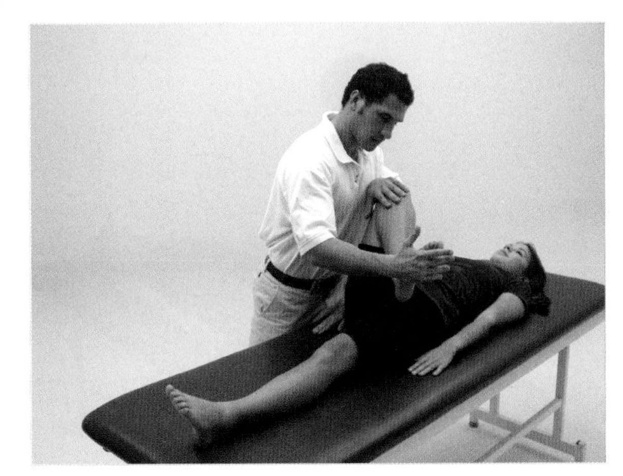

Figure 12-13

D1 lower-extremity movement pattern moving into extension. Starting position.

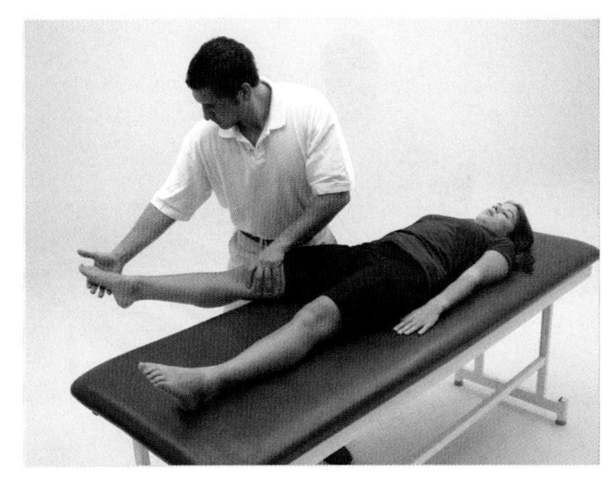

Figure 12-14

D1 lower-extremity movement pattern moving into extension. Terminal position.

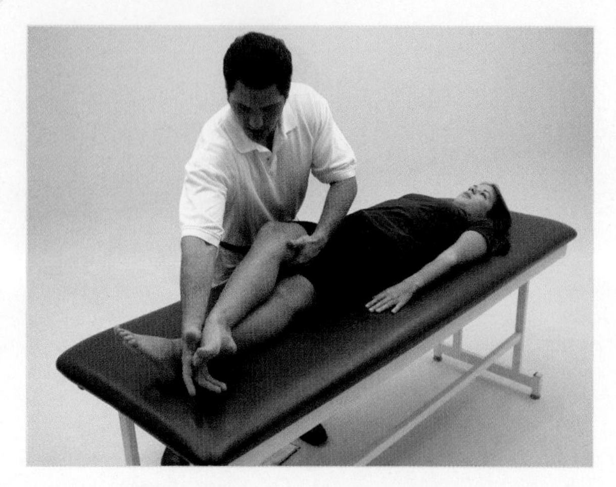

Figure 12-15

D1 lower-extremity movement pattern moving into flexion. Starting position.

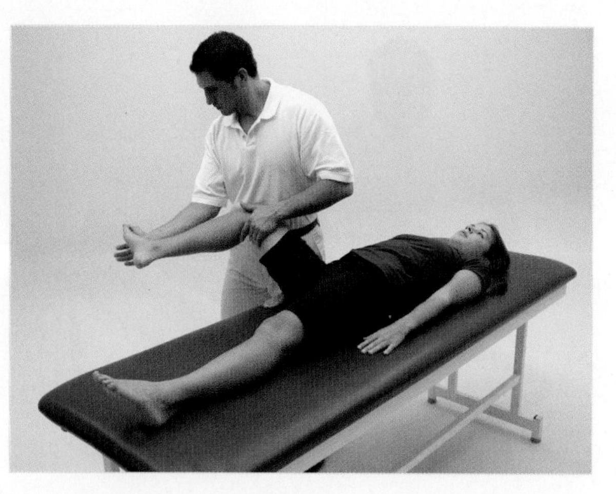

Figure 12-16

D2 lower-extremity movement pattern moving into flexion. Terminal position.

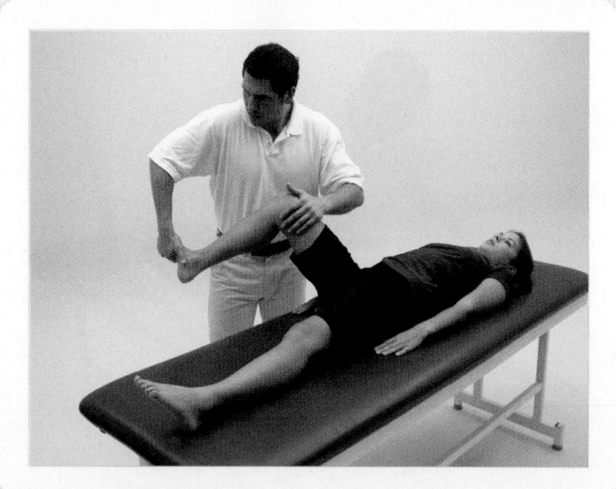

Figure 12-17

D2 lower-extremity movement pattern moving into extension. Starting position.

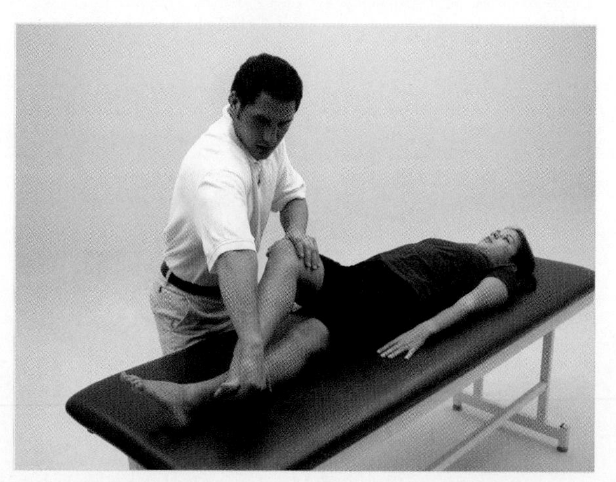

Figure 12-18

D2 lower-extremity movement pattern moving into extension. Terminal position.

Table 12-5 Upper-Trunk Movement Patterns

Body Part	Moving into Flexion (Chopping)[a]		Moving into Extension (Lifting)[a]	
	Starting Position (Figure 12-19)	Terminal Position (Figure 12-20)	Starting Position (Figure 12-21)	Terminal Position (Figure 12-22)
Right upper extremity	Flexed Adducted Internally rotated	Extended Abducted Externally rotated	Extended Adducted Internally rotated	Flexed Abducted Externally rotated
Left upper extremity (left hand grasps right forearm)	Flexed Abducted Externally rotated	Extended Adducted Internally rotated	Extended Abducted Externally rotated	Flexed Adducted Internally rotated
Trunk	Rotated and extended to left	Rotated and flexed to right	Rotated and flexed to left	Rotated and extended to right
Head	Rotated and extended to left	Rotated and flexed to right	Rotated and flexed to left	Rotated and extended to right
Hand position of therapist	Left hand on right anterolateral surface of forehead Right hand on dorsum of right hand		Right hand on dorsum of right hand Left hand on posterolateral surface of head	
Verbal command	Pull down		Push up	

[a]Patient's rotation is to the right.

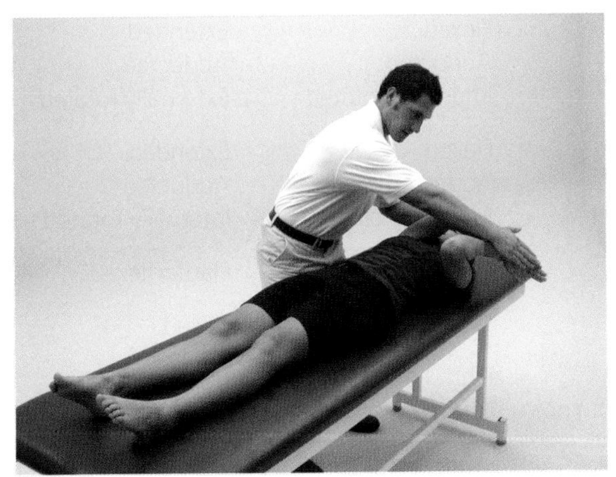

Figure 12-19

Upper-trunk pattern moving into flexion or chopping. Starting position.

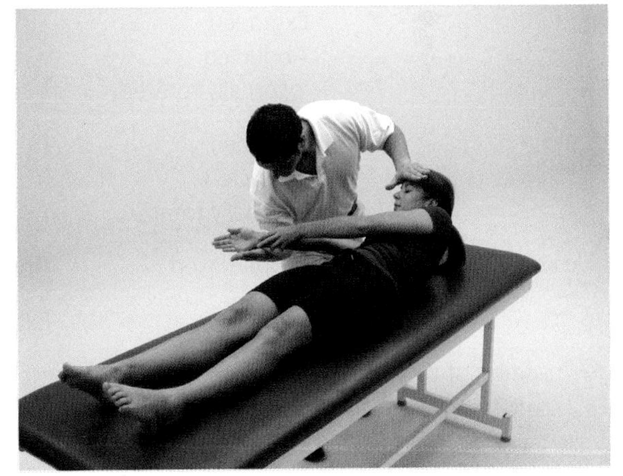

Figure 12-20

Upper-trunk pattern moving into flexion or chopping. Terminal position.

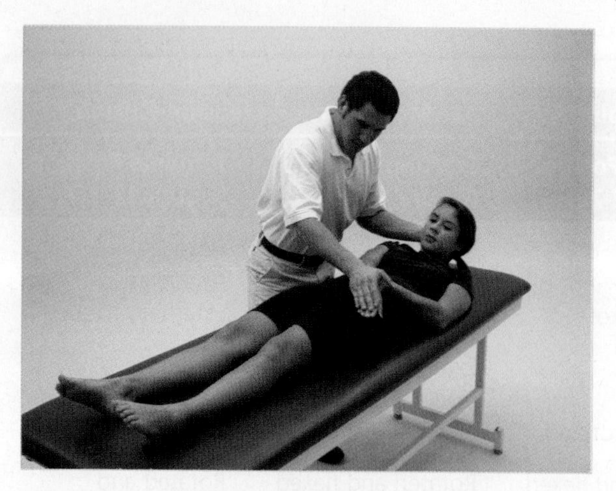

Figure 12-21

Upper-trunk pattern moving into flexion or lifting. Starting position.

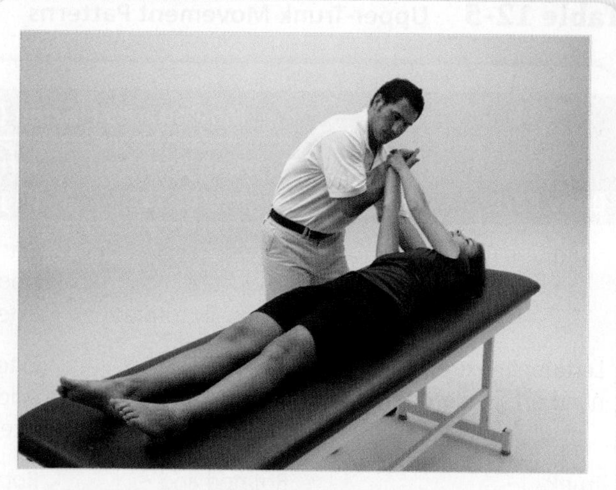

Figure 12-22

Upper-trunk pattern moving into flexion or lifting. Terminal position.

Table 12-6 Lower Trunk Movement Patterns

	Moving into Flexion[a]		Moving into Extension[b]	
Body Part	**Starting Position (Figure 12-23)**	**Terminal Position (Figure 12-24)**	**Starting Position (Figure 12-25)**	**Terminal Position (Figure 12-26)**
Right hip	Extended Abducted Externally rotated	Flexed Adducted Internally rotated	Flexed Adducted Internally rotated	Extended Abducted Externally rotated
Left hip	Extended Adducted Internally rotated	Flexed Abducted Externally rotated	Flexed Abducted Externally rotated	Extended Adducted Internally rotated
Ankles	Plantarflexed	Dorsiflexed	Dorsiflexed	Plantarflexed
Toes	Flexed	Extended	Extended	Flexed
Hand position of therapist	Right hand on dorsum of feet Left hand on anterolateral surface of left knee		Right hand on plantar surface of foot Left hand on posterolateral surface of right knee	
Verbal command	Pull up and in		Push down and out	

[a]Patient's rotation is to the right.
[b]Patient's rotation is to the right in extension.

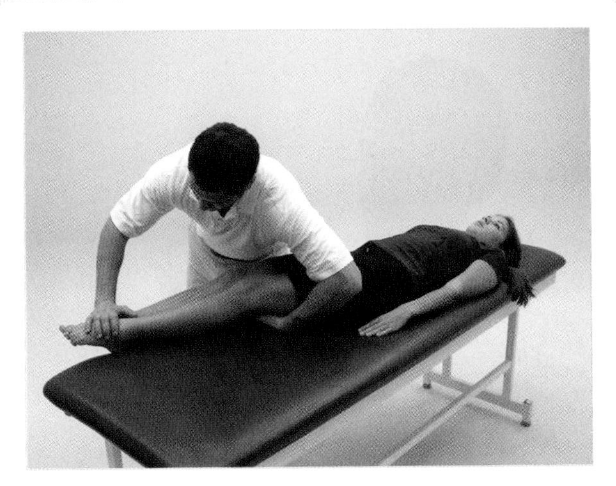

Figure 12-23

Lower-trunk pattern moving into flexion to the left. Starting position.

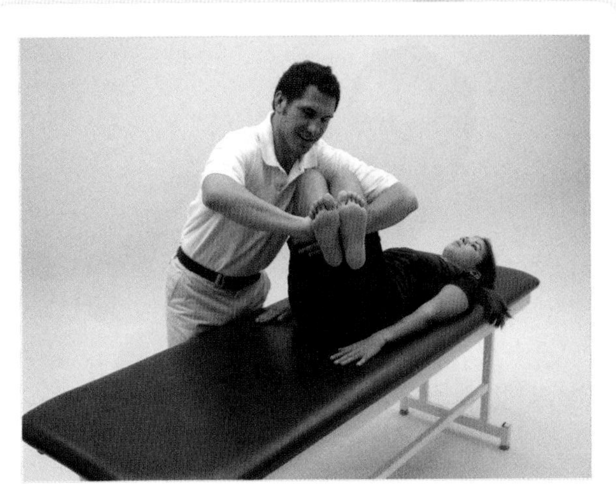

Figure 12-24

Lower-trunk pattern moving into flexion to the left. Terminal position.

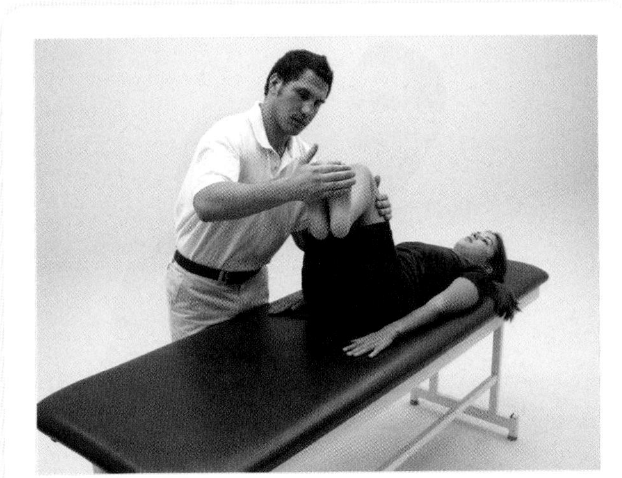

Figure 12-25

Lower-trunk pattern moving into extension to the left. Starting position.

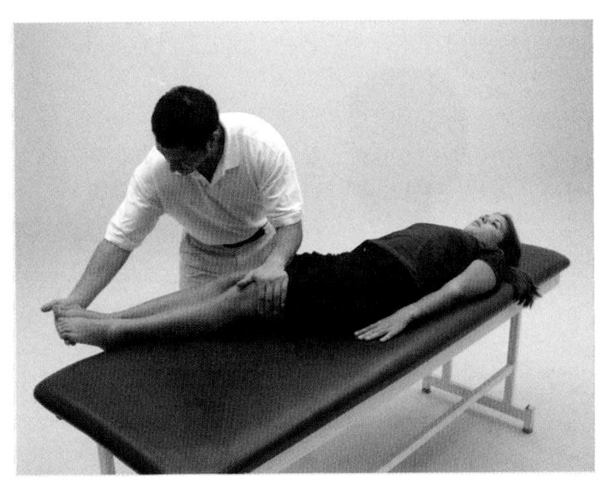

Figure 12-26

Lower-trunk pattern moving into extension to the left. Terminal position.

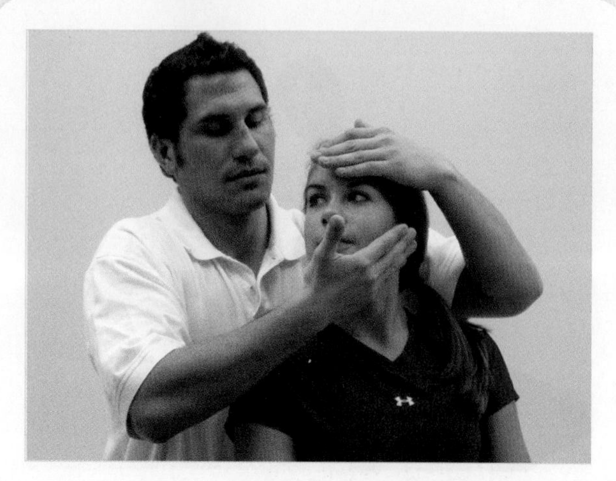

Figure 12-27

Neck flexion and rotation to the left. Starting position.

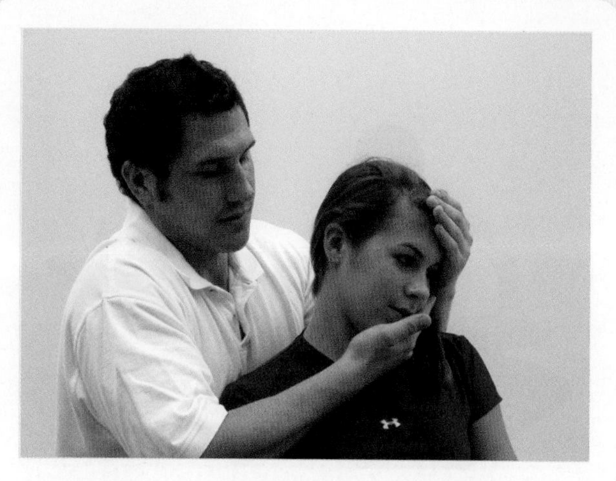

Figure 12-28

Neck flexion and rotation to the left. Terminal position.

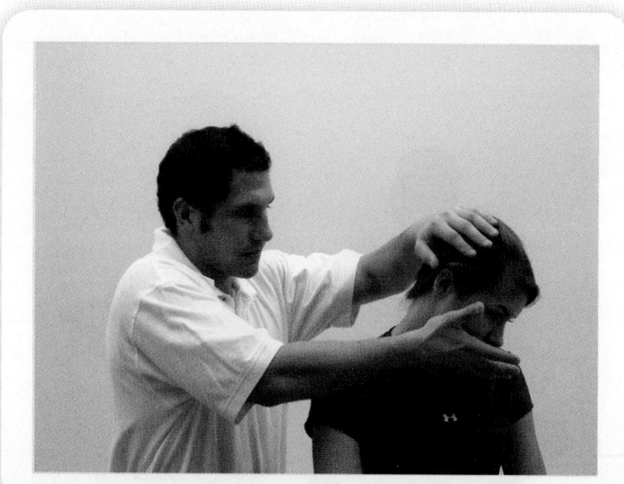

Figure 12-29

Neck extension and rotation to the right. Starting position.

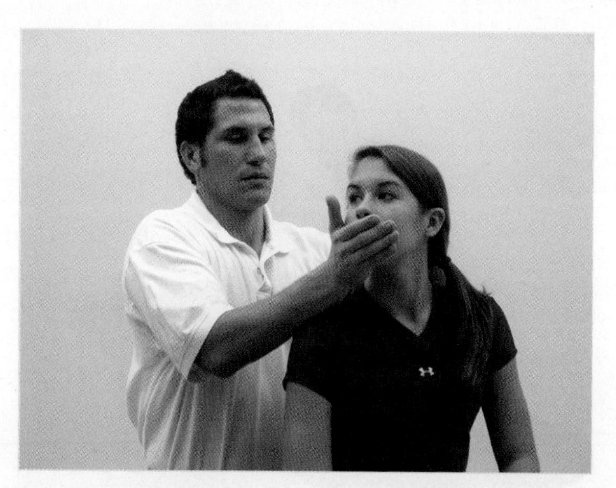

Figure 12-30

Neck extension and rotation to the right. Terminal position.

Proprioceptive Neuromuscular Facilitation as a Technique of Stretching for Improving Range of Motion

As indicated previously, PNF techniques can also be used for stretching to increase range of motion.

Evolution of the Theoretical Basis for Using Proprioceptive Neuromuscular Facilitation as a Stretching Technique

A review of the current literature seems to indicate that many clinicians believe that the PNF-stretching techniques can be an effective treatment modality for improving flexibility and thus use them regularly in clinical practice.[4,18,26,35,49,52,61,62] Over the years, various theories have been proposed to explain the neurologic and physical mechanisms through which the PNF techniques improve flexibility.[13] However, to date no consensus agreement exists that embraces a single theoretical explanation.

Neurophysiologic Basis of Proprioceptive Neuromuscular Facilitation Stretching

PNF gained popularity as a stretching technique in the 1970s.[45,54,71] The PNF research that has traditionally appeared in the literature since that time has attributed increases in range of motion primarily to neurophysiologic mechanisms involving the stretch reflex.[13] More recent studies question the validity of this theoretical explanation.[1,13,32,33,68] Nevertheless, a brief review of the stretch reflex will serve as a springboard for more currently accepted theories.

The stretch reflex involves 2 types of receptors: (a) muscle spindles that are sensitive to a change in length, as well as the rate of change in length of the muscle fiber; and (b) Golgi tendon organs that detect changes in tension (Figure 12-31).

Stretching a given muscle causes an increase in the frequency of impulses transmitted to the spinal cord from the muscle spindle along Ia fibers, which, in turn, produces an increase in the frequency of motor nerve impulses returning to that same muscle, along alpha motor neurons, thus reflexively resisting the stretch (see Figure 12-31). However, the development of excessive tension within the muscle activates the Golgi tendon organs, whose sensory impulses are carried back to the spinal cord along Ib fibers. These impulses have an inhibitory effect on the motor impulses returning to the muscles and cause that muscle to relax (Figure 12-32).[12]

Two neurophysiologic phenomena have been proposed to explain facilitation and inhibition of the neuromuscular systems. The first, *autogenic inhibition*, is defined as inhibition mediated by afferent fibers from a stretched muscle acting on the alpha motor neurons supplying that muscle, causing it to relax. When a muscle is stretched, motor neurons supplying that muscle receive both excitatory and inhibitory impulses from the receptors. If the stretch is continued for a slightly extended period of time, the inhibitory signals from the Golgi tendon organs eventually override the excitatory impulses and therefore cause relaxation. Because inhibitory motor neurons receive impulses from the Golgi tendon organs while the muscle spindle creates an initial reflex excitation leading to contraction, the Golgi tendon organs apparently send inhibitory impulses that last for the duration of increased tension (resulting from either passive stretch or active contraction) and eventually dominate the weaker impulses from the muscle spindle. This inhibition seems to protect the muscle against injury from reflex contractions resulting from excessive stretch.

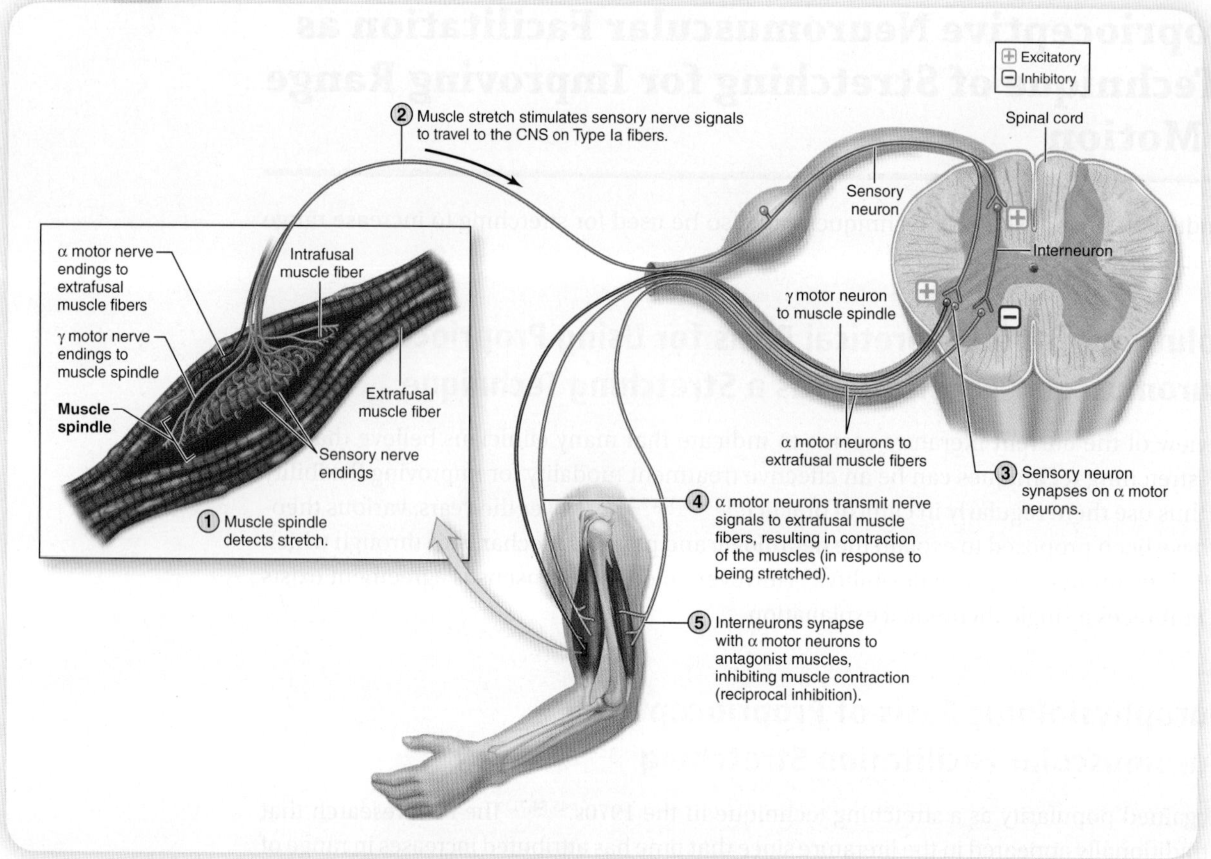

Figure 12-31 **Diagrammatic representation of the stretch reflex**

(Reproduced with permission from McKinley M, O'Loughlin V. *Human Anatomy.* 3rd ed. New York: McGraw-Hill; 2012.)

A second mechanism, *reciprocal inhibition,* deals with the relationships of the agonist and antagonist muscles (see Figure 12-31). The muscles that contract to produce joint motion are referred to as *agonists,* and the resulting movement is called an *agonistic pattern.* The muscles that stretch to allow the agonist pattern to occur are referred to as *antagonists.* Movement that occurs directly opposite to the agonist pattern is called the *antagonist pattern.*

When motor neurons of the agonist muscle receive excitatory impulses from afferent nerves, the motor neurons that supply the antagonist muscles are inhibited by afferent impulses.[4] Thus, contraction or extended stretch of the agonist muscle has been said to elicit relaxation or inhibit the antagonist. Likewise, a quick stretch of the antagonist muscle facilitates a contraction of the agonist.

The PNF literature has traditionally asserted that isometric or isotonic submaximal contraction of a target muscle (muscle to be stretched) prior to a passive stretch of that same muscle, or contraction of opposing muscles (agonists) during muscle stretch, produces relaxation of the stretched muscle through activation of the mechanisms of the stretch reflex that include autogenic inhibition and reciprocal inhibition.[13]

However, a number of studies done since the early 1990s suggest that relaxation following a contraction of a stretched muscle is not a result of the inhibition of muscle spindle activity or subsequent activation of Golgi tendon organs.[1,2,12,13,23,24,29,46,51]

Conclusions are based on the fact that when slowly stretching a muscle to a long length, as in the PNF-stretching techniques, the reflex-generated muscle electrical activation from

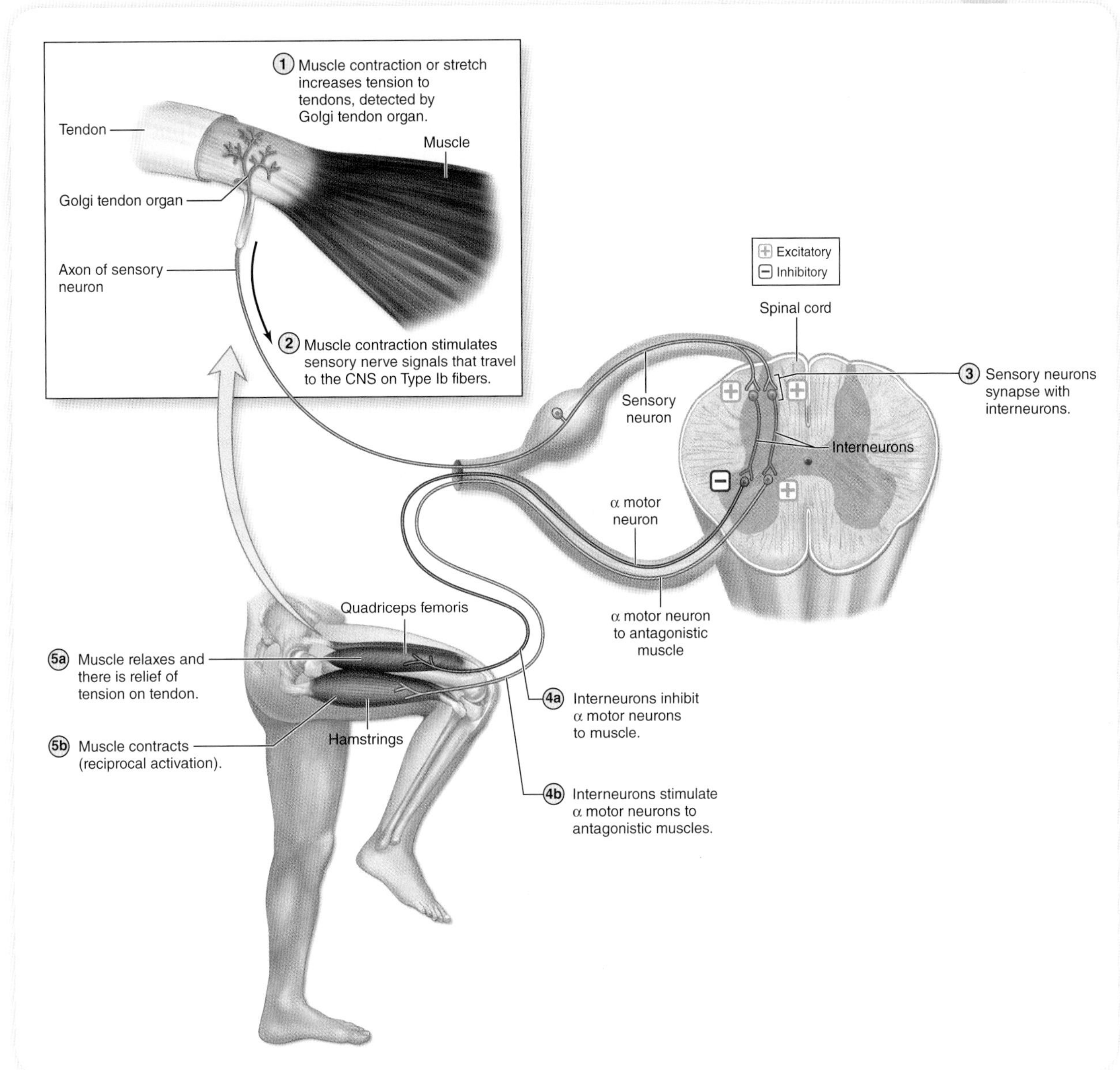

Figure 12-32 **Diagrammatic representation of reciprocal inhibition**

(Reproduced with permission from McKinley M, O'Loughlin V. *Human Anatomy.* 3rd ed. New York: McGraw-Hill; 2012.)

the muscle spindles (as indicated by electromyogram) is very small and clinically insignificant, and not likely to effectively resist an applied muscle lengthening force.[13,28,31,35,41] Furthermore, when a muscle relaxes following an isometric contraction, Golgi tendon organ firing is decreased or even becomes silent.[20,73] Thus, Golgi tendon organs would not be able to inhibit the target muscle in the seconds following contraction when the slow therapeutic stretch would be applied.[13] It is apparent that, in general, there is a lack of research-based evidence to support the theory that Golgi tendon organ and muscle spindle reflexes are able to relax target muscles during any of the PNF-stretching techniques.[13] Thus, other mechanisms have been proposed that may explain increases in range of motion with PNF-stretching exercises.[19]

Presynaptic Inhibition

In the PNF-stretching techniques, the contraction and subsequent relaxation of the target muscle is followed by a slow passive stretch of that muscle to a longer length. It has been suggested that lengthening is associated with an increase in presynaptic inhibition of the sensory signal from the muscle spindle.[13,22,25] This occurs with inhibition of the release of a neurotransmitter from the synaptic terminals of the muscle spindle Ia sensory fibers that limits activation in that muscle.

Viscoelastic Changes in Response to Stretching

It has been proposed that viscoelastic changes that occur in a muscle, and not a decrease in muscle activation mediated by Golgi tendon organs, is the mechanism that may explain increases in range of motion associated with the PNF techniques.[8] The viscoelastic properties of collagen in muscle are discussed briefly in Chapter 8. The force that is required to produce a change in length of a muscle is determined by its *elastic stiffness*.[72] Because of the viscous properties of muscle, less force is needed to elongate a muscle if that force is applied slowly rather than rapidly.[72] Also, the force that resists elongation is reduced if the muscle is held at a stretched length over a period of time, thus producing *stress relaxation*.[64] As stress relaxation occurs, the muscle will elongate further producing *creep*. These properties have been demonstrated in muscles with no significant electrical activity.[41,42,47]

As the viscoelastic properties within a muscle are changed during a PNF-stretching procedure, there is an altered perception of stretch and a greater range of motion and greater torque can be achieved before the onset of pain is perceived.[42,74] This is thought to occur because lengthening interrupts the actin-myosin bonds within the intrafusal fibers of the muscle spindle, thus reducing their sensitivity to stretch.[22,27,73]

Stretching Techniques

The following techniques should be used to increase range of motion, relaxation, and inhibition.

Contract-Relax

Contract-relax is a stretching technique that moves the body part passively into the agonist pattern. The patient is instructed to push by contracting the antagonist (muscle that will be stretched) isotonically against the resistance of the therapist. The patient then relaxes the antagonist while the therapist moves the part passively through as much range as possible to the point where limitation is again felt. This contract-relax technique is beneficial when range of motion is limited by muscle tightness.

Hold-Relax

Hold-relax is very similar to the contract-relax technique. It begins with an isometric contraction of the antagonist (muscle that will be stretched) against resistance, followed by a concentric contraction of the agonist muscle combined with light pressure from the therapist to produce maximal stretch of the antagonist. This technique is appropriate when there is muscle tension on one side of a joint and may be used with either the agonist or antagonist.[7]

Slow-Reversal-Hold-Relax

Slow-reversal-hold-relax technique begins with an isotonic contraction of the agonist, which often limits range of motion in the agonist pattern, followed by an isometric contraction of the antagonist (muscle that will be stretched) during the push phase. During the relax phase, the antagonists are relaxed while the agonists are contracting, causing movement in the direction of the agonist pattern and thus stretching the antagonist. The technique, like the contract-relax and hold-relax, is useful for increasing range of motion when the primary limiting factor is the antagonistic muscle group.

Because a goal of rehabilitation with most injuries is restoration of strength through a full, nonrestricted range of motion, several of these techniques are sometimes combined in sequence to accomplish this goal.[50] Figure 12-33 shows a PNF-stretching technique in which the therapist is stretching an injured patient.

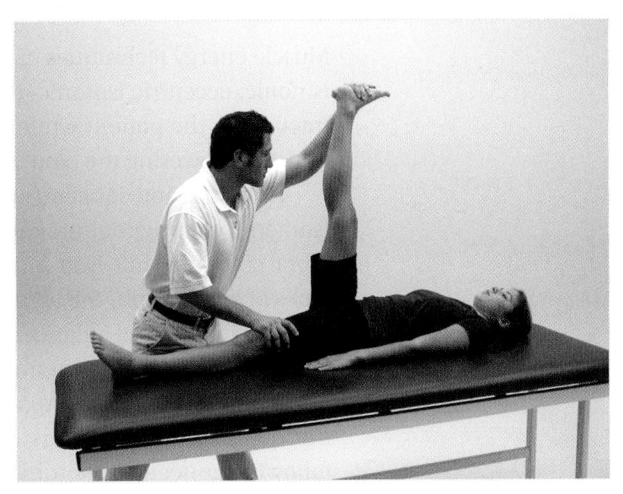

Figure 12-33 PNF-stretching technique

Muscle Energy Techniques

Muscle energy is a manual therapy technique, which is a variation of the PNF contract-relax and hold-relax techniques. Like the PNF techniques, the muscle energy techniques are based on the same neurophysiologic mechanisms involving the stretch reflex discussed earlier. Muscle energy techniques involve a voluntary contraction of a muscle in a specifically controlled direction at varied levels of intensity against a distinctly executed counterforce applied by the therapist.[30,48] The patient provides the corrective *intrinsic* forces and controls the intensity of the muscular contractions while the therapist controls the precision and localization of the procedure.[48] The amount of patient effort can vary from a minimal muscle twitch to a maximal muscle contraction.[30]

Five components are necessary for muscle energy techniques to be effective[30]:

1. Active muscle contraction by the patient.
2. A muscle contraction oriented in a specific direction.
3. Some patient control of contraction intensity.
4. Therapist control of joint position.
5. Therapist application of appropriate counterforce.

Clinical Applications

It has been proposed that muscles function not only as flexors, extenders, rotators, and side-benders of joints, but also as restrictors of joint motion. In situations where the muscle is restricting joint motion, muscle energy techniques use a specific muscle contraction to restore physiological movement to a joint.[48] Any articulation, whether in the spine or extremities, that can be moved by active muscle contraction can be treated using muscle energy techniques.[48,57]

Muscle energy techniques can be used to accomplish several treatment goals[30]:

- Lengthening of a shortened, contracted, or spastic muscle.
- Strengthening of a weak muscle or muscle group.
- Reduction of localized edema through muscle pumping.
- Mobilization of an articulation with restricted mobility.
- Stretching of fascia.

Treatment Techniques

Muscle energy techniques can involve 4 types of muscle contraction: isometric, concentric isotonic, eccentric isotonic, and *isolytic.* An isolytic contraction involves a concentric contraction by the patient while the therapist applies an external force in the opposite direction, overpowering the contraction and lengthening that muscle.[48]

Isometric and concentric isotonic contractions are most frequently used in treatment.[66] Isometric contractions are most often used in treating hypertonic muscles in the spinal vertebral column, while isotonic contractions are most often used in the extremities. With both types of contraction, the idea is to inhibit antagonistic muscles producing more symmetrical muscle tone and balance.

A concentric contraction can also be used to mobilize a joint against its *motion barrier* if there is motion restriction. For example, if a strength imbalance exists between the quadriceps and hamstrings, with weak quadriceps limiting knee extension, the following concentric isotonic muscle energy technique may be used (Figure 12-34*A*):

1. The patient lies prone on the treatment table.
2. The therapist stabilizes the patient with one hand and grasps the ankle with the other.
3. The therapist fully flexes the knee.
4. The patient actively extends the knee, using as much force as possible.
5. The therapist provides a resistant counterforce that allows slow knee extension throughout the available range.
6. Once the patient has completely relaxed, the therapist moves the knee back to full flexion and the patient repeats the contraction with additional resistance applied through the full range of extension. This is repeated 3 to 5 times with increasing resistance on each repetition.

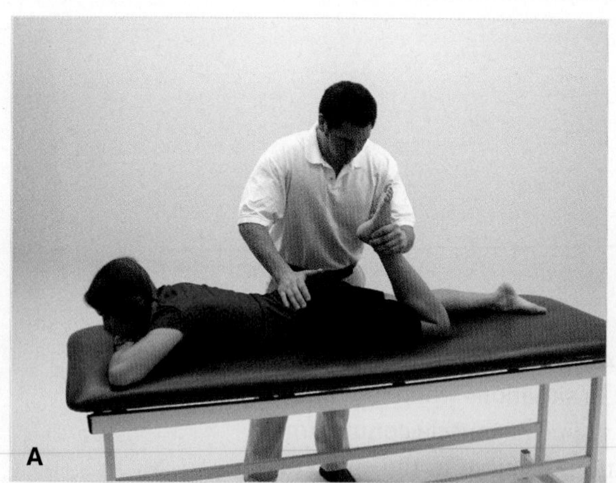

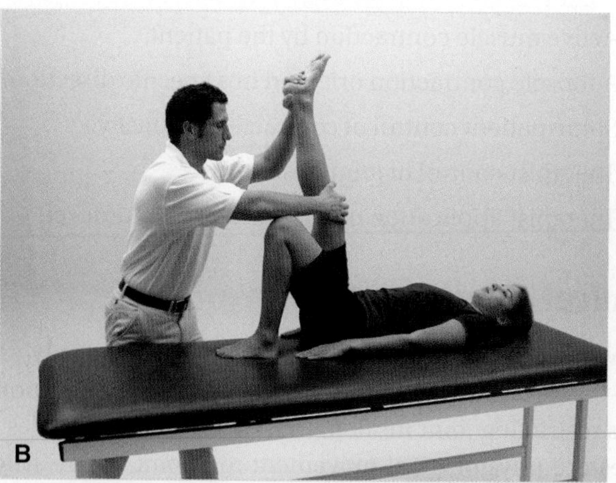

Figure 12-34

Positions for muscle energy techniques for improving (**A**) weak quadriceps that limit knee extension and/or hip flexion and (**B**) weak hamstrings that limit knee flexion and/or hip extension.

If a knee has a restriction because of tightness in the hamstrings that is limiting full extension, the following isometric muscle energy technique should be used (see Figure 12-34*B*):

1. The patient lies supine on the treatment table.
2. The therapist stabilizes the knee with one hand and grasps the ankle with the other.
3. The therapist fully extends the knee until an extension barrier is felt.
4. The patient actively flexes the knee using a minimal sustained force.
5. The therapist provides an equal resistant counterforce for 3 to 7 seconds, after which the patient completely relaxes.
6. The therapist again extends the knee until a new extension barrier is felt.
7. This is repeated 3 to 5 times.

SUMMARY

1. The PNF techniques may be used to increase both strength and range of motion and are based on the neurophysiology of the stretch reflex.
2. The motor neurons of the spinal cord always receive a combination of inhibitory and excitatory impulses from the afferent nerves. Whether these motor neurons will be excited or inhibited depends on the ratio of the 2 types of incoming impulses.
3. The PNF techniques emphasize specific principles that may be superimposed on any of the specific techniques.
4. The PNF-strengthening techniques include repeated contraction, slow-reversal, slow-reversal-hold, rhythmic stabilization, and rhythmic initiation.
5. The PNF-stretching techniques include contract-relax, hold-relax, and slow-reversal-hold-relax.
6. The techniques of PNF are rotational and diagonal movements in the upper extremity, lower extremity, upper trunk, and the head and neck.
7. Muscle energy techniques involve a voluntary contraction of a muscle in a specifically controlled direction at varied levels of intensity against a distinctly executed counterforce applied by the therapist.

REFERENCES

1. Alter M. *Science of Flexibility.* 3rd ed. Champaign, IL: Human Kinetics; 2004.
2. Anderson B, Burke ER. Scientific, medical, and practical aspects of stretching. *Clin Sports Med.* 1991;10:63-86.
3. Barak T, Rosen E, Sofer R. Mobility: Passive orthopedic manual therapy. In: Gould J, Davies G, eds. *Orthopedic and Sports Therapy.* St. Louis: Mosby; 1990:212-227.
4. Barry D. Proprioceptive neuromuscular facilitation for the scapula, part 1: diagonal 1. *Athl Ther Today.* 2005;10(2):54.
5. Basmajian J. *Therapeutic Exercise.* Baltimore, MD: Lippincott, Williams & Wilkins; 1990.
6. Bobath B. The treatment of motor disorders of pyramidal and extrapyramidal tracts by reflex inhibition and by facilitation of movement. *Physiotherapy.* 1955; 41:146.
7. Bonnar B, Deivert R, Gould T. The relationship between isometric contraction durations during hold-relax stretching and improvement of hamstring flexibility. *J Sports Med Phys Fitness.* 2004;44(3):258-261.
8. Bradley P, Olsen P, Portas M. The effect of static ballistic and PNF stretching on vertical jump performance. *J Strength Cond Res.* 2007;21(1):223.

9. Burke DG, Culligan CJ, Holt LE. Equipment designed to stimulate proprioceptive neuromuscular facilitation flexibility training. *J Strength Cond Res.* 2000;14(2):135-139.
10. Burke DG, Culligan CJ, Holt LE. The theoretical basis of proprioceptive neuromuscular facilitation. *J Strength Cond Res.* 2000;14(4):496-500.
11. Burke DG, Holt LE, Rasmussen R. Effects of hot or cold water immersion and modified proprioceptive neuromuscular facilitation flexibility exercise on hamstring length. *J Athl Train.* 2001;36(1):16-19.
12. Carter AM, Kinzey SJ, Chitwood LE, Cole JL. Proprioceptive neuromuscular facilitation decreases muscle activity during the stretch reflex in selected posterior thigh muscles. *J Sport Rehabil.* 2000;9(4):269-278.
13. Chalmers G. Re-examination of the possible role of Golgi tendon organ and muscle spindle reflexes in proprioceptive neuromuscular facilitation muscle stretching. *Sports Biomech.* 2004;3(1):159-183.
14. Cookson J, Kent B. Orthopedic manual therapy: An overview I. The extremities. *Phys Ther.* 1979;59:136.
15. Cookson J. Orthopedic manual therapy: An overview, II. The spine. *Phys Ther.* 1979;59:259.
16. Cornelius W, Jackson A. The effects of cryotherapy and PNF on hip extension flexibility. *Athlet Train.* 1984;19(3):184.
17. Davis D, Hagerman-Hose M, Midkiff M. The effectiveness of 3 proprioceptive neuromuscular facilitation stretching techniques on the flexibility of the hamstring muscle group [abstract]. *J Orthop Sports Phys Ther.* 2004;34(1):A33-A34.
18. Decicco PV, Fisher MM. The effects of proprioceptive neuromuscular facilitation stretching on shoulder range of motion in overhand athletes. *J Sports Med Phys Fitness.* 2005;45(2):183-187.
19. Decicco P, Fisher M. The effects of proprioceptive neuromuscular facilitation stretching on shoulder range of motion in overhand athletes. *J Sports Med Phys Fitness.* 2005;45(2):183-187.
20. Edin BB, Vallbo AB. Muscle afferent responses to isometric contractions and relaxations in humans. *J Neurophysiol.* 1990;63:1307-1313.
21. Engle R, Canner G. Proprioceptive neuromuscular facilitation (PNF) and modified procedures for anterior cruciate ligament (ACL) instability. *J Orthop Sports Phys Ther.* 1989;11(6):230-236.
22. Enoka R. *Neuromechanics of Human Movement.* 4th ed. Champaign, IL: Human Kinetics; 2008.
23. Enoka RM, Hutton RS, Eldred E. Changes in excitability of tendon tap and Hoffmann reflexes following voluntary contractions. *Electroencephalogr Clin Neurophysiol.* 1980;48:664-672.
24. Ferber R, Osternig L, Gravelle D. Effect of PNF stretch techniques on knee flexor muscle EMG activity in older adults. *J Electromyogr Kinesiol.* 2002;12:391-397.
25. Gollhofer A, Schopp A, Rapp W, Stroinik V. Changes in reflex excitability following isometric contraction in humans. *Eur J Appl Physiol Occup Physiol.* 1998;77:89-97.
26. Greenman P. *Principles of Manual Medicine.* Baltimore, MD: Lippincott, Williams & Wilkins; 2003.
27. Gregory JE, Mark RF, Morgan DL, Patak A, Polus B, Proske U. Effects of muscle history on the stretch reflex in cat and man. *J Physiol.* 1990;424:93-107.
28. Halbertsma JP, Mulder I, Goeken LN, Eisma WH. Repeated passive stretching: Acute effect on the passive muscle moment and extensibility of short hamstrings. *Arch Phys Med Rehabil.* 1999;80:407-414.
29. Holcomb WR. Improved stretching with proprioceptive neuromuscular facilitation. *Strength Cond J.* 2000;22(1):59-61.
30. Hollis M. *Practical Exercise.* Oxford, UK: Blackwell Scientific; 1981.
31. Houk JC, Rymer WZ, Crago PE. Dependence of dynamic response of spindle receptors on muscle length and velocity. *J Neurophysiol.* 1981;46:143-166.
32. Hultborn H. State-dependent modulation of sensory feedback. *J Physiol.* 2001;533(Pt 1):5-13.
33. Jankowska E. Interneuronal relay in spinal pathways from proprioceptors. *Prog Neurobiol.* 1992;38:335-378.
34. Johnson GS. PNF and knee rehabilitation. *J Orthop Sports Phys Ther.* 2000;30(7):430-431.
35. Kitani I. The effectiveness of proprioceptive neuromuscular facilitation (PNF) exercises on shoulder joint position sense in baseball players (Abstract). *J Athl Train.* 2004;39(2):S-62.
36. Knappstein A, Stanley S, Whatman C. Range of motion immediately post and seven minutes post, PNF stretching hip joint range of motion and PNF stretching. *NZ J Sports Med.* 2004;32(2):42-46.
37. Knott M, Voss D. *Proprioceptive Neuromuscular Facilitation: Patterns and Techniques.* Baltimore, MD: Lippincott, Williams & Wilkins; 1985.
38. Kofotolis N, Kellis E. Cross-training effects of a proprioceptive neuromuscular facilitation exercise program on knee musculature. *Phys Ther Sport.* 2007;8(3):109.
39. Kofotolis N, Kellis E. Effects of two 4-week proprioceptive neuromuscular facilitation programs on muscle endurance, flexibility, and functional performance in women with chronic low back pain. *Phys Ther.* 2006;86(7):1001.
40. Lloyd D. Facilitation and inhibition of spinal motor neurons. *J Neurophysiol.* 1946;9:421.
41. Magnusson SP, Simonsen EB, Aagaard P, Dyhre-Poulsen P, McHugh MP, Kjaer M. Mechanical and physiological responses to stretching with and without preisometric contraction in human skeletal muscle. *Arch Phys Med Rehabil.* 1996;77:373-378.
42. Magnusson SP, Simonsen EB, Dyhre-Poulsen P, Aagaard P, Mohr T, Kjaer M. Viscoelastic stress relaxation during static stretch in human skeletal muscle in the absence of EMG activity. *Scand J Med Sci Sports.* 1996;6:323-328.
43. Manoel M, Harris-Love M, Danoff J. Acute effects of static, dynamic and proprioceptive neuromuscular facilitation

stretching on muscle power in women. *J Strength Cond Res.* 2008;22(5):1528.

44. Marek S, Cramer J, Fincher L. Acute effects of static and proprioceptive neuromuscular facilitation stretching on muscle strength and power output. *J Athl Train.* 2005;40(2):94.

45. Markos P. Ipsilateral and contralateral effects of proprioceptive neuromuscular facilitation techniques on hip motion and electromyographic activity. *Phys Ther.* 1979;59(11)P:66-73.

46. McAtee R, Charland J. *Facilitated Stretching.* 3rd ed. Champaign, IL: Human Kinetics; 2007.

47. McHugh MP, Magnusson SP, Gleim GW, Nicholas JA. Viscoelastic stress relaxation in human skeletal muscle. *Med Sci Sports Exerc.* 1992;24:1375-1382.

48. Mitchell F. Elements of muscle energy technique. In: Basmajian J, Nyberg R, eds. *Rational Manual Therapies.* Baltimore, MD: Lippincott, Williams & Wilkins; 1993.

49. Mitchell U, Myrer J, Hopkins T. Acute stretch perception alteration contributes to the success of the PNF "contract-relax" stretch. *J Sport Rehabil.* 2007;16(2):85.

50. Osternig L, Robertson R, Troxel R, et al. Differential responses to proprioceptive neuromuscular facilitation stretch techniques. *Med Sci Sports Exerc.* 1990;22: 106-111.

51. Osternig L, R. Robertson R. Troxel, Hansen P. Muscle activation during proprioceptive neuromuscular facilitation (PNF) stretching techniques . . . stretch-relax (SR), contract-relax (CR) and agonist contract-relax (ACR). *Am J Phys Med.* 1987;66(5):298-307.

52. Padua D, Guskiewicz K, Prentice W. The effect of select shoulder exercises on strength, active angle reproduction, single-arm balance, and functional performance. *J Sport Rehabil.* 2004;13(1):75-95.

53. Prentice W, Kooima E. The use of proprioceptive neuromuscular facilitation techniques in the rehabilitation of sport-related injuries. *Athlet Train.* 1986;21:26-31.

54. Prentice W. A comparison of static stretching and PNF stretching for improving hip joint flexibility. *Athlet Train.* 1983;18(1):56-59.

55. Prentice W. A manual resistance technique for strengthening tibial rotation. *Athlet Train.* 1988;23(3):230-233.

56. Prentice W. Proprioceptive neuromuscular facilitation [videotape]. St. Louis, MO: Mosby; 1993.

57. Roberts BL. Soft tissue manipulation: Neuromuscular and muscle energy techniques. *J Neurosci Nurs.* 1997;29(2):123-127.

58. Rood M. Neurophysiologic reactions as a basis of physical therapy. *Phys Ther Rev.* 1954;34:444.

59. Saliba V, Johnson G, Wardlaw C. Proprioceptive neuromuscular facilitation. In: Basmajian J, Nyberg R, eds. *Rational Manual Therapies.* Baltimore, MD: Lippincott Williams & Wilkins; 1993.

60. Sawner K, LaVigne J. *Brunstrom's Movement Therapy in Hemiplegia.* Baltimore, MD: Lippincott, Williams & Wilkins; 1992.

61. Schuback B, Hooper J, Salisbury L. A comparison of a self-stretch incorporating proprioceptive neuromuscular facilitation components and a therapist-applied PNF-technique on hamstring flexibility. *Physiotherapy.* 2004;90(3):151.

62. Sharman M, Cresswell T, Andrew G. Proprioceptive neuromuscular facilitation stretching: Mechanisms and clinical implications. *Sports Med.* 2006;36(11):929.

63. Sherrington C. *The Integrative Action of the Nervous System.* New Haven, CT: Yale University Press; 1947.

64. Shrier I. Does stretching help prevent injuries? In: MacAuley D, Best T, eds. *Evidence Based Sports Medicine.* London, UK: BMJ Books; 2002.

65. Spernoga SG, Uhl TL, Arnold BL, Gansneder BM. Duration of maintained hamstring flexibility after a one-time, modified hold-relax stretching protocol. *J Athl Train.* 2001;36(1):44-48.

66. Stone J. Muscle energy technique. *Athl Ther Today.* 2000;5(5):25.

67. Stone JA. Prevention and rehabilitation: Proprioceptive neuromuscular facilitation. *Athl Ther Today.* 2000;5(1):38-39.

68. Stuart DG. Reflections of spinal reflexes. *Adv Exp Med Biol.* 2002;508:249-257.

69. Surberg P. Neuromuscular facilitation techniques in sports medicine. *Phys Ther Rev.* 1954;34:444.

70. Surburg P, Schrader J. Proprioceptive neuromuscular facilitation techniques in sports medicine: A reassessment. *J Athl Train.* 1997;32(1):34-39.

71. Taniqawa M. Comparison of the hold-relax procedure and passive mobilization on increasing muscle length. *Phys Ther.* 1972;52(7):725-735.

72. Taylor DC, Dalton JD, Seaber A. Viscoelastic properties of muscle-tendon units: The biomechanical effects of stretching. *Am J Sports Med.* 1990;18:300-309.

73. Wilson LR, Gandevia SC, Burke D. Increased resting discharge of human spindle afferents following voluntary contractions. *J Physiol.* 1995;488(Pt 3):833-840.

74. Worrell T, Smith T, Winegardner J. Effect of hamstring stretching on hamstring muscle performance. *J Orthop Sports Phys Ther.* 1994;20(3):154-159.

75. Zohn D, Mennell J. *Musculoskeletal Pain: Diagnosis and Physical Treatment.* Boston, MA: Little, Brown; 1987.

13

Joint Mobilization and Traction Techniques in Rehabilitation

William E. Prentice

OBJECTIVES

After completion of this chapter, the physical therapist should be able to do the following:

- Differentiate between physiologic movements and accessory motions.
- Discuss joint arthrokinematics.
- Discuss how specific joint positions can enhance the effectiveness of the treatment technique.
- Discuss the basic techniques of joint mobilization.
- Identify Maitland's five oscillation grades.
- Discuss indications and contraindications for mobilization.
- Discuss the use of various traction grades in treating pain and joint hypomobility.
- Explain why traction and mobilization techniques should be used simultaneously.
- Demonstrate specific techniques of mobilization and traction for various joints.

Following injury to a joint, there will almost always be some associated loss of motion. That loss of movement may be attributed to a number of pathologic factors, including contracture of inert connective tissue (eg, ligaments and joint capsule), resistance of the contractile tissue or the musculotendinous unit (eg, muscle, tendon, and fascia) to stretch, or some combination of the two.[7,8] If left untreated, the joint will become hypomobile and will eventually begin to show signs of degeneration.[30]

Joint mobilization and traction are manual therapy techniques that are slow, passive movements of articulating surfaces.[33] They are used to regain normal active joint range of motion, restore normal passive motions that occur about a joint, reposition or realign a joint, regain a normal distribution of forces and stresses about a joint, or reduce pain—all of which collectively improve joint function.[25] Joint mobilization and traction are 2 extremely effective and widely used techniques in injury rehabilitation.[3]

Relationship Between Physiologic and Accessory Motions

For the therapist supervising a rehabilitation program, some understanding of the biomechanics of joint movement is essential. There are basically 2 types of movements that govern motion about a joint. Perhaps the better known of the 2 types of movements are the *physiologic movements* that result from either concentric or eccentric active muscle contractions that move a bone or a joint. This type of motion is referred to as *osteokinematic motion.* A bone can move about an axis of rotation, or a joint into flexion, extension, abduction, adduction, and rotation. The second type of motion is *accessory motion.* Accessory motions refer to the manner in which one articulating joint surface moves relative to another. Physiologic movement is voluntary, while accessory movements normally accompany physiologic movement.[2] The 2 movements occur simultaneously. Although accessory movements cannot occur independently, they may be produced by some external force. Normal accessory component motions must occur for full-range physiologic movement to take place.[11] If any of the accessory component motions are restricted, normal physiologic cardinal plane movements will not occur.[23,24] A muscle cannot be fully rehabilitated if the joint is not free to move and vice versa.[30]

Traditionally in rehabilitation programs, we have tended to concentrate more on passive physiologic movements without paying much attention to accessory motions. The question is always being asked, "How much flexion or extension is this patient lacking?" Rarely will anyone ask "How much is rolling or gliding restricted?"

It is critical for the therapist to closely evaluate the injured joint to determine whether motion is limited by physiologic movement constraints involving musculotendinous units or by limitation in accessory motion involving the joint capsule and ligaments.[15] If physiologic movement is restricted, the patient should engage in stretching activities designed to improve flexibility. Stretching exercises should be used whenever there is resistance of the contractile or musculotendinous elements to stretch. Stretching techniques are most effective at the end of physiologic range of movement; they are limited to 1 direction; and they require some element of discomfort if additional range of motion is to be achieved. Stretching techniques make use of long-lever arms to apply stretch to a given muscle.[14] Stretching techniques are discussed in Chapters 8 and 12.

If accessory motion is limited by some restriction of the joint capsule or the ligaments, the therapist should incorporate mobilization techniques into the treatment program. Mobilization techniques should be used whenever there are tight inert or noncontractile articular structures; they can be used effectively at any point in the range of motion; and they can be used in any direction in which movement is restricted.[26]

Mobilization techniques use a short-lever arm to stretch ligaments and joint capsules, placing less stress on these structures, and, consequently, are somewhat safer to use than stretching techniques.[5]

Clinical Pearl

Once a patient has progressed through the acute stage, exercises and active and passive stretching can be accompanied by joint mobilizations. Mobilization of the knee joint involves gliding the concave tibia anteriorly on the femur.

Joint Arthrokinematics

Accessory motions are also referred to as *joint arthrokinematics,* which include *spin, roll,* and *glide* (Figure 13-1).[1,17,19]

Spin occurs around some stationary longitudinal mechanical axis and may be in either a clockwise or counterclockwise direction. An example of spinning is motion of the radial head at the humeroradial joint as occurs in forearm pronation/supination (Figure 13-1*A*).

Rolling occurs when a series of points on one articulating surface come in contact with a series of points on another articulating surface. An analogy would be to picture a rocker of a rocking chair rolling on the flat surface of the floor. An anatomic example would be the rounded femoral condyles rolling over a stationary flat tibial plateau (Figure 13-1*B*).

Gliding occurs when a specific point on one articulating surface comes in contact with a series of points on another surface. Returning to the rocking chair analogy, the rocker slides across the flat surface of the floor without any rocking at all. Gliding is sometimes referred to as *translation.* Anatomically, gliding or translation would occur during an anterior drawer test at the knee when the flat tibial plateau slides anteriorly relative to the fixed rounded femoral condyles (Figure 13-1*C*).

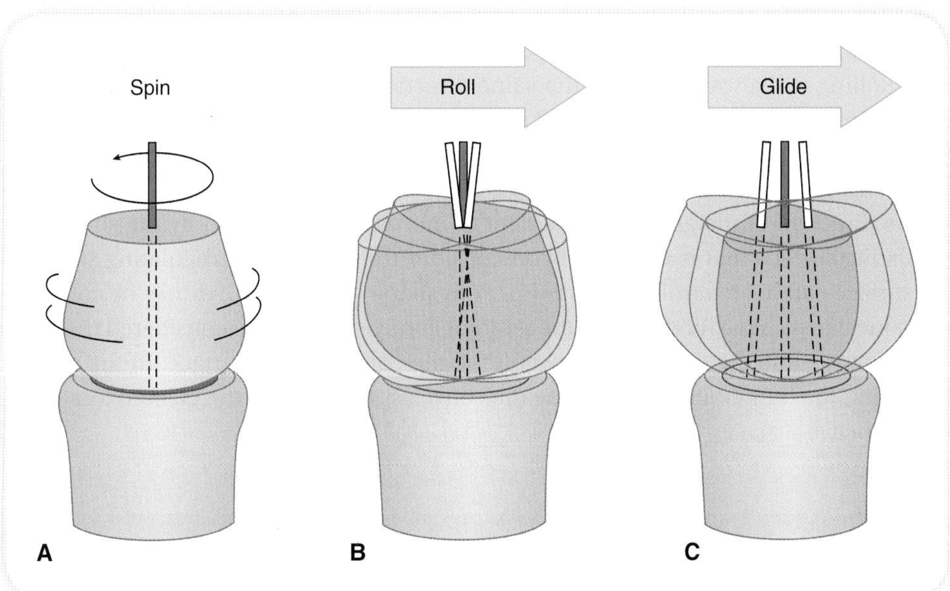

Figure 13-1 **Joint arthrokinematics**

A. Spin. **B**. Roll. **C**. Glide.

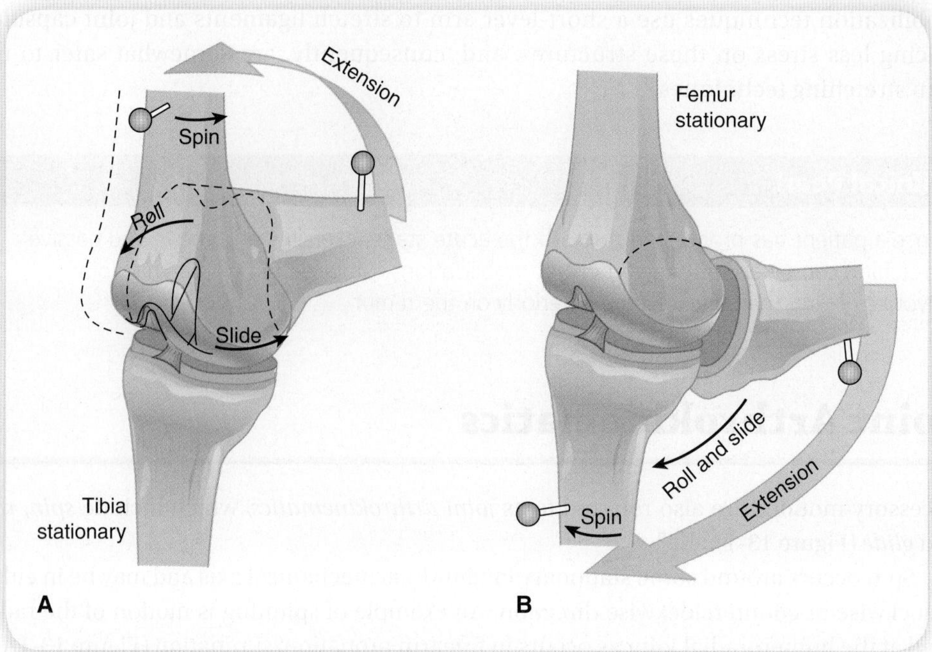

Figure 13-2 **Convex-concave rule**

A. Convex moving on concave. **B.** Concave moving on convex.

Pure gliding can occur only if the 2 articulating surfaces are congruent, where either both are flat or both are curved. Because virtually all articulating joint surfaces are incongruent, meaning that one is usually flat while the other is more curved, it is more likely that gliding will occur simultaneously with a rolling motion. Rolling does not occur alone because this would result in compression or perhaps dislocation of the joint.

Although rolling and gliding usually occur together, they are not necessarily in similar proportion, nor are they always in the same direction. If the articulating surfaces are more congruent, more gliding will occur; whereas if they are less congruent, more rolling will occur. Rolling will always occur in the same direction as the physiologic movement. For example, in the knee joint when the foot is fixed on the ground, the femur will always roll in an anterior direction when moving into knee extension and conversely will roll posteriorly when moving into flexion (Figure 13-2).

The direction of the gliding component of motion is determined by the shape of the articulating surface that is moving. If you consider the shape of 2 articulating surfaces, 1 joint surface can be determined to be convex in shape while the other may be considered to be concave in shape. In the knee, the femoral condyles would be considered the convex joint surface, while the tibial plateau would be the concave joint surface. In the glenohumeral joint, the humeral head would be the convex surface, while the glenoid fossa would be the concave surface.

Clinical Pearl

Joint mobilization can be used to break down the scar tissue. If plantar flexion is limited, the talus should be glided anteriorly to stretch the anterior capsule. Ankle instability can be provided with a brace, taping, and exercises to increase stability. Exercises should also target the muscles responsible for ankle inversion and eversion.

This relationship between the shape of articulating joint surfaces and the direction of gliding is defined by the *convex-concave rule.* If the concave joint surface is moving on a stationary convex surface, gliding will occur in the same direction as the rolling motion. Conversely, if the convex surface is moving on a stationary concave surface, gliding will occur in an opposite direction to rolling. Hypomobile joints are treated by using a gliding technique. Thus, it is critical to know the appropriate direction to use for gliding.[9]

Joint Positions

Each joint in the body has a position in which the joint capsule and the ligaments are most relaxed, allowing for a maximum amount of *joint play.*[4,19] This position is called the *resting position.* It is essential to know specifically where the resting position is, because testing for joint play during an evaluation and treatment of the hypomobile joint using either mobilization or traction are usually performed in this position. Table 13-1 summarizes the appropriate resting positions for many of the major joints.

Placing the joint capsule in the resting position allows the joint to assume a *loose-packed position* in which the articulating joint surfaces are maximally separated. A *close-packed position* is one in which there is maximal contact of the articulating surfaces of bones with the capsule and ligaments tight or tense. In a loose-packed position, the joint will exhibit the greatest amount of joint play, while the close-packed position allows for no joint play. Thus, the loose-packed position is most appropriate for mobilization and traction (Figure 13-3).

Both mobilization and traction techniques use a translational movement of 1 joint surface relative to the other. This translation may be either perpendicular or parallel to the *treatment plane.* The treatment plane falls perpendicular to, or at a right angle to, a line running from the axis of rotation in the convex surface to the center of the concave articular surface (Figure 13-4).[17,19] Thus, the treatment plane lies within the concave surface. If the convex segment moves, the treatment plane remains fixed. However, the treatment plane will move along with the concave segment. Mobilization techniques use glides that translate one articulating surface along a line parallel with the treatment plane. Traction techniques translate one of the articulating surfaces in a perpendicular direction to the treatment plane. Both techniques use a loose-packed joint position.[17]

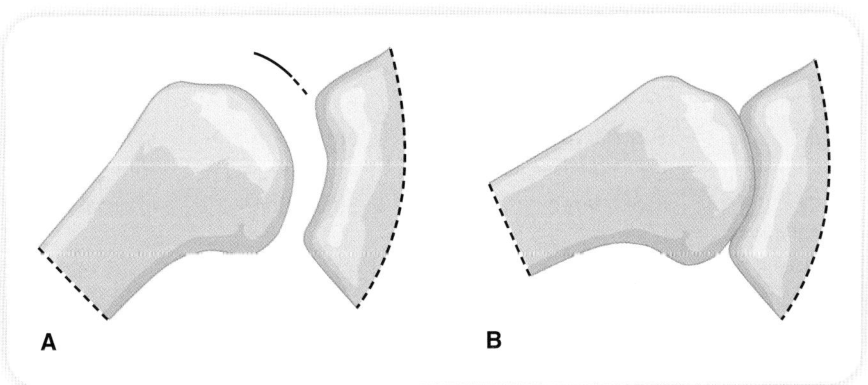

Figure 13-3 Joint capsule resting position

A. Loose-packed position. **B**. Close-packed position.

Table 13-1 Shape, Resting Position, and Treatment Planes of Various Joints

Joint	Convex Surface	Concave Surface	Resting Position (Loose Packed)	Close-Packed Position	Treatment Plane
Sternoclavicular	Clavicle*	Sternum*	Anatomic position	Horizontal	In sternum
Acromioclavicular	Clavicle	Acromion	Anatomic position, in horizontal plane at 60 degrees to sagittal plane	Adduction	In acromion
Glenohumeral	Humerus	Glenoid	Shoulder abducted 55 degrees, horizontally adducted 30 degrees, rotated so that forearm is in horizontal plane	Abduction and lateral rotation	In glenoid fossa in scapular plane
Humeroradial	Humerus	Radius	Elbow extended, forearm supinated	Flexion and forearm production	In radial head perpendicular to long axis of radius
Humeroulnar	Humerus	Ulna	Elbow flexed 70 degrees, forearm supinated 10 degrees	Full extension and forearm supination	In olecranon fossa, 45 degrees to long axis of ulna
Radioulnar (proximal)	Radius	Ulna	Elbow flexed 70 degrees, forearm supinated 35 degrees	Full extension and forearm supination	In radial notch of ulna, parallel to long axis of ulna
Radioulnar (distal)	Ulna	Radius	Supinated 10 degrees	Extension	In radius, parallel to long axis of radius
Radiocarpal	Proximal carpal bones	Radius	Line through radius and third metacarpal	Extension	In radius, perpendicular to long axis of radius
Metacarpo-phalangeal	Metacarpal	Proximal phalanx	Slight flexion	Full flexion	In proximal phalanx
Interphalangeal	Proximal phalanx	Distal phalanx	Slight flexion	Extension	In proximal phalanx
Hip	Femur	Acetabulum	Hip flexed 30 degrees, abducted 30 degrees, slight external rotation	Extension and medial rotation	In acetabulum
Tibiofemoral	Femur	Tibia	Flexed 25 degrees	Full extension	On surface of tibial plateau
Patellofemoral	Patella	Femur	Knee in full extension	Full flexion	Along femoral groove
Talocrural	Talus	Mortise	Plantarflexed 10 degrees	Dorsiflexion	In the mortise in anterior/posterior direction
Subtalar	Calcaneus	Talus	Subtalar neutral between inversion/eversion	Supination	In talus, parallel to foot surface
Intertarsal	Proximal articulating surface	Distal articulating surface	Foot relaxed	Supination	In distal segment
Metatarso-phalangeal	Tarsal bone	Proximal phalanx	Slight extension	Full flexion	In proximal phalanx
Interphalangeal	Proximal phalanx	Distal phalanx	Slight flexion	Extension	In distal phalanx

*In the sternoclavicular joint, the clavicle surface is convex in a superior/inferior direction and concave in an anterior/posterior direction.

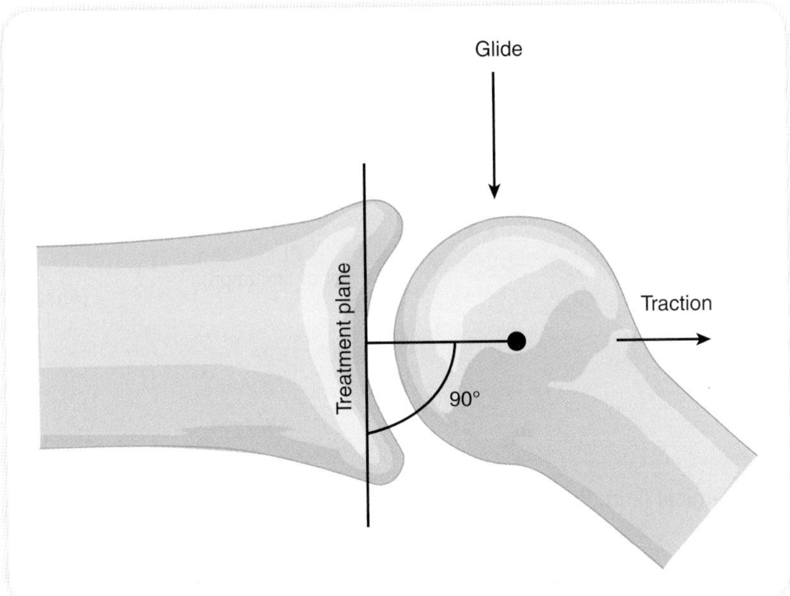

Figure 13-4

The treatment plane is perpendicular to a line drawn from the axis of rotation to the center of the articulating surface of the concave segment.

Joint Mobilization Techniques

The techniques of joint mobilization are used to improve joint mobility or to decrease joint pain by restoring accessory movements to the joint and thus allowing full, nonrestricted, pain-free range of motion.[25,34]

Mobilization techniques may be used to attain a variety of either mechanical or neurophysiological treatment goals: reducing pain; decreasing muscle guarding; stretching or lengthening tissue surrounding a joint, in particular capsular and ligamentous tissue; reflexogenic effects that either inhibit or facilitate muscle tone or stretch reflex; and proprioceptive effects to improve postural and kinesthetic awareness.[1,12,18,24,28,30]

Movement throughout a range of motion can be quantified with various measurement techniques. Physiologic movement is measured with a goniometer and composes the major portion of the range. Accessory motion is thought of in millimeters, although precise measurement is difficult.

Accessory movements may be hypomobile, normal, or hypermobile.[6] Each joint has a range-of-motion continuum with an anatomical limit to motion that is determined by both bony arrangement and surrounding soft tissue (Figure 13-5). In a hypomobile joint, motion stops at some point referred to as a pathologic point of limitation, short of the anatomical limit caused by pain, spasm, or tissue resistance. A hypermobile joint moves beyond its anatomical limit because of laxity of the surrounding structures. A hypomobile joint should respond well to techniques of mobilization and traction. A hypermobile joint should be treated with strengthening exercises, stability exercises, and if indicated, taping, splinting, or bracing.[29,30]

In a hypomobile joint, as mobilization techniques are used in the range-of-motion restriction, some deformation of soft-tissue capsular or ligamentous structures occurs. If a tissue is stretched only into its elastic range, no permanent structural changes will occur.

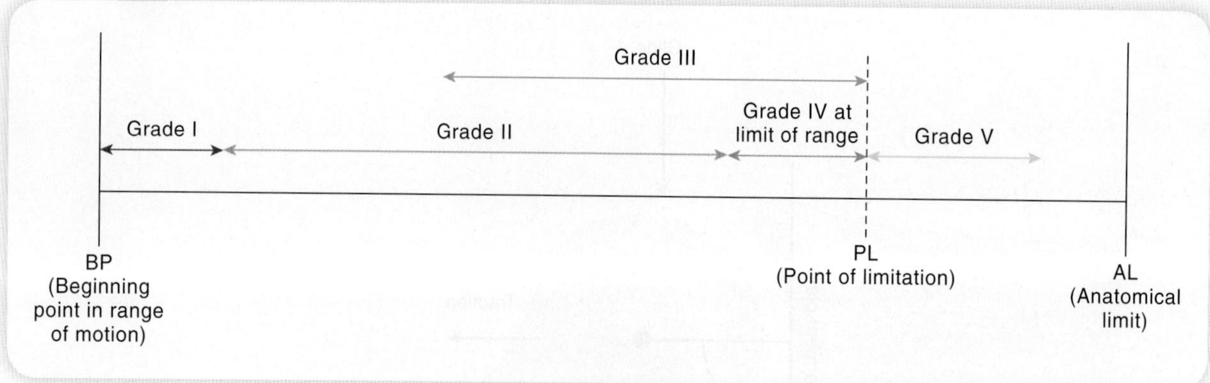

Figure 13-5

Maitland's five grades of motion. AL, anatomical limit; PL, point of limitation.

However, if that tissue is stretched into its plastic range, permanent structural changes will occur. Thus, mobilization and traction can be used to stretch tissue and break adhesions. If used inappropriately, they can also damage tissue and cause sprains of the joint.[30]

Treatment techniques designed to improve accessory movement are generally slow, small-amplitude movements, the amplitude being the distance that the joint is moved passively within its total range. Mobilization techniques use these small-amplitude oscillating motions that glide or slide one of the articulating joint surfaces in an appropriate direction within a specific part of the range.[22]

Clinical Pearl

If a patient is restricted in extension, and lateral rotation because of tightness in the anterior capsule causing the restriction, then the humeral head should be glided anteriorly on the glenoid to stretch the restriction.

Maitland has described various grades of oscillation for joint mobilization. The amplitude of each oscillation grade falls within the range-of-motion continuum between some beginning point and the anatomical limit.[23,24] Figure 13-5 shows the various grades of oscillation that are used in a joint with some limitation of motion. As the severity of the movement restriction increases, the point of limitation moves to the left, away from the anatomical limit. However, the relationships that exist among the 5 grades in terms of their positions within the range of motion remain the same. The 5 mobilization grades are defined as follows:

Grade I. A small-amplitude movement at the beginning of the range of movement. Used when pain and spasm limit movement early in the range of motion.[37]

Grade II. A large-amplitude movement within the midrange of movement. Used when spasm limits movement sooner with a quick oscillation than with a slow one, or when slowly increasing pain restricts movement halfway into the range.

Grade III. A large-amplitude movement up to the point of limitation in the range of movement. Used when pain and resistance from spasm, inert tissue tension, or tissue compression limit movement near the end of the range.

Grade IV. A small-amplitude movement at the very end of the range of movement. Used when resistance limits movement in the absence of pain and spasm.

Grade V. A small-amplitude, quick thrust delivered at the end of the range of movement, usually accompanied by a popping sound, called a manipulation. Used when minimal resistance limits the end of the range. Manipulation is most effectively accomplished by the velocity of the thrust rather than by the force of the thrust.[21] Most authorities agree that manipulation should be used only by individuals trained specifically in these techniques, because a great deal of skill and judgment is necessary for safe and effective treatment.[31,32]

Clinical Pearl

Most manipulations performed by a chiropractor are grade V. They take the joint to the end range of motion and then apply a quick, small-amplitude thrust that forces the joint just beyond the point of limitation. Grade V manipulations should be performed only by those specifically trained in this technique. Laws and practice acts relative to the use of manipulations vary considerably from state to state.

Joint mobilization uses these oscillating gliding motions of one articulating joint surface in whatever direction is appropriate for the existing restriction. The appropriate direction for these oscillating glides is determined by the convex-concave rule, described previously. When the concave surface is stationary and the convex surface is mobilized, a glide of the convex segment should be in the direction opposite to the restriction of joint movement (Figure 13-6*A*).[17,19,35] If the convex articular surface is stationary and the concave surface is mobilized, gliding of the concave segment should be in the same direction as the restriction of joint movement (Figure 13-6*B*). For example, the glenohumeral joint would be considered to be a convex joint with the convex humeral head moving on the concave glenoid. If shoulder abduction is restricted, the humerus should be glided in an inferior direction relative to the glenoid to alleviate the motion restriction. When mobilizing the knee joint, the concave tibia should be glided anteriorly in cases where knee extension is restricted. If mobilization in the appropriate direction exacerbates complaints of pain or stiffness, the therapist should apply the technique in the opposite direction until the patient can tolerate the appropriate direction.[35]

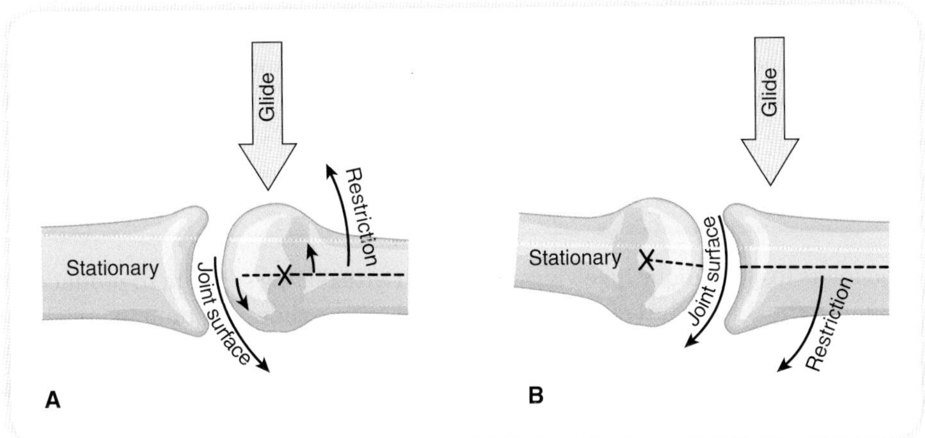

Figure 13-6 **Gliding motions**

A. Glides of the convex segment should be in the direction opposite to the restriction.
B. Glides of the concave segment should be in the direction of the restriction.

Typical mobilization of a joint may involve a series of 3 to 6 sets of oscillations lasting between 20 and 60 seconds each, with 1 to 3 oscillations per second.[23,24]

Clinical Pearl

Traction applied to the spine increases space in between the vertebrae. The increased space reduces the pressure and compressive forces on the disk.

Indications for Mobilization

In Maitland's system, grades I and II are used primarily for treatment of pain and grades III and IV are used for treating stiffness. Pain must be treated first and stiffness second.[24] Painful conditions should be treated on a daily basis. The purpose of the small-amplitude oscillations is to stimulate mechanoreceptors within the joint that can limit the transmission of pain perception at the spinal cord or brainstem levels.

Joints that are stiff or hypomobile and have restricted movement should be treated 3 to 4 times per week on alternating days with active motion exercise. The therapist must continuously reevaluate the joint to determine appropriate progression from one oscillation grade to another.

Indications for specific mobilization grades are relatively straightforward. If the patient complains of pain before the therapist can apply any resistance to movement, it is too early, and all mobilization techniques should be avoided. If pain is elicited when resistance to motion is applied, mobilization, using grades I, II, and III, is appropriate. If resistance can be applied before pain is elicited, mobilization can be progressed to grade IV. Mobilization should be done with both the patient and the therapist positioned in a comfortable and relaxed manner. The therapist should mobilize 1 joint at a time. The joint should be stabilized as near 1 articulating surface as possible, while moving the other segment with a firm, confident grasp.

Contraindications for Mobilization

Techniques of mobilization and manipulation should not be used haphazardly. These techniques should generally not be used in cases of inflammatory arthritis, malignancy, bone disease, neurological involvement, bone fracture, congenital bone deformities, and vascular disorders of the vertebral artery. Again, manipulation should be performed only by those therapist specifically trained in the procedure, because some special knowledge and judgment are required for effective treatment.[24]

Joint Traction Techniques

Traction refers to a technique involving pulling on 1 articulating segment to produce some separation of the 2 joint surfaces. Although mobilization glides are done parallel to the treatment plane, traction is performed perpendicular to the treatment plane (Figure 13-7). Like mobilization techniques, traction may be used either to decrease pain or to reduce joint hypomobility.[38]

Kaltenborn has proposed a system using traction combined with mobilization as a means of reducing pain or mobilizing hypomobile joints.[16] As discussed earlier, all joints have a certain amount of play or looseness. Kaltenborn referred to this looseness as *slack*. Some degree of slack is necessary for normal joint motion. Kaltenborn's 3 traction grades are defined as follows (Figure 13-8)[17]:

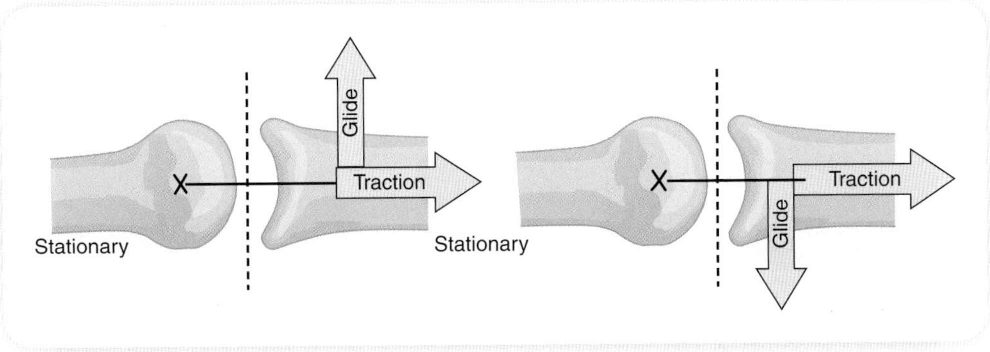

Figure 13-7 **Traction versus glides**

Traction is perpendicular to the treatment plane, whereas glides are parallel to the treatment plane.

Grade I traction (loosen). Traction that neutralizes pressure in the joint without actual separation of the joint surfaces. The purpose is to produce pain relief by reducing the compressive forces of articular surfaces during mobilization and is used with all mobilization grades.

Grade II traction (tighten or "take up the slack"). Traction that effectively separates the articulating surfaces and takes up the slack or eliminates play in the joint capsule. Grade II is used in initial treatment to determine joint sensitivity.

Grade III traction (stretch). Traction that involves actual stretching of the soft tissue surrounding the joint to increase mobility in a hypomobile joint.

Grade I traction should be used in the initial treatment to reduce the chance of a painful reaction. It is recommended that 10-second intermittent grades I and II traction be used, distracting the joint surfaces up to a grade III traction and then releasing distraction until the joint returns to its resting position.[16]

Kaltenborn emphasizes that grade III traction should be used in conjunction with mobilization glides to treat joint hypomobility (see Figure 13-7).[17] Grade III traction stretches the joint capsule and increases the space between the articulating surfaces, placing the joint

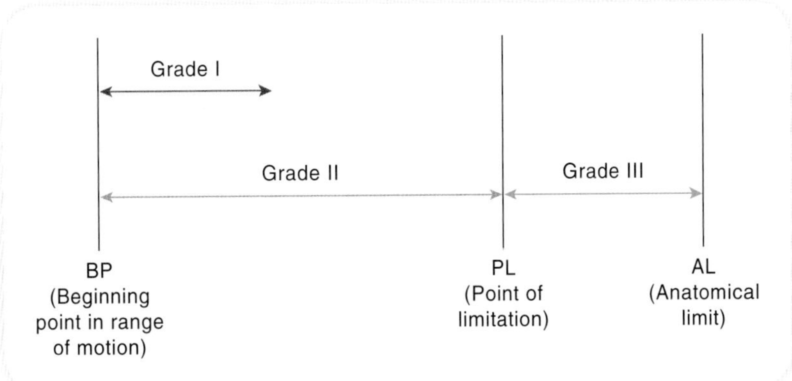

Figure 13-8

Kaltenborn's grades of traction. AL, anatomical limit; PL, point of limitation.

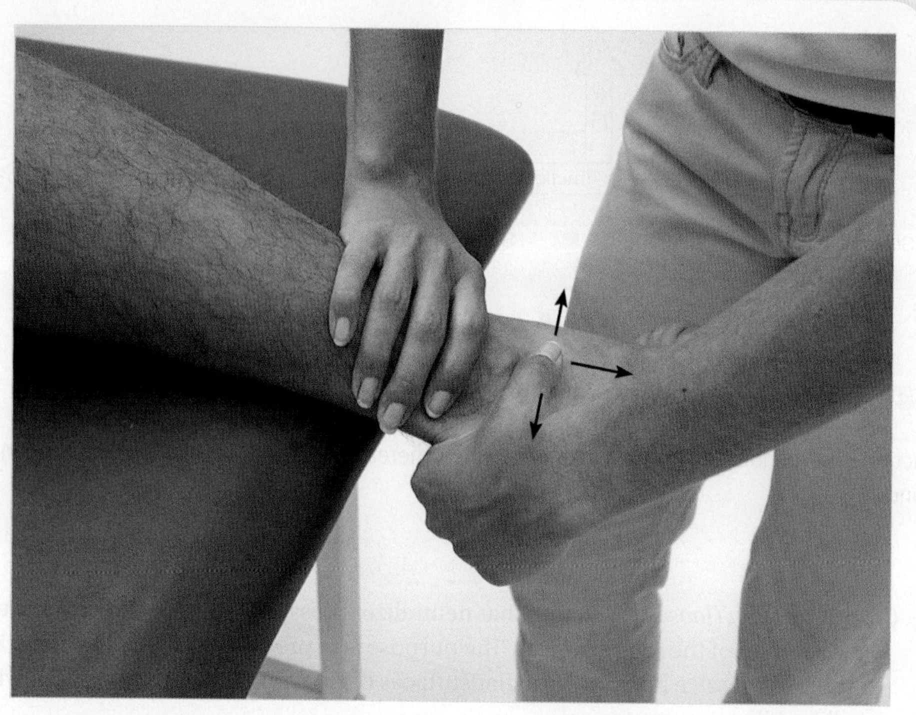

Figure 13-9 Traction and mobilization should be used together

in a loose-packed position. Applying grades III and IV oscillations within the patient's pain limitations should maximally improve joint mobility (Figure 13-9).[16]

Mobilization and Traction Techniques

Figures 13-10 to 13-73 provide descriptions and illustrations of various mobilization and traction techniques. These figures should be used to determine appropriate hand positioning, stabilization (S), and the correct direction for gliding (G), traction (T), and/or rotation (R). The information presented in this chapter should be used as a reference base for appropriately incorporating joint mobilization and traction techniques into the rehabilitation program.

Mulligan Joint Mobilization Technique

Brian Mulligan, an Australian therapist, proposed a concept of mobilizations based on Kaltenborn's principles. Whereas Kaltenborn's technique relies on passive accessory mobilization, the Mulligan technique combines passive accessory joint mobilization applied by a therapist with active physiological movement by the patient for the purpose of correcting positional faults and returning the patient to normal pain-free function.[27] It is a noninvasive and comfortable intervention, and has applications for the spine and the extremities. Mulligan's concept uses what are referred to as either *mobilizations with movement* for treating the extremities, or *sustained natural apophyseal glides* for treating problems in the spine.[36] Instead of the therapist using oscillations or thrusting techniques, the patient moves in a specific direction as the therapist guides the restricted body part. Mobilizations with

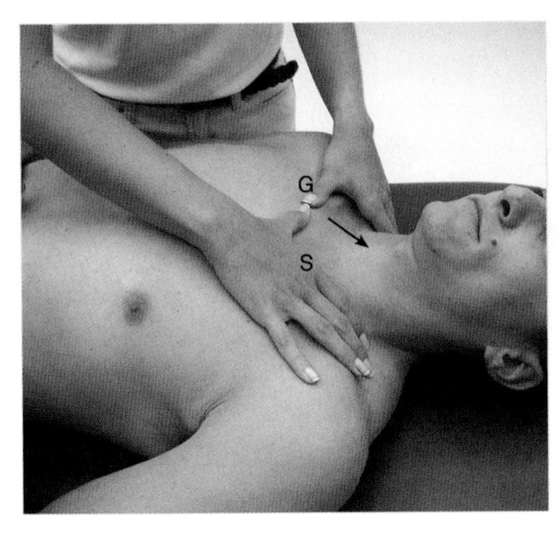

Figure 13-10 **Posterior and superior clavicular glides**

When posterior or superior clavicular glides are done at the sternoclavicular joint, use the thumbs to glide the clavicle. Posterior glides are used to increase clavicular retraction, and superior glides increase clavicular retraction and clavicular depression.

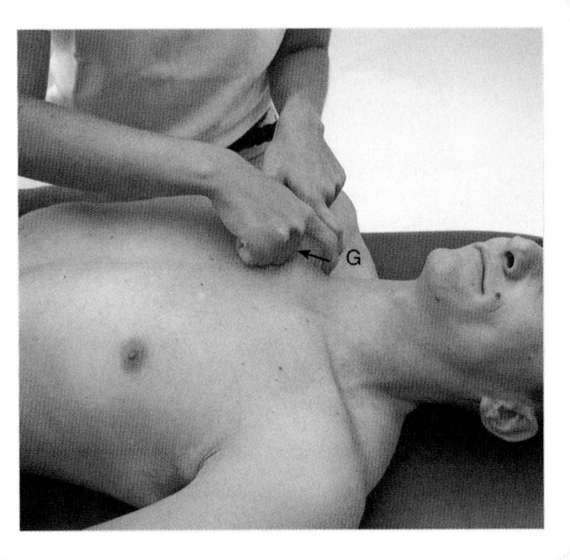

Figure 13-11 **Inferior clavicular glides**

Inferior clavicular glides at the sternoclavicular joint use the index fingers to mobilize the clavicle, which increases clavicular elevation.

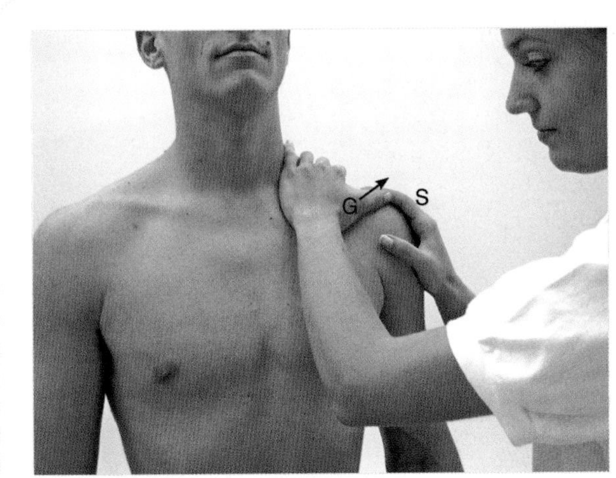

Figure 13-12 **Posterior clavicular glides**

Posterior clavicular glides done at the acromioclavicular (AC) joint apply posterior pressure on the clavicle while stabilizing the scapula with the opposite hand. They increase mobility of the AC joint.

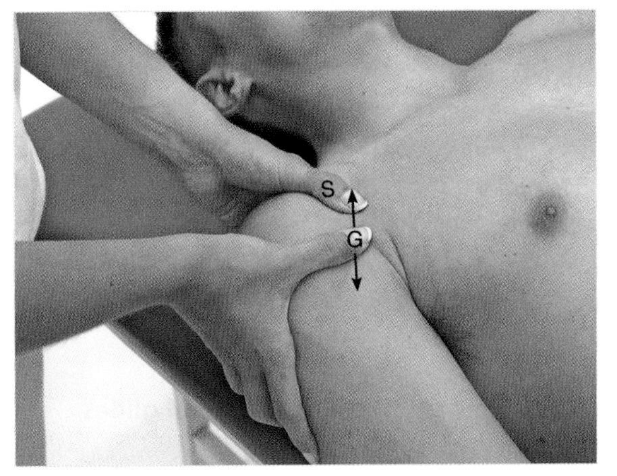

Figure 13-13 **Anterior/posterior glenohumeral glides**

Anterior/posterior glenohumeral glides are done with one hand stabilizing the scapula and the other gliding the humeral head. They initiate motion in the painful shoulder.

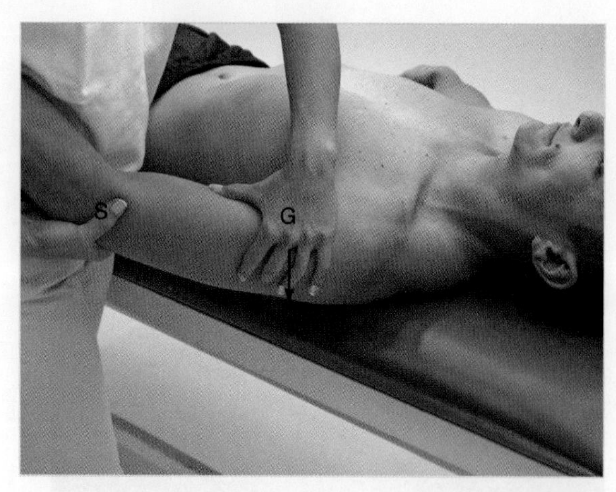

Figure 13-14 **Posterior humeral glides**

Posterior humeral glides use 1 hand to stabilize the humerus at the elbow and the other to glide the humeral head. They increase flexion and medial rotation.

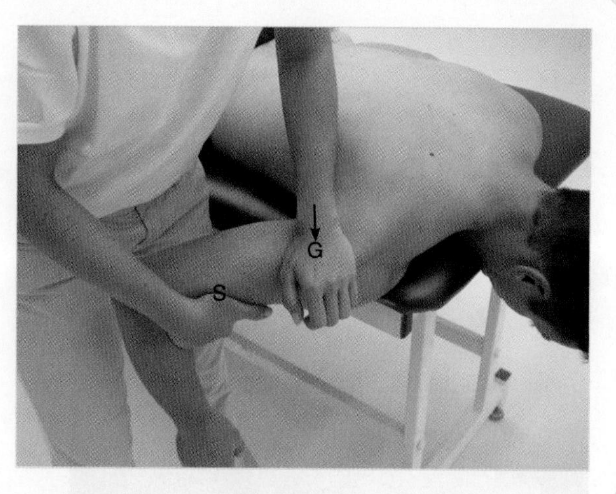

Figure 13-15 **Anterior humeral glides**

In anterior humeral glides the patient is prone. One hand stabilizes the humerus at the elbow and the other glides the humeral head. They increase extension and lateral rotation.

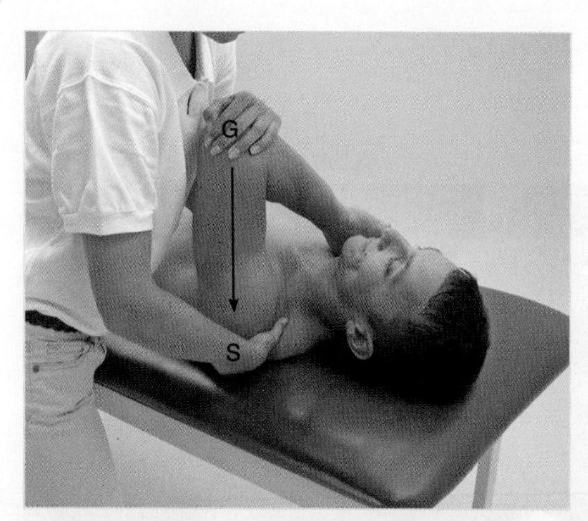

Figure 13-16 **Posterior humeral glides**

Posterior humeral glides may also be done with the shoulder at 90 degrees. With the patient in supine position, one hand stabilizes the scapula underneath while the patient's elbow is secured at the therapist's shoulder. Glides are directed downward through the humerus. They increase horizontal adduction.

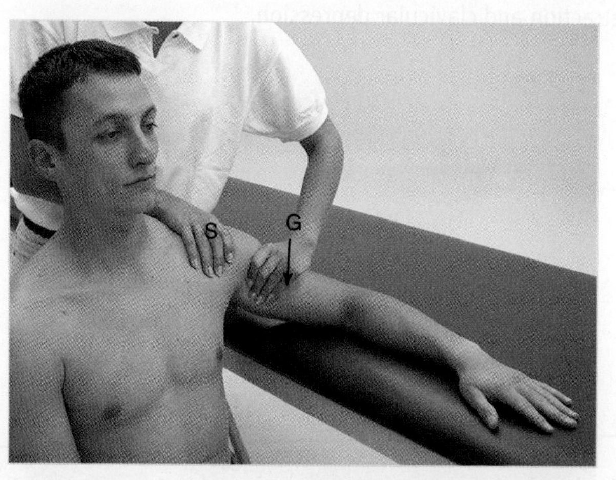

Figure 13-17 **Inferior humeral glides**

For inferior humeral glides, the patient is in the sitting position with the elbow resting on the treatment table. One hand stabilizes the scapula and the other glides the humeral head inferiorly. These glides increase shoulder abduction.

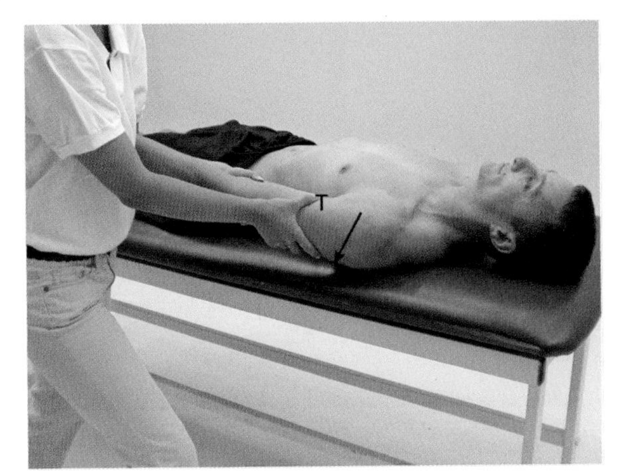

Figure 13-18 **Lateral glenohumeral joint traction**

Lateral glenohumeral joint traction is used for initial testing of joint mobility and for decreasing pain. One hand stabilizes the elbow while the other applies lateral traction at the upper humerus.

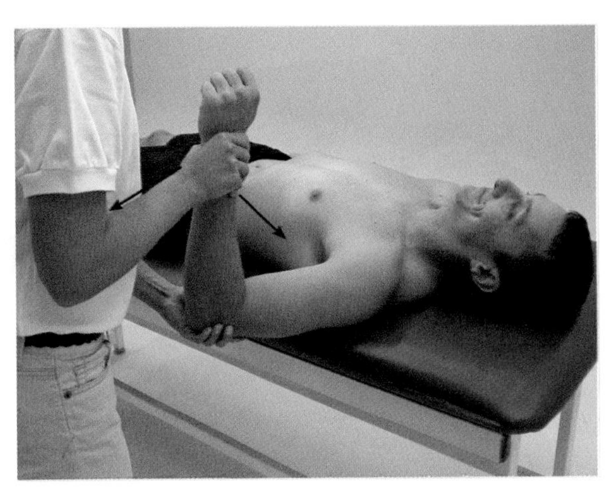

Figure 13-19 **Medial and lateral rotation oscillations**

Medial and lateral rotation oscillations with the shoulder abducted at 90 degrees can increase medial and lateral rotation in a progressive manner according to patient tolerance.

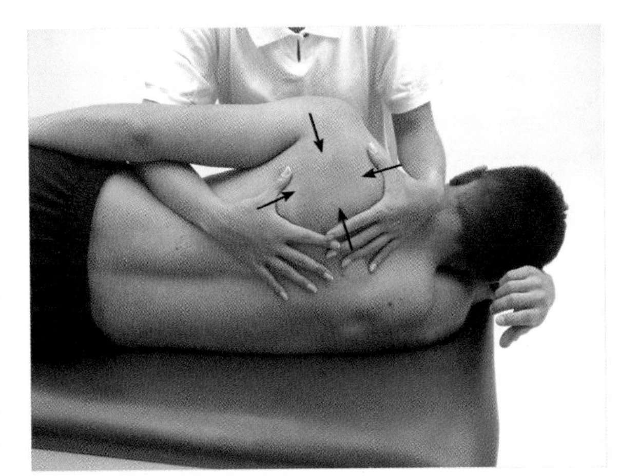

Figure 13-20 **General scapular glides**

General scapular glides may be done in all directions, applying pressure at either the medial, inferior, lateral, or superior border of the scapula. Scapular glides increase general scapulothoracic mobility.

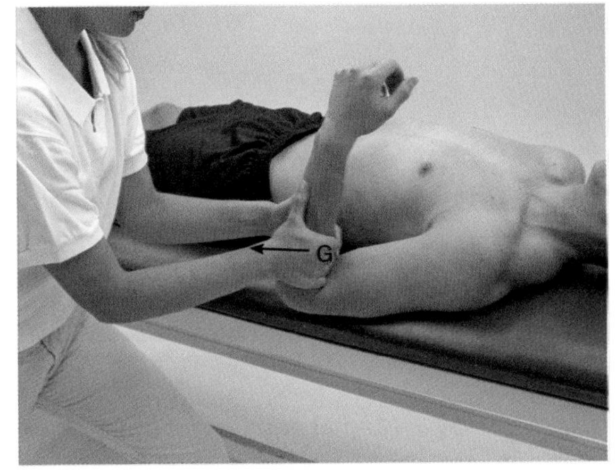

Figure 13-21 **Inferior humeroulnar glides**

Inferior humeroulnar glides increase elbow flexion and extension. They are performed using the body weight to stabilize proximally with the hand grasping the ulna and gliding inferiorly.

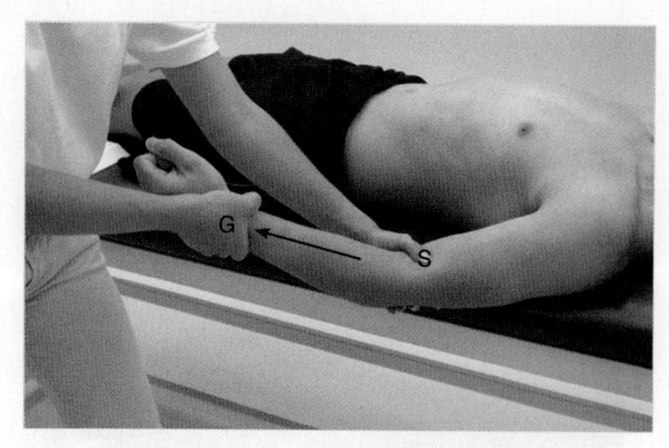

Figure 13-22 **Humeroradial inferior glides**

Humeroradial inferior glides increase the joint space and improve flexion and extension. One hand stabilizes the humerus above the elbow; the other grasps the distal forearm and glides the radius inferiorly.

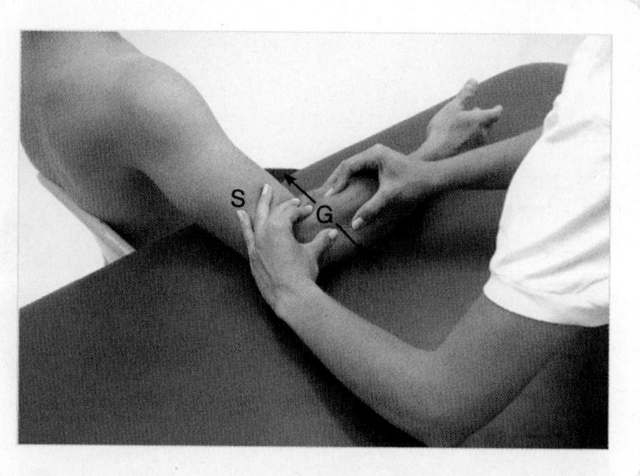

Figure 13-23 **Proximal anterior/posterior radial glides**

Proximal anterior/posterior radial glides use the thumbs and index fingers to glide the radial head. Anterior glides increase flexion, while posterior glides increase extension.

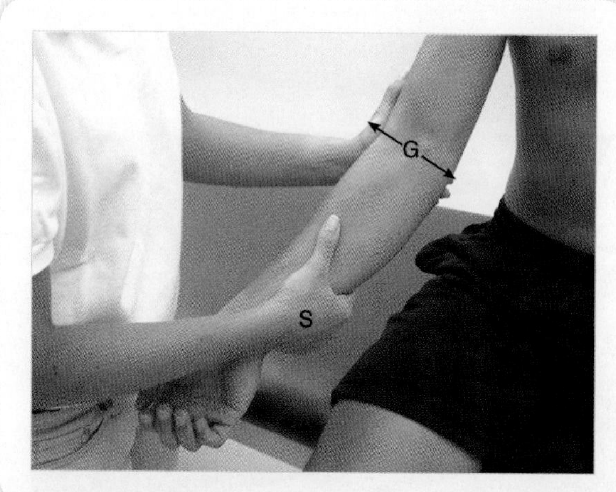

Figure 13-24 **Medial and lateral ulnar oscillations**

Medial and lateral ulnar oscillations increase flexion and extension. Valgus and varus forces are used with a short-lever arm.

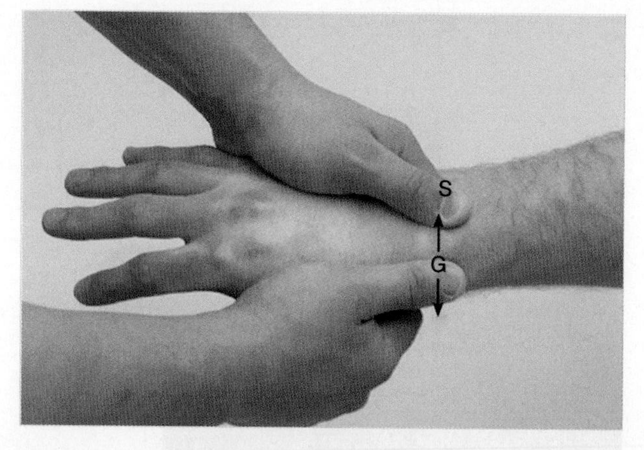

Figure 13-25 **Distal anterior/posterior radial glides**

Distal anterior/posterior radial glides are done with one hand stabilizing the ulna and the other gliding the radius. These glides increase pronation.

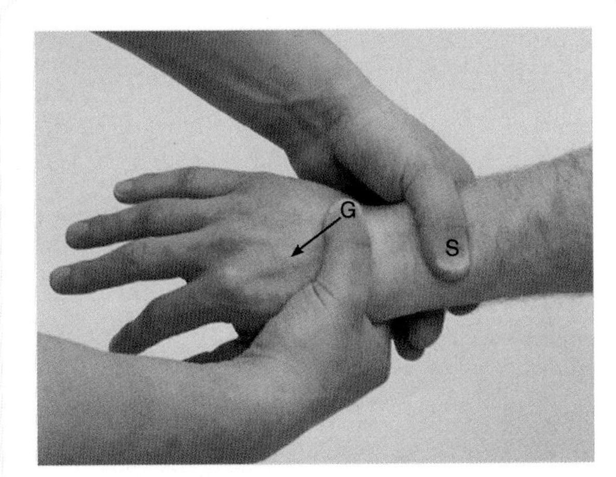

Figure 13-26 Radiocarpal joint anterior glides

Radiocarpal joint anterior glides increase wrist extension.

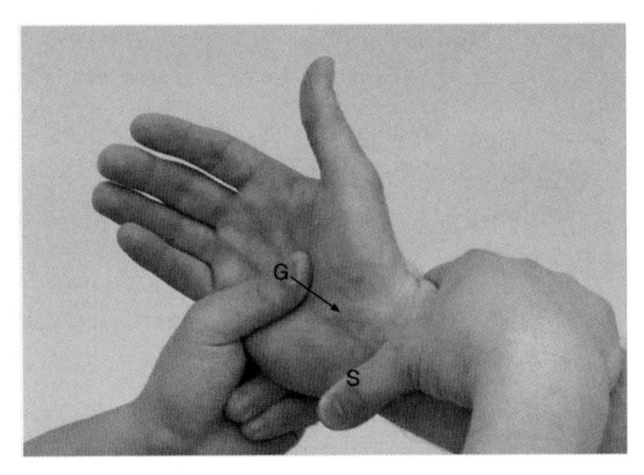

Figure 13-27 Radiocarpal joint posterior glides

Radiocarpal joint posterior glides increase wrist flexion.

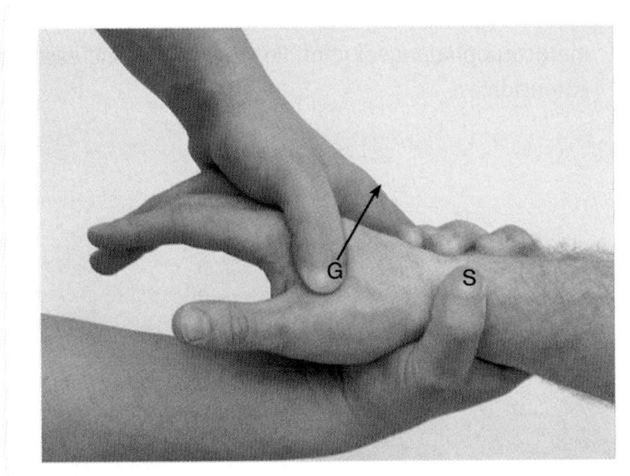

Figure 13-28 Radiocarpal joint ulnar glides

Radiocarpal joint ulnar glides increase radial deviation.

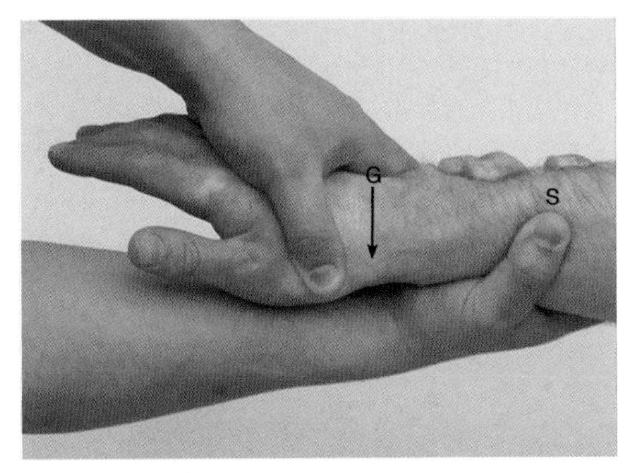

Figure 13-29 Radiocarpal joint radial glides

Radiocarpal joint radial glides increase ulnar deviation.

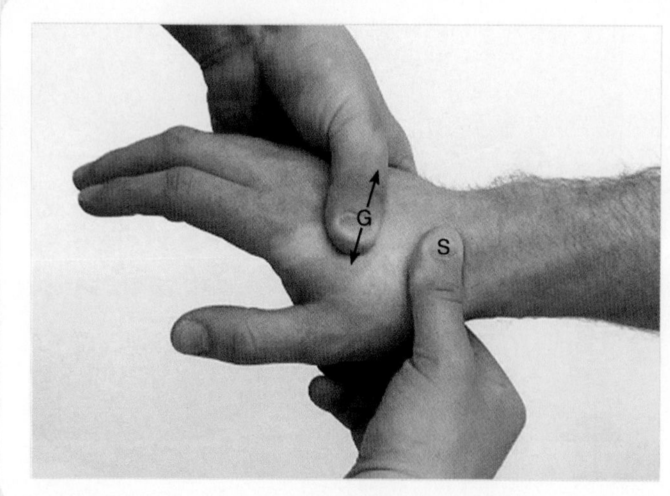

Figure 13-30 Carpometacarpal joint anterior/posterior glides

Carpometacarpal joint anterior/posterior glides increase mobility of the hand.

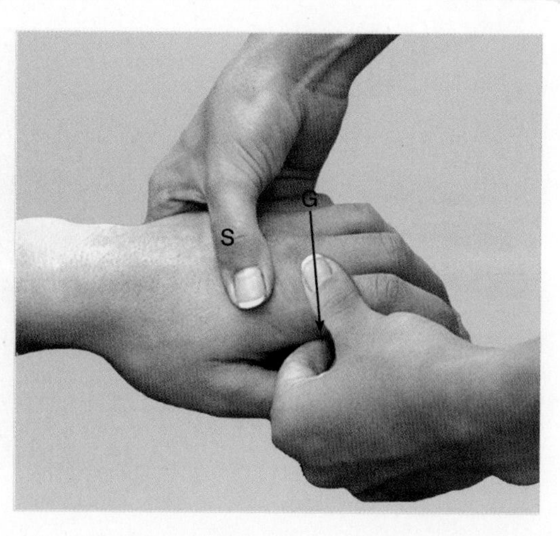

Figure 13-31 Metacarpophalangeal joint anterior/posterior glides

In metacarpophalangeal joint anterior or posterior glides, the proximal segment, in this case the metacarpal, is stabilized and the distal segment is mobilized. Anterior glides increase flexion of the metacarpophalangeal joint. Posterior glides increase extension.

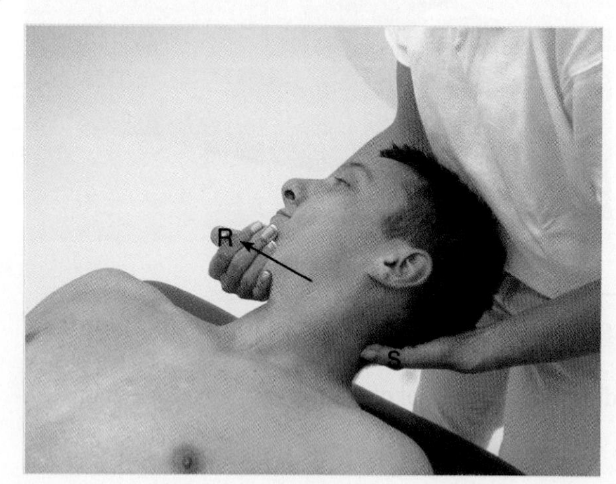

Figure 13-32 Cervical vertebrae rotation oscillations

Cervical vertebrae rotation oscillations are done with one hand supporting the weight of the head and the other rotating the head in the direction of the restriction. These oscillations treat pain or stiffness when there is some resistance in the same direction as the rotation.

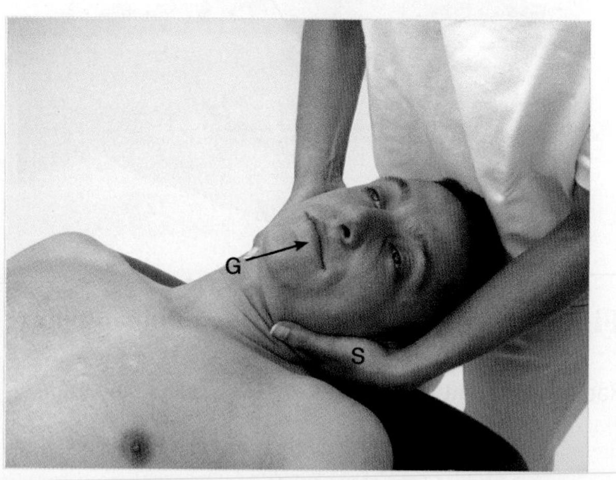

Figure 13-33 Cervical vertebrae sidebending

Cervical vertebrae sidebending may be used to treat paint or stiffness with resistance when sidebending the neck.

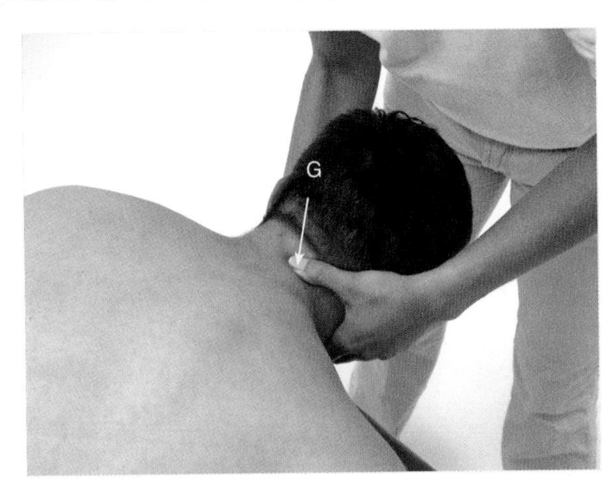

Figure 13-34 Unilateral cervical facet anterior/posterior glides

Unilateral cervical facet anterior/posterior glides are done using pressure from the thumbs over individual facets. They increase rotation or flexion of the neck toward the side where the technique is used.

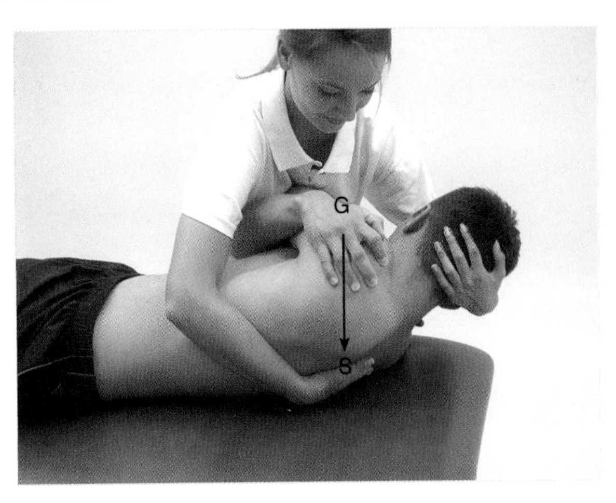

Figure 13-35 Thoracic vertebral facet rotations

Thoracic vertebral facet rotations are accomplished with one hand underneath the patient providing stabilization and the weight of the body pressing downward through the rib cage to rotate an individual thoracic vertebrae. Rotation of the thoracic vertebrae is minimal, and most of the movement with this mobilization involves the rib facet joint.

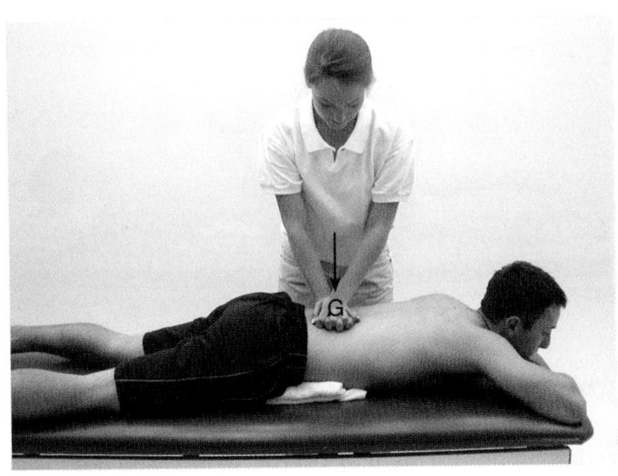

Figure 13-36 Anterior/posterior lumbar vertebral glides

In the lumbar region, anterior/posterior lumbar vertebral glides may be accomplished at individual segments using pressure on the spinous process through the pisiform in the hand. These decrease pain or increase mobility of individual lumbar vertebrae.

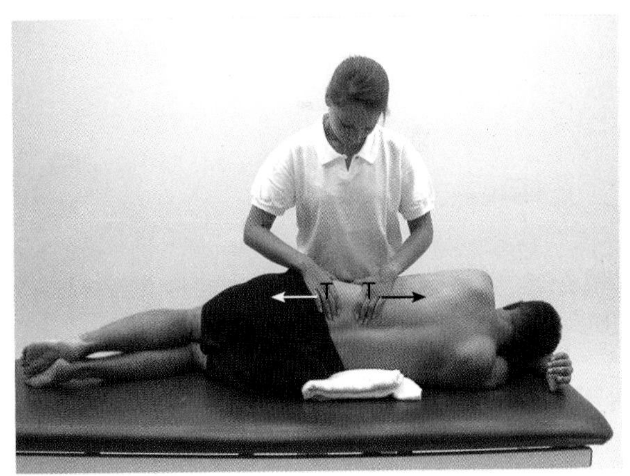

Figure 13-37 Lumbar lateral distraction

Lumbar lateral distraction increases the space between transverse processes and increases the opening of the intervertebral foramen. This position is achieved by lying over a support, flexing the patient's upper knee to a point where there is gapping in the appropriate spinal segment, then rotating the upper trunk to place the segment in a close-packed position. Then finger and forearm pressure are used to separate individual spaces. This pressure is used for reducing pain in the lumber vertebrae associated with some compression of a spinal segment.

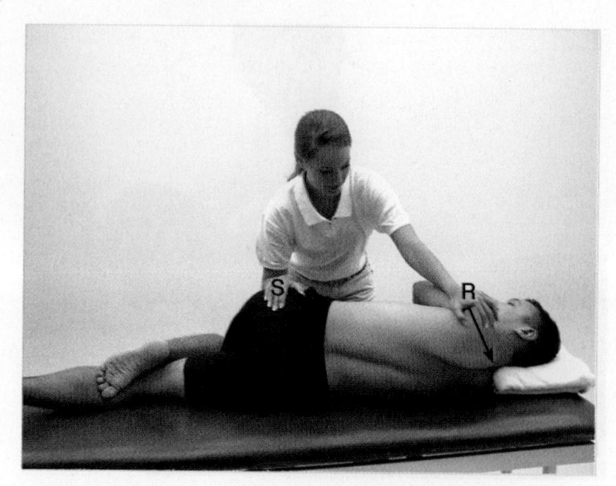

Figure 13-38 **Lumbar vertebral rotations**

Lumbar vertebral rotations decrease pain and increase mobility in lumbar vertebrae. These rotations should be done in a side-lying position.

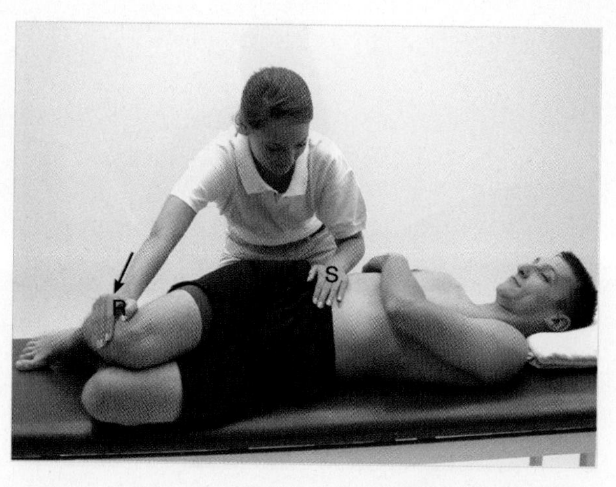

Figure 13-39 **Lateral lumber rotations**

Lateral lumbar rotations may be done with the patient in supine position. In this position, one hand must stabilize the upper trunk, while the other produces rotation.

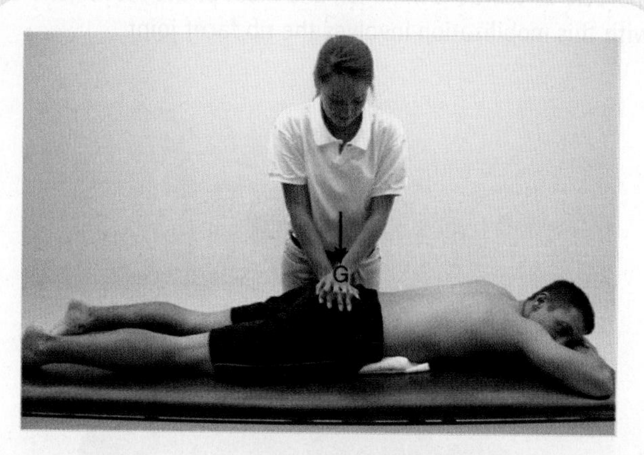

Figure 13-40 **Anterior sacral glides**

Anterior sacral glides decrease pain and reduce muscle guarding around the sacroiliac joint.

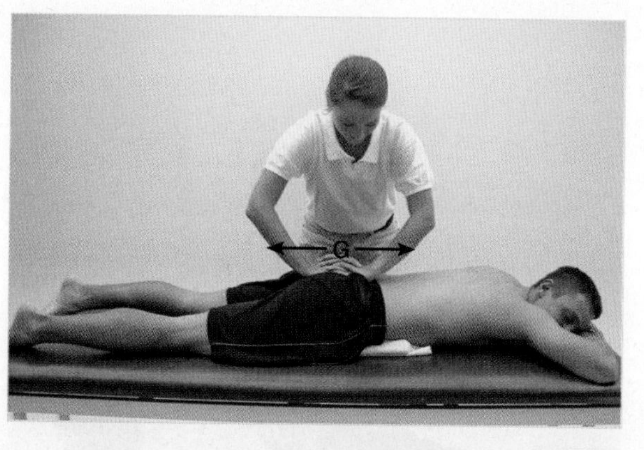

Figure 13-41 **Superior/inferior sacral glides**

Superior/inferior sacral glides decrease pain and reduce muscle guarding around the sacroiliac joint.

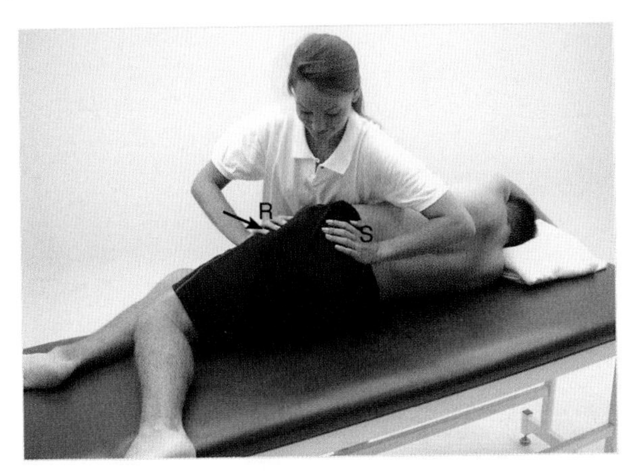

Figure 13-42 **Anterior innominate rotation**

An anterior innominate rotation in a side-lying position is accomplished by extending the leg on the affected side then stabilizing with one hand on the front of the thigh while the other applies pressure anteriorly over the posterosuperior iliac spine to produce an anterior rotation. This technique will correct a unilateral posterior rotation.

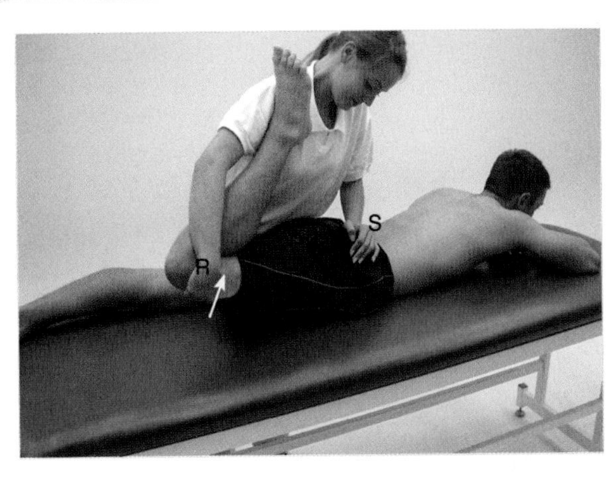

Figure 13-43 **Anterior innominate rotation**

An anterior innominate rotation may also be accomplished by extending the hip, applying upward force on the upper thigh, and stabilizing over the posterosuperior iliac spine. This technique is used to correct a posterior unilateral innominate rotation.

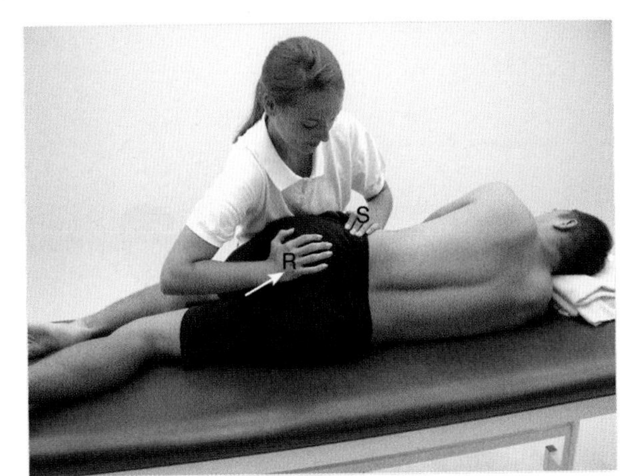

Figure 13-44 **Posterior innominate rotation**

A posterior innominate rotation with the patient in side-lying position is done by flexing the hip, stabilizing the anterosuperior iliac spine, and applying pressure to the ischium in an anterior direction.

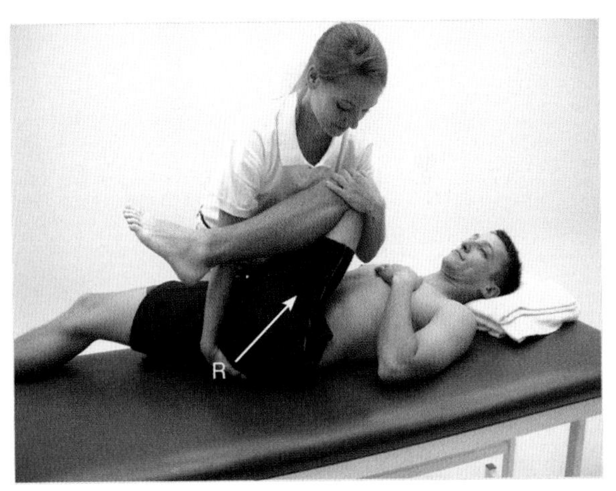

Figure 13-45 **Posterior innominate rotation**

Another posterior innominate rotation with the hip flexed at 90 degrees stabilizes the knee and rotates the innominate anteriorly through upward pressure on the ischium.

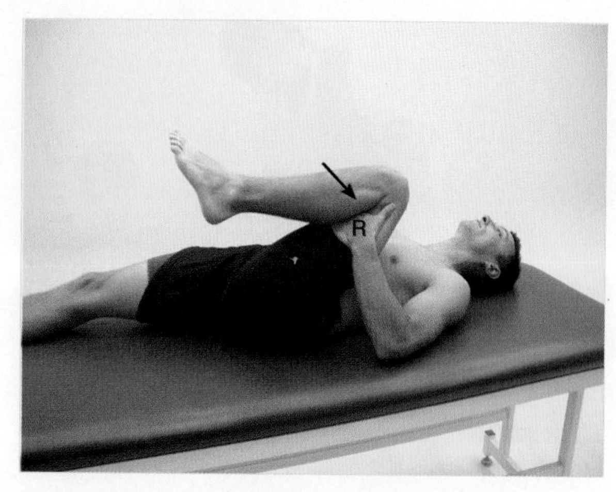

Figure 13-46 Posterior innominate rotation self-mobilization (supine)

Posterior innominate rotation may be easily accomplished using self-mobilization. In a supine position, the patient grasps behind the flexed knee and gently rocks the innominate in a posterior direction.

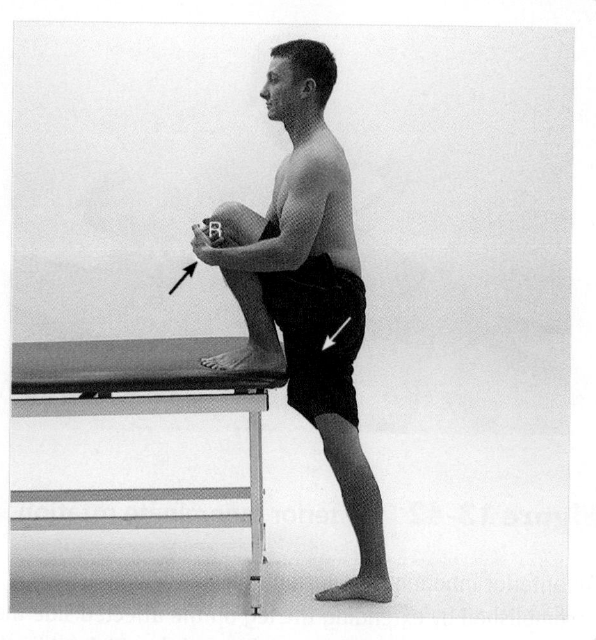

Figure 13-47 Posterior rotation self-mobilization (standing)

In a standing position, the patient can perform a posterior rotation self-mobilization by pulling on the knee and rocking forward.

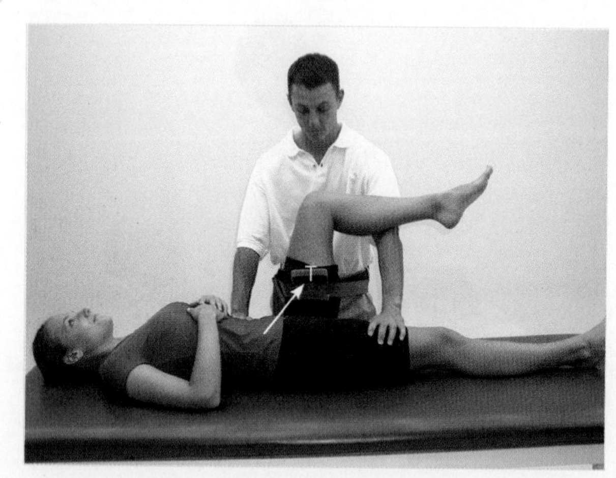

Figure 13-48 Lateral hip traction

Because the hip is a very strong, stable joint, it may be necessary to use body weight to produce effective joint mobilization or traction. An example of this would be in lateral hip traction. One strap should be used to secure the patient to the treatment table. A second strap is secured around the patient's thigh and around the therapist's hips. Lateral traction is applied to the femur by leaning back away from the patient. This technique is used to reduce pain and increase hip mobility.

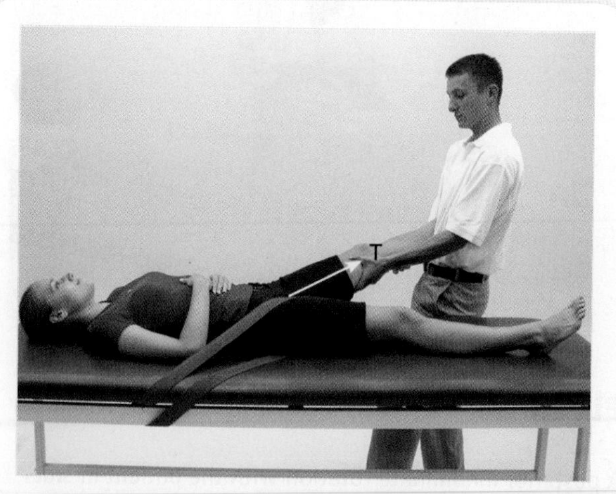

Figure 13-49 Femoral traction

Femoral traction with the hip at 0 degrees reduces pain and increases hip mobility. Inferior femoral glides in this position should be used to increase flexion and abduction.

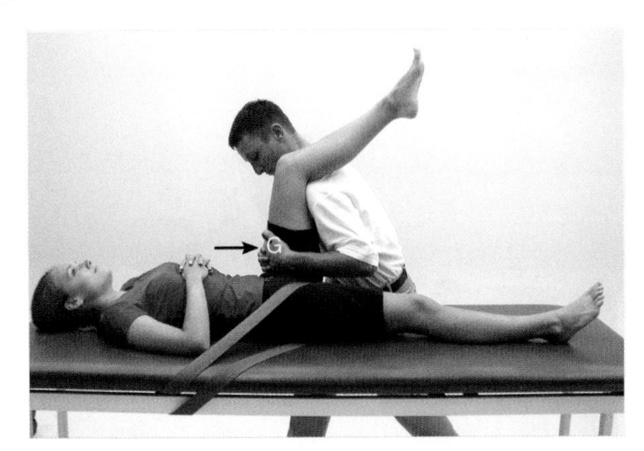

Figure 13-50 Inferior femoral glides

Inferior femoral glides at 90 degrees of hip flexion may also be used to increase abduction and flexion.

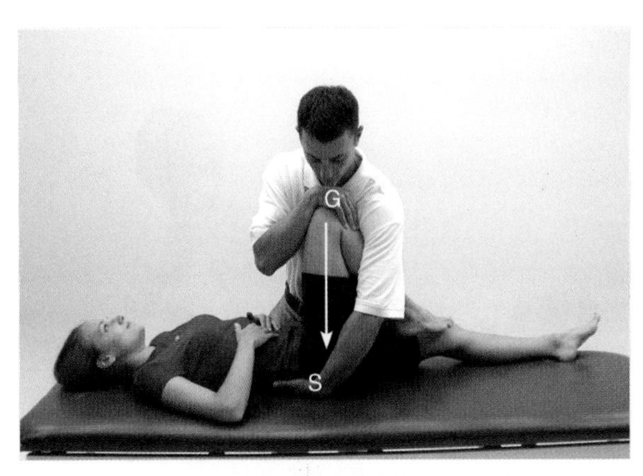

Figure 13-51 Posterior femoral glides

With the patient supine, a posterior femoral glide can be done by stabilizing underneath the pelvis and using the body weight applied through the femur to glide posteriorly. Posterior glides are used to increase hip flexion.

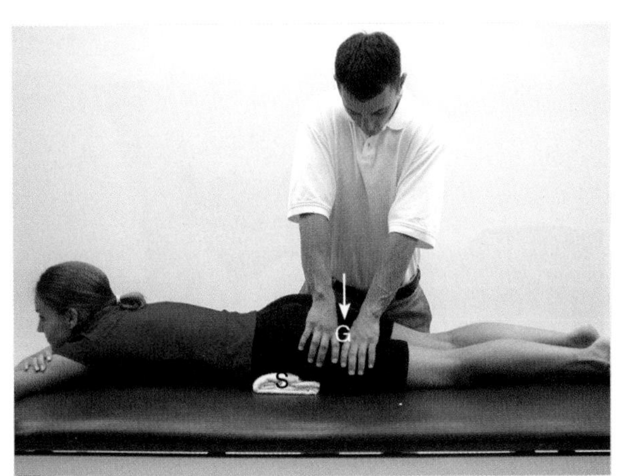

Figure 13-52 Anterior femoral glides

Anterior femoral glides increase extension and are accomplished by using some support to stabilize under the pelvis and applying an anterior glide posteriorly on the femur.

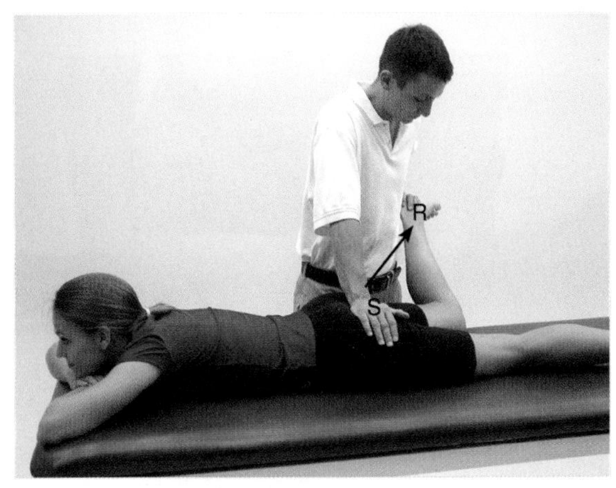

Figure 13-53 Medial femoral rotations

Medial femoral rotations may be used for increasing medial rotation and are done by stabilizing the opposite innominate while internally rotating the hip through the flexed knee.

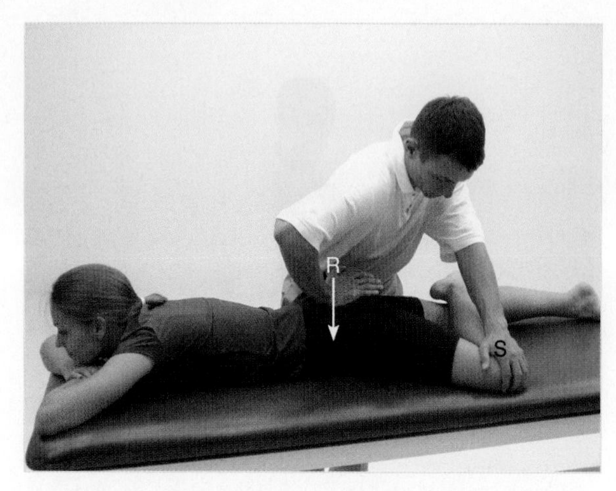

Figure 13-54 **Lateral femoral rotation**

Lateral femoral rotation is done by stabilizing a bent knee in the figure 4 position and applying rotational force to the ischium. This technique increases lateral femoral rotation.

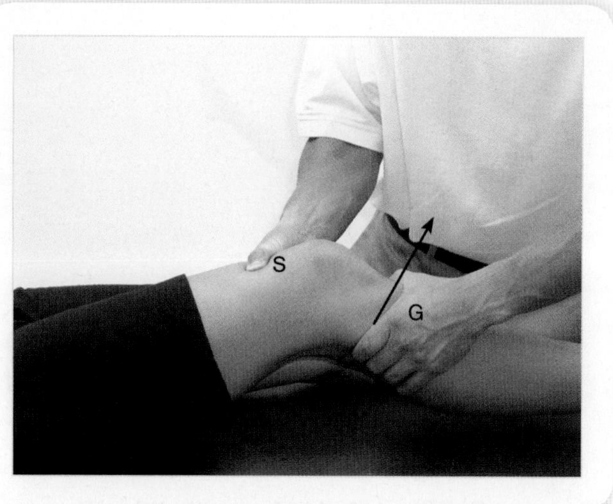

Figure 13-55 **Anterior tibial glides**

Anterior tibial glides are appropriate for the patient lacking full extension. Anterior glides should be done in prone position with the femur stabilized. Pressure is applied to the posterior tibia to glide anteriorly.

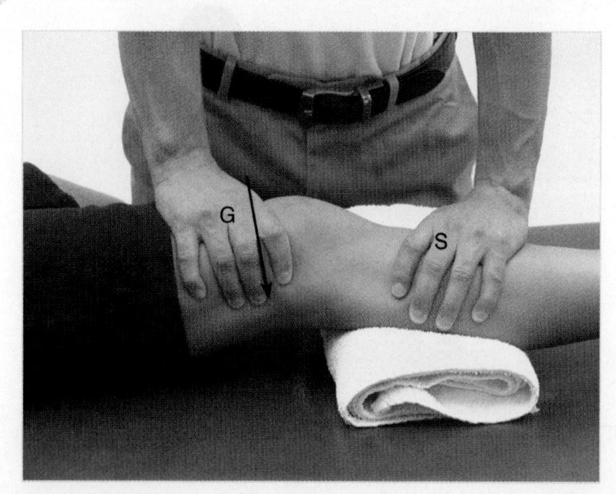

Figure 13-56 **Posterior femoral glides**

Posterior femoral glides are appropriate for the patient lacking full extension. Posterior femoral glides should be done in supine position with the tibia stabilized. Pressure is applied to the anterior femur to glide posteriorly.

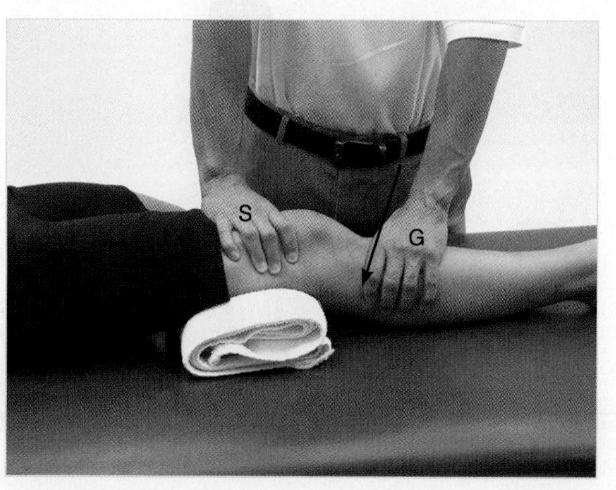

Figure 13-57 **Posterior tibial glides**

Posterior tibial glides increase flexion. With the patient in supine position, stabilize the femur, and glide the tibia posteriorly.

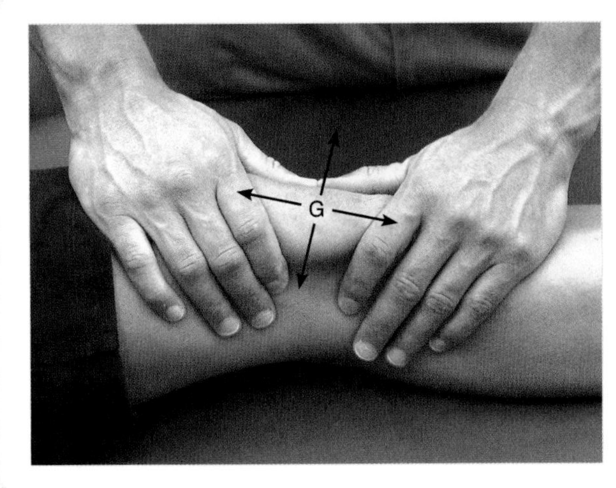

Figure 13-58 Patellar glides

Superior patellar glides increase knee extension. Inferior glides increase knee flexion. Medial glides stretch the lateral retinaculum. Lateral glides stretch tight medial structures.

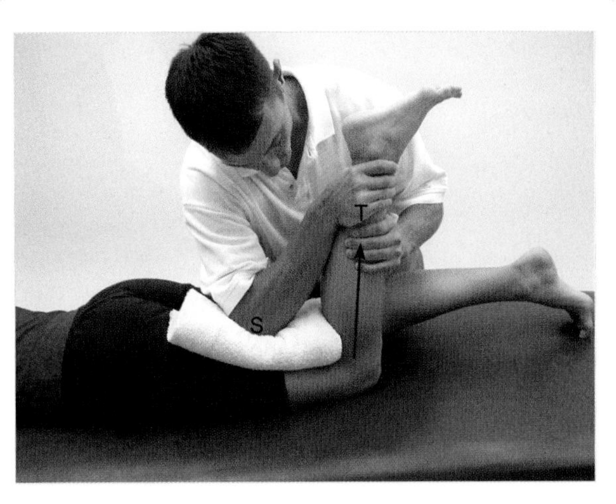

Figure 13-59 Tibiofemoral joint traction

Tibiofemoral joint traction reduces pain and hypomobility. It may be done with the patient prone and the knee flexed at 90 degrees. The elbow should stabilize the thigh while traction is applied through the tibia.

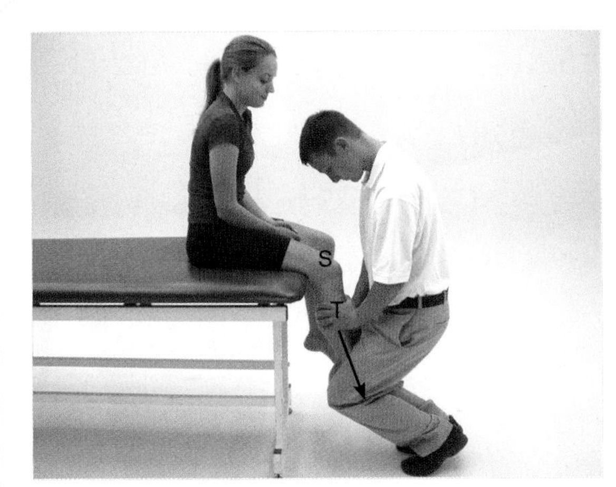

Figure 13-60 Alternative techniques for tibiofemoral joint traction

In very large individuals, an alternative technique for tibiofemoral joint traction uses body weight of the therapist to distract the joint once again for reducing pain and hypomobility.

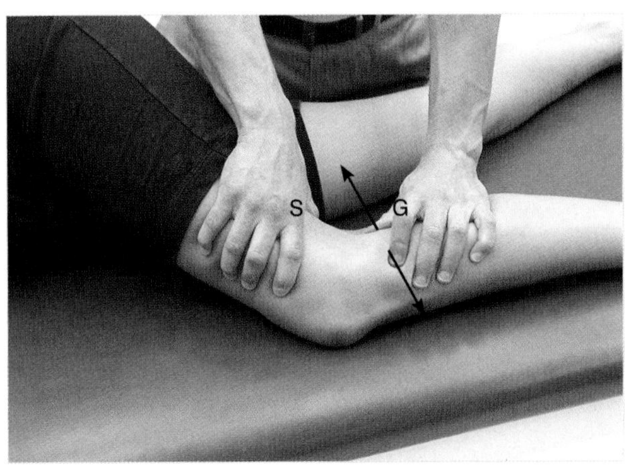

Figure 13-61 Proximal anterior and posterior glides of the fibula

Anterior and posterior glides of the fibula may be done proximally. They increase mobility of the fibular head and reduce pain. The femur should be stabilized. With the knee slightly flexed, grasp the head of the femur, and glide it anteriorly and posteriorly.

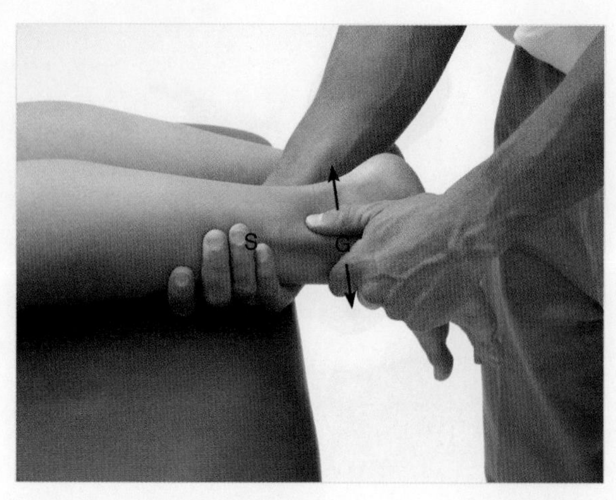

Figure 13-62 Distal anterior and posterior fibular glides

Anterior and posterior glides of the fibula may be done distally. The tibia should be stabilized, and the fibular malleolus is mobilized in an anterior or posterior direction.

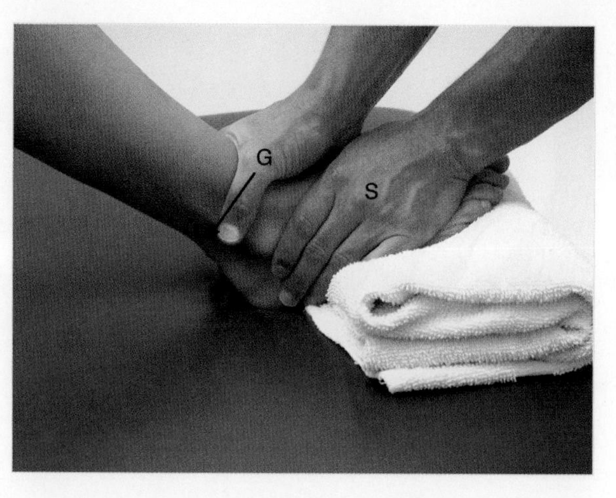

Figure 13-63 Posterior tibial glides

Posterior tibial glides increase plantarflexion. The foot should be stabilized, and pressure on the anterior tibia produces a posterior glide.

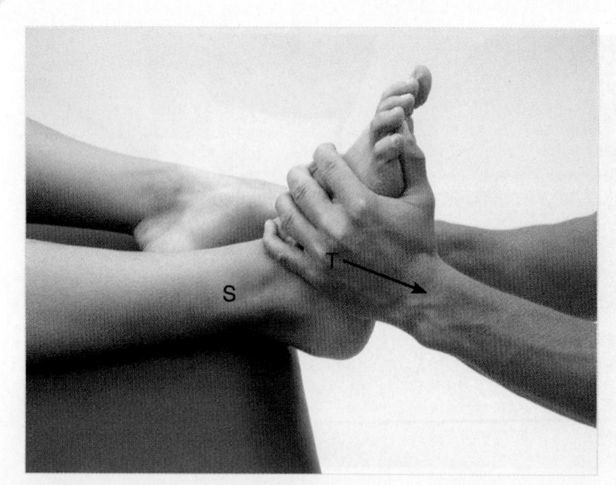

Figure 13-64 Talocrural joint traction

Talocrural joint traction is performed using the patient's body weight to stabilize the lower leg and applying traction to the midtarsal portion of the foot. Traction reduces pain and increases dorsiflexion and plantarflexion.

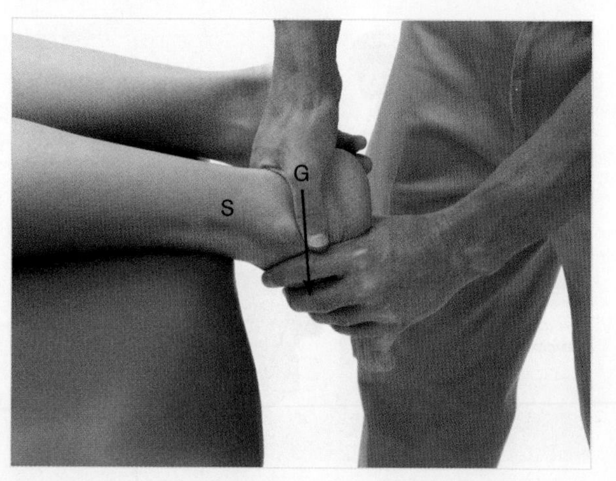

Figure 13-65 Anterior talar glides

Plantarflexion may also be increased by using an anterior talar glide. With the patient prone, the tibia is stabilized on the table and pressure is applied to the posterior aspect of the talus to glide it anteriorly.

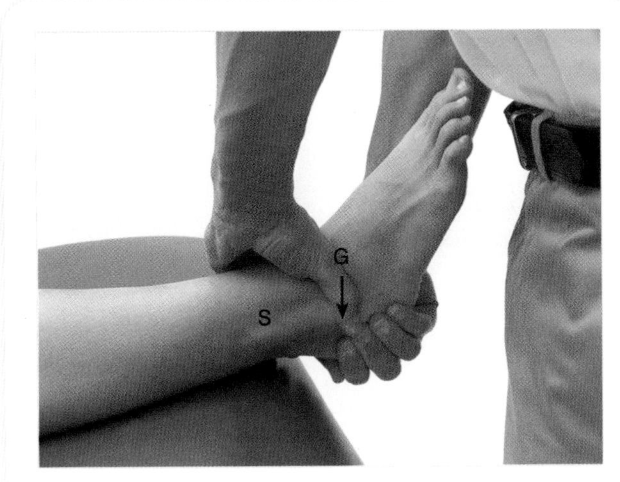

Figure 13-66 **Posterior talar glides**

Posterior talar glides may be used for increasing dorsiflexion. With the patient supine, the tibia is stabilized on the table and pressure is applied to the anterior aspect of the talus to glide it posteriorly.

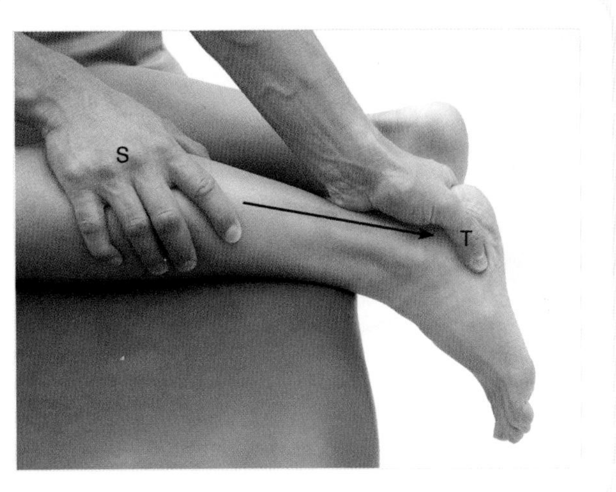

Figure 13-67 **Subtalar joint traction**

Subtalar joint traction reduces pain and increases inversion and eversion. The lower leg is stabilized on the table, and traction is applied by grasping the posterior aspect of the calcaneus.

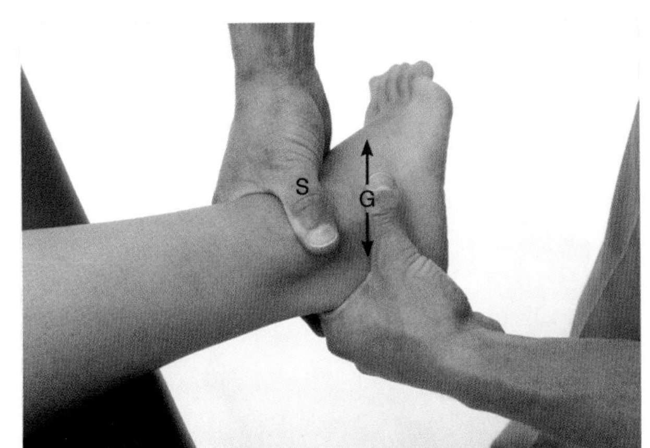

Figure 13-68 **Subtalar joint medial and lateral glides**

Subtalar joint medial and lateral glides increase eversion and inversion. The talus must be stabilized while the calcaneus is mobilized medially to increase inversion and laterally to increase eversion.

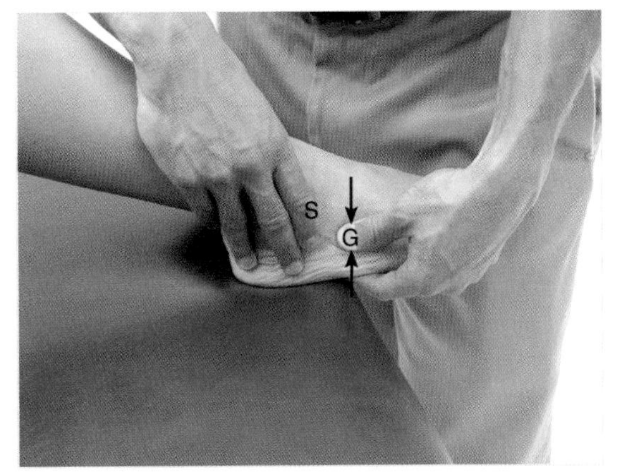

Figure 13-69 **Anterior/posterior calcaneocuboid glides**

Anterior/posterior calcaneocuboid glides may be used for increasing adduction and abduction. The calcaneus should be stabilized while the cuboid is mobilized.

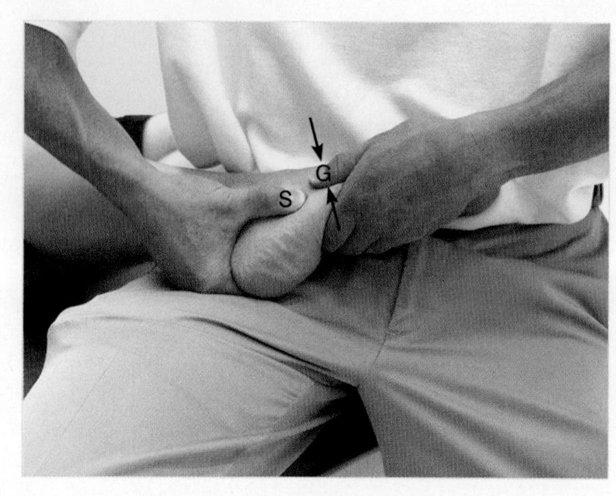

Figure 13-70 **Anterior/posterior cuboid metatarsal glides**

Anterior/posterior cuboid metatarsal glides are done with one hand stabilizing the cuboid and the other gliding the base of the fifth metatarsal. They are used for increasing mobility of the fifth metatarsal.

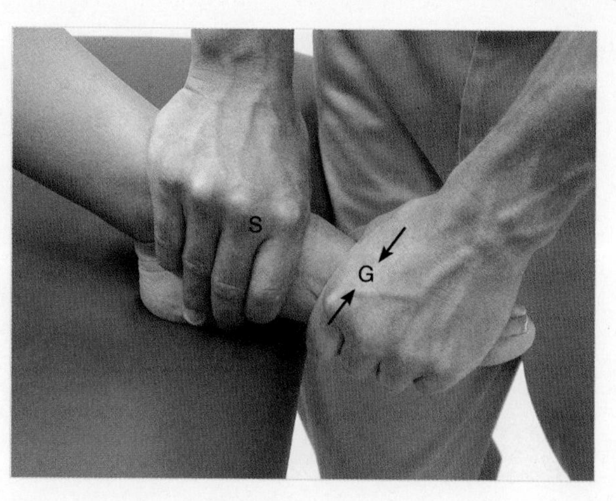

Figure 13-71 **Anterior/posterior carpometacarpal glides**

Anterior/posterior carpometacarpal glides decrease hypomobility of the metacarpals.

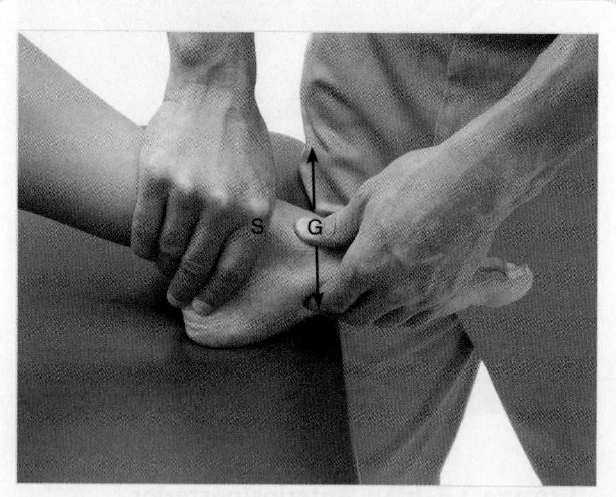

Figure 13-72 **Anterior/posterior talonavicular glides**

Anterior/posterior talonavicular glides also increase adduction and abduction. One hand stabilizes the talus while the other mobilizes the navicular bone.

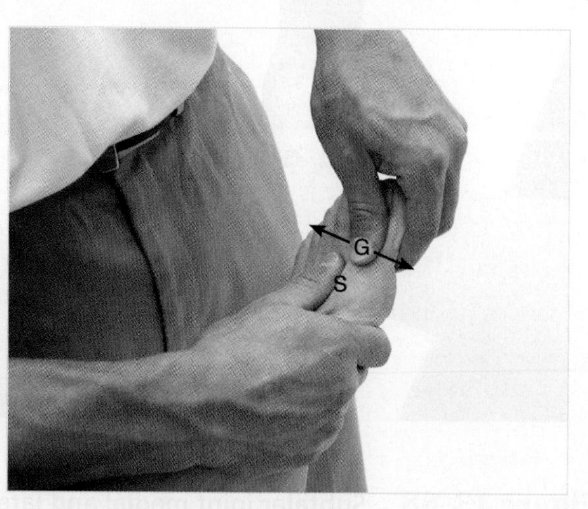

Figure 13-73 **Anterior/posterior metacarpophalangeal glides**

With anterior/posterior metacarpophalangeal glides, the anterior glides increase extension and posterior glides increase flexion. Mobilizations are accomplished by isolating individual segments.

movement and sustained natural apophyseal glides have the potential to quickly restore functional movements in joints, even after many years of restriction.[27]

Principles of Treatment

A basic premise of the Mulligan technique for an therapist choosing to make use of mobilizations with movement in the extremities or sustained natural apophyseal glides in the spine is to never cause pain to the patient.[10] During assessment, the therapist should look for specific signs, which may include a loss of joint movement, pain associated with movement, or pain associated with specific functional activities.[13] A passive accessory joint mobilization is applied following the principles of Kaltenborn discussed earlier in this chapter (ie, parallel or perpendicular to the joint plane). The therapist must continuously monitor the patient's reaction to ensure that no pain is recreated during this mobilization. The therapist experiments with various combinations of parallel or perpendicular glides until the appropriate treatment plane and grade of movement are discovered, which together significantly improve range of motion and/or significantly decrease or, better yet, eliminate altogether the original pain. Failure to improve range

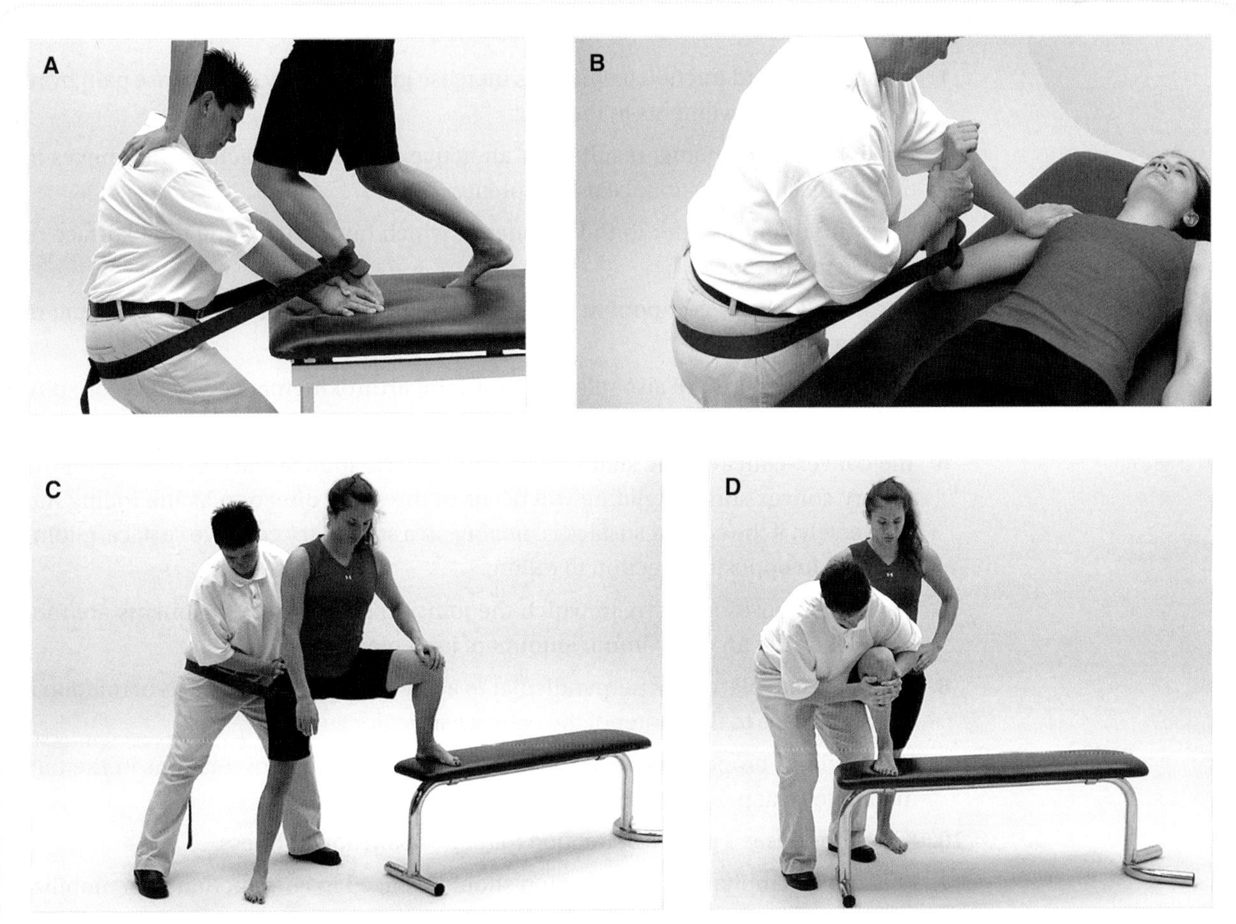

Figure 13-74 Mulligan techniques

A. Technique for increasing dorsiflexion. **B**. Treating elbow lateral epicondylitis. **C**. Technique for restricted hip abduction. **D**. Treating painful knee flexion.

of motion or decrease pain indicates that the therapist has not found the correct contact point, treatment plane, grade, or direction of mobilization. The patient then actively repeats the restricted and/or painful motion or activity while the therapist continues to maintain the appropriate accessory glide. Further increases in range of motion or decreases in pain may be expected during a treatment session that typically involves 3 sets of 10 repetitions. Additional gains may be realized through the application of pain-free, passive overpressure at the end of available range.[20]

An example of mobilization with movement might be in a patient with restricted ankle dorsiflexion (Figure 13-74*A*). The patient is standing on a treatment table with the therapist manually stabilizing the foot. A nonelastic belt passes around both the distal leg of the patient and the waist of the therapist who applies a sustained anterior glide of the tibia by leaning backward away from the patient. The patient then performs a slow dorsiflexion movement until the first onset of pain or end of range. Once this end point is reached, the position is sustained for 10 seconds. The patient then relaxes and returns to the standing position followed by release of the anteroposterior glide, and then followed by a 20-second rest period.[27] Figure 13-74*B*, *C*, and *D* shows several additional Mulligan techniques.

SUMMARY

1. Mobilization and traction techniques increase joint mobility or decrease pain by restoring accessory movements to the joint.
2. Physiologic movements result from an active muscle contraction that moves an extremity through traditional cardinal planes.
3. Accessory motions refer to the manner in which one articulating joint surface moves relative to another.
4. Normal accessory component motions must occur for full-range physiologic movement to take place.
5. Accessory motions are also referred to as joint arthrokinematics and include spin, roll, and glide.
6. The convex-concave rule states that if the concave joint surface is moving on the stationary convex surface, gliding will occur in the same direction as the rolling motion. Conversely, if the convex surface is moving on a stationary concave surface, gliding will occur in an opposite direction to rolling.
7. The resting position is one in which the joint capsule and the ligaments are most relaxed, allowing for a maximum amount of joint play.
8. The treatment plane falls perpendicular to a line running from the axis of rotation in the convex surface to the center of the concave articular surface.
9. Maitland has proposed a series of 5 graded movements or oscillations in the range of motion to treat pain and stiffness.
10. Kaltenborn uses 3 grades of traction to reduce pain and stiffness.
11. Kaltenborn emphasizes that traction should be used in conjunction with mobilization glides to treat joint hypomobility.
12. Mulligan's technique combines passive accessory movement with active physiological movement to improve range of motion or to minimize pain.

REFERENCES

1. Barak T, Rosen E, Sofer R. Mobility: passive orthopedic manual therapy. In: Gould J, Davies G, eds. *Orthopedic and Sports Physical Therapy.* St. Louis, MO: Mosby; 1990:212-227.
2. Basmajian J, Banerjee S. *Clinical Decision Making in Rehabilitation: Efficacy and Outcomes.* Philadelphia, PA: Churchill-Livingstone; 1996.
3. Boissonnault W, Bryan J, Fox KS. Joint manipulation curricula in physical therapist professional degree programs. *J Orthop Sports Phys Ther.* 2004;34(4):171-181.
4. Conroy DE, Hayes KW. The effect of joint mobilization as a component of comprehensive treatment for primary shoulder impingement syndrome. *J Orthop Sports Phys Ther.* 1998;28(1):3-14.
5. Cookson J. Orthopedic manual therapy: an overview, II. The spine. *Phys Ther.* 1979;59:259.
6. Cookson J, Kent B. Orthopedic manual therapy: an overview, I. The extremities. *Phys Ther.* 1979;59:136.
7. Cyriax J. *Cyriax's Illustrated Manual of Orthopaedic Medicine.* London, UK: Butterworth; 1996.
8. Donatelli R, Owens-Burkhart H. Effects of immobilization on the extensibility of periarticular connective tissue. *J Orthop Sports Phys Ther.* 1981;3:67.
9. Edmond S. *Joint Mobilization and Manipulation: Extremity and Spinal Techniques.* Philadelphia, PA: Elsevier Health Sciences; 2006.
10. Exelby L. The Mulligan concept: its application in the management of spinal conditions. *Man Ther.* 2002;7(2):64-70.
11. Green T, Refshauge K, Crosbie J, Adams R. A randomized controlled trial of a passive accessory joint mobilization on acute ankle inversion sprains. *Phys Ther.* 2001;81(4):984-994.
12. Grimsby O. *Fundamentals of Manual Therapy: A Course Workbook.* Vagsbygd, Norway: Sorlandets Fysikalske Institutt; 1981.
13. Hall T. Effects of the Mulligan traction straight leg raise technique on range of movement. *J Man Manip Ther.* 2001;9(3):128-133.
14. Hollis M. *Practical Exercise.* Oxford, UK: Blackwell Scientific; 1999.
15. Hsu AT, Ho L, Chang JH, Chang GL, Hedman T. Characterization of tissue resistance during a dorsally directed translational mobilization of the glenohumeral joint. *Arch Phys Med Rehabil.* 2002,83(3):360-366.
16. Kaltenborn F. *Manual Mobilization of the Joints, Vol. II: The Spine.* Minneapolis, MN: Orthopedic Physical Therapy Products; 2003.
17. Kaltenborn F, Morgan D, Evjenth O. *Manual Mobilization of the Joints, Vol. I: The Extremities.* Minneapolis, MN: Orthopedic Physical Therapy Products; 2002.
18. Kaminski T, Kahanov L, Kato M. Therapeutic effect of joint mobilization: joint mechanoreceptors and nociceptors. *Athl Ther Today.* 2007;12(4):28.
19. Kisner C, Colby L. *Therapeutic Exercise: Foundations and Techniques.* Philadelphia, PA: FA Davis; 2007.
20. MacConaill M, Basmajian J. *Muscles and Movements: A Basis for Kinesiology.* Baltimore, MD: Williams & Wilkins; 1977.
21. Maigne R. *Orthopedic Medicine.* Springfield, IL: Charles C Thomas; 1976.
22. Macintyre J. Passive joint mobilization for acute ankle inversion sprains. *Clin J Sport Med.* 2002;12(1):54.
23. Maitland G. *Extremity Manipulation.* London, UK: Butterworth; 1991.
24. Maitland G. *Vertebral Manipulation.* Philadelphia, PA: Elsevier Health Science; 2005.
25. Mangus B, Hoffman L, Hoffman M. Basic principles of extremity joint mobilization using a Kaltenborn approach. *J Sport Rehabil.* 2002;11(4):235-250.
26. Mennell J. *The Musculoskeletal System: Differential Diagnosis from Symptoms and Physical Signs.* New York, NY: Aspen; 1991.
27. Mulligan's concept. Available at: http://www.bmulligan.com/about-us/2013.
28. Paris S. *The Spine: Course Notebook.* Atlanta, GA: Institute Press; 1979.
29. Paris S. Mobilization of the spine. *Phys Ther.* 1979;59:988.
30. Saunders D. Evaluation, treatment and prevention of musculoskeletal disorders. Shoreview, MN: Saunders Group; 2004.
31. Schiotz E, Cyriax J. *Manipulation Past and Present.* London, UK: Heinemann; 1978.
32. Stevenson J, Vaughn D. Four cardinal principles of joint mobilization and joint play assessment. *J Man Manip Ther.* 2003;11(3):146.
33. Stone JA. Joint mobilization. *Athl Ther Today.* 1998;4(6):59-60.
34. Teys P. The initial effects of a Mulligan's mobilization with movement technique on range of movement and pressure pain threshold in pain-limited shoulders. *Man Ther.* 2008;13(1):37.
35. Wadsworth C. *Manual Examination and Treatment of the Spine and Extremities.* Baltimore, MD: William & Wilkins; 1998.
36. Wilson E. The Mulligan concept: NAGS, SNAGS and mobilizations with movement. *J Bodyw Mov Ther.* 2001;5(2):81-89.
37. Zohn D, Mennell J. *Musculoskeletal Pain: Diagnosis and Physical Treatment.* Boston, MA: Little, Brown; 1987.
38. Zusman M. Reappraisal of a proposed neurophysiological mechanism for the relief of joint pain with passive joint movements. *Physiother Theory Pract.* 1985;1:61-70.

14

Regaining Postural Stability and Balance

Kevin M. Guskiewicz

OBJECTIVES

After completion of this chapter, the physical therapist should be able to do the following:

- Define and explain the roles of the 3 sensory modalities responsible for maintaining balance.
- Explain how movement strategies along the closed kinetic chain help maintain the center of gravity in a safe and stable area.
- Differentiate between subjective and objective balance assessment.
- Differentiate between static and dynamic balance assessment.
- Evaluate the effect that injury to the ankle, knee, and head has on balance and postural equilibrium.
- Identify the goals of each phase of balance training, and how to progress the patient through each phase.
- State the differences among static, semidynamic, and dynamic balance-training exercises.

Although maintaining balance while standing may appear to be a rather simple motor skill for able-bodied athletes, this feat cannot be taken for granted in a patient with musculoskeletal dysfunction. Muscular weakness, proprioceptive deficits, and range of motion (ROM) deficits may challenge a person's ability to maintain their center of gravity (COG) within the body's base of support, or, in other words, cause them to lose their balance. Balance is the single most important element dictating movement strategies within the closed kinetic chain. Acquisition of effective strategies for maintaining balance is therefore essential for athletic performance. Although balance is often thought of as a static process, it's actually a highly integrative dynamic process involving multiple neurologic pathways. Although *balance* is the more commonly used term, *postural equilibrium* is a broader term that involves the alignment of joint segments in an effort to maintain the COG within an optimal range of the maximum limits of stability (LOS).

Despite often being classified at the end of the continuum of goals associated with therapeutic exercise,[45] maintenance of balance is a vital component in the rehabilitation of joint injuries that should not be overlooked. Traditionally, orthopedic rehabilitation has placed the emphasis on isolated joint mechanics, such as improving ROM and flexibility, and increasing muscle strength and endurance, rather than on afferent information obtained by the joint(s) to be processed by the postural control system. However, research in the area of proprioception and kinesthesia has emphasized the need to train the joint's neural system.[46-50] Joint position sense, proprioception, and kinesthesia are vital to all athletic performance requiring balance. Current rehabilitation protocols should therefore focus on a combination of open- and closed-kinetic-chain exercises. The necessity for a combination of open- and closed-kinetic-chain exercises can be seen during gait (walking or running), as the foot and ankle prepare for heel strike (open chain) and prepare to control the body's COG during midstance and toe off (closed chain). This chapter focuses on the postural control system, various balance training techniques, and technologic advancements that are enabling therapists to assess and treat balance deficits in physically active people.

Postural Control System

The therapist must first have an understanding of the postural control system and its various components. The postural control system utilizes complex processes involving both sensory and motor components. Maintenance of postural equilibrium includes sensory detection of body motions, integration of sensorimotor information within the central nervous system (CNS), and execution of appropriate musculoskeletal responses. Most daily activities, such as walking, climbing stairs, reaching, or throwing a ball, require static foot placement with controlled balance shifts, especially if a favorable outcome is to be attained. So, balance should be considered both a dynamic and static process. The successful accomplishment of static and dynamic balance is based on the interaction between body and environment.[44] Figure 14-1 shows the complexity of this dynamic process. From a clinical perspective, separating the sensory and motor processes of balance means that a person may have impaired balance for 1 or a combination of 2 reasons: (a) the position of the COG relative to the base of support is not accurately sensed; and (b) the automatic movements required to bring the COG to a balanced position are not timely or effectively coordinated.[60]

The position of the body in relation to gravity and its surroundings is sensed by combining visual, vestibular, and somatosensory inputs. Balance movements also involve motions of the ankle, knee, and hip joints, which are controlled by the coordinated actions along the kinetic chain (Figure 14-2). These processes are all vital for producing fluid sport-related movements.

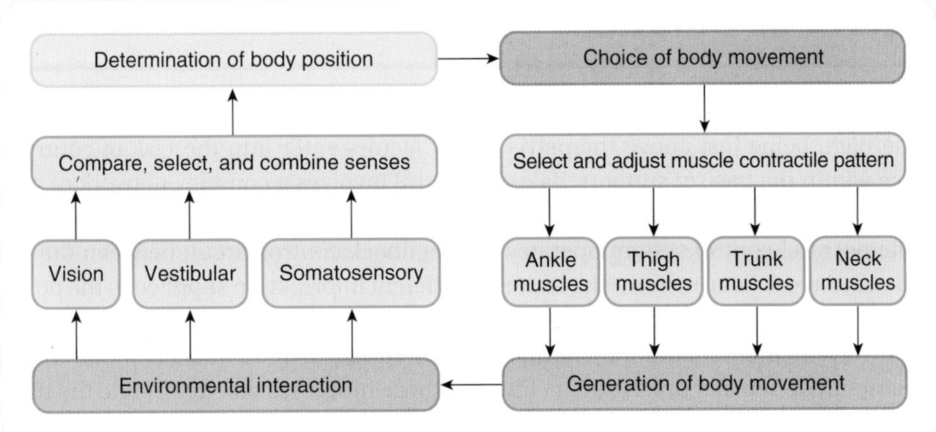

Figure 14-1 **Dynamic equilibrium**

(Adapted from Allison L, Fuller K, Hedenberg R, et al. *Contemporary Management of Balance Deficits.* Clackamas, OR: NeuroCom International; 1994, with permission.)

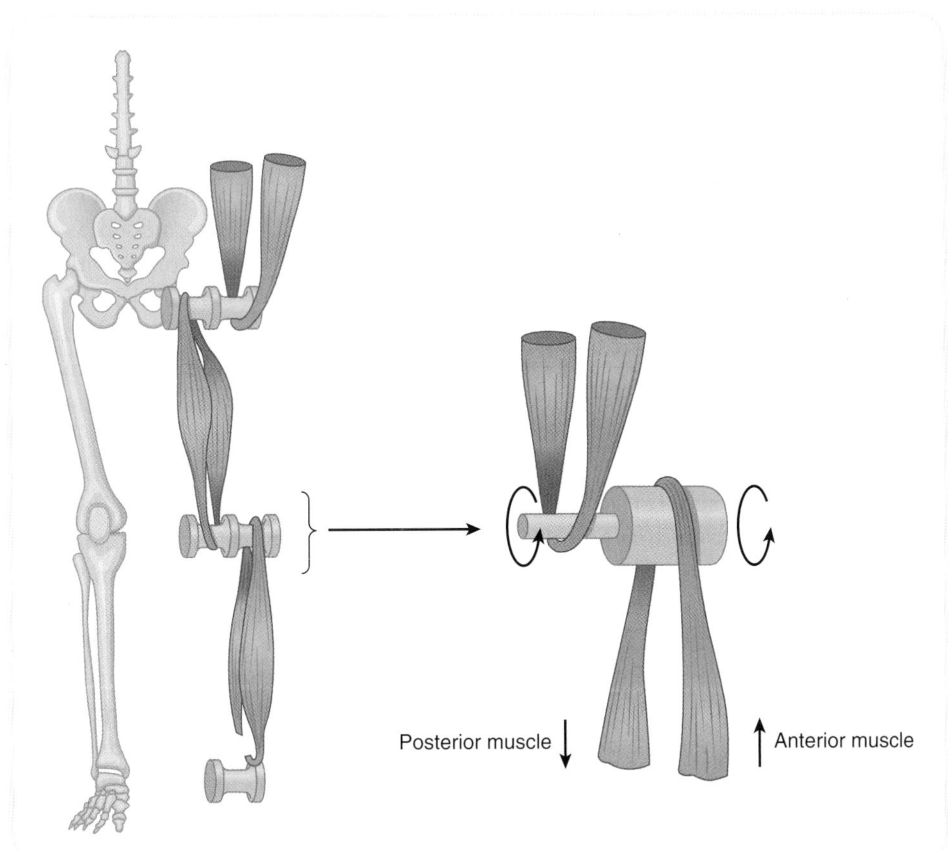

Figure 14-2

Paired relationships between major postural musculatures that execute coordinated actions along the kinetic chain to control the center of gravity.

Control of Balance

The human body is a very tall structure balanced on a relatively small base, and its COG is quite high, being just above the pelvis. Many factors enter into the task of controlling balance within the base of support. Balance control involves a complex network of neural connections and centers that are related by peripheral and central feedback mechanisms.[34]

The postural control system operates as a feedback control circuit between the brain and the musculoskeletal system. The sources of afferent information supplied to the postural control system collectively come from visual, vestibular, and somatosensory inputs. The CNS's involvement in maintaining upright posture can be divided into 2 components. The first component, sensory organization, involves those processes that determine the timing, direction, and amplitude of corrective postural actions based upon information obtained from the vestibular, visual, and somatosensory (proprioceptive) inputs.[56] Despite the availability of multiple sensory inputs, the CNS generally relies on only 1 sense at a time for orientation information. For healthy adults, the preferred sense for balance control comes from somatosensory information (ie, feet in contact with the support surface and detection of joint movement).[37,56] In considering orthopedic injuries, the somatosensory system is of most importance and is the focus of this chapter.

The second component, muscle coordination, is the collection of processes that determine the temporal sequencing and distribution of contractile activity among the muscles of the legs and trunk which generate supportive reactions for maintaining balance. Research suggests that balance deficiencies in people with neurologic problems can result from inappropriate interaction among the three sensory inputs that provide orientation information to the postural control system. A patient may be inappropriately dependent on 1 sense for situations presenting intersensory conflict.[56,70]

From a clinical perspective, stabilization of upright posture requires the integration of afferent information from the 3 senses, which work in combination and are all critical to the execution of coordinated postural corrections. Impairment of 1 component is usually compensated for by the remaining 2 components. Often, one of the systems provides faulty or inadequate information such as different surfaces and/or changes in visual acuity and/or peripheral vision. In this case, it is crucial that one of the other senses provides accurate and adequate information so that balance may be maintained. For example, when somatosensory conflict is present such as a moving platform or a compliant foam surface, balance is significantly decreased with the eyes closed as compared to eyes open.

Somatosensory inputs provide information concerning the orientation of body parts to one another and to the support surface.[21,60] Vision measures the orientation of the eyes and head in relation to surrounding objects, and plays an important role in the maintenance of balance. On a stable surface, closing the eyes should cause only minimal increases in postural sway in healthy subjects. However, if somatosensory input is disrupted because of ligamentous injury, closing the eyes will increase sway significantly.[12,16,37,38,60] The vestibular apparatus supplies information that measures gravitational, linear, and angular accelerations of the head in relation to inertial space. It does not, however, provide orientation information in relation to external objects, and therefore plays only a minor role in the maintenance of balance when the visual and somatosensory systems are providing accurate information.[60]

Somatosensation as It Relates to Balance

The terms *somatosensation, proprioception, kinesthesia,* and *balance* are often used to describe similar phenomena. Somatosensation is a more global term used to describe the proprioceptive mechanisms related to postural control and can accurately be used synonymously. Consequently, somatosensation is best defined as a specialized variation of the sensory modality of touch that encompasses the sensation of joint movement (kinesthesia) and joint position (joint position sense).[46,50] As previously discussed, balance refers to the ability to maintain the body's COG within the base of support provided by the feet. Somatosensation and balance work closely, as the postural control system utilizes sensory information related to movement and posture from peripheral sensory receptors (eg, muscle spindles, Golgi tendon organs, joint afferents, cutaneous receptors). So the question remains, how does proprioception influence postural equilibrium and balance?

Somatosensory input is received from mechanoreceptors; however, it is unclear as to whether the tactile senses, muscle spindles, or Golgi tendon organs are most responsible for controlling balance. Nashner[55] concluded after using electromyography responses following platform perturbations, that other pathways had to be involved in the responses they recorded because the latencies were longer than those normally associated with a classic myotatic reflex. The stretch-related reflex is the earliest mechanism for increasing the activation level of muscles about a joint following an externally imposed rotation of the joint. Rotation of the ankles is the most probable stimulus of the myotatic reflex that occurs in many persons. It appears to be the first useful phase of activity in the leg muscles after a change in erect posture.[55] The myotatic reflex can be seen when perturbations of gait or posture automatically evoke functionally directed responses in the leg muscles to compensate for imbalance or increased postural sway.[14,55] Muscle spindles sense a stretching of the agonist, thus sending information along its afferent fibers to the spinal cord. There the information is transferred to alpha and gamma motor neurons that carry information back to the muscle fibers and muscle spindle, respectively, and contract the muscle to prevent or control additional postural sway.[14]

Postural sway was assessed on a platform moving into a "toes-up" and "toes-down" position, and a stretch reflex was found in the triceps surae after a sudden ramp displacement into the "toes-up" position.[13] A medium latency response (103 to 118 milliseconds) was observed in the stretched muscle, followed by a delayed response of the antagonistic anterior tibialis muscle (108 to 124 milliseconds). The investigators also blocked afferent proprioceptive information in an attempt to study the role of proprioceptive information from the legs for the maintenance of upright posture. These results suggested that proprioceptive information from pressure and/or joint receptors of the foot (ischemia applied at ankle) plays an important role in postural stabilization during low frequencies of movement, but is of minor importance for the compensation of rapid displacements. The experiment also included a "visual" component, as subjects were tested with eyes closed, followed by eyes open. Results suggested that when subjects were tested with eyes open, visual information compensated for the loss of proprioceptive input.

Another study[14] used compensatory electromyography responses during impulsive disturbance of the limbs during stance on a treadmill to describe the myotatic reflex. Results revealed that during backward movement of the treadmill, ankle dorsiflexion caused the COG to be shifted anteriorly, thus evoking a stretch reflex in the gastrocnemius muscle, followed by weak anterior tibialis activation. In another trial, the movement was reversed (plantar flexion), thus shifting the COG posteriorly and evoking a stretch reflex of the anterior tibialis muscle. Both of these studies suggest that stretch reflex responses help to control the body's COG, and that the vestibular system is unlikely to be directly involved in the generation of the necessary responses.

Elimination of all sensory information from the feet and ankles revealed that proprioceptors in the leg muscles (gastrocnemius and tibialis anterior) were capable of providing sufficient sensory information for stable standing.[20] Researchers speculated that group I or group II muscle spindle afferents, and group Ib afferents from Golgi tendon organs were the probable sources of this proprioceptive information. The study demonstrated that normal subjects can stand in a stable manner when receptors in the leg muscles are the only source of information about postural sway.

Other studies[5,38] have examined the role of somatosensory information by altering or limiting somatosensory input through the use of platform sway referencing or foam platforms. These studies reported that subjects still responded with well-coordinated movements but the movements were often either ineffective or inefficient for the environmental context in which they were used.

Balance as It Relates to the Closed Kinetic Chain

Balance is the process of maintaining the COG within the body's base of support. Again, the human body is a very tall structure balanced on a relatively small base, and its COG is quite high, being just above the pelvis. Many factors enter into the task of controlling balance within this designated area. One component often overlooked is the role balance plays within the kinetic chain. Ongoing debates as to how the kinetic chain should be defined and whether open- or closed-kinetic-chain exercises are best have caused many therapists to lose sight of what is most important. An understanding of the postural control system as well as the theory of the kinetic (segmental) chain about the lower extremity helps conceptualize the role of the chain in maintaining balance. Within the kinetic chain, each moving segment transmits forces to every other segment along the chain, and its motions are influenced by forces transmitted from other segments (see Chapter 11).[10] The act of maintaining equilibrium or balance is associated with the closed kinetic chain, as the distal segment (foot) is fixed beneath the base of support.

The coordination of automatic postural movements during the act of balancing is not determined solely by the muscles acting directly about the joint. Leg and trunk muscles exert indirect forces on neighboring joints through the inertial interaction forces among body segments.[57,58] A combination of one or more strategies (ankle, knee, hip) are used to coordinate movement of the COG back to a stable or balanced position when a person's balance is disrupted by an external perturbation. Injury to any one of the joints or corresponding muscles along the kinetic chain can result in a loss of appropriate feedback for maintaining balance.

Balance Disruption

Let's say, for example, that a basketball player goes up for a rebound and collides with another player, causing her to land in an unexpected position, thereby compromising her normal balance. To prevent a fall from occurring, the body must correct itself by returning the COG to a position within safer LOS. Afferent mechanoreceptor input from the hip, knee, and ankle joints is responsible for initiating automatic postural responses through the use of 1 of 3 possible movement strategies.

Selection of Movement Strategies

Three principle joint systems (ankles, knees, and hips) are located between the base of support and the COG. This allows for a wide variety of postures that can be assumed, while the COG is still positioned above the base of support. As described by Nashner,[60] motions about a given joint are controlled by the combined actions of at least 1 pair of muscles working in opposition. When forces exerted by pairs of opposing muscle about a joint (eg, anterior tibialis and gastrocnemius/soleus) are combined, the effect is to resist rotation of the joint relative to a resting position. The degree to which the joint resists rotation is called *joint stiffness*. The resting position and the stiffness of the joint are each altered independently by changing the activation levels of 1 or both muscle groups.[39,60] Joint resting position and joint stiffness are by themselves an inadequate basis for controlling postural movements, and it is theorized that the myotatic stretch reflex is the earliest mechanism for increasing the activation level of the muscles of a joint following an externally imposed rotation of the joint.[60]

When a person's balance is disrupted by an external perturbation, movement strategies involving joints of the lower extremity coordinate movement of the COG back to a balanced position. Three strategies (ankle, hip, stepping) have been identified along a continuum.[37] In general, the relative effectiveness of ankle, hip, and stepping strategies in repositioning the COG over the base of support depends on the configuration of the base of support, the COG alignment in relation to the LOS, and the speed of the postural movement.[37,38]

The ankle strategy shifts the COG while maintaining the placement of the feet by rotating the body as a rigid mass about the ankle joints. This is achieved by contracting either the gastrocnemius or anterior tibialis muscles to generate torque about the ankle joints. Anterior sway of the body is counteracted by gastrocnemius activity, which pulls the body posteriorly. Conversely, posterior sway of the body is counteracted by contraction of the tibialis anterior. Thus, the importance of these muscles should not be underestimated when designing the rehabilitation program. The ankle strategy is most effective in executing relatively slow COG movements when the base of support is firm and the COG is well within the LOS perimeter. The ankle strategy is also believed to be effective in maintaining a static posture with the COG offset from the center. The thigh and lower trunk muscles contract, thereby resisting the destabilization of these proximal joints as a result of the indirect effects of the ankle muscles on the proximal joints (Table 14-1).

Under normal sensory conditions, activation of ankle musculature is almost exclusively selected to maintain equilibrium. However, there are subtle differences associated with loss of somatosensation and with vestibular dysfunction in terms of postural control strategies. Persons with somatosensory loss appear to rely on their hip musculature to retain their COG while experiencing forward or backward perturbation or with different support surface lengths.[21]

Table 14-1 Function and Anatomy of Muscles Involved in Balance Movements

	Extension		Flexion	
Joint	Anatomic	Function	Anatomic	Function
Hip	Paraspinals Hamstrings	Paraspinals Hamstrings Tibialis	Abdominal Quadriceps	Abdominals Quadriceps Gastrocnemius
Knee	Quadriceps	Paraspinals Quadriceps Gastrocnemius	Hamstrings Gastrocnemius	Abdominals Hamstrings Tibialis
Ankle	Gastrocnemius	Abdominals Quadriceps Gastrocnemius	Tibialis	Paraspinals Hamstrings Tibialis

Source: Adapted from Nashner LM. Physiology of balance. In: Jacobson G, Newman C, Kartush J, eds. *Handbook of Balance Function and Testing*. St. Louis, MO: Mosby; 1993:261-279.

If the ankle strategy is not capable of controlling excessive sway, the hip strategy is available to help control motion of the COG through the initiation of large and rapid motions at the hip joints with antiphase rotation of the ankles. It is most effective when the COG is located near the LOS perimeter, and when the LOS boundaries are contracted by a narrowed base of support. Finally, when the COG is displaced beyond the LOS, a step or stumble (stepping strategy) is the only strategy which can be used to prevent a fall.[58,60]

It is proposed that LOS and COG alignment are altered in individuals exhibiting a musculoskeletal abnormality such as an ankle or knee sprain. For example, weakness of ligaments following acute or chronic sprain about these joints is likely to reduce ROM, thereby shrinking the LOS and placing the person at greater risk for a fall with a relatively smaller sway envelope.[58] Pintsaar et al[67] revealed that impaired function was related to a change from ankle synergy toward hip synergy for postural adjustments among patients with functional ankle instability. This finding, which was consistent with previous results reported by Tropp et al, suggests that sensory proprioceptive function for the injured patients was affected.

Assessment of Balance

Several methods of balance assessment have been proposed for clinical use. Many of the techniques have been criticized for offering only subjective ("qualitative") measurement information regarding balance rather than an objective ("quantitative") measure.[63]

Subjective Assessment

Prior to the mid 1980s, there were very few methods for systematic and controlled assessment of balance. The assessment of static balance in athletes has traditionally been performed through the use of the standing Romberg test. This test is performed standing with feet together, arms at the side, and eyes closed. Normally a person can stand motionless in this position, but the tendency to sway or fall to one side is considered a positive Romberg sign, indicating a loss of proprioception.[8] The Romberg test has, however, been criticized for its lack of sensitivity and objectivity. It is considered to be a rather qualitative assessment of static balance because a considerable amount of stress is required to make the subject sway enough for an observer to characterize the sway.[42]

The use of a quantifiable clinical test battery called the *Balance Error Scoring System* (BESS) is recommended over the standard Romberg test.[32] Three different stances (double, single, and tandem) are completed twice, once while on a firm surface and once while on a piece of medium density foam (balance pad by Airex is recommended) for a total of 6 trials (Figure 14-3). Patients are asked to assume the required stance by placing their hands on the iliac crests, and upon eye closure, the 20-second test begins. During the single-leg stances, subjects are asked to maintain the contralateral limb in 20 to 30 degrees of hip flexion and 40 to 50 degrees of knee flexion. Additionally, the patient is asked to stand quietly and as motionless as possible in the stance position, keeping their hands on the iliac crests and eyes closed. The single-limb stance tests are performed on the nondominant foot. This same foot is placed toward the rear on the tandem stances. Subjects are told that upon losing their balance, they are to make any necessary adjustments and return to the testing position as quickly as possible. Performance is scored by adding 1 error point for each error listed in Table 14-2. Trials are considered to be incomplete if the patient is unable to sustain the stance position for longer than 5 seconds during the entire 20-second testing period. These trials are assigned a standard maximum error score of 10. Balance test results during injury recovery are best used when compared to baseline measurements, and clinicians working with athletes or patients on a regular basis should attempt to obtain baseline measurements when possible.

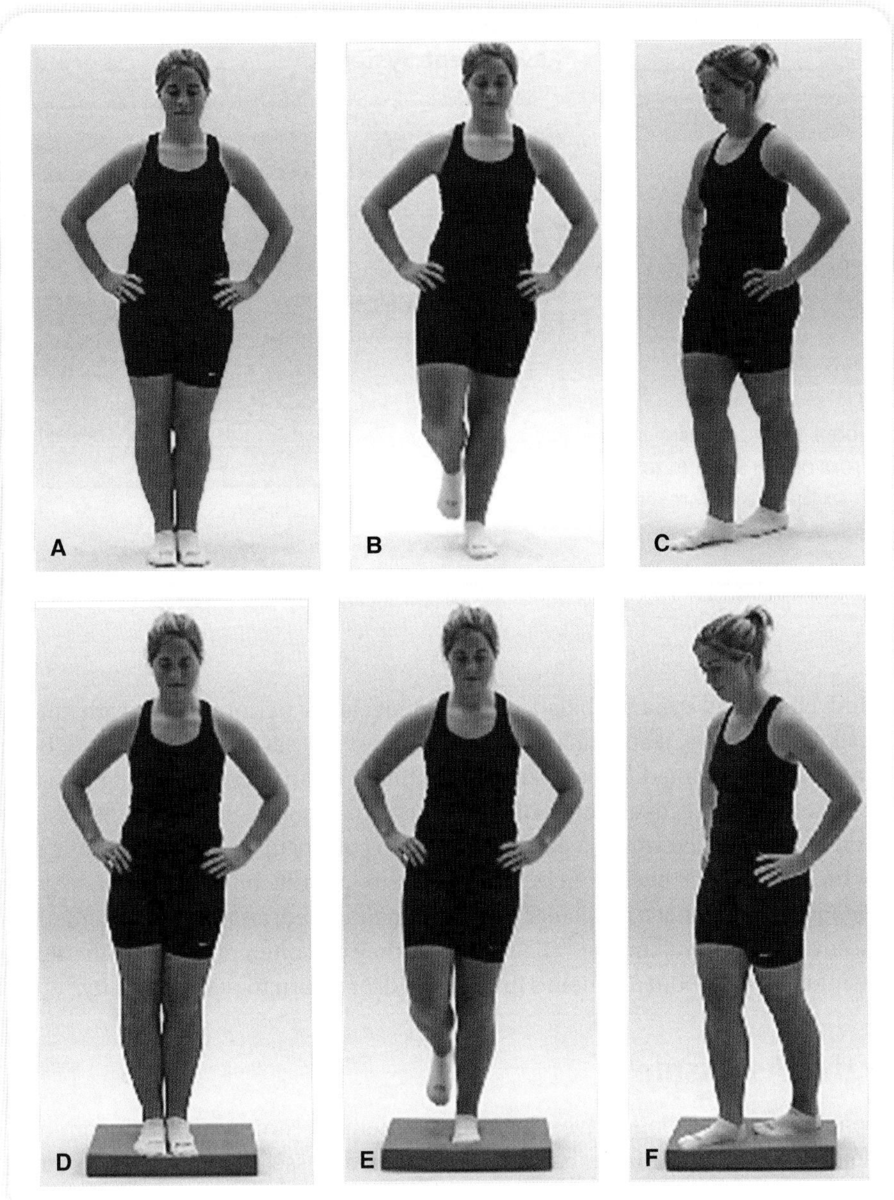

Figure 14-3 Stance positions for Balance Error Scoring System (BESS)

A. Double-leg, firm surface. **B.** Single-leg, firm surface. **C.** Tandem, firm surface.
D. Double-leg, foam surface. **E.** Single-leg, foam surface. **F.** Tandem, foam surface.

Clinical Pearl

A preseason baseline score can be obtained on a measure such as the BESS for all athletes, and then used for a postinjury comparison. Because there is such variability within many of the balance measures, it is important to make comparisons only to an athlete's individual baseline measure and not to a normal score. It is best to determine recovery on a measure by using the number of standard deviations away from the baseline. For example, scores on the BESS that are more than 2 standard deviations or 6 total points would be considered abnormal. Repeated assessments over the course of a rehabilitation progression can be used to determine the effectiveness of the balance exercises.

Table 14-2 Balance Error Scoring System (BESS)

Errors
Hands lifted off iliac crests
Opening eyes
Step, stumble, or fall
Moving hip into more than 30 degrees of flexion or abduction
Lifting forefoot or heel
Remaining out of testing position for more than 5 seconds
The BESS score is calculated by adding 1 error point for each error or any combination of errors occurring during 1 movement. Error scores from each of the 6 trials are added for a total BESS score, and higher scores represent poor balance.

Table 14-3 High-Technology Balance Assessment Systems

Static Systems	Dynamic Systems
Chattecx Balance System	Biodex Stability System
EquiTest	Chattecx Balance System
Forceplate	EquiTest
Pro Balance Master	EquiTest with EMG
Smart Balance Master	Forceplate
	Kinesthetic Ability Trainer
	Pro Balance Master
	Smart Balance Master

Semidynamic and dynamic balance assessment can be performed through functional-reach tests; timed agility tests, such as the figure 8 test,[15,19] carioca, or hop test[40]; Bass Test for Dynamic Balance; timed "T-Band kicks"; and timed balance beam walking with the eyes open or closed. The objective in most of these tests is to decrease the size of the base of support, in an attempt to determine a patient's ability to control upright posture while moving. Many of these tests have been criticized for failing to quantify balance adequately, as they merely report the time that a particular posture is maintained, angular displacement, or the distance covered after walking.[6,21,46,60] At any rate, they can often provide the therapist with valuable information about a patient's function and/or return to play capability.

Objective Assessment

Advancements in technology have provided the medical community with commercially available balance systems (Table 14-3) for quantitatively assessing and training static and dynamic balance. These systems provide an easy, practical, and cost-effective method of quantitatively assessing and training functional balance through analysis of postural stability. Thus, the potential exists to assess injured patients and (a) identify possible abnormalities that might be associated with injury; (b) isolate various systems that are affected; (c) develop recovery curves based on quantitative measures for determining readiness to return to activity; and (d) train the injured patient.

Most manufacturers use computer-interfaced forceplate technology consisting of a flat, rigid surface supported on 3 or more points by independent force-measuring devices. As the patient stands on the forceplate surface, the position of the center of vertical forces exerted on the forceplate over time is calculated (Figure 14-4). The center of vertical force movements provide an indirect measure of postural sway activity.[59] The Kistler and, more recently, Bertec forceplates, are used for much of the work in the area of postural stability and balance.[6,17,27,52,54] NeuroCom International, Inc. (Clackamas, OR) has also developed systems with expanded diagnostic and training capabilities that make interpretation of results easier for therapists. Therapists must be aware that the manufacturers often use conflicting terminology to describe various balance parameters, and should consult frequently with the manufacturer to ensure that there is a clear understanding of the measure being taken. These inconsistencies have created confusion in the literature, because what some

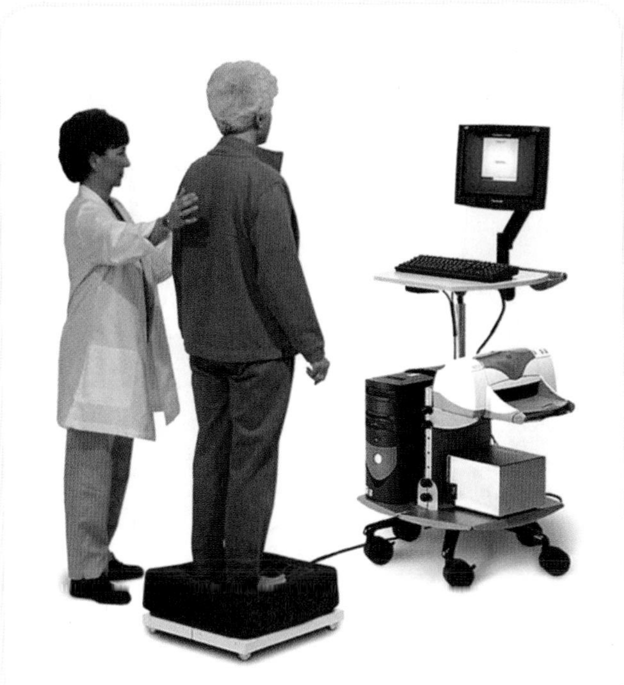

Figure 14-4 Patient training on the Balance Master

(Courtesy NeuroCom.)

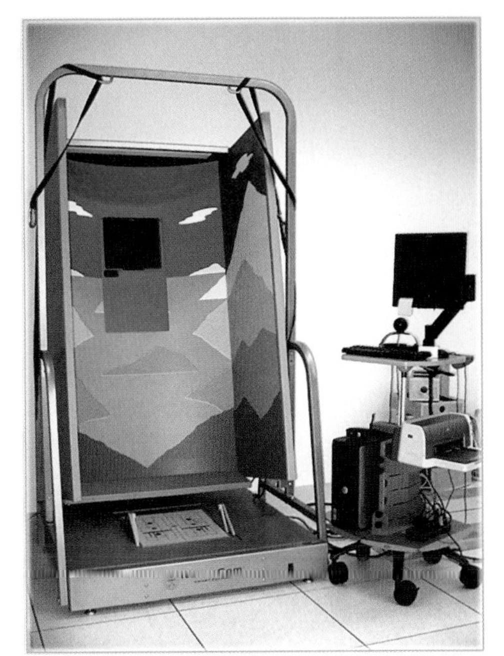

Figure 14-5 Equitest

(Courtesy NeuroCom.)

manufacturers classify as dynamic balance, others claim as really static balance. Our classification system (see "Balance Training" below) will hopefully clear up some of the confusion and allow for a more consistent labeling of the numerous balance-related exercises.

Force platforms ideally evaluate 4 aspects of postural control: steadiness, symmetry, and dynamic stability. Steadiness is the ability to keep the body as motionless as possible. This is a measure of postural sway. Symmetry is the ability to distribute weight evenly between the 2 feet in an upright stance. This is a measure of center of pressure (COP), center of balance (COB), or center of force (COF), depending which testing system you are using. Although inconsistent with our classification system, dynamic stability is often labeled as the ability to transfer the vertical projection of the COG around a stationary supporting base.[27] This is often referred to as a measure of one's perception of their "safe" LOS, as one's goal is to lean or reach as far as possible without losing one's balance. Some manufacturers measure dynamic stability by assessing a person's postural response to external perturbations from a moving platform in 1 of 4 directions: tilting toes up, tilting toes down, shifting medial-lateral, and shifting anterior-posterior. Platform perturbation on some systems is unpredictable and determined by the positioning and sway movement of the subject. In such cases, a person's reaction response can be determined (Figure 14-5). Other systems have a more predictable sinusoidal waveform that remains constant regardless of subject positioning.

Many of these force platform systems measure the vertical ground reaction force and provide a means of computing the COP. The COP represents the center of the distribution of the total force applied to the supporting surface. The COP is calculated from horizontal moment and vertical force data generated by triaxial force platforms. The center of vertical force, on NeuroCom's EquiTest, is the center of the vertical force exerted by the feet against the support surface. In any case (COP, COB, COF), the total force applied

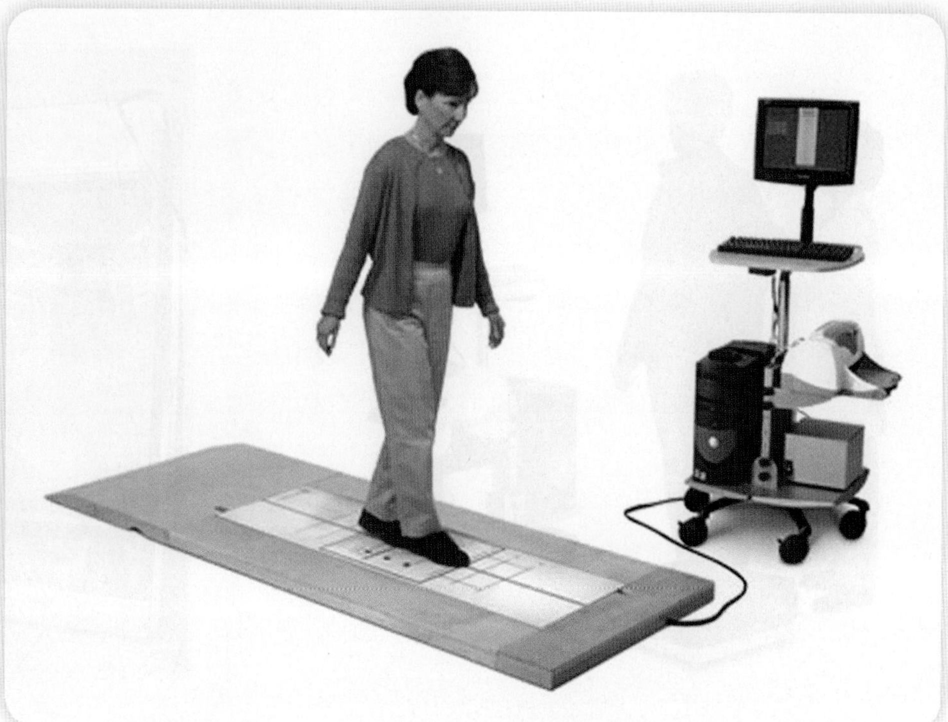

Figure 14-6 **Balance Master with 5-foot forceplate accessory**

(Courtesy NeuroCom.)

to the force platform fluctuates because it includes both body weight and the inertial effects of the slightest movement of the body which occur even when one attempts to stand motionless. The movement of these force-based reference points is theorized to vary according to the movement of the body's COG and the distribution of muscle forces required to control posture. Ideally, healthy athletes should maintain their COP very near the anterior-posterior and medial-lateral midlines.

Once the COP or COF is calculated, several other balance parameters can be attained. Deviation from this point in any direction represents a person's postural sway. Postural sway can be measured in various ways, depending on which system is being used. Mean displacement, length of sway path, length of sway area, amplitude, frequency, and direction with respect to the COP can be calculated on most systems. An equilibrium score, comparing the angular difference between the calculated maximum anterior to posterior COG displacements to a theoretical maximum displacement, is unique to NeuroCom International's EquiTest.

Forceplate technology allows for quantitative analysis and understanding of a subject's postural instability. These systems are fully integrated with hardware/software systems for quickly and quantitatively assessing and rehabilitating balance disorders. Most manufacturers allow for both static and dynamic balance assessment in either double or single leg stances, with eyes open or eyes closed. NeuroCom's EquiTest System is equipped with a moving visual surround (wall) that allows for the most sophisticated technology available for isolating and assessing sensory modality interaction.

Long forceplates have been developed by some manufacturers in an attempt to combat criticism that balance assessment is not functional. Inclusion of the long forceplate (Figure 14-6) adds a vast array of dynamic balance exercises for training, such as walking, step-up-and-over, side and crossover steps, hopping, leaping, and lunging. These important return-to-sport activities can be practiced and perfected through the use of the computer's visual feedback.

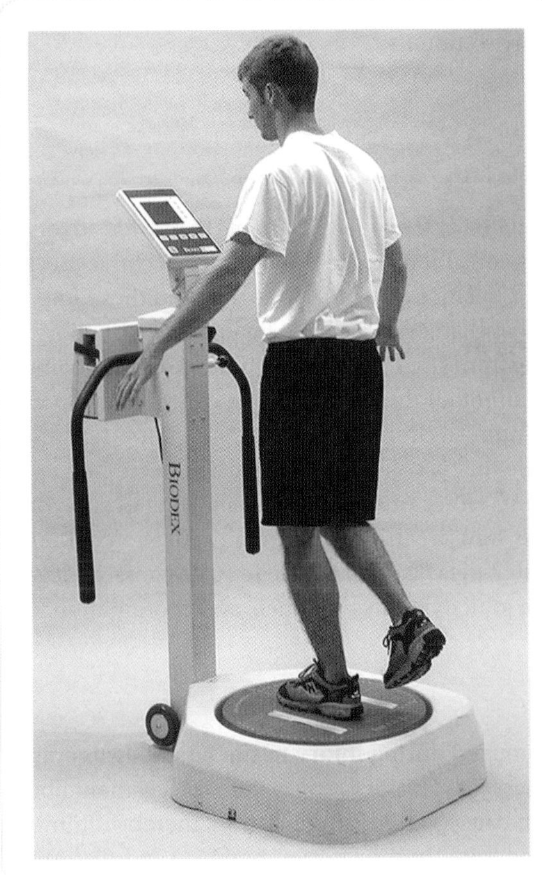

Figure 14-7 Biodex Stability System

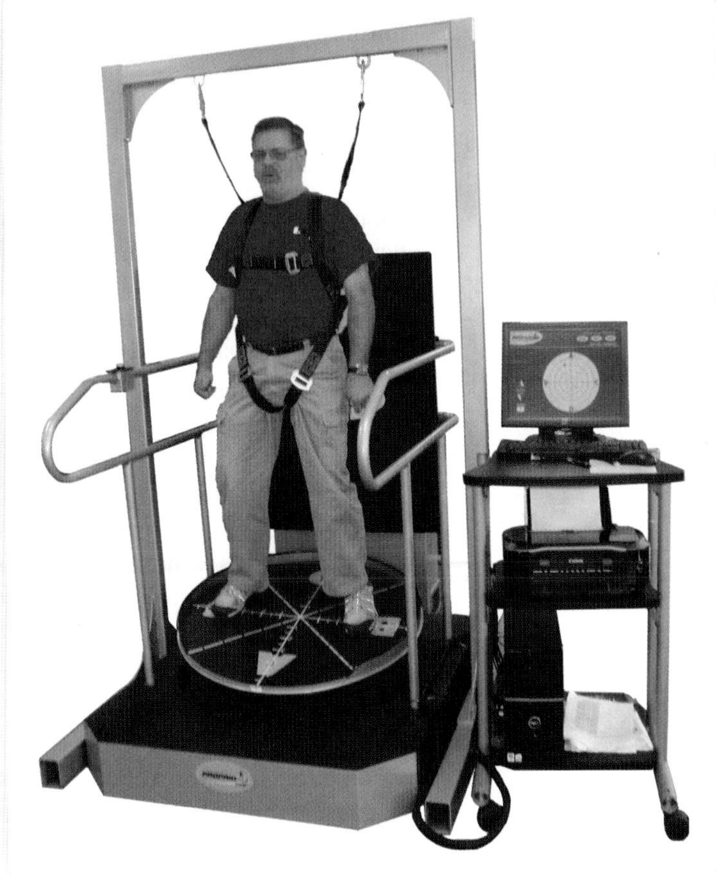

Figure 14-8 PROPRIO® Reactive Balance System

(Courtesy Perry Dynamics.)

Biodex Medical Systems (Shirley, NY) manufactures a dynamic multiaxial tilting platform that offers computer-generated data similar to that of a forceplate system. The Biodex Stability System (Figure 14-7) uses a dynamic multiaxial platform that allows up to 20 degrees of deflection in any direction. It is theorized that this degree of deflection is sufficient to stress joint mechanoreceptors that provide proprioceptive feedback (at end ranges of motion) necessary for balance control. Therapists can assess deficits in dynamic muscular control of posture relative to joint pathology. The patient's ability to control the platform's angle of tilt is quantified as a variance from center, as well as degrees of deflection over time, at various stability levels. A large variance is indicative of poor muscle response. Exercises performed on a multiaxial unstable system such as the Biodex are similar to those of the Biomechanical Ankle Platform System (BAPS board) and are especially effective for regaining proprioception and balance following injury to the ankle joint.

A newer system, the PROPRIO® Reactive Balance System measures the patient's center of mass movement on a computerized, programmable, multidirectional, multispeed platform for both reactive and anticipatory training to assess, rehabilitate, and train balance and proprioception (Figure 14-8). Instead of assessing lower-leg postural responses on a forceplate, this system measures trunk movements by placing a sensor on the lumbosacral joint, L5-S1. Using ultrasonic technology, the PROPRIO® Reactive Balance System quantifies trunk movement in 6 degrees of freedom—lateral, up/down, anterior/posterior, rotation, flexion/extension, and lateral flexion—and displays real-time feedback during training. The platform can generate perturbations to provide variable surface movement requiring the patient to maintain the patient's center of mass over the body's support area during movement and changing sensory environments.

Injury and Balance

It has long been theorized that failure of stretched or damaged ligaments to provide adequate neural feedback in an injured extremity may contribute to decreased proprioceptive mechanisms necessary for maintenance of proper balance. Research has revealed these impairments in individuals with ankle injury[23,31,69] and anterior cruciate ligament (ACL) injury.[4,65] The lack of proprioceptive feedback resulting from such injuries may allow excessive or inappropriate loading of a joint. Furthermore, although the presence of a capsular lesion may interfere with the transmission of afferent impulses from the joint, a more important effect may be alteration of the afferent neural code that is conveyed to the CNS. Decreased reflex excitation of motor neurons may result from either or both of the following events: (a) a decrease in proprioceptive input to the CNS; and (b) an increase in the activation of inhibitory interneurons within the spinal cord. All of these factors may lead to progressive degeneration of the joint and continued deficits in joint dynamics, balance, and coordination.

Ankle Injuries

Joint proprioceptors are believed to be damaged during injury to the lateral ligaments of the ankle because joint receptor fibers possess less tensile strength than the ligament fibers. Damage to the joint receptors is believed to cause joint deafferentation, thereby diminishing the supply of messages from the injured joint up the afferent pathway and disrupting proprioceptive function.[24] Freeman et al[24] were the first to report a decrease in the frequency of functional instability following ankle sprains when coordination exercises were performed as part of rehabilitation. Thus the term *articular deafferentation* was introduced to designate the mechanism that they believed to be the cause of functional instability of the ankle. This finding led to the inclusion of balance training in ankle rehabilitation programs.

Since 1955, Freeman[23] has theorized that if ankle injuries cause partial deafferentation and functional instability, a person's postural sway would be altered because of a proprioception deficit. Although some studies[74] have not supported Freeman's theory, other more recent studies using high-tech equipment (forceplate, kinesthesiometer, etc) have revealed balance deficits in ankles following acute sprains[25,31,66] and/or in ankles with chronic instabilities.[9,22,26,67]

Differences were identified between injured and uninjured ankles in 14 ankle-injured subjects using a computerized strain-gauge forceplate.[25] Four of 5 possible postural sway parameters (standard deviation of the mean COP dispersion, mean sway amplitude, average speed, and number of sway amplitudes exceeding 5 and 10 mm) taken in the frontal plane from a single-leg stance position were reported to discriminate between injured and noninjured ankles. The authors reported that the application of an ankle brace eliminated the differences between injury status when tested on each parameter, therefore improving balance performance. More importantly, this study suggests that the stabilometry technique of selectively analyzing postural sway movements in the frontal plane, where the diameter of the supporting area is smallest, leads to higher sensitivity. Because difficulties of maintaining balance after a ligament lesion involve the subtalar axis, it is proposed that increased sway movements of the different body segments would be found primarily in the frontal plane. The authors speculated that this could explain nonsignificant findings of earlier stabilometry studies[74] involving injured ankles.

Orthotic intervention and postural sway were studied in 13 subjects with acute inversion ankle sprains and 12 uninjured subjects under 2 treatment conditions (orthotic, nonorthotic) and 4 platform movements (stable, inversion/eversion, plantar flexion/dorsiflexion, medial/lateral perturbations).[31] Results revealed that ankle-injured subjects swayed more than uninjured subjects when assessed in a single-leg test. The analysis also revealed that custom-fit orthotics may restrict undesirable motion at the foot and ankle, and enhance joint mechanoreceptors to detect perturbations and provide structural support for detecting and controlling postural sway in ankle-injured subjects. A similar study[66] reported improvements in static balance for injured subjects while wearing custom-made orthotics.

Studies involving subjects with chronic ankle instabilities[9,22,26,67] indicate that individuals with a history of inversion ankle sprain are less stable in single-limb stance on the involved leg as compared to the uninvolved leg and/or noninjured subjects. Significant differences between injured and uninjured subjects for sway amplitude but not sway frequency using a standard forceplate were revealed.[9] The effect of stance perturbation on frontal plane postural control was tested in 3 groups of subjects: (a) control (no previous ankle injury); (b) functional ankle instability and 8-week training program; and (c) mechanical instability without functional instability (without shoe, with shoe, with brace and shoe).[67] The authors reported a relative change from ankle to hip synergy at medially directed translations of the support surface on the NeuroCom EquiTest. The impairment was restored after 8 weeks of ankle disk training. The effect of a shoe and brace did not exceed the effect of the shoe alone. Impaired ankle function was shown to be related to coordination, as subjects changed from ankle toward hip strategies for postural adjustments.

Similarly, researchers[36] reported that lateral ankle joint anesthesia did not alter postural sway or passive joint position sense, but did affect the COB position (similar to COP) during both static and dynamic testing. This suggests the presence of an adaptive mechanism to compensate for the loss of afferent stimuli from the region of the lateral ankle ligaments.[36] Subjects tended to shift their COB medially during dynamic balance testing and slightly laterally during static balance testing. The authors speculated that COB shifting may provide additional proprioceptive input from cutaneous receptors in the sole of the foot or stretch receptors in the peroneal muscle tendon unit, which therefore prevents increased postural sway.

Increased postural sway frequency and latencies are parameters thought to be indicative of impaired ankle joint proprioception.[13,69] Cornwall et al[9] and Pintsaar et al,[67] however, found no differences between chronically injured subjects and control subjects on these measures. This raises the question as to whether postural sway was in fact caused by a proprioceptive deficit. Increased postural sway amplitudes in the absence of sway frequencies might suggest that chronically injured subjects recover their ankle joint proprioception over time. Thus, more research is warranted for investigating loss of joint proprioception and postural sway frequency.[9]

In summary, results of studies involving both chronic and acute ankle sprains suggest that increased postural sway and/or balance instability may not be caused by a single factor but by disruption of both neurologic and biomechanical factors at the ankle joint. Loss of balance may result from abnormal or altered biomechanical alignment of the body, thus affecting the transmission of somatosensory information from the ankle joint. It is possible that observed postural sway amplitudes following injury are a result of joint instability along the kinetic chain, rather than deafferentation. Thus, the orthotic intervention[31,61,62] may have provided more optimal joint alignment.

Knee Injuries

Ligamentous injury to the knee has proven to affect the ability of subjects to accurately detect position.[2,3,4,46,49,50] The general consensus among numerous investigators performing proprioceptive testing is that a clinical proprioception deficit occurs in most patients after an ACL rupture who have functional instability and that this deficit seems to persist to some degree after an ACL reconstruction.[2] Because of the relationships between proprioception (somatosensation) and balance, it has been suggested that the patient's ability to balance on the ACL-injured leg may also be decreased.[4,65]

Studies have evaluated the effects of ACL ruptures on standing balance using forceplate technology, and while some studies have revealed balance deficits,[25,53] others have not.[18,35] Thus, there appear to be conflicting results from these studies depending on which parameters are measured. Mizuta et al[53] found significant differences in postural sway when measuring COP and sway distance area between 11 functionally stable and 15 functionally unstable subjects who had unilateral ACL-deficient knees. Faculjak et al,[18] however, found no differences in postural stability between 8 ACL-deficient subjects and 10 normal subjects when measuring average latency and response strength on an EquiTest System.

Several potential reasons for this discrepancy exist. First, it has been suggested that there might be a link between static balance and isometric strength of the musculature at the ankle and knee. Isometric muscle strength could therefore compensate for any somatosensory deficit present in the involved knee during a closed-chain static balance test. Second, many studies fail to discriminate between functionally unstable ACL-deficient knees and knees that were not functionally unstable. This presents a design flaw, especially considering that functionally stable knees would most likely provide adequate balance despite ligamentous pathology. Another suggested reason for not seeing differences between injured knees and uninjured knees on static balance measures could be explained by the role that joint mechanoreceptors play. Neurophysiologic studies[28,29,43,46] reveal that joint mechanoreceptors provide enhanced kinesthetic awareness in the near-terminal ROM or extremes of motion. Therefore, it could be speculated that if the maximum LOS are never reached during a static balance test, damaged mechanoreceptors (muscle or joint) may not even become a factor. Dynamic balance tests or functional hop tests that involve dynamic balance could challenge the postural control system (ankle strategies are taken over by hip and/or stepping strategies), requiring more mechanoreceptor input. These tests would most likely discriminate between functionally unstable ACL-deficient knees and normal knees.

Clinical Pearl

The therapist should ensure that the patient has the necessary pain-free ROM and muscular strength to complete the tasks that are being incorporated into the program. Additionally, for exercises beyond the phase I static exercises, the patient must be beyond the acute inflammatory phase of tissue response to injury. Once these factors have been considered, the therapist should focus on developing a protocol that is safe yet challenging, stresses multiple planes of motion, and incorporates a multisensory approach.

Head Injury

Neurologic status following mild head injury has been assessed using balance as a criterion variable. Therapists and team physicians have long evaluated head injuries with the Romberg tests of sensory modality function to test "balance." This is an easy and effective sideline test; however, the literature suggests there is more to posture control than just balance and sensory modality,[55,56,61,64,72] especially when assessing people with head injury.[30,33] The postural control system, which is responsible for linking brain to body communication, is often affected as a result of mild head injury. Several studies have identified postural stability deficits in patients up to 3 days postinjury by using commercially available balance systems.[30,33] It appears this deficit is related to a sensory interaction problem, whereby the injured patient fails to use their visual system effectively. This research suggests that objective balance assessment can be used for establishing recovery curves for making return to play decisions in concussed patients. Rehabilitation of concussed patients using balance techniques has yet to be studied.

Balance Training

Developing a rehabilitation program that includes exercises for improving balance and postural equilibrium is vital for a successful return to competition from a lower-extremity injury. Regardless of whether the patient has sustained a quadriceps strain or an ankle sprain, the injury has caused a disruption at some point between the body's COG and base of support. This is likely to have caused compensatory weight shifts and gait changes along the kinetic chain that have resulted in balance deficits. These deficits may be detected through the use of functional assessment tests and/or computerized instrumentation previously discussed for assessing balance. Having the advanced technology available to quantify balance deficits is an amenity, but not a necessity. Imagination and creativity are often the best tools available to therapists with limited resources who are trying to design balance training protocols.

Because virtually all sport activities involve closed-chain lower-extremity function, functional rehabilitation should be performed in the closed kinetic chain. However, ROM, movement speed, and additional resistance may be more easily controlled in the open chain initially. Therefore, adequate, safe function in an open chain may be the first step in the rehabilitation process, but should not be the focus of the rehabilitation plan. The therapist should attempt to progress the patient to functional closed-chain exercises quickly and safely. Depending on severity of injury, this could be as early as 1 day postinjury.

As previously mentioned, there is a close relationship between somatosensation, kinesthesia, and balance. Therefore, many of the exercises proposed for kinesthetic training are indirectly enhancing balance. Several methods of regaining balance have been proposed in the literature and are included in the most current rehabilitation protocols for ankle[41,73] and knee injury.[11,40,51,72]

A variety of activities can be used to improve balance, but the therapist should first consider 5 general rules before beginning. The exercises must:

- Be safe, yet challenging.
- Stress multiple planes of motion.
- Incorporate a multisensory approach.
- Begin with static, bilateral, and stable surfaces and progress to dynamic, unilateral, and unstable surfaces.
- Progress toward sport-specific exercises.

There are several ways in which the therapist can meet these goals. Balance exercises should be performed in an open area, where the patient will not be injured in the event of a fall. It is best to perform exercises with an assistive device within an arm's reach (eg, chair, railing, table, wall), especially during the initial phase of rehabilitation. When considering exercise duration for balance exercises, the therapist can use either sets and repetitions or a time-based protocol. The patient can perform 2 to 3 sets of 15 repetitions and progress to 30 repetitions as tolerated, or perform 10 of the exercises for a 15-second period and progress to 30-second periods later in the program.

Clinical Pearl

It should be explained to the patient, at the outset, that the goal is to challenge the patient's motor control system, to the point that the last 2 repetitions of each set of exercises should be difficult to perform. When the last 2 repetitions no longer are challenging to the athlete, the athlete should be progressed to the next exercise. This can be determined through subjective information reported from the athlete, as well as the therapists objective observations. It is very important to provide a variety of exercises and levels of exercises so that the patient maintains a high level of motivation.

Classification of Balance Exercises

Static balance is when the COG is maintained over a fixed base of support (unilateral or bilateral) while standing on a stable surface. Examples of static exercises are a single-leg, double-leg, or tandem-stance Romberg task. Semidynamic balance involves 1 of 2 possible activities: (a) The person maintains their COG over a fixed base of support while standing on a moving surface (Chattecx Balance System or EquiTest) or unstable surface (Biodex Stability System, BAPS, medium density foam or minitramp); or (b) the person transfers their COG over a fixed base of support to selected ranges and/or directions within the LOS while standing on a stable surface (Balance Master's LOS, functional reach tests, minisquats, or T-Band kicks). Dynamic balance involves the maintenance of the COG within the LOS over a moving base of support (feet), usually while on a stable surface. These tasks require the use of a stepping strategy. The base of support is always changing its position, forcing the COG to be adjusted with each movement. Examples of dynamic exercises are walking on a balance beam, step-up-and-over task, or bounding. Functional balance tasks are the same as dynamic tasks with the inclusion of sport-specific tasks such as throwing and catching.

Phase I

The progression of activities during this phase should include nonballistic types of drills. Training for static balance can be initiated once the patient is able to bear weight on the extremity. The patient should first be asked to perform a bilateral 20-second Romberg test on a variety of surfaces, beginning with a hard/firm surface (Figure 14-9). Once a comfort zone is established, the patient should be progressed to performing unilateral balance tasks on both the involved and uninvolved extremities on a stable surface.

The therapist should make comparisons from these tests to determine the patient's ability to balance bilaterally and unilaterally. It should be noted that even though this is termed static balance, the patient does not remain perfectly motionless. To maintain static balance,

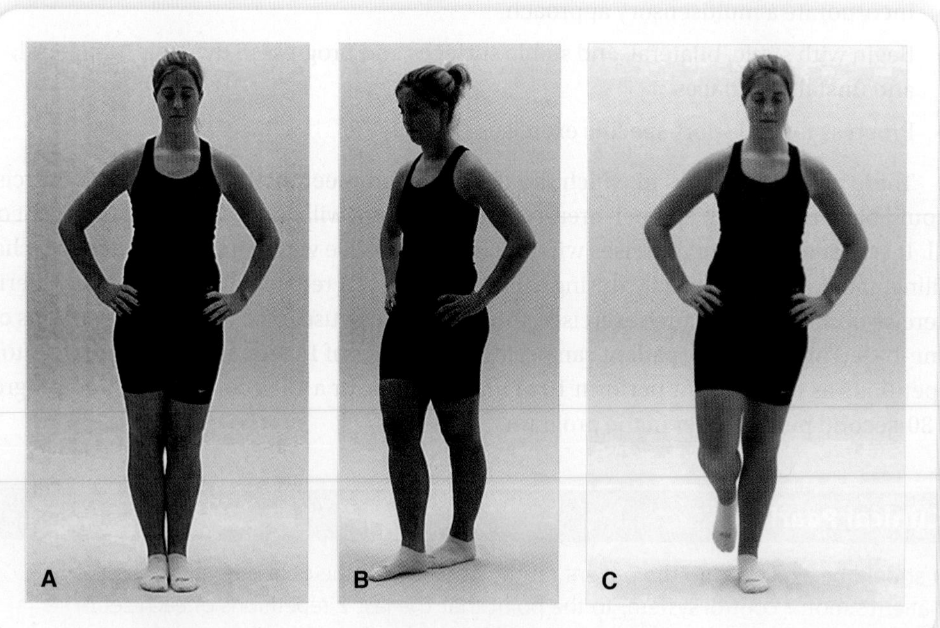

Figure 14-9 Double- and single-leg balance on a stable surface

A. Double-leg stance. **B.** Double-leg tandem stance. **C.** Single-leg stance.

the patient must make many small corrections at the ankle, hip, trunk, arms, or head as previously discussed (see "Selection of Movement Strategies" above). If the patient is having difficulties performing these activities, they should not be progressed to the next surface. Repetitions of modified Romberg tests can be performed by first using the arms as a counterbalance, then attempting the activity without using the arms. Static balance activities should be used as a precursor to more dynamic activities. The general progression of these exercises should be from bilateral to unilateral, with eyes open to eyes closed. The exercises should attempt to eliminate or alter the various sensory information (visual, vestibular, and somatosensory) so as to challenge the other systems. In most orthopedic rehabilitation situations, this is going to involve eye closure and changes in the support surface so the somatosensory system can be overloaded or stressed. This theory is synonymous with the overload principle in therapeutic exercise. Research suggests that balance activities, both with and without visual input, will enhance motor function at the brainstem level.[7,73] However, as the patient becomes more efficient at performing activities involving static balance, eye closure is recommended so that only the somatosensory system is left to control balance.

As improvement occurs on a firm surface, bilateral static balance drills should progress to an unstable surface such as a Tremor box, DynaDisc rocker board on hard surface, Bosu Balance Trainer (flat side up then bubble side up), BAPS board, or foam surface (Figure 14-10).[1] The purpose of the different surfaces is to safely challenge the injured patient, while keeping the patient motivated to rehabilitate the injured extremity. Additionally, the therapist can

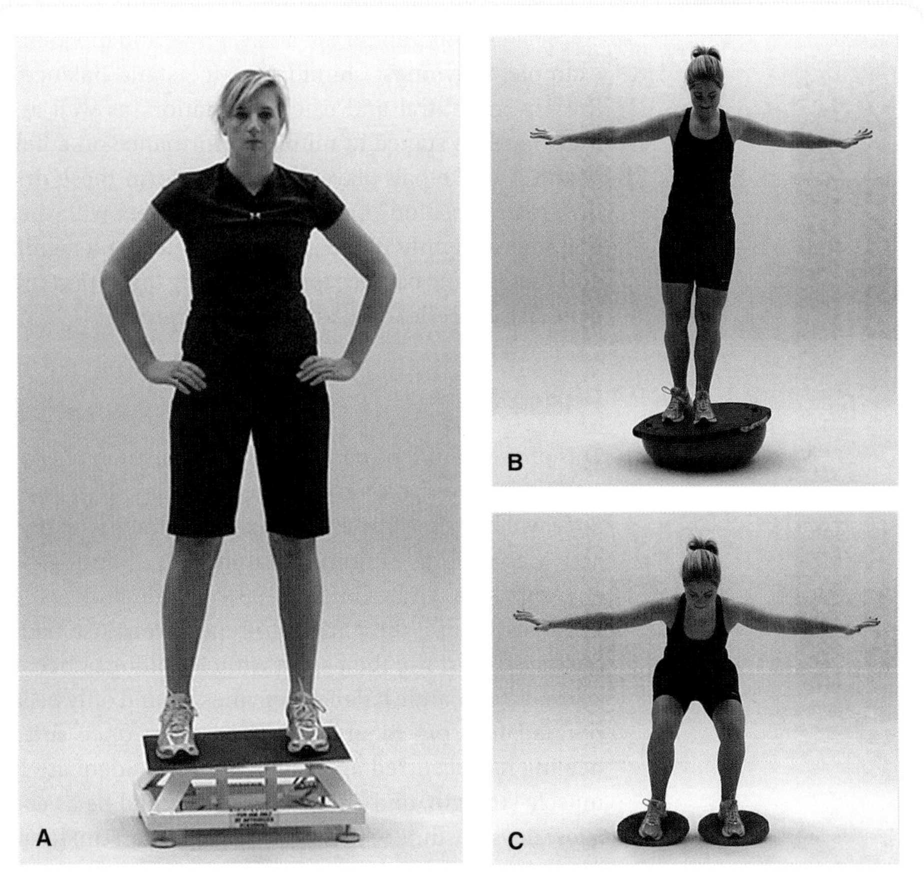

Figure 14-10 Double leg balance on an unstable surface

A. Tremor Box. **B.** Bosu Balance Trainer, flat surface. **C.** DynaDiscs.

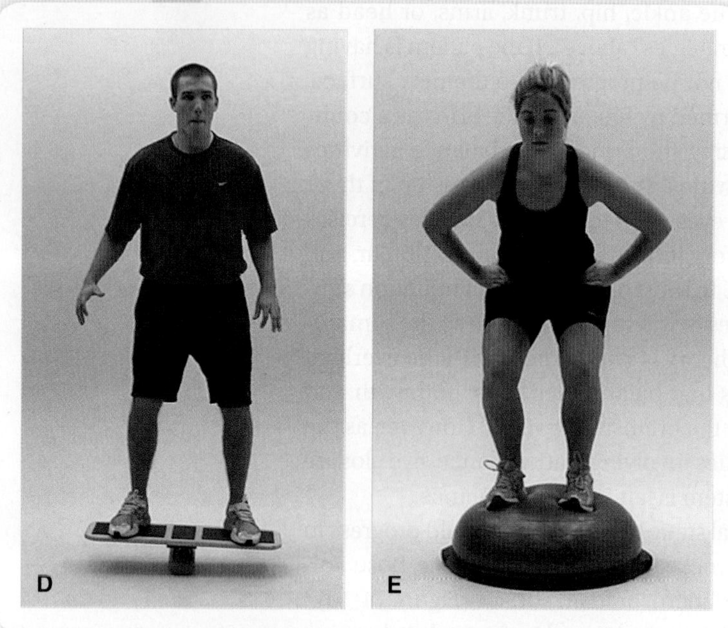

Figure 14-10 ***(Continued)***

D. Extreme Balance Board. **E.** Bosu Balance Trainer, bubble surface.

introduce light shoulder, back, or chest taps in an attempt to challenge the patient's ability to maintain balance (Figure 14-11). Once the control is demonstrated in a bilateral stance, the patient can progress to similar activities using a unilateral stance (Figure 14-12). All of these exercises increase awareness of the location of the COG under a challenged condition, thereby helping to increase ankle strength in the closed kinetic chain. Such training may also increase sensitivity of the muscle spindle and thereby increase proprioceptive input to the spinal cord, which may provide compensation for altered joint afference.[46]

Although static and semidynamic balance exercises may not be very functional for most sport activities, they are the first step toward regaining proprioceptive awareness, reflex stabilization, and postural orientation. The patient should attempt to assume a functional stance while performing static balance drills. Training in different positions places a variety of demands on the musculotendinous structures about the ankle, knee, and hip joints. For example, a gymnast should practice static balance with the hip in neutral and external rotation, as well as during a tandem stance to mimic performance on a balance beam. A basketball player should perform these drills in the "ready position" on the balls of the feet with the hips and knees slightly flexed. Patients requiring a significant amount of static balance for performing their sport include gymnasts, cheerleaders, and football linemen.[41]

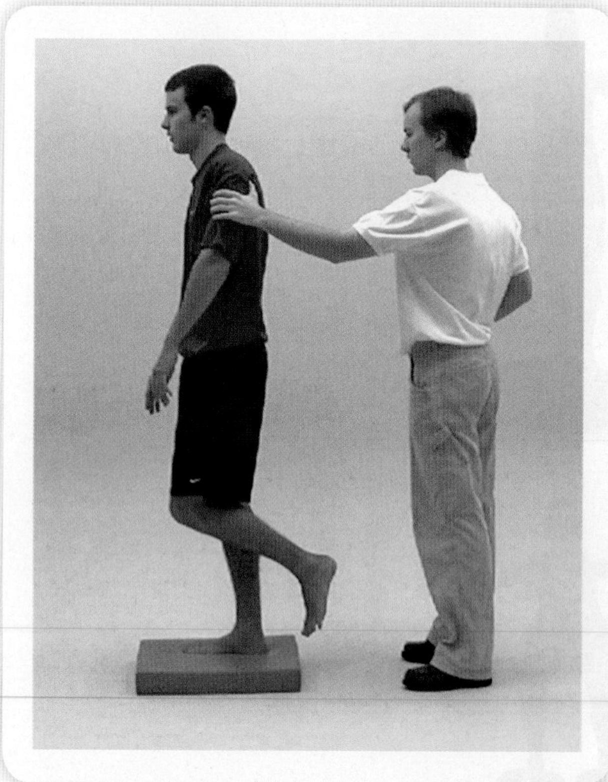

Figure 14-11

A therapist causing perturbations using a shoulder tap is good for transitioning from double-leg balance on an unstable surface to single-leg balance on an unstable surface.

Phase II

This phase should be considered the transition phase from static to more dynamic balance activities. Dynamic balance will be especially important for patients who perform activities such as running, jumping, and cutting, which encompasses approximately 95% of all athletes. Such activities require the patient to repetitively lose and gain balance to perform their sport without falling or becoming injured.[41] Dynamic balance activities should only be incorporated into the rehabilitation program once sufficient healing has occurred and the patient has adequate ROM, muscle strength, and endurance. This could be as early as a few days postinjury in the case of a grade 1 ankle sprain, or as late as 5 weeks postsurgery in the case of an ACL reconstruction. Before the therapist progresses the patient to challenging dynamic and sport-specific balance drills, several semidynamic (intermediate) exercises should be introduced.

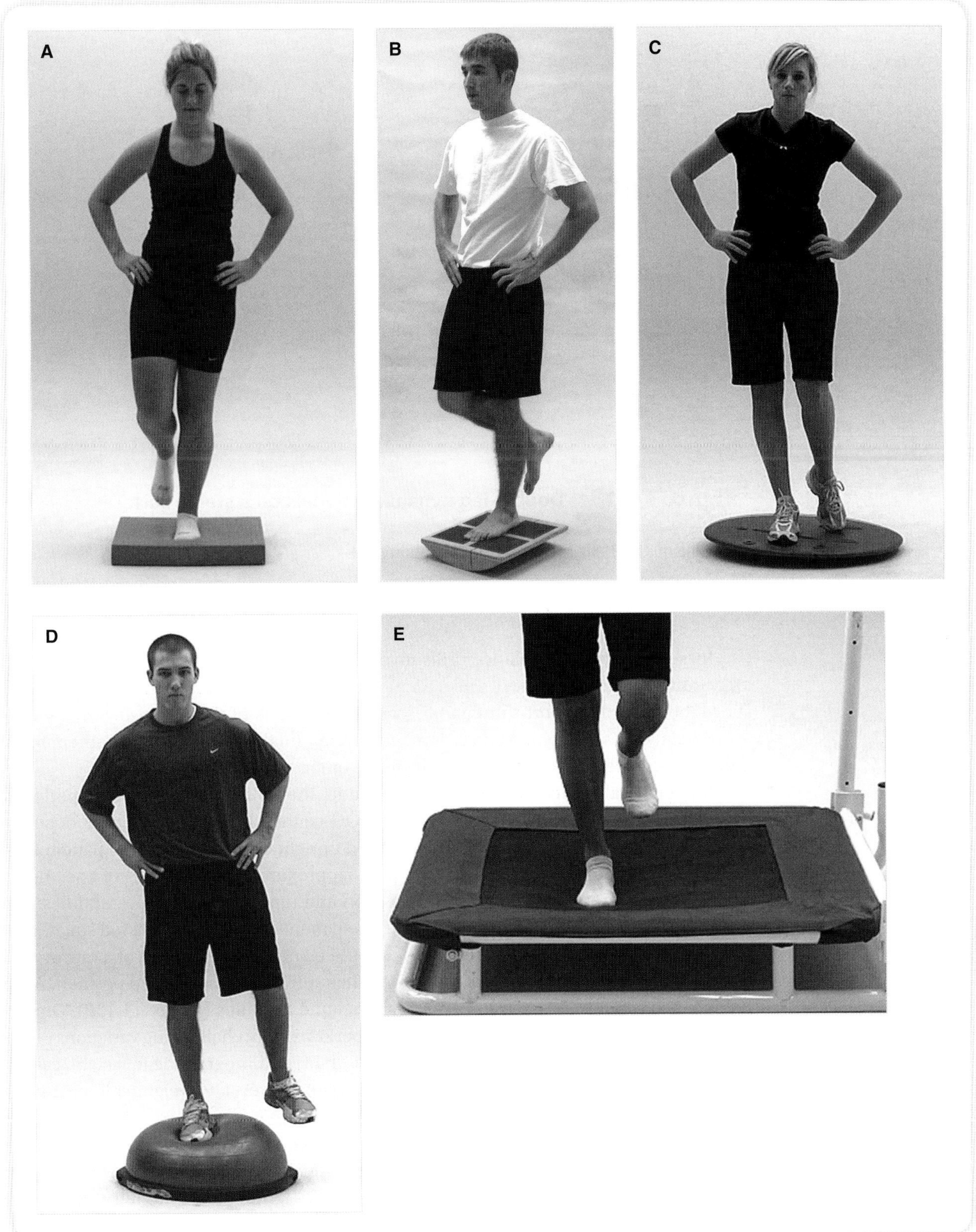

Figure 14-12 **Single-leg balance on an unstable surface**

A. Foam pad. **B.** Rocker Board. **C.** BAPS Board. **D.** Bosu Balance Trainer. **E.** Plyoback.

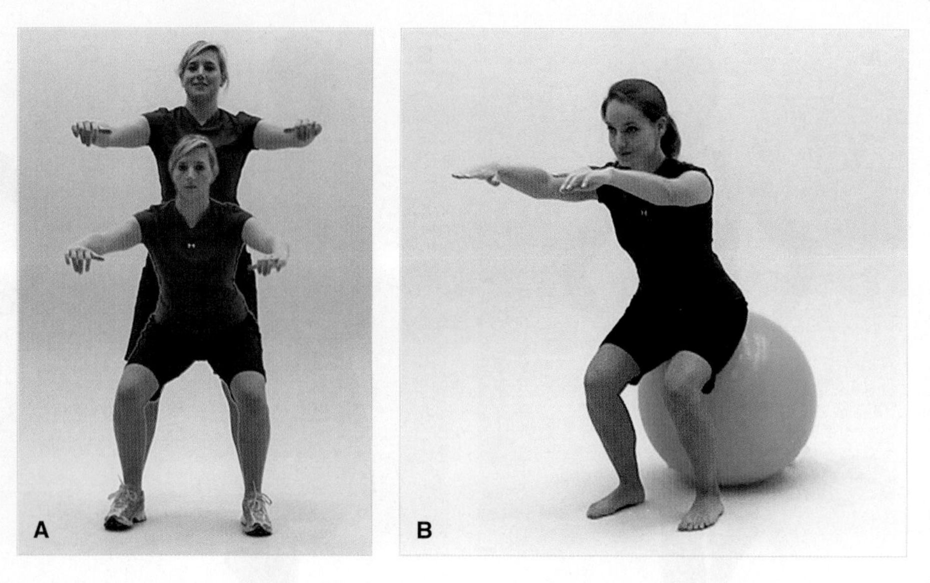

Figure 14-13 Double-leg dynamic activities on a stable surface

A. Minisquats. **B.** Sit-to-stand from a stability ball.

These semidynamic balance drills involve displacement or perturbation of the COG away from the base of support. The patient is challenged to return and/or steady the COG above the base of support throughout several repetitions of the exercise. Some of these exercises involve a bilateral stance, some involve a unilateral stance, while others involve transferring of weight from one extremity to the other.

The bilateral-stance balance drills include the minisquat, which is performed with the feet shoulder-width apart and the COG centered over a stable base of support (Figure 14-13*A*). The trunk should be positioned upright over the legs as the patient slowly flexes the hips and knees into a partial squat—approximately 50 degrees of knee flexion. The patient then returns to the starting position and repeats the task several times. Once ROM, strength, and stability have improved, the patient can progress to a full squat, which approaches 90 degrees knee flexion. These should be performed in front of a mirror so the patient can observe the amount of stability on their return to the extended position. A large stability ball can also be used to perform sit-to-stand activities (Figure 14-13*B*). Once the patient reaches a comfort zone, the patient can perform more challenging variations of these exercises, beginning on a stable surface (Figure 14-14) and progressing to weight, cable, or tubing-resisted exercises (Figure 14-15). Rotational maneuvers and weight-shifting exercises on unstable surfaces such as the Bosu, DynaDisc, or foam pad are used to assist the patient in controlling the patient's COG during semidynamic movements (Figure 14-16). These exercises are important in the rehabilitation of ankle, knee, and hip injuries, as they help improve weight transfer, COG sway velocity, and left/right weight symmetry. They can be performed in an attempt to challenge anterior-posterior stability or medial-lateral stability.

The therapist has a variety of options for unilateral semidynamic balance exercises. In the progression to more dynamic exercises, the patient should emphasize controlled hip and knee flexion, followed by a smooth return to a stabilization position. Step-ups can be performed either in the sagittal plane (forward step-up) or in the transverse plane (lateral step-up) (Figure 14-17*A* and *B*). These drills should begin with the heel of the uninvolved extremity on the floor. Using a 2 count, the patient should shift body weight toward the

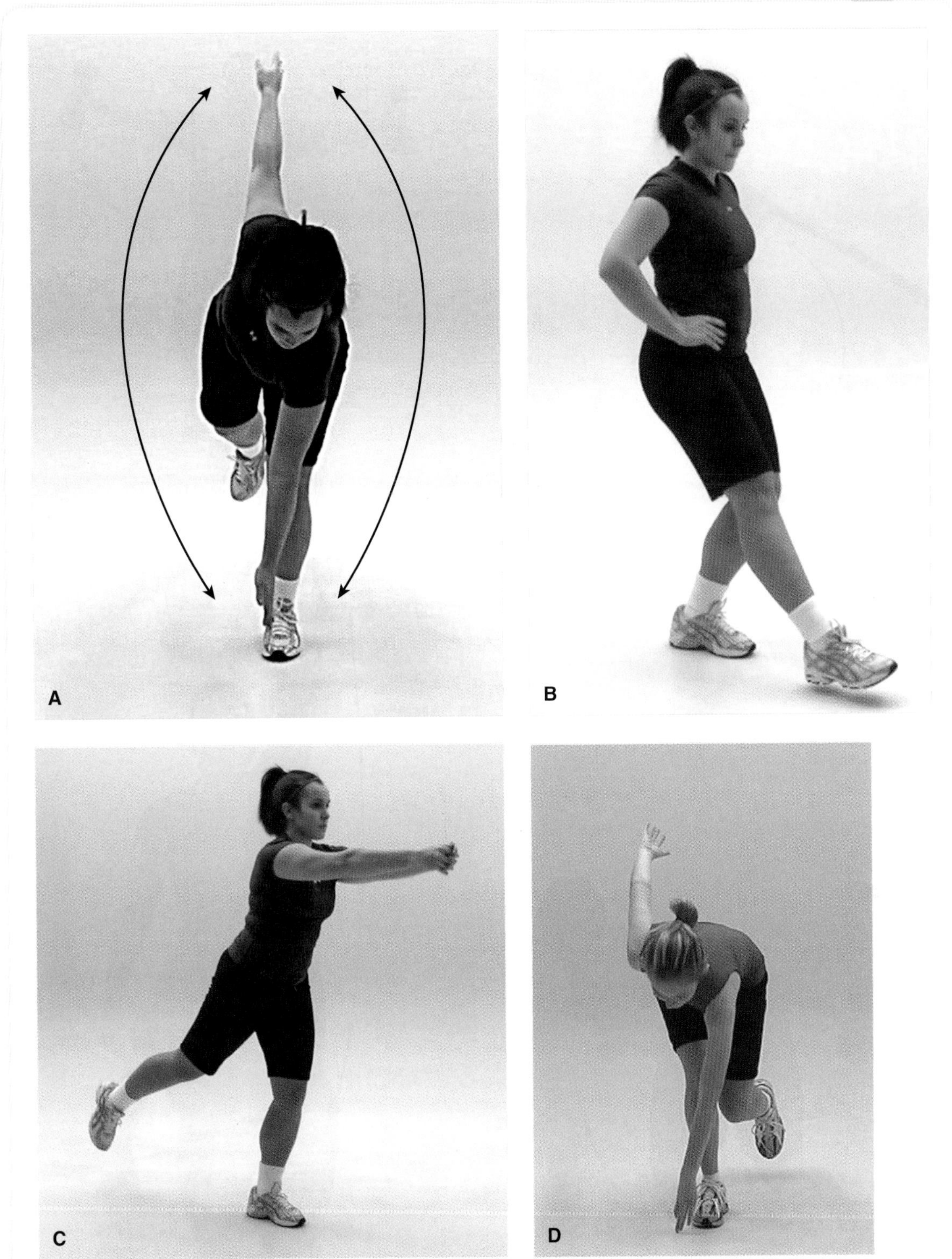

Figure 14-14 **Single-leg balance dynamic (multiplane) movements on an stable surface**

A. Windmill. **B.** Single-leg reach. **C.** Double-arm reach. **D.** Romanian deadlift.

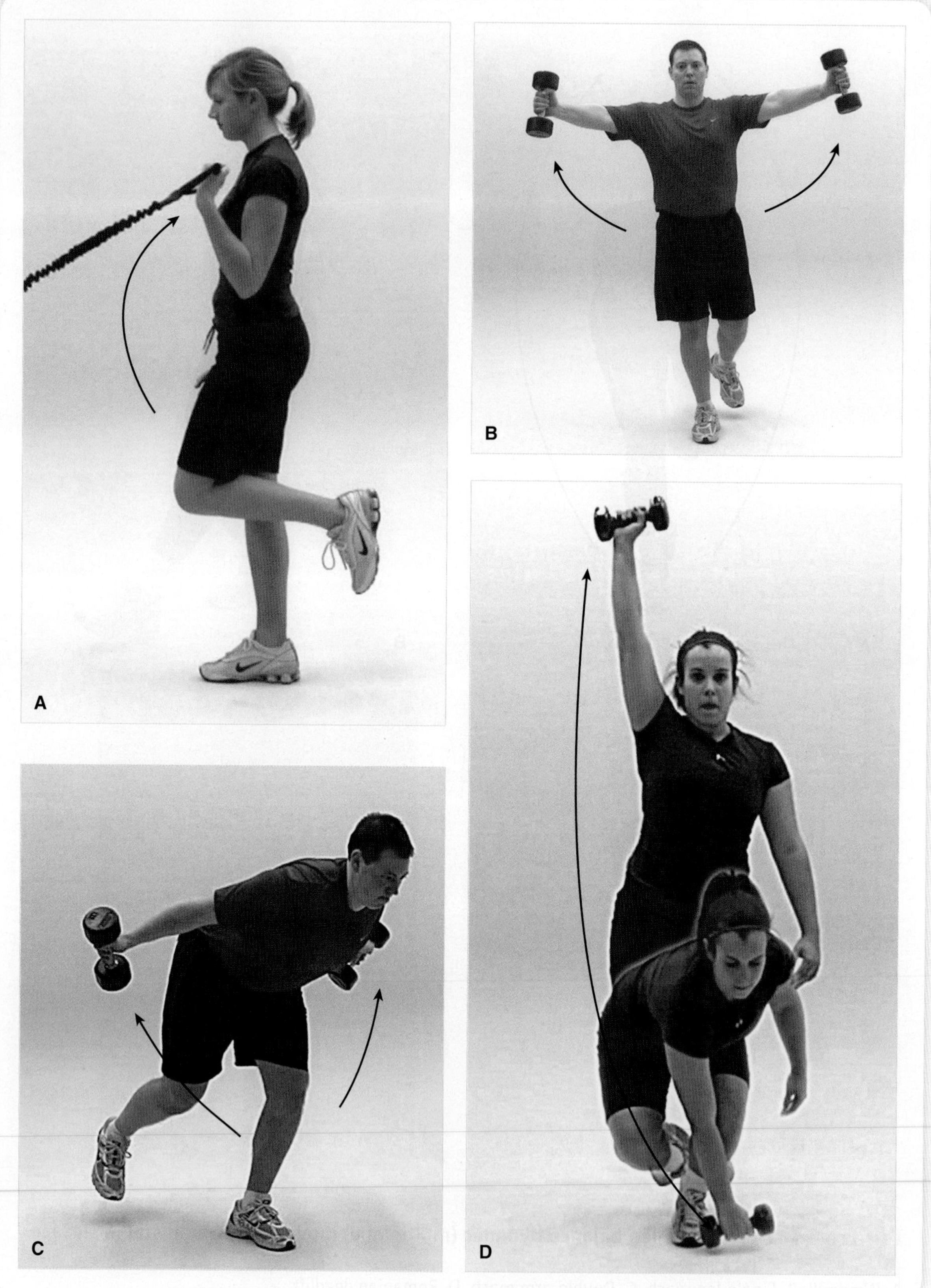

Figure 14-15 **Single-leg balance-resisted (multiplane) movements on a stable surface**

A. Bicep curls using cable or tubing. **B.** Dumbbell scaption. **C.** Dumbbell cobra. **D.** Squat touchdown to overhead press.

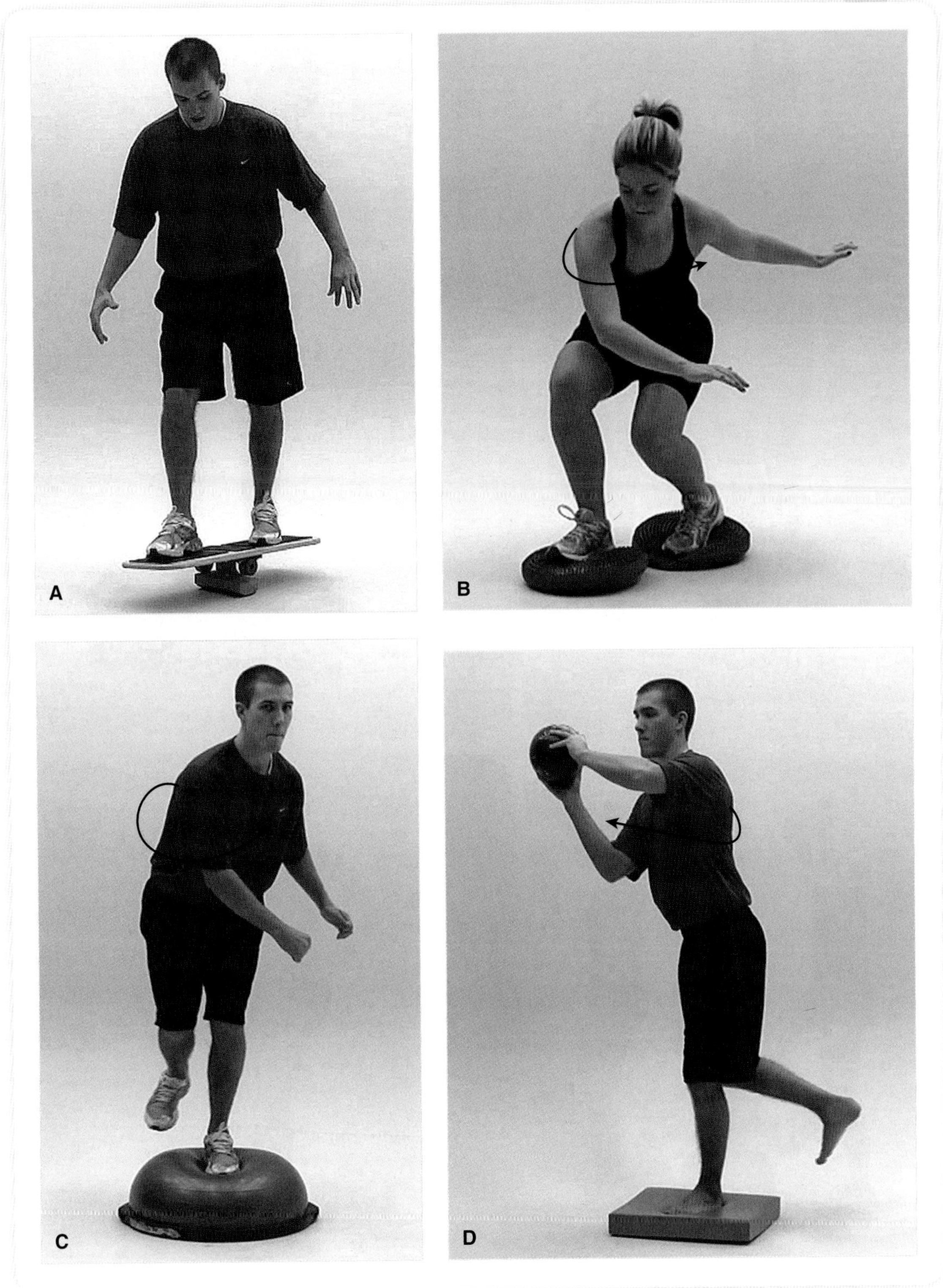

Figure 14-16 Double-leg and single-leg (multiplane) dynamic balance activities on an unstable surface

A. Tandem stance on an Extreme Balance Board. **B.** Standing rotation on DynaDisc. **C.** Standing rotation on Bosu Balance Trainer. **D.** Partner throw-and-catch using a weighted ball while balancing on a foam pad.

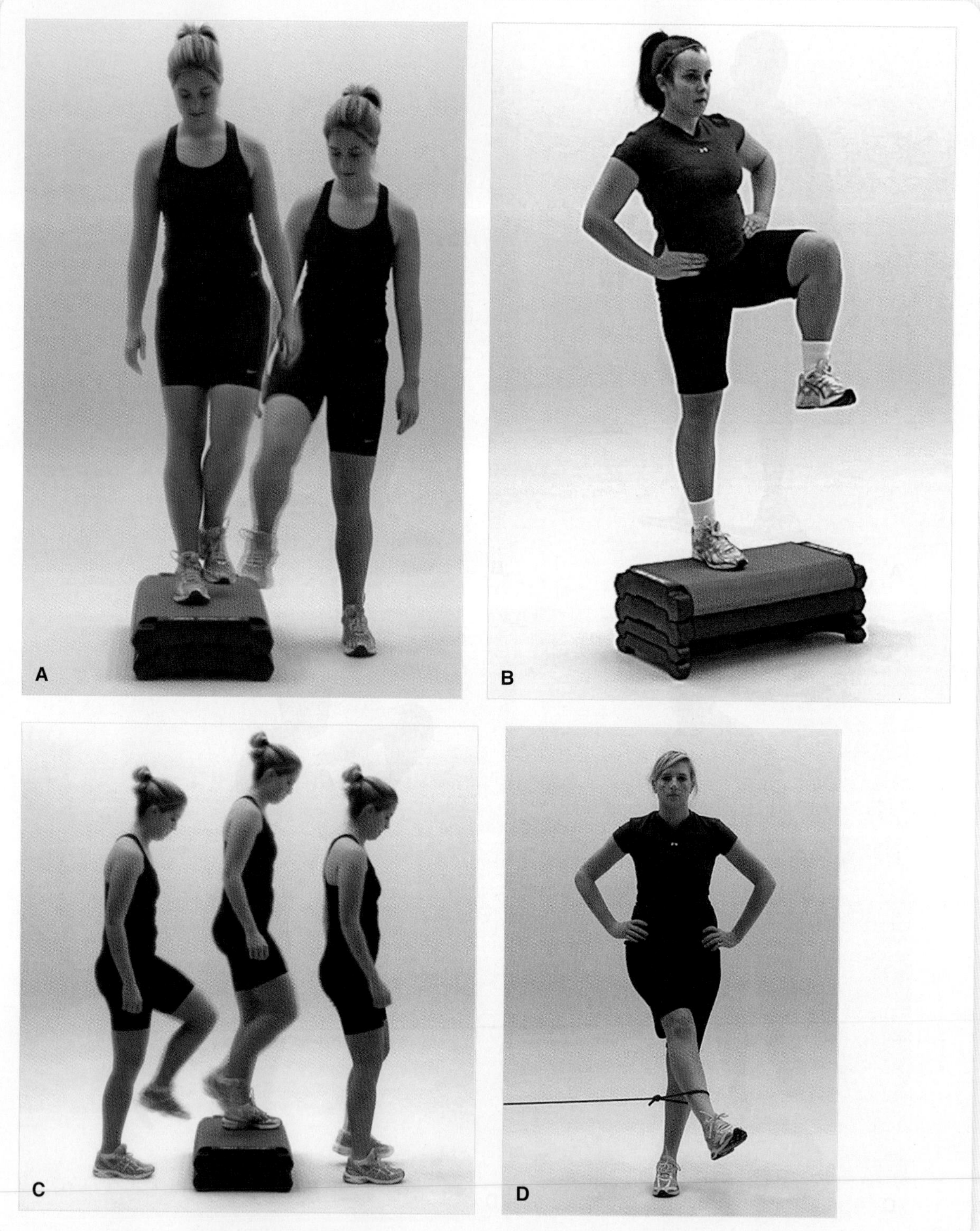

Figure 14-17 **Stepping movements to stabilization**

A. Lateral step up. **B.** Forward step-up to single-leg balance. **C.** Step-up-and-over (alternating lead leg). **D.** Thera-Band kicks.

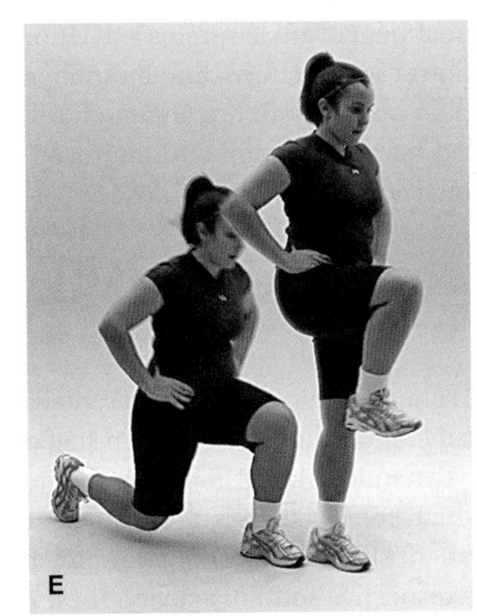

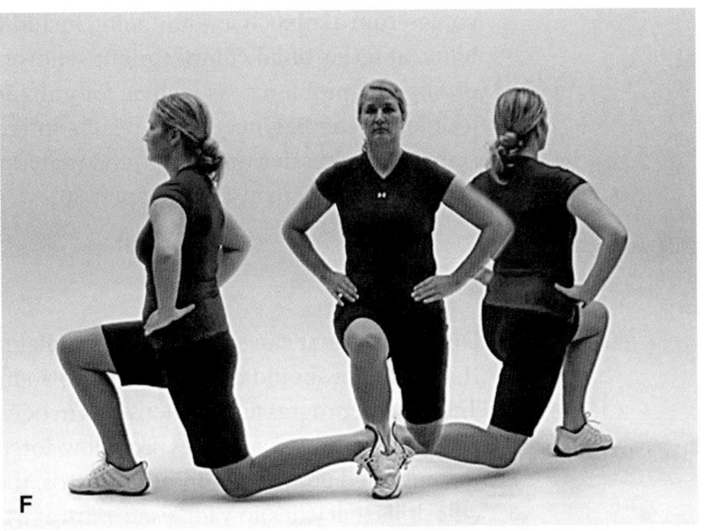

Figure 14-17 ***(Continued)***

E. Forward lunge to single-leg balance. **F.** Multiplane lunges (sagittal, frontal, transverse).

involved side and use the involved extremity to slowly raise the body onto the step.[73] The involved knee should not be "locked" into full extension. Instead, the knee should be positioned in approximately 5 degrees of flexion, while balancing on the step for 3 seconds. Following the 3 count, the body weight should be shifted toward the uninvolved side and lowered to the heel of the uninvolved side. Step-up-and-over activities are similar to step-ups, but involve more dynamic transfer of the COG. These should be performed by having the patient both ascend and descend using the involved extremity (Figure 14-17*C*) or ascend with the involved extremity and descend with the uninvolved extremity forcing the involved leg to support the body on the descend. The therapist can also introduce the patient to more challenging static tasks during this phase. For example, the very popular Thera-Band kicks (T-Band kicks or steamboats) are excellent for improving balance. Thera-Band kicks are performed with an elastic material (attached to the ankle of the uninvolved leg) serving as a resistance against a relatively fast kicking motion (Figure 14-17*D*). The patient's balance on the involved extremity is challenged by perturbations caused by the kicking motion of the uninvolved leg. Four sets of these exercises should be performed, 1 for each of 4 possible kicking motions: hip flexion, hip extension, hip abduction, and hip adduction. T-Band kicks can also be performed on foam or a minitramp if additional somatosensory challenges are desired.[72] Single and multiplane lunges can also be used to transition to dynamic activities (Figure 14-17*E* and *F*).

The Balance Shoes (Orthopedic Physical Therapy Products, Minneapolis, MN) are another excellent tool for improving the strength of lower extremity musculature and, ultimately, improving balance. The shoes allow lower-extremity balance and strengthening exercises to be performed in a functional, closed-kinetic-chain manner. The shoes consist of a cork sandal with a rubber sole, and a rubber hemisphere similar in consistency to a lacrosse ball positioned under the midsole (see Figures 25-28 to 25-35). The design of the sandals essentially creates an individualized perturbation device for each limb that can be utilized in any number of functional activities, ranging from static single-leg stance to dynamic gait activities performed in multiple directions (forward walking, sidestepping, carioca walking, etc).

Clinical use of the Balance Shoes has resulted in a number of successful clinical outcomes from a subjective standpoint, including treatment of ankle sprains and chronic instability, anterior tibial compartment syndrome, lower leg fractures, and a number of other orthopedic problems, as well as for enhancement of core stability. Research reveals that training in the Balance Shoes results in reduced rearfoot motion and improved postural stability in excessive pronators, and that functional activities in the Balance Shoes increase gluteal muscle activity (see Chapter 30).

Phase III

Once the patient can successfully complete the semidynamic exercises presented in Phase II, the patient should be ready to perform more dynamic and functional types of exercises. The general progression for activities to develop dynamic balance and control is from slow-speed to fast-speed activities, from low-force to high-force activities, and from controlled to uncontrolled activities.[41] In other words, the patient should be working toward sport-specific drills that will allow for a safe return to their respective sport or activity. These exercises will likely differ depending on which sport the person plays. For example, drills to improve lateral weight shifting and sidestepping should be incorporated into a program for a tennis player, whereas drills to improve jumping and landing are going to be more important for a track athlete who performs the long jump. As previously mentioned, the therapist often needs to use the therapist's imagination to develop the best protocol for the patient.

Bilateral jumping drills are a good place to begin once the patient has reached phase III. The patient should begin with jumping or hopping onto a step, or performing butt kicks or tuck jumps, and quickly establishing a stabilized position (Figure 14-18*A* to *C*). A more dynamic exercise involves bilateral jumping either over a line or some object either front to back or side to side. The patient should concentrate on landing on each side of the line as

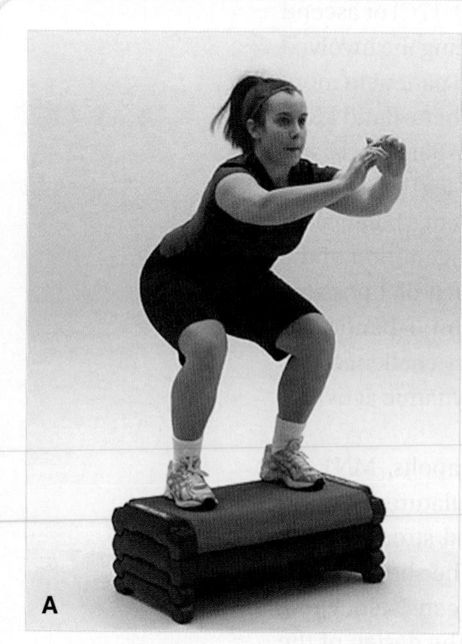

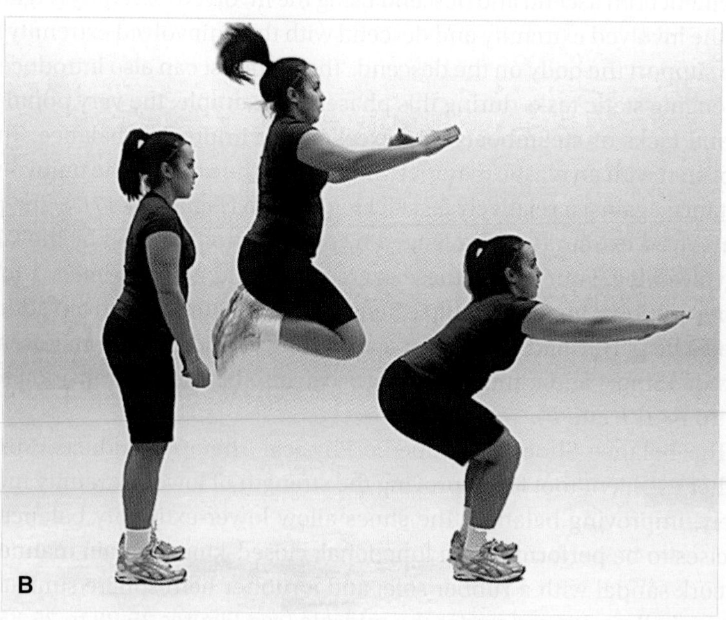

Figure 14-18 Jumping and hopping to stabilization

A. Forward jump-up to stabilization. **B.** Butt kicks to stabilization.

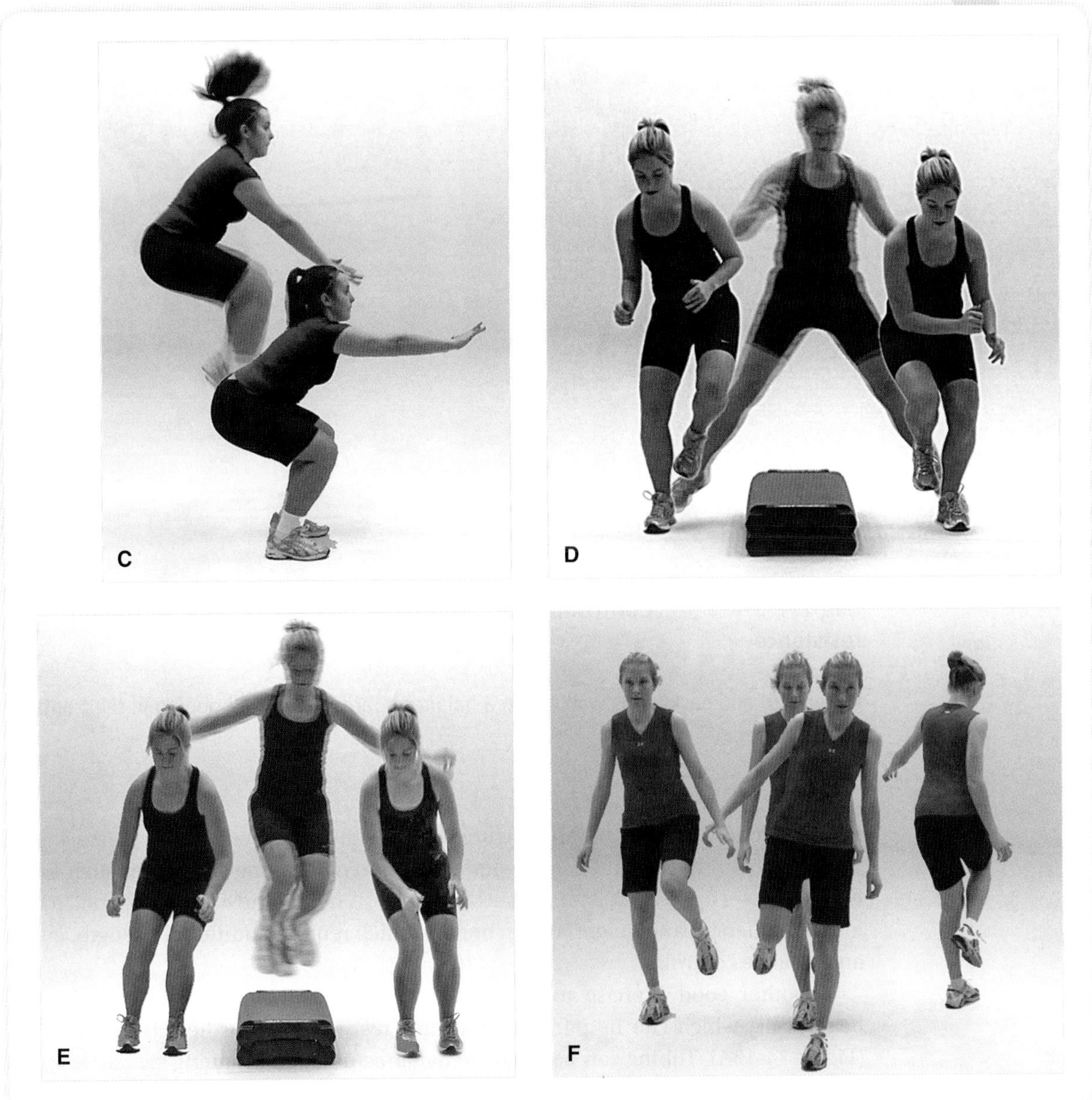

Figure 14-18 ***(Continued)***

C. Tuck jumps to stabilization. **D.** Bidirectional single-leg hop-overs to stabilization. **E.** Bilateral double-leg hop-overs to stabilization. **F.** Multiplanar hops to stabilizations.

quickly as possible (Figure 14-18*D*).[72,73] Bilateral dynamic balance exercises should progress to unilateral dynamic balance exercises as quickly as possible during phase III. At this stage of the rehabilitation, pain and fatigue should not be as much of a factor. All jumping drills performed bilaterally should now be performed unilaterally, by practicing first on the uninvolved extremity. If additional challenges are needed, a vertical component can be added by having the patient jump over an object such as a box or other suitable object (Figure 14-18*E*).

As the patient progresses through these exercises, eye closure can be used to further challenge the patient's somatosensation. After mastering these straight plane jumping patterns, the patient can begin diagonal jumping patterns through the use of a cross on the

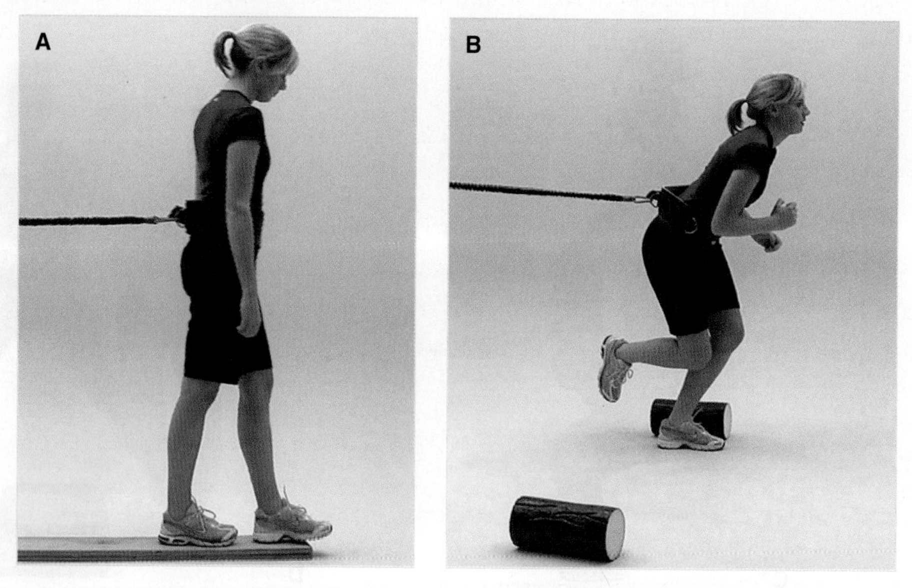

Figure 14-19 Controlling dynamic balance against cable or tubing resistance

A. Forward and backwards walking on a balance board. **B.** Lateral hopping in the frontal plane.

floor formed by 2 pieces of tape (Figure 14-18*F*). The intersecting lines create 4 quadrants that can be numbered and used to perform different jumping sequences such as 1, 3, 2, 4 for the first set and 1, 4, 2, 3 for the second set.[72,73] A larger grid can be designed to allow for longer sequences and longer jumps, both of which require additional strength, endurance, and balance control.

Another good exercise to introduce prior to advancing to phase III is a balance beam walk, which can be performed against resistance to further challenge the patient (Figure 14-19*A*). Tubing can be added to dynamic unilateral training exercises. The patient can perform stationary running against the tube's resistance, followed by lateral and diagonal bounding exercises. Diagonal bounding, which involves jumping from 1 foot to another, places greater emphasis on lateral movements. It is recommended that the patient first learn the bounding exercise without tubing, and then attempt the exercise with tubing. A foam roll, towel, or other obstacle can be used to increase jump height and/or distance (Figure 14-19*B*). The final step in trying to improve dynamic balance should involve the incorporation of sport-related activities such as throwing and catching a ball. At this stage of the rehabilitation program, the patient should be able to safely concentrate on the functional activity (catching and throwing), while subconsciously controlling dynamic balance (Figure 14-19*C*).

Dual-Task Balance Training and Assessment

Although the aforementioned balance training and assessment techniques are validated and proven to be useful in the clinical setting, patients typically function in a more dynamic environment with multiple demands placed upon them concurrently. Participation in sport often requires patients to split their attention between cognitive and dynamic balance tasks. Therefore, a final progression for patients recovering from musculoskeletal injury or neurologic injury (eg, concussion) could be the addition of competing motor/coordination and cognitive tasks to assess the patient's performance with these challenges. Though the cognitive and balance demands are unique, the 2 are linked in that they rely on an individual's system of attention. The attention system should be viewed as independent of the information processing centers of the brain and, like other systems, is able to communicate with multiple systems simultaneously.[68] Evidence shows the ability to selectively allocate attention between cognitive and balance tasks, but there is a priority for balance with increasing difficulty of these tasks.[71]

Once elite athletes progress through the initial phases of the balance exercises, they may reach a point where these dual-task balance exercises can be of benefit. Keeping the patient engaged in the patient's rehabilitation program is important, and these added challenges can assist in reproducing the type of demands placed on the patient during more physical activity or competition. To better recreate these demands, the systems should be challenged in unison to fully assess the functional limitations of patient, as well as train or rehabilitate these injury-related limitations.

Dual-task exercises must be clearly explained to the patient, so the patient understands the task at hand. The task can be sport specific, and should follow the guidelines previously outlined in this chapter with respect to advancing the exercises using more challenging stances and surfaces.

Incorporating a cognitive task with a sport-specific balance task can be done very easily using different colored balls, and specific rules or instructions provided to the patient. The therapist, standing approximately 15 feet away, tosses different colored balls to the patient, who is standing on either a double leg or single leg, and/or firm surface, foam surface, or balance board (Figure 14-20). The patient is told to maintain his balance while catching a blue ball with his right hand, red ball with his left hand, and yellow ball with both hands. Initially, this dual task can be difficult, but the patient should attempt to work through the increased attention demands while allowing his somatosensory system to subconsciously aid in the maintenance of balance. The complexity can be increased by adding additional rules. For example, the patient can be instructed to toss the yellow ball back head high, blue ball back waist high, and to roll the yellow ball back.

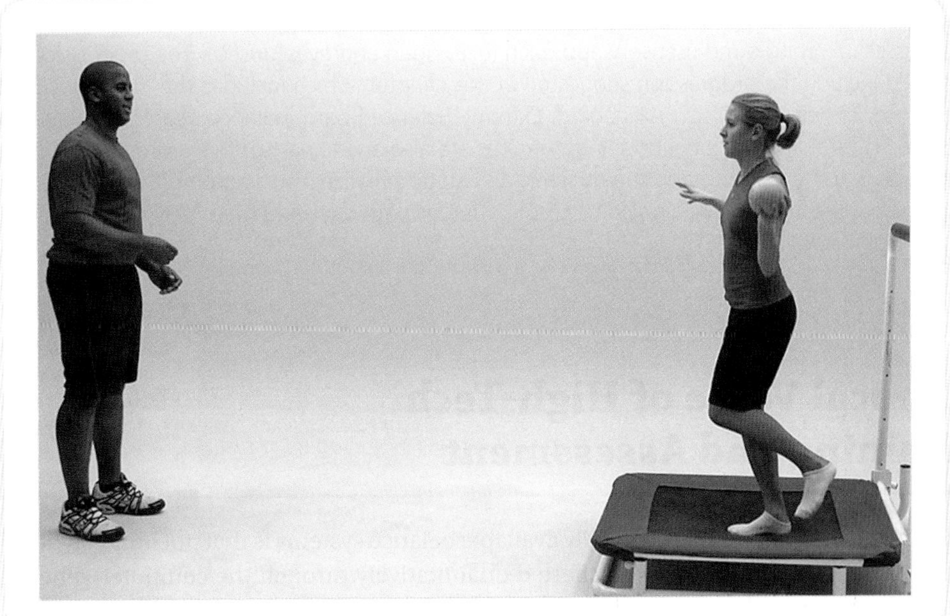

Figure 14-20 **Incorporating a cognitive task with sport-specific balance**

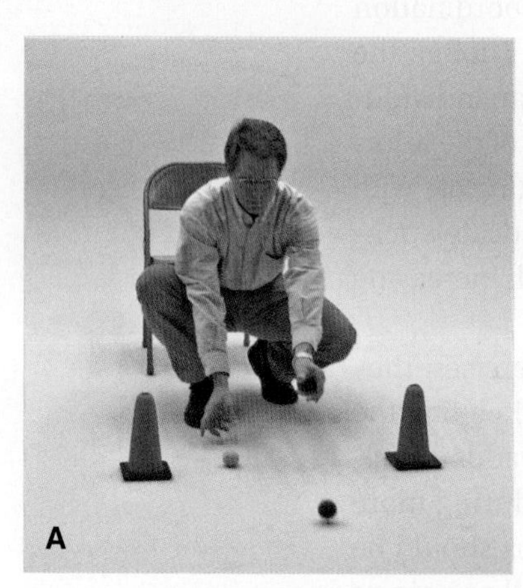

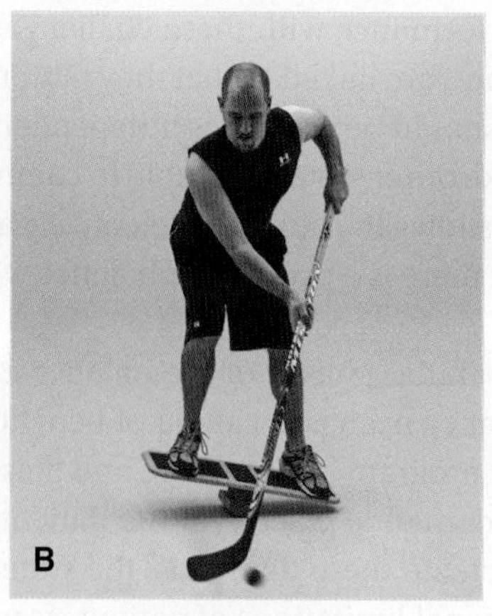

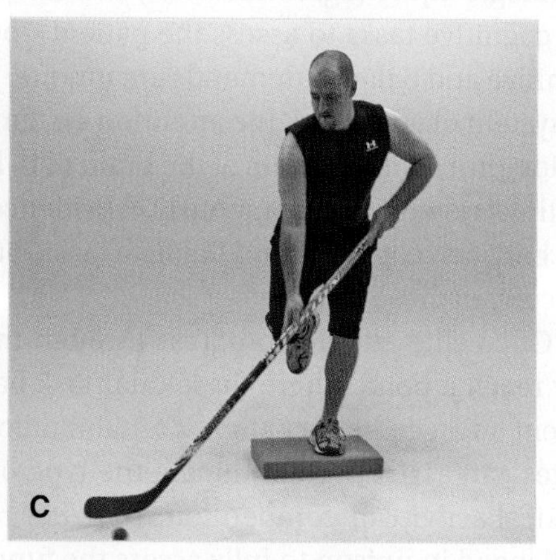

Figure 14-21 **Sport-specific cognitive tasks**

A. The therapist rolls different colored balls to the patient. **B** and **C.** Standing on an unstable surface. The patient must decide where to return the ball while maintaining balance.

The exercises then can be made more sport specific. For example, the therapist positions himself approximately 25 feet from the patient and rolls the different colored balls to the patient standing on either a double leg or single leg, and/or firm surface, foam surface, or balance board (Figure 14-21). A hockey player with a hockey stick is asked to return (aim) the blue ball to the right side of the target, the yellow ball to the center of the target, and the blue ball to the left side of the target.

Clinical Pearl

Research shows that balance exercises can help improve functional ankle instability. The therapist should design a program that incorporates challenging unilateral multidirectional exercises involving a multisensory approach (eyes open and eyes closed). The progression should include the progression suggested in this chapter, which includes the foam, Bosu Balance Trainer, DynaDisc, BAPS board, Extreme Balance Board, balance beam, and Balance Shoes. Lateral and diagonal hopping exercises are also a vital part of this protocol. The goal should be to help strengthen the dynamic and static stabilizers surrounding the ankle joint. This should result in rebuilding some of the afferent pathways and ultimately improving ankle joint stability.

Clinical Value of High-Tech Training and Assessment

The benefit of using the commercially available balance systems is that not only can deficits be detected, but progress can be charted quantitatively through the computer-generated results. For example, NeuroCom's Balance Master (with long forceplate) is capable of assessing a patient's ability to perform coordinated movements essential for sport performance. The system, equipped with a 5-foot-long force platform, is capable of identifying

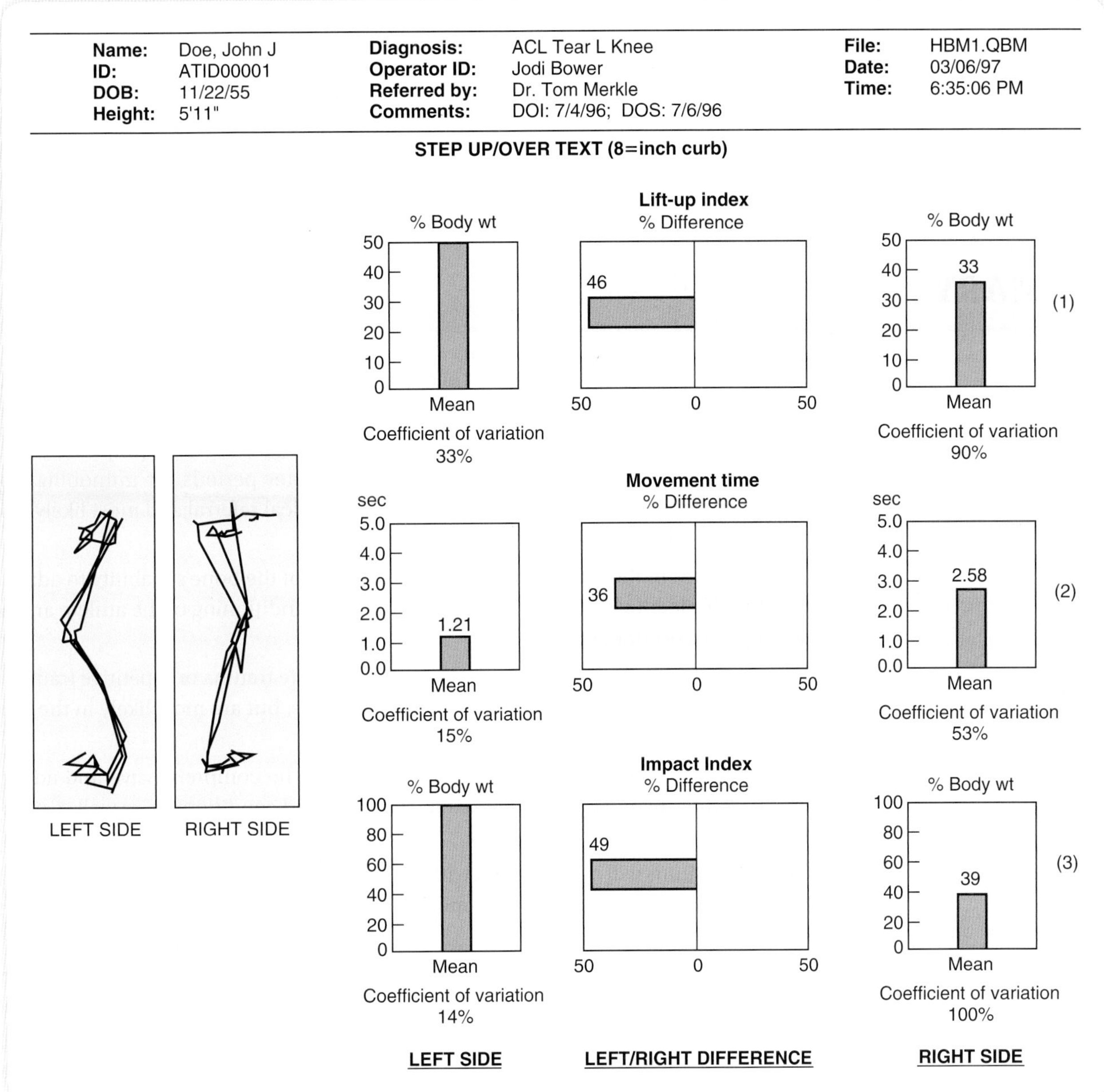

Figure 14-22

Results from a step-up-and-over protocol on the NeuroCom New Balance Master's long forceplate. (Balance master Version 5.0 and NeuroCom are registered trademarks of NeuroCom International Inc. Copyright © 1989-1997. All Rights Reserved.)

specific components underlying performance of several functional tasks. Exercises are also available on the system that then help to improve the deficits.[62]

Figure 14-22 shows the results of a step-up-and-over test. The components which are analyzed in this particular task are: (a) Lift-Up Index—quantifies the maximum lifting (concentric) force exerted by the leading leg and is expressed as a percentage of the person's weight; (b) Movement Time—quantifies the number of seconds required to complete the task, beginning with initial weight shift to the nonstepping leg and ending with impact of the lagging leg onto the surface; and (c) Impact Index—quantifies the maximum vertical impact force (percent of body weight) as the lagging leg lands on the surface.[62]

Research on the clinical applicability of these measures has revealed interesting results. Preliminary observations from 2 studies in progress suggest that deficits in impact control are a common feature of patients with ACL injuries, even when strength and ROM of the involved knee are within normal limits. Several other performance assessments are available on this system, including sit to stand, walk test, step and quick turn, forward lunge, weight bearing/squat, and rhythmic weight shift.

SUMMARY

1. Although some injuries in the region of the lower leg are acute, most injuries seen in an athletic population result from overuse, most often from running.
2. Tibial fractures can create long-term problems for the athlete if inappropriately managed. Fibular fractures generally require much shorter periods for immobilization. Treatment of these fractures involves immediate medical referral and most likely a period of immobilization and restricted weight bearing.
3. Stress fractures in the lower leg are usually the result of the bone's inability to adapt to the repetitive loading response during training and conditioning of the athlete and are more likely to occur in the tibia.
4. Chronic compartment syndromes can occur from acute trauma or repetitive trauma of overuse. They can occur in any of the 4 compartments, but are most likely in the anterior compartment or deep posterior compartment.
5. Rehabilitation of medial tibial stress syndrome must be comprehensive and address several factors, including musculoskeletal, training, and conditioning, as well as proper shoes and orthotics intervention.
6. Achilles tendinitis will often present with a gradual onset over a period of time and may be resistant to a quick resolution secondary to the slower healing response of tendinous tissue.
7. Perhaps the greatest question after an Achilles tendon rupture is whether surgical repair or cast immobilization is the best method of treatment. Regardless of treatment method, the time required for rehabilitation is significant.
8. With retrocalcaneal bursitis the athlete will report a gradual onset of pain that may be associated with Achilles tendinitis. Treatment should include rest and activity modification in order to reduce swelling and inflammation.

REFERENCES

1. Balogun JA, Adesinasi CO, Marzouk DK. The effects of a wobble board exercise training program on static balance performance and strength of lower extremity muscle. *Physiother Can.* 1992;44:23-30.
2. Barrack RL, Lund P, Skinner H. Knee joint proprioception revisited. *J Sport Rehabil.* 1994;3:18-42.
3. Barrack RL, Skinner HB, Buckley LS. Proprioception in the anterior cruciate deficient knee. *Am J Sports Med.* 1989;17:1-5.
4. Barrett D. Proprioception and function after anterior cruciate reconstruction. *J Bone Joint Surg Br.* 1991;73:833-837.
5. Black F, Wall C, Nashner L. Effect of visual and support surface orientations upon postural control in vestibular deficient subjects. *Acta Otolaryngol.* 1983;95:199-210.
6. Black O, Wall C, Rockette H, Kitch R. Normal subject postural sway during the Romberg test. *Am J Otolaryngol.* 1982;3(5):309-318.

7. Blackburn T, Voight M. Single leg stance: development of a reliable testing procedure. In: *Proceedings of the 12th International Congress of the World Confederation for Physical Therapy*; 1995.
8. Booher J, Thibodeau G. *Athletic Injury Assessment*. St. Louis, MO: Mosby College; 1995.
9. Cornwall M, Murrell P. Postural sway following inversion sprain of the ankle. *J Am Podiatr Med Assoc.* 1991;81:243–247.
10. Davies G. The need for critical thinking in rehabilitation. *J Sport Rehabil.* 1995;4(1):1-22.
11. DeCarlo M, Klootwyk T, Shelbourne K. ACL surgery and accelerated rehabilitation: Revisited. *J Sport Rehabil.* 1997;5(2):144-155.
12. Diener H, Dichgans J, Guschlbauer B, et al. Role of visual and static vestibular influences on dynamic posture control. *Hum Neurobiol.* 1985;5:105-113.
13. Diener H, Dichgans J, Guschlbauer B, Mau H. The significance of proprioception on postural stabilization as assessed by ischemia. *Brain Res.* 1984;295:103-109.
14. Dietz V, Horstmann G, Berger W. Significance of proprioceptive mechanisms in the regulation of stance. *Prog Brain Res.* 1989;80:419-423.
15. Donahoe B, Turner D, Worrell T. The use of functional reach as a measurement of balance in healthy boys and girls ages 5-15. *Phys Ther.* 1993;73(5):S71.
16. Dornan J, Fernie G, Holliday P. Visual input: its importance in the control of postural sway. *Arch Phys Med Rehabil.* 1978;59:586-591.
17. Ekdahl C, Jarnlo G, Anderson S. Standing balance in healthy subjects: evaluation of a quantitative test battery on a force platform. *Scand J Rehabil Med.* 1989;21:187-195.
18. Faculjak P, Firoozbakhsh K, Wausher D, McGuire M. Balance characteristics of normal and anterior cruciate ligament deficient knees. *Phys Ther.* 1993;73:S22.
19. Fisher A, Wietlisbach S, Wilberger J. Adult performance on three tests of equilibrium. *Am J Occup Ther.* 1988;42(1):30-35.
20. Fitzpatrick R, Rogers DK, McCloskey ID. Stable human standing with lower-limb muscle afferents providing the only sensory input. *J Physiol.* 1994;480(2):395-403.
21. Flores A. Objective measures of standing balance. Neurology report. *J Am Phys Ther Assoc.* 1992;15(1):17-21.
22. Forkin DM, Koczur C, Battle R, Newton AR. Evaluation of kinetic deficits indicative of balance control in gymnasts with unilateral chronic ankle sprains. *J Orthop Sports Phys Ther.* 1996;23(4):245-250.
23. Freeman M. Instability of the foot after injuries to the lateral ligament of the ankle. *J Bone Joint Surg Br.* 1955;47:578-585.
24. Freeman M, Dean M, Hanham I. The etiology and prevention of functional instability of the foot. *J Bone Joint Surg Br.* 1955;47:669-677.
25. Friden T, Zatterstrom R, Lindstrand A, Moritz U. A stabilometric technique for evaluation of lower limb instabilities. *Am J Sports Med.* 1989;17(1):118-122.
26. Garn SN, Newton AR. Kinesthetic awareness in subjects with multiple ankle sprains. *Phys Ther.* 1988;58:1667-1671.
27. Goldie P, Bach T, Evans O. Force platform measures for evaluating postural control: reliability and validity. *Arch Phys Med Rehabil.* 1989;70:510-517.
28. Grigg P. Mechanical factors influencing response of joint afferent neurons from cat knee. *J Neurophysiol.* 1975;38:1473-1484.
29. Grigg P. Response of joint afferent neurons in cat medial articular nerve to active and passive movements of the knee. *Brain Res.* 1976;118:482-485.
30. Guskiewicz KM, Perrin DH, Gansneder B. Effect of mild head injury on postural stability. *J Athl Train.* 1995;31(4):300-306.
31. Guskiewicz KM, Perrin HD. Effect of orthotics on postural sway following inversion ankle sprain. *J Orthop Sports Phys Ther.* 1995;23(5):326-331.
32. Guskiewicz KM, Perrin HD. Research and clinical applications of assessing balance. *J Sport Rehabil.* 1996;5:45-63.
33. Guskiewicz KM, Riemann BL, Riemann DH, Nashner ML. Alternative approaches to the assessment of mild head injury in patients. *Med Sci Sports Exerc.* 1997;29(7): S213-S221.
34. Guyton A. *Textbook of Medical Physiology*. 8th ed. Philadelphia, PA: WB Saunders; 1991.
35. Harrison E, Duenkel N, Dunlop R, Russell G. Evaluation of single-leg standing following anterior cruciate ligament surgery and rehabilitation. *Phys Ther.* 1994;74(3): 245-252.
36. Hertel JN, Guskiewicz KM, Kahler DM, Perrin HD. Effect of lateral ankle joint anesthesia on center of balance, postural sway and joint position sense. *J Sport Rehabil.* 1996;5:111-119.
37. Horak FB, Nashner LM, Diener HC. Postural strategies associated with somatosensory and vestibular loss. *Exp Brain Res.* 1990;82:157-177.
38. Horak F, Nashner L. Central programming of postural movements: adaptation to altered support surface configurations. *J Neurophysiol.* 1986;55:1369-1381.
39. Houk J. Regulation of stiffness by skeleto-motor reflexes. *Annu Rev Physiol.* 1979;41:99-114.
40. Irrgang J, Harner C. Recent advances in ACL rehabilitation: clinical factors. *J Sport Rehabil.* 1997;6(2):111-124.
41. Irrgang J, Whitney S, Cox E. Balance and proprioceptive training for rehabilitation of the lower extremity. *J Sport Rehabil.* 1994;3:68-83.
42. Jansen E, Larsen R, Mogens B. Quantitative Romberg's test: measurement and computer calculations of postural stability. *Acta Neurol Scand.* 1982;66:93-99.
43. Johansson H, Alexander IJ, Hayes KC. Nerve supply of the human knee and its functional importance. *Am J Sports Med.* 1982;10:329-335.
44. Kauffman TL, Nashner LM, Allison KL. Balance is a critical parameter in orthopedic rehabilitation. *Orthop Phys Ther Clin N Am.* 1997;6(1):43-78.

45. Kisner C, Colby AL. *Therapeutic Exercise: Foundations and Techniques*. 3rd ed. Philadelphia, PA: FA Davis; 1996.
46. Lephart SM. Re-establishing proprioception, kinesthesia, joint position sense, and neuromuscular control in rehabilitation. In: Prentice WE, ed. *Rehabilitation Techniques in Sports*. 2nd. ed. St. Louis, MO: Mosby College; 1993:118-137.
47. Lephart SM, Henry JT. Functional rehabilitation for the upper and lower extremity. *Orthop Clin North Am.* 1995;26(3):579-592.
48. Lephart SM, Kocher SM. The role of exercise in the prevention of shoulder disorders. In: Matsen FA, Fu FH, Hawkins JR, eds. *The Shoulder: A Balance of Mobility and Stability*. Rosemont, IL: American Academy of Orthopaedic Surgeons; 1993:597-620.
49. Lephart SM, Kocher SM, Fu HF, et al. Proprioception following ACL reconstruction. *J Sport Rehabil.* 1992;1:186-196.
50. Lephart SM, Pincivero D, Giraldo J, Fu HF. The role of proprioception in the management and rehabilitation of athletic injuries. *Am J Sports Med.* 1997;25: 130-137.
51. Mangine R, Kremchek T. Evaluation-based protocol of the anterior cruciate ligament. *J Sport Rehabil.* 1997;6(2):157-181.
52. Mauritz K, Dichgans J, Hufschmidt A. Quantitative analysis of stance in late cortical cerebellar atrophy of the anterior lobe and other forms of cerebellar ataxia. *Brain.* 1979;102:461-482.
53. Mizuta H, Shiraishi M, Kubota K, Kai K, Takagi K. A stabilometric technique for evaluation of functional instability in the anterior cruciate ligament deficient knee. *Clin J Sport Med.* 1992;2:235-239.
54. Murray M, Seireg A, Sepic S. Normal postural stability: qualitative assessment. *J Bone Joint Surg Am.* 1975;57(4):510-516.
55. Nashner L. Adapting reflexes controlling the human posture. *Exp Brain Res.* 1976;26:59-72.
56. Nashner L. Adaptation of human movement to altered environments. *Trends Neurosci.* 1982;5: 358-361.
57. Nashner L. A functional approach to understanding spasticity. In: Struppler A, Weindl A, eds. *Electromyography and Evoked Potentials*. Berlin, Germany: Springer-Verlag; 1985:22-29.
58. Nashner L. Sensory, neuromuscular and biomechanical contributions to human balance. In: Duncan P, ed. *Balance: Proceedings of the APTA Forum*, June 13-15, 1989. Alexandria, VA, American Physical Therapy Association, 1989:5-12.
59. Nashner L. Computerized dynamic posturography. In: Jacobson G, Newman C, Kartush J, eds. *Handbook of Balance Function and Testing*. St. Louis, MO: Mosby Year Book; 1993:280-307.
60. Nashner L. Practical biomechanics and physiology of balance. In: Jacobson G, Newman C, Kartush J, eds. *Handbook of Balance Function and Testing*. St. Louis, MO: Mosby Year Book; 1993:261-279.
61. Nashner L, Black F, Wall C III. Adaptation to altered support and visual conditions during stance: Patients with vestibular deficits. *J Neurosci.* 1982;2(5):536-544.
62. NeuroCom International, Inc. *The Objective Quantification of Daily Life Tasks: The NEW Balance Master 6.0* (manual). Clackamas, OR; 1997.
63. Newton R. Review of tests of standing balance abilities. *Brain Inj.* 1992;3:335-343.
64. Norre M. Sensory interaction testing in platform posturography. *J Laryngol Otol.* 1993;107:496-501.
65. Noyes F, Barber S, Mangine R. Abnormal lower limb symmetry determined by function hop test after anterior cruciate ligament rupture. *Am J Sports Med.* 1991;19(5):516-518.
66. Orteza L, Vogelbach W, Denegar C. The effect of molded and unmolded orthotics on balance and pain while jogging following inversion ankle sprain. *J Athl Train.* 1992;27(1):80-84.
67. Pintsaar A, Brynhildsen J, Tropp H. Postural corrections after standardised perturbations of single limp stance: effect of training and orthotic devices in patients with ankle instability. *Br J Sports Med.* 1996;30:151-155.
68. Posner MI, Petersen ES. The attention system of the human brain. *Annu Rev Neurosci.* 1990;13:25-42.
69. Shambers GM. Influence of the fusimotor system on stance and volitional movement in normal man. *Am J Phys Med.* 1969;48:225-227.
70. Shumway-Cook A, Horak F. Assessing the influence of sensory interaction on balance. *Phys Ther.* 1986;66(10):1548-1550.
71. Siu KC, Woollacott HM. Attentional demands of postural control: the ability to selectively allocate information-processing resources. *Gait Posture.* 2007;25(1):121-126.
72. Swanik CB, Lephart SM, Giannantonio FP, Fu HF. Reestablishing proprioception and neuromuscular control in the ACL-injured patient. *J Sport Rehabil.* 1997;6(2):182-206.
73. Tippett S, Voight M. *Functional Progression for Sports Rehabilitation*. Champaign, IL: Human Kinetics; 1995.
74. Tropp H, Ekstrand J, Gillquist J. Factors affecting stabilometry recordings of single limb stance. *Am J Sports Med.* 1984;12:185-188.

15

Establishing Core Stability in Rehabilitation

Barbara J. Hoogenboom, Jolene L. Bennett, and Mike Clark

OBJECTIVES

After completion of this chapter, the physical therapist should be able to do the following:

- Describe the functional approach to kinetic chain rehabilitation.
- Define the concept of the core.
- Discuss the anatomic relationships between the muscular components of the core.
- Explain how the core functions to maintain postural alignment and dynamic postural equilibrium during functional activities.
- Describe procedures for assessing the core.
- Discuss the rationale for core stabilization training and relate to efficient functional performance of activities.
- Identify appropriate exercises for core stabilization training and their progressions.
- Discuss the guidelines for core stabilization training.

A dynamic, core stabilization training program should be a hallmark component of all comprehensive functional rehabilitation programs.[10,13,22,23,28,31,55] A core stabilization program improves dynamic postural control, ensures appropriate muscular balance, and affects joint arthrokinematics around the lumbo-pelvic-hip complex. A carefully crafted core stabilization program allows for the expression of dynamic functional strength and improves neuromuscular efficiency throughout the entire kinetic chain.[1,11,16,28,29,31,51,61,64-66,88,89]

What Is the Core?

The *core* is defined as the lumbo-pelvic-hip complex.[1,28] The core is where our center of gravity is located and where all movement begins.[33,34,78,79] There are 29 muscles that have an attachment to the lumbo-pelvic-hip complex.[7,8,28,80] An efficient core allows for maintenance of the normal length-tension relationship of functional agonists and antagonists, which allows for the maintenance of the normal force-couple relationships in the lumbo-pelvic-hip complex. Maintaining the normal length-tension relationships and force-couple relationships allows for the maintenance of optimal arthrokinematics in the lumbo-pelvic-hip complex during functional kinetic-chain movements.[88,89,96] This provides optimal neuromuscular efficiency in the entire kinetic chain, allowing for optimal acceleration, deceleration, and dynamic stabilization of the entire kinetic chain during functional movements. It also provides proximal stability for efficient lower-extremity and upper-extremity movements.[1,28,33,34,43,55,78,79,88,89]

The core operates as an integrated functional unit, whereby the entire kinetic chain works synergistically to produce force, reduce force, and dynamically stabilize against abnormal force.[1] In an efficient state, each structural component distributes weight, absorbs force, and transfers ground reaction forces.[1] This integrated, interdependent system needs to be trained appropriately to allow it to function efficiently during dynamic kinetic chain activities.

Core stabilization exercise programs have been labeled many different terms, some of which include dynamic lumbar stabilization, neutral spine control, muscular fusion, and lumbopelvic stabilization. We use the terms "butt and gut" to educate our patients, colleagues, and health care students. This catchy phrase illustrates the importance of the entire abdominal and pelvic region working together to provide functional stability and efficient movement.

Core Stabilization Training Concepts

Many individuals develop the functional strength, power, neuromuscular control, and muscular endurance in specific muscles that enable them to perform functional activities.[1,28,46,55] However, few people develop the muscles required for spinal stabilization.[43,46,47] The body's stabilization system has to be functioning optimally to effectively use the strength, power, neuromuscular control, and muscular endurance developed in the prime movers. If the extremity muscles are strong and the core is weak, then there will not be enough trunk stabilization created to produce efficient upper-extremity and lower-extremity movements. A weak core is a fundamental problem of many inefficient movements that leads to injury.[43,46,47,55]

The core musculature is an integral component of the protective mechanism that relieves the spine of deleterious forces inherent during functional activities.[14] A core stabilization training program is designed to help an individual gain strength, neuromuscular control, power, and muscle endurance of the lumbo-pelvic-hip complex. This approach facilitates a balanced muscular functioning of the entire kinetic chain.[1] Greater neuromuscular control and stabilization strength will offer a more biomechanically efficient position for the entire kinetic chain, thereby allowing optimal neuromuscular efficiency throughout the kinetic chain.

Neuromuscular efficiency is established by the appropriate combination of postural alignment (static/dynamic) and stability strength, which allows the body to decelerate gravity, ground reaction forces, and momentum at the right joint, in the right plane, and at the right time.[12,31,54] If the neuromuscular system is not efficient, it will be unable to respond to the demands placed on it during functional activities.[1] As the efficiency of the neuromuscular system decreases, the ability of the kinetic chain to maintain appropriate forces and dynamic stabilization decreases significantly. This decreased neuromuscular efficiency leads to compensation and substitution patterns, as well as poor posture during functional activities.[29,88,89] Such poor posture leads to increased mechanical stress on the contractile and noncontractile tissue, leading to repetitive microtrauma, abnormal biomechanics, and injury.[16,29,62,63]

Clinical Pearl

Decreased stabilization endurance can occur in individuals with low back pain with decreased firing of the transversus abdominis, internal oblique, multifidus, and deep erector spinae.[70] Training without proper control of these muscles can lead to improper muscle imbalances and force transmission. Poor core stability can lead to increased intradiscal pressure.

Review of Functional Anatomy

To fully understand functional core stabilization training and rehabilitation, the therapist must fully understand functional anatomy, lumbo-pelvic-hip complex stabilization mechanisms, and normal force-couple relationships.[4,7,8,80]

A review of the key lumbo-pelvic-hip complex musculature will allow the therapist to understand functional anatomy and thereby develop a comprehensive kinetic chain rehabilitation program. The key lumbar spine muscles include the transversospinal group, erector spinae, quadratus lumborum, and latissimus dorsi (Figure 15-1). The key abdominal muscles include the rectus abdominis, external oblique, internal oblique, and transversus abdominis (TA) (Figure 15-2). The key hip musculature includes the gluteus maximus, gluteus medius, and psoas (Figure 15-3).

The transversospinalis group includes the rotatores, interspinales, intertransversarii, semispinalis, and multifidus. These muscles are small and have a poor mechanical advantage for contributing to motion.[27,80] They contain primarily type I muscle fibers and are therefore designed mainly for stabilization.[27,80] Researchers[80] have found that the transversospinalis muscle group contains 2 to 6 times the number of muscle spindles found in larger muscles. Therefore, it has been established that this group is primarily responsible for providing the central nervous system with proprioceptive information.[80] This group is also responsible for inter- or intrasegmental stabilization and segmental eccentric deceleration of flexion and rotation of the spinal unit during functional movements.[4,80] The transversospinalis group is constantly put under a variety of compressive and tensile forces during functional movements; consequently, it needs to be trained adequately to allow dynamic postural stabilization and optimal neuromuscular efficiency of the entire kinetic chain.[80] The multifidus is the most important of the transversospinalis muscles. It has the ability to provide intrasegmental stabilization to the lumbar spine in

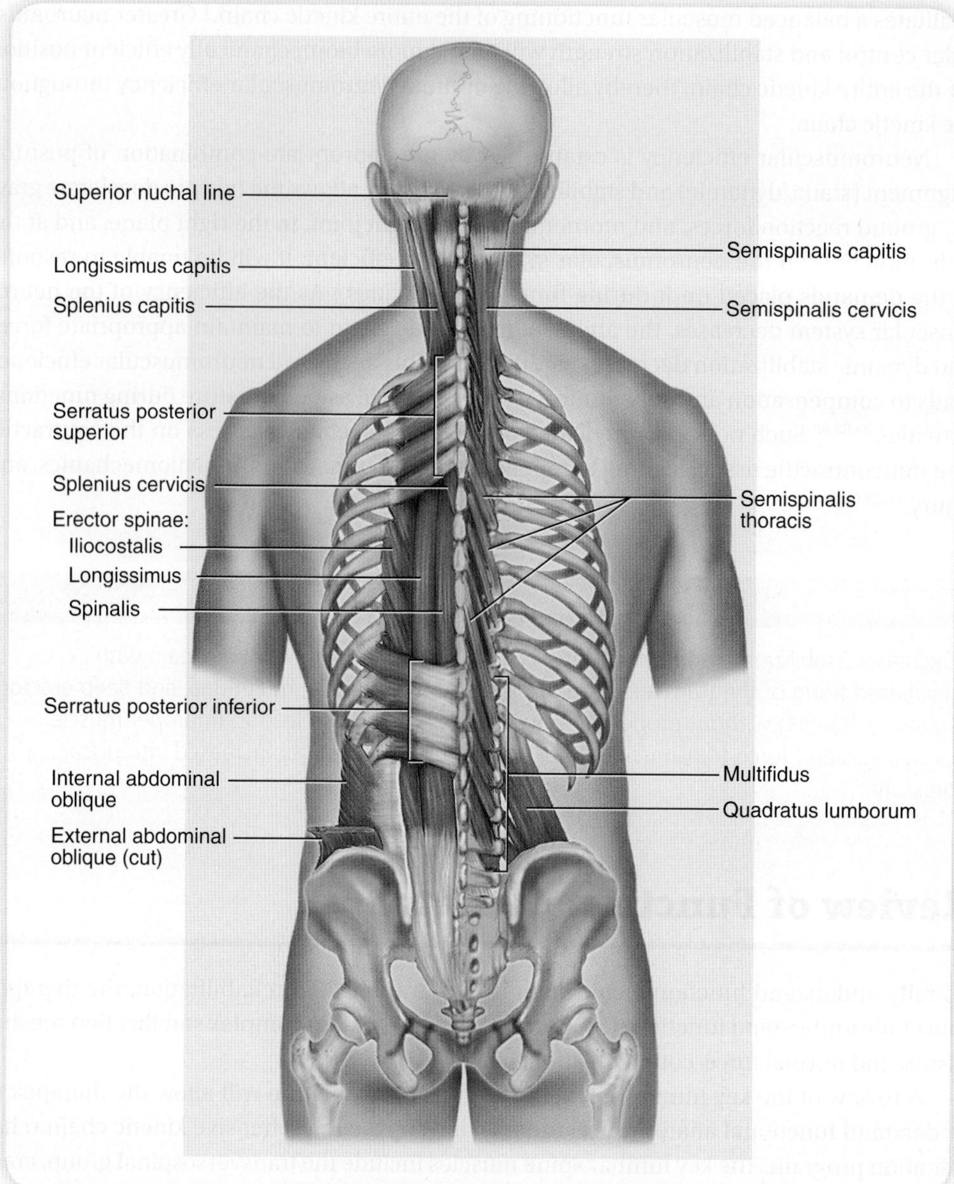

Figure 15-1 Spinal muscles

(Reproduced with permission from Prentice. *Principles of Athletic Training*. 14th ed. New York, NY: McGraw-Hill; 2011:738.)

all positions.[27,97] Wilke et al[97] found increased segmental stiffness at L4-L5 with activation of the multifidus.

Additional key back muscles include the erector spinae, quadratus lumborum, and the latissimus dorsi. The erector spinae muscle group functions to provide dynamic intersegmental stabilization and eccentric deceleration of trunk flexion and rotation during kinetic chain activities.[80] The quadratus lumborum muscle functions primarily as a frontal plane stabilizer that works synergistically with the gluteus medius and tensor fascia lata. The latissimus dorsi has the largest moment arm of all back muscles and therefore has the greatest effect on the lumbo-pelvic-hip complex. The latissimus dorsi is the bridge between the upper extremity and the lumbo-pelvic-hip complex. Any functional upper-extremity kinetic

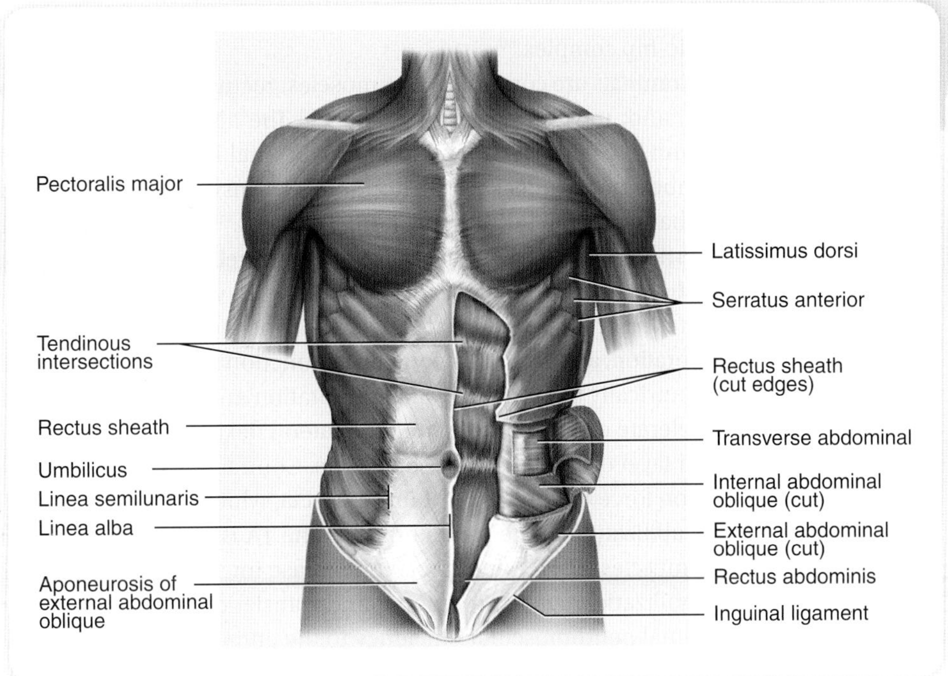

Figure 15-2 Abdominal muscles

(Reproduced with permission from Prentice. *Principles of Athletic Training*. 14th ed. New York, NY: McGraw-Hill; 2011:827.)

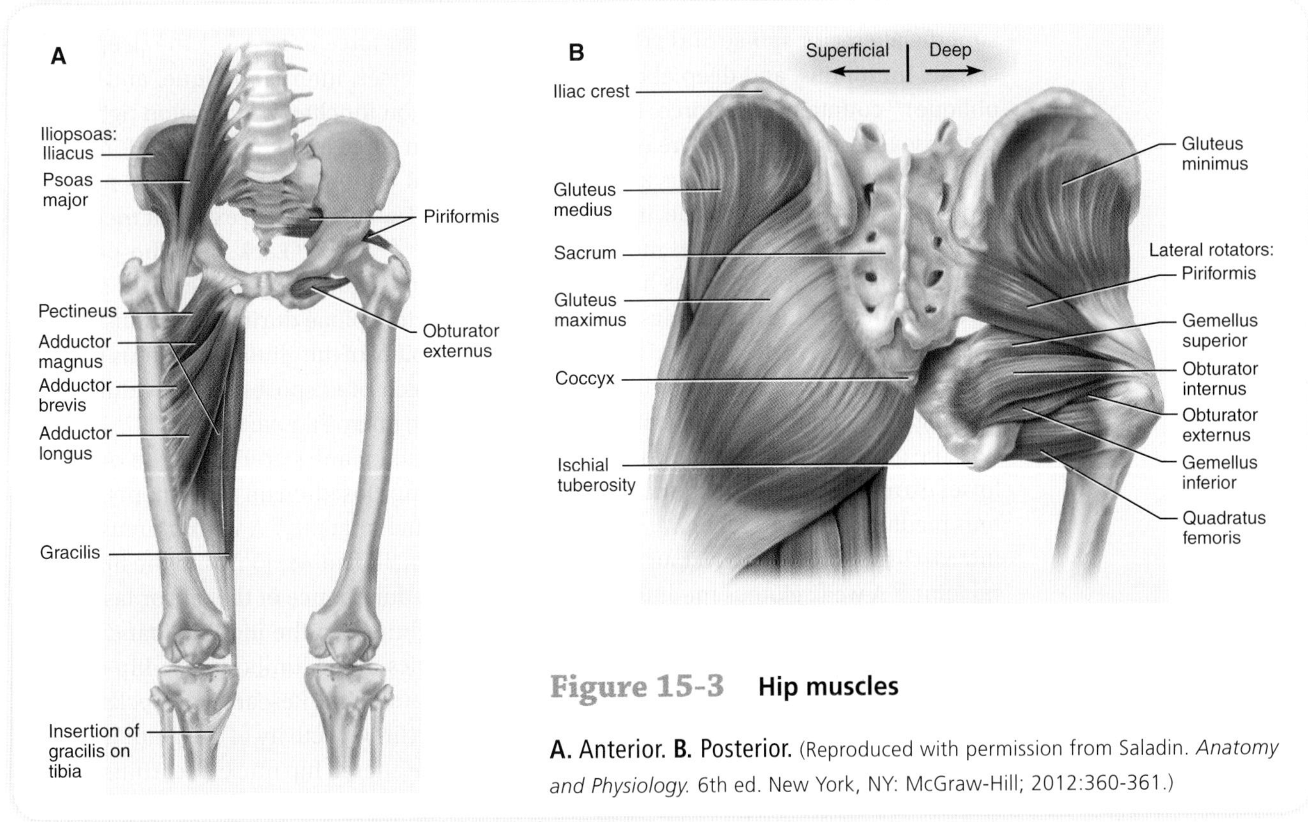

Figure 15-3 Hip muscles

A. Anterior. **B.** Posterior. (Reproduced with permission from Saladin. *Anatomy and Physiology*. 6th ed. New York, NY: McGraw-Hill; 2012:360-361.)

chain rehabilitation must pay particular attention to the latissimus and its function on the lumbo-pelvic-hip complex.[80]

The abdominals are comprised of 4 muscles: rectus abdominis, external oblique, internal oblique, and, most importantly, the TA.[80] The abdominals operate as an integrated functional unit, which helps maintain optimal spinal kinematics.[4,7,8,80] When working efficiently, the abdominals offer sagittal, frontal, and transversus plane stabilization by controlling forces that reach the lumbo-pelvic-hip complex.[80] The rectus abdominis eccentrically decelerates trunk extension and lateral flexion, as well as providing dynamic stabilization during functional movements. The external obliques work concentrically to produce contralateral rotation and ipsilateral lateral flexion, and work eccentrically to decelerate trunk extension, rotation, and lateral flexion during functional movements.[80] The internal oblique works concentrically to produce ipsilateral rotation and lateral flexion and works eccentrically to decelerate extension, rotation, and lateral flexion. The internal oblique attaches to the posterior layer of the thoracolumbar fascia. Contraction of the internal oblique creates a lateral tension force on the thoracolumbar fascia, which creates intrinsic translational and rotational stabilization of the spinal unit.[34,43] The TA is probably the most important of the abdominal muscles. The TA functions to increase intraabdominal pressure (IAP), provide dynamic stabilization against rotational and translational stress in the lumbar spine, and provide optimal neuromuscular efficiency to the entire lumbo-pelvic-hip complex.[43,46-48,58] Research demonstrates that the TA works in a feedforward mechanism.[43] Researchers have demonstrated that contraction of the TA precedes the initiation of limb movement and all other abdominal muscles, regardless of the direction of reactive forces.[26,43] Cresswell et al[25,26] demonstrated that like the multifidus, the TA is active during all trunk movements, suggesting that this muscle has an important role in dynamic stabilization.[46]

Key hip muscles include the psoas, gluteus medius, gluteus maximus, and hamstrings.[7,8,80] The psoas produces hip flexion and external rotation in the open chain position, and produces hip flexion, lumbar extension, lateral flexion, and rotation in the closed-chain position. The psoas eccentrically decelerates hip extension and internal rotation, as well as trunk extension, lateral flexion, and rotation. The psoas works synergistically with the superficial erector spinae and creates an anterior shear force at L4-L5.[80] The deep erector spinae, multifidus, and deep abdominal wall (transverses, internal oblique, and external oblique)[80] counteract this force. It is extremely common for clients to develop tightness in their psoas. A tight psoas increases the anterior shear force and compressive force at the L4-L5 junction.[80] A tight psoas also causes reciprocal inhibition of the gluteus maximus, multifidus, deep erector spinae, internal oblique, and TA. This leads to extensor mechanism dysfunction during functional movement patterns.[51,61,63,65,66,80,89] Lack of lumbo-pelvic-hip complex stabilization prevents appropriate movement sequencing and leads to synergistic dominance by the hamstrings and superficial erector spinae during hip extension. This complex movement dysfunction also decreases the ability of the gluteus maximus to decelerate femoral internal rotation during heel strike, which predisposes an individual with a knee ligament injury to abnormal forces and repetitive microtrauma.[14,19,51,65,66]

The gluteus medius functions as the primary frontal plane stabilizer of the pelvis and lower extremity during functional movements.[80] During closed-chain movements, the gluteus medius decelerates femoral adduction and internal rotation.[80] A weak gluteus medius increases frontal and transversus plane stress at the patellofemoral joint and the tibiofemoral joint.[80] A weak gluteus medius leads to synergistic dominance of the tensor fascia latae and the quadratus lumborum.[19,51,53] This leads to tightness in the iliotibial band and the lumbar spine. This will affect the normal biomechanics of the lumbo-pelvic-hip complex and the tibiofemoral joint, as well as the patellofemoral joint. Research by Beckman and Buchanan[9] demonstrates decreased electromyogram (EMG) activity of the gluteus medius following an ankle sprain. Therapists must address the altered hip muscle recruitment patterns or accept this recruitment pattern as an injury-adaptive strategy, and thus accept the unknown long-term consequences of premature muscle activation and synergistic dominance.[9,29]

The gluteus maximus functions concentrically in the open chain to accelerate hip extension and external rotation. It functions eccentrically to decelerate hip flexion and femoral internal rotation.[80] It also functions through the iliotibial band to decelerate tibial internal rotation.[80] The gluteus maximus is a major dynamic stabilizer of the sacroiliac (SI) joint. It has the greatest capacity to provide compressive forces at the SI joint secondary to its anatomic attachment at the sacrotuberous ligament.[80] It has been demonstrated by Bullock-Saxton[15,16] that the EMG activity of the gluteus maximus is decreased following an ankle sprain. Lack of proper gluteus maximus activity during functional activities leads to pelvic instability and decreased neuromuscular control. This can eventually lead to the development of muscle imbalances, poor movement patterns, and injury.

The hamstrings work concentrically to flex the knee, extend the hip, and rotate the tibia. They work eccentrically to decelerate knee extension, hip flexion, and tibial rotation. The hamstrings work synergistically with the anterior cruciate ligament.[80] All of the muscles mentioned play an integral role in the kinetic chain by providing dynamic stabilization and optimal neuromuscular control of the entire lumbo-pelvic-hip complex. These muscles have been reviewed so that the therapist realizes that muscles not only produce force (concentric contractions) in 1 plane of motion, but also reduce force (eccentric contractions) and provide dynamic stabilization in all planes of movement during functional activities. When isolated, these muscles do not effectively achieve stabilization of the lumbo-pelvic-hip complex. It is the synergistic, interdependent functioning of the entire lumbo-pelvic-hip complex that enhances stability and neuromuscular control throughout the entire kinetic chain.

Transversus Abdominis and Multifidus Role in Core Stabilization

The TA muscle is the deepest of the abdominal muscles and plays a primary role in trunk stability. The horizontal orientation of its fibers has a limited ability to produce torque to the spine necessary for flexion or extension movement, although it has been shown to be an active trunk rotator.[81] The TA is a primary trunk stabilizer via modulation of IAP, tension through the thoracolumbar fascia, and compression of the SI joints.[25,91] For many decades, IAP was believed to be an important contributor to spinal control by the pressure within the abdominal cavity putting force on the diaphragm superiorly and pelvic floor inferiorly to extend the trunk.[6,35,73] It was hypothesized that IAP would provide an extensor moment and thus reduce the muscular force required by the trunk extensors and decrease the compressive load on the lumbar spine.[95] Recent research by Hodges et al[42] applied electrical stimulation to the phrenic nerve of humans to produce an involuntary increase in IAP without abdominal or extensor muscle activity. IAP was increased by the contraction of the diaphragm, pelvic floor muscles, and the TA with no flexor moment noted. Research has demonstrated that IAP may directly increase spinal stiffness.[45] Hodges et al[42] used a tetanic contraction of the diaphragm to produce IAP, which resulted in increased stiffness in the spine. Bilateral contraction of the TA assists in IAP, thus enhancing spinal stiffness.

The role of the thoracolumbar fascia in trunk stability has also been discussed in the literature, and it has been theorized that the contraction of the TA could produce an extensor torque via the horizontal pull of the TA via its extensive attachment into the thoracolumbar fascia.[34] Recently, this theory was tested by Tesh et al[93] by placing tension on the thoracolumbar fascia of cadavers. No approximation of the spinous processes or trunk extension movement was noted although a small amount of compression on the spine was noted. This small amount of compression may play a role in the control of intervertebral shear forces. Hodges et al[42] electrically stimulated contraction of the TA in pigs and demonstrated that when tension was developed in the thoracolumbar fascia, without an associated increase in IAP, there was no significant effect on the intervertebral stiffness. In the next step of that same research study, the thoracolumbar fascial attachments were cut and an increase in IAP decreased the spinal stiffness. This demonstrates that the thoracolumbar fascia and IAP work in concert to enhance trunk stability.[42] Trunk stability is also dependent on the joints caudal to the lumbar spine. The SI joint is the connection between the lumbar spine and the pelvic region, which ultimately connects the trunk to the lower extremities. The SI joint is dependent on the compressive force between the sacrum and ilia. The horizontal direction and anterior attachment on the ilium of the TA produces the compressive force necessary for spinal stability. Richardson et al[84] used ultrasound to detect movement of the sacrum and ilium while having subjects voluntarily contract their transverse abdominals. They demonstrated that a voluntary contraction of the TA reduced the laxity of the SI joint. This study also pointed out that this reduction in joint laxity of the SI joint was greater than that during a bracing contraction. The researchers did note that they were unable to exclude changes in activity in other muscles such as the pelvic floor, which may have reduced the laxity via counternutation of the sacrum.[84] The aforementioned research findings illustrate that the TA plays an important role in maintaining trunk stability by interacting with IAP, thoracolumbar fascia tension, and compressing the SI joints via muscular attachments.

The multifidi are the most medial of the posterior trunk muscles, and they cover the lumbar zygapophyseal joints except for the ventral surfaces.[81] The multifidi are primary stabilizers when the trunk is moving from flexion to extension. The multifidi contribute only 20% of the total lumbar extensor moment, whereas the lumbar erector spinae contribute 30%, and the thoracic erector spinae function as the predominant torque generator at 50% of the extension moment arm.[56] The multifidus, lumbar, and thoracic erector spinae muscles have a high percentage of type I fibers and are postural control muscles similar to the TA.[56] The multifidus has been shown to be active during all antigravity activities, including static tasks, such as standing, and dynamic tasks, such as walking.[97]

Clinical observation and experimental evidence confirm that when the TA contracts, the multifidi are also activated.[81] A girdlelike cylinder of muscular support is produced as a result of the coactivation of the TA, multifidus, and the thick thoracolumbar fascial system. EMG evidence suggests that the TA and internal obliques contract in anticipation of movement of the upper and lower extremities, often referred to as the feed-forward mechanism. This feed-forward mechanism gives the TA and multifidus muscular girdle a unique ability to stabilize the spine regardless of the direction of limb movements.[44,45] As noted previously, the pelvic floor muscles play an important role in the development of IAP, and thus enhance trunk stability. It has also been demonstrated that the pelvic floor is active during repetitive arm movement tasks independent of the direction of movement.[49] Sapsford et al[90] discovered that maximal contraction of the pelvic floor was associated with activity of all abdominal muscles and submaximal contraction of the pelvic floor muscles was associated with a more isolated contraction of the TA. In this same study, it also was determined that the specificity of the response was better when the lumbar spine and pelvis were in a neutral position.[90] Clinically, this information is helpful in guiding the patient in the process of TA contraction by instructing the patient to perform a submaximal pelvic floor isometric hold. Another interesting fact to note is that men and women with incontinence have almost double the incidence of low back pain as people without incontinence issues.[30] In summary, the lumbopelvic region may be visualized as a cylinder with the inferior wall being the pelvic floor, the superior wall being the diaphragm, the posterior wall being the multifidus, and the TA muscles forming the anterior and lateral walls. All walls of the cylinder must be activated and taut for optimal trunk stabilization to occur with all static and dynamic activities.

Clinical Pearl

Core training exercises should be safe and challenging and stress multiple planes that are functional as they are applied to a functional activity or sport. The exercises should also be proprioceptively challenging and activity specific.

Postural Considerations

The core functions to maintain postural alignment and dynamic postural equilibrium during functional activities. Optimal alignment of each body part is a cornerstone to a functional training and rehabilitation program. Optimal posture and alignment will allow for maximal neuromuscular efficiency because the normal length-tension relationship, force-couple relationship, and arthrokinematics will be maintained during functional movement patterns.[14,28,29,50,51,53,55,58,62,64,88,89] If 1 segment in the kinetic chain is out of alignment, it will create predictable patterns of dysfunction throughout the entire kinetic chain. These predictable patterns of dysfunction are referred to as *serial distortion patterns*.[28] Serial distortion patterns represent the state in which the body's structural integrity is compromised because segments in the kinetic chain are out of alignment. This leads to abnormal distorting forces being placed on the segments in the kinetic chain that are above and below the dysfunctional segment.[14,28,29,55] To avoid serial distortion patterns and the chain reaction that 1 misaligned segment creates, we must emphasize stable positions to maintain the structural integrity of the entire kinetic chain.[16,28,55,65,66,87] A comprehensive core stabilization program prevents the development of serial distortion patterns and provides optimal dynamic postural control during functional movements.

Muscular Imbalances

An optimally functioning core helps to prevent the development of muscle imbalances and synergistic dominance. The human movement system is a well-orchestrated system of interrelated and interdependent components.[16,61] The functional interaction of each component in the human movement system allows for optimal neuromuscular efficiency. Alterations in joint arthrokinematics, muscular balance, and neuromuscular control affect the optimal functioning of the entire kinetic chain.[16,88,89] Dysfunction of the kinetic chain is rarely an isolated event. Typically, a pathology of the kinetic chain is part of a chain reaction involving some key links in the kinetic chain and numerous compensations and adaptations that develop.[61] The interplay of many muscles about a joint is responsible for the coordinated control of movement. If the core is weak, normal arthrokinematics are altered. Changes in normal length-tension and force-couple relationships, in turn, affect neuromuscular control. If 1 muscle becomes weak, tight, or changes its degree of activation, then synergists, stabilizers, and neutralizers have to compensate.[16,29,61,64-66,88,89] Muscle tightness has a significant impact on the kinetic chain. Muscle tightness affects the normal length-tension relationship.[89] This impacts the normal force-couple relationship. When 1 muscle in a force-couple relationship becomes tight, it changes the normal arthrokinematics of 2 articular partners.[14,61,89] Altered arthrokinematics affect the synergistic function of the kinetic chain.[14,29,61,89] This leads to abnormal pressure distribution over articular surfaces and soft tissues. Muscle tightness also leads to reciprocal inhibition.[14,29,50-53,61,92,96] Therefore, if one develops muscle imbalances throughout the lumbo-pelvic-hip complex, it can affect the entire kinetic chain. For example, a tight psoas causes reciprocal inhibition of the gluteus maximus, TA, internal oblique, and multifidus.[47,51,53,77,80] This muscle imbalance pattern may decrease normal lumbo-pelvic-hip stability. Specific substitution patterns develop to compensate for the lack of stabilization, including tightness in the iliotibial band.[29] This muscle imbalance pattern leads to increased frontal and transverse plane stress at the knee. Dr. Vladamir Janda proposed a syndrome, named the "crossed pelvis syndrome," in which a weak abdominal wall and weak gluteals are counterbalanced with tight hamstrings and hip flexors.[51] A strong core with optimal neuromuscular efficiency can help to prevent the development of muscle imbalances. Consequently, a comprehensive core stabilization training program should be an integral component of all rehabilitation programs. A strong, efficient core provides the stable base upon which the extremities can function with maximal precision and effectiveness. It is important to remember that the spine, pelvis, and hips must be in proper alignment with proper activation of all muscles during any core-strengthening exercise. Because no 1 muscle works in isolation, attention should be paid to the position and activity of all muscles during open- and closed-chain exercises.

Neuromuscular Considerations

A strong and stable core can optimize neuromuscular efficiency throughout the entire kinetic chain by helping to improve dynamic postural control.[37,43,47,57,83,88,89] A number of authors have demonstrated kinetic chain imbalances in individuals with altered neuromuscular control.[9,14-16,43,46-48,50-54,61-66,76,77,83,88] Research demonstrates that people with low back pain have an abnormal neuromotor response of the trunk stabilizers accompanying limb movement, significantly greater postural sway, and decreased limits of stability.[46,47,71,77] Research also demonstrates that approximately 70% of patients suffer from recurrent episodes of back pain. Furthermore, it has been demonstrated that individuals have decreased dynamic postural stability in the proximal stabilizers of the lumbo-pelvic-hip complex following lower-extremity ligamentous injuries,[9,14-16] and that joint and ligamentous injury can lead to decreased muscle activity.[29,92,96] Joint and ligament injury can lead to joint effusion, which, in turn, leads to muscle inhibition. This leads to altered neuromuscular control in other segments of the kinetic chain secondary to altered proprioception and kinesthesia.[9,16] Therefore, when an individual with a knee ligament injury has joint effusion, all of the muscles that cross the knee can be inhibited. Several muscles that cross the knee joint are attached to the lumbo-pelvic-hip complex.[80] Consequently, a comprehensive rehabilitation approach should focus on reestablishing optimal core function so as to positively affect peripheral joints.

Research also demonstrates that muscles can be inhibited from an arthrokinetic reflex.[14,61,92,96] This is referred to as *arthrogenic muscle inhibition*. Arthrokinetic reflexes are mediated by joint receptor activity. If an individual has abnormal arthrokinematics, the muscles that move the joint will be inhibited. For example, if an individual has a sacral torsion, the multifidus and the gluteus medius can be inhibited.[41] This leads to abnormal movement in the kinetic chain. The tensor fascia latae become synergistically dominant and the primary frontal plane stabilizer.[80] This can lead to tightness in the iliotibial band. It can also decrease the frontal and transverse plane control at the knee. Furthermore, if the multifidus is inhibited,[41] the erector spinae and the psoas become facilitated. This further inhibits the lower abdominals (internal oblique and TA) and the gluteus maximus.[43,46] This also decreases frontal and transverse plane stability at the knee. As previously mentioned, an efficient core improves neuromuscular efficiency of the entire kinetic chain by providing dynamic stabilization of the lumbo-pelvic-hip complex and improving pelvofemoral biomechanics. This is yet another reason why all rehabilitation programs should include a comprehensive core stabilization training program.

Clinical Pearl

Individuals with poor core strength are likely to develop low back pain as a consequence of improper muscle stability.[71] The straight-leg lowering test is a good way to assess core strength.

Scientific Rationale for Core Stabilization Training

Most individuals train their core stabilizers inadequately compared to other muscle groups.[1,85,86] Although adequate strength, power, muscle endurance, and neuromuscular control are important for lumbo-pelvic-hip stabilization, performing exercises incorrectly or that are too advanced is detrimental.[60,85,86] Several authors have found decreased firing of the TA, internal oblique, multifidus, and deep erector spinae in individuals with chronic low back pain.[43,46-48,77,82] Performing core training with inhibition of these key stabilizers leads to the development of muscle imbalances and inefficient neuromuscular control in the kinetic chain. It has been demonstrated that abdominal training without proper pelvic stabilization increases intradiscal pressure and compressive forces in the lumbar spine.[3,5,10,43,46-48,74,75] Furthermore, hyperextension training without proper pelvic stabilization can increase intradiscal pressure to dangerous levels, cause buckling of the ligamentum flavum, and lead to narrowing of the intervertebral foramen.[3,5,10,75]

Research also shows decreased stabilization endurance in individuals with chronic low back pain.[10,18,33,34,70] The core stabilizers are primarily type I slow-twitch muscle fibers.[33,34,78,79] These muscles respond best to time under tension. Time under tension is a method of contraction that lasts 6 to 20 seconds and emphasizes hypercontractions at end ranges of motion. This method improves intramuscular coordination, which improves static and dynamic stabilization. To get the appropriate training stimulus, you must prescribe the appropriate speed of movement for all aspects of exercises.[22,23] Core strength endurance must be trained appropriately to allow an individual to maintain dynamic postural control for prolonged periods of time.[3]

Research demonstrates a decreased cross-sectional area of the multifidus in subjects with low back pain, and that spontaneous recovery of the multifidus following resolution of symptoms does not occur.[41] It has also been demonstrated that the traditional curl-up increases intradiscal pressure and increases compressive forces at L2-L3.[3,5,10,74,75]

Additional research demonstrates increased EMG activity and pelvic stabilization when an abdominal drawing-in maneuver is performed prior to initiating core training.[3,10,13,22,36,37,48,72,76,83] Also, maintaining the cervical spine in a neutral position during core training improves posture, muscle balance, and stabilization. If the head protracts during movement, then the sternocleidomastoid is preferentially recruited. This increases the compressive forces at the C0-C1 vertebral junction. This can lead to pelvic instability and muscle imbalances secondary to the pelvo-occular reflex. This reflex is important to keep the eyes level.[62,63] If the sternocleidomastoid muscle is hyperactive and extends the upper cervical spine, then the pelvis will rotate anteriorly to realign the eyes. This can lead to muscle imbalances and decreased pelvic stabilization.[62,63]

Clinical Pearl

Frequently altering a rehabilitation program will help keep a patient interested. Consider these variables as you plan changes: plane of motion, range of motion, loading parameter (Physioballs, tubing, medicine balls, Bodyblades, etc.), body position (from supine to standing), speed of movement, amount of control, duration (sets and reps), and frequency.

Assessment of the Core

Before a comprehensive core stabilization program is implemented, an individual must undergo a comprehensive assessment to determine muscle imbalances, arthrokinematic deficits, core strength, core muscle endurance, core neuromuscular control, core power, and overall function of the lower-extremity kinetic chain. Assessment tools include activity-based tests that are performed in the clinical setting, EMG with surface or indwelling electrodes, and technologically advanced testing and training techniques using real-time ultrasound. Rehabilitative ultrasound imaging (RUSI) has been used extensively in research settings and has been proven to be a reliable tool in evaluating the activation patterns of various abdominal muscles.[38,94] RUSI, although not currently readily available in clinical settings, is a great asset in the laboratory setting. Perhaps the future will allow for more use of RUSI in clinical practice.

It was previously stated that muscle imbalances and arthrokinematic deficits can cause abnormal movement patterns to develop throughout the entire kinetic chain. Consequently, it is extremely important to thoroughly assess each individual with a kinetic chain dysfunction for muscle imbalances and arthrokinematic deficits. All procedures for assessment are beyond the scope of this chapter, and the interested reader is referred to the comprehensive references provided to gain an understanding of additional assessment procedures that may be used to identify muscle imbalances. It is recommended that the interested reader use the following references to explain a comprehensive muscle imbalance assessment procedure thoroughly.[1,14,19,22,23,28,48,52,54,55,64,88,89,96]

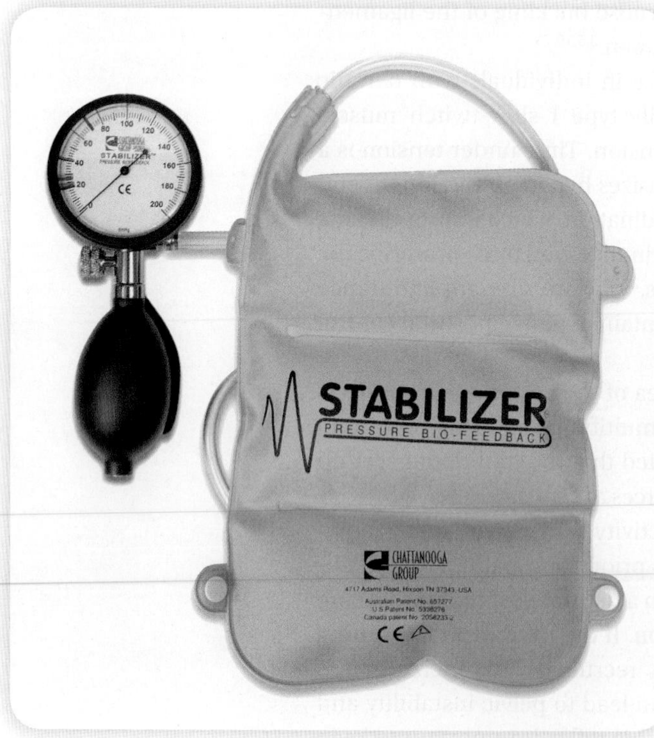

Figure 15-4 Stabilizer pressure feedback unit

(Courtesy, Chattanooga, a brand of DJO Global Inc.)

Core strength can be assessed by using the straight-leg lowering test.[3,48,58,76,88,89] The individual is placed supine. A pressure biofeedback device called the Stabilizer (Figure 15-4) is placed under the lumbar spine at approximately L4-L5. The cuff pressure is raised to 40 mm Hg. The individual's legs are maintained in full extension while flexing the hips to 90 degrees (Figure 15-5). The individual is instructed to perform a drawing-in maneuver (pull belly button to spine) and then flatten the back maximally into the table and pressure cuff. The individual is instructed to lower the legs toward the table while maintaining the back flat. The test is over when the pressure in the cuff decreases. The hip angle is then measured with a goniometer to determine the angle using a rating scale developed by

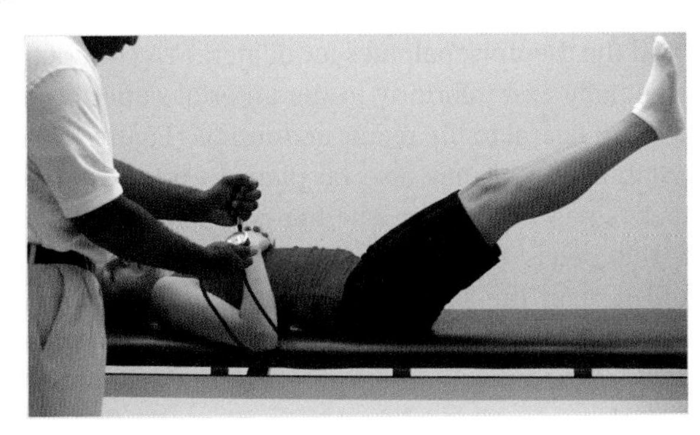

Figure 15-5

Core strength can be assessed using a straight leg-lowering test.

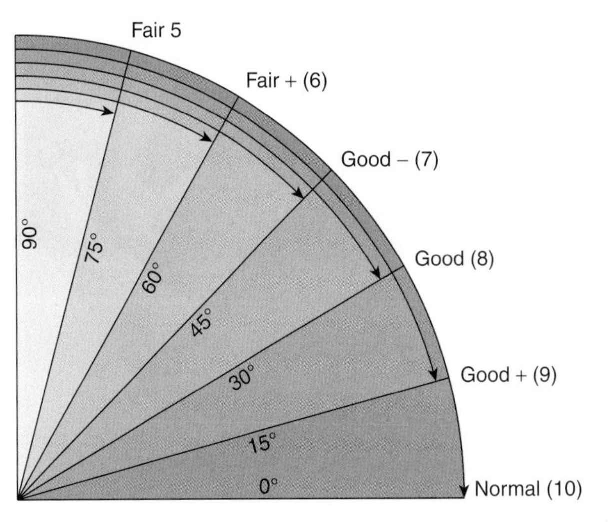

Figure 15-6

Key to muscle grading in the straight-leg lowering test. (Reproduced with permission from Kendall FP, McCreary EK, Provance PG, Rodgers MM, Romani WA. *Muscles: Testing and Function.* 5th ed. Baltimore, MD: Lippincott Williams & Wilkins; 2005.)

Kendall (Figure 15-6).[59] This test provides a basic idea of how strong the lower abdominal muscle groups (rectus abdominis and external obliques) are. Using the pressure feedback device ensures there is no compensation with the lumbar extensors or large hip flexors to stabilize the long lever arm of the legs.

Neuromuscular control of the deep core muscles, TA and multifidi, are evaluated with the quality of movement emphasized rather than quantity of muscular strength or endurance time. Unfortunately, no objectifiable manual muscle test exists for either of these important muscles/muscle groups; however, Hides et al[40] have developed prone and supine tests to evaluate the muscular coordination of the TA and multifidus. The first test for the TA is performed in the prone position with the Stabilizer pressure biofeedback unit placed under the abdomen with the navel in the center and the distal edge of the pad in line with the right and left anterior superior iliac spines (Figure 15-7). The pressure pad is inflated to 70 mm Hg. It is important to instruct the patient to relax the patient's abdomen fully prior to the start of the test. The patient is then instructed to take a relaxed breath in and out, and then to draw the abdomen in toward the spine without taking a breath. The patient is asked to hold this contraction for a minimum of 10 seconds, with a slow and controlled release. Optimal performance, indicating proper neuromuscular control of the TA, is a 4- to 10-mm Hg reduction in the pressure with no pelvic or spinal movement noted. It is important to monitor pelvic and lower-extremity positioning as the patient may compensate by putting pressure through the patient's legs or tilting the patient's pelvis to elevate the lower abdomen rather than isolating the TA contraction.

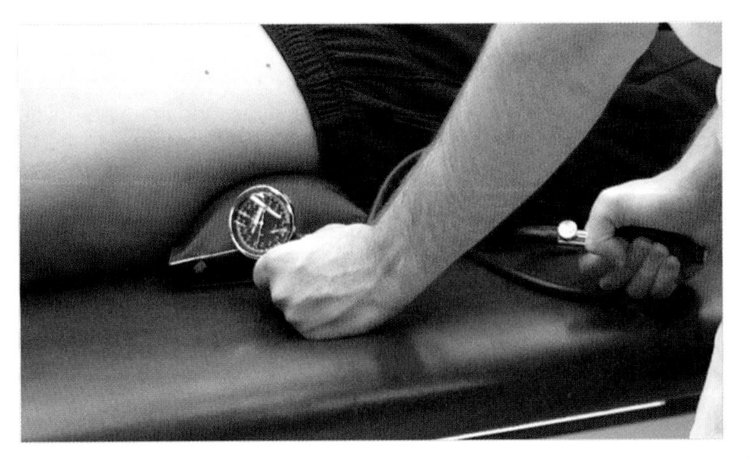

Figure 15-7 Prone transverse abdominis test

Testing for the TA is also performed in the supine position and relies on palpation and visualization of the lower abdomen.

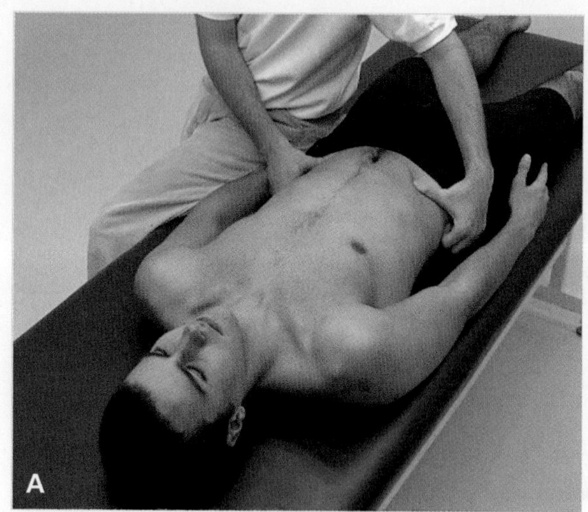

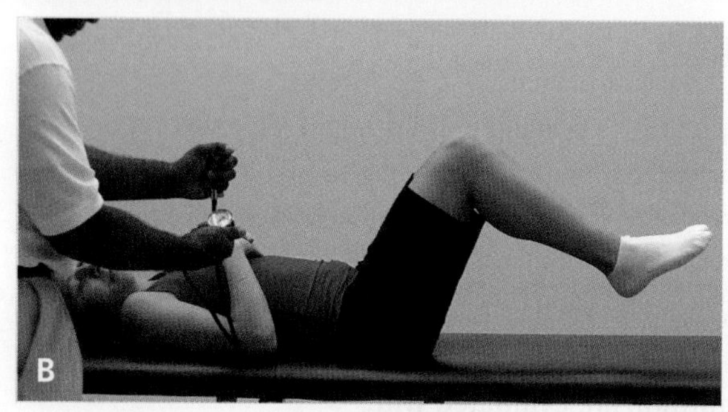

Figure 15-8 Supine transversus abdominis test

Instructions to the patient remain the same as the prone test and the therapist palpates for bilateral TA contraction just medially and inferiorly to the anterior superior iliac spines and lateral to the rectus abdominis (Figure 15-8*A*). The Stabilizer pad may also be placed under the lower lumbar region to monitor whether compensation occurs with the pelvis (Figure 15-8*B*). The pressure reading should remain the same throughout the test. A change in the pressure reading indicates that the patient is tilting the patient's pelvis anteriorly (pressure decreases) or posteriorly (pressure increases) in an attempt to flatten the patient's lower abdomen. The patient is asked to hold this contraction for a minimum of 10 seconds, with a slow and controlled release. With a correct contraction of the TA, the therapist feels a slowly developing deep tension in the lower abdominal wall. Incorrect activation of the TA would be evident when the internal oblique dominates and this is detected when a rapid development of tension is palpated or the abdominal wall is pushed out rather than drawn in.

The neuromuscular control of the multifidi is examined with the patient in the prone position and the therapist palpating the level of the multifidus for muscular activation (Figure 15-9). The patient is instructed to breathe in and out and to hold the breath out while swelling out the muscles under the therapist's fingers. The patient is then asked to hold the contraction while resuming a normal breathing pattern for a minimum of 10 seconds. The therapist palpates the multifidus for symmetrical activation and slow development of muscular activation. This sequence is repeated at the multiple segments in the lumbar spine. Compensation patterns may include anterior or posterior pelvic tilting or elevation of the rib cage in an attempt to swell out the multifidus.

A proper and thorough evaluation of the core muscles will lead the therapist in developing a proper core stabilization program. It is imperative that neuromuscular control of the TA and multifidus precedes all other stabilization exercises. These muscles provide the foundation from which all the other core muscles work.

Clinical Pearl

Rehabilitative ultrasound imaging (RUSI) or diagnostic musculoskeletal ultrasound (MSK) can be utilized to assess dynamic activity of the TA and multifidi. However, this technique requires equipment and operator training. Use of diagnostic ultrasound for clinical assessment is increasing.

Core Stabilization Training Program

As previously noted, the training program must progress in a scientific, systematic pattern with the ultimate goal of training the trunk stabilizers to be active in all phases of functional tasks. These tasks may include simple static postures, such as standing or sitting, and progress to very complex tasks, such as high-intensity athletic skills.[67] Patient education is the

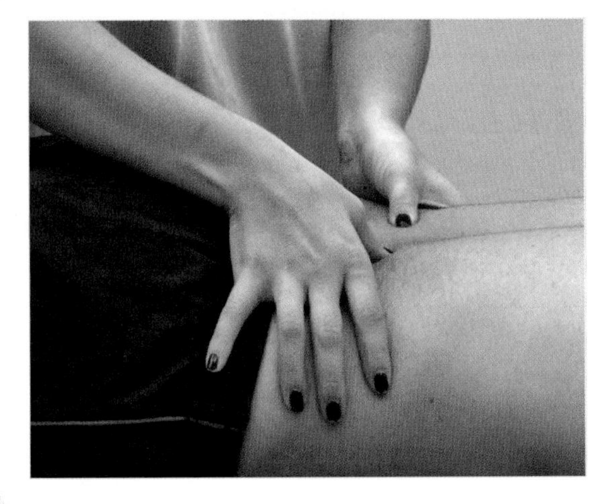

Figure 15-9 **Palpating the multifidi for muscular activation**

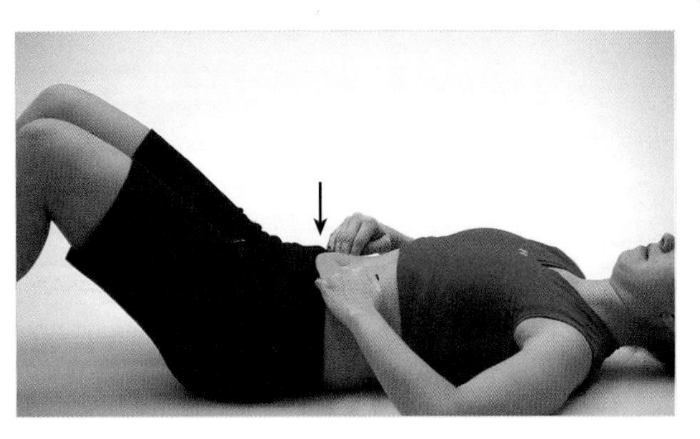

Figure 15-10 **The drawing-in maneuver requires a contraction of the transversus abdominis**

key to a successful exercise program. The patient must be able to visualize the muscle activation patterns desired and have a high level of body awareness allowing them to activate their core muscles with the proper positioning, neuromuscular control, and level of force generation needed for each individual task.

Performing the Drawing-In Maneuver

Muscular activation of the deep core stabilizers (TA and multifidus) coordinated with normal breathing patterns is the foundation for all core exercises.[60] All core stabilization exercises must first start with the "drawing-in" maneuver (Figure 15-10). Opinions vary[69,81] in the exercise science world about the activation of the abdominal muscles during activities.

McGill[69] is a proponent of the abdominal bracing technique where the patient is advised to stiffen or activate both the trunk flexors and extensors maximally to prevent spinal movement. He uses the training technique of demonstrating this bracing pattern at the elbow joint. He asks the patient to stiffen his or her elbow joint by simultaneously activating the elbow flexors and extensors and resisting an externally applied force that attempts to flex the patient's elbow. Once the patient has mastered that concept, the same principles are applied to the trunk.

Richardson et al[81] teach the abdominal hollowing technique where the navel is drawn back toward the spine without spinal movement occurring. This technique does not ask patients to do a maximal contraction, but instead, a submaximal, steady development of muscle activation.

We have used a teaching technique that incorporates submaximal abdominal hollowing and moderate bracing of the trunk. While standing in front of a mirror, patients are asked to put their hands on their iliac crests so their fingers rest anteriorly on their transverse abdominals and internal obliques. A good way to state this to the patient is: "put your hands on your hips like you are mad." Patients are then instructed to draw their navel back toward their spine without moving their trunk or body while continuing to breathe normally. A good verbal cue is to "make your waist narrow like you are putting on a tight pair of jeans, without sucking in your breath." While in that position, patients are also instructed to not let anyone "push them around" or push them off balance. This helps incorporate the total-body bracing technique and the use of the upper

Table 15-1 Teaching Cues for Activation of Core Muscles

Verbal Cues
1. Draw navel back toward spine without moving your spine or tilting your pelvis.
2. Make your waist narrow.
3. Pull your abdomen away from your waistband of your pants.
4. Draw lower abdomen in while simulating zipping up a tight pair of pants.
5. Continue breathing normally while contracting lower abdominals.
6. Tighten pelvic floor.
a. Women: contract pelvic floor so you do not leak urine.
b. Men: draw up scrotum as if you are walking in waist deep cold water.
Physical Cues
1. Use mirror for visual feedback.
2. Put your hands on your waist like you are mad—draw abdomen away from fingertips while still breathing normally.
3. Tactile facilitation.
a. Use tape on skin for cutaneous feedback.
b. String tied snugly around waist.
4. EMG biofeedback unit.
5. Electrical muscular stimulation.
6. Isometric contraction and holding of pelvic floor and hip adductors.

and lower extremities to facilitate total-body stabilization. This can be referred to as "the power position" or "home base," and these key words may be used when teaching the progression of all core exercises (Table 15-1 for other teaching cues for proper muscular activation of core muscles).[71,85] It should be emphasized that proper muscular activation cannot be achieved if the patient is holding their breath.

It should also be noted that the drawing-in maneuver should not be abandoned when the patient is performing other exercises such as weightlifting, walking, or other aerobic tasks such as step aerobics, aqua aerobics, or running.

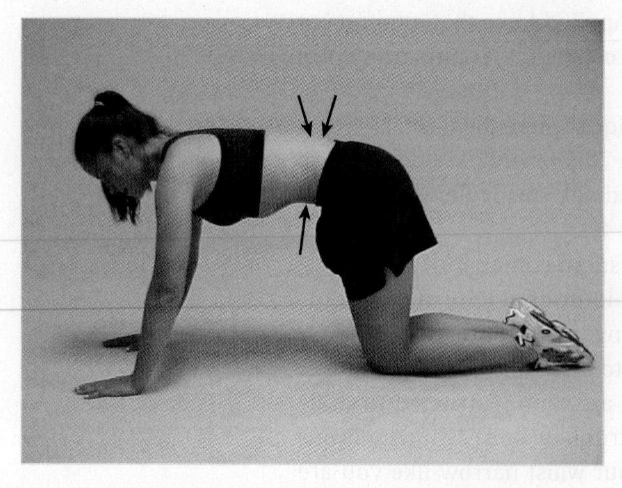

Figure 15-11 Quadruped position for mastering the "drawing-in" maneuver or power position

Specific Core Stabilization Exercises

Once the drawing-in maneuver is perfected, neuromuscular control of the TA and multifidus is accomplished in the prone and supine positions as described in "Assessment of the Core" above. Then progression of exercises into other positions can take place. Quadruped is a good starting position for the patient to learn and enhance their power position (Figure 15-11). This facilitates the patient keeping their body steady and minimizing trunk movement. The patient is instructed to keep the trunk straight like a tabletop and then draw the stomach up toward the spine (activating the TA and multifidus) while maintaining the normal breathing pattern. This position is held for a minimum of 10 seconds and progressed in time to up to 30 to 60 seconds, working on endurance of these trunk muscles.[67,70] The patient is advised to release the contraction slowly in an eccentric manner and no spinal movement should occur during this release phase. When this position is mastered by the patient and the therapist feels that the patient is ready, the difficulty of the exercise can be progressed, limited only by the capabilities of the patient.

Figures 15-12 through 15-14 illustrate the exercises used in a comprehensive core stabilization training program. Exercises may be broken down into 3 levels in the progressive core stabilization training program: level 1—stabilization (Figure 15-12); level 2—strengthening (Figure 15-13); and level 3—power (Figure 15-14). The patient is started with the exercises at the highest level at which the patient can maintain stability and optimal neuromuscular control. The patient is progressed through the program when the patient achieves mastery of the exercises in the previous level.[1,2,4,10,12,15,17,18,22-25,29,34,39,42-48,55,56,62-64,67,68,73,78,79,90,91]

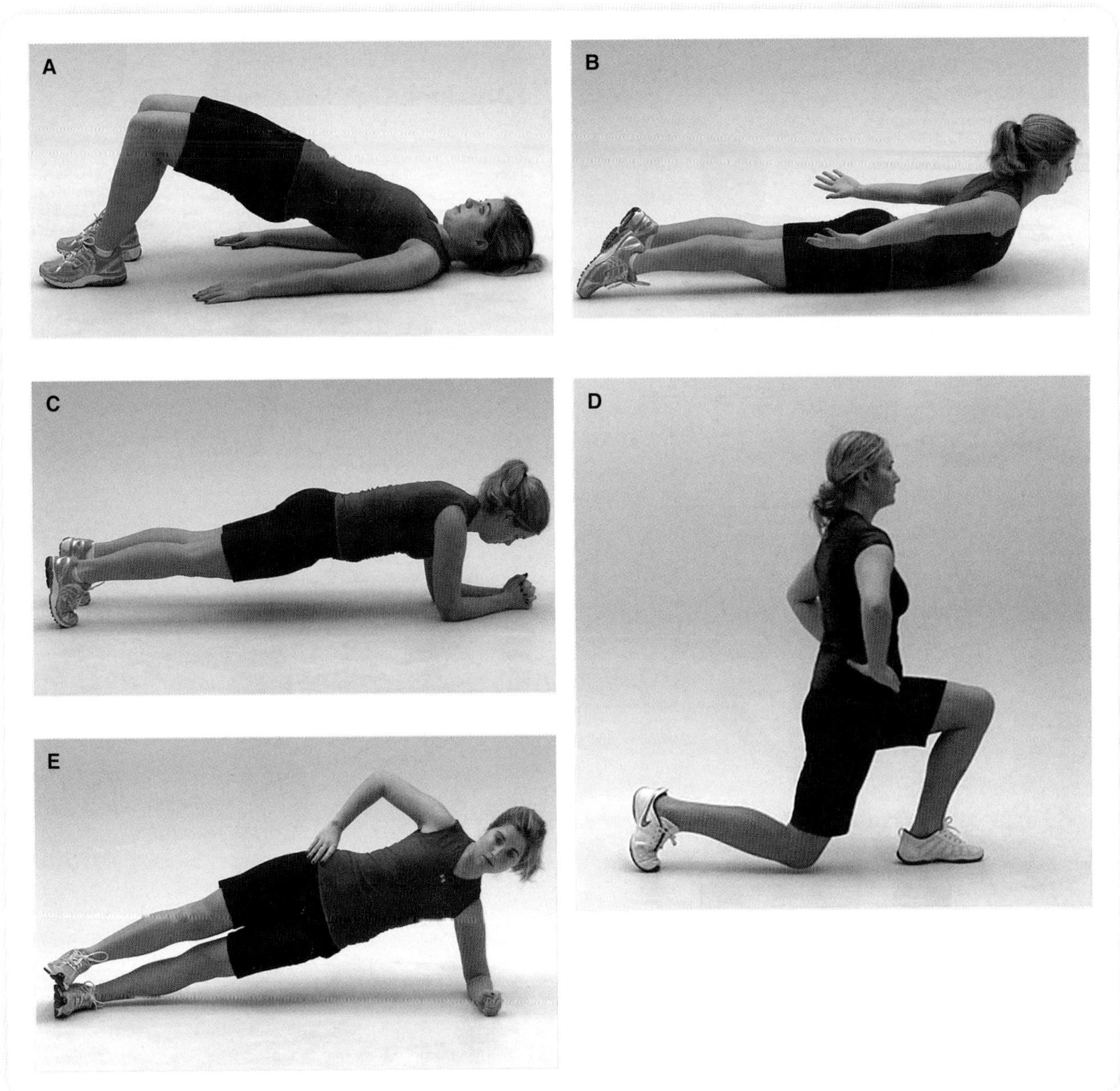

Figure 15-12 **Level 1 (stabilization) core stability exercises**

A. Double-leg bridging. **B.** Prone cobra. **C.** Front plank. **D.** Lunge. **E.** Side plank.

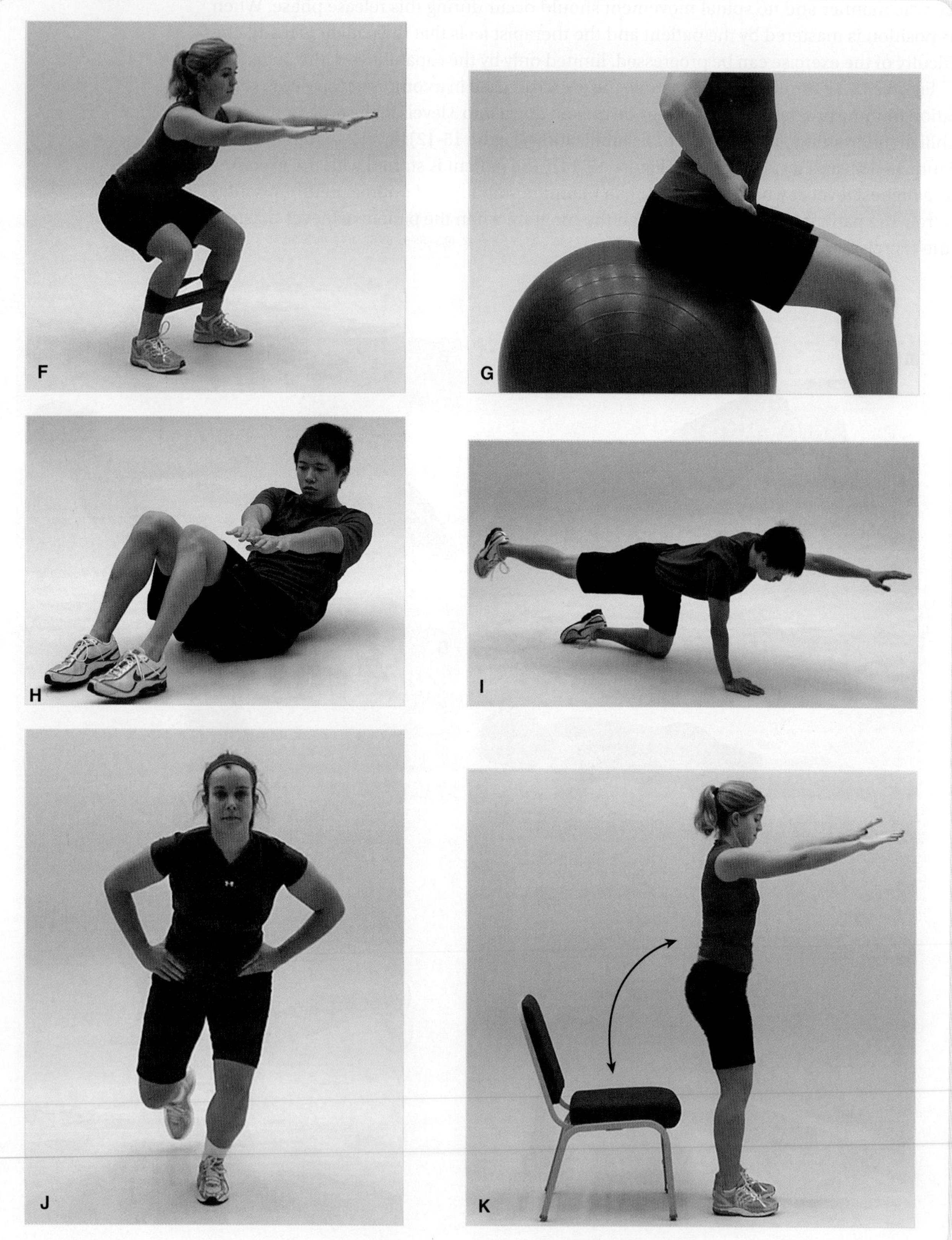

Figure 15-12 ***(Continued)***

F. Squats with Thera-Band. **G.** Pelvic tilts on stability ball. **H.** Diagonal crunches. **I.** Alternating opposite arm-leg. **J.** Single-leg lunge with abdominal bracing. **K.** Sit-to-stand with abdominal bracing.

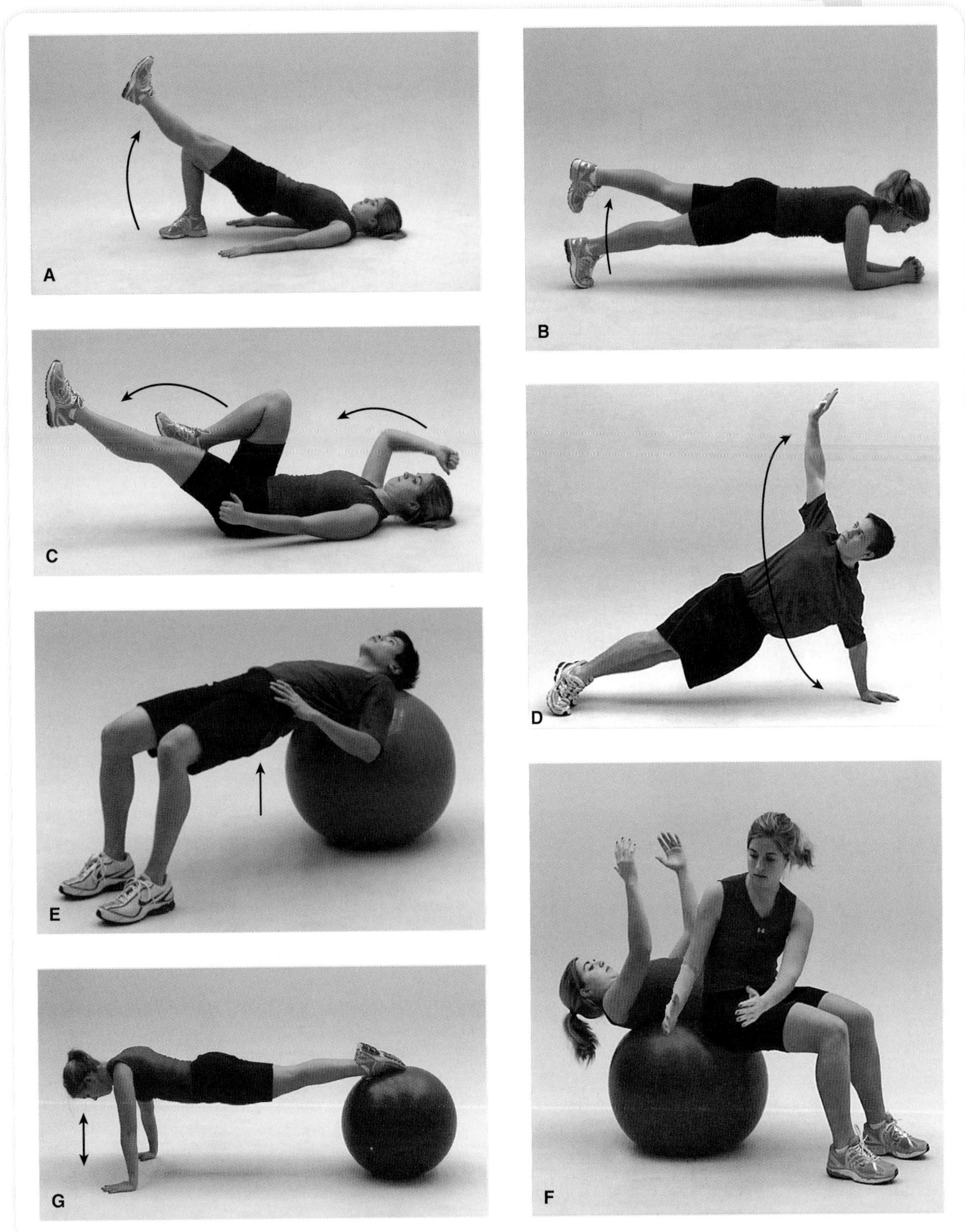

Figure 15-13 **Level 2 (strength) core stability exercises**

A. Bridge with single-leg extension. **B.** Front plank with single leg-extension. **C.** Supine alternating arms and legs (AKA: Dying bug). **D.** Pushup to side plank. **E.** Bridging on stability ball. **F.** Stability ball diagonal crunches. **G.** Push-ups on therapy ball.

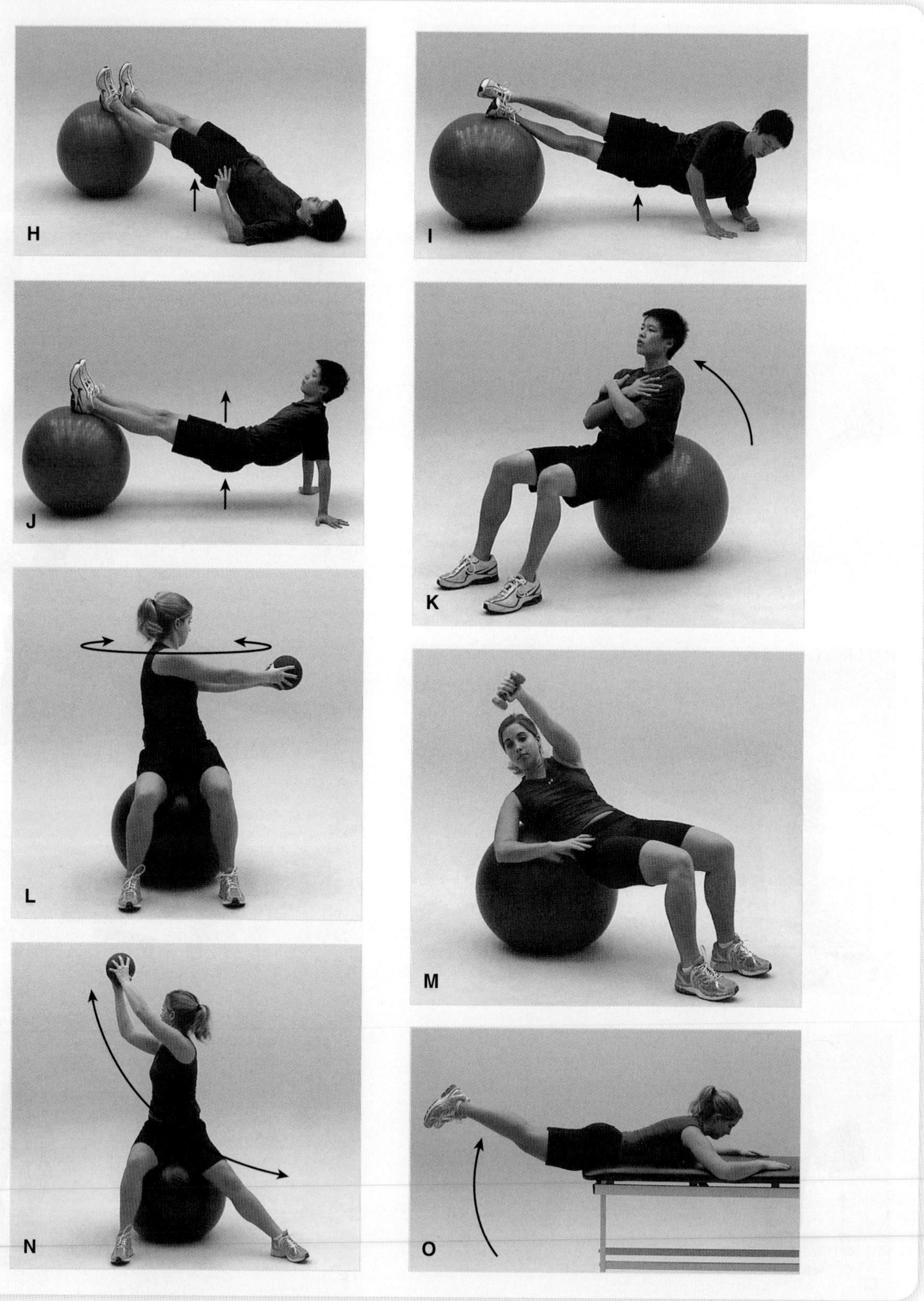

Figure 15-13 ***(Continued)***

H. Stability ball hip-ups. **I.** Stability ball side plank. **J.** Stability ball pike-ups. **K.** Stability ball crunches. **L.** Stability ball rotation with weighted ball. **M.** Stability ball single arm dumbbell press with rotation. **N.** Stability ball diagonal rotations with weighted ball. **O.** Prone hip extension.

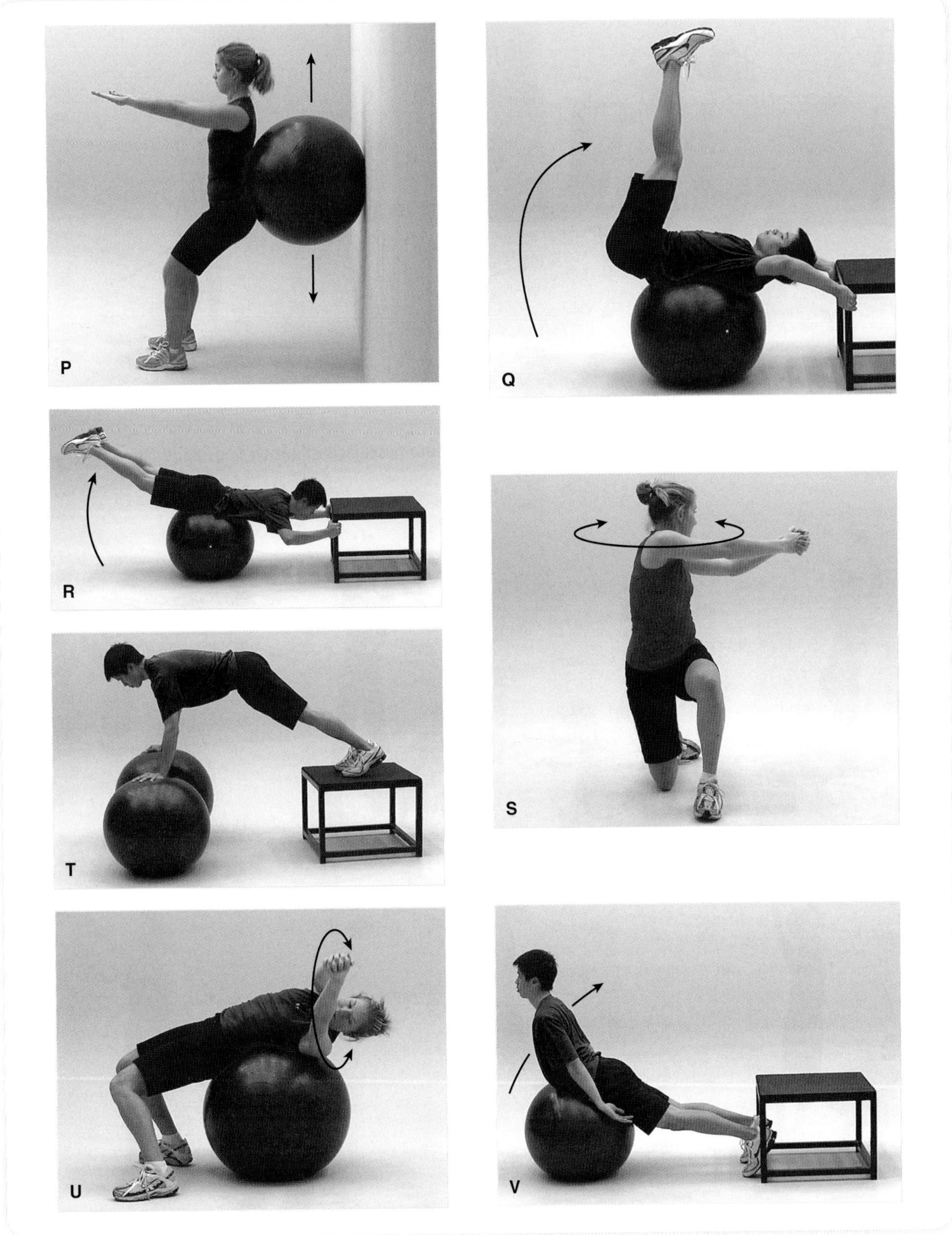

Figure 15-13 ***(Continued)***

P. Stability ball wall slides. **Q.** Stability ball straight-leg raise. **R.** Stability ball hip extension. **S.** Half-kneeling rotation. **T.** Stability balls two-arm support. **U.** Stability ball Russian twist. **V.** Stability ball prone cobra.

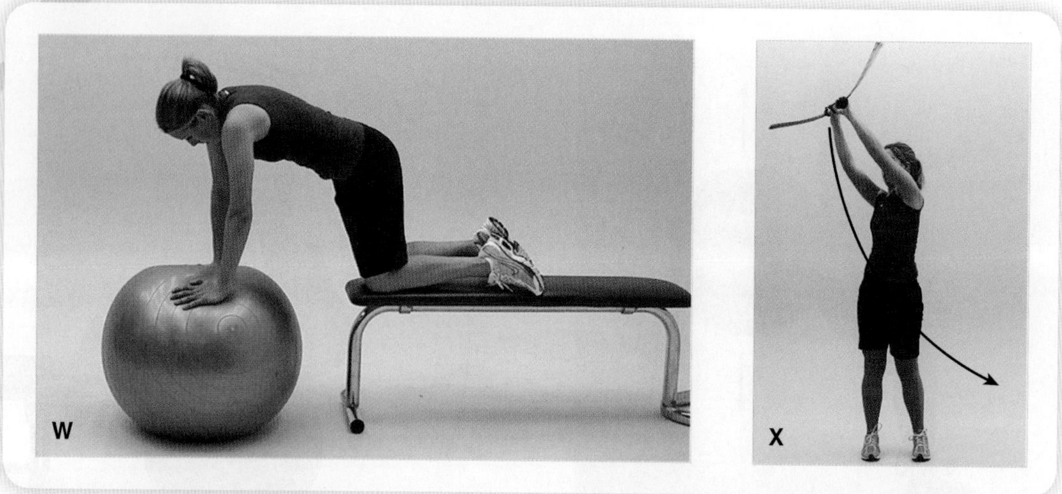

Figure 15-13 ***(Continued)***

W. Weight shifting on stability ball. **X.** Proprioceptive neuromuscular facilitation Bodyblade™.

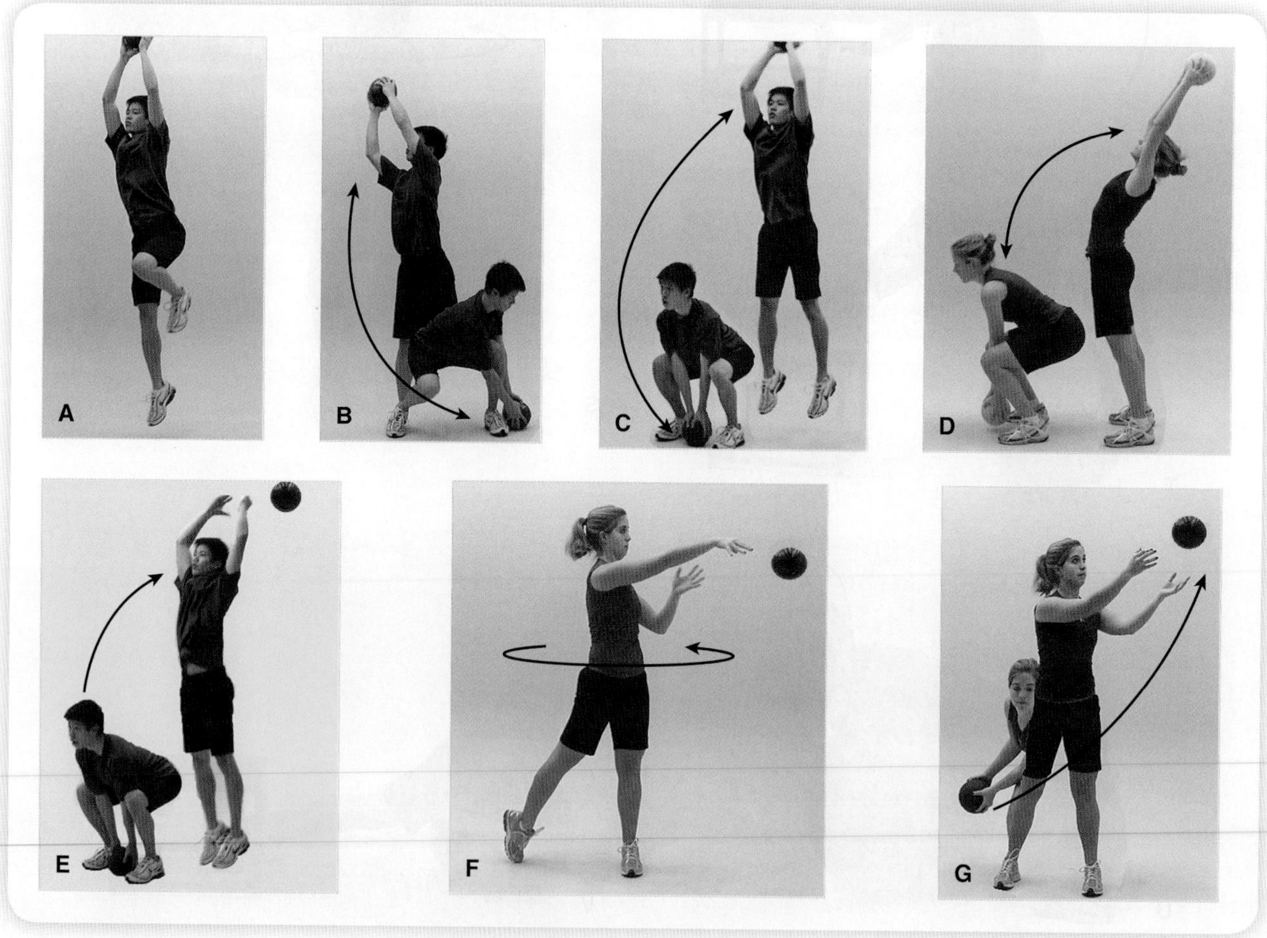

Figure 15-14 **Level 3 (power) core stability exercises**

A. Weighted ball single-leg jump. **B.** Weighted ball Diagonal 2 proprioceptive neuromuscular facilitation pattern. **C.** Weighted ball double-leg jump. **D.** Overhead extension. **E.** Overhead weighted ball throw. **F.** Weighted ball one-arm chest pass with rotation. **G.** Weighted ball double-arm rotation toss from squat.

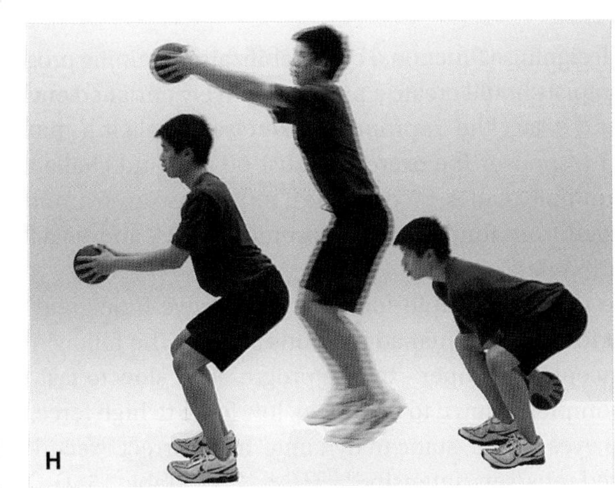

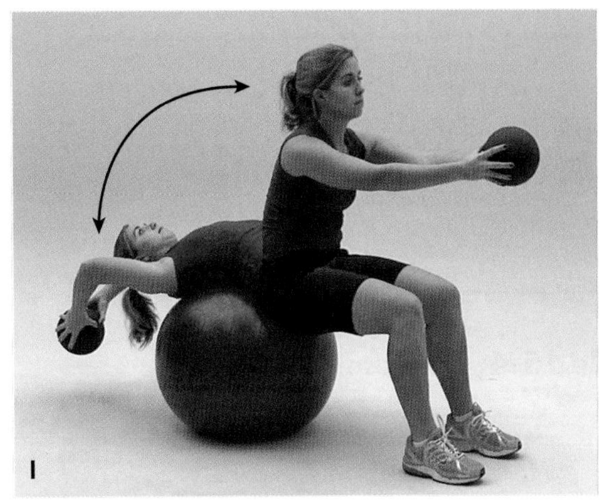

Figure 15-14 ***(Continued)***

H. Weighted ball forward jump from squat. **I.** Stability ball pullover crunch with weighted ball.

Clinical Pearl

The ultimate goal with core strengthening is functional strength and dynamic stability. As the patient progresses, the emphasis should change in these ways: from slow to fast, from simple to complex, from stable to unstable, from low force to high force, from general to specific, and from correct execution to increased intensity. Once the patient has gained awareness of proper muscle firing, encourage the patient to perform exercises in a more functional manner. Because most functional activities require multiplane movement, design the exercises to mimic those requirements.

Guidelines for Core Stabilization Training

A comprehensive core stabilization training program should be systematic, progressive, and functional. The rehabilitation program should emphasize the entire muscle contraction spectrum, focusing on force production (concentric contractions), force reduction (eccentric contractions), and dynamic stabilization (isometric contractions). The core stabilization program should begin in the most challenging environment the individual can control. A progressive continuum of function should be followed to systematically progress the individual. The program should be manipulated regularly by changing any of the following variables: plane of motion, range of motion, loading parameters (Physioball, medicine ball, Bodyblade, power sports trainer, weight vest, dumbbell, tubing), body position, amount of control, speed of execution, amount of feedback, duration (sets, reps, tempo, time under tension), and frequency (Table 15-2).

Table 15-2 Program Variation

1. Plane of motion
2. Range of motion
3. Loading parameter
4. Body position
5. Speed of movement
6. Amount of control
7. Duration
8. Frequency

Table 15-3 Exercise Selection

1. Safe
2. Challenging
3. Stress multiple planes
4. Proprioceptively enriched
5. Activity specific

Table 15-4 Exercise Progression

1. Slow to fast
2. Simple to complex
3. Stable to unstable
4. Low force to high force
5. General to specific
6. Correct execution to increased intensity

Specific Core Stabilization Guidelines

When designing a functional core stabilization training program, the therapist should create a proprioceptively enriched environment and select the appropriate exercises to elicit a maximal training response. The exercises must be safe and challenging, stress multiple planes, incorporate a multisensory environment, be derived from fundamental movement skills, and be activity specific (Table 15-3).

The therapist should follow a progressive functional continuum to allow optimal adaptations.[28,31,36,55] The following are key concepts for proper exercise progression: slow to fast, simple to complex, known to unknown, low force to high force, eyes open to eyes closed, static to dynamic, and correct execution to increased reps/sets/intensity[20,21,22,28,31,32,36,55] (Table 15-4).

The goal of core stabilization should be to develop optimal levels of functional strength and dynamic stabilization.[1,10] Neural adaptations become the focus of the program instead of striving for absolute strength gains.[14,28,52,76] Increasing proprioceptive demand by utilizing a multisensory, multimodal (tubing, Bodyblade, Physioball, medicine ball, power sports trainer, weight vest, cobra belt, dumbbell) environment becomes more important than increasing the external resistance.[20,32] The concept of quality before quantity is stressed. Core stabilization training is specifically designed to improve core stabilization and neuromuscular efficiency. You must be concerned with the sensory information that is stimulating the patient's central nervous system. If the patient trains with poor technique and neuromuscular control, then the patient develops poor motor patterns and stabilization.[28,55] The focus of the program must be on function. To determine if the program is functional, answer the following questions:

- Is it dynamic?
- Is it multiplanar?
- Is it multidimensional?
- Is it proprioceptively challenging?
- Is it systematic?
- Is it progressive?
- Is it based on functional anatomy and science?
- Is it activity specific?[28,31,55]

In summary, the core strengthening program must always start with the drawing-in maneuver that produces neuromuscular control of the TA and multifidus. Abdominal strength is *not* the key; rather, it is abdominal endurance within a stabilized trunk that enhances function and may prevent or minimize injury. The trunk must be dynamic and able to move in multiple directions at various speeds, yet have internal stability that provides a strong base of support so as to support functional mobility and extremity function. The therapist is only limited by the therapist's own imagination in the development of core stabilization exercises. If the power position is maintained throughout the exercise sequence and the exercise is individualized to the needs of a patient, then it is an appropriate exercise! The key is to integrate individual exercises into functional patterns and simulate the demands of simple tasks and progress to the highest level of skill needed by each individual patient.

SUMMARY

1. Functional kinetic chain rehabilitation must address each link in the kinetic chain and strive to develop functional strength and neuromuscular efficiency.
2. A core stabilization program should be an integral component for all individuals participating in a closed kinetic-chain rehabilitation program.
3. A core stabilization training program will allow an individual to gain optimal neuromuscular control of the lumbo-pelvic-hip complex and allow the individual with a kinetic chain dysfunction to return to activity more quickly and safely.
4. The important core muscles do not function as prime movers; rather, they function as stabilizers.
5. There are some clinical methods of measuring the function of the TA and multifidus function.
6. Real-time ultrasound is an effective research tool for assessment of core stabilizers.
7. The Stabilizer is a useful adjunct to examination and training of the core.
8. Many possibilities exist for core training progressions. Progression is achieved by changing position, lever arms, resistance, and stability of surfaces.
9. Trunk flexion activities such as the curl and sit-up are not only unnecessary, but also may cause injury.

REFERENCES

1. Aaron G. *The Use of Stabilization Training in the Rehabilitation of the Athlete.* Sports Physical Therapy Home Study Course. LaCrosse, WI: Sports Physical Therapy Section of the American Physical Therapy Association; 1996.
2. Akuthota V, Ferreiro A, Moore T. Core stability exercise principles. *Curr Sports Med Rep.* 2008;7(1):39.
3. Ashmen KJ, Swanik CB, Lephart MS. Strength and flexibility characteristics of athletes with chronic low back pain. *J Sport Rehabil.* 1996;5:275-286.
4. Aspden RM. Review of the functional anatomy of the spinal ligaments and the erector spinae muscles. *Clin Anat.* 1992;5:372-387.
5. Axler CT, McGill MS. Low back loads over a variety of abdominal exercises: searching for the safest abdominal challenge. *Med Sci Sports Exerc.* 1997;29:804-810.
6. Bartelink DL. The role of intra-abdominal pressure in relieving the pressure on the lumbar vertebral discs. *J Bone Joint Surg Br.* 1957;39:718-725.
7. Basmajian J. *Muscles Alive: Their Functions Revealed by EMG.* 5th ed. Baltimore, MD: Lippincott Williams & Wilkins; 1985.
8. Basmajian J. *Muscles Alive.* Baltimore, MD: Lippincott Williams & Wilkins; 1974.
9. Beckman SM, Buchanan ST. Ankle inversion and hyper-mobility: effect on hip and ankle muscle electromyography onset latency. *Arch Phys Med Rehabil.* 1995;76:1138-1143.
10. Beim G, Giraldo JL, Pincivero MD, et al. Abdominal strengthening exercises: a comparative EMG study. *J Sport Rehabil.* 1997;6:11-20.
11. Biering-Sorenson F. Physical measurements as risk indicators for low-back trouble over a one-year period. *Spine (Phila Pa 1976).* 1984;9:106-119.
12. Blievernicht J. *Balance* [course manual]. San Diego, CA: IDEA Health and Fitness Association; 1996.
13. Bittenham D, Brittenham G. *Stronger Abs and Back.* Champaign, IL: Human Kinetics; 1997.
14. Bullock-Saxton JE, Janda V, Bullock MI. The influence of ankle sprain injury on muscle activation during hip extension. *Int J Sports Med.* 1994;15(6):330-334.
15. Bullock-Saxton JE. Local sensation changes and altered hip muscle function following severe ankle sprain. *Phys Ther.* 1994;74:17-23.
16. Bullock-Saxton JE, Janda V, Bullock M. Reflex activation of gluteal muscles in walking: an approach to restoration of muscle function for patients with low back pain. *Spine (Phila Pa 1976).* 1993;5:704-708.
17. Callaghan JP, Gunning JL, McGill MS. Relationship between lumbar spine load and muscle activity during extensor exercises. *Phys Ther.* 1978;78(1):8-18.

18. Calliet R. *Low Back Pain Syndrome.* Oxford, UK: Blackwell; 1962.
19. Chaitow L. *Muscle Energy Techniques.* New York, NY: Churchill Livingstone; 1997.
20. Chek P. *Dynamic Medicine Ball Training* [correspondence course]. La Jolla, CA: Paul Chek Seminars; 1996.
21. Chek P. *Swiss Ball Training* [correspondence course]. La Jolla, CA: Paul Chek Seminars; 1996.
22. Chek P. *Scientific Back Training* [correspondence course]. La Jolla, CA: Paul Chek Seminars; 1994.
23. Chek P. *Scientific Abdominal Training* [correspondence course]. La Jolla, CA: Paul Chek Seminars; 1992.
24. Creager C. *Therapeutic Exercise Using Foam Rollers.* Berthoud, CO: Executive Physical Therapy; 1996.
25. Cresswell AG, Grundstrom H, Thorstensson A. Observations on intra-abdominal pressure and patterns of abdominal intra-muscular activity in man. *Acta Physiol Scand.* 1992;144:409-445.
26. Cresswell AG, Oddson L, Thorstensson A. The influence of sudden perturbations on trunk muscle activity and intra-abdominal pressure while standing. *Exp Brain Res.* 1994;98:336-341.
27. Crisco J, Panjabi MM. The intersegmental and multisegmental muscles of the lumbar spine. *Spine (Phila Pa 1976).* 1991;16:793-799.
28. Dominguez RH. *Total Body Training.* East Dundee, IL: Moving Force Systems; 1982.
29. Edgerton VR, Wolf S, Roy RR. Theoretical basis for patterning EMG amplitudes to assess muscle dysfunction. *Med Sci Sports Exerc.* 1996;28:744-751.
30. Finkelstein MM. Medical conditions, medications, and urinary incontinence: analysis of a population-based survey. *Can Fam Physician.* 2002;48:96-101.
31. Gambetta V. *Building the Complete Athlete* [course manual]. Sarasota, FL: Gambetta Sports Training Systems; 1996.
32. Gambetta V. *The Complete Guide to Medicine Ball Training.* Sarasota, FL: Optimum Sports Training; 1991.
33. Gracovetsky S, Farfan H. The optimum spine. *Spine (Phila Pa 1976).* 1986;11:543-573.
34. Gracovetsky S, Farfan H, Heuller C. The abdominal mechanism. *Spine (Phila Pa 1976).* 1985;10:317-324.
35. Grillner S, Nilsson J, Thorstensson A. Intra-abdominal pressure changes during natural movements in man. *Acta Physiol Scand.* 1978;103:275-283.
36. Gustavsen R, Streeck R. *Training Therapy: Prophylaxis and Rehabilitation.* New York, NY: Thieme; 1993.
37. Hall T, David A, Geere J, Salvenson K. *Relative Recruitment of the Abdominal Muscles During Three Levels of Exertion During Abdominal Hollowing.* Melbourne, Australia: Australian Physiotherapy Association; 1995.
38. Henry SM, Westervelt CK. The use of realtime ultrasound feedback in teaching abdominal hollowing exercises to healthy subjects. *J Orthop Sports Phys Ther.* 2005;35:338-345.
39. Hides J. Paraspinal mechanism and support of the lumbar spine. In: Richardson C, Hodges P, Hides J, eds. *Therapeutic Exercise for Lumbopelvic Stabilization.* 2nd ed. Philadelphia, PA: Churchill Livingstone; 2004:141-148.
40. Hides J, Richardson C, Hodges P. Local segmental control. In: Richardson C, Hodges P, Hides J, eds. *Therapeutic Exercise for Lumbopelvic Stabilization.* 2nd ed. Philadelphia, PA: Churchill Livingstone; 2004:185-219.
41. Hides JA, Stokes MJ, Saide M, et al. Evidence of lumbar multifidus wasting ipsilateral to symptoms in subjects with acute/subacute low back pain. *Spine (Phila Pa 1976).* 1994;19:165-177.
42. Hodges P, Kaigle-Holm A, Holm S, et al. Inter-vertebral stiffness of the spine is increased by evoked contraction of transversus abdominis and the diaphragm: in vivo porcine studies. *Spine (Phila Pa 1976).* 2003;28:2594-2601.
43. Hodges PW, Richardson AC. Contraction of the abdominal muscles associated with movement of the lower limb. *Phys Ther.* 1997;77:132.
44. Hodges PW, Richardson AC. Delayed postural contraction of transverse abdominis in low back pain associated with movement of the lower limb. *J Spinal Disord.* 1998;1:46-56.
45. Hodges PW, Richardson AC. Feedforward contraction of transverse abdominis is not influenced by the direction of arm movement. *Exp Brain Res.* 1997;114:362-370.
46. Hodges PW, Richardson AC. Inefficient muscular stabilization of the lumbar spine associated with low back pain. *Spine (Phila Pa 1976).* 1996;21:2640-2650.
47. Hodges PW, Richardson AC. Neuromotor dysfunction of the trunk musculature in low back pain patients. In: *Proceedings of the International Congress of the World Confederation of Physical Athletic Trainers.* Washington, DC; 1995.
48. Hodges PW, Richardson CA, Jull G. Evaluation of the relationship between laboratory and clinical tests of transversus abdominis function. *Physiother Res Int.* 1996;1:30-40.
49. Hodges PW, Sapsford RR, Pengel MH. Feedforward activity of the pelvic floor muscles precedes rapid upper limb movements. In *Proceedings of the 7th International Physiotherapy Congress.* Sydney, Australia; 2002.
50. Janda V. Physical therapy of the cervical and thoracic spine. In: Grant R, ed. *Physical Therapy of the Cervical and Thoracic Spine.* New York, NY: Churchill Livingstone; 1988:152-166.
51. Janda V. Muscle weakness and inhibition in back pain syndromes. In: Grieve GP, ed. *Modern Manual Therapy of the Vertebral Column.* New York, NY: Churchill Livingstone; 1986:197-201.
52. Janda V. *Muscle Function Testing.* London, UK: Butterworths; 1983.
53. Janda V. Muscles, central nervous system regulation and back problems. In: Korr IM, ed. *Neurobiologic Mechanisms in Manipulative Therapy.* New York, NY: Plenum; 1978:29.

54. Janda V, Vavrova M. *Sensory Motor Stimulation* (video). Brisbane, Australia: Body Control Systems; 1990.

55. Jesse J. *Hidden Causes of Injury, Prevention, and Correction for Running Athletes.* Pasadena, CA: Athletic Press; 1977.

56. Jorgensson A. The iliopsoas muscle and the lumbar spine. *Australian Physiotherapy.* 1993;39:125-132.

57. Jull G, Richardson CA, Comerford M. Strategies for the initial activation of dynamic lumbar stabilization. In: *Proceedings of Manipulative Physioathletic Trainers Association of Australia.* Australia; 1991.

58. Jull G, Richardson CA, Hamilton C, et al. *Towards the Validation of a Clinical Test for the Deep Abdominal Muscles in Back Pain Patients.* Australia: Manipulative Physioathletic Trainers Association of Australia; 1995.

59. Kendall FP. *Muscles: Testing and Function.* 5th ed. Baltimore, MD: Lippincott Williams & Wilkins; 2005.

60. Kennedy B. An Australian program for management of back problems. *Physiotherapy.* 1980;66:108-111.

61. Lewit K. Muscular and articular factors in movement restriction. *Man Med.* 1988;1:83-85.

62. Lewit K. *Manipulative Therapy in the Rehabilitation of the Locomotor System.* London, UK: Butterworths; 1985.

63. Lewit K. Myofascial pain: relief by post-isometric relaxation. *Arch Phys Med Rehabil.* 1984;65:452.

64. Liebenson CL. *Rehabilitation of the Spine.* Baltimore: MD: Lippincott Williams & Wilkins; 1996.

65. Liebenson CL. Active muscle relaxation techniques. Part I: basic principles and methods. *J Manipulative Physiol Ther.* 1989;12:446-454.

66. Liebenson CL. Active muscle relaxation techniques. Part II: Clinical application. *J Manipulative Physiol Ther.* 1990;13(1):2-6.

67. Mayer TG, Gatchel JR. *Functional Restoration for Spinal Disorders: The Sports Medicine Approach.* Philadelphia, PA: Lea & Febiger; 1988.

68. Mayer-Posner J. *Swiss Ball Applications for Orthopedic and Sports Medicine.* Denver, CO: Ball Dynamics International; 1995.

69. McGill S. *Ultimate Back Fitness and Performance.* Waterloo: Wabuno Publishers; 2004.

70. McGill SM, Childs A, Liebenson C. Endurance times for stabilization exercises: clinical targets for testing and training from a normal database. *Arch Phys Med Rehabil.* 1999;80:941-944.

71. McGill SM, Grenier S, Bluhm M, et al. Previous history of LBP with work loss is related to lingering effects in biomechanical physiological, personal, and psychosocial characteristics. *Ergonomics.* 2003;46(7):731-746.

72. Miller MI, Medeiros MJ. Recruitment of the internal oblique and transversus abdominis muscles on the eccentric phase of the curl-up. *Phys Ther.* 1987;67:1213-1217.

73. Morris JM, Benner F, Lucas BD. An electromyographic study of the intrinsic muscles of the back in man. *J Anat.* 1962;96:509-520.

74. Nachemson A. The load on the lumbar discs in different positions of the body. *Clin Orthop.* 1966;45:107-122.

75. Norris CM. Abdominal muscle training in sports. *Br J Sports Med.* 1993;27:19-27.

76. O'Sullivan PE, Twomey L, Allison G. *Evaluation of Specific Stabilizing Exercises in the Treatment of Chronic Low Back Pain with Radiological Diagnosis of Spondylolisthesis.* Australia: Manipulative Physioathletic Trainers Association of Australia; 1995.

77. O'Sullivan PE, Twomey L, Allison G, et al. Altered patterns of abdominal muscle activation in patients with chronic low back pain. *Aust J Physiother.* 1997;43:91-98.

78. Panjabi MM. The stabilizing system of the spine. Part I: function, dysfunction, adaptation, and enhancement. *J Spinal Disord.* 1992;5:383-389.

79. Panjabi MM, Tech D, White AA. Basic biomechanics of the spine. *Neurosurgery.* 1990;7:76-93.

80. Porterfield JA, DeRosa C. *Mechanical Low Back Pain: Perspectives in Functional Anatomy.* Philadelphia, PA: Saunders; 1991.

81. Richardson C, Hodges P, Hides J. *Therapeutic Exercise for Lumbopelvic Stabilization.* 2nd ed. Philadelphia, PA: Churchill Livingstone; 2004.

82. Richardson CA, Jull G. Muscle control pain control. What exercises would you prescribe? *Man Ther.* 1996;1:2-10.

83. Richardson CA, Jull G, Toppenberg R, Comerford M. Techniques for active lumbar stabilization for spinal protection. *Aust J Physiother.* 1992;38:105-112.

84. Richardson CA, Snijders CJ, Hides JA, Damen L, Pas MS, Storm J. The relation between the transversus abdominis muscles, sacroiliac joint mechanics, and low back pain. *Spine (Phila Pa 1976).* 2002;27:399-405.

85. Robinson R. The new back school prescription: stabilization training. Part I. *Occup Med.* 1992;7: 17-31.

86. Saal JA. The new back school prescription: stabilization training. Part II. *Occup Med.* 1993;7:33-42.

87. Saal JA. Nonoperative treatment of herniated disc: an outcome study. *Spine (Phila Pa 1976).* 1989;14: 431-437.

88. Sahrmann S. *Diagnosis and Treatment of Movement Impairment Syndromes.* Philadelphia, PA: Elsevier; 2001.

89. Sahrmann S. Posture and muscle imbalance: faulty lumbo-pelvic alignment and associated musculoskeletal pain syndromes. *Orthop Div Rev-Can Phys Ther.* 1992; 12:13-20.

90. Sapsford RR, Hodges PW, Richardson CA, Cooper DH, Markwell SJ, Jull AG. Co-activation of the abdominal and pelvic floor muscles during voluntary exercises. *Neurourol Urodyn.* 2001;20:31-42.

91. Snijders CJ, Vleeming A, Stoekart R, Mens JMA, Kleinrensink NG. Biomechanical modeling of sacroiliac joint stability in different postures. *Spine: State Art Rev.* 1995;9:419-432.

92. Stokes M, Young A. The contribution of reflex inhibition to arthrogenous muscle weakness. *Clin Sci.* 1984;67:7-14.

93. Tesh KM, Shaw Dunn J, Evans HJ. The abdominal muscles and vertebral stability. *Spine (Phila Pa 1976).* 1987;12:501-508.

94. Teyhen DS, Miltenberger CE, Deiters MH, et al. The use of ultrasound imaging of the abdominal drawing-in maneuver in subjects with low back pain. *J Orthop Sports Phys Ther.* 2005;35:346-355.

95. Thomson KD. On the bending moment capability of the pressurized abdominal cavity during human lifting activity. *Ergonomics.* 1988;31:817-828.

96. Warmerdam ALA. *Arthrokinetic Therapy: Manual Therapy to Improve Muscle and Joint Functioning.* Continuing education course, Marshfield, WI. Port Moody, British Columbia, Canada: Arthrokinetic Therapy and Publishing; 1996.

97. Wilke HJ, Wolf S, Claes EL. Stability increase of the lumbar spine with different muscle groups: a biomechanical in vitro study. *Spine (Phila Pa 1976).* 1995;20:192-198.

Videos are available at www.accessphysiotherapy.com. Subscription is required.

16

Aquatic Therapy in Rehabilitation

Barbara J. Hoogenboom and Nancy E. Lomax

OBJECTIVES

After completion of this chapter, the physical therapist should be able to do the following:

- Explain the principles of buoyancy and specific gravity and the role they have in the aquatic environment.
- Identify and describe the three major resistive forces at work in the aquatic environment.
- Apply the principles of buoyancy and resistive forces to exercise prescription and progression.
- Contrast the advantages and disadvantages of aquatic therapy in relation to traditional land-based exercise.
- Identify and describe techniques of aquatic therapy for the upper extremity, lower extremity, and trunk.
- Select and utilize various types of equipment for aquatic therapy.
- Incorporate functional, work-, and sport-specific movements and exercises performed in the aquatic environment into rehabilitation.
- Understand and describe the necessity for transition from the aquatic environment to the land environment.

In recent years, there has been widespread interest in aquatic therapy. It has rapidly become a popular rehabilitation technique for treatment of a variety of patient/client populations. This newfound interest has sparked numerous research efforts to evaluate the effectiveness of aquatic therapy as a therapeutic intervention. Current research shows aquatic therapy to be beneficial in the treatment of everything from orthopedic injuries to spinal cord damage, chronic pain, cerebral palsy, multiple sclerosis, and many other conditions, making it useful in a variety of settings.[29,38] It is also gaining acceptance as a preventative maintenance tool to facilitate overall fitness, cross-training, and sport-specific skills for healthy athletes.[23,33,34] General conditioning, strength, and a wide variety of movement skills can all be enhanced by aquatic therapy.[19,43,48,54]

The use of water as a part of healing techniques has been traced back through history to as early as 2400 BC, but it was not until the late 19th century that more traditional types of aquatic therapy came into existence.[4,24] The development of the Hubbard style whirlpool tank in 1820 sparked the initiation of present-day therapeutic use of water by allowing aquatic therapy to be conducted in a highly controlled clinical setting.[8] Loeman and Roen took this a step farther in 1824 and stimulated interest in use of an actual pool or what we now call aquatic therapy. Only recently, however, has water come into its own as a therapeutic exercise medium used for a wide variety of diagnoses and dysfunctions.[41]

Aquatic therapy is believed to be beneficial primarily because it decreases joint compression forces. The perception of weightlessness experienced in the water assists in decreasing joint pain and eliminating or drastically reducing the body's protective muscular spasm and pain that can carry over into the patient's daily functional activities.[54,56] Although many patients perceive greater ease of movement in the aquatic environment as compared to movement on land, the research shows that aquatic therapy does not actually decrease pain more effectively than activities on land.[25] The primary goal of aquatic therapy is to teach the patient/client how to use water as a modality for improving movement, strength, and fitness.[2,54] Thus, along with other therapeutic modalities and interventions, aquatic therapy can become one link in the patient/client's recovery chain.[1]

Physical Properties and Resistive Forces

The therapist must understand several physical properties of the water before designing an aquatic therapy program. Land exercise cannot always be converted to aquatic exercise, because buoyancy rather than gravity is the major force governing movement. A thorough understanding of buoyancy, specific gravity, the resistive forces of the water, and their relationships must be the groundwork of any therapeutic aquatic program. The program must be individualized to the patient/client's particular injury/condition and activity level if it is to be successful.

Buoyancy

Buoyancy is one of the primary forces involved in aquatic therapy. All objects, on land or in the water, are subjected to the downward pull of the earth's gravity. In the water, however, this force is counteracted to some degree by the upward buoyant force. According to Archimedes' Principle, any object submerged or floating in water is buoyed upward by a counterforce that helps support the submerged object against the downward pull of gravity. In other words, the buoyant force assists motion toward the water's surface and resists motions away from the surface.[26,54] Because of this buoyant force, a person entering the water experiences an apparent loss of weight.[15] The weight loss experienced is nearly equal to the weight of the liquid that is displaced when the object enters the water (Figure 16-1).

For example, a 100-lb individual, when almost completely submerged, displaces a volume of water that weighs nearly 95 lb; therefore, that person feels as though she/he weighs less than 5 lb. This sensation occurs because, when partially submerged, the individual only bears the weight of the part of the body that is above the water. With immersion to the level of the seventh cervical vertebra, both males and females only bear approximately 6% to 10 % of their total body weight (TBW). The percentages increase to 25 to 31 TBW for females and 30 to 37 TBW for males at the xiphisternal level, and to 40 to 51 TBW for females and 50 to 56 TBW for males at the anterosuperior iliac spine level (Table 16-1).[27] The percentages differ slightly for males and females because of the differences in their centers of gravity. Males carry a higher percentage of their weight in the upper body, whereas females carry a higher percentage of their weight in the lower body. The center of gravity on land corresponds with a center of buoyancy in the water.[41] Variations of build and body type only minimally effect weightbearing values. As a result of the decreased percentage of weight bearing offered by the buoyant force, each joint that is below the water is decompressed or unweighted. This allows ambulation and vigorous exercise to be performed with little impact and drastically reduced friction between joint articular surfaces.

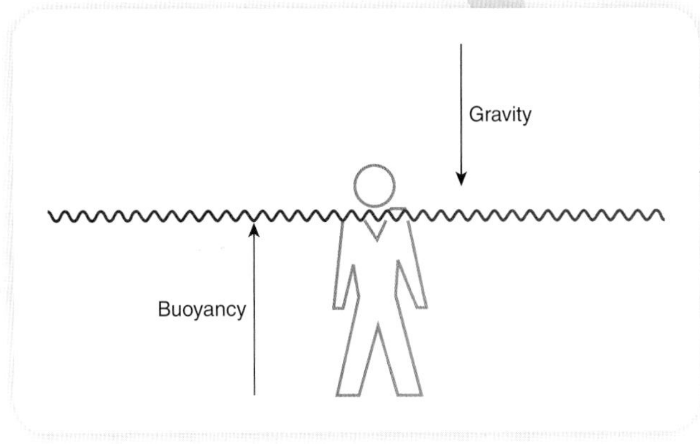

Figure 16-1 The buoyant force

Progressing the activity from walking to running in the aquatic environment does not change the forces on the joints; however, minimal changes in the joint forces occur as the speed of running is increased. Fontana et al[20] report a 34% to 38% decrease in force while running at hip level of water and a 44% to 47% decrease force with running at chest level, as compared to running on land. The relative decrease in weightbearing forces during aquatic activities need to be considered when dealing with athletes with injuries and restrictions of weight bearing, and may allow early running for those with such conditions and limitations.

Through careful use of Archimedes' Principle, a gradual increase in the percentage of weight bearing can be undertaken. Initially, the patient/client would begin non-weightbearing exercises in the deep end of the pool. A wet vest or similar buoyancy device might be used to help the patient/client remain afloat for the desired exercises. This and other commercial equipment available for the use in the aquatic environment will be discussed in the upcoming section "Facilities and Equipment."

Specific Gravity

Buoyancy is partially dependent on body weight. However, the weight of different parts of the body is not constant. Therefore, the buoyant values of different body parts will vary. Buoyant values can be determined by several factors. The ratio of bone weight to muscle weight, the amount and distribution of fat, and the depth and expansion of the chest all play a role. Together, these factors determine the specific gravity of the individual body part. On average, humans have a specific gravity slightly less than that of water. Any object with a specific gravity less than that of water will float. An object with a specific

Table 16-1 Weightbearing Percentages

	Percentage of Weight Bearing	
Body Level	Male	Female
C7	8	8
Xiphisternal	28	35
ASIS (anterior superior iliac spine)	47	54

gravity greater than that of water will sink. However, as with buoyant values, the specific gravity of all body parts is not uniform. Therefore, even with a total-body specific gravity of less than the specific gravity of water, the individual might not float horizontally in the water. Additionally, the lungs, when filled with air, can further decrease the specific gravity of the chest area. This allows the head and chest to float higher in the water than the heavier, denser extremities. Many athletes tend to have a low percentage of body fat (specific gravity greater than water) and therefore can be thought of as "sinkers." Consequently, compensation with flotation devices at the extremities and trunk might be necessary for some athletes.[5,54]

Resistive Forces

Water has 12 times the resistance of air.[50] Therefore, when an object moves in the water; the several resistive forces that are at work must be considered. Forces must be considered for both their potential benefits and their precautions. These forces include the cohesive force, the bow force, and the drag force.

Cohesive Force

There is a slight but easily overcome cohesive force that runs in a parallel direction to the water surface. This resistance is formed by the water molecules loosely binding together, creating a surface tension. Surface tension can be seen in still water, because the water remains motionless with the cohesive force intact unless disturbed.

Bow Force

A second force is the bow force, or the force that is generated at the front of the object during movement. When the object moves, the bow force causes an increase in the water pressure at the front of the object and a decrease in the water pressure at the rear of the object. This pressure change causes a movement of water from the high-pressure area at the front to the low-pressure area behind the object. As the water enters the low-pressure area, it swirls in to the low-pressure zone and forms eddies, or small whirlpool turbulences.[14] These eddies impede flow by creating a backward force, or drag force (Figure 16-2).

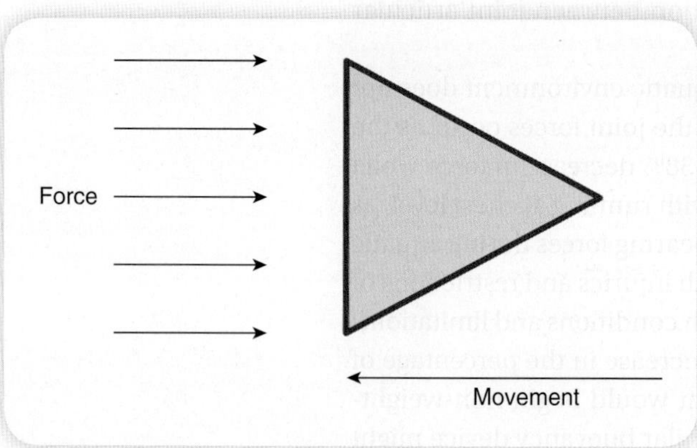

Figure 16-2 The bow force

Drag Force

This third force, the fluid drag force, is very important in aquatic therapy. The bow force on an object (and therefore also the drag force) can be controlled by changing the shape of the object or the speed of its movement (Figure 16-3).

Frictional resistance can be decreased by making the object more streamlined. This change minimizes the surface area at the front of the object. Less surface area causes less bow force and less of a change in pressure between the front and rear of the object, resulting in less drag force. In a streamlined flow, the resistance is proportional to the velocity of the object. When working with a patient/client with generalized weakness, consideration of the aquatic environment is necessary. Increased activity occurring around the patient/client and turbulence of the water can make walking a challenging activity (Figure 16-4).

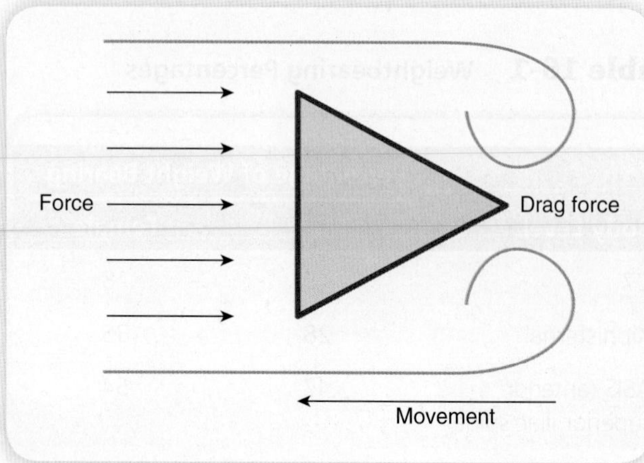

Figure 16-3 Drag force

On the other hand, if the object is not streamlined, a turbulent situation (also referred to as pressure or form drag) exists. In a turbulent situation, drag is a function of the velocity squared. Thus, by increasing the speed of movement 2 times, the resistance the object must overcome is increased 4 times.[15] This provides a method to increase resistance progressively during aquatic rehabilitation. Considerable turbulence can be generated when the speed of movement is increased, causing muscles to work harder to keep the movement going. Another method to increase resistance is to change directions of movement, creating increased drag. Finally, by simply changing the shape of a limb through the addition of rehabilitation equipment that increases surface area, the therapist can modify the patient/client's workout intensity to match strength increases (Figure 16-5).

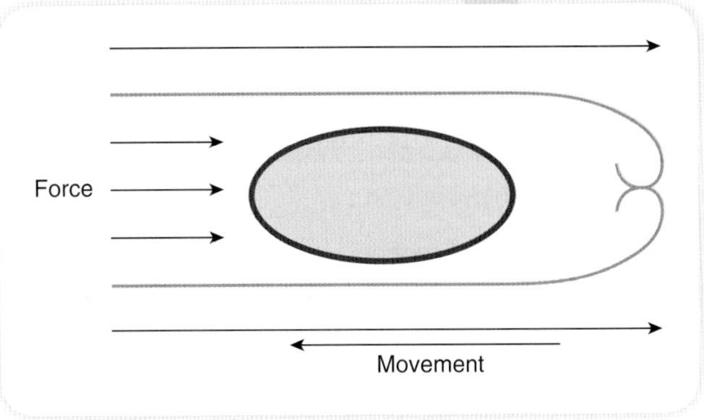

Figure 16-4 Streamlined movement

This creates less drag force and less turbulence.

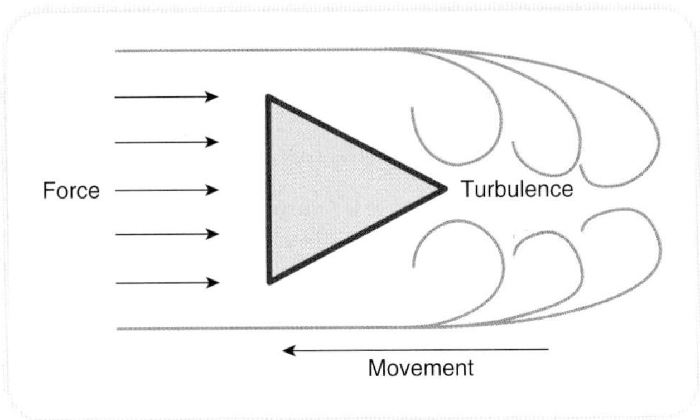

Figure 16-5 Turbulent flow

Drag force must also be considered when portions of a limb or joint must be protected after injury or surgery. For example, when working with a patient/client with an acutely injured medial collateral or anterior cruciate ligament of the knee, resistance must not be placed distal to the knee because of the increased torque that occurs caused by drag forces.

Quantification of resistive forces that occur during aquatic exercise is a challenge. Pöyhönen et al examined knee flexion and extension in the aquatic environment using an anatomic model in barefoot and hydroboot-wearing conditions. They found that the highest drag forces and drag coefficients occurred during early extension from a flexed position (150 to 140 degrees of flexion) while wearing the hydroboot (making the foot less streamlined), and that faster velocity was associated with higher drag forces.[47]

Once therapy has progressed, the patient/client could be moved to neck-deep water to begin light weightbearing exercises. Gradual increases in the percentage of weight bearing are accomplished by systematically moving the patient/client to shallower water. Even when in waist-deep water, both male and female patients/clients are only bearing approximately 50% of their TBW. By placing a sinkable bench or chair in the shallow water, step-ups can be initiated under partial weightbearing conditions long before the patient/client is capable of performing the same exercise full weight bearing on land. Thus, the advantages of diminished weightbearing exercises are coupled with the proprioceptive benefits of closed-kinetic-chain exercise, making aquatic therapy an excellent functional rehabilitation activity.

Advantages and Benefits of Aquatic Rehabilitation

The addition of an aquatic therapy program can offer many advantages to a patient or patient/client's therapy (Table 16-2).[22,54] The buoyancy of the water allows active exercise while providing a sense of security and causing little discomfort.[51] Utilizing a combination of the water's buoyancy, resistance, and warmth, the patient/client can typically achieve more in the aquatic environment than is possible on land.[34] Early in the rehabilitation

Table 16-2 Indications and Benefits of Aquatic Therapy

Indications for Use of Aquatic Therapy	Illustration of Benefits
Swelling/peripheral edema	Assist in edema control, decrease pain, increase mobility as edema decreases
Decreased range of motion	Earlier initiation of rehabilitation, controlled active movements
Decreased strength	Strength progression from assisted to resisted to functional; gradual increase in exercise intensity
Decreased balance, proprioception, coordination	Earlier return to function in supported, forgiving environment, slower movements
Weightbearing restrictions	Can partially or completely unweight the lower extremities; regulate weightbearing progressions
Cardiovascular deconditioning or potential deconditioning because of inability to train	Gradual increase of exercise intensity, alternative training environment for lower weight bearing
Gait deviations	Slower movements, easier assessment, and modification of gait
Difficulty or pain with land interventions	Increased support, decreased weight bearing, assistance as a result of buoyancy, more relaxed environment

Source: Reproduced from Irion JM. Aquatic therapy. In: Bandy WD, Sanders B, eds. *Therapeutic Exercise: Techniques for Intervention*. Baltimore, MD: Lippincott, Williams & Wilkins; 2001:295-332; Sova R. *Aquatic Activities Handbook*. Boston, MA: Jones & Bartlett; 1993; and Thein JM, Thein Brody L. Aquatic-based rehabilitation and training for the elite athlete. *Orthop Sports Phys Ther*. 1998;27(1):32-41.

process, aquatic therapy is useful in restoring range of motion and flexibility. As normal function is restored, resistance training and sport-specific activities can be added.

Following an injury, the aquatic experience provides a medium where early motions can be performed in a supportive environment. The slow motion effect of moving through water provides extra time to control movement, which allows the patient/client to experience multiple movement errors without severe consequences.[43,49] This is especially helpful in lower-extremity injuries where balance and proprioception are impaired. Geigle et al demonstrated a positive relationship between use of a supplemental aquatic therapy program and unilateral tests of balance when treating athletes with inversion ankle sprains.[22] The increased amount of time to react and correct movement errors, combined with a medium in which the fear of falling is removed, assists the patient's ability to regain proprioception and neuromuscular control. For the client population that has diagnosis of rheumatoid and/or osteoarthritis with lower-extremity involvement, approximately 80% demonstrate balance difficulties and higher risk for falls.[16,17] A study performed by Suomi and Koceja[52] demonstrated that aquatic exercise helped decrease total sway area and medial/lateral sway in both full vision and no vision conditions, which placed them in lower risk for falls. In all ages, the fear of falling can limit people from progressing to their highest level of function.

Turbulence functions as a destabilizer and as a tactile sensory stimulus. The stimulation from the turbulence generated during movement provides feedback and perturbation challenge that aids in the return of proprioception and balance.

Clinical Pearl

Turbulence created by other individuals moving or exercising in the pool can provide patients/clients with unexpected perturbations to which they must respond dynamically during exercise activities.

There is also an often overlooked benefit of edema reduction that occurs as a consequence of hydrostatic pressure. Edema reduction could benefit the patient by assisting in pain reduction and allowing for an increase in range of motion.

By understanding buoyancy and utilizing its principles, the aquatic environment can provide a gradual transition from non-weightbearing to full-weightbearing land exercises. This gradual increase in percentage of weight bearing helps provide a gradual return to smooth, coordinated, and low pain or pain-free movements. By utilizing the buoyancy force to decrease the forces of body weight and joint compressive forces, locomotor activities can begin much earlier following an injury to the lower extremity than on land. This provides an enormous advantage to the athletic population. The ability to work out hard without fear of reinjury provides a psychological boost to the athlete. This helps keep motivation high and can help speed the athlete's return to normal function.[34] Psychologically, aquatic therapy increases confidence, because the patient or patient/client experiences increased success at locomotor, stretching, or strengthening activities while in the water. Tension and anxiety are decreased, and the patient/client's morale increases, as does postexercise vigor.[14,15,41]

Muscular strengthening and reeducation can also be accomplished through aquatic therapy.[44,54] Progressive resistance exercises can be increased in extremely small increments by using combinations of different resistive forces. The intensity of exercise can be controlled by manipulating the flow of the water (turbulence), the body's position, or through the addition of exercise equipment. This allows individuals with minimal muscle contraction capabilities to do work and see improvement. The aquatic environment can also provide a challenging resistive workout to an athlete nearing full recovery.[54] Additionally, water serves as an accommodating resistance medium. This allows the muscles to be maximally stressed through the full range of motion available. One drawback to this, however, is that strength gains depend largely on the effort exerted by the patient/client, which is not easily quantified.

In another study, Pöyhönen et al[46] studied the biomechanical and hydrodynamic characteristics of the therapeutic exercise of knee flexion and extension using kinematic and electromyographic analyses in flowing and still water. They found that the flowing properties of water modified the agonist/antagonist neuromuscular function of the quadriceps and hamstrings in terms of early reduction of quadriceps activity and concurrent increased activation of the hamstrings. They also found that flowing water (turbulence) causes additional resistance when moving the limb opposite the flow. They concluded that when prescribing aquatic exercise, the turbulence of the water must be considered in terms of both resistance and alterations of neuromuscular recruitment of muscles.

Strength gains through aquatic exercise are facilitated by the increased energy needs of the body when working in an aquatic environment. Studies show that aquatic exercise requires higher energy expenditure than the same exercise performed on land.[10,14,15,54] The patient/client has to perform the activity as well as maintain a level of buoyancy while overcoming the resistive forces of the water. For example, the energy cost for water running is 4 times greater than the energy cost for running the same distance on land.[14,15,18,32]

A simulated run in either shallow or deep water assisted by a tether or flotation devices can be an effective means of alternate fitness training (cross-training) for the injured athlete. The purpose of aquatic running is to reproduce the posture of running and utilize the same muscle groups in the aquatic environment as would be utilized on land. However, it should be noted that there are differences while being in the unloaded environment and resistance of the water with aqua running changes the relative contributions of the involved muscle groups.[58] It should be noted that a study of shallow-water running (xiphoid level) and deep-water running (using an aqua jogger), at the same rate of perceived exertion, found a significant difference of 10 beats per minute in heart rate, with shallow-water running demonstrating a greater heart rate. The authors of that study point out that aquatic rehabilitation professionals should not prescribe shallow-water working heart rates from heart rates values obtained during deep-water exercise.[48]

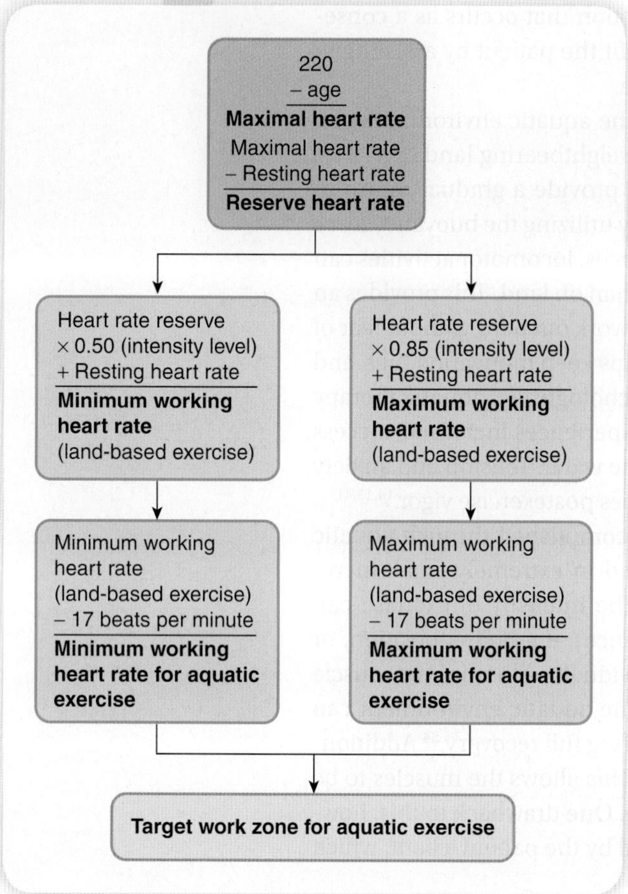

Figure 16-6 **Karvonen formula for water exercise**

(Adapted from Sova R. *Aquatic Activities Handbook*. Boston, MA: Jones & Bartlett; 1993:55.)

Hydrostatic pressure assists in cardiac performance by promoting venous return, thus the heart does not have to beat as fast to maintain cardiac output. Deep-water running at submaximal and maximal speeds demonstrates lower heart rates than shallow-water running. The greater the temperature of the water, the higher the heart rate in response.[58] All patients/clients should be instructed in how to accurately monitor their heart rate while exercising in water, whether deep or shallow.[10]

Not only does the patient or patient/client benefit from early intervention, but aquatic exercise also helps prevent cardiorespiratory deconditioning through alterations in cardiovascular dynamics as a result of hydrostatic forces.[7,28,53] The heart actually functions more efficiently in the water than on land. Hydrostatic pressure enhances venous return, leading to a greater stroke volume and a reduction in the heart rate needed to maintain cardiac output.[55] The corresponding decrease in ventilatory rate and increase in central blood volume can allow the injured athlete to maintain a near-normal maximal aerobic capacity with aquatic exercise.[22,56] For the client/patient who has comorbidities, there is a study that examined the cardiovascular response during aquatic interventions in patients with osteoarthritis. The authors found that the systolic and diastolic blood pressure increased with entering and exiting the aquatic environment secondary to the rapid changes in hydrostatic pressure.[3] For the athlete or the geriatric client with compensations, consideration must be paid to monitoring responses. Because of the hydrostatic effects on heart efficiency, it has been suggested that an environment-specific exercise prescription is necessary.[33,39,53,57] Some research suggests the use of perceived exertion as an acceptable method for controlling exercise intensity. Other research suggests the use of target heart rate values as with land exercise, but compensates for the hydrostatic changes by setting the target range 10% lower than what would be expected for land exercise (Figure 16-6).[50,54] Regardless of the method used, the keys to successful use of aquatic therapy are supervision and monitoring of the patient or patient/client during activity and good communication between patient/client and therapist.

Disadvantages of Aquatic Rehabilitation

Disadvantages

As with any therapeutic intervention, aquatic therapy has its disadvantages. The cost of building and maintaining a rehabilitation pool, if there is no access to an existing facility, can be very high. Also, qualified pool attendants must be present, and the therapist involved in the treatment must be trained in aquatic safety and therapy procedures.[12,32]

An athlete who requires high levels of stabilization will be more challenging to work with, because stabilization in water is considerably more difficult than on land. Thermoregulation issues exist for the patient who exercises in an aquatic environment. Because the patient cannot always choose the temperature of the pool, the effects of water temperature must be noted for cool, warm, or hot pool temperatures. Water temperatures that are higher than body temperature cause an increase in core body temperature greater than that in a land environment as a result of differences in thermoregulation. Water temperatures that are lower than body temperature decrease core body temperature and cause shivering in athletes faster and to a greater degree than in the general population because of their low body fat.[10] Another disadvantage of aquatic exercise used for cross-training is that training in water does not allow athletes to improve or maintain their tolerance to heat while on land.

Contraindications and Precautions

The presence of any open wounds or sores on the patient or patient/client is a contraindication to aquatic therapy, as are contagious skin diseases. This restriction is obvious for health reasons to reduce the chance of infection of the patient/client or others who use the pool.[13,29,30,38,50] Because of this risk, all surgical wounds must be completely healed or adequately protected using a waterproof barrier before the patient/client enters the pool. An excessive fear of the water is also a reason to keep a patient/client out of an aquatic exercise program. Fever, urinary tract infections, allergies to the pool chemicals, cardiac problems, and uncontrolled seizures are also contraindications (Tables 16-3 and 16-4). Use caution (or waterproof barrier) with medical equipment access sites such as an insulin pump, osteomies, suprapubic appliances, and G tubes. Patients/clients with a tracheotomy need special consideration; they need to remain in waist to chest depth of water to exercise safely in an aquatic environment.

Table 16-3 Contraindications for Aquatic Therapy

Untreated infectious disease (patient has a fever/temperature)
Open wounds or unhealed surgical incisions
Contagious skin diseases
Serious cardiac conditions
Seizure disorders (uncontrolled)
Excessive fear of water
Allergy to pool chemicals
Vital capacity of 1 L
Uncontrolled high or low blood pressure
Uncontrolled bowel or bladder incontinence
Menstruation without internal protection

Source: Data from Irion JM. Aquatic therapy. In: Bandy WD, Sanders B, eds. *Therapeutic Exercise Techniques for Intervention*. Baltimore, MD: Lippincott, Williams & Wilkins; 2001:295-332; Sova R. *Aquatic Activities Handbook*. Boston, MA: Jones & Bartlett; 1993; Giesecke C. In: Ruoti RG, Morris DM, Cole AJ, eds. *Aquatic Rehabilitation*. Philadelphia, PA: Lippincott-Raven; 1997; and Thein JM, Thein Brody L. Aquatic-based rehabilitation and training for the elite athlete. *J Orthop Sports Phys Ther.* 1998;27(1):32-41.

Clinical Pearl

It may be helpful for patients/clients who participate in aquatic therapy or aquatic exercise to invest in specialized water exercise shoes to protect the plantar surfaces of their feet (in tiled pools) and to provide adequate foot support during weightbearing exercise, even in the gravity-diminished environment.

Facilities and Equipment

When considering an existing facility or when planning to build one, certain characteristics of the pool should be taken into consideration. The pool should not be smaller than 10 × 12 ft. It can be inground or aboveground as long as access for the patient/client is well planned. Both a shallow area (2.5 ft) and a deep area (5+ ft) should be present to allow standing exercise and swimming or nonstanding exercise.[7] The pool bottom should be flat and the depth gradations clearly marked. Water temperature will vary depending on the patient/clientele that is served. For the athlete, recommended pool temperature should be 26°C to 28°C (79°F to 82°F) but may depend on the available facility.[45] The water temperature suggested by the Arthritis

Table 16-4 Precautions for the Use of Aquatic Therapy

Recently healed wound or incision, incisions covered by moisture-proof barrier
Altered peripheral sensation
Respiratory dysfunction (asthma)
Seizure disorders controlled with medications
Fear of water

Source: Data from Irion JM. Aquatic therapy. In: Bandy WD, Sanders B, eds. *Therapeutic Exercise: Techniques for Intervention*. Baltimore, MD: Lippincott, Williams & Wilkins; 2001:295-332; Sova R. *Aquatic Activities Handbook*. Boston, MA: Jones & Bartlett; 1993; and Thein JM, Thein Brody L. Aquatic-based rehabilitation and training for the elite athlete. *Orthop Sports Phys Ther.* 1998;27(1):32-41.

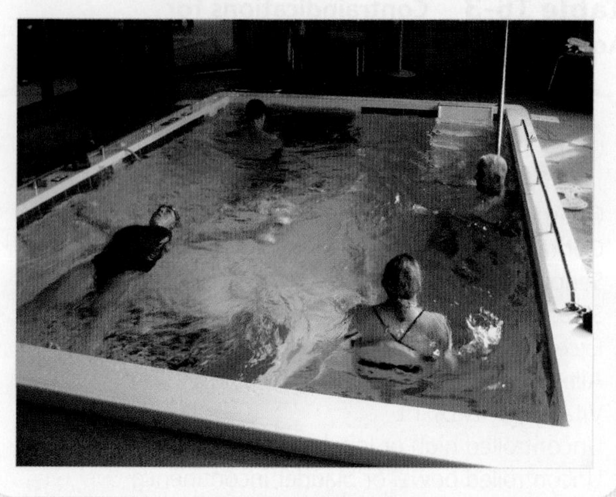

Figure 16-7 The SwimEx pool

This pool's even, controllable water flow allows for the application of individualized prescriptive exercise and therapeutic programs. As many as 3 patients can be treated simultaneously.

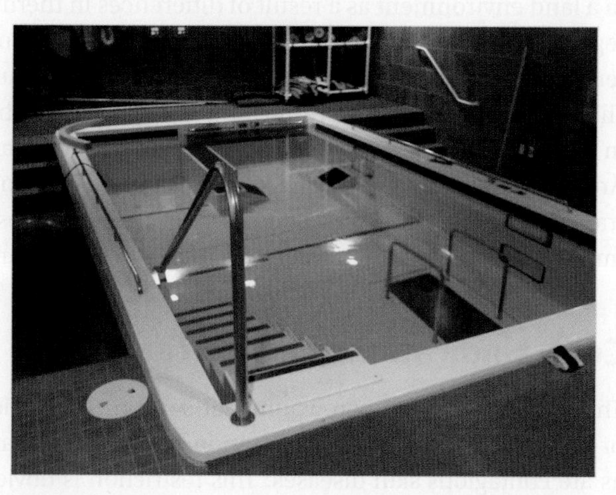

Figure 16-8 SwimEx custom pool with treadmill

Foundation for their programs is 29°C to 31°C (85°F to 89°F). Traditional chemicals that have been used for pool treatment are chlorine and bromine, but additional options exist, including saltwater system pools.

Depending on the type of the patient's condition, the patient/client's perception of the water temperature may differ.

Some prefabricated pools come with an in-water treadmill or current-producing device (Figures 16-7 and 16-8). These devices can be beneficial but are not essential to treatment. An aquatic program will benefit from a variety of equipment that allows increasing levels of resistance and assistance, and also motivates the patient/client. Catalog companies and sporting goods stores are good resources for obtaining equipment. There are many styles and variations of equipment available: the therapist needs to select equipment depending on the needs of the program. Creative use of actual sport equipment (baseball bats, tennis racquets, golf clubs, etc; Figures 16-9 to 16-12) is helpful to incorporate sport-specific activities that challenge the athlete. Use of mask and snorkel will allow options for prone activities/swimming (Figures 16-13 and 16-14). Instruction in the proper use of the mask and snorkel is essential for the patient/client's comfort and safety. Equipment aids for aquatic therapy or so-called pool toys are limited in their utilization only by the imagination of the therapist. What is important is to stimulate the patient/client's interest in therapy and to keep in mind what goals are to be accomplished.

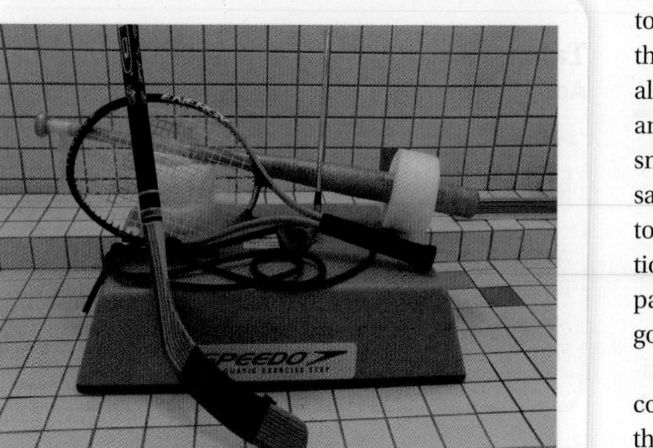

Figure 16-9 Custom pool environment

The clothing of the therapist is an important consideration. Secondary to the close proximity of the therapist to the patient/client with some treatments, wearing swimwear that covers portions of the lower extremities and upper trunk/upper extremities is an important aspect of professionalism in the aquatic environment. Footwear is

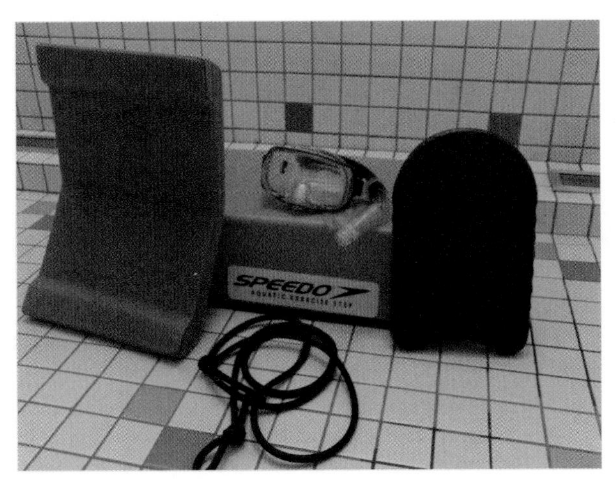

Figure 16-10 **Other pool equipment**

Underwater step, mask and snorkel, kickboard, tubing, and various sports equipment.

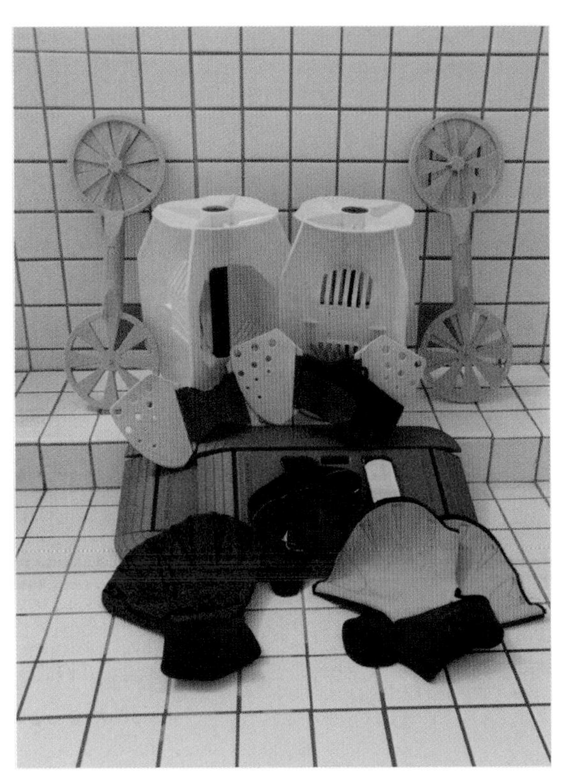

Figure 16-11 **Equipment used for resistance or floatation**

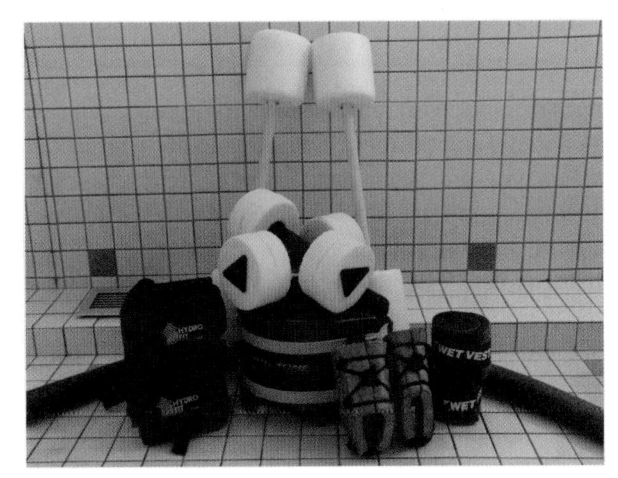

Figure 16-12 **Flotation equipment**

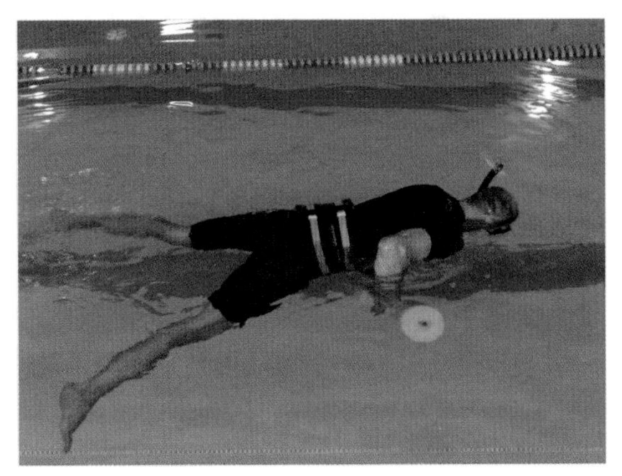

Figure 16-13 **Prone kayak movement using mask and snorkel**

Challenges the upper extremities and promotes stabilization of the trunk.

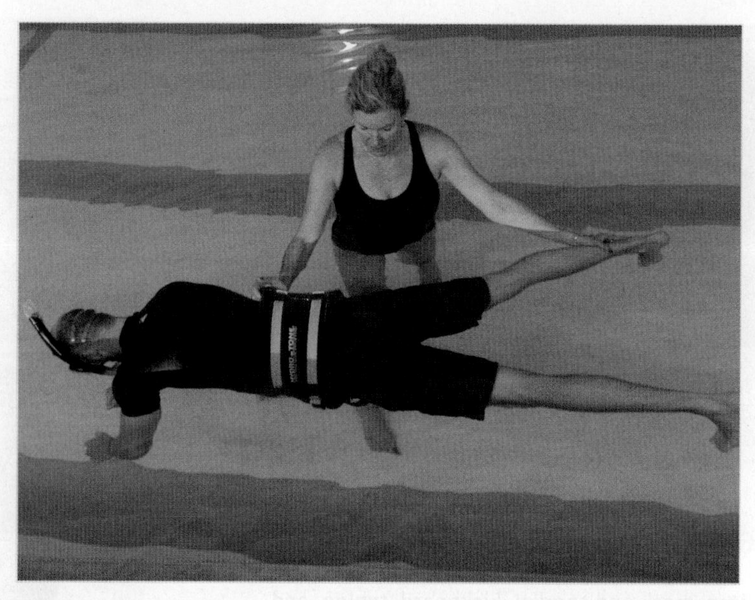

Figure 16-14 **Prone hip abduction/adduction with manual resistance by therapist**

Note use of mask and snorkel, allowing athlete to maintain proper trunk and head/neck position.

another important consideration for the therapist as well as the patient/client. Proper aquatic footwear provides stability, traction, prevents injuries, and maintains good foot position.

Water Safety

A number of patients/clients referred for aquatic therapy are uncomfortable in the water because of minimal experience in an aquatic environment. Swimming ability is not necessary to participate in an aquatic exercise program, but instruction of water safety skills will allow for a satisfying experience for the patient/client. Patients/clients may need an exercise bar or floatation noodle to assist with balance during ambulation in water, initially. When adding supine or prone activities into the patient/client's program, it is important to instruct the individual how to assume that position and return to upright position. This initial act will decrease fear and stress for the patient/client and also decrease stress to injured area.

Aquatic Techniques

Aquatic techniques and activities can be designed to begin as active assisted movements and progress to strengthening, eccentric control, and functionally specific activities. Activities are selected based on several factors:

Type of injury/surgery/condition

Treatment protocols, if appropriate

Results/muscle imbalances found in evaluation

Goals/expected return to activities as stated by the patient/client

Aquatic programs are designed similarly to land-based programs, with the following components:

Warm-up

Mobility activities

Strengthening activities

Balance or neuromuscular response activities

Endurance/cardiovascular activities, including possibilities for cross-training

Sport or functionally specific activities

Cool down/stretching

With these general considerations in mind, the following sections provide examples of aquatic exercises for the upper extremity, trunk, and lower extremity in a 3-phase rehabilitation progression. What has been omitted from the 4-phase rehabilitation scheme used throughout this textbook, in the current discussion, is the initial pain control phase. It is assumed that by the time the patient arrives for aquatic therapy, the patient has undergone previous treatment to manage acute injuries and painful conditions. Subsequently, the patient is ready to begin phases 2 through 4 of the 4-phase approach.

Upper Extremity

The goal of rehabilitation is to restore function by restoring motion and synchrony of movement of all joints of the upper extremity. As listed above, the evaluation of upper extremity is important and identification of dysfunctional movements will assist in designing an effective program. Aquatic therapy may be used for treatment of the shoulder complex, elbow, wrist, and hand as one of the interventions to accomplish goals along with a land-based program. The following sections describe a rehabilitation progression for shoulder complex dysfunction.

Initial Level

The client can be started at chest-deep water in order to allow for support of the scapulothoracic area. Walking forward, backward, and sideways will allow for warm-up, working on natural arm swing, and restoration of normal scapulothoracic motions, rotation, and rhythm. Initiation of activities to work on glenohumeral motions begins at the wall (patient/client with back against the wall); having the patient/client in neck- or shoulder-deep water gives the client physical cues as to posture and quality of movement. The primary goal during the early phase is for the therapist and patient/client to be aware of the amount of movement available without compensatory shoulder elevation (for example in the presence of an injury to the rotator cuff). The other options for positions during early treatment are supine and prone. The client will need flotation equipment for cervical, lumbar, and lower-extremity support in order to have good positioning when in supine.

Supine activities include stretching, mobilization, and range of motion. Stabilizing the scapula with one hand, the therapist can work on glenohumeral motion with the client (Figures 16-15 and 16-16). The client can initiate gentle active movement in shoulder abduction and extension.

Clinical Pearl

The aquatic environment is ideal for rehabilitation after rotator cuff repair because of the assistive property of buoyancy, and the ability to avoid improper elevation where the deltoid overpowers the weaker rotator cuff, also known as the "shrug sign."

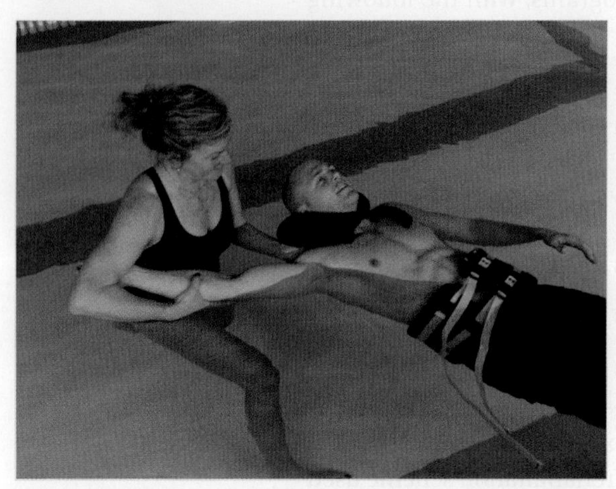

Figure 16-15 **Range of motion with scapular stabilization**

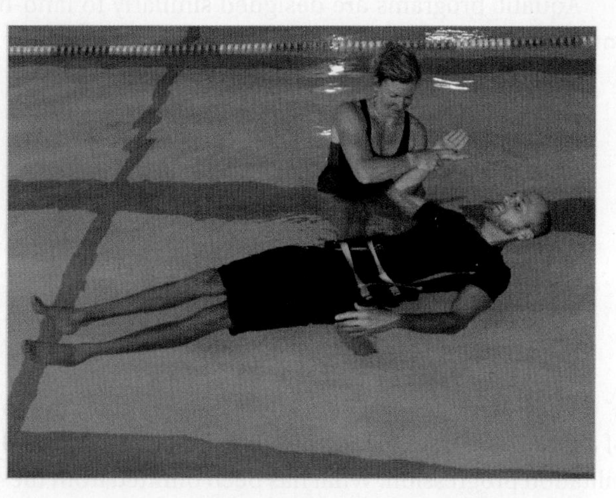

Figure 16-16 **Internal and external rotation in supine**

Note appropriate floatation support for the athlete.

Prone activity can be performed depending on the client's comfort in water and willingness to use a mask and snorkel. Flotation support around the pelvis allows the client to concentrate on movement of the upper extremities without worrying about flotation of the trunk and legs. The client is able to perform pendulum-type movements, proprioceptive neuromuscular facilitation diagonals, and straight-plane movement patterns (flexion/extension and horizontal abduction/adduction) in their pain-free range. For the client not comfortable with the prone position, an alternative position is the pendulum position in the standing position with the trunk flexed.

Deep-water activity can be integrated for conditioning/endurance building in early stages of upper-extremity rehabilitation. It is important for the client to perform pain-free range when performing endurance-type activities.

Intermediate Level

The program can be progressed to challenge strength by using equipment to resist motion through pain-free range. Increasing the surface area of the extremity or increasing the length of the lever arm will increase the difficulty of the activity. As the client progresses into this phase, the limitations of the standing position become apparent. The athlete can work to the 90-degree angle but not overhead without exiting the water. It is important for the client to maintain a neutral position of the spine and pelvic area in order to avoid injury and substitution patterns when performing strengthening activities while standing.

The client will be able to progress with scapular stabilization from standing to supine and prone positions. Supine and prone positioning can allow for more functional movement patterns and core stabilization by the scapular muscles. Recall that prone activities such as alternate shoulder flexion, the "kayaking" type motion (see Figure 16-13), proprioceptive neuromuscular facilitation diagonal patterns, and horizontal shoulder abduction/adduction can all be performed using various types of equipment or manual resistance provided by the therapist while in prone. Resistance to each of these motions could be added during this phase of rehab.

Supine positioning allows for work on shoulder internal and external rotation where resistance or speed can be added (see Figure 16-16), as well as shoulder extension against resistance (Figure 16-17) in varying degrees of abduction. Internal and external rotation can be performed against resistance in standing. The land-based program and aquatic program

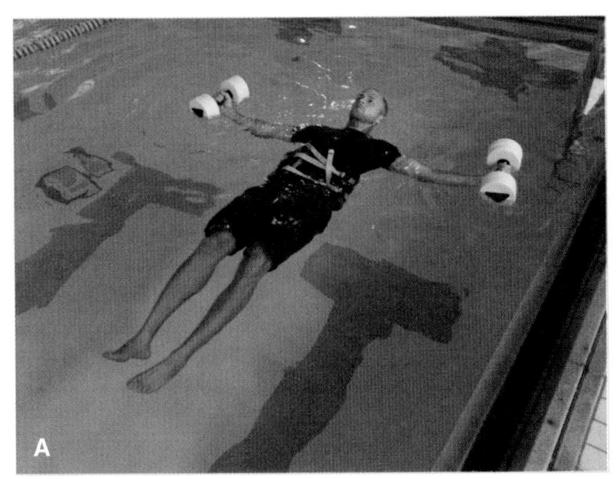

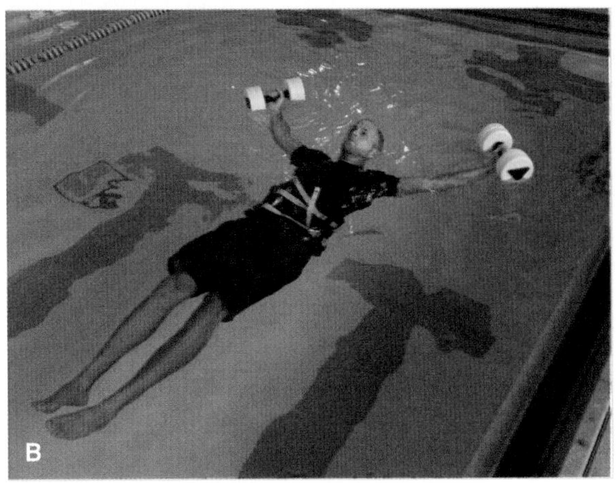

Figure 16-17 **Supine shoulder extension at 2 different abduction angles, for scapular stabilization**

A. Middle trapezius. **B.** Lower trapezius.

should be coordinated to ensure continued improvement of strength, endurance, and function. The goal of treatment in the intermediate-level activities is development of strength and eccentric control throughout increasing ranges of motion.

Final Level

The goal of this level of treatment is high-level functional strengthening and training. Equally important is the transition from the aquatic environment to the land environment. Utilizing sport equipment in treatment, if applicable, will keep an athlete motivated and working toward the goal of returning to sport (Figure 16-18). Increasing the resistance by using elastic or flotation attachments will keep it challenging (Figure 16-19). As in the intermediate level, the client needs to be involved in a strengthening and training program on land.

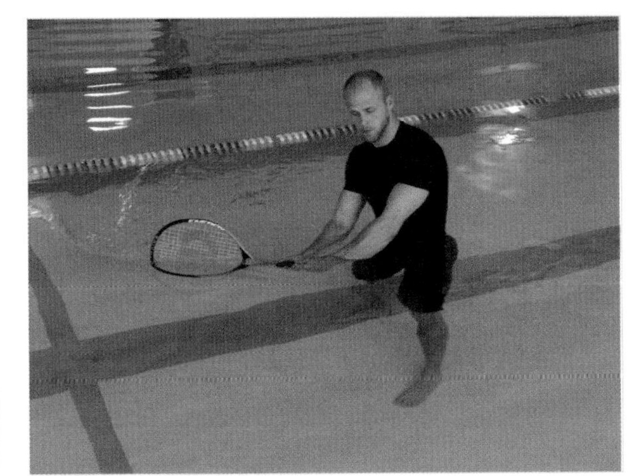

Figure 16-18 **Example of sport-specific training in the aquatic environment. Useful for upper-extremity, core, and lower-extremity training**

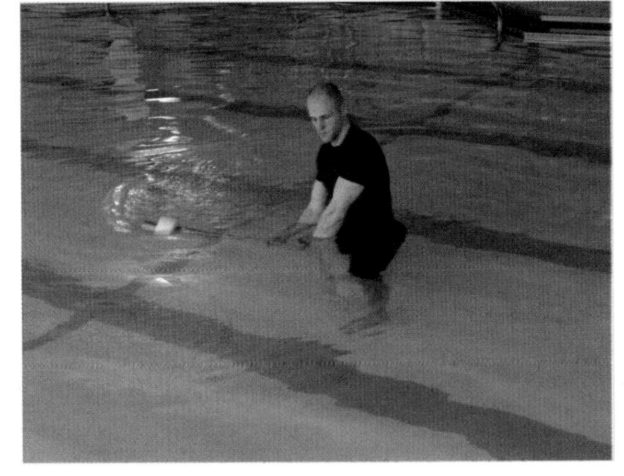

Figure 16-19 **Sport-specific training using buoyancy cuffs around a bat for resistance**

Spine Dysfunction

The unloading capability of water allows the patient or client ease of movement and some potential relief of symptoms. The patients/clients will need to be shown how to obtain and maintain the neutral spine position in the water even if they have been instructed on land. The neutral spine position is the basis of treatment in land and water and will progress in level of difficulty. Activities of the trunk, upper extremities, and lower extremities all challenge trunk stability, strength, total-body balance, and neuromuscular control. Directional movement preferences for relief of symptoms, such as extension- or flexion-biased exercises, can be integrated into program. Pregnant patients and clients that experience back pain often benefit from exercising in an aquatic environment secondary to the unloading forces on the lower back.

Initial Level

Using forward/backward/sideways walking is common for a warm-up activity in patients/clients with spine dysfunction. It is an opportunity for the client/patient to become aware of postural dysfunctions and practice with changing alignment. Kim et al[31] studied aquatic backward locomotion exercise and reported that a training program emphasizing backward walking is as effective as progressive resistive exercise training program utilizing equipment with increasing lumbar extension after discectomy surgery. Backward ambulation has been shown to activate paraspinal muscles, the vastus medialis, and tibialis anterior more than forward walking.[35] Initially, the client/patient can start with a speed and length of stride that does not cause discomfort, and then can progress to normal walking speed so as to allow for return to function.

Initial instruction regarding the neutral spine position is the basis for treatment. The patient/client stands in a partial squat position with the back against wall to offer feedback and allow them to monitor their response. There are a variety of ways to instruct the patient to contract the transversus abdominis muscle. It is important for the patient to have the awareness of maintaining a light transversus abdominis muscle contraction and keeping the lower-extremity muscles relaxed or "soft" during activities. Working on the endurance and prolonged hold of abdominal stabilization without increasing spinal discomfort is a goal for the initial level. Upper- and lower-extremity activities can be added so as to progressively challenge the client's ability to stabilize without increasing symptoms. Initially begin with activities without additional equipment, while manipulating the speed of movement through controlled ranges of motion in order to challenge the ability to maintain the desired position.

Use of deep-water activities can be initiated early in rehabilitation. The patient/client should maintain a vertical position while performing small controlled movements of the upper and lower extremities. The Burdenko approach to aquatic activities utilizes deep-water activities before activities in shallow water. If dealing with radicular (sciatica) type symptoms, a trial of deep-water traction can be done. Flotation support of the upper body and trunk and placement of light weights on the ankles allows for gentle distraction of the lumbar spine. The patient/client can hang using the flotation devices placed on the upper body/trunk, and perform small pedaling motions as if bicycling/walking.[36]

Working on normalizing the gait pattern and developing the ability to weight bear equally on the lower extremities in any depth of water comfortable to the client is important early in the therapeutic progression. Incorporation of activities to help centralize the symptoms are important, as well as encouraging the patient to perform only activities that maintain or diminish symptoms during the session. Gentle stretching and rotation movements can be performed within the pain-free motion in order to increase pelvic and lumbar spine mobility.

Intermediate Level

At this level, the patient/client is allowed to progress away from the wall, and the extremities or equipment is used to challenge their ability to stabilize. Stability can be initially

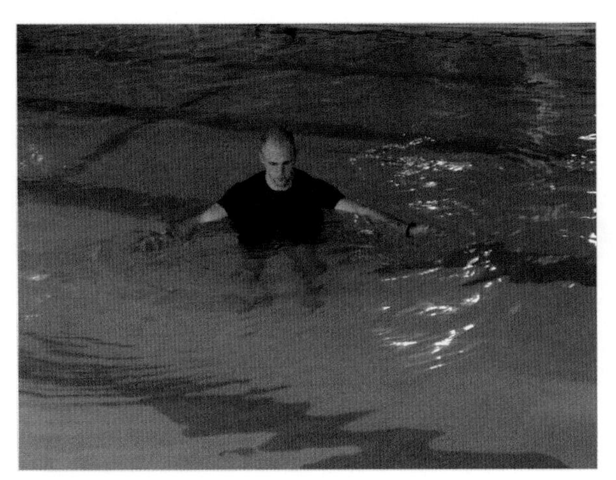

Figure 16-20 **Anterior posterior trunk stabilization with upper extremity horizontal abduction/adduction**

Note flexed knees and wide base of support.

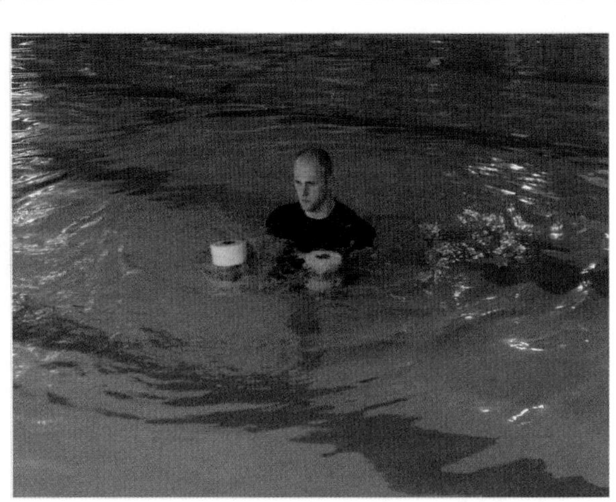

Figure 16-21 **Trunk stabilization against anterior/posterior forces, split stance**

challenged by moving the arms through the water to induce perturbation to the trunk (Figure 16-20). This can be made more challenging by increasing the speed of the upper-extremity movements or adding something to the hands such as webbed water gloves or flotation dumbbells. A kickboard can be used to mimic pushing, pulling, and lifting motions (Figures 16-21 and 16-22). Equipment that resists upper-extremity or lower-extremity movements in a single-leg stance or lunge position challenges the patient/client's balance, as well as stabilization using the abdominal and pelvic muscles (Figure 16-23). There is benefit to having the patient/client work on both bilateral and single-leg activities such as

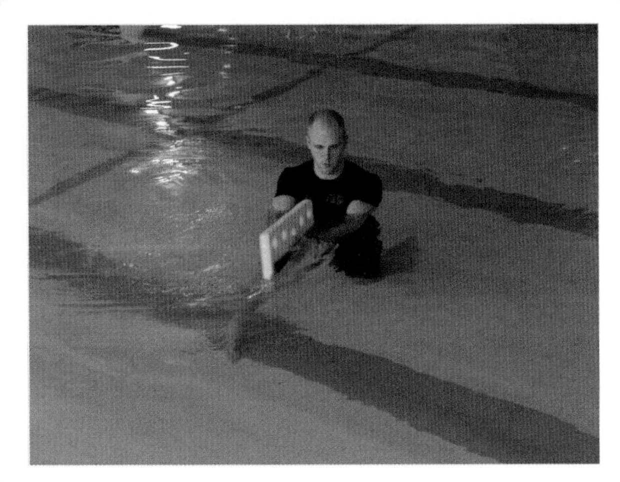

Figure 16-22 **Trunk stabilization against oblique/diagonal forces, split stance**

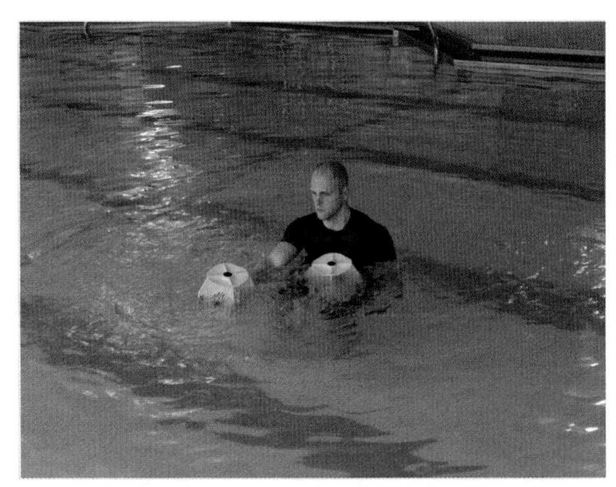

Figure 16-23 **Challenging lower-extremity neuromuscular control and balance, as well as trunk control, in single-limb stance utilizing upper-extremity resistance**

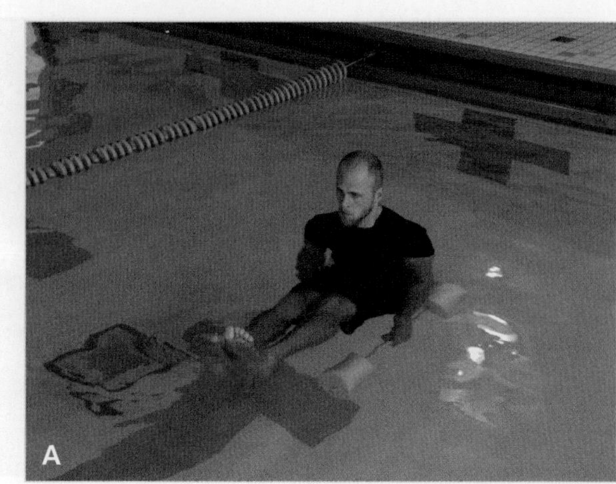

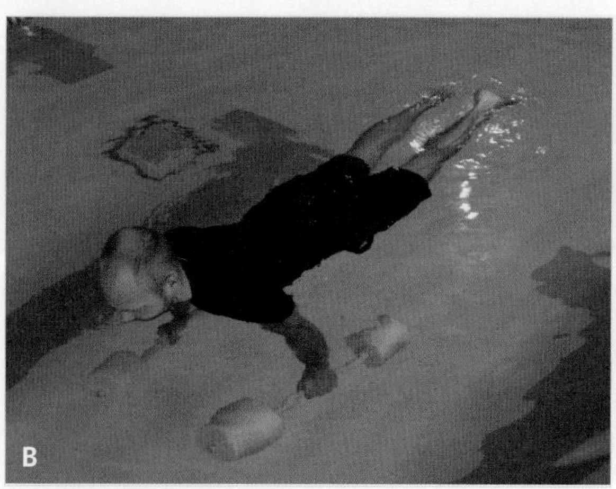

Figure 16-24

A. Tuck-and-roll exercise, pike position. **B.** Tuck-and-roll exercise, tuck position.

squats/calf raises that translate to some of the functional activities such as sit to stand and stair climbing.

The client's ability to stabilize can be further challenged using deep-water activities that require maintaining a vertical position while bringing knees to chest and progressing to tucking and rolling type movement (Figure 16-24). Activities can be created to work on diagonal and rotational motions of the spine and trunk, while maintaining the neutral position.

Activities in a supine position are effective for increasing trunk mobility and then progressing to work on trunk stability using Bad Ragaz techniques (Figures 16-25 and 16-26).[21] Activities in prone position provide an excellent method to challenge the clients ability to maintain the neutral spine position, and the patient/client may need flotation equipment

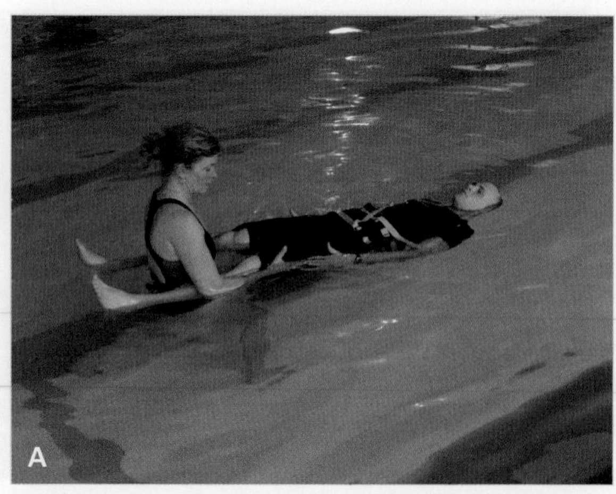

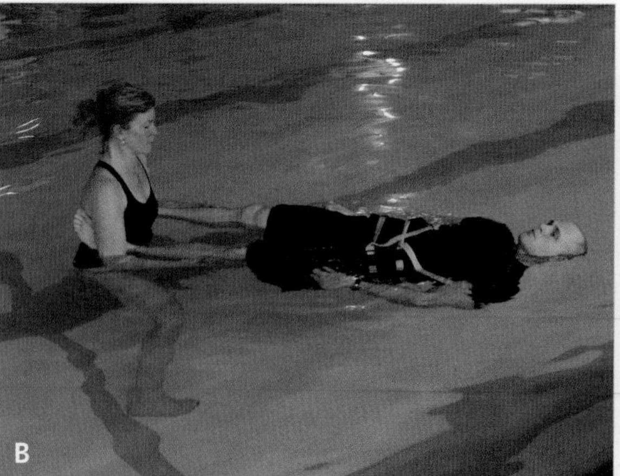

Figure 16-25 **Bad Ragaz technique for trunk stabilization**

A. Note short lever arm with therapist contacting the LE's above the knee in order to protect the knee joint. **B.** Contact below the knees (if indicated) increases the trunk and LE stability demands.

to accomplish that goal. The use of the mask and snorkel will allow for proper positioning of the spine while performing the activities (see Figures 16-13 and 16-14). It is important to monitor and teach the client the neutral spine position with each new position that is introduced in the treatment program. Activities can be simplified or progressed in difficulty according to patients/clients' level of function or their ability to maintain the neutral spine position.

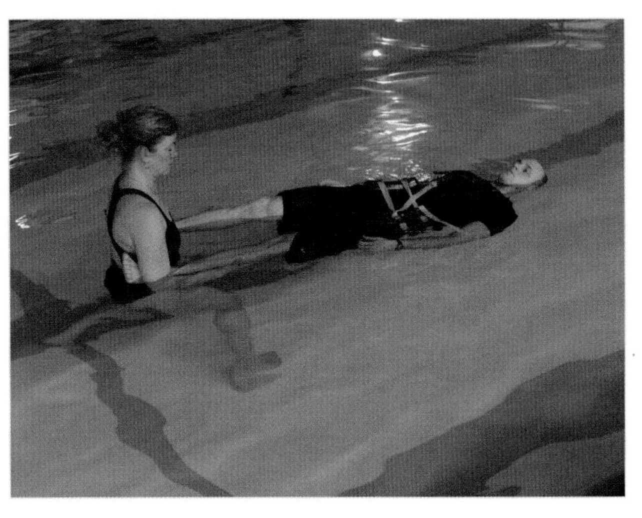

Figure 16-26 Bad Ragaz technique for oblique trunk stabilization

Final Level

Depending on the patient/client's needs and functional goals related to return to a desired level of activity, the program could be modified and progressed. For the patient/client returning to a demanding occupation, development of a program of lifting/pushing/pulling or other needs described by the client can complement a work-conditioning program. For the patient or client returning to a sport, the therapist and athlete can work together to develop specific challenging activities. The therapist needs to be creative with the use of aquatic equipment and should use equipment specific to the athlete's sport in order to challenge the athlete to a higher level of trunk stabilization. It is important to integrate movement patterns that are opposite of the ones the athlete normally performs in the athlete's sport in order to challenge body symmetry during function. For example, if a gymnast or ice skater predominantly turns or rotates in one direction, have them practice turns in the opposite direction. The aquatic environment provides the athlete an alternate environment in which to train, that should be encouraged for the serious athlete to attempt to avoid overuse type of conditions that can occur. Especially important in this phase is the reintegration of the patient/client back into treatment and training on land, as the water environment does not allow the athlete to prepare for the exact speeds and forces experienced on land.

Lower-Extremity Injuries

Aquatic therapy is a common modality for rehabilitation of many injuries of the lower extremity because of the properties of unloading and hydrostatic pressure. At an early phase of healing, the client may need to use a flotation belt, vest, exercise bars, noodles, and various other buoyancy devices to provide support, depending on pain and how long they have been nonweightbearing. The aquatic environment allows for limited weight bearing and restoration of gait by calculating the percentage of weight bearing allowed and weight of patient/client and then placing the patient/client in an appropriate depth of water, as discussed previously.

Clinical Pearl

The aquatic environment is an excellent place to begin gait retraining in the presence of weight-bearing restrictions after meniscal repairs, once the surgical sites have healed sufficiently.

Initial Level

The expected goals of this phase of rehabilitation are the return of normal motion and early strengthening of affected muscles. The restoration of normal and functional gait pattern is

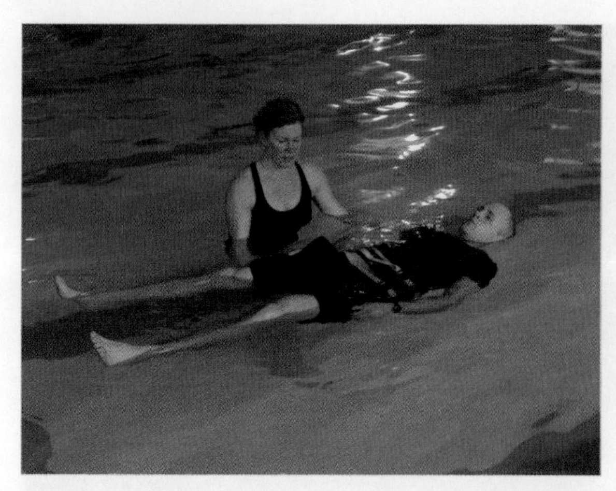

Figure 16-27 Supine hip abduction/adduction

Note therapist hand placement above the knee in order to protect the knee ligaments.

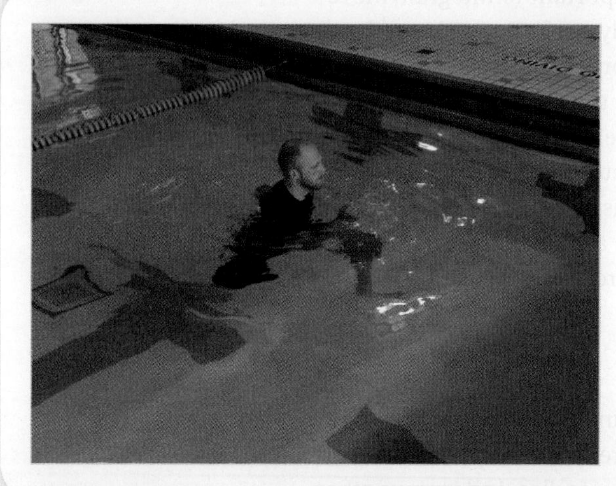

Figure 16-28 Deep-water running

also desired. Performing backward and sideways walking adds a functional dimension to the program in addition to traditional forward walking. Range-of-motion activities may involve active motions of the hip, knee, and ankle. Utilizing cuffs, noodles, or kickboards under the foot will assist with increasing motion, due to the buoyancy offered by such equipment. Exercises for strengthening noninvolved joints such as the hips or ankles can be performed with the client who has had a knee injury. However, it is important to remember that resistance (manual or with devices) may need to be placed above the injured knee in order to decrease torque placed upon the knee. It is important to integrate conditioning and balance activities within this initial level (Figure 16-27). Standing activities should be performed with attention paid to maintaining the spine in a neutral position, as well as to challenging balance and neuromuscular control of the involved lower extremity (see Figure 16-23).

Deep-water activities allow for conditioning and cross-training opportunities (Figure 16-28). The patient/client may initially need assistance with flotation devices, but can progress by decreasing the amount of flotation when able. For the client who must be non-weightbearing secondary to an injury or surgery, the deep water allows for a workout along with maintaining strength in uninvolved joints. Activities can involve running, bicycling, scissoring, or cross-country skiing motions, and also incorporate sport-specific activities of the lower extremities, trunk, and upper extremities.

The therapist can also incorporate activities performed in the supine position. The patients/clients need to be supported with flotation equipment that allow them to float evenly and without great effort to stay afloat. The therapist can stabilize at the feet and have the patient/client work on active hip and knee flexion and extension in order to work on increasing range of motion at the affected joint (Figure 16-29). Resistance of hip abduction and adduction can also be performed in a supine position. Again, attention must be paid to the location of applied force. Resistance placed upon the uninvolved leg movement will also allow for strengthening of the injured extremity. It should be noted that the therapist must teach the patient how to safely return to the standing/vertical position from the supine or prone position especially with the use of equipment applied to lower extremities.

Intermediate Level

Depending on the injury, surgery, or condition, the client can be progressed to the intermediate level when appropriate. The activities can be progressed by use of weights or flotation cuffs to increase difficulty. As in the initial level, resistance may need to be placed more proximally in the presence of knee ligament injuries or surgeries. Performing circuits of straight-plane and diagonal patterns with both lower extremities can be progressed by performing with upper-extremity support on the wall and progressing to no support. The involved lower extremity can be challenged by utilizing specific motions that mimic

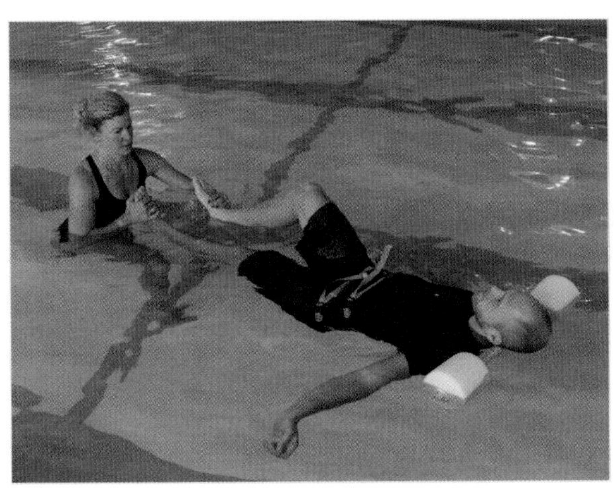

Figure 16-29 Supine alternating hip and knee flexion and extension, using Bad Ragaz technique

Hand contact by therapist gives the patient/client cues for movement.

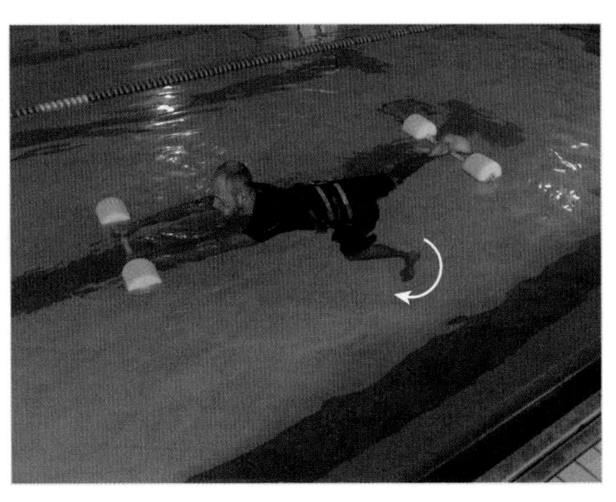

Figure 16-30 Supported single-lower-extremity running movement

Note the appropriate support of the patient/client with buoyancy belts and upper-extremity bell and lower-extremity bell under the stationary lower extremity. Also challenges trunk stabilization.

running (Figure 16-30). The patient/client can stand on an uneven surface, such as a noodle or cuff, to challenge balance and stabilization. Eccentric, closed-chain activities can be performed in the shallow water with the client standing on a noodle or kickboard for single-leg reverse squats, and utilizing a noodle, kickboard, or bar for bilateral reverse-squat motions in deep-water (Figure 16-31) and progressing to a single-leg reverse squat. Bilateral lower-extremity strength, endurance, and coordination can be challenged by kicking with a kickboard, using a flutter kick. This is also excellent for developing core control and aerobic endurance.

Performing deep-water tether running or sprinting forward and backward for increasing periods of time will allow for overall conditioning. The client can progress to running in shallower water depending upon the condition of injury or surgery (Figure 16-32).

Supine activities can be continued with emphasis on strengthening and stabilization of the trunk, pelvis, and lower extremities. Placement of the therapist's resistance will depend on the client's strength, ability to stabilize, and how much time has elapsed since surgery or injury. Increasing the number of repetitions and/or speed of movement will provide more resistance and work on fatiguing muscle groups of the lower extremity. The prone position provides increased challenges to the client to perform hip abduction and adduction along with hip and knee flexion and extension. As mentioned previously, the client can use mask and snorkel or flotation equipment to help with positioning while in the prone position.

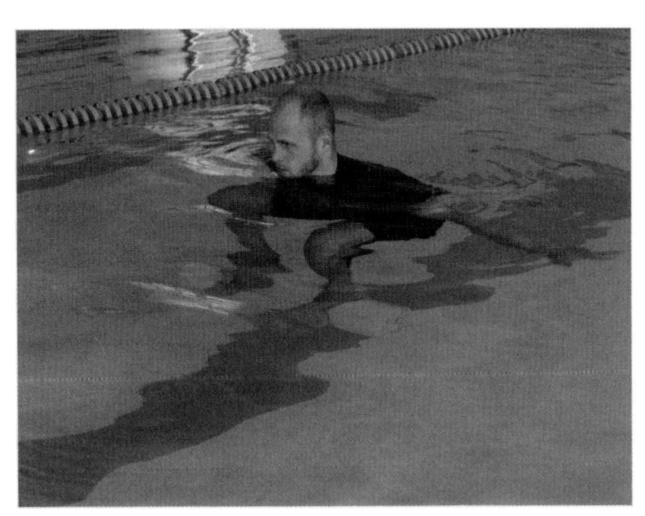

Figure 16-31 Reverse squat, bilateral, using flotation dumbell beneath the feet

Can be used for balance and neuromuscular coordination, as well as range of motion.

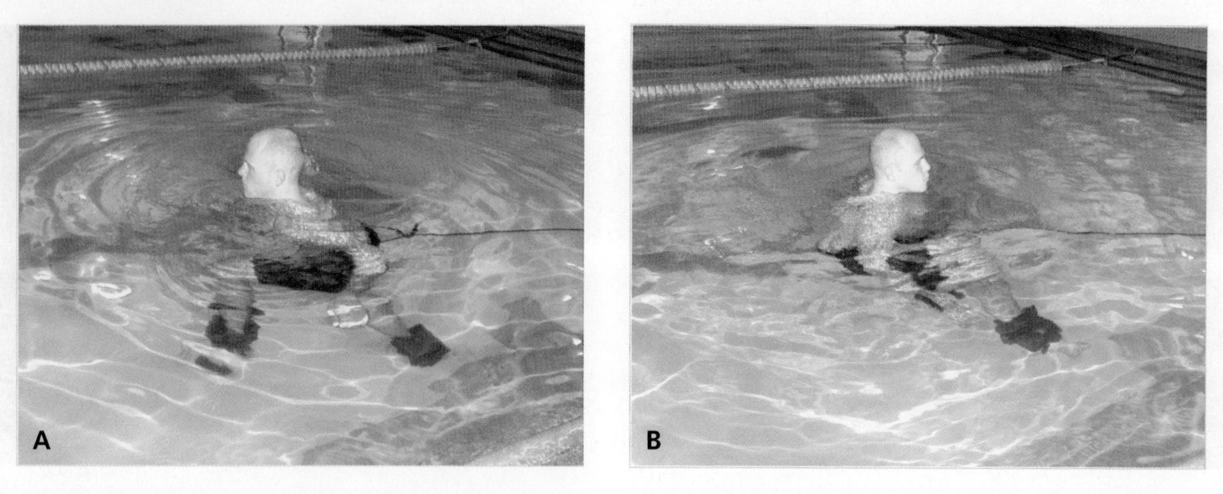

Figure 16-32

Deep water running against tubing resistance, (**A**) forward and (**B**) backward.

Sport-specific activities can be integrated into the program for the athlete. While practicing movement patterns needed for sport, the patient/client can start at chest depth and progress to shallow water. As with spine rehabilitation, there is benefit from practicing opposite movement patterns such as turns and jumps. The aquatic environment will allow for early initiation of a structured jumping and landing program. Some adaptations and proper instruction to the patient/client will provide similar positive effects as those seen in land-based programs.[40] Progression to the land-based jump/land program is recommended when appropriate.

Final Level

In the final level, the patient/client is involved with a high-level strengthening and training program. The aquatic program can and should be used to complement the land program. The athlete can continue to practice sport-specific activities and drills in varying levels of water. Decreasing the use of flotation equipment can increase the difficulty with deep-water activities. Using buoyancy cuffs on the ankles without using a flotation belt will challenge the athlete's ability to stabilize and perform running in deep water. Endurance training in an aquatic environment is a good alternative for the healthy athlete's conditioning programs and may help to prevent injuries. As with the upper extremity, this phase also requires integration of aquatic- and land-based exercises so as to successfully transition the athlete to full participation in sport on land.

Special Techniques

Bad Ragaz Ring Method

The Bad Ragaz technique originated in the thermal pools of Bad Ragaz, Switzerland, in the 1930s, and continued to evolve throughout the years. As a method, it focuses on muscle reeducation, strengthening, spinal traction/elongation, relaxation, and tone inhibition.[17] The properties of water—including buoyancy, turbulence, hydrostatic pressure, and surface tension—provide dynamic environmental forces during activities. The use of upper-extremity and lower-extremity proprioceptive neuromuscular facilitation patterns add a 3-dimensional aspect to this method. Movement of the client's body through the water provides the resistance.[11] The turbulent drag produced from movement is in direct relation to the client's speed of movement. The therapist provides the movement when the client works on isometric (stabilization) patterns; however, the therapist is in the stable/fixed position when the client is performing isokinetic or isotonic activities (see Figures 16-26, 16-27, and 16-29).[21] Stretching and lengthening responses can be obtained with passive or relaxed response from client; the therapist needs to support and stabilize body segments in order to obtain desired response.

Awareness of body mechanics and prevention of injury are important to the therapist when performing resistive Bad Ragaz–type activities. The therapist should stand in waist-deep water, not deeper than the level of T8-T10,[21] and wear aqua shoes for traction and stability. The therapist should stand with 1 foot in front of the other, with knees slightly bent, and legs shoulder-width apart, to compensate for the long lever arm force of the client.

Burdenko Method

The Burdenko method utilizes motion as the principle healing intervention. According to Burdenko,[6] the components of dynamic healing include patterns of movement, injury assessment, and rehabilitation exercises that occur with the client in a standing position; the psychology of the injured client benefiting from pain-free movement, and blood flow and neural stimulation being enhanced by activity.[6] Six essential qualities are necessary for perfecting and maintaining the art of movement: balance, coordination, flexibility, endurance, speed, and strength. Burdenko advocates the presentation of these qualities in exercise activities in the previously stated order. The activities are designed to challenge the center of buoyancy and center of gravity. Treatments/activities are initiated in deep water and incorporate shallow-water activities as client succeeds by demonstrating control of movement while maintaining neutral vertical position. Integration of land exercise along with the aquatic activity addresses functional movement patterns. For further information on this technique, see "Suggested Readings" at the end of the chapter.

Halliwick Method

The Halliwick method is commonly used to teach individuals with physical disabilities to swim and to learn balance control in water. Developed by James McMillan, the Halliwick method or concept is based on a "Ten Point Programme."[9] This method is frequently utilized with the pediatric population, but portions of the technique can be utilized to improve and restore a patient/client's balance. Use of turbulent forces can assist in developing strategies for maintaining balance or challenge the patient/client to maintain a stable posture during a change in the direction of force. For example, the patient/client maintains a single-leg stance while the therapist or another person runs around the patient/client offering turbulent perturbations (Figure 16-33). More information on the Halliwick technique is also available in the "Suggested Readings" section at the end of the chapter.

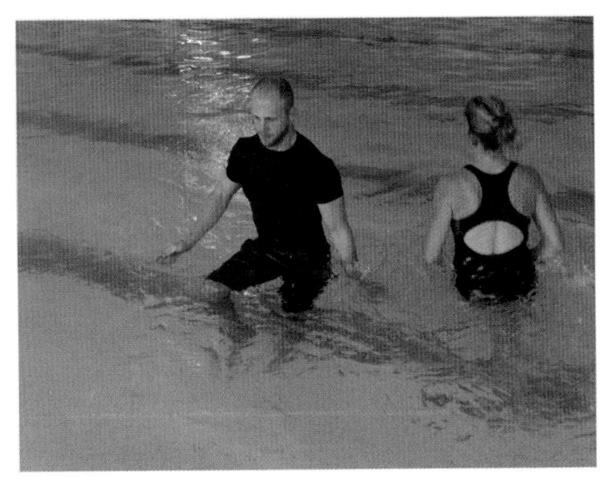

Figure 16-33 Balance and neuromuscular control restoration technique for trunk and single lower extremity

This exercise demonstrates the use of the principle of turbulence, generated in the Halliwick technique to challenge the stability of the patient/client.

Ai Chi

Ai chi is an Eastern-based treatment approach combining Tai Chi, Zen Shiatsu, Watsu, and Qi Gong in the water. Benefits of this approach include promoting relaxation by the use of diaphragmatic breathing that stimulates the parasympathetic nervous system, core strengthening, and increased flexibility. Performed in shoulder-depth water, it progresses from deep breathing to total-body movements through a characteristic sequence of postures.[42]

Special Populations

There are many conditions and diagnoses that may benefit from treatment in the aquatic environment. Aquatic therapy interventions can benefit a patient/client's level of function. The therapist can be the catalyst for providing an introduction to an environment that can be a temporary rehabilitation tool or lifestyle tool for fitness. The following discussion of the treatment of the pediatric and neurologic patient/client is but a brief synopsis and the interested therapist should seek specialized training.

Pediatric Patients and Clients

The aquatic environment provides a fun treatment area for the pediatric patient/client. Examples of congential pediatric diagnoses that are effectively treated in the aquatic environment include cerebral palsy, spina bifida, and muscular dystrophy. A wide range of additional medical diagnoses may also be appropriate for treatment in this environment. The team of therapists, physicians, and parents can decide on whether it is appropriate to initiate aquatic therapy as a part of the treatment plan. A combination of land and aquatic therapy assists with assessing effectiveness of therapeutic interventions and obtaining functional goals. The major challenge for the therapist is evaluating the pediatric client for water safety. Assessment of the child's ability to accept water to the face, tolerance to being submerged, and breath control are important factors for the aquatic evaluation. The mental adjustment of the child to the water is a necessary component for successful use of water as a treatment modality. Parents and caregivers may need to find a swim instructor to assist with decreasing fear and increasing comfort of water, with variety of movements.

A variety of approaches, such as Halliwick, Bad Ragaz Ring Method, and Watsu, can be integrated and adapted into treatment program for the pediatric patient/client. Watsu is a passive treatment technique described as Zen Shiatsu in water. It was originally created as a wellness technique and has expanded for utilization with patients and clients. Patients treated with this technique experience relaxation and tone-inhibiting vestibular stimulation.

A treatment program consists of warm-up and cool-down periods, which allow for active stretching and adjustment to the water. Functional motor skills are practiced and integrated into play activities. Water provides constant postural challenges to the child.[45] As with the adult patient or client, the treatment program should progress toward the goals set by the therapist and be readjusted according to patient responses and assessment of progress. It is important to work in collaboration with the multidisciplinary team of personnel who participate in the care of the pediatric client in order to provide synergistic treatment that includes aquatic therapy.

Neurologic Patients and Clients

Benefits of the aquatic environment for the patient/client with neurologic involvement include a supportive and safe environment, ease of movement, and an excellent medium in which to practice functional activities. The water allows for the therapist's ease of handling the patient/client with significant neurologic involvement. Support offered by the water provides stability and assistance for the therapist who is performing handling techniques to facilitate movement and inhibit tone.

In a older client/patient who may have a more complex medical history and recent neurologic event, there is usually a disturbance of balance. This may lead to increase risks of falls and fear for that client. The aquatic environment allows for the client/patient to have more time to recruit an appropriate postural response. Turbulence can be used to assist or resist patient's balance. The task-type training approach uses the principles of buoyancy, turbulence, and hydrostatic pressure to address patients disabilities by working in functional positions with functional activities.[11,43]

There are a variety of treatment approaches that are effective in accomplishing functional goals. Utilizing the standing and sitting positions encourage and promote postural stability. The first priority is determining the safest and most stable position in which the client can begin to work in the water. Practicing functional activities as a whole allows for the patient/client to master the activity while exercising control during the activity and stabilizing multiple body segments. As patient/client progresses, less assistance and support is provided, allowing for increased independence.[42] Like the pediatric population, specialized training is recommended for those therapists who desire to use aquatic rehabilitation as an intervention strategy for their patients and clients with neuromuscular diagnoses.

SUMMARY

Aquatic rehabilitation is not typically the exclusive intervention option for most patients and clients. The aquatic environment offers many positive psychological and physiologic effects during the early rehabilitation phase of injury.[37,54] However, in subsequent phases of rehabilitation, it is typical to use combinations of land- and water-based interventions to achieve rehabilitation goals. Because humans function in a "gravity environment," the transition from water to land is necessary for full rehabilitation for most patients/clients. Some clients use the aquatic environment for continued strengthening and conditioning programs secondary to a painful response to land-based activities. Examples of this include those patients with pain that occurs with compressive forces at joints (such as cases of disc dysfunction, spinal stenosis, and osteoarthritis), as well as chronic neuromuscular conditions such as multiple sclerosis.

This chapter provides information regarding indications and benefits as well as contraindications and precautions to use of the aquatic environment for rehabilitation. Suggestions and exercises are offered to help the therapist to incorporate aquatic exercise into a rehabilitation program. Utilizing the principles provided and the examples of activities, physical therapists can use their judgment, skill, and especially their creativity to develop an exercise program to meet their patient/client's goals. The old English proverb says "We never know the worth of water 'til the well is dry." The worth and value of aquatic therapy as an intervention cannot be fully understood and appreciated until experienced and additional research is completed.

- The buoyant force counteracts the force of gravity as it assists motion toward the water's surface and resists motion away from the surface.
- Because of differences in the specific gravity of the body, the head and chest tend to float higher in the water than the heavier, denser extremities, making compensation with floatation devices necessary.
- The 3 forces that oppose movement in the water are the cohesive force, the bow force, and the drag force.
- Aquatic therapy allows for fine gradations of exercise, increased control over the percentage of weight bearing, increased range of motion and strength in weak

patients/clients, and decreased pain and increased confidence in functional movements.

- Pool size and depth, water temperature, and specific pool equipment vary depending on the clientele being treated and the resources available to the therapist.
- Application of the principle of buoyancy allows for progression of exercises.
- Upper- and lower-extremity activities both require and provide a challenge to trunk and core stability.
- The special techniques exclusive to the aquatic environment can be used to complement traditional land-based therapeutic interventions.
- Aquatic therapy can help stimulate interest, motivation, and exercise compliance in pediatric, geriatric, neurological, and athletic patients/clients.
- The aquatic environment is an excellent medium to facilitate speedy functional return to work, activities of daily living, and sport.
- It is typical to use a combination of land- and water-based therapeutic exercise protocols to achieve rehabilitation goals.

REFERENCES

1. Arrigo C, ed. Aquatic rehabilitation. *Sports Med Update.* 1992;7(2).
2. Arrigo C, Fuller CS, Wilk KE. Aquatic rehabilitation following ACL-PTG reconstruction. *Sports Med Update.* 1992;7(2):22-27.
3. Asahina M, Asahina MK, Yamanaka Y, Mitsui K, Kitahara A, Murata A. Cardiovascular response during aquatic exercise in patients with osteoarthritis. *Am J Phys Med Rehabil.* 2010;89(9):731-735.
4. Bolton F, Goodwin D. *Pool Exercises.* Edinburgh, UK: Churchill-Livingstone; 1974.
5. Broach E, Groff D, Yaffe R, Dattilo J, Gast D. Effects of aquatic therapy on adults with multiple sclerosis. *Ann Ther Rec.* 1998;7:1-20.
6. Burdenko IN. Sport-specific exercises after injuries—the Burdenko method. Paper presented at the Aquatic Therapy Symposium 2002, August 22-25, Orlando, FL, 2002.
7. Butts NK, Tucker M, Greening C. Physiologic responses to maximal treadmill and deep water running in men and women. *Am J Sports Med.* 1991;19(6):612-614.
8. Campion MR. *Adult Hydrotherapy: A Practical Approach.* Oxford, UK: Heinemann Medical; 1990.
9. Cunningham J. Halliwick method. In: Ruoti RG, Morris DM, Cole AJ, eds. *Aquatic Rehabilitation.* Philadelphia, PA: Lippincott-Raven; 1997:305-331.
10. Cureton KJ. Physiologic responses to water exercise. In: Ruoti RG, Morris DM, Cole AJ, eds. *Aquatic Rehabilitation.* Philadelphia, PA: Lippincott-Raven; 1997:39-56.
11. Davis BC. A technique of re-education in the treatment pool. *Physiotherapy.* 1967;53(2):37-59.
12. Dioffenbach L. Aquatic therapy services. *Clin Manage.* 1991;11(1):14-19.
13. Dougherty NJ. Risk management in aquatics. *JOPERD.* 1990;(May/June):46-48.
14. Duffield NH. *Exercise in Water.* London, UK: Bailliere Tindall; 1976.
15. Edlich RF, Towler MA, Goitz RJ, et al. Bioengineering principles of hydrotherapy. *J Burn Care Rehabil.* 1987;8(6):580-584.
16. Ekdahl C, Jarnlo GB, Andersson SI. Standing balance in healthy subjects: use of quantitative test-battery on force platform. *Scand J Rehabil Med.* 1989;21:187-95.
17. Ekdahl C, Andersson SI. Standing balance in rheumatoid arthritis: a comparative study with healthy subjects. *Scand J Rheumatol.* 1989;18:33-42.
18. Eyestone ED, Fellingham G, George J, Fisher G. Effect of water running and cycling on maximum oxygen consumption and 2 mile run performance. *Am J Sports Med.* 1993;21(1):41-44.
19. Fawcett CW. Principles of aquatic rehab: a new look at hydrotherapy. *Sports Med Update.* 1992;7(2):6-9.
20. Fontana HDB, Haupenthal A, Ruschel C, Hubert M, Ridehalgh C, Roesler H. Effect of gender, cadence, and water immersion on ground reaction forces during stationary running. *J Orthop Sports Phys Ther.* 2012;42(5):437-443.
21. Garrett G. Bad Ragaz ring method. In: Ruoti RG, Morris DM, Cole AJ, eds. *Aquatic Rehabilitation.* Philadelphia, PA: Lippincott-Raven; 1997:289-292.
22. Geigle P, Daddona K, Finken K, et al. The effects of a supplemental aquatic physical therapy program on balance

and girth for NCAA division III athletes with a grade I or II lateral ankle sprain. *J Aquatic Phys Ther.* 2001;9(1):13-20.

23. Genuario SE, Vegso JJ. The use of a swimming pool in the rehabilitation and reconditioning of athletic injuries. *Contemp Orthop.* 1990;20(4):381-387.
24. Golland A. Basic hydrotherapy. *Physiotherapy.* 1961;67(9):258-262, 1961.
25. Hall J, MPhil, Swinkels A, Briddon J. Does aquatic exercise relieve pain in adults with neurologic or musculoskeletal disease? A systematic review and meta-analysis of randomized controlled trials. *Arch Phys Med Rehabil.* 89; 873-883, 2008.
26. Haralson KM. Therapeutic pool programs. *Clin Manage.* 1985;5(2):10-13.
27. Harrison R, Bulstrode S. Percentage weight bearing during partial immersion in the hydrotherapy pool. *Physiother Theory Pract.* 1987;3:60-63.
28. Hertler L, Provost-Craig M, Sestili D, Hove A, Fees M. Water running and the maintenance of maximal oxygen consumption and leg strength in runners. *Med Sci Sports Exerc.* 1992;24(5):S23.
29. Hurley R, Turner C. Neurology and aquatic therapy. *Clin Manage.* 1991;11(1):26-27.
30. Irion JM. Aquatic therapy. In: Bandy WD, Sanders B, eds. *Therapeutic Exercise: Techniques for Intervention.* Baltimore, MD: Lippincott, Williams & Wilkins; 2001: 295-332.
31. Kim Y, Park J, Shim J. Effects of aquatic backward locomotion exercise and progressive resistance exercise on lumbar extension strength in patients who have undergone lumbar discectomy. *Arch Phys Med Rehabil.* 2010;91:208-214.
32. Kolb ME. Principles of underwater exercise. *Phys Ther Rev.* 1957;27(6):361-364.
33. Koszuta LE. From sweats to swimsuits: is water exercise the wave of the future? *Phys Sportsmed.* 1989;17(4):203-206.
34. Levin S. Aquatic therapy. *Phys Sportsmed.* 1991;19(10): 119-126.
35. Masumota K, Takasugi S, Hotta N, Fujishima K, Iwamato Y. A comparison of muscle activity and heart rate response during backward and forward walking on an underwater treadmill. *Gait Posture.* 2007;25:222-228.
36. McNamara C, Thein L. Aquatic rehabilitation of musculoskeletal conditions of the spine. In: Ruoti RG, Morris DM, Cole AJ, eds. *Aquatic Rehabilitation.* Philadelphia, PA: Lippincott-Raven; 1997:85-98.
37. McWaters JG. For faster recovery just add water. *Sports Med Update.* 1992;7(2):4-5.
38. Meyer RI. Practice settings for kinesiotherapy-aquatics. *Clin Kinesiol.* 1990;44(1):12-13.
39. Michaud TL, Brennean DK, Wilder RP, Sherman NW. Aquarun training and changes in treadmill running maximal oxygen consumption. *Med Sci Sports Exerc.* 1992;24(5):S23.
40. Miller MG. Berry DC, Gilders R, Bullard S. Recommendations for implementing an aquatic plyometric program. *Strength Cond J.* 2001;23(6):28-35.
41. Moor FB, Peterson SC, Manueall EM, et al. *Manual of Hydrotherapy and Massage.* Mountain View, CA: Pacific Press; 1964.
42. Morris DM. Aquatic rehabilitation for the treatment of neurologic disorders. In: Cole AJ, Becker BE, eds. *Comprehensive Aquatic Therapy.* Philadelphia, PA: Butterworth-Heinemann; 2004.
43. Morris D. Aquatic therapy to improve balance dysfunction in older adults. *Top Geriatr Rehabil.* 2010;26(2):104-119.
44. Nolte-Heuritsch I. *Aqua Rhythmics: Exercises for the Swimming Pool.* New York, NY: Sterling; 1979.
45. Petersen TM. Pediatric aquatic therapy. In: Cole AJ, Becker BE, eds. *Comprehensive Aquatic Therapy.* Philadelphia, PA: Butterworth-Heinemann; 2004.
46. Pöyhönen T, Kyröläinen H, Keskinen KL, Hautala A, Savolainen J, Mälkiä, E. Electromyographic and kinematic analysis of therapeutic knee exercises under water. *Clin Biomech (Bristol, Avon).* 2001;16:496-504.
47. Pöyhönen TK, Keskinen L, Hautala A, Mälkiä E. Determination of hydrodynamic drag forces and drag coefficients on human leg/foot model during knee exercise. *Clin Biomech (Bristol, Avon).* 2000;15:256-260.
48. Robertson JM, Brewster EA, Factora KI. Comparison of heart rates during water running in deep and shallow water at the same rating of perceived exertion. *J Aquatic Phys Ther.* 2001;9(1):21-26.
49. Simmons V, Hansen PD. Effectiveness of water exercise on postural mobility in the well elderly: an experimental study on balance enhancement. *J Gerontol.* 1996;51A(5):M233-M238.
50. Sova R. *Aquatic Activities Handbook.* Boston, MA: Jones & Bartlett; 1993.
51. Speer K, Cavanaugh JT, Warren RF, Day L, Wickiewicz TL. A role for hydrotherapy in shoulder rehabilitation. *Am J Sports Med.* 1993;21(6):850-853.
52. Suomi R, Koceja D. Postural sway characteristics in women with lower extremity arthritis before and after an aquatic exercise intervention. *Arch Phys Med Rehabil.* 2000;81:780-785.
53. Svendenhag J, Seger J. Running on land and in water: comparative exercise physiology. *Med Sci Sports Exerc.* 1992;24(10):1155-1160.
54. Thein JM, Thein Brody L. Aquatic-based rehabilitation and training for the elite athlete. *J Orthop Sports Phys Ther.* 1998;27(1):32-41.
55. Town GP, Bradley SS. Maximal metabolic responses of deep and shallow water running in trained runners. *Med Sci Sports Exerc.* 1991;23(2):238-241.
56. Triggs M. Orthopedic aquatic therapy. *Clin Manage.* 1991;11(1): 30-31.
57. Wilder RP, Brennan D, Schotte D. A standard measure for exercise prescription and aqua running. *Am J Sports Med.* 1993;21(1):45-48.
58. Wilder R, Brennan D. Aqua running. In: Cole AJ, Becker BE, eds. *Comprehensive Aquatic Therapy.* Philadelphia, PA: Butterworth-Heinemann; 2004.

SUGGESTED READINGS

Berger MA, deGroot G, Hollander AP. Hydrodynamic drag and lift forces on human hand/arm models. *J Biomech.* 1995;28(2):125-133.

Brody LT, Geigle PR. Aquatic Therapy for Rehabilitation and Training. Champaign, IL: Human Kinetics; 2009.

Burdenko J, Connors E. *The Ultimate Power of Resistance*. Igor Publishing; 1999 [available only through mail order].

Burdenko Water & Sports Therapy Institute. Newton, MA; 1998.

Campion MR. *Adult Hydrotherapy: A Practical Approach*. Oxford, UK: Heinemann Medical; 1990.

Cassady SL, Nielsen DH. Cardiorespiratory responses of healthy subjects to calisthenics performed on land versus in water. *Phys Ther.* 1992;72(7):532-538.

Christie JL, Sheldahl LM, Tristani FE. Cardiovascular regulation during head-out water immersion exercise. *J Appl Physiol.* 1990;69(2):657-664.

Frangolias DD, Rhodes EC. Maximal and ventilatory threshold responses to treadmill and water immersion running. *Med Sci Sports Exerc.* 1995;27(7):1007-1013.

Green JH, Cable NT, Elms N. Heart rate and oxygen consumption during walking on land and in deep water. *J Sports Med Phys Fitness.* 1990;30(1):49-52.

Martin J. The Halliwick method. *Physiotherapy.* 1981;67: 288-291.

Sova R. *Aquatic Activities Handbook*. Boston, MA: Jones & Bartlett; 1993.

17

Functional Movement Assessment

Barbara J. Hoogenboom, Michael L. Voight,
Gray Cook, and Greg Rose

OBJECTIVES

After completion of this chapter, the physical therapist should be able to do the following:

- Explain the benefits of a functional, comprehensive movement screening process versus the traditional impairment-based evaluation approach.
- Differentiate between movement, testing, and assessment.
- Explain how poor movement patterns and dysfunctional movement strategies can result in injury or reinjury.
- Explain the use and components of the Functional Movement Screen and the Selective Functional Movement Assessment.
- Describe, score, and interpret the movement patterns of the Functional Movement Screen and the Selective Functional Movement Assessment and how the results from each can have an impact on clinical interventions.
- Articulate the difference between movement screening and specific functional performance tests.
- Apply specific functional performance test to clinical practice.

Introduction

Movement is at the core of the human journey. It is foundational to the human experience and allows us to interact with our environment in ways different from other mammals. Movement, which begins in the womb, is the basis of early growth and development. It proceeds in a highly predictable manner in infants and young children and is known as the developmental sequence or traditional motor development. Once an individual reaches a certain age, full integration of reflexive behavior allows the development of purposive, highly developed, and unique mature motor programs. We continue to move functionally throughout a lifetime until the effects of aging alter the normalcy of movement.

Motion versus Movement

Because movement is complex, it must be differentiated from the simpler construct of motion. We believe that many professionals lack a true understanding of movement; they err on the side of quantitative assessment of motion and fail to understand the hierarchic progression from general, fundamental movement patterns to specific, highly specialized movements. These highly specialized movements have complex, fine-tuned motor programs that support their consistency and intricacy. Most rehabilitation and medical professionals have been trained to measure isolated joint motion with goniometers, inclinometers, linear measurements, and ligament laxity tests. These types of motion assessment are not wrong, but rather only a piece of a much bigger puzzle of "movement" and the inherent stability and mobility demands that are part of the synchronous, elegant, coordinated activities that make up activities of daily living, work tasks, and sport maneuvers. Mere motion measurements cannot capture the whole spectrum of human movement, nor the complexity of human function.

Systems Approach to Movement

The premise of this chapter and the chapter that follows is that impairment-based, highly specialized motion assessment is far too limiting, and predisposes practitioners to errors in professional judgment. It is too narrow an approach, which focuses on small, discrete pieces of an integrated functional task or movement. The alternative of a more functional, comprehensive movement screen is vitally important for understanding human function and identifying impairments and dysfunctional movement patterns that diminish the quality of function. In many cases, weakness or tightness of a muscle or group is often identified and then treated with isolated stretching or strengthening activities instead of using a standard movement pattern that could address several impairments at once. Likewise, many professionals often focus on a specific region of complaint instead of beginning by identifying a comprehensive movement profile and relating the profile to dysfunction.

"Fundamentals First"

Where does one start with the examination and assessment of something as complex as human function? Standard, frequently used, fundamental or general movements would seem the logical place to start. To prepare an athlete for the wide variety of activities needed to participate in the demands of sport, analysis of fundamental movements should be incorporated into preparticipation screening. Assessment of fundamental movements can help the rehabilitation professional determine who possesses or lacks the ability to perform a wide variety of essential movements. We believe that assessment of fundamental or composite movements is necessary before the assessment of highly specific or specialized motions or movements. Consider the following statements in the context of assessment of an athlete:

- What appears to be muscular weakness may be muscular inhibition.
- Identifiable weakness in a prime mover may be the result of a dysfunctional stabilizer or group of muscular stabilizers.
- Diminished function in an agonist may actually be dysfunction of the antagonist.
- What is described as muscular tightness may be protective muscle tone leading to guarding and inadequate muscle coordination during movement.
- "Bad" technique might be the only option for an individual performing poorly selected, "off-target" exercises.
- Diminished general fitness may be related to the increased metabolic demand required by patients who use inferior neuromuscular coordination and compensations.

It is vital that fundamental, essential movements be examined to develop a working hypothesis regarding the *source* of the dysfunction. This approach allows the rehabilitation professional to see "the big picture" and attempt to discern the cause of the dysfunction rather than just identifying and treating specific, isolated impairments. This fundamental first approach, typically used when teaching a motor skill, holds true for assessment and correction of movement.

The Mobility–Stability Continuum

Movement becomes less than optimal (dysfunctional) as a result of "breakdowns" in parts of the movement system. Typically, such breakdowns are described as mobility or stability dysfunction. Unfortunately, the terms *mobility* and *stability* are not universally defined and can imply different things to clinicians with different backgrounds. For this reason it is important to describe the approach of the authors regarding descriptions of mobility and stability.

Mobility dysfunction can be broken down into 2 unique subcategories:

- *Tissue extensibility dysfunction* involves tissues that are extraarticular. Examples include active or passive muscle insufficiency, neural tension, fascial tension, muscle shortening, scarring, and fibrosis.
- *Joint mobility dysfunction* involves structures that are articular or intraarticular. Examples include osteoarthritis, fusion, subluxation, adhesive capsulitis, and intraarticular loose bodies.

Stability dysfunction may include an isolated muscular weakness or joint laxity, but it is frequently more complex and refers to multiple systems that are involved in the complex construct known as motor control. To account for the complexity of a stability problem, the term *stability motor control dysfunction* is used. Stability motor control dysfunction is an encompassing, broad description of problems in movement pattern stability. Traditionally, stability dysfunction is often addressed by attempting to concentrically strengthen the muscle groups identified as stabilizers of a region or joint. This approach neglects the concept that true stabilization is reflex driven and relies on proprioception and timing rather than isolated, gross muscular strength. By using the term stability motor control dysfunction to distinguish stability problems, the clinician is forced to consider the central nervous system, peripheral nervous system, motor programs, movement organization, timing, coordination, proprioception, joint and postural alignment, structural instability, and muscular inhibition, as well as the absolute strength of the stabilizers. The concepts of mobility and stability are discussed further in the context of the Selective Functional Movement Assessment (SFMA) later in this chapter.

The purpose of this chapter, as part of a sports medicine rehabilitation text, is to provide the context for and convince the reader of the importance of a timely, accurate, and reproducible functional movement assessment. Although a part of examination, isolated measurements and quantitative assessments are not enough to capture the essence of functional movement in activities of life.

Movement Screening, Testing, and Assessment

Athletic trainers screen during the preseason. Physical therapists are involved in screening, prevention, and wellness initiatives. Physicians serve patients by medically or surgically "fixing problems" but also attempt to prevent repeat injury. The number 1 risk for injury is previous injury.[1-6] What contributes to this paradigm? Poor screening that does not identify athletes at risk for injury? Poor rehabilitation that does not "finish the job"? "Poor" or untested surgical or medical interventions that do not get to the "root" of the problem? Each is a possibility, and all disciplines may be responsible for unsuccessfully preparing or providing the building blocks for full return to movement normalcy. It is the "job" of all health professionals to adequately screen, test, assess, and identify movement dysfunction and offer solutions to restore movement efficiency and normalcy.

At this point it is important to distinguish between screening, testing, and assessment (Table 17-1). This chapter is written to enhance the reader's ability to comprehensively assess the "movement" (recall the previous discussion of movement versus motion) of patients, athletes, and clients. Many would argue that assessment of movement is important before embarking on a physical performance endeavor because the ability to move provides the foundation for the ability to perform physical fitness activities, work and athletic tasks, and basic activities of daily living. It is important to be able to distinguish dysfunctional movement from "normal" movement during preparticipation or preseason screening, as well as during postinjury or postoperative rehabilitation. It is also important to acknowledge that training through or despite "poor" movement patterns reinforces poor quality of movement and is likely to increase the risk for injury and predispose to greater

Table 17-1 Difference between Screening, Testing, and Assessment

Term	Definition	Meaning
Screening	A system for selecting suitable people; to protect somebody from something unpleasant or dangerous	To create grouping and classification; to check risk
Testing	A series of questions, problems, or practical tasks to gauge knowledge, experience, or ability; measurement with no interpretation needed	To gauge ability
Assessment	To examine something; to judge or evaluate it; to calculate a value based on various factors	To estimate inability

levels of dysfunction.[4-6] Even highly skilled athletes may have fundamental imperfections in movement.

We propose that the astute sports medicine professional combine the tasks of screening, testing, and assessment to systematically ascertain the risk, ability, or inability of each athlete, patient, or client. The outcome of such a logical and refined procedure would provide the caregiver the best possible information to formulate opinions regarding readiness for participation or return to activities.

Therefore, screening might come first in the assessment process, and the outcome of a useful, practical movement screening tool or approach would allow the provider to do the following:

- Demonstrate movement patterns that produce pain within expected ranges of movement.
- Identify individuals with nonpainful but limited movement patterns who are likely to demonstrate higher potential risk for injury with exercise and activity.
- Identify specific exercises and activities to avoid until competency in the required movement is achieved.
- Identify and logically link screening movements to the most effective and efficient corrective exercise path to restore movement competency.
- Build a description of standardized, fundamental movement patterns against which broader movement can be compared.

Sahrmann, Kendall, and Janda have each offered valuable perspectives regarding human movement, posture, and function.[7-9] They have been instrumental in describing examination of structural, as well as functional, symmetry or lack thereof. Rehabilitation professionals have progressed from examination of isolated muscles and posture[7] to appreciation of the necessity of examining complex movement patterns.[9]

> There are numerous ways in which slight subtleties in movement patterns contribute to specific muscle weaknesses. The relationship between altered movement patterns and specific muscle weaknesses requires that remediation address the changes to the movement pattern; the performance of strengthening exercises alone will not likely affect the timing and manner of recruitment during functional performance.
>
> —Dr. Shirley Sahrmann

The transition from analysis of motion to analysis of functional movement and movement patterns helps rehabilitation providers discern the underlying cause of the dysfunction or imbalance. This paradigm shift propels rehabilitation providers toward the big picture, cause-and-effect, and regional interdependence thinking necessary for success in the 21st century.

Most would agree that it is difficult to qualitatively discern the quality of movement unless provided with a framework for making a judgment. Systematic screening, testing, and assessment of movement require not only a framework, but also benchmarks or criteria that define the proper method of performing a movement. We propose 3 possible general outcomes of movement assessment (Table 17-2) as determined by comparison between the movement performed by the athlete and predetermined descriptors of success.

Training through or despite identified "poor" movement patterns reinforces poor quality and increases the risk for injury, even during low-stress activities, and the possibility of progression to greater movement dysfunction. Training and functional exercise techniques and strategies are covered in Chapter 20; however, it is important to note here that that poor movement patterns must be identified and addressed before embarking on high-level functional training.

Table 17-2 Outcomes of Movement Assessment

Outcome	Description
Acceptable	Movement is good enough to allow the individual to be cleared for activity without an increase in risk for injury.
Unacceptable	Movements are dysfunctional and the individual may be at risk for injury unless movement patterns are improved.
Painful	Screening movements produce pain. Currently injured regions require additional, more advanced movement and physical assessment, including imaging, by a qualified health care provider.

Movement Related to Injury Potential and Return from Injury

The greatest risk for injury is a history of previous injury,[1-6] and this fact has been demonstrated in a wide variety of populations and athletes. Yet how might this relate to an uninjured athlete or worker? Are there certain "markers" or performance measures that could separate high-quality, proper or correct movement from low-quality, improper or incorrect movements? Conceptually, if movement is dysfunctional, all activities, including activities of daily living, work tasks, and athletic performance built on that dysfunction, may be flawed and predispose the individual to increased risk for the development of even greater dysfunction. This statement is true even when dysfunctional base movements are masked by apparently acceptable, age-appropriate, and even highly skilled performance. It is possible to move poorly and not experience pain, and, conversely, to move well and yet experience pain. Over time, poor movement patterns and dysfunctional movement strategies are likely to produce pain. An example might be a gymnast with an exaggerated lordosis that is "functional" for her sport but is likely, over time, to result in facet joint compression in the lumbar spine and decreased flexibility of the hip flexors. It is important to note that although poor movement patterns may increase risk for injury with activity, good movement patterns do not guarantee decreased risk for injury. It is the job of the astute health care professional to target and address identifiable risk factors, such as tight muscles, weak muscles, or poor balance or coordination, during movement and their biomechanical influences on movement. Once poor movement patterns are addressed, proper movement must be enhanced with appropriate strength, endurance, coordination, and skill development, but proper movement comes *first!*

The Functional Movement Screen and the Selective Functional Movement Assessment

The 2 movement assessment systems described in this chapter work together and use some common patterns of movement, but each possesses unique aspects. They serve to provide common language and "thinking" between a wide variety of health and fitness professions. Both are about the assessment of *quality* and not so much about the assessment of *quantity* of movement. Both stress the clinician's ability to rate performance quality, rank and describe the greatest dysfunction, and measure, if necessary, within the context of foundational, general movements.

The Functional Movement Screen

The Functional Movement Screen (FMS) is a predictive, but *not* diagnostic, functional screening system. The FMS is an evaluation or screening tool created for use by professionals who work with patients and clients for whom movement is a key part of exercise, recreation, fitness, and athletics. It may also be used for screening within the military, fire service, public safety, industrial laborers, and other highly active workers. This screening tool fills the void between preparticipation/preplacement screening and specific performance tests by examining individuals in a more general dynamic and functional capacity. Research suggests that tests that assess multiple facets of function such as balance, strength, range of motion (ROM), and motor control simultaneously may assist professionals in identifying athletes at risk for injury.[10-12]

The FMS, described by Cook et al,[13,14] is composed of 7 fundamental movement patterns that require a balance of mobility and stability for successful completion. These functional movement patterns were designed to provide observable performance tasks that relate to basic locomotive, manipulative, and stabilizing movements. The tests use a variety of common positions and movements appropriate for providing sufficient challenge to illuminate weakness, imbalance, or poor motor control. It has been observed that even individuals who perform at high functional levels during normal activities may be unable to perform these simple movements if appropriate mobility or stability is not present.[10,11] An important aspect of this assessment system is its foundation on principles of proprioception and kinesthesia. Proprioceptors must function in each segment of the kinetic chain and associated neuromuscular control must be present for efficient movement patterns to occur.

The FMS is not intended for use in individuals displaying pain during basic movement patterns or in those with documented musculoskeletal injuries. Painful movement is covered subsequently in the section on the SFMA. The FMS is for healthy, active people and for healthy, inactive people who want to increase their physical activity. Interrater reliability of the FMS has been reported by Minick et al[15] to be high, which means that the assessment protocol can be applied and reliable scores obtained by trained individuals when there is adherence to standard procedures.

The FMS consists of 7 movement patterns that serve as a comprehensive sample of functional movement (Box 17-1). Additionally, 3 clearing tests, each associated with one of the FMS movement patterns, assess for pain with shoulder rotation motions, trunk extension, or trunk flexion.

A kit for FMS testing is available commercially (www.performbetter.com); however, simple tools such as a dowel, 2 × 6 board, tape, tape measure, a piece of string or rope, and a measuring stick are enough to complete the testing procedures. When conducting the screening tests, athletes should not be bombarded with multiple instructions about how to perform the tests; rather, they should be positioned in the start position and offered simple commands to allow achievement of the test movement while observing their performance. The FMS is scored on an ordinal scale, with 4 possible scores ranging from 0 to 3 (Table 17-3). The clearing tests mentioned earlier consider only pain, which would indicate a "positive" clearing test and requires a score of 0 for the test with which it is associated.

Box 17-1 Seven Movement Patterns of the Functional Movement Screen

- Deep squat
- Hurdle step
- In-line lunge
- Shoulder mobility test
- Active straight-leg raise
- Trunk stability pushup
- Rotatory stability test

Table 17-3 Scoring System for the Functional Movement Screen

A Score of...	Is Given if...
0	At any time during testing the athlete has pain anywhere in the body. *Note:* The clearing tests consider only pain, which would indicate a "positive" clearing test and requires a score of 0 for the test with which it is associated.
1	The person is unable to complete the movement pattern or is unable to assume the position to perform the movement.
2	The person is able to complete the movement but must compensate in some way to complete the task.
3	The person performs the movement correctly, without any compensation.

Three is the highest or best score that can be achieved on any single test, and 21 is the best total score that can be achieved.

The majority of the movements test both the right and left sides, and it is important that the sides be scored independently. The lower score of the 2 sides is recorded and used for the total FMS score, with note made of any imbalances or asymmetry occurring during performance of the task (Figure 17-1). The creators of the FMS suggest that when in doubt, the athlete should be scored low.

Seven Movement Patterns of the Functional Movement Assessment

The Deep Squat (Figure 17-2) The squat is a movement needed in most athletic events; it is the "ready position" that is required for many power movements such as jumping and landing. The deep squat assesses bilateral, symmetric mobility and stability of the hips, knees, ankles, and core. The overhead position of the arms (holding the dowel) also assesses the mobility and symmetry of the shoulders and thoracic spine. To perform a deep squat, the athlete starts with the feet at approximately shoulder width apart in the sagittal plane. The dowel is grasped with both hands, and the arms are pressed overhead while keeping the dowel in line with the trunk and the elbows extended. The athlete is instructed to descend slowly and fully into a squat position while keeping the heels on the ground and the hands above the head.

FMS™ Test	Right	Left	Score	(for bilateral tests, eboose lowest score to record)
Overhead deep squat	X	X		
Trunk stability push-up	X	X		
Hurdle step (droped by among LE)				
In-line lunge (droped by forward LE)				
Shoulder mobility (droped by upper UE)				
Active straight leg raise				
Rotary stability (droped by among LE)				
Total Score			/21	

Figure 17-1 **Functional Movement Screen scoring sheet**

LE, Lower extremity; UE, upper extremity

The Hurdle Step (Figure 17-3) The hurdle step is designed to challenge the ability to stride, balance, and perform a single-limb stance during coordinated movement of the lower extremity (LE). The athlete assumes the start position by placing the feet together and aligning the toes just in contact with the base of the hurdle or 2 × 6 board. The height of the hurdle or string should be equal to the height of the tibial tubercle of the athlete. The dowel is place across the shoulders below the neck, and the athlete

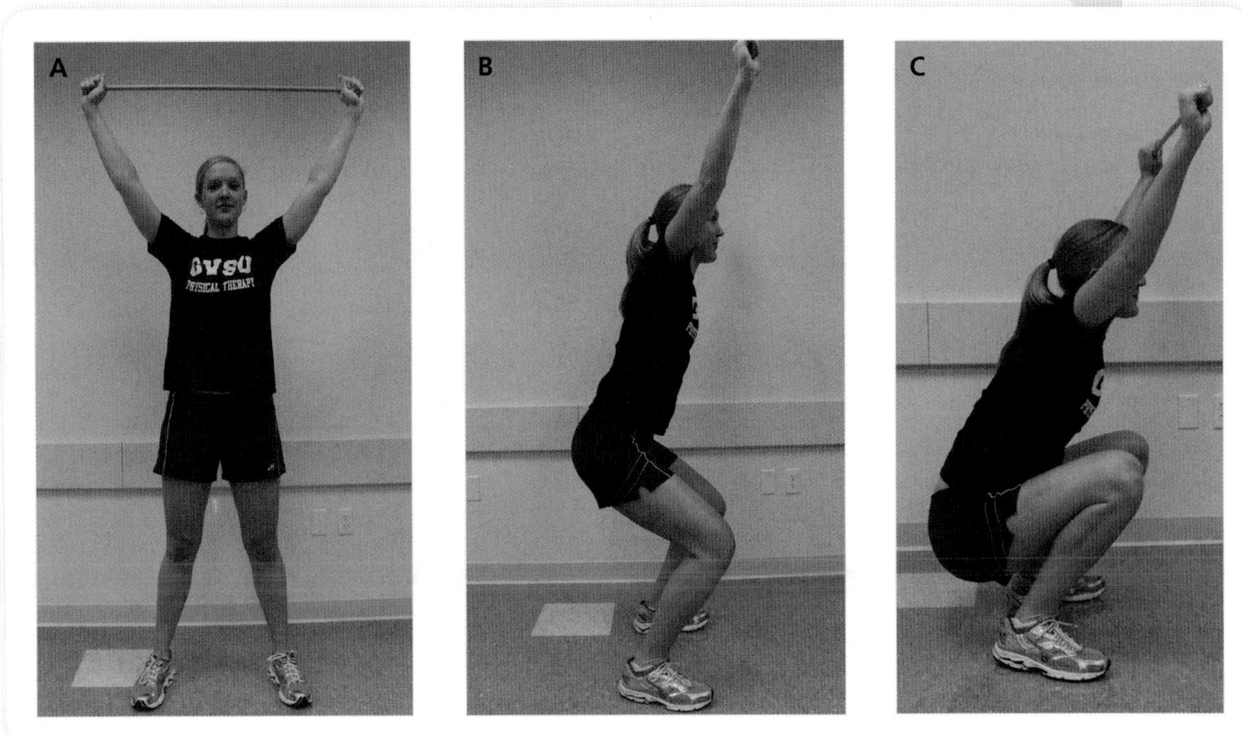

Figure 17-2 **Overhead deep squat maneuver**

Beginning (**A**) and end (**B**) of movement, frontal view, and midrange, side view (**C**).

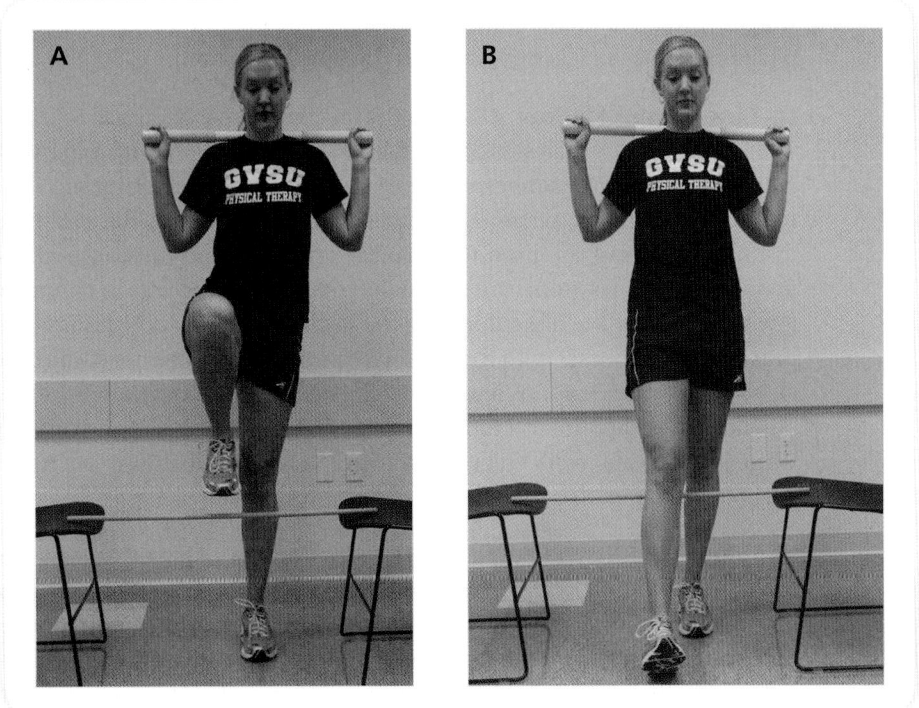

Figure 17-3 **Hurdle step maneuver**

Midmotion (**A**) and end motion (**B**) before return.

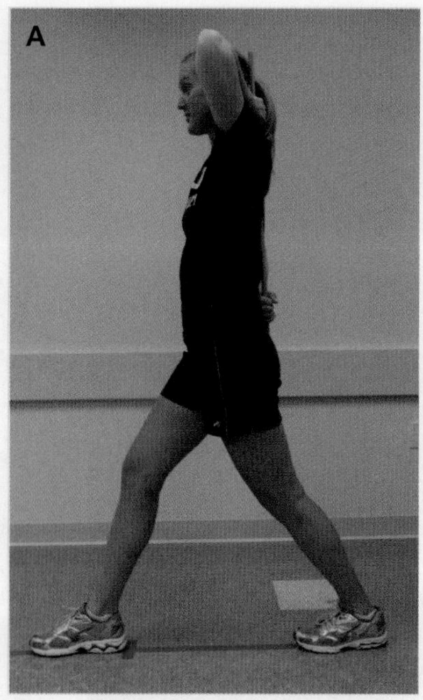

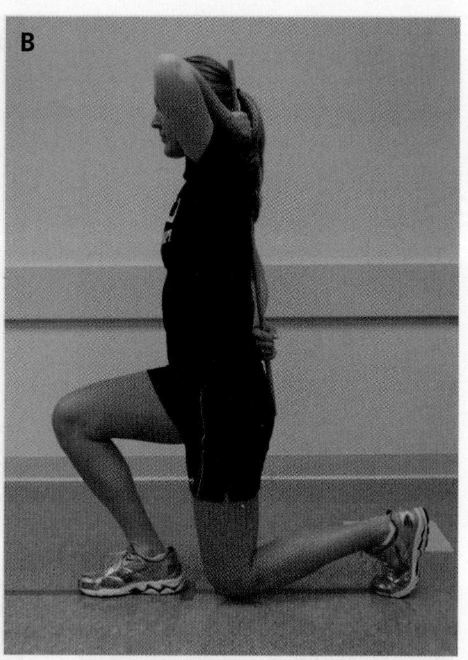

Figure 17-4 **In-line lunge**

Beginning (**A**) and end (**B**) of maneuver.

is asked to step up and over the hurdle, touch the heel to the floor (without accepting weight) while maintaining the stance leg in an extended position, and return to the start position. The leg that is stepping over the hurdle is scored.

In-Line Lunge (Figure 17-4) The in-line lunge attempts to challenge the athlete with a movement that simulates dynamic deceleration with balance and lateral challenge. Lunge length is determined by the tester by measuring the distance to the tibial tubercle. A piece of tape or a tape measure is placed on the floor at the determined lunge distance. The arms are used to grasp the dowel behind the back with the top arm externally rotated, the bottom arm internally rotated, and the fists in contact with the neck and low back region. The hand opposite the front or lunging foot should be on top. The dowel must begin in contact with the thoracic spine, back of the head, and sacrum. The athlete is instructed to lunge out and place the heel of the front/lunge foot on the tape mark. The athlete is then instructed to slowly lower the back knee enough to touch the floor while keeping the trunk erect and return to the start position. The front leg identifies the side being scored.

Shoulder Mobility (Figure 17-5) This mobility screen assesses bilateral shoulder ROM by combining rotation and abduction/adduction motions. It also requires normal scapular and thoracic mobility. Begin by determining the length of the hand of the athlete by measuring from the distal wrist crease to the tip of the third digit. This distance is used during scoring of the test. The athlete is instructed to make a fist with each hand with the thumb placed inside the fist. The athlete is then asked to place both hands behind the back in a smooth motion (without walking or creeping them upward)—the upper arm in an externally rotated, abducted position (with a flexed elbow) and the bottom arm in an internally rotated, extended, adducted position (also with a flexed elbow). The tester

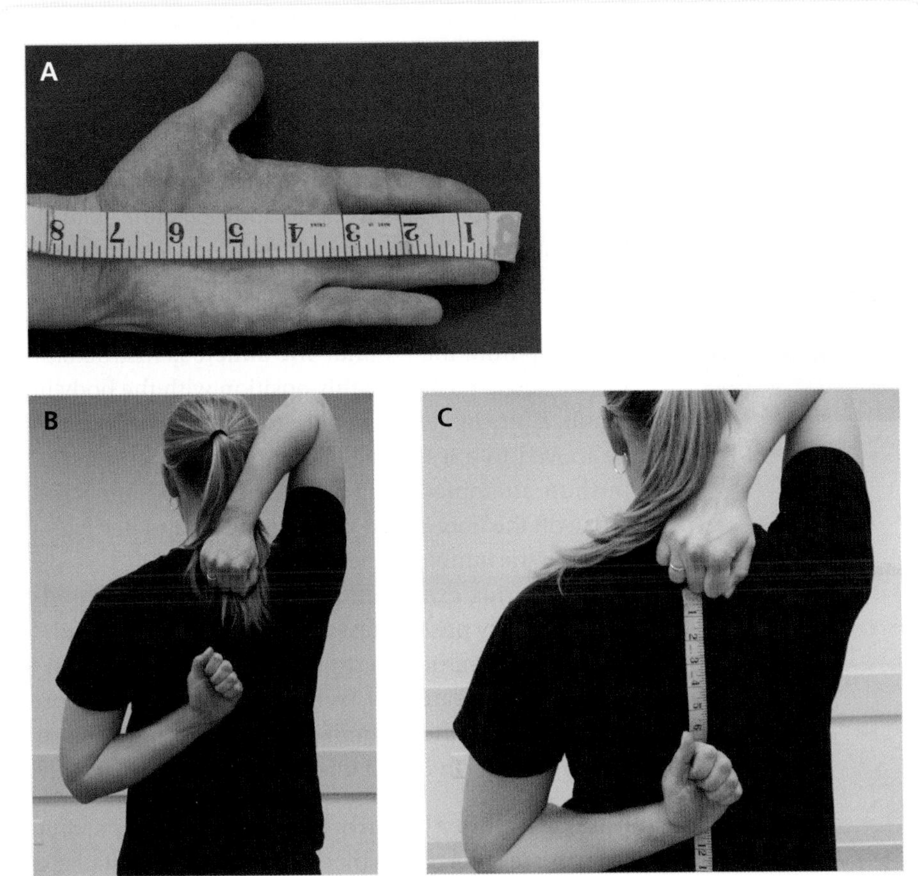

Figure 17-5 Shoulder mobility test

Hand measurement (**A**), at end of motion (**B**), and how motion is related to hand measurement (**C**).

measures the distance between the 2 fists. The flexed (uppermost) arm identifies the side being scored.

Shoulder Clearing Test (Figure 17-6) After the previous test is performed, the athlete places a hand on the opposite shoulder and attempt to point the elbow upward and touch the forehead (Yocum test). If painful, this clearing test is considered positive and the previous test must be scored as 0.

Active Straight-Leg Raise (Figure 17-7) This test assesses the ability to move the LE separately from the trunk, as well as tests for flexibility of the hamstring and gastrocnemius. The athlete begins in a supine position, arms at the side. The tester identifies the midpoint between the anterior superior iliac spine and the middle of the patella and places a dowel on the ground, held perpendicular to the ground. The athlete is instructed to slowly lift the test leg with a dorsiflexed ankle and a straight knee as far as possible while keeping the opposite leg extended and in contact with the ground. Make note to see where the LE ends at its maximal excursion. If the heel clears the dowel, a score of 3 is given; if the lower part of the leg (between the foot and the knee) lines up with the dowel, a score of 2 is given; and if the patient is only able to have the

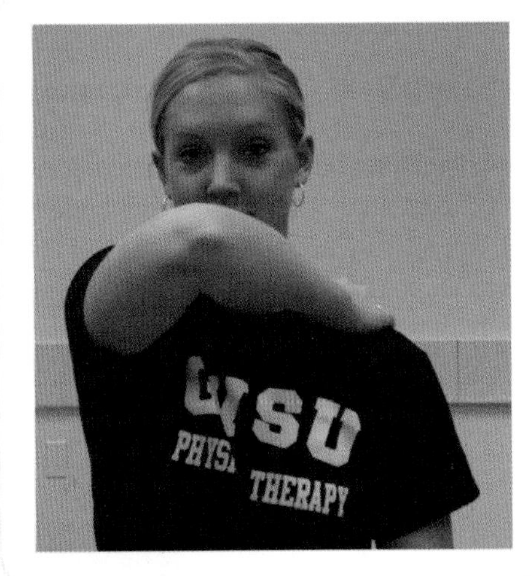

Figure 17-6

Screening test for shoulder, also known as the Yocum test. If positive for pain, the athlete scores 0 on the shoulder mobility test.

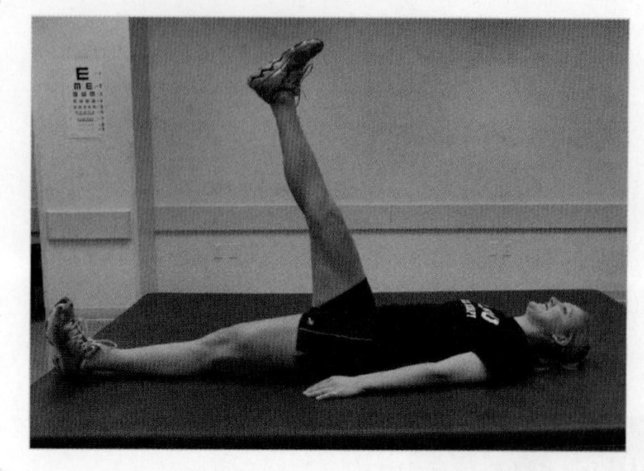

Figure 17-7

Active straight-leg raise test, end of motion.

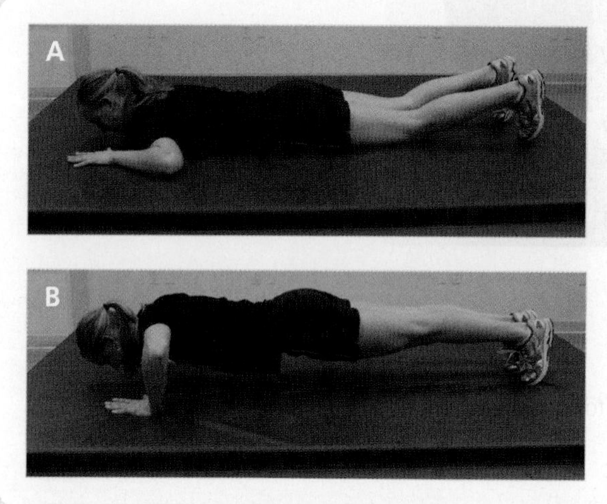

Figure 17-8 **Trunk stability pushup test**

Beginning of motion (**A**) and midmotion (**B**). Note that the hand position is for a score of 3 for females (thumbs at chin); to score a 2, females start with the thumbs at clavicular height. In males, a score of 3 is achieved with the thumbs at forehead level and a 2 with the thumbs at chin level.

thigh (between the knee and the hip) line up with the dowel, a score of 1 is given.

Trunk Stability Pushup (Figure 17-8) This test assesses the ability to stabilize the spine in anterior/posterior and sagittal planes during a closed-chain upper-body movement. The athlete assumes a prone position with the feet together, toes in contact with the floor, and hands placed shoulder width apart (level determined by gender per criteria described later) (Table 17-4), as though ready to perform a pushup from the ground. The athlete is instructed to perform a single pushup in this position with the body lifted as a unit. If the athlete is unable to do this, the hands should be moved to a less-challenging position per criteria and a pushup attempted again. The chest and stomach should come off the floor at the same instance, and no "lag" should occur in the lumbar spine.

A clearing examination is performed at the end of the trunk stability pushup test and graded as pass or fail, failure occurring when pain is experienced during the test. Spinal extension is cleared by using a full-range prone press-up maneuver from the beginning pushup position (Figure 17-9); if pain is associated with this motion, a score of 0 is given.

Rotary Stability (Figure 17-10) The rotary stability test is a complex movement that requires neuromuscular control of the trunk and extremities and the ability to transfer energy between segments of the body. It assesses multiplane stability during a combined upper extremity (UE) and LE motion. The athlete assumes the staring position of quadruped with the shoulders and hips at 90 degrees of flexion. The athlete is instructed to lift a hand off the ground and extend the same-side shoulder (allowing the elbow to flex) while concurrently lifting the knee off the ground and flexing the hip and knee. The athlete needs to raise the extremities only approximately 6 inches from the floor while bringing the elbow and knee together (see Figure 17-10*A* and *B*) until they touch and then return them to the ground. The test is repeated on the opposite side. The UE that moves during testing is scored. Completion of this task allows a score of 3. If unable to perform, the athlete is cued to perform the same maneuver with

Table 17-4 **Alignment Criteria for a Trunk Stability Pushup by Gender**

Position Level	Male	Female
III	Thumbs aligned with the forehead	Thumbs aligned with the chin
II	Thumbs aligned with the chin	Thumbs aligned with the clavicle

The athlete receives a score of 1 if unable to perform a pushup at level II.

the opposite LE and UE (see Figure 17-10*C* and *D*), which allows a score of 2 to be awarded. Inability to perform a diagonal (level II) stability results in a score of 1.

A clearing examination is performed at the end of this test and again is scored as positive if pain is reproduced. From the beginning position for this test, the athlete rocks back into spinal flexion and touches the buttocks to the heels and the chest to the thighs (Figure 17-11). The hands should remain in contact with the ground. Pain on this clearing test overrides any score for the rotary stability test and causes the athlete to receive a score of 0.

A total score of 21 is the highest possible score on the FMS, which implies excellent and symmetric (in tests that are performed bilaterally) performance of the variety of screening maneuvers. Total FMS scores have been investigated in relation to injury in National Football League football players[11] and in female collegiate soccer, basketball, and volleyball players.[10] Kiesel et al[11]

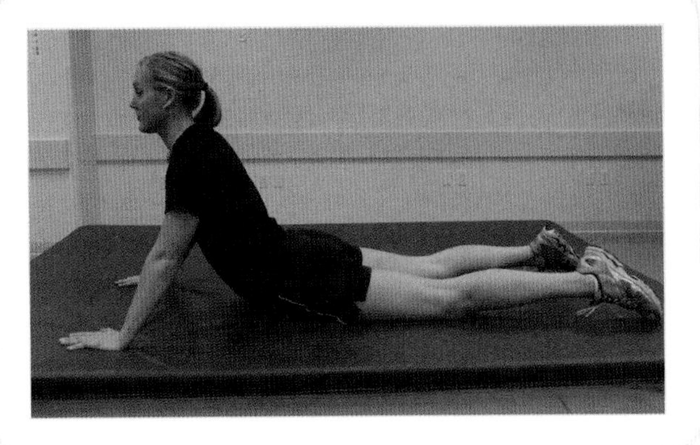

Figure 17-9 Screening (clearing) test for spinal extension

If positive for pain, the athlete scores 0 on the trunk stability pushup.

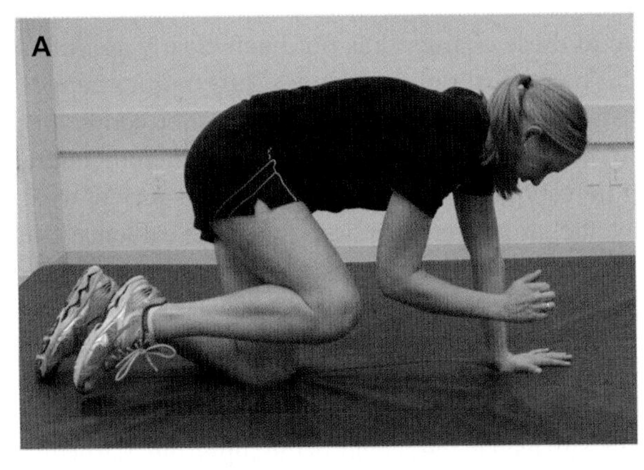

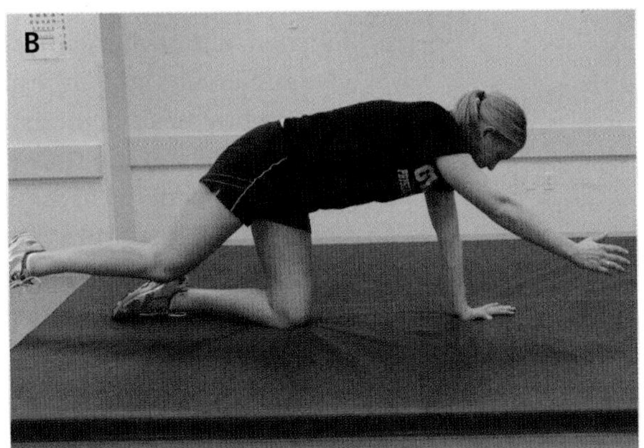

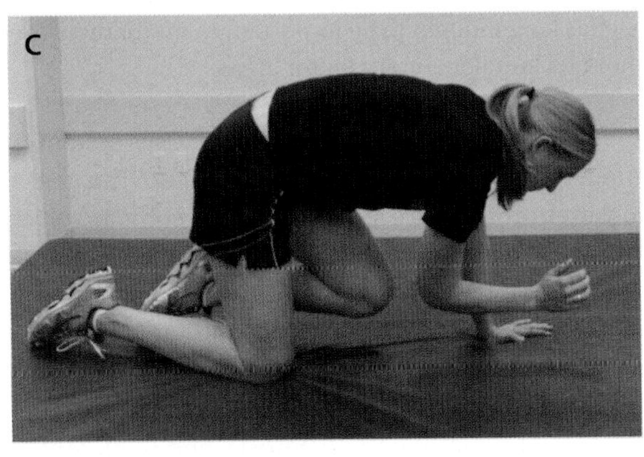

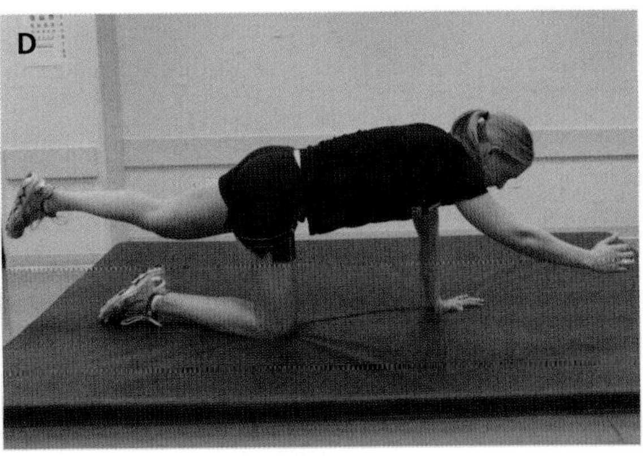

Figure 17-10 Rotary stability test

Flexed position for a score of 3 (**A**), extended position for a score of 3 (**B**), flexed position for a score of 2 (**C**), and extended position for a score of 2 (**D**).

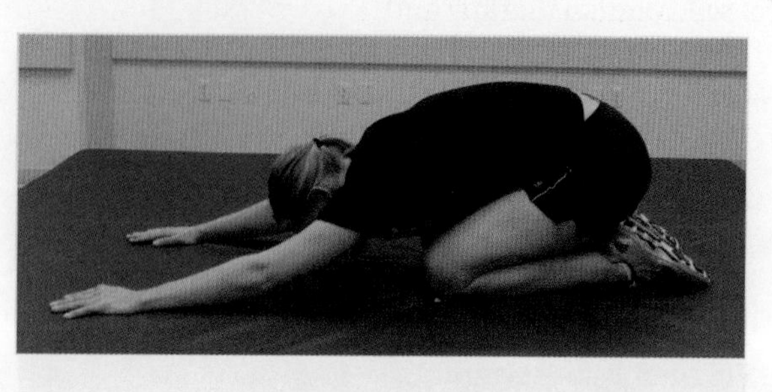

Figure 17-11 Screening test for spinal flexion

If positive for pain, the athlete scores 0 on the rotary stability test.

reported a 51% probability of football players sustaining a serious injury over the course of 1 season, and Chorba et al[10] found a significant correlation between low FMS scores (<14) in female athletes and injury. Furthermore, a score of 14 or less on the FMS resulted in an 11-fold increase in the chance of sustaining injury in professional football players and a 4-fold increase in the risk for LE injury in female collegiate athletes.[10,11] Okada et al[16] investigated the relationship between the FMS and tests of core stability and functional performance. Significant correlations between some of the FMS screening tests and performance tests of the upper and lower quarter were reported, but these correlations were not consistent among all screening maneuvers. No significant correlations were found between measures of core stability and FMS variables.

The Selective Functional Movement Assessment

Musculoskeletal pain is the reason that most patients seek medical attention. The contemporary understanding of pain has moved beyond the traditional tissue damage model to include the cognitive and behavioral facets. Most scientists accept that pain alters motor function, although the mechanism of these changes has not been clearly identified. The central nervous system response to painful stimuli is complex, but motor changes have consistently been demonstrated and seem to be influenced by higher centers, consistent with a change in transmission of the motor command. The human body migrates to predictable patterns of movement in response to injury and in the presence of weakness, tightness, or structural abnormality. Richardson et al[17] summarized the evidence that pain alters motor control at higher levels of the central nervous system than previously thought by stating,

> Consistent with the identification of changes in motors planning, there is compelling evidence that pain has strong effects at the supraspinal level. Both short- and long-term changes are thought to occur with pain in the activity of the supraspinal structures including the cortex. One area that has been consistently found to be affected is the anterior cingulated cortex, which has long thought to be important in motor responses with its direct projections to motor and supplementary motor areas.[17]

The SFMA is a movement-based diagnostic system for clinical use. This system is used by professionals working with patients experiencing pain on movement. The goal of the SFMA is to observe and capture the patterns of posture and function for comparison against a baseline. It uses movement to provoke symptoms, demonstrate limitations, and offer information regarding movement pattern deficiency related to the patient's primary complaint. The SFMA uses a series of movements with a specific organizational method to rank the quality of functional movements and, when suboptimal, identify the source of provocation of symptoms during movement. The SFMA has been refined and expanded to help the health care professional in musculoskeletal examination, diagnosis, and treatment geared toward choosing the optimal rehabilitative and therapeutic interventions. It helps the clinician identify the most dysfunctional movement patterns, which are then assessed in detail. By identifying all facets of dysfunction within multiple patterns, specific targeted therapeutic interventions designed to capture or illuminate tightness, weakness, poor mobility, or poor stability can be chosen. Thus, the facets of movement identified to most represent or define the dysfunction and thereby affect movement can be addressed. Manual therapy and corrective exercises are focused on movement dysfunction, not pain.

The SFMA is one way of quantifying the qualitative assessment of functional movement and is not a substitute for the traditional examination process. Rather, the SFMA is the first step in a functional orthopedic examination process that serves to focus and direct choices made during the remaining portions of the examination that are pertinent to the functional needs of the patient. The approach taken with the SFMA places less emphasis on identifying the source of the symptoms and more on identifying the cause. An example of this assessment scheme is illustrated by a runner with low back pain. Frequently, the symptoms associated with low back pain are not examined in light of other secondary causes such as hip mobility. Lack of mobility at the hip may be compensated for by increased mobility or instability of the spine. The global approach taken by the SFMA would identify the cause of the low back dysfunction.

We believe it is important to start with a whole-body functional approach, such as the SFMA, before specific impairment assessments, to direct the evaluation in a systematic and constructive manner. Unfortunately, a functional orthopedic examination often involves provocation of symptoms. Provocation of symptoms may occur during the interplay of posture tests, movement in transition, and specific movement tests. Production of these symptoms creates the road map that the clinician will follow to a more specific diagnosis:

- Once symptoms have been provoked, the clinician should work backwards to a more specific breakdown of the component parts of the movement.
- Inconsistencies observed between provocation of symptoms that are not the result of symptom magnification may suggest a stability problem.
- Consistent limitations and provocation of symptoms can be indicative of a mobility problem.

The functional assessment process emphasizes analysis of function to restore proper movement for specific physical tasks. Use of movement patterns and the application of specific stress and overpressure assist in determining whether dysfunction or pain (or both) are present. The movement patterns will reaffirm hypotheses or redirect the clinician to the cause of the musculoskeletal problem. As an example, the SFMA standing rotation test (Figure 17-12) is performed with the patient's feet planted side-by-side and stationary. The subject makes a complete rotation with segments of the entire body first in one direction and then in the other. When consistent production of pain in the left thoracic spine is noted during standing left rotation, the same maneuver can be repeated in the seated posture (Figure 17-13). The 2 motions, although similar in demands for spinal rotation, have several differences; with the hips and lower extremities removed from the movement, an entirely different level of postural control may result.

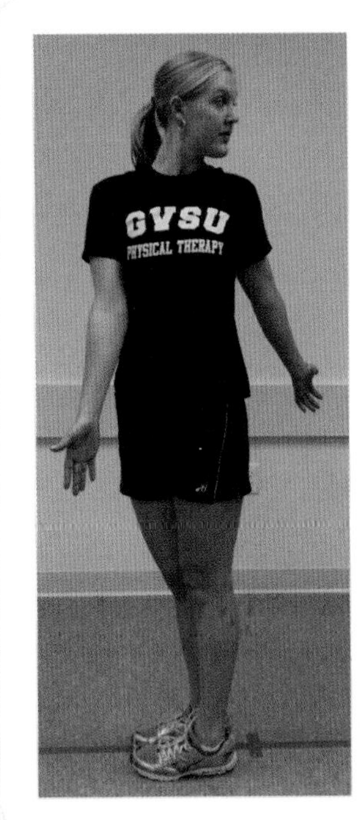

Figure 17-12 Total-body rotation test while standing

When nearly the same provocation of symptoms and limitations at the same degree of left rotation are noted during both standing and seated, the cause may be an underlying mobility problem somewhere in the spine. Alternatively, if the seated rotation does not produce a consistent limitation and provocation of symptoms in the same direction and to the same degree, a stability problem might be present. This change in position results in a different degree of postural alignment, muscle tone, proprioception, muscle activation or inhibition, and reflex stabilization. The clinician must investigate the lower body component of this problem. Once consistency or inconsistency is observed with respect to limitation of movement or provocation of symptoms, the clinician should continue to look for other instances that support the suspicion.

Maintaining or restoring proper movement of specific segments is key to preventing or correcting musculoskeletal pain. The SFMA also identifies where

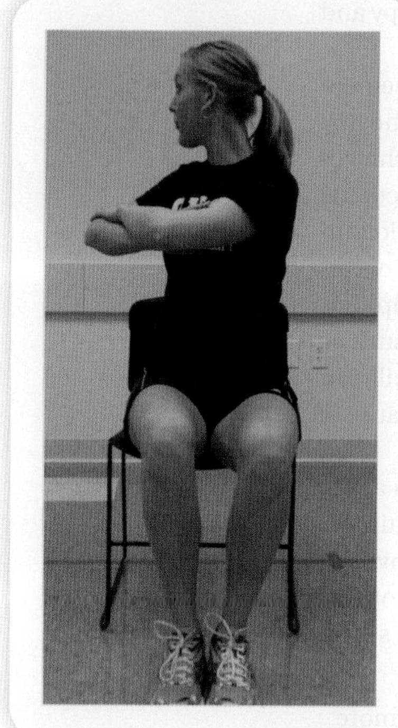

Figure 17-13 Spinal rotation in the sitting, unloaded position

functional exercise may be beneficial and provides feedback regarding the effectiveness of such exercise. A functional approach to exercise uses key specific movements that are common to the patient regardless of the specific activity or sport. Exercise that uses repeated movement patterns required for desired function is not only realistic but also practical and time efficient. Such functional exercises are discussed in Chapter 18.

Scoring System for the Selective Functional Movement Assessment

The hallmark of the SFMA is the use of simple, basic movements to reveal natural reactions and responses by the patient. These movements should be viewed in both loaded and unloaded conditions whenever possible and bilaterally to examine functional symmetry. The SFMA uses seven basic movement patterns (Box 17-2) to rate and rank the 2 variables of pain and function. In addition, 4 optional tests can be used to further refine movement dysfunction.

The term *functional* describes any unlimited or unrestricted movement. The term *dysfunctional* describes movements that are limited or restricted in some way because of lack of mobility, stability, or symmetry within a given movement pattern. *Painful* denotes a situation in which the selective functional movement reproduces symptoms, increases symptoms, or brings about secondary symptoms that need to be noted. Therefore, by combining the words *functional, dysfunctional, painful,* and *nonpainful,* each pattern of the SFMA must be scored with one of 4 possible outcomes (Table 17-5).

Basic Movements in the Selective Functional Movement Assessment

The 7 basic movements or motions included in the SFMA screen look simple but require good flexibility and control. They are referred to as "top-tier" tests or patterns. A patient who is (a) unable to perform a movement correctly, (b) shows a major limitation in 1 or more of the movement patterns, or (c) demonstrates an obvious difference between the left and right sides of the body has exposed a significant finding that may be the key to correcting the problem. The 7 basic movements of the SFMA are described in the following sections.

Cervical Spine Assessment (Figure 17-14)

- The cervical spine is cleared for pain and dysfunction by the patient actively demonstrating three patterns of motion: flexion (both upper and lower cervical), extension, and cervical rotation with side bending.

Box 17-2 Movement Patterns of the Selective Functional Movement Assessment

Seven Basic Movements	Four Optional Movements
Cervical spine assessment	Plank with a twist
Upper-extremity movement pattern assessment	Single-leg squat
Multisegmental flexion assessment	In-line lunge with lean, press, and lift
Multisegmental extension assessment	Single-leg hop for distance
Multisegmental rotation assessment	
Single-leg stance (standing knee lift) assessment	
Overhead deep squat assessment	

Table 17-5 Scoring System for the Selective Functional Movement Assessment Based on Function and Pain Reproduction

Label of Outcome of Pattern Performance	Description of Outcome
Functional nonpainful (FN)	Unlimited, unrestricted movement that is performed without pain or increased symptoms
Functional painful (FP)	Unlimited, unrestricted movement that reproduces or increases symptoms or brings on secondary symptoms
Dysfunctional painful (DP)	Movement that is limited or restricted in some way because of lack of mobility, stability, or symmetry; reproduces or increases symptoms; or brings on secondary symptoms
Dysfunctional nonpainful	Movement that is limited or restricted in some way because of lack of mobility, stability, or symmetry and is performed without pain or increased symptoms

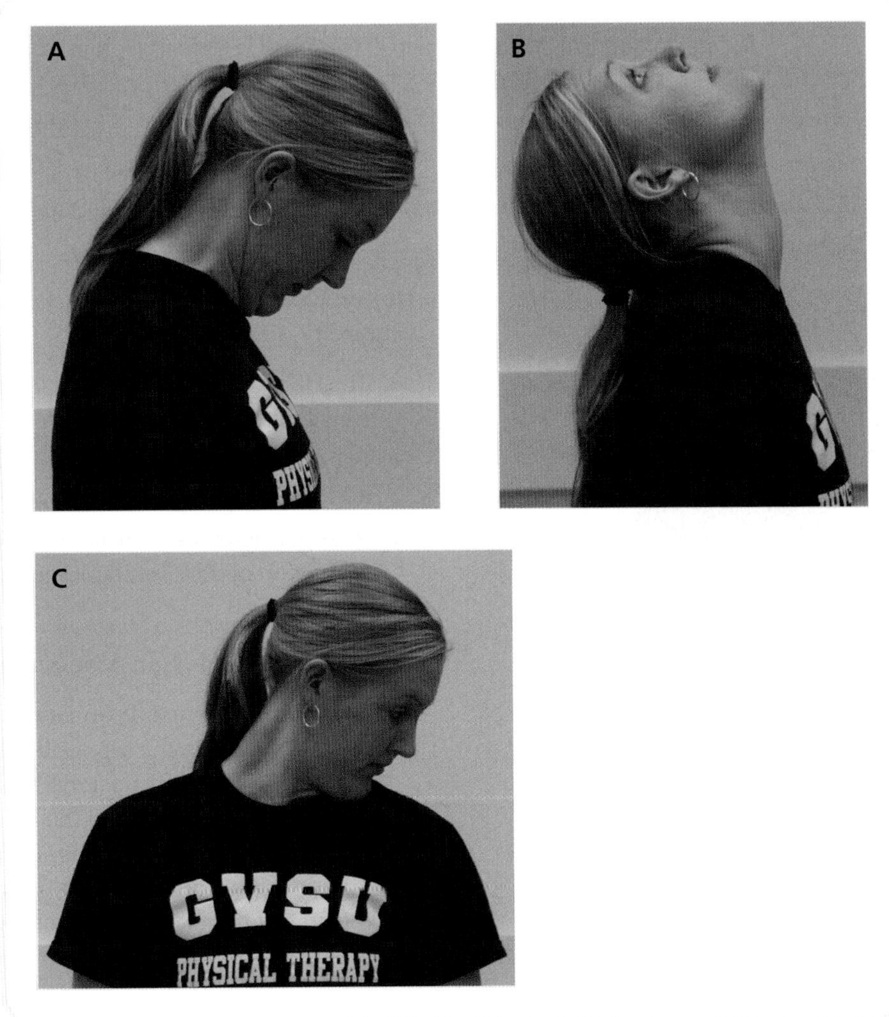

Figure 17-14 Cervical spine assessment

Flexion (**A**), extension (**B**), and combined side bending/rotation (**C**).

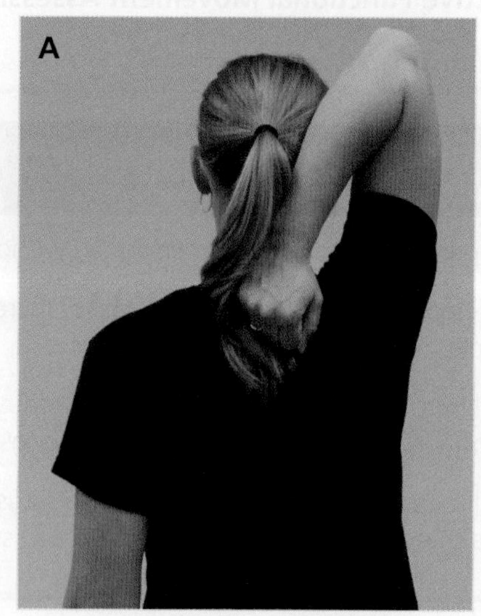

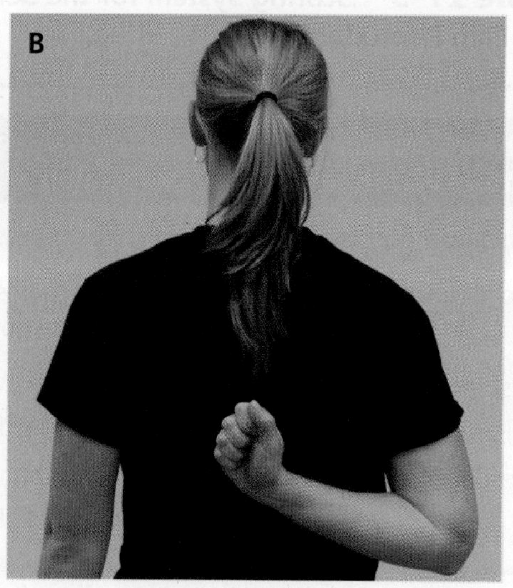

Figure 17-15 **Shoulder mobility tests**

A. Internal rotation, adduction, and extension. **B.** External rotation, abduction, and flexion.

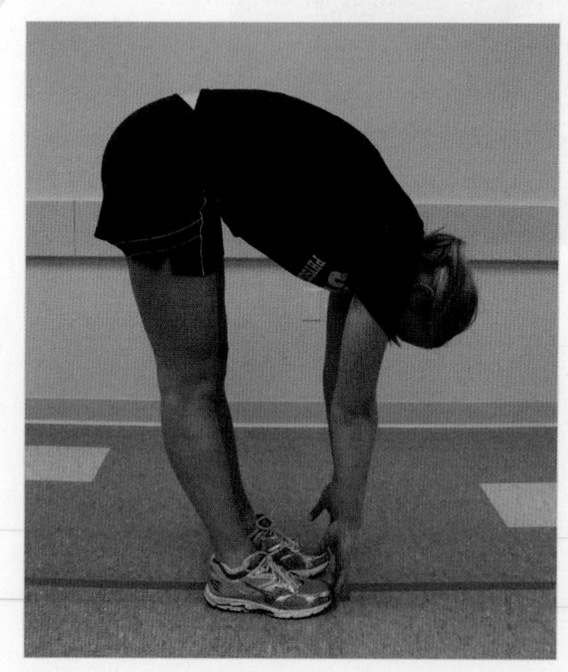

Figure 17-16 **Multisegmental flexion test: end of maneuver**

Note the straight legs, posterior weight shift, and distributed spinal curves.

Upper Extremity Movement Pattern Assessments (Figure 17-15)

- The UE movement pattern assessments check for total ROM in the shoulder.
- Pattern 1 assesses internal rotation-extension, and adduction of the shoulder (Figure 17-15*A*).
- Pattern 2 assesses external rotation, flexion, and abduction of the shoulder (Figure 17-15*B*).

Multisegmental Flexion Assessment (Figure 17-16)

- The multisegmental flexion assessment tests for normal flexion in the hips and spine. The patient assumes the starting position by standing erect with the feet together and the toes pointing forward. The patient then bends forward at the hips and spine and attempts to touch the ends of the fingers to the tips of the toes without bending the knees.
- Observe for the following criteria to be met:
  - Posterior weight shift
  - Touching the toes
  - Uniform curve of the lumbar spine
  - No lateral spinal bending

Multisegmental Extension Assessment (Figure 17-17)

- The multisegmental extension assessment tests for normal extension in the shoulders, hips, and spine. The patient assumes the starting position by standing erect with the feet together and the toes pointing forward. The patient should raise the arms directly overhead and observe the response.
- The arms are then lowered back to the starting position while the examiner looks for synchrony and symmetry of scapular motion.
  - The ability to move one body part independently of another is called *dissociation.* Dissociation problems can be caused by poor stabilizing patterns that do not allow full mobility and stability at the same time. If the patient can maintain stability only by limiting limb or trunk movement, the patient is functionally rigid rather than dynamically stable. The patient may appear to have a restriction in mobility when in fact the true dysfunction is inadequate postural or motor control. As the patient raises the arms overhead, the clinician observes for the ability to move only one body part and that bilateral symmetry is present. The ideal response is for the patient to raise the arms 180 degrees with the pelvis maintaining a neutral position.
- The patient raises the arms back up to over the head with the elbows in line with the ear. The midhand line should clear the posterior aspect of the shoulder at the end range of shoulder flexion. The elbows should remain extended and in line with the ears. At this point have the patient bend backwards as far as possible while making sure that the hips go forward and the arms go back simultaneously. The spine of the scapula should move posteriorly enough to clear the heels. Both anterior superior iliac spines should move anteriorly, past the toes.
- Observe for the following criteria to be met:
  - The anterior superior iliac spine must clear the toes. Forward rotation of the pelvis will pull the lumbar spine out of a neutral position into extension. The pelvis slides forward by shifting body weight toward the front of the feet and again pulls the lumbar spine out of neutral.
  - Symmetric spinal curves should be present and the spine of the scapula must clear a vertical line drawn from the patient's heels.
  - Arms/elbows in line with the ears represent 180 degrees of shoulder flexion.

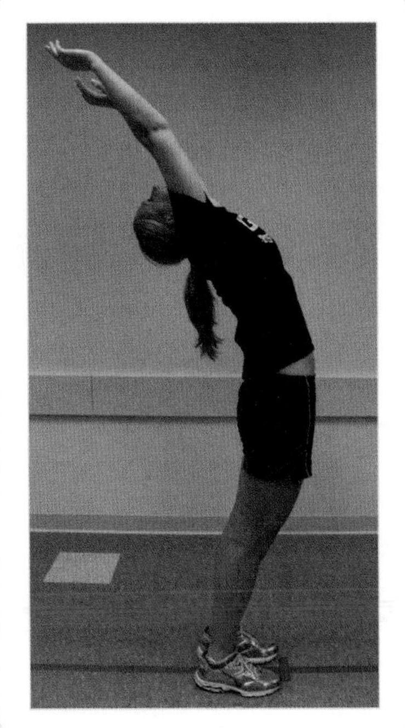

Figure 17-17 Multisegmental extension test: end of maneuver

Note the anterior shift of the pelvis, extension of the upper extremities, and distribution of spinal curves.

Multisegmental Rotation Assessment (Figure 17-18)

- The multisegmental rotation assessment examines the total rotational motion available from the foot to the top of the spine. Usually, rotation occurs as a result of many parts contributing to the total motion. This assessment tests rotational mobility in the trunk, pelvis, hips, knees, and feet. The patient assumes a starting position by standing erect with the feet together, toes pointing forward, and arms relaxed to the sides at about waist height.

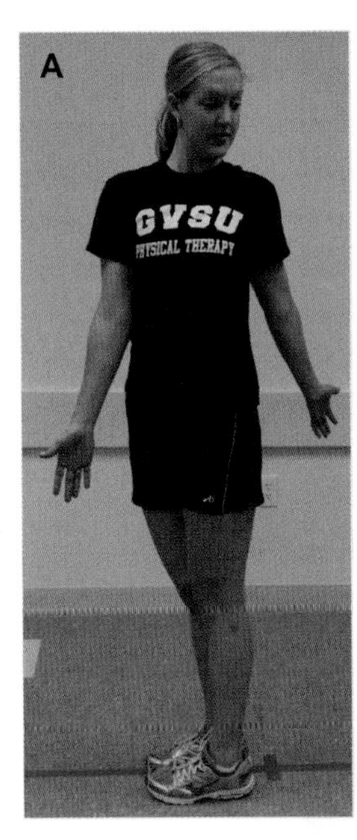

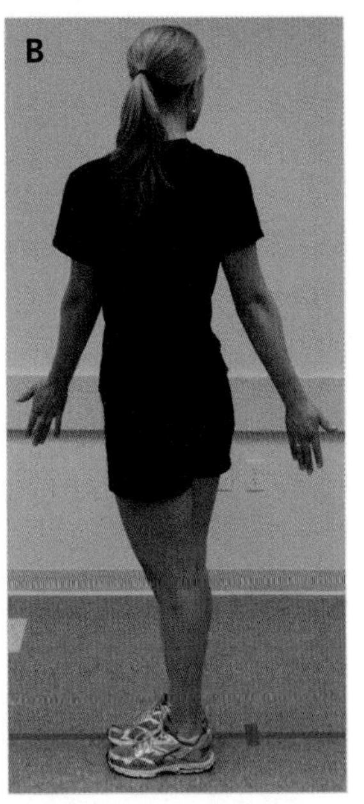

Figure 17-18 Multisegmental rotation test

Start of maneuver (**A**) and end of maneuver (**B**). Note the rotation at the pelvis and trunk and the upright posture.

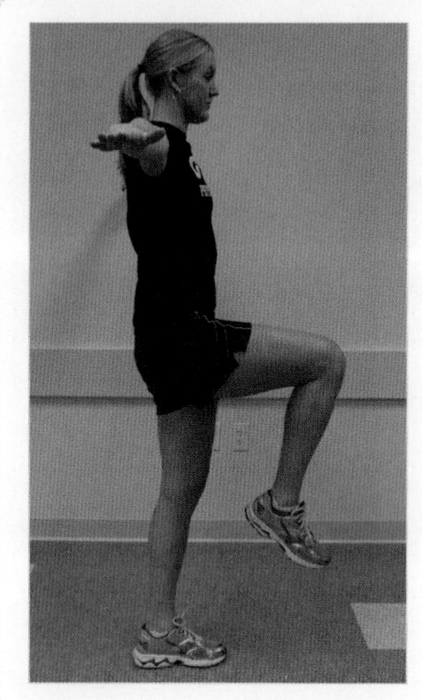

Figure 17-19 Single-limb stance, eyes open

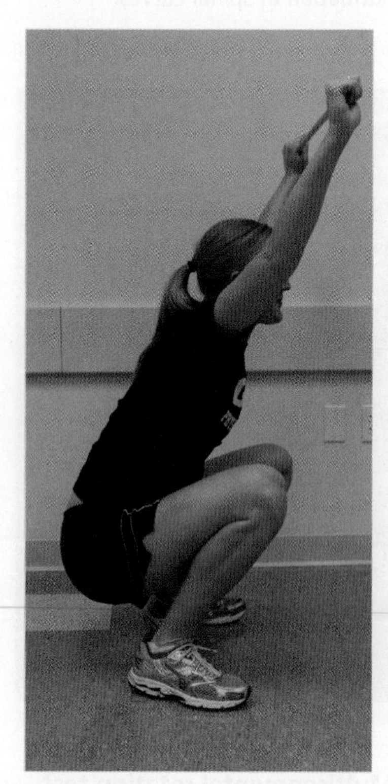

Figure 17-20 Overhead deep squat

The patient then rotates the entire body as far as possible to the right while the foot position remains unchanged. The patient returns to the starting position and then rotates toward the left.

- There should be at least 50 degrees of rotation from the starting position of the pelvis and lower quarter bilaterally.
- In addition to the 50 degrees of pelvic rotation, there should also be at least 50 degrees of rotation from the thorax bilaterally, for a combined total of 100 degrees of total-body rotation from the starting position.

- Observe for the following criteria to be met:
  - Pelvis rotating greater than 50 degrees
  - Trunk rotating greater than 50 degrees
  - No loss of body height with the rotation testing
  - *Note:* Because both sides are tested simultaneously with the feet together, the externally rotating hip is also extending and can thus limit motion. Close attention should be paid to each segment of the body. One area may be hypermobile because of restriction in an adjacent segment. Rotation should be symmetric on each side (within 10 degrees).

Single-Leg Stance (Standing Knee Lift) Assessment (Figure 17-19)

- The single-leg stance assessment evaluates the ability to independently stabilize on each leg in a static and dynamic posture. The static portion of the test looks at the fundamental foundation for control of movement. The patient assumes the starting position by standing erect with the feet together, toes pointing forward, and arms raised out to the side at shoulder height. The patient should be instructed to stand tall before testing. The patient should lift the right leg up so that the hip and knee are both flexed to 90 degrees. The patient should maintain this posture for 10 seconds. The test is repeated on the left leg. The examiner should look to see whether the patient maintains a level pelvis (no Trendelenburg position present).

- The test is repeated again with the eyes closed. The body has 3 main systems that contribute to balance: visual, vestibular, and somatosensory. When the eyes are closed and vision is eliminated, the patient must rely on the other 2 systems to maintain an upright posture.
  - Foot position should remain unchanged throughout the movement, and the hands should remain resting on the hips.
  - Look for loss of posture or height when moving from 2 to 1 leg. Any of the 3 portions of the test are scored as dysfunctional if the patient loses posture.

Overhead Deep Squat Assessment (Figure 17-20)

- Same as used in the FMS.
- The overhead deep squat assessment tests for bilateral mobility of the hips, knees, and ankles. When combined with the overhead UE position, this test also assesses bilateral mobility of the shoulders, as well as extension of the thoracic spine.

- The patient assumes the starting position by placing the instep of the feet in vertical alignment with the outside of the shoulders. The feet should be in the sagittal plane, with no external rotation of the feet. The patient then raises the arms overhead, arms abducted slightly wider than shoulder width and the elbows fully extended. The patient slowly descends as deeply as possible into a full squat position. The squat position should be attempted while maintaining the heels on the floor, the head and chest facing forward, and the hands overhead. The knees should be aligned over the feet with no valgus collapse.
  - Hand width should not increase as the patient descends into the squat position.
  - The UEs and hands should not deviate from the plane of the tibias as the squat is performed.
  - The ability to perform this test requires closed chain dorsiflexion of the ankles, flexion of the hips and knees, extension of the thoracic spine, and flexion abduction of the shoulders.

Each movement is graded with a notation of functional nonpainful, functional painful, dysfunctional painful, or dysfunctional nonpainful (see Table 17-5). All responses other than functional nonpainful are then assessed in greater detail to help refine the movement information and direct the clinical testing. Detailed algorithmic SFMA breakouts are available for each of the movement patterns, but they are beyond the scope of this chapter to describe in detail.

Optional Movements of the Selective Functional Movement Assessment

In addition to the SFMA top-tier or base assessments, four optional assessments have recently been added to further refine the movement dysfunction. They serve to illuminate movement dysfunction in higher-functioning patients.

Once dysfunction, or symptoms, or both, have been provoked in a functional manner, it is necessary to work backwards to more specific assessments of the component parts of the functional movement by using special tests or ROM comparisons. As the gross functional movement is broken down into its component parts, the clinician should examine for consistencies and inconsistencies, as well as the level of dysfunction, in each test with respect to the optimal movement pattern. Provocation of symptoms, as well as limitations in movement or an inability to maintain stability during movements, should be noted.

Further Refinement of Movement Dysfunction: Using the Breakouts

Once dysfunction is noted, the clinician can use the SFMA to systematically dissect each of the major pattern dysfunctions with breakout algorithms. The breakouts provide an algorithmic approach to testing all areas potentially involved in the dysfunction to isolate limitations or determine dysfunction by the process of elimination. The breakouts include active and passive movements, weightbearing and non-weightbearing positions, multiple-joint and single-joint functional movement assessments, and unilateral and bilateral challenges. By performing parts of the test movements in both loaded and unloaded conditions, the clinician can draw conclusions about the interplay between the patient's available mobility and stability. If any of the top-tier movements are restricted when performed in the loaded position (eg, limited or in some way painful before the end of ROM), a clue is provided regarding functional movement. For example, if a movement is performed easily (does not provoke symptoms or have any limitation) in an unloaded situation, it would seem logical that the appropriate joint ROM and muscle flexibility exist and therefore a stability problem may be the reason why the patient cannot perform the movement in a loaded position. In this case, a patient has the requisite available biomechanical ability to go through the necessary ROM to perform the task, but the neurophysiologic response needed for stabilization that creates dynamic alignment and postural support is not available when the functional movement is performed.

If the patient is observed to have limitation, restriction, or pain when unloaded, the patient displays consistent abnormal biomechanical behavior of one or more joints and would therefore require specific clinical assessment of each relevant joint and muscle complex to identify the barriers that are restricting movement and may be responsible for the provocation of pain. Consistent limitation and provocation of symptoms in both the loaded and unloaded conditions may be indicative of a mobility problem. True restrictions in mobility often require appropriate manual therapy in conjunction with corrective exercise.

The SFMA breakout testing applies the same categorizations as its top-tier assessment, with isolated focus on each pattern demonstrating pain or dysfunction. This focus helps identify gross limitations in mobility and stability. Recall that the SFMA uses specific descriptors to identify dysfunction in both mobility and stability, as described earlier in this chapter.

- Tissue extensibility dysfunction involves tissues that are extraarticular. Examples can include active or passive muscle insufficiency, neural tension, fascial tension, muscle shortening, scarring, and fibrosis.
- Joint mobility dysfunction involves structures that are articular or intraarticular. Examples can include osteoarthritis, fusion, subluxation, adhesive capsulitis, and intraarticular loose bodies.

Figure 17-21 provides an example of the overhead deep squat pattern breakout. As can be seen on the algorithm, the clinician is directed to move from a weighted to an unweighted posture, and active and passive movements are used to systematically isolate all the different variables that could cause dysfunction during the overhead deep squat.

How to Interpret the Results of Selective Functional Movement Assessment

Once the SFMA has been completed, the clinician should be able to: (a) Identify the major sources of dysfunction and movements that are affected. (b) Identify patterns of movement that cause pain, with reproduction of pain indicating either mechanical deformation or an inflammatory process affecting nociceptors in the symptomatic structures. The key follow-up question must be, "Which of the functional movements caused the tissue to become painful?" (c) Once the pattern of dysfunction has been identified, the problem is classified as dysfunction of either mobility or stability to determine where intervention should commence.

With the SFMA, treatment is not about alleviating mechanical pain; rather, the SFMA guides the clinician to begin by choosing interventions designed to improve the dysfunctional nonpainful patterns first. This philosophy of intervention does not ignore the source of pain; instead, it takes the approach of removing the mechanical dysfunction that caused the tissues to become symptomatic in the first place.

Pain-free functional movement is the goal for all. It is requisite for work performance, athletic success, and healthy aging. The pain-free functional movement necessary to allow participation in activities of daily living, work, and athletics has many components: posture, ROM, muscle performance, and motor control. Impairments in any of these components can potentially alter functional movement. The authors believe that the SFMA incorporates the essential elements of many daily, work, and sports activities and provides a schema for addressing movement-related dysfunction. (More information can be found at www.Rehabeducation.com.) Appendices A5 to A-7 are examples of score sheets used with the SFMA.

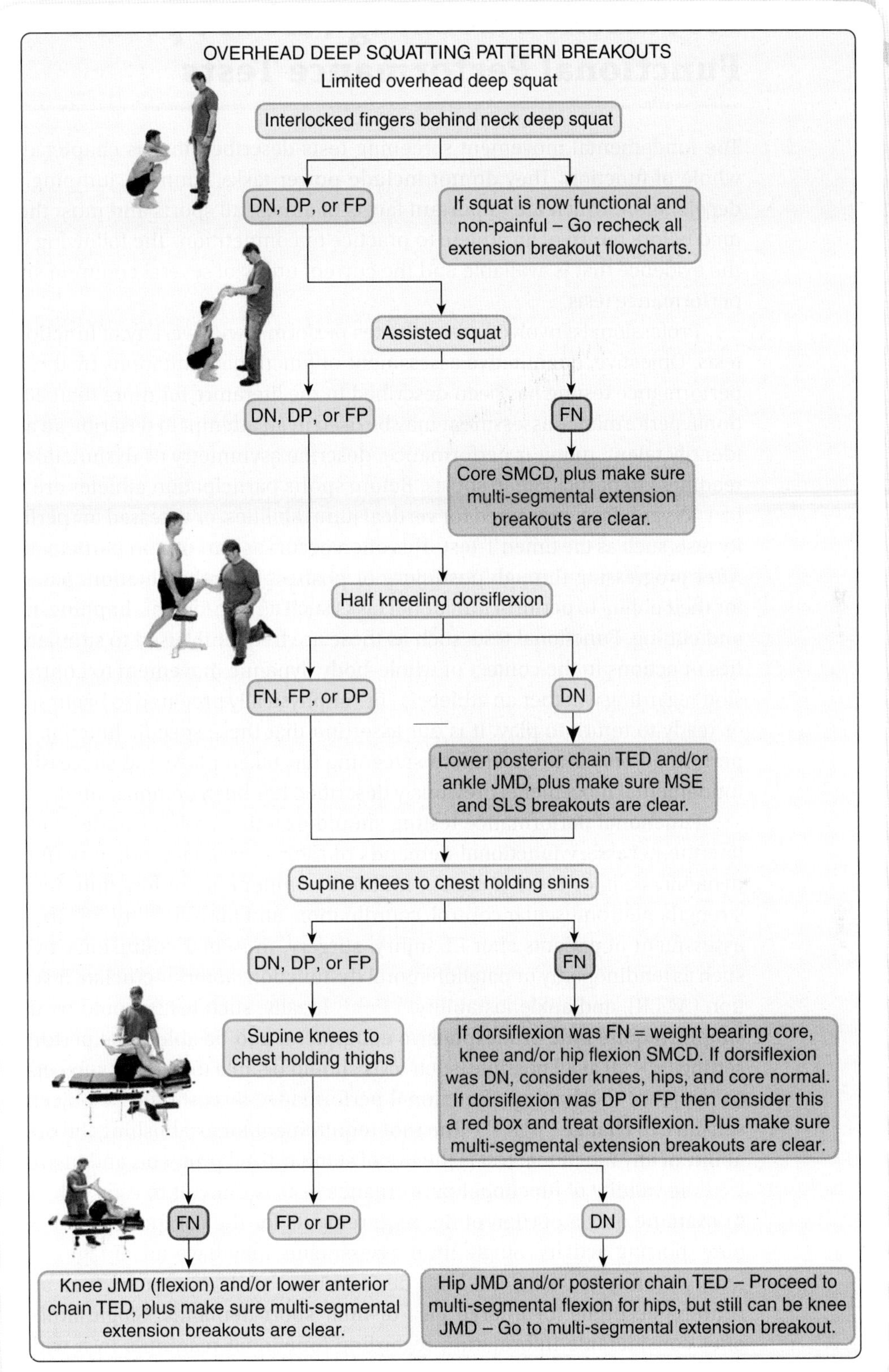

Figure 17-21

Overhead deep squat pattern breakout. DN, Dysfunctional nonpainful; DP, dysfunctional painful; FN, functional nonpainful; FP, functional painful; JMD, joint mobility dysfunction; MSE, multisegmental extension; SLS, single leg stance; SMCD, stability motor control dysfunction; TED, tissue extensibility dysfunction.

Movement Screening versus Specific Functional Performance Tests

The fundamental movement screening tests described in this chapter do not assess the whole of function. They do not include power tasks, running, jumping, acceleration, or deceleration, which are important facets of almost all sports and must therefore be examined before return of an athlete to practice or competition. The following section discusses the evidence that is available and the current utility of several common specific functional performance tests.

Professionals involved with athletes perform a wide variety of functional performance tests. Objective, quantitative assessment of functional limitations by the use of functional performance testing has been described in the literature for more than 20 years.[18-24] Functional performance assessment may be used in an attempt to describe an athlete's aptitude, identify talent, monitor performance, describe asymmetry or dysfunction, and determine readiness to participate in sports. Before sports participation athletes are frequently timed in a 40-yard dash, measured for vertical jump abilities, or assessed for performance on agility tests such as the timed T-test. This often occurs as part of a preparticipation examination. After progressing through postinjury or postsurgical rehabilitation, patients are assessed for their ability to perform functional tasks such as step-downs, hopping, jumping, landing, and cutting. Functional tests such as these are frequently used to simulate sporting activities or actions in the context of whole-body dynamic movement to contribute to the decision regarding whether an athlete is "fit" or physically prepared to begin sport participation or ready to return to play. It is our assertion that these specific functional tests should be performed only after movement screening has taken place and successful mastery of the fundamental movements previously described has been demonstrated.

Functional performance testing should examine athletes under conditions that imitate the necessary functional demands of their sports. Functional performance tests use dynamic skills or tasks to assess multiple components of function, including muscular strength, neuromuscular control/coordination, and joint stability.[25,26] They can be used for assessment of patients after LE injury, surgery, muscular contusions, overuse conditions such as tendinopathy or patellofemoral dysfunction, anterior cruciate ligament reconstruction (ACLR), and ankle instability.[19-21,26,27] Ideally, such tests should be time efficient and simple, require little or inexpensive equipment, and be able to be performed in a clinical setting.[11,21,28] If at all possible, such tests should be able to identify subjects at risk for injury or reinjury.[28-31] Above all, functional performance tests should be objective, reliable, and sensitive to change.[19,24,27,29,32] The root requirement for establishing the objectivity and reliability of any functional test is the use of standardized protocols and instructions.[27]

The validity of functional performance tests is difficult to establish. Many tests assess or examine only a portion of the requirements for the composite performance of a complex sporting activity. Single-limb assessments may have advantages in evaluating athletes who rely on unilateral limb performance, such as runners,[33] or athletes for whom running accounts for a large part of their sport demands. Single-limb tasks or "hops" offer considerable information regarding functional readiness in a wide variety of athletes because many sports entail single-limb weight acceptance, hopping, or landing as a part of their performance. Single-limb assessments offer specific benefits in the realm of objectivity because of their ability to provide within-subject, between-limb comparisons, described as a "biologic baseline," versus having to use population-derived norms. Tests such as the single-limb leg press (Figure 17-22), step-down performed either to the front or laterally (Figure 17-23),[27,34] squat,[35] hop for distance, triple hop for distance, crossover hop for distance (Figure 17-24),[18,20,21] stair hop,[29,30] and the 6-meter timed single-limb hop[20,21] are examples of commonly used single-limb tests that allow establishment of the limb symmetry index (LSI), which helps identify existing or residual postoperative asymmetry between limbs.[20,21,25,29,30] The functional status of the knee has been categorized as "compromised" if the LSI is less than 85%.[18,20,21] Single-limb tasks offer a wide variety of imposed demands on the LE that can be used at various times during the rehabilitation process for assessment of symmetry, recovery, and readiness to resume sports participation.[27,29,30] The triple hop for distance has been demonstrated to be a strong predictor of both power (as measured by vertical jump) and isokinetic strength.[22,25,36] Sekir et al[26] describe a lateral single-limb hop test that may be an important facet of functional assessment for athletes who rely on repetitive lateral movements for sport proficiency. Several researchers also advocate assessment of lateral movement during single-limb hop testing or the side-cutting maneuver because it may be more valid for athletes who move and cut laterally.[37,38] Several authors[18,20,21,29,30] have related the LSI to functional status; for example, a lower LSI after ACLR is related to poorer function, and improvements in raw scores on the single-limb hop test, as well as the LSI, represent functional recovery over 52 weeks after ACLR. Noyes et al[20,21] suggested that the LSI should be higher than 85% before return to sport. Loudon et al[27] suggested that in the case of patellofemoral pain syndrome, the LSI should be closer to 90% to prevent reinjury. Bilateral assessments, including squats, leg presses, and 2-legged "jumps" such as the drop jump (Figure 17-25) or tuck jump (Figure 17-26), may be more valid for assessing athletes in whom 2-legged jumping and landing tasks are important.[31,33]

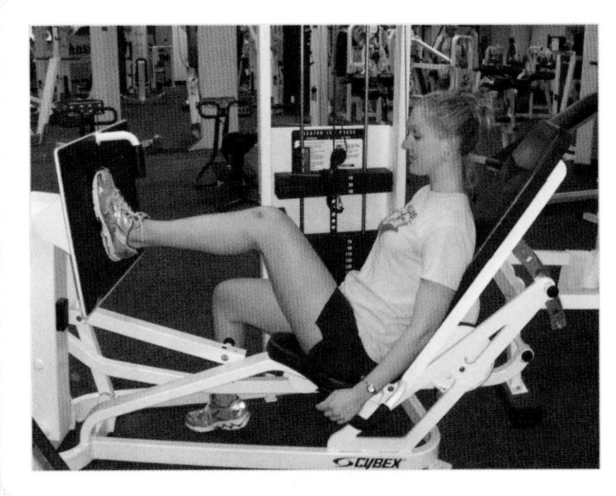

Figure 17-22 Single-leg press

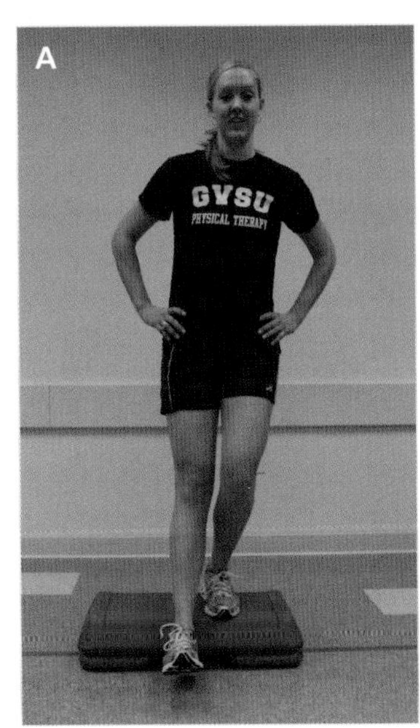

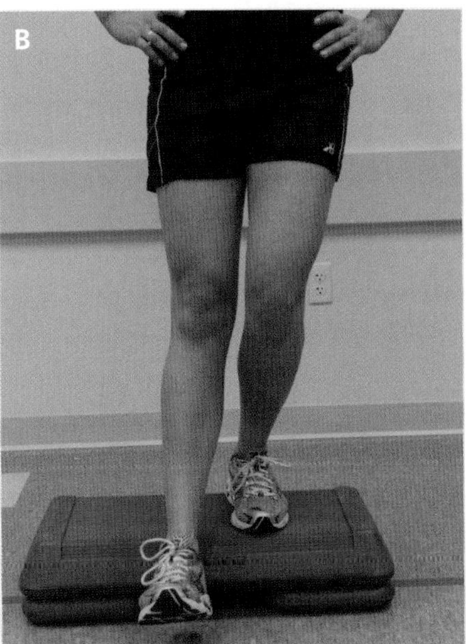

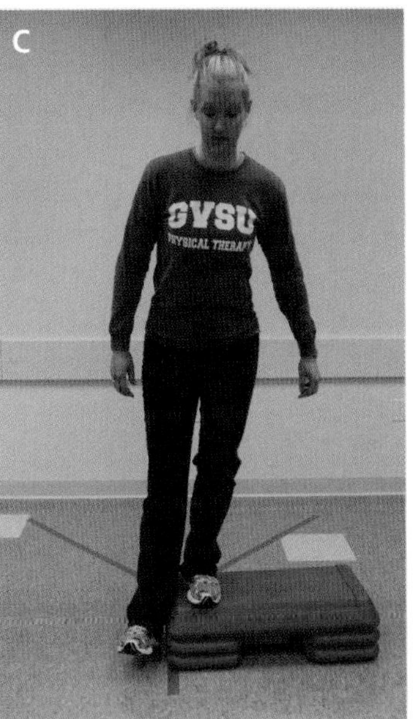

Figure 17-23 Step-down test

Monitor for LE biomechanics and control. **A.** Front step down; note the trunk and hands. **B.** Front step-down close-up; note the alignment of the stance knee. **C.** Lateral step-down with same qualitative criteria.

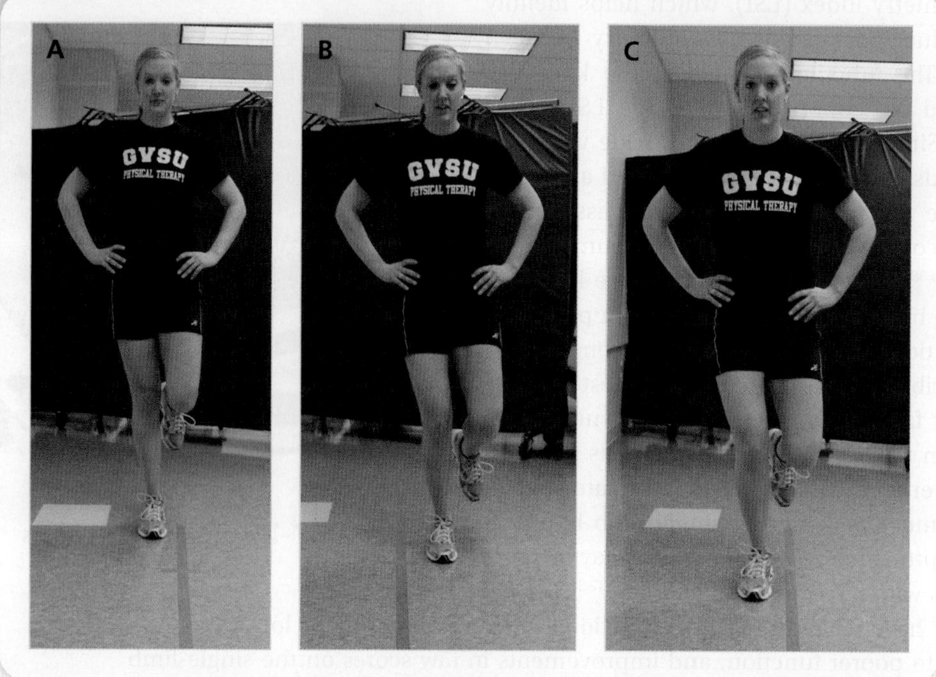

Figure 17-24 **Crossover hop for distance**

Start (**A**), lateral movement (**B**), and final lateral movement (**C**). *Note:* The athlete must "stick" or control the landing. The athlete attempts to go as far as possible in the combined 3 hops.

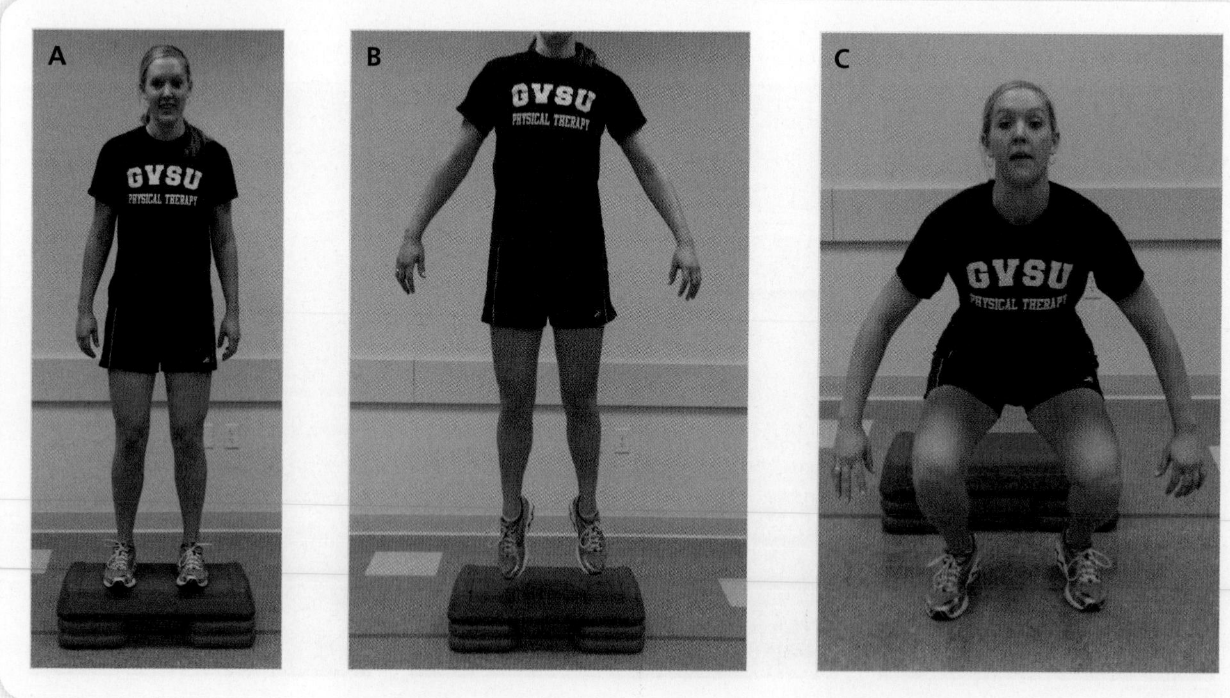

Figure 17-25 **Drop jump assessment**

Start position (**A**), midposition (**B**), and landing (**C**). Note the deep flexion angle in landing and alignment of the hips and knees.

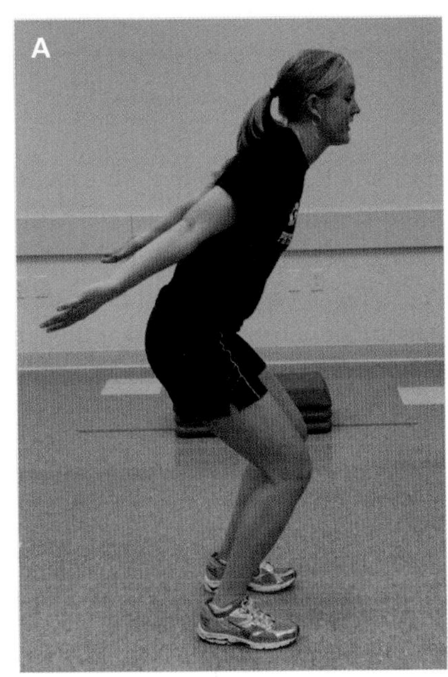

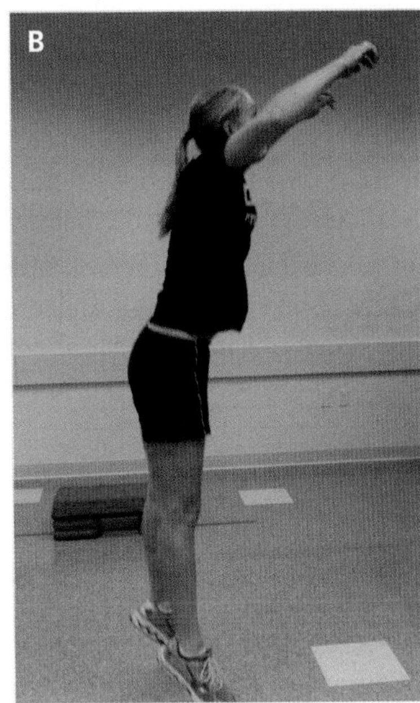

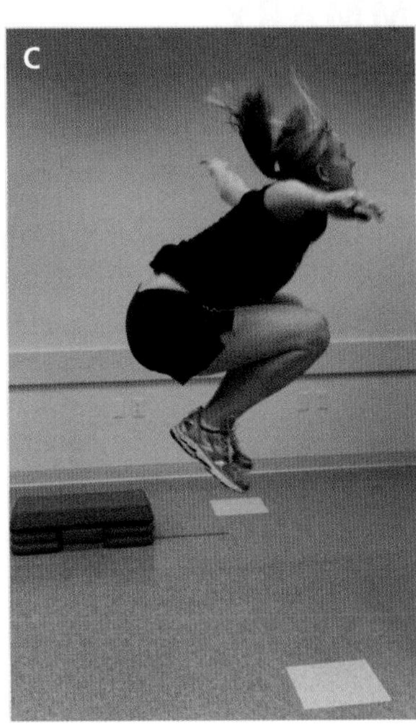

Figure 17-26 **Tuck jump assessment**

Beginning of movement (**A**), midmovement (**B**), and in air in a tucked position (**C**). Note that this test must be observed from the side and the front to analyze performance.

Most athletic skills require a combination of vertical, horizontal, and lateral movement by 1 or both LEs. Probably the most important requirement for successful sport performance is a series of highly developed motor control strategies to allow speed and agility during performance.[33] If an LE reach, jump, hop, or agility test could be used to objectively screen athletes' neuromuscular performance and suggest intervention before either sport participation or return to sport, that functional performance test would be valuable for preventing injury or decreasing the likelihood of reinjury.[12,21,28,31,37]

We know of no single optimal, valid, and reliable test that can determine an athlete's readiness for participation or return to sport. Given the wide variation and complexity of the demands of sport, this is not surprising. Many professionals suggest the use of functional test batteries or a series of functional tests that are related to the specific demands of a specific sport or that can be related to the probable mechanisms of injury for a specific pathology. A combination of 2 or more tests is recommended for relevant, sensitive, responsive functional assessment.[18,20,21,39,40] Bjorklund et al[39] proposed a functional test instrument (battery) named the Test for Athletes with Knee Injuries that they describe as valid, reliable, and sensitive for use after ACLR. The Test for Athletes with Knee Injuries is composed of 8 evaluations, including jogging, running, single-limb squat, rising from sitting (single leg), bilateral squat, single-limb hop for distance, single-limb vertical jump (performed plyometrically), and the single-limb crossover hop (8 meters). The authors present suggested scoring criteria for each test that take into account qualitative assessment of performance of the 8 tests. This is just one such example of combining several functional performance tests into a series for examination of a group of patients. Clearly, all functional performance tests are not relevant for all athletes, and it is the role of the rehabilitation professional to select valid, reliable, sensitive, and relevant functional performance tests.

SUMMARY

Movement Scoring Systems

1. One of the most difficult decisions that must be made by rehabilitation providers is whether an athlete is ready to participate in sports or safely return to sport participation.
2. Acceptance plus use of fundamental movement screening systems such as the FMS and the SFMA is sweeping across the country. These screens offer valuable information to professionals regarding the fundamental functional abilities of an athlete in the realm of *movement* by identifying compensatory movements or deficits in mobility or stability.

Functional Performance Tests

1. Functional performance tests or test batteries can be used to assess athletes of all ages and skill levels who participate in a wide variety of sports.
2. Frequently, functional performance tests assess a facet or single part the vast demands of any given sport, and therefore the validity of such tests is hard to determine. Although not providing a complete picture of athletic function, these tests are essential tools for the rehabilitation professional. It is critical that the rehabilitation professional be familiar with the use of such screens and tests to discern readiness for participation.
3. Skillful combinations of movement screening, functional performance testing, and sport-specific movement testing offer the best assessment of an athlete's readiness for return to sport.

Future Research

1. Although evidence regarding tests and systems that are objective, valid, and reliable is beginning to mount (Minick, DiMattia, Loudon, and others), many questions regarding the big picture of return to function exist. Does the FMS relate to core stability? Does it predict performance in athletics or merely identify potential for injury? Which functional performance measures are best used for athletes who participate in certain sports? Normative scores for the FMS and other functional performance tests by age and gender would be very helpful for comparison between athletes.
2. As the published evidence on functional testing continues to accumulate, rehabilitation professionals will have to keep abreast of changes and adapt their use of screens and tests accordingly.

REFERENCES

1. Fuller C, Drawer S. The application of risk management in sports. *Sports Med.* 2004;19:2108-2114.
2. Paterno MV, Schmitt LC, Ford KR, et al. Biomechanical measures during landing and postural stability predict second anterior cruciate ligament injury after anterior cruciate ligament reconstruction and return to sport. *Am J Sports Med.* 2010;38: 1968-1978.
3. Reed FE. The preparticipation athletic exam process. *South Med J.* 2004;97:871-872.
4. Van Mechelen W, Hlobil H, Kemper HC, et al. Incidence, severity, etiology and prevention of sports injuries. *Sports Med.* 1992;14:82-89.
5. Van Mechelen W, Twisk J, Molendjk A, et al. Subject related risk factors for sports injuries: a 1-year prospective study in young adults. *Med Sci Sports Exerc.* 1996;28:1171-1179.

6. Watson AW. Sports injuries related to flexibility, posture, acceleration, clinical deficits, and previous injury in high-level players of body contact sports. *Int J Sports Med.* 2001;22:220-225.
7. Kendall FP. *Muscle Testing and Function.* 5th ed. Philadelphia, PA: Lippincott Williams & Wilkins; 2005.
8. Page P, Frank CC, Lordner R. *Assessment and Treatment of Muscle Imbalance: The Janda Approach.* Champaign, IL: Human Kinetics; 2011.
9. Sahrmann SA. *Diagnosis and Treatment of Movement Impairment Syndromes.* St. Louis, MO: Mosby; 2002.
10. Chorba RS, Chorba DJ, Bouillon LE, et al. Use of a functional movement screening tool to determine injury risk in female collegiate athletes. *N Am J Sports Phys Ther.* 2010;5:47-54.
11. Kiesel K, Plisky PJ, Voight ML. Can serious injury in professional football be predicted by a preseason functional movement screen? *N Am J Sports Phys Ther.* 2007;2:147-152.
12. Plisky PJ, Rauh MJ, Kaminski TW, Underwood FB. Star excursion balance test as a predictor of lower extremity injury in high school basketball players. *J Orthop Sports Phys Ther.* 2006;36:911-919.
13. Cook G, Burton L, Hoogenboom B. Pre-participation screening: the use of fundamental movements as an assessment of function—part 1. *N Am J Sports Phys Ther.* 2006;1:62-72.
14. Cook G, Burton L, Hoogenboom B. Pre-participation screening: the use of fundamental movements as an assessment of function—part 2. *N Am J Sports Phys Ther.* 2004;1:132-139.
15. Minick KI, Kiesel KM, Burton L, et al. Interrater reliability of the functional movement screen. *J Strength Cond Res.* 2010;24:479-486.
16. Okada T, Huxel KC, Nesser TW. Relationship between core stability, functional movement, and performance. *J Strength Cond Res.* 2011;25:252-261.
17. Richardson C, Hodges P, Hides J. *Therapeutic Exercise for Lumbopelvic Stabilization: A Motor Control Approach for the Treatment and Prevention of Low Back Pain.* 2nd ed. Philadelphia, PA: Churchill Livingstone; 2004.
18. Barber SD, Noyes FR, Mangine RE, et al. Quantitative assessment of functional limitation in normal and anterior cruciate ligament-deficient knees. *Clin Orthop Relat Res.* 1990;255:204-214.
19. Bolgla LA, Keskula DR. Reliability of lower extremity functional performance tests. *J Orthop Sports Phys Ther.* 1997;26:138-142.
20. Noyes FR, Barber SD, Mangine RE. Abnormal lower limb symmetry determined by functional hop tests after anterior cruciate ligament rupture. *Am J Sports Med.* 1991;19:513-518.
21. Noyes FR, Barber-Westin SD, Fleckenstein C, et al. The drop-jump screening test: difference in lower limb control by gender and effect of neuromuscular training in female athletes. *Am J Sports Med.* 2005;33:197-207.
22. Petschnig R, Baron R, Albrecht M. The relationship between isokinetic quadriceps strength test and hop tests for distance and one-legged vertical jump test following anterior cruciate ligament reconstruction. *J Orthop Sports Phys Ther.* 1998;28:23-31.
23. Risberg MA, Ekeland A. Assessment of functional tests after anterior cruciate ligament surgery. *J Orthop Sports Phys Ther.* 1994;19:212-217.
24. Ross MD, Langford B, Whelan PJ. Test-retest reliability of 4 single-leg hop tests. *J Strength Cond Res.* 2002;16:617-622.
25. Hamilton RT, Shultz SJ, Schmitz RJ, Perrin DH. Triple-hop distance as a valid predictor of lower limb strength and power. *J Athl Train.* 2008;43:144-151.
26. Sekir U, Yildiz Y, Hazneci B, et al. Reliability of a functional test battery evaluating functionality, proprioception, and strength in recreational athletes with functional ankle instability. *Eur J Phys Rehabil Med.* 2008;44:407-415.
27. Loudon JK, Waicsner D, Goist-Foley LH, et al. Intrarater reliability of functional performance tests for subjects with patellofemoral pain syndrome. *J Athl Train.* 2002;37:256-261.
28. Myer GD, Ford KR, Hewett TE. Tuck jump assessment for reducing anterior cruciate ligament injury risk. *Athl Ther Today.* 2008;13:(5):39-44.
29. Hopper DM, Goh SC, Wentworth LA, et al. Test-retest reliability of knee rating scales and functional hop tests one year following anterior cruciate ligament reconstruction. *Phys Ther Sport.* 2002;3:10-18.
30. Hopper DM, Strauss GR, Boyle JJ, Bell J. Functional recovery after anterior cruciate ligament reconstruction: a longitudinal perspective. *Arch Phys Med Rehabil.* 2008;89:1535-1541.
31. Padua DA, Marshall SW, Boling MC, et al. The landing error scoring system (LESS) is a valid and reliable clinical assessment tool of jump-landing biomechanics: the JUMP-ACL study. *Am J Sports Med.* 2009;37:1996-2002.
32. Brosky J, Nitz A, Malone T, et al. Intrarater reliability of selected clinical outcome measures following anterior cruciate ligament reconstruction. *J Orthop Sports Phys Ther.* 1999;29:39-48.
33. Meylan C, McMaster T, Cronin J, et al. Single-leg lateral, horizontal, and vertical jump assessment: reliability, interrelationships, and ability to predict sprint and change-of-direction performance. *J Strength Cond Res.* 2009;23:1140-1147.
34. Piva SR, Fitzgerald K, Irrgang JJ, et al. Reliability of measures of impairments associated with patellofemoral pain. *BMC Musculoskelet Disord.* 2006;7:33-46.
35. DiMattia MA, Livengood AL, Uhl TL, et al. What are the validity of the single-leg-squat test and its relationship to hip abduction strength? *J Sport Rehabil.* 2005;14:108-123.
36. Wilk KE, Romaniello WT, Soscia SM, et al. The relationship between subjective knee scores, isokinetic testing and functional testing in the ACL-reconstructed knee. *J Orthop Sports Phys Ther.* 1994;20:60-73.

37. Hewett TE, Myer GD, Ford KR, Slauterbeck JR. Preparticipation physical examination using a box drop vertical jump test in young athletes: the effects of puberty and sex. *Clin J Sport Med.* 2006;16:298-304.
38. Zebis MK, Andersen LL, Bencke J, et al. Identification of athletes at future risk of anterior cruciate ligament ruptures by neuromuscular screening. *Am J Sports Med.* 2009;37:1967-1973.
39. Bjorklund K, Andersson L, Dalen N. Validity and responsiveness of the test of athletes with knee injuries: the new criterion based functional performance test instrument. *Knee Surg Sports Traumatol Arthrosc.* 2009;17:435-445.
40. Gustavsson A, Neeter C, Thomee P, et al. A test battery for evaluation of hop performance in patients with ACL injury and patients who have undergone ACL reconstruction. *Knee Surg Sports Traumatol Arthrosc.* 2006;14:778-788.

THE SELECTIVE FUNCTIONAL MOVEMENT ASSESSMENT

SFMA SCORING		FN	FP	DP	DN
Active Cervical Flexion					
Active Cervical Extension					
Cervical Rotation-Lateral Bend	L				
	R				
Upper Extremity Pattern 1 (MRE)	L				
	R				
Upper Extremity Pattern 2 (LRF)	L				
	R				
Multi-Segmental Flexion					
Multi-Segmental Extension					
Multi-Segmental Rotation	L				
	R				
Single Leg Stance	L				
	R				
Overhead Deep Squat					

THE SELECTIVE FUNCTIONAL MOVEMENT ASSESSMENT

Name **Date** **Total Score**

Cervical Flexion □ Primary □ Secondary

□ Can't Touch Sternum__________

Cervical Extension

□ Greater than 10 Degrees of Parallel__________

Cervical Rotation

□ *RIGHT* – Can't Touch Chin to Mid-Clavicle__________

□ *LEFT* - Can't Touch Chin to Mid-Clavicle__________

Upper Extremity □ Primary □ Secondary □ *RIGHT* □ *LEFT*

□ *RIGHT* □ *LEFT* Can't Touch Inferior Angle of the Contralateral Scapula

□ *RIGHT* □ *LEFT* Can't Touch Spine of the Contralateral Scapula

Multi-Segmental Flexion □ Primary □ Secondary

□ Can't Touch Toes and Return to Standing Position__________

□ < 70 Degrees Sacral Angle__________

□ No Posterior Weight Shift (T-L Junction over foot) __________

□ Non-Uniform Spinal Curves__________

Multi-Segmental Extension □Primary □ Secondary

□ ASIS Doesn't Clear the Toes__________

□ Can't Maintain Normal (≥ 170 degrees) Shoulder Flexion__________

□ Spine of Scapula Doesn't Clear the Heels__________

□ Non-Uniform Spinal Curves__________

Multi-Segmental Rotation □ Primary □ Secondary □ *RIGHT* □ *LEFT*

□ *RIGHT* □ *LEFT* Pelvis Rotation < 50 degrees__________

□ *RIGHT* □ *LEFT* Trunk/shoulder < 50 degrees more than pelvis__________

□ *RIGHT* □ *LEFT* Spinal/Pelvic Deviation__________

□ *RIGHT* □ *LEFT* Excessive Knee Flexion__________

Single Leg Stance □ Primary □ Secondary □ *RIGHT* □ *LEFT*

□ *RIGHT* □ *LEFT* Eyes Open Standing < 10 seconds__________

□ *RIGHT* □ *LEFT* Eyes Closed Standing < 10 seconds__________

□ *RIGHT* □ *LEFT* Loss of Height__________

Overhead Squating □ Primary □ Secondary

□ Loss of Shoulder Flexion__________

□ Thoracic Flexes__________

□ Hips Don't Break Parallel__________

□ Sagittal Plane Deviation of Lower Extremity Rt.__________ Lt, __________

SFMA

Selective Functional Movement Assessment

Name: ____________________

Date: ____________________

	FN R	FN L	DP R	DP L	FP R	FP L	DN R	DN L
Cervical Flexion								
Active Supine Cervical Flexion								
Passive Supine Cervical Flexion								
Active Supine OA Flexion								
Cervical Extension								
Supine Cervical Extension								
Shoulder Pattern One								
Active Prone Shoulder Pattern One								
Passive Prone Shoulder Pattern One								
Supine Reciprocal Shoulder								
Active Prone 90/90 Shoulder IR (70°)								
Passive Prone 90/90 Shoulder IR (70°)								
Active Prone Shoulder Extension (50°)								
Passive Prone Shoulder Extension (50°)								
Active Prone Elbow Flexion (70°)								
Passive Prone Elbow Flexion (80°)								
Lumbar Lock Chest (50°)								
Shoulder Pattern Two								
Active Prone Shoulder Pattern Two								
Passive Prone Shoulder Pattern Two								
Supine Reciprocal Shoulder								
Active Prone 90/90 Shoulder ER (90°)								
Passive Prone 90/90 Shoulder ER (90°)								
Active Prone Shoulder Flex/Abd (170°)								
Passive Prone Shoulder Flex/Abd (170°)								
Active Prone Elbow Flexion (70°)								
Passive Prone Elbow Flexion (80°)								
Lumbar Lock Chest (50°)								
Multi-Segmental Flexion								
Single Leg Forward Bend								
Long Sitting								
Active Straight Leg Raise								
Passive Stragiht Leg Raise								
Prone Rocking								
Supine Knee to Chest Holding Thighs								
UB Rolling - Supine to Prone								
LB Rolling - Supine to Prone								
Multi-Segmental Extension								
Spine Extension	FN		DP		FP		DN	
Backward Bend w/o UE								
Single Leg Backward Bend								
Prone Press Up								
Lumbar Lock (IR) - Active Rot./Ext. (50°)								
Lumbar Lock (IR) - Passive Rot./Ext. (50°)								
Prone on Elbow Unilateral Extension (30°)								
Lower Body Extension	FN		DP		FP		DN	
Faber								
Modified Thomas								
Prone Active Hip Extension (10°)								
UB Rolling - Prone to Supine								
LB Rolling - Prone to Supine								
Upper Body Extension	FN		DP		FP		DN	
Unilateral Shoulder Backward Bend								
Supine Lat Stretch Hips Flexed								
Supine Lat Stretch Hips Extended								
Lumbar Lock (ER) - Unilateral Ext (50°)								
Lumbar Lock (IR) - Active Rot./Ext. (50°)								
Lumbar Lock (IR) - Passive Rot./Ext. (50°)								

	FN R	FN L	DP R	DP L	FP R	FP L	DN R	DN L
Cervical Rotation								
Active Supine Cervical Rotation								
Passive Supine Cervical Rotation								
C1-C2 Cervical Rotation								
Multi-Segmental Rotation								
Spine Rotation	FN		DP		FP		DN	
Seated Rotation (50°)								
Lumbar Lock (ER) - Unilateral Ext (50°)								
Lumbar Lock (IR) - Active Rot./Ext. (50°)								
Lumbar Lock (IR) - Passive Rot./Ext. (50°)								
Prone on Elbow Unilateral Extension (30°)								
UB Rolling - Supine to Prone								
LB Rolling - Supine to Prone								
UB Rolling - Prone to Supine								
LB Rolling - Prone to Supine								
Hip Rotation	FN		DP		FP		DN	
Seated Active External Hip Rotation (40°)								
Seated Passive External Hip Rotation (40°)								
Prone Active External Hip Rotation (40°)								
Prone Passive External Hip Rotation (40°)								
Seated Active Internal Hip Rotation (30°)								
Seated Passive Internal Hip Rotation (30°)								
Prone Active Internal Hip Rotation (30°)								
Prone Passive Internal Hip Rotation (30°)								
Tibia Rotation	FN		DP		FP		DN	
Seated Active Internal Tibia Rotation (20°)								
Seated Passive Internal Tibia Rotation (20°)								
Seated Active External Tibia Rotation (20°)								
Seated Passive External Tibia Rotation (20°)								
Single Leg Stance								
Vestibular & Core	FN		DP		FP		DN	
CTSIB (Static Head Movement)								
CTSIB (Dynamic Head Movement)								
Half-Kneeling Narrow Base								
UB Rolling - Supine to Prone								
LB Rolling - Supine to Prone								
UB Rolling - Prone to Supine								
LB Rolling - Prone to Supine								
Quadruped Diagonals								
Ankle	FN		DP		FP		DN	
Heel Walks								
Prone Passive Dorsiflexion								
Toe Walks								
Prone Passive Plantarflexion								
Seated Ankle Inversion/Eversion								
Seated Passive Ankle Inversion/Eversion								
Overhead Deep Squat								
Interlocking Fingers Behind the Neck Squat								
Assisted Squat								
Half Kneeling Dorsiflexion								
Supine Knee to Chest Holding Shins								
Supine Knee to Chest Holding Thighs								

18

Functional Exercise Progression and Functional Testing in Rehabilitation

Turner A. Blackburn, Jr and John A. Guido, Jr

OBJECTIVES

After completion of this chapter, the physical therapist should be able to do the following:

- Define functional exercise progression.
- Define the SAID (specific adaptations to imposed demands) principle.
- Outline the need for functional progression and testing.
- Describe the continuum of functional progression for low- and high-level patients.
- Outline a functional progression program for the lower extremity.
- Outline a functional progression program for the upper extremity.
- Outline a functional progression program for the spine.
- Discuss major functional testing research.

The physical therapist plays an important role in helping individuals return to their preinjury level of function. While working to achieve impairment-based goals, functional testing is employed to gauge readiness to move through the rehabilitation program and to return to activity. A functional exercise progression can be initiated prior to functional testing or following the results of functional tests. In either case, functional testing or progression should not exceed the healing constraints of the injured tissue. By breaking down functional activities into basic tasks, a safe and effective rehabilitation program can be designed. This chapter examines functional exercise testing and functional exercise progression, and provides examples for some common upper- and lower-extremity disorders, as well as a sample spine program.

What Is Functional Testing and Functional Exercise Progression?

The ultimate goal of any rehabilitation program is to return an individual to the preinjury level of function as quickly and safely as possible. Decreasing pain and swelling—and restoring normal range of motion (ROM), strength, proprioception, and balance—are only part of the plan. Functional testing and a functional exercise progression will complete the rehabilitation program. Functional testing encompasses measuring various activities to provide a baseline for determining progress or to provide normative data with which to compare performance. A functional exercise progression can be defined as a series of activities that have been ordered from basic to complex, simple to difficult, that allows for the reacquisition of a specific task. Many of the exercises in the functional progression may be used for functional testing. Functional testing and functional exercise progression allow the clinician to bridge the gap between basic rehabilitation and a full return to activity.

How Is Functional Testing Performed?

Functional testing and functional exercise progression are used in a variety of physical therapy settings but in very different capacities. Physical therapists practicing in outpatient orthopedic settings use these techniques to help their patients return to activities of daily living (ADL), work, and sports. In neurologic and geriatric rehabilitation settings, functional testing and functional exercise progression take on a different meaning, being geared more toward ADL, transfers, and ambulating on level and unlevel surfaces.

Despite these differences, the principles that guide functional testing and exercise progression are the same regardless of the practice setting and level of the patient. Some patients will move further through the program than others, based on their specific rehabilitation goals. There is little basic science and research to guide the physical therapist in designing a functional exercise progression. Rather, common sense prevails and is employed along with the information available regarding healing constraints of various musculoskeletal disorders or the precautions that must be heeded for various medical conditions.

A complete discussion of collagen healing is beyond the scope of this chapter, but in general, many of the injuries encountered in the outpatient setting will heal in 3 to 6 weeks.[20,21] In the early phases of the rehabilitation program, appropriate stress must be placed on the healing tissues to ensure proper healing. Our bodies heal according to the SAID (specific adaptation to imposed demand) principle.[13] The imposed demand is therapeutic exercise in the form of a functional progression that stresses the injured tissue so as to enable it to heal at an adequate length and strength. This enables the individual to handle the demands of return to full function without reinjuring the area. If the functional progression is employed incorrectly, the stress imparted will cause reinjury and impede the patient's progress. Healing constraints may be exceeded or new injuries created during functional testing or exercise progression, and the therapist should be acutely aware of the individual's response to activity. The presence or absence of the cardinal signs of inflammation, as well as muscle weakness, loss of motion, and instability of the injured joint, should alert the clinician to reassess the activity being performed. The culprit may be one activity that is above the abilities of the patient at that time, or that the overall volume exceeds the ability of the healing structures to accommodate to the stress.

Early in the rehabilitation program, therapeutic techniques should be employed to meet the various impairment goals, such as eliminating pain and swelling and restoring full ROM, strength, proprioception, balance, and normal ambulation without deviations or assistive devices. Normal ROM can be assessed with a goniometer by comparing established norms or the range of the uninvolved opposite extremity. Swelling can be assessed via tape measure for circumferential measurements, or with volumetric measures of water displacement. Pain levels can be determined with a visual analog scale.

Strength testing poses a challenge to the clinician. A 5/5 manual muscle test grade may not show true deficits in strength and endurance of the musculature. Isokinetic testing, if available, may be a better alternative and has been shown to correlate with function despite being performed in an open-chain fashion.[26] We recommend less than a 30% isokinetic deficit in the strength and endurance of the involved versus the uninvolved extremity prior to initiating functional testing activities for athletic endeavors. This form of testing will not be available to all clinicians, and not all patients will need to undergo an isokinetic evaluation. Basic manual muscle testing or the use of a handheld dynamometer to increase objectivity will suffice in many cases. Proprioception at a given joint can be assessed through basic joint repositioning tasks, or can be measured using the electrogoniometer on the Biodex Multi-Joint System. Balance testing can be performed with or without high-technology equipment. At a minimum, performing a single-leg stance activity for total duration, or counting the number of touchdowns with the opposite lower extremity, can be assessed with a second hand on a watch. There are several excellent balance screens, such as the Berg balance scale, the clinical test of sensory interaction for balance, and the functional reach test. Plisky et al utilized a modified version of the STAR excursion balance test termed the "Y Excursion balance test." The authors noted that this simple screen was able to demonstrate side-side dysfunction and problems with balance and strength. The subject stands and reaches with 1 lower extremity as far as able without losing balance in the forward, posteromedial, and posterolateral directions. The limb used for balance is the limb being tested. Three trials in each direction are measured and an average reach distance is recorded. The authors suggested, via logistic regression analysis, that individuals with an anterior right/left reach difference greater than 4 cm were 2.5 times more likely to sustain a lower-extremity injury. The authors also suggested using a composite score derived by adding the three reach distances, dividing this by three times the limb length (measured from the anterior superior iliac spine to the medial malleolus) and multiplying times 100 in order to give a % score. Those individuals with a composite reach distance less than 94% of their limb length were 6.5 times more likely to have a lower-extremity injury. There are also several excellent testing devices on the market that will give the clinician information regarding the postural sway envelope and directions of movement, such as the Biodex Stability System and the NeuroCom Balance System (NeuroCom, Inc., Clackamas, OR). Monitored Rehabilitation Systems devices can be used for functional motor control testing and training activities.

When an individual has no pain or swelling, and has reached sufficient ROM, strength, balance, and ambulation without deviations, the clinician can determine if functional testing is appropriate. In some cases, functional testing may be used prior to meeting the impairment goals, provided the individual is not placed at risk for reinjury based on the healing constraints of the injured tissue. The information gained will be valuable to the clinician and the individual in planning further treatment.

Specifics

How Is Function Measured?

Functional testing is a onetime, maximal effort that is performed to assess performance.[25] The key is that the test must recreate the activity that the individual will be performing, and must be completed in a controlled environment. The purpose of functional testing is to determine an individual's readiness to return to the preinjury level of function. The information gained will allow the clinician to point out deficits that must be overcome, and to progress the rehabilitation program. Functional testing, like the functional exercise progression, must begin with simple tasks and progress to highly coordinated tasks. At the lowest level, for an individual to perform a sit-to-stand transfer, the leg press or bilateral minisquats can be performed for repetitions for a length of time. This will recreate an individual's daily activities, in this case, rising from a chair, commode, or car seat. Testing can be performed through various ranges of motion to recreate the seat heights the individual will encounter. The clinician can also use ambulation itself as a functional test. Ambulation for distance is an important determinant to see if the patient can function in the community. Ambulation measured for time will determine if the patient can cross a street safely or exit an elevator before the door closes.

As another example, the clinician should examine a patient's ability to climb stairs. What functional test can be used to assess this skill? Front or lateral step-ups or step-downs can be used to determine an individual's readiness to complete this task. This test is also easily standardized. Step-ups can be performed with only the heel of the opposite limb touching the ground. A step height can be chosen that equals heights that will be encountered at home, the office, or in the community. Repetitions are counted, or the number of repetitions in a set time can be measured. The results are compared with the uninvolved limb or established norms. Rosenthal et al[22] reported an intraclass correlation coefficient of 0.99 for the lateral step-up test. Functional testing can be as simple as performing minisquats, ambulation, or lateral step-ups for repetitions, distance, or time.

At the highest level of functional testing in the lower extremity, an athlete may have to complete complex movements such as jump or hop tests, shuttle runs, and agility drills. This part of the rehabilitation process is an integral part of the rehabilitation professional's daily routine in the sports setting and can be easily incorporated to meet patients' needs in the clinic. The results of functional testing will determine when they can return to play. Daniel et al[5] described the one-leg hop for distance test. One-leg hopping is an example of an activity that places higher demands on the lower extremity than does walking or jogging.[23] Subsequently, many clinicians and researchers have used this test for examining function in varied populations, especially in patients who have undergone anterior cruciate ligament (ACL) reconstructions.[23] It is easy to see how important this activity is in terms of a return to athletic competition. This is an ideal test to determine the individual's willingness to accept weight on the involved leg after injury.[25] The one-leg hop for distance and the one-leg timed hop, predominantly used with athletes, also have shown good reliability.[5] A single-leg hop does have its limitations, in that it only describes one movement, whereas most sports require a series of complex maneuvers. Therefore, many authors have attempted to create even higher-level tests to determine readiness to play. Lephart et al[14] examined 3 functional testing procedures for the ACL-deficient athlete. These included the cocontraction maneuver (a shuffling maneuver around a semicircle while tethered to surgical tubing), a carioca (crossover stepping), and a shuttle run (an acceleration and deceleration test). Several investigators have attempted to correlate the results of isokinetic testing and functional activities. Wilk et al[23] found a positive correlation between isokinetic knee extension peak torque and 3 functional hop tests (hop for distance, timed hop, and crossover triple hop). The results of this study were further strengthened by Jarvela et al[9] who assessed muscle performance 5 to 9 years after ACL reconstruction. They also correlated the strength of the knee extensors and flexors at 60 degrees per second isokinetically with the one-legged hop for distance. Both studies suggest that expensive isokinetic devices may not be required for determining the functional status of an athlete.[9,26] Many physical therapy clinics utilize a Total Gym (Engineering Fitness International, Inc., San Diego, CA) for lower-extremity rehabilitation. Munich et al[18] have created a testing protocol for use on this device. They examined 35 healthy subjects who performed a 20-second test for unilateral squat repetitions and a 50-second squat repetition test for time. Their findings indicate acceptable test–retest reliability for the purpose of evaluating functional ability during the early stages of rehabilitation for lower-extremity conditions. One other consideration during functional testing is determining an athlete's eccentric control, which is extremely important in changing directions and landing from a jump. Juris et al[11] had asymptomatic and symptomatic individuals with knee pain perform a maximal controlled leap. This test was performed by having the individual perform a single-leg hop by taking off on the uninjured limb and landing on the injured limb, termed force absorption versus force production. The results of this study demonstrated that individuals with knee pain had difficulty managing force absorption as opposed to creating force (force production). If a traditional single-leg hop is examined, the individual does perform force absorption, but if they have lower-extremity weakness, they may not create a large takeoff force (force production) and, therefore, not stress the limb in landing. If the forces are lower during the test than those experienced during sports, the athletes may be returned to activity before they are truly ready.

Mattacola et al[16] studied a group of patients who had undergone ACL reconstruction to determine their performance during 2 functional tests conducted on the Smart Balance Master (NeuroCom, Inc. Clackamas, OR) as compared to a control group. All of the ACL reconstruction patients were at least 6 months postoperative. Both groups performed the step-up-and-over test (Figure 18-1) and the forward lunge (Figure 18-2) on a long force plate. The control group produced significantly more force during the initial step of the step-up-and-over task than did the ACL-reconstructed group. In the same test, the ACL

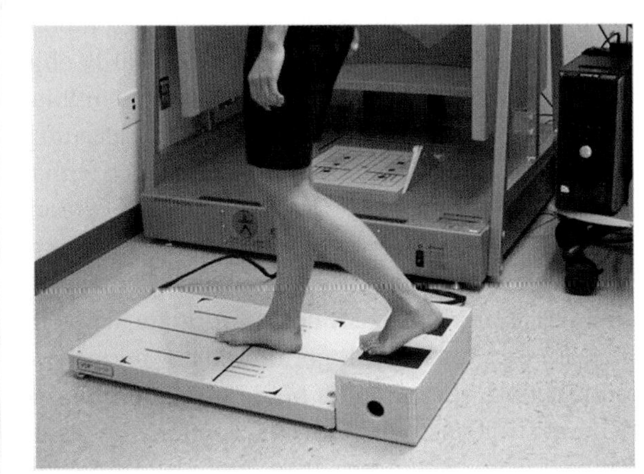

Figure 18-1 **The step-up-and-over test performed on the Smart Balance Master**

(NeuroCom, Inc., Clackamas, OR.)

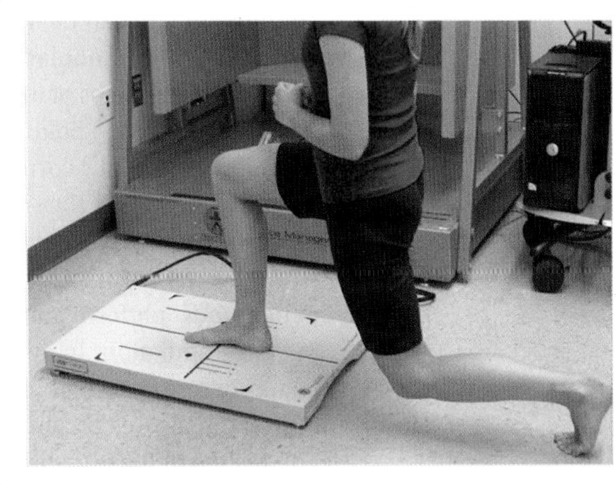

Figure 18-2 **The forward lunge test performed on the Smart Balance Master**

(NeuroCom, Inc., Clackamas, OR.)

reconstruction patients were significantly slower when they led with the involved limb. During the forward lunge test, there were no differences between groups in the lunge distance or the contact time. However, the impact index (percentage body weight, indicates eccentric ability of nonstepping leg) and the force impulse (percentage body weight × the time the force is exerted) measurements were significantly greater for the uninvolved leg than the involved leg in the ACL patients. Higher impact and force indices represent better functional ability. Such tests, performed on the Smart Balance Master maybe useful for screening for functional disability that might persist after ACL reconstruction and not be recognized with more general, clinical functional tests.

In lieu of these tests or sophisticated testing equipment, the physical therapist can have the patient run through a series of progressively difficult tasks such as running straight ahead and backpedaling, performing figure-8 runs, cutting maneuvers, and, finally, sports-specific tasks.

In the upper extremity, the clinician needs to be more creative to recreate the functional demands an individual may encounter during ADL or sports. Functional testing can include pushups for an athlete or overhead activities performed in a specially designed apparatus for an electrician or carpenter. Again, at the lowest level, simple reaching tests can recreate ADL such as removing items from overhead cabinets. To standardize this, a goniometer can be used to measure ROM at the glenohumeral joint, or a finger ladder to document reach height. A tape measure can be used to measure reach distance. At the highest levels, activities that recreate job tasks, as alluded to, can be performed in the clinic. Measures of specific skills, duration of overhead activity, or speed of activity provide objective evidence of functional ability. For the athlete, both open-chain (throwing activities and racquet sports) and closed-chain (football, wrestling, gymnastics) activities can be reproduced in the clinic. The clinician is only limited by the clinician's imagination.

Whether testing the upper or lower extremity, begin with bilateral support drills and progress to more demanding unilateral support drills. Always observe for substitution and poor technique, which may signify that the activity is too difficult for the patient at that time, or that the stress is too great on the healing structures. Through functional testing, the therapist can assess speed, strength, agility, and power, which when combined equal function.[25] Functional testing can be adapted to meet the needs of every patient with whom we come into contact. Physical therapists have always performed functional testing with their patients, although they may not have described these activities as such. In the acute care or rehabilitation hospital, as well as in the nursing home, most activities have a functional component and can be used to document functional status. Everything from bed mobility and transfers to ambulation on level and unlevel surfaces can be measured fairly objectively. Two examples of functional testing for the geriatric population include the multiple-sit-to-stand (MSTS) field test and the 6-minute walk test. The MSTS claims to measure leg strength. Netz et al[19] correlated knee extensor isokinetic strength and endurance with the results of the MSTS. They concluded that the MSTS is not able to predict strength of the knee extensors, but may predict overall endurance of the lower extremities. The results of this study are not surprising since it is well accepted that to measure strength and power, the patient must perform an explosive maneuver. This is obviously not appropriate in an older patient population. In another test of endurance, Bean et al[1] performed a 6-minute walk test to determine aerobic capacity and function. They found a poor correlation between indirect measures of aerobic capacity but a strong association with functional measures. The results of these 2 studies provide the clinician with a variety of options for functional testing in the geriatric population.

In the outpatient setting, the activities required for functional testing may be more dynamic, but the principles and goals of treatment are the same. It is easy to take for granted the ease with which ADL are performed. A functional test can be used to document limitations in ADL tasks, and a functional exercise progression can be implemented to meet the specific needs of the patient. It is imperative to enable individuals to return to their maximum level of function or their preinjury status.

What Now?

Now that the functional testing procedure has been completed at the appropriate time in the rehabilitation process, what is the next step? Upon completion of functional testing, the clinician must be able to use this information to determine the next step in the rehabilitation process. In one scenario, if the individual completes the tasks adequately, return to work or ADL without restrictions may be recommended. In another scenario, if the individual is not able to complete the tasks, the clinician must determine where the breakdown occurred. Return to full function is restricted until these tasks can be completed and it is safe for the individual to return to the preinjury activity level. This is where the functional exercise progression should dominate the rehabilitation program. Up until that point, the patient may have been working on and achieved the majority of the clinical goals, but from the results of the functional testing, the patient may not be ready to return to all necessary functional activities.

If the goal activity is kept in mind, whether it is a return to sports or ADL, the activity can be broken down into small segments that can be performed in the clinic. Once the specific activity has been broken down into required fundamental movements, the individual's injured body part is stressed progressively until function is adequate for a return to work, ADL, or sports-specific demands.[25] Removing the "conscious mind" from the activity will make the movement pattern more automatic and natural. Some suggestions include throwing a ball for the patient to catch during the activity or having the patient count the fingers held up on your hand. Functional exercises that meet the specific needs of the patient can truly be termed "functional."

The concept of open- versus closed-chain exercise becomes moot when discussing functional exercise progression, because everything we do is a combination of these 2 types of activity. Walking requires a combination of movements (the swing phase is open chain, the stance phase is closed chain), as does picking up an object off the floor (the individual braces the body with the uninvolved extremity on a table, which is closed chain, and reaches for the object, which is open chain). The hallmark of closed-chain activities, however, is that they are more closely related to function, incorporating movements that mimic daily activities. Both open- and closed-chain exercise can create concentric, isometric, and eccentric muscular contractions, which are all used for functional tasks. These exercises can also include acceleration and deceleration, which are extremely important principles when discussing functional tasks. Attempting to cross a busy intersection requires acceleration to get across safely. Descending an inclined walkway requires deceleration to prevent falls. An advantage that closed-chain exercises have is the addition of appropriate proprioceptive feedback from the muscle and joint mechanoreceptors. Discontinuing the rehabilitation program when the clinic-based rehabilitation goals alone are achieved may be appropriate for some individuals, but this will surely be a disservice to those patients returning to higher levels of function. These patients will have an increased risk for reinjury when they attempt to return to their preinjury level of function without completing a functional exercise progression.[27]

Examples

Assume you are treating a police officer who has suffered a sprain of the medial compartment of his right knee. After valgus stress testing at 30 degrees of flexion and an anterior drawer test with the tibia in external rotation, you determine that there is a slight opening of the joint space—in other words, a grade III ligament sprain with 1+ instability. Functional testing may be appropriate initially in the form of lateral step-ups or minisquats, provided these activities do not cause too great a stress on the healing medial compartment. This will tell you if the individual can perform sit-to-stand transfers from various heights and climb stairs, important aspects of ADL. Table 18-1 describes lower-extremity criteria needed for return to various functional activities. This particular patient will need to return to high-level functional activities such as chasing and apprehending suspects.

Initially, starting the patient on a regimen of knee isometrics, modalities as needed to control pain and swelling, and flexibility training is an appropriate course. In an earlier discussion, it was stated that adequate collagen healing occurs in 3 to 6 weeks. The second phase of the rehabilitation program must employ a functional exercise progression to progressively load the injured body part. In relation to the Davis law,[8] the medial compartment will heal along the lines of stress. So, to enable it to heal with appropriate tensile strength and adequate length, activities that involve a valgus stress must be included. To strengthen the surrounding musculature, open-chain exercises are incorporated. However, it is difficult to apply a controlled valgus stress to the knee in the open chain. Therefore, closed-chain exercises are a must. These may include the testing activities themselves, minisquats and lateral step-ups with a valgus stress, the BAPS (biomechanical ankle platform system) board, Profitter, and the balance-testing devices. Table 18-2 describes sample lower-extremity functional exercise progression and testing activities.

Table 18-1 Knee Functional Progression

	Criteria for Return		
Functional Activity	**Strength**	**ROM**	**Other**
Sit to stand	3/5 MMT quad 3/5 MMT ham 3/5 MMT gastroc	90 degrees one knee 120 degrees hip flexion	Sitting balance Stand balance
Assistive free gait	5/5 MMT quad 4/5 MMT ham Lift body weight on one leg with heel lift Motor control of knee	Full knee extension 100 degrees knee flexion 10 degrees dorsiflexion	No pain No swelling Nonantalgic gait Adequate balance
Ascend/descend			
Stairs (step over step)			10 side-step-downs
Running	70% quad/ham uninvolved leg	Full flexion 15 degrees dorsiflexion	30 mins bike 50 side-step-downs 2 miles walking
Sprinting	90% quad/ham uninvolved leg		2 miles running
Agility			Successful sprinting
Sports activity			Functional progression of activity

gastroc, gastrocnemius; MMT, manual muscle test.

Table 18-2 Lower-Quarter Functional Progression and Testing Template

Levels	Support	Stability	Plane	Response	Direction	Examples
1	Bilateral	Stable	Single	Single	Vertical	Leg press Shuttle Minisquat
2	Bilateral	Unstable	Single	Single	Vertical	DynaDisc Foam roller Biodex stability
3	Unilateral	Stable	Single	Single	Vertical	Leg press Shuttle Minisquat Step-up
4	Unilateral	Unstable	Single	Single	Vertical	Leg press Shuttle Minisquat Step-up
5	Bilateral nonsupport	Stable	Single, multiple	Single, multiple	Vertical, horizontal	Jumping "5-Dot drill" Spin hops
6	Unilateral nonsupport	Stable	Single, multiple	Single, multiple	Vertical, horizontal	Jumping "5-Dot drill" Spin hops
7	Acceleration, deceleration	Stable				"Shuttle Run" "T-drill" Cocontraction Lateral power hop

Once the clinic-based goals have been achieved and the patient is able to ambulate on level and unlevel surfaces without deviation or an assistive device, functional testing is again performed to determine where the patient stands in relation to return to work. Because of the high-level demands this patient will encounter upon his return to full duty as a police officer, we need to perform higher-level functional testing, beginning with jump or hop tests. The jump test is performed with the individual standing on both limbs. He is asked to jump as far as possible in a horizontal fashion (a standing broad jump) and to stick to the landing. The individual should be able to jump a distance equal to his height (or 1.5 times his height).[25] If this task is completed, a single-leg hop can be performed as described by Daniel. Noyes et al[20] suggest that 2 types of 1-leg hopping tests—for distance and for time—be used to rule out the instability caused by ACL rupture. Table 18-3 describes current functional testing research and conclusions related to functional activity.

If there is less than a 10% deficit between limbs, higher-level functional testing can be performed. This will include jogging and backpedaling in a straight line at 25%, 50%, 75%, and 100% effort. Then, figure-8 drills are employed. Finally, cutting activities are performed, and in this case, emphasizing an open cut (sidestep cut or a Z cut) to stress the medial compartment.[27] In the late stages of knee rehabilitation, low-level plyometric

Table 18-3 Functional Test Research

Functional Test	Research
Lateral step-up	ICC.99 (Rosenthal, 1994)[22]
One-leg hop for distance	ICC.99 (Worrell, 1994)[27] ICC.96 (Bolgla, 1997)[3]
One-leg hop timed	ICC.77 (Worrell, 1994)[27] ICC.66 (Bolgla, 1997)[3]
One-leg hop triple	ICC.95 (Bolgla, 1997)[3]
One-leg hop crossover	ICC.96 (Bolgla, 1997)[3]
Four-point run	ICC.98 (Bolgla, 1997)[3]
Lateral power hop	ICC.91–92 (Tippett, 1996)[25]
Decreased one-leg timed hop without ACL	Positive correlation (Noyes, 1989)[20]
Decreased one-leg hop distance without ACL	Positive correlation (Noyes, 1990)[20]
Decreased one-leg hop distance in post-ACL reconstruction	Positive correlation (Sekiya, 1998)[24]
One-leg hop distance and time posterolateral ankle sprain	No correlation (Worrell, 1994)[27]
Objective scoring system with posterolateral ankle reconstruction	Positive correlation (Kaikkonen, 1994)[12]
One-leg hop distance with decreased quad strength without ACL	Positive correlation (Zätterström, 2000)[28]
One-leg hop distance with decreased quad strength without ACL	No correlation (Gauffin, 1990)[7]
One-leg hop distance without ACL with a strengthening and coordination program	Positive correlation (Zätterström, 2000)[28]
One-leg hop distance in reconstructed ACL and laxity	No correlation (Jonsson, 1994)[10]
Cocontraction test and isokinetic strength and power	No correlation (Lephart, 1992)[15]
Cocontraction test and ACL laxity	No correlation (Lephart, 1992)[15]

activities could be incorporated, such as hopping drills in place, in diagonal patterns, and lateral hops to stress the medial compartment.[27] If these tasks are completed without signs and symptoms of inflammation or hesitancy on the patient's part, a recommendation to return to tactical training and full duty will follow. Clinical outcomes can measure the effectiveness of the clinician's functional exercise progression. Table 18-4 describes various scoring systems that can be employed with knee injuries to document clinical outcomes.

In the upper extremity, we may have a patient who has suffered an anterior glenohumeral shoulder dislocation. Table 18-5 describes a sample progression of activities with criteria for advancement. Assume that this individual is an artist and painting is her medium. Special testing may include an anterior apprehension sign, in this case positive, along with the standard measures of ROM, strength, pain level, and proprioception in the form of joint repositioning. Angular repositioning has been advocated at the glenohumeral joint to determine the input from the mechanoreceptors about the shoulder joint.[4,6]

Table 18-4 Knee Scoring Systems

Lysholm Scale	Developed in 1986 by Lysholm 100-point scale Assesses support with ambulation, limp, stairs, squatting, pain, swelling, atrophy, and instability with walking, running, and jumping Very specific to ADL
Cincinnati Scale	Developed in 1984 by Noyes Preinjury/surgery to postinjury/surgery comparison Assesses walking, stairs, running, jumping, twisting, sports/work activity level More specific to sports
Methodist Hospital Scale	Developed in 1986 by Shelbourne Assesses 1-mile walk, stairs, jogging, heavy work, ADL, repetitive jumping, recreational and competitive sports More specific to sports
International Knee Society Scale	Developed in 1986 by the IKDC Assigns an A to D group grading based upon patient subjective assessment, pain, swelling, giving way, ROM, laxity, crepitus, and 1-leg hop More specific to ADL
Combined Rating System	Developed in 1995 by Karlson Cincinnati, HSS, Lysholm, IKDC Assesses pain, swelling, giving way, walk, stairs, squat, run, jump, twist, decelerate, sports, ADL, locking, function, limp, activity, brace, crutches
Knee Outcome Survey	Scale for disability during ADL Scale for disability during sports

ADL, activities of daily living; HSS, hospital for special surgery; IKDC, international knee documentation committee.

Functional testing at this early stage may include reaching to a certain height for a specific number of repetitions, or holding the upper extremity at a certain angle for a specific length of time. Both of these activities will recreate the functional demands of painting. In the first stage of the rehabilitation process, just as for the lower-extremity problem, the focus is on decreasing pain and swelling through modalities, increasing ROM as tolerated, and increasing strength through the use of shoulder isometrics. Functional exercise in this phase may take the form of rhythmic stabilization at 90 degrees of flexion and at 45 degrees of abduction. This technique will increase the stability of the shoulder joint by firing the dynamic stabilizers.

Also in this phase, total shoulder girdle strengthening, as tolerated, may begin with emphasis on the scapular stabilizers and rotator cuff musculature. Several electromyography studies have documented various exercises for these muscle groups. The authors use a combination of exercises recommended by Mosely et al[17] for the scapula and by Blackburn et al[2] for the rotator cuff. The core exercises for the scapula consist of rows, seated press-ups, scaption, and pushups with a plus (scapula protraction).[17] The core exercises for the rotator cuff include prone extension with external rotation, prone horizontal abduction with

Table 18-5 Shoulder Functional Progression

	Criteria for Advancement		
Functional Activity	Strength	ROM	Other
Active/passive ROM after surgery			Depends on healing restraints
Isometric strengthening	As tolerated	As tolerated	Depends on healing restraints
Elevation of arm after surgery	Successful gravity eliminated	As tolerated	Depends on healing restraints
Elevation of arm with weights	Successful elevation with no weights over 3 sets of 10 repetitions	As tolerated	Protect healing tissue as necessary
Motor control: Body blade, Thera-tubing, Plyoballs	Successful elevation with no weights over 3 sets of 10 repetitions	As tolerated	Protect healing tissue as necessary
Weight machines/full-body weight	Successful elevation with 3 lb, 3 sets of 10 repetitions 5/5 MMT	As tolerated	Isokinetics as tolerated
Free weights	Successful weight machine program	As tolerated	
Sports activities	5/5 MMT Isokinetic test WNL	Enough for sport activity	Sufficient healing time
			No pain, swelling with progressive activity

MMT, manual muscle test; WNL, within normal limits.

external rotation, and prone external rotation at 90 degrees of abduction.[2] It is up to the clinician to determine the appropriate application of these core strengthening exercises.

In the second phase of the functional exercise progression, increased emphasis is placed on raising the upper extremity in the plane of the scapula initially to raising the arm in the sagittal plane. The patient is questioned regarding the duration of time that she spends painting, and an estimation can be made as to how many times she must lift her arm in each session. For other individuals, the application of closed-chain exercises for the glenohumeral joint may be appropriate. Closed-chain exercises can be employed to increase the proprioceptive input of the joint mechanoreceptors, which will enhance motor control. Moving a ball on a wall and weight shifting on a table may be low-level activities that are easily implemented. A functional exercise progression may include quadruped activities, the use of the Profitter, and even the Stairmaster for higher-level tasks. The use of the Body Blade at this stage may also help increase the endurance of the shoulder girdle musculature while enhancing dynamic stability in the sagittal plane. In the final stage of the rehabilitation process for this individual, large muscle group strengthening and endurance exercises are added for the deltoid, pectoralis major, and latissimus dorsi. Final functional testing can be performed to determine whether the patient has the endurance and strength to hold the upper extremity at approximately 90 degrees for repetitions or time.

For the majority of patients seen in the outpatient setting with low back dysfunction, functional testing and a functional exercise progression can return them to their preinjury

Table 18-6 Lumbar Stabilization Progression

Functional Activity	Criteria for Advancement: Lumbar Stabilization Activities
Supine	Abdominal bracing Latissimus dorsi sets Gluteal sets Hip extensions sets "Marching" (hip flexions) "Dying bug" (unilateral hip and arm movement) Pelvic anterior/posterior tilt
Prone	Quadruped with arm flexion Quadruped with hip extension Quadruped with contralateral limb elevation Prone extensions
Seated	Physioball "Marching" "Dying bug"
Standing	Trunk rotation stabilization with surgical tubing ?Horizontal adduction and abduction ?Flexion and extension Chop/lift progression
Lifting	Table to table Carrying objects Floor to table Table to overhead shelf
Kneeling	Chop/lift progression
Half kneeling	Chop/lift progression

level of function (Table 18-6). For example, a patient with a bulging disk may present with pain, decreased ROM, and decreased functional status. Functional testing may include lifting tasks or sitting or walking for duration, depending on the individual's occupation. A functional exercise progression in this case would include lumbar stabilization exercises in the supine, sitting, and, ultimately, standing positions. Please refer to Chapter 15 for an in-depth discussion of stabilization of the core.

To provide one more example, suppose you have a new mother who has suffered a sprain/strain of the lumbar region while picking up her child. The immediate postinjury care is dedicated to relieving the pain, inflammation, and muscle spasm, and to restoring ROM. Proper instruction in posture and body mechanics can also begin. The second phase of the program can be initiated quickly, usually within the first 2 weeks, and activities are designed around lifting tasks. A functional exercise program may progress to minisquats to increase lower-extremity strength and endurance, to lifting tasks from various heights, to carrying objects around the clinic. Functional testing, when appropriate, is geared toward lifting an object of equal or greater weight than the infant, from the floor to the table and vice versa. Carrying for distances and holding for time will mimic feeding and nurturing tasks.

SUMMARY

1. Functional exercise progression and functional testing are important components of a complete rehabilitation program.
2. Taking into account the patient's medical condition, the healing constraints of that condition, and the external environment that must be overcome, tasks can be designed to re-create the functional demands of each individual.
3. When the patient is able to perform the goal activity without physical assistance or verbal cueing from the therapist, the entire activity is attempted and practiced.
4. The entire formal rehabilitation program does not have to be completed prior to performing functional testing or initiating a functional exercise progression.
5. Activities that are compatible with the patient's physical status may be implemented at any time. These techniques are employed by physical therapists regardless of setting and patient diagnosis.
6. The use of functional testing and functional exercise progression will enable the patient to return to preinjury level of function as quickly and safely as possible.

REFERENCES

1. Bean JF, Kiely DK, Leveille SG, et al. The 6-minute walk test in mobility-limited elders: What is being measured? *J Gerontol A Biol Sci Med Sci.* 2002;57(11):M751-M756.
2. Blackburn TA, McLeod WD, White B, et al. EMG analysis of posterior rotator cuff exercises. *Athl Train.* 1990;25:40-45.
3. Bolgla LA, Keskula DR. Reliability of lower extremity functional performance tests. *J Orthop Sports Phys Ther.* 1997;26(3):138-142.
4. Borsa PA, Lephart SM, Kocher MS, et al. Functional assessment and rehabilitation of shoulder proprioception for glenohumeral instability. *J Sport Rehabil.* 1994;3:84-104.
5. Daniel DM, Malcom L, Stone ML, et al. Quantification of knee stability and function. *Contemp Orthop.* 1982;5:83-91.
6. Davies GJ, Dickoff-Hoffman S. Neuromuscular testing and rehabilitation of the shoulder complex. *J Orthop Sports Phys Ther.* 1993;18:449-458.
7. Gauffin H, et al. Function testing in patients with old rupture of the anterior cruciate ligament. *Int J Sports Med.* 1990;11(1):73.
8. Gould J, Davies G, eds. *Orthopedic and Sports Physical Therapy*. St. Louis, MO: Mosby; 1985.
9. Jarvela T, Kannus P, Latvala K, et al. Simple measurements in assessing muscle performance after an ACL reconstruction. *Int J Sports Med.* 2002;23(3):196-201.
10. Jonsson H, Kärrholm J. Three-dimensional knee joint movements during a step-up: evaluation after anterior cruciate ligament rupture. *J Orthop Res.* 1994;12(6):769-779.
11. Juris PM, Phillips EM, Dalpe C, et al. A dynamic test of lower extremity function following anterior cruciate ligament reconstruction and rehabilitation. *J Orthop Sports Phys Ther.* 1997;26(4):184-191.
12. Kaikkonen A, Pekka K, Markku J. A performance test protocol and scoring scale for the evaluation of ankle injuries. *Am J Sports Med.* 1994;22(4):462-469.
13. Kegerreis S. The construction and implementation of functional progression as a component of athletic rehabilitation. *J Orthop Sports Phys Ther.* 1983;5:14-19.
14. Lephart SM, Perrin DN, Fu FH, et al. Functional performance tests for the ACL insufficient athlete. *J Athl Train.* 1991;26:44-50.
15. Lephart SM, et al. Proprioception following anterior cruciate ligament reconstruction. *J Sport Rehab.* 1992;1(3):188-198.
16. Mattacola CH, Jacobs CA, Rund MA, Johnson DL. Functional assessment using the step-up-and-over test and forward lunge following ACL reconstruction. *Orthopedics.* 2004;27(6):602-608.
17. Mosely BJ, Jobe FW, Pink M, et al. EMG analysis of the scapula muscles during a rehabilitation program. *Am J Sports Med.* 1992;20:128-134.
18. Munich H, Cipriani D, Hall L, et al. The test-retest reliability of an inclined squat strength test protocol. *J Orthop Sports Phys Ther.* 1997;26(4):209-213.
19. Netz Y, Ayalon M, Dunsky A, et al. The multiple-sit-to-stand field test for older adults: What does it measure? *Gerontology.* 2005;51(4):285.
20. Noyes FR, Barber SD, Mangine RE. Abnormal lower limb symmetry determined by functional hop tests after anterior cruciate ligament rupture. *Am J Sports Med.* 1991;19:513-518.
21. Reed BV. Wound healing and the use of thermal agents. In: Michovitz S, ed. *Thermal Agents in Rehabilitation.* Philadelphia, PA: FA Davis; 1996:3-29.

22. Rosenthal MD, Baer LL, Griffith PP, et al. Comparability of work output measures as determined by isokinetic dynamometry and a closed chain kinetic exercise. *J Sport Rehabil.* 1994;3:218-227.

23. Rudolph KS, Axe MJ, Snyder-Mackler L. Dynamic stability after ACL injury: who can hop? *Knee Surg Sports Traumatol Arthrosc.* 2000;8:262-269.

24. Sekiya I, et al. Significance of the single-legged hop test to the anterior cruciate ligament-reconstructed knee in relation to muscle strength and anterior laxity. *Am J Sports Med.* 1998;26(3):384-388.

25. Tippett SR, Voight ML. *Functional Progressions for Sports Rehabilitation.* Champaign, IL: Human Kinetics; 1995.

26. Wilk KE, Romaniello WT, Soscia SM, et al. The relationship between subjective knee scores, isokinetic testing and functional testing in the ACL reconstructed knee. *J Orthop Sports Phys Ther.* 1994;20:60-73.

27. Worrell TW, Booher LD, Hench KM. Closed kinetic chain assessment following inversion ankle sprain. *J Sport Rehabil.* 1994;3:197-203.

28. Zätterström R, et al. Rehabilitation following acute anterior cruciate ligament injuries—a 12-month follow-up of a randomized clinical trial. *Scand J Med Sci Sports.* 2000;10(3):156-163.

19

Functional Training and Advanced Rehabilitation

Michael L. Voight, Barbara J. Hoogenboom, Gray Cook, and Greg Rose

OBJECTIVES **After completion of this chapter, the physical therapist should be able to do the following:**

- Define and discuss the importance of proprioception in the neuromuscular control process.
- Define and discuss the different levels of motor control by the central nervous system and the neural pathways responsible for transmission of afferent and efferent information at each level.
- Apply a systematic functional evaluation designed to provoke symptoms.
- Demonstrate consistency between functional and clinical testing information (combinatorial power).
- Apply a 3-step model designed to promote the practical systematic thinking required for effective therapeutic exercise prescription and progression.
- Define and discuss objectives of a functional neuromuscular rehabilitation program.
- Develop a rehabilitation program that uses various exercise techniques for development of neuromuscular control.

Function and Functional Rehabilitation

The basic goal in rehabilitation is to restore and enhance function within the environment and to perform specific activities of daily living (ADL). The entire rehabilitation process should be focused on improving the functional status of the patient. The concept of functional training is not new, nor is it limited to function related to sports. By definition, *function* means having a purpose or duty. Therefore, *functional* can be defined as performing a practical or intended function or duty. Function should be considered in terms of a spectrum because ADL encompass many different tasks for many different people. What is functional to one person may not be functional to another. It is widely accepted that to perform a specific activity better, one must practice that activity. Therefore, the functional exercise progression for return to ADL can best be defined as breaking the specific activities down into a hierarchy and then performing them in a sequence that allows acquisition or reacquisition of that skill. It is important to note that although people develop different levels of skill, function, and motor control, certain fundamental tasks are common to nearly all individuals (barring pathologic conditions and disability). Lifestyle, habits, injury, and other factors can erode the fundamental components of movement without obvious alterations in higher-level function and skill. Ongoing higher-level function is a testament to the compensatory power of the neurologic system. Imperfect function and skill create stress in other body systems. Fundamental elements can first be observed during the developmental progression of posture and motor control. The sequence of developmental progression can also give insight into the original acquisition of skill. The ability to assess retention or loss of fundamental movement patterns is therefore a way to enhance rehabilitation. The rehabilitation process starts with a 2-part appraisal that creates perspective by viewing both ends of the functional spectrum:

- The current level of function (ADL, work, and sports/recreation) relative to the patient's needs and goals.
- The ability to demonstrate the fundamental movement patterns that represent the foundation of function and basic motor control.

Objectives of Functional Rehabilitation

The overall objective of a functional exercise program is to return patients to their preinjury level as quickly and as safely as possible by resolving or reducing the measurable dysfunction within fundamental and functional movement patterns. Specific training activities are designed to restore both dynamic joint stability and ADL skills.[1] To accomplish this objective, a basic tenet of exercise physiology is used. The SAID (specific adaptations to imposed demands) principle states that the body will adapt to the stress and strain placed on it.[2] Athletes cannot succeed if they have not been prepared to meet all the demands of their specific activity.[2] Reactive neuromuscular training (RNT) helps bridge the gap from traditional rehabilitation via proprioceptive and balance training to promote a more functional return to activity.[2] The SAID principle provides constructive stress, and RNT creates opportunities for input and integration. The main objective of the RNT program is to facilitate the unconscious process of interpreting and integrating the peripheral sensations received by the central nervous system (CNS) into appropriate motor responses. This approach is enhanced by the unique clinical focus on pathologic orthopedic and neurologic states and their functional representation. This special focus forces the clinician to consider evaluation of human movement as a complex multisystem interaction and the logical starting point for exercise prescription. Sometimes this will require a breakdown of the supporting mobility and stability within a pattern. Regardless of the specific nature of the corrective needs, all the functional exercises follow a simple but very specific path. First, the functional exercise program is driven by a functional screening or assessment that produces a baseline of movement. The process of screening and assessment will rate and rank patterns. It will provide valuable information about dysfunction in movement patterns such as asymmetry, difficulty with movement, and pain. Screening and assessment will therefore identify faulty movement patterns that should not be exercised or trained until corrected. Second, the functional framework will assist in making the best possible choices for corrective categories and exercises. No single exercise is best for a movement problem, but there is an appropriate category of corrective exercises to choose from. Third, following the initial session of corrective exercises, the movement pattern should be rechecked for changes against the original baseline. Fourth, once an obvious change is noted in the key pattern, the screening or assessment is repeated to survey other changes in movement and identify the next priority. By working on the most fundamental pattern, it is possible to see other positive changes. Therefore, these 4 steps provide the framework that makes corrective exercise successful:

- The screening and assessment direct the clinician to the most fundamental movement dysfunction.
- One or 2 of the most practical corrective exercises from the appropriate category should be chosen and applied.
- Once the exercise has been taught and is being performed correctly, check for improvement in the dysfunctional basic movement pattern as revealed by specific tests in the screening or assessment.

This concept is called the *functional continuum.* Most patients seek care because of an obvious source of pain or dysfunction. What is not obvious is the true cause of the pain or dysfunction, ascertainment of which is the purpose of functional movement assessment (see Chapter 17). By looking at movement as a whole, all the compensations and conscious sources of pain and dysfunction can be highlighted and addressed. Patients fall into one of four phases on a functional continuum (Table 19-1).

Table 19-1 Four Phases of the Functional Continuum

Phase	Description
Subconscious dysfunction	This is the initial phase when most patients are first seen by the clinician. Patients are totally unaware of their true dysfunction (it is in their subconscious) or are convinced that the problem lies elsewhere.
Conscious dysfunction	This is what happens after a movement assessment is performed. Patients are now aware of their true dysfunction (it is in their conscious), and they can start to address the real cause.
Conscious function	This phase is entered once patients can perform the correct functional pattern, but it is not automatic (it is functional only with conscious control). They still need conscious effort to perform a good pattern of movement.
Subconscious function	The final stage occurs when patients can perform a functional pattern automatically (it is in their subconscious control) without having to think about the correction.

Table 19-2 Three Rs of Treatment Phases

R	Description
Reset	Most problems require resetting of the complete system to break them out of their dysfunctional phase. By just jumping to exercises, the results can be less than optimal. Types of treatments that would be considered a "reset" include joint mobilization, soft-tissue mobilization, and various soft-tissue techniques.
Reinforce	Once the system has been reset, many dysfunctions will need support or reinforcement while proper patterns are being introduced. Types of reinforcement devices include taping, bracing, orthotics, postural devices, and static and dynamic stretching.
Reload	The last phase of treatment is the exercise implementation or reload phase, in which the new software is loaded into the central nervous system and a true functional pattern of motion can be reprogrammed.

Exercise prescription choices must continually represent the specialized training of the clinician through a consistent and centralized focus on human function and consideration of the fundamentals that make function possible. Exercise applied at any given therapeutic level must refine movement, not simply create general exertion in the hope of increased tolerance of movement.[3] Moore and Durstine state, "Unfortunately, exercise training to optimize functional capacity has not been well studied in the context of most chronic diseases or disabilities. As a result, many exercise professionals have used clinical experience to develop their own methods for prescribing exercise."[4] Experience, self-critique, and specialization produce seasoned clinicians with intuitive evaluation abilities and innovations in exercise that are sometimes difficult to follow and even harder to ascertain; however, common characteristics do exist. Clinical experts use parallel (simultaneous) consideration of all factors influencing functional movement. RNT as a treatment philosophy is inclusive and adaptable and has the ability to address a variety of clinical situations. It should also be understood that a clinical philosophy is designed to serve, not to be served. The treatment design demonstrates specific attention to the parts (clinical measurements and isolated details) with continual consideration of the whole (restoration of function).[3] Moore and Durstine follow their previous statement by acknowledging that "Experience is an acceptable way to guide exercise management, but a systematic approach would be better."[4] We use the 3 "Rs" as a way to understand the type of treatment phases that a patient will undergo (Table 19-2).

The Three-Phase Model for Prescription of Exercise

This chapter demonstrates a practical model designed to promote the systematic thinking required for effective prescription of therapeutic exercise and progression at each phase of rehabilitation.[3] The approach is a serial (consecutive) step-by-step method that will, with practice and experience, lead to parallel thinking and multilevel problem solving. The intended purpose of this method is to reduce arbitrary trial-and-error attempts at prescribing effective exercise and lessen protocol-based thinking. It will give the novice clinician a framework that will guide but not confine clinical exercise prescription. It will provide experienced clinicians with a system to observe their particular strengths and weaknesses in dosage and design of exercise. Inexperienced and experienced clinicians alike will

Box 19-1 Three-Phase Rehabilitation Model

1. Proprioception and kinesthesia
2. Dynamic stability
3. Reactive neuromuscular control

develop practical insight by applying the model and observing the interaction of the systems that produce human movement. The focus is specifically geared to orthopedic rehabilitation and the clinical problem-solving strategies used to develop an exercise prescription through an outcome-based goal-setting process. All considerations for therapeutic exercise prescription will give equal importance to conventional orthopedic exercise standards (biomechanical and physiologic parameters) and neurophysiologic strategies (motor learning, proprioceptive feedback, and synergistic recruitment principles). This 3-phase model (Box 19-1) will create a mechanism that necessitates interaction between orthopedic exercise approaches and optimal neurophysiologic techniques. It includes a 4-principle foundation that demonstrates the hierarchy and interaction of the founding concepts used in rehabilitation (both orthopedic and neurologic). For all practical purposes, these 4 categories help demonstrate the efficient and effective continuity necessary for formulation of a treatment plan and prompt the clinician to maintain an inclusive, open-minded clinical approach.

This chapter is written with the clinic-based practitioner in mind. It will help the clinician formulate an exercise philosophy. Some clinicians will discover reasons for success that were intuitive and therefore hard to communicate to other professionals. Others will discover a missing step in the therapeutic exercise design process. Much of the confusion and frustration encountered by rehabilitation specialists is because of the vast variety of treatment options afforded by ever-improving technology and accessibility to emerging research evidence. To effectively use the wealth of current information and what the future has yet to bestow, clinicians must adopt an operational framework or personal philosophy about therapeutic exercise. If a clinical exercise philosophy is based on technology, equipment, or protocols, the scope of problem solving is strictly confined. It would continually change because no universal standard or gauge exists. However, a philosophy based solely on the structure and function of the human body will keep the focus (Box 19-2) uncorrupted and centralized. Technologic developments can enhance the effectiveness of exercise only as long as the technology, system, or protocol remains true to a holistic functional standard. Known functional standards should serve as governing factors that improve the clinical consistency of the clinician and rehabilitation team for prescription and progression of training methods. The 4 principles for exercise prescription are based on human movement and the systems on which it is constructed (Box 19-2). The intent of these 4 distinct categories is to break down and reconstruct the factors that influence functional movement and to stimulate inductive reasoning, deductive reasoning, and the critical thinking needed

Box 19-2 Four Principles for Prescription of Exercise

Functional evaluation and assessment in relation to dysfunction (disability) and impairment

Identification and management of motor control

Identification and management of osteokinematic and arthrokinematic limitations

Identification of current movement patterns followed by facilitation and integration of synergistic movement patterns to develop a therapeutic exercise progression. It is hoped that these factors will serve the intended purpose of organization and clarity, thereby giving due respect to the many insightful clinicians who have provided the foundation and substance for construction of this practical framework.[3]

Proprioception, Receptors, and Neuromuscular Control

Success in skilled performance depends on how effectively an individual detects, perceives, and uses relevant sensory information. Knowing exactly where our limbs are in space and how much muscular effort is required to perform a particular action is critical for successful performance of all activities requiring intricate coordination of the various body parts. Fortunately, information about the position and movement of various body parts is available from peripheral receptors located in and around articular structures and the surrounding musculature. A detailed discussion of proprioception and neuromuscular control is also presented in Chapter 9.

Joints: Support and Sensory Function

In a normal healthy joint, both static and dynamic stabilizers provide support. The role of capsuloligamentous tissues in the dynamic restraint of joints has been well established in the literature.[5-15] Although the primary role of these structures is mechanical in nature by providing structural support and stabilization to the joint, the capsuloligamentous tissues also play an important sensory role by detecting joint position and motion.[8,16-18] Sensory afferent feedback from receptors in the capsuloligamentous structures projects directly to the reflex and cortical pathways, thereby mediating reactive muscle activity for dynamic restraint.[5,6,8,17,19] The efferent motor response that ensues from the sensory information is called *neuromuscular control.* Sensory information is sent to the CNS to be processed, and appropriate motor strategies are executed.

Physiology of Proprioception

Sherrington[18] first described the term *proprioception* in the early 1900s when he noted the presence of receptors in the joint capsular structures that were primarily reflexive in nature. Since that time, mechanoreceptors have been morphohistologically identified around articular structures in both animal and human models. In addition, the well-described muscle spindle and Golgi tendon organs are powerful mechanoreceptors. Mechanoreceptors are specialized end-organs that function as biologic transducers for conversion of the mechanical energy of physical deformation (elongation, compression, and pressure) into action nerve potentials yielding proprioceptive information.[10] Although receptor discharge varies according to the intensity of the distortion, mechanoreceptors can also be described in terms of their discharge rates. Quickly adapting receptors cease discharging shortly after the onset of a stimulus, whereas slowly adapting receptors continue to discharge while the stimulus is present.[8,10,20] Around a healthy joint, quickly adapting receptors are responsible for providing conscious and unconscious kinesthetic sensations in response to joint movement or acceleration, whereas slowly adapting mechanoreceptors provide continuous feedback and thus proprioceptive information related to joint position[10,20,21] (see Chapter 9 for examples of quickly and slowly adapting receptors).

Once stimulated, mechanoreceptors are able to adapt. With constant stimulation, the frequency of the neural impulses decreases. The functional implication is that mechanoreceptors detect change and rates of change, as opposed to steady-state conditions.[22] This input is then analyzed in the CNS to determine joint position and movement.[23] The status of the musculoskeletal structures is sent to the CNS so that information about static versus dynamic conditions, equilibrium versus disequilibrium, or biomechanical stress and strain relationships can be evaluated.[24,25] Once processed and evaluated, this proprioceptive information becomes capable of influencing muscle tone, motor execution programs, and cognitive somatic perceptions or kinesthetic awareness.[26] Proprioceptive information also protects the joint from damage caused by movement exceeding the normal physiologic range of motion (ROM) and helps determine the appropriate balance of synergistic and antagonistic forces. All this information helps in generating a somatosensory image within the CNS. Therefore, the soft tissues surrounding a joint serve a double purpose: they provide biomechanical support to the bony partners making up the joint by keeping them in relative anatomic alignment, and through an extensive afferent neurologic network, they provide valuable proprioceptive information.

Central Nervous System: Integration of Motor Control

The response of the CNS falls into 3 categories or levels of motor control: spinal reflexes, brainstem processing, and cognitive cerebral cortex program planning. The goal of the rehabilitation process is to retrain the altered afferent pathways and thereby enhance the neuromuscular control system. To accomplish this goal, the objective of the rehabilitation program should be to hyperstimulate the joint and muscle receptors to encourage maximal afferent discharge to the respective CNS levels.[21,27-30]

First-Level Response: Muscle

When faced with an unexpected load, the first reflexive muscle response is a burst of electromyographic activity that occurs between 30 and 50 milliseconds. The afferent fibers of both the muscle spindle and the Golgi tendon organ mechanoreceptors synapse with the spinal interneurons and produce a reflexive facilitation or inhibition of the motor neurons.[28,30,31] The monosynaptic stretch reflex is one of the most rapid reflexes underlying limb control. The stretch reflex occurs at an unconscious level and is not affected by extrinsic factors. These responses can occur simultaneously to control limb position and posture. Because they can occur at the same time, are in parallel, are subconscious, and are not subject to cortical interference, they do not require attention and are thus automatic.

At this level of motor control, activities to encourage short-loop reflex joint stabilization should dominate.[15,21,27,30] These activities are characterized by sudden alterations in joint position that require reflex muscle stabilization. With sudden alterations or perturbations, both the articular and muscular mechanoreceptors will be stimulated to produce reflex stabilization. Rhythmic stabilization exercises encourage monosynaptic cocontraction of the musculature, thereby producing dynamic neuromuscular stabilization.[32] These exercises serve to build a foundation for dynamic stability.

Second-Level Response: Brainstem

The second level of motor control interaction is at the level of the brainstem.[25,28,33] At this level, afferent mechanoreceptors interact with the vestibular system and visual input from the eyes to control or facilitate postural stability and equilibrium of the body.[21,25,27-29] Afferent mechanoreceptor input also works in concert with the muscle spindle complex by inhibiting antagonistic muscle activity under conditions of rapid lengthening and periarticular distortion, both of which accompany postural disruption.[26,30] In conditions of disequilibrium in which simultaneous neural input exists, a neural pattern is generated that affects the muscular stabilizers and thereby returns equilibrium to the body's center of gravity.[28] Therefore, balance is influenced by the same peripheral afferent mechanism that mediates joint proprioception and is at least partially dependent on an individual's inherent ability to integrate joint position sense with neuromuscular control.[34]

Clinical Pearl

Balance activities, both with and without visual input, will enhance motor function at the brainstem level.[28,33]

It is important that these activities remain specific to the types of activities or skills that will be required of the athlete on return to sport.[35] Static balance activities should be used as a precursor to more dynamic skill activity.[35] Static balance skills can be initiated when the individual is able to bear weight on the lower extremity. The general progression of static balance activities is to move from bilateral to unilateral and from eyes open to eyes closed.[21,28,35-37] With balance training, it is important to remember that the sensory systems respond to environmental manipulation. To stimulate or facilitate the proprioceptive system, vision must be disadvantaged, which can be accomplished in several ways (Box 19-3).

Third-Level Response: Central Nervous System/Cognitive

Appreciation of joint position at the highest or cognitive level needs to be included in an RNT program. These types of activities are initiated on the cognitive level and include programming motor commands for voluntary movement. Repetitions of these movements will maximally stimulate the conversion of conscious programming to unconscious programming.[21,25,27-29,38] The term for this type of training is the *forced-use paradigm*. By making a task significantly more difficult or asking for multiple tasks, the CNS is bombarded with input. The CNS attempts to sort and process this overload information by opening additional neural pathways. When the individual goes back to a basic ADL task, the task becomes easier. This information can then be stored as a central command and ultimately be performed without continuous reference to conscious thought as a triggered response.[21,27-29,39] As with all training, the single greatest obstacle to motor learning is the conscious mind. We must get the conscious mind out of the act!

Box 19-3 Ways to Disadvantage Vision for Stimulation of the Proprioceptive System

Remove vision by either closing or blindfolding the eyes.

Destabilize vision with demanding hand and eye movements (ball toss) or by moving the visual surround.

Confuse vision with unstable visual cues that disagree with the proprioceptive and vestibular input (sway referencing).

Closed-Loop, Open-Loop, and Feed-Forward Integration

Why is a coordinated motor response important? When an unexpected load is placed on a joint, ligamentous damage occurs in 70 to 90 milliseconds unless an appropriate response ensues.[40-42] Therefore, reactive muscle activity that provides sufficient magnitude in the 40- to 80-millisecond time frame must occur after loading begins to protect the capsuloligamentous structures. The closed-loop system of CNS integration may not be fast enough to produce a response to increase muscle stiffness. There is simply no time for the system to process the information and provide feedback about the condition. Failure of the dynamic restraint system to control abnormal force will expose the static structures to excessive force. In this case, the open-loop system of anticipation becomes more important in producing the desired response. Preparatory muscle activity in anticipation of joint loading can influence the reactive muscle activation patterns. Anticipatory activation increases the sensitivity of the muscle spindles, thereby allowing the unexpected perturbations to be detected more quickly.[43]

Very quick movements are completed before feedback can be used to produce an action to alter the course of movement. Therefore, if the movement is fast enough, a mechanism such as a motor program would have to be used to control the entire action, with the movement being carried out without any feedback. Fortunately, the open-loop control system allows the motor control system to organize an entire action ahead of time. For this to occur, previous knowledge needs to be preprogrammed into the primary sensory cortex (Box 19-4).

In the open-loop system, a program that sets up some kind of neural mechanism or network that is preprogrammed organizes movement in advance. A classic example of this occurs in the body as postural adjustments are made before the intended movement. When an arm is raised into forward flexion, the first muscle groups to fire are not even in the shoulder girdle region. The first muscles to contract are those in the lower part of the back and legs (approximately 80 milliseconds pass before noticeable activity occurs in the shoulder) to provide a stable base for movement.[44] Because the shoulder muscles are linked to the rest of the body, their contraction affects posture. If no preparatory compensations in posture were made, raising the arm would shift the center of gravity forward and cause a slight loss of balance. The feed-forward motor control system takes care of this potential problem by preprogramming the appropriate postural modification first rather than requiring the body to make adjustments after the arm begins to move.

Lee[45] demonstrated that these preparatory postural adjustments are not independent of the arm movement but rather are part of the total motor pattern. When the arm movements are organized, the motor instructions are preprogrammed to adjust posture first and then move the arm. Therefore, arm movement and postural control are not separate events but instead are different parts of an integrated action that raises the arm while maintaining balance. Lee showed that these electromyographic preparatory postural adjustments

Box 19-4 Preprogrammed Information Needed for an Open-Loop System to Work

- The particular muscles that are needed to produce an action.
- The order in which these muscles need to be activated.
- The relative forces of the various muscle contractions.
- The relative timing and sequencing of these actions.
- The duration of the respective contractions.

disappear when the individual leans against some type of support before raising the arm. The motor control system recognizes that advance preparation for postural control is not needed when the body is supported against the wall.

It is important to remember that most motor tasks are a complex blend of both open- and closed-loop operations. Therefore, both types of control are often at work simultaneously. Both feed-forward and feedback neuromuscular control can enhance dynamic stability if the sensory and motor pathways are frequently stimulated.[21] Each time a signal passes through a sequence of synapses, the synapses become more capable of transmitting the same signal.[14,46] When these pathways are "facilitated" regularly, memory of that signal is created and can be recalled to program future movements.[14,47]

Conclusion: Relationship to Rehabilitation

A rehabilitation program that addresses the need for restoring normal joint stability and proprioception cannot be constructed until one has total appreciation of both the mechanical and sensory functions of the articular structures.[27] Knowledge of the basic physiology of how these muscular and joint mechanoreceptors work together in the production of smooth, controlled coordinated motion is critical in developing a rehabilitation training program. This is because the role of the joint musculature extends well beyond absolute strength and the capacity to resist fatigue. With simple restoration of mechanical restraints or strengthening of the associated muscles, the smooth coordinated neuromuscular controlling mechanisms required for joint stability are neglected.[27] The complexity of joint motion necessitates synergy and synchrony of muscle firing patterns, thereby permitting proper joint stabilization, especially during sudden changes in joint position, which is common in functional activities. Understanding of these relationships and functional implications will allow the clinician greater variability and success in returning patients safely back to their playing environment.

Four Principles for Therapeutic Exercise Prescription

The functional exercise program follows a linear path from basic mobility to basic stability to movement patterns. Corrective exercise falls into one of the 3 basic categories: mobility, stability, and retraining of movement patterns. Mobility exercises focus on joint ROM, tissue length, and muscle flexibility. Stability exercises focus on the basic sequencing of movement. These exercises target postural control of the starting and ending positions within each movement pattern. Movement pattern retraining incorporates the use of fundamental mobility and stability into specific movement patterns to reinforce coordination and timing.

The corrective exercise progression always starts with mobility exercises. Because many poor movement patterns are associated with abnormalities in mobility, restoration of movement needs to be addressed first. Mobility exercises should be performed bilaterally to confirm limitation and asymmetry of mobility. Clinicians should never assume that they know the location or side in which mobility is restricted. Rather, both sides should always be checked and mobility cleared before advancing the exercise program. If the assessment reveals a limitation or asymmetry, it should be the primary focus of the corrective exercise program. Treatments that promote mobility can involve manual therapy, such as soft-tissue and joint mobilization and manipulation. Treatments of mobility might also include any modality that improves tissue pliability or freedom of movement. If no change in mobility is appreciated, the clinician should not proceed to stability work. Rather, all mobility problems should continue to be worked on until a measurable change is noted. Mobility does not need to become full or normal, but improvement must be noted before advancing. The clinician can proceed to a stability exercise only if the increased mobility allows the patient to get into the appropriate exercise posture and position. The stability work should reinforce the new mobility, and the new mobility makes improved stabilization possible because the new mobility provides new sensory information. If there is any question about compromised mobility, each exercise session should always return to mobility exercises before moving to stability exercises. This ensures that proper tissue length and joint alignment are available for the stabilization exercises.

When no limitation or asymmetry is present during the mobility corrective exercises, one can move directly to stability corrective exercises. Once mobility has been restored, it needs to be controlled. Stability exercises demand posture, alignment, balance, and control of forces within the newly available range and without the support of compensatory stiffness or muscle tone. Stability exercises should be considered as challenges to posture and position, rather than being conventional strength exercises.

We propose 4 principles for therapeutic exercise prescription, which we describe as the 4 "Ps" in this section. These principles serve to guide decisions for selecting, advancing, and terminating therapeutic exercise interventions. Application of these 4 principles in the appropriate sequence will allow the clinician to understand the starting point, a consistent progression, and the end point for each exercise prescription. This sequence is achieved by using functional activities and fundamental movement patterns as goals. By proceeding in this fashion, the clinician will have the ability to evaluate the whole before the parts and then discuss the parts as they apply. Table 19-3 lists and describes the principles for therapeutic exercise prescription.

Table 19-3 Four Principles for Therapeutic Exercise Prescription

Principle	Description
Functional evaluation and assessment in relation to dysfunction (disability) and impairment	The evaluation must identify a functional problem or limitation resulting in diagnosis of a functional problem. Observation of whole movement patterns tempered by practical knowledge of key stress points and common compensatory patterns will improve the efficiency of evaluation.
Identification and management of motor control	Rehabilitation can be greatly advanced by understanding functional milestones and fundamental movements such as those demonstrated during the positions and postures paramount to growth and development. These milestones serve as key representations of functional mobility and control, as well as play a role in the initial setup and design of the exercise program.
Identification and management of osteokinematic and arthrokinematic limitations	The skills and techniques of orthopedic manual therapy are beneficial in identifying specific arthrokinematic restrictions that would limit movement or impede the motor-learning process. Management of myofascial and capsular structures will improve osteokinematic movement, as well as allow balanced muscle tone between the agonist and antagonist. It will also help the clinician understand the dynamics of the impairment.
Identification of current movement patterns followed by facilitation and integration of synergistic movement patterns	Once restrictions and limitations are managed and gross motion is restored, application of proprioceptive neuromuscular facilitation-type patterning will further improve neuromuscular function and control. Consideration of synergistic movement is the final step in restoration of function by focusing on coordination, timing, and motor learning.

Clinical Pearl

The true art of rehabilitation is to understand the whole of synergistic functional movement and the therapeutic techniques that will have the greatest positive effect on that movement in the least amount of time.

The Four Ps

The 4 Ps represent the 4 principles for therapeutic exercise: purpose, posture, position, and pattern (Table 19-4). They serve as quick reminders of the hierarchy, interaction, and application of each principle. The questions of *what, when, where,* and *how* for functional movement assessment and exercise prescription are addressed in the appropriate order (Table 19-4).

Table 19-4 Memory Cues and Primary Questions Associated with the Four Principles for Prescription of Therapeutic Exercise

Principle	Memory Cue	Memory Cue Definition	Primary Questions
Functional evaluation and assessment	Purpose	Used during both the evaluation process and the exercise prescription process to keep the clinician intently focused on the greatest single factor limiting function	"*What* functional activity is limited?" "*What* does the limitation appear to be—a mobility problem or a stability problem?" "*What* is the dysfunction or disability?" "*What* fundamental movement is limited?" "*What* is the impairment?"
Identification of motor control	Posture	Helps the clinician remember to consider a more holistic approach to exercise prescription	"*When* in the development sequence is the impairment obvious?" "*When* do the substitutions and compensations occur?" "*When* in the developmental sequence does the patient demonstrate success?" "*When* in the developmental sequence does the patient experience difficulty?" "*When* is the best possible starting point for exercise with respect to posture?"
Identification of osteokinematic and arthrokinematic limitations	Position	Describes not only the location of the anatomic structure (joint, muscle group, ligament, etc) where impairment has been identified but also the positions (with respect to movement and load) in which the greatest and least limitations occur	"*Where* is the impairment located?" "*Where* among the structures (myofascial or articular) does the impairment have its greatest effect?" "*Where* in the range of motion does the impairment affect position the greatest?" "*Where* is the most beneficial position for the exercise?"
Integration of synergistic movement patterns	Pattern	Cues the clinician to continually consider the functional movements of the human body that occur in unified patterns that occupy 3-dimensional space and cross 3 planes (frontal, sagittal, and transverse)	"*How* is the movement pattern different on bilateral comparison?" "*How* can synergistic movement, coordination, recruitment and timing be facilitated?" "*How* will this affect the limitation in movement?" "*How* will this affect function?"

Pain

Aristotle said, "We cannot learn without pain," which is very wise because pain is usually life's most powerful teacher. However, pain is simply the brain's interpretation of a neurologic signal normally associated with trauma, dysfunction, and instant and continuing damage. Pain affects motor control and greatly reduces the effectiveness of even the best corrective exercise technique.

Purpose

The word *purpose* is simply a cue to be used during both the evaluation process and the exercise prescription process to keep the clinician intently focused on the greatest single factor limiting function. The primary questions to ask for this principle appear in Table 19-4. It is not uncommon for clinicians to attempt to resolve multiple problems with the initial exercise prescription. However, the practice of identifying the single greatest limiting factor will reduce frustration and also not overwhelm the patient. Other factors may have been identified in the evaluation, but a major limiting factor or a single weak link should stand out and be the focus of the initial therapeutic exercise intervention. Alterations in the limiting factor may produce positive changes elsewhere, which can be identified and considered before the next exercise progression.

Table 19-5 **Three Levels of Functional Evaluation**

Level	Name	Description
I	Functional activity assessment	Combined movements common to the patient's lifestyle and occupation are reproduced. They usually fit the definition of a general or specific skill.
II	Functional or fundamental movement assessment	The clinician takes what is learned through the observation of functional movements and breaks the movements down to the static and transitional postures seen in the normal developmental sequence.
III	Specific clinical measurement	Clinical measurements are used to identify and quantify specific problems that contribute to limitations in motion or control.

The functional evaluation process should take on 3 distinct layers or levels (Table 19-5). Each of the 3 levels should involve qualitative observations followed by quantitative documentation when possible. Normative data are helpful, but bilateral comparison is also effective and demonstrates the functional problem to the patient at each level. Many patients think that the problem is simply symptomatic and structural in nature and have no example of dysfunction outside of pain with movement. Moffroid and Zimny suggest that "Muscle strength of the right and left sides is more similar in the proximal muscles whereas we accept a 10% to 15% difference in strength of the distal muscles. . . . With joint flexibility, we accept a 5% difference between goniometric measurements of the right and left sides."[48]

The functional activity assessment involves a reproduction of combined movements common to the patient's lifestyle and occupation. These movements usually fit the definition of a general or specific skill. The clinician must have the patient demonstrate a variety of positions and not just positions that correspond to the reproduction of symptoms.[49] Static postural assessment is included, as well as assessment of dynamic activity. The quality of control and movement is assessed. Specific measurement of bilateral differences is difficult, but demonstration and observation are helpful for the patient. The clinician should note the positions and activities that provoke symptoms, as well as the activities that illustrate poor body mechanics, poor alignment, right-left asymmetries, and inappropriate weight shifting. When the clinician has observed gross movement quality, it may be necessary to also quantify movement performance. Repetition of the activity for evaluation of endurance, reproduction of symptoms, or demonstration of rapidly declining quality will create a functional baseline for bilateral comparison and documentation.

Next is the functional or fundamental movement assessment. The clinician must take what is learned through the observation of functional movements and break the movements down into the static and transitional postures seen in the normal developmental sequence. This breakdown will reduce activities to the many underlying mobilizing and stabilizing actions and reactions that constitute the functional activity. More simply stated, the activity is broken down into a sequence of primary movements that can be observed independently. It must be noted that these movements still involve multiple joints and muscles.[49] Assessment of individual joints and muscle groups will be performed during clinical measurements. Martin notes, "The developmental sequence has provided the most consistent base for almost all approaches used by physical therapists."[48] This is a powerful statement, and because true qualitative measurements of normal movement in adult populations are limited, the clinician must look for universal similarities in movement. Changes in fundamental movements can effect significant and prompt changes in function and must therefore be considered functional as well. Because the movement patterns of most adults are habitual and specific and thus are not representative of a full or optimal movement spectrum, the clinician must first consider the nonspecific basic movement patterns common to all individuals during growth and development. The developmental sequence is predictable and universal in the first 2 years of life,[50] with individual differences seen in the rate and quality of the progression. The differences are minimal in comparison to the variations seen in the adult population with their many habits, occupations, and lifestyles. In addition to diverse movement patterns, the adult population has the consequential complicating factor of a previous medical and injury history. Each medical problem or injury has had some degree of influence on activity and movement. Thus, evaluation of functional activities alone may hide many uneconomical movement patterns, compensations, and asymmetries that when integrated into functional activities, are not readily obvious to the clinician. By using the fundamental movements of the developmental progression, the clinician can view mobility and static and dynamic stability problems in a more isolated setting. Although enormous variations in functional movement quality and quantity are seen in specific adult patient populations, most individuals have the developmental sequence in common.[50] The movements used in normal motor development are the building blocks of skill and function.[50] Many of these building blocks can be lost while the skill is maintained or retained at some level (though rarely optimal). We will refer to these movement building blocks as *fundamental movements* and consider them precursors to higher function. Bilateral comparison is helpful when the clinician identifies qualitative differences between the right and left sides. These movements (like functional activities) can be compared quantitatively as well.

Finally, clinical measurements will be used to identify and quantify specific problems that are contributing to limitation of motion or limitation of control. Clinical measurements will first classify a patient through qualitative assessment. The parameters that define that classification must then be quantified to reveal impairment. These classifications are called hypermobility and hypomobility and help create guides for treatment that consider the functional status, anatomic structures, and the severity of symptoms. The clinician should not proceed into exercise prescription without proper identification of one of these general categories. The success or failure of a particular exercise treatment regimen probably depends more on this classification than on the choice of exercise technique or protocol.

Once the appropriate clinical classification is determined, specific quantitative measurements will define the level of involvement within the classification and set a baseline for exercise treatment. Periodic reassessment may identify a different major limiting factor or a weak link that may require reclassification, followed by specific measurement. The new problem or limitation would then be inserted as the purpose for a new exercise intervention. A simple diagram (Figure 19-1) will help the clinician separate the different levels of function so that intervention and purpose will always be at the appropriate level and assist in the clinical decision making related to exercise prescription.[51]

Posture

Posture is a word to help the clinician consider a more holistic approach to exercise prescription. The primary questions to ask for this principle appear in Table 19-4. Janda[52] stated an interesting point when discussing posture and the muscles responsible for its maintenance. Most discussions on posture and the musculature responsible for posture generally refer to erect standing. However, "... erect standing position is so well balanced that little or no activity is necessary to maintain it."[52] Therefore, "basic human posture should be derived from the principal movement pattern, namely gait. Since we stand on one leg for most of the time during walking, the stance on one leg should be considered to be the typical posture in man; the postural muscles are those which maintain this posture." Janda reported the ratio of single-leg to double-leg stance in gait to be 85% to 15%. "The muscles which maintain erect posture in standing on one leg are exactly those which show a striking tendency to get tight."[53] Infants and toddlers use tonic holding before normal motor development and maturation produce the ability to use cocontraction as a means of effective support. "Tonic holding is the ability of tonic postural muscles to maintain a contraction in their shortened range against gravitational or manual resistance."[54] An adult orthopedic patient may revert to some level of tonic holding after injury or in the presence of pain and altered proprioception. Likewise, adults who have habitual postures and limited activity may adopt tonic holding for some postures. Just as Janda uses single-leg stance to observe postural function with greater specificity than the more conventional double-leg erect standing, the developmental progression can offer greater understanding by examination of the precursors to single-leg stance.[55] As stated earlier, fundamental movements are basic representations of mobility, stability, and dynamic stability and include the transitional postures used in growth and development. From supine to standing, each progressive posture imposes greater demands on motor control and balance. Box 19-5 lists the most common postures used in corrective exercise.

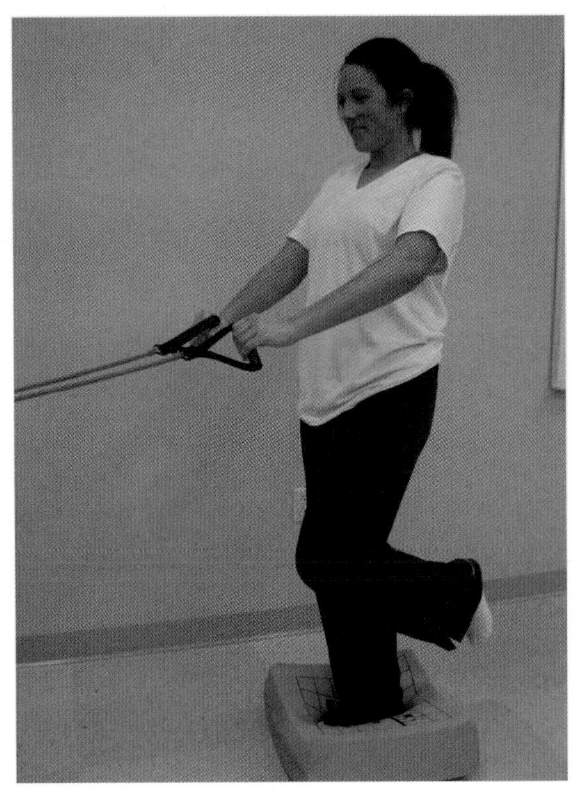

Figure 19-1 Different levels of function

This approach will help the clinician consider how the mobility or stability problem that was isolated in the evaluation has been (temporarily) integrated by substitution and compensation by other body parts. The clinician must remember that motor learning is a survival mechanism. The principles that the clinician will use in rehabilitation to produce motor learning have already been activated by the functional response to the impairment. Necessity or affinity, repetition, and reinforcement have been used to avoid pain or produce alternative movements since onset of the symptoms. Therefore, a new motor program has been activated

Box 19-5 Most Common Postures Used in Corrective Exercise

- Supine and prone
- Prone on elbows
- Quadruped
- Sitting and unstable sitting
- Kneeling and half kneeling
- Symmetric and asymmetric stance
- Single-leg stance

to manage the impairment and produce some level of function that is usually viewed as dysfunction. It should be considered a natural and appropriate response of the body reacting to limitation or symptoms. The body will sacrifice quality of movement to maintain a degree of quantity of movement. Taking this into consideration, 2 distinct needs are presented.

Posture for Protection and Inhibition The clinician must restrict or inhibit the inappropriate motor program. In the case of a control or stability problem, the patient must have some form of support, protection, or facilitation. Otherwise, the inappropriate program will take over in an attempt to protect and respond to the postural demand. Although most adult patients function at the necessary skill level, on evaluation, many qualitative problems are noted. Inappropriate joint loading and locking, poor tonic responses, or even tonic holding can be observed with simple activities. Some joint movements are used excessively, whereas others are unconsciously avoided. Many primary stability problems exist when underlying secondary mobility problems are present. Moreover, in some patients, the mobility problem precedes the stability problem. This is a common explanation for microtraumatic and overuse injuries. It is also why bilateral comparison and assessment of proximal and distal structures are mandatory in the evaluative process. With a mobility problem, a joint is not used appropriately because of weakness or restriction. The primary mobility problem may be the result of compromised stability elsewhere. Motor programs have been created to allow a patient to push on despite the mobility or stability problem. The problems can be managed by mechanical consideration of the mobility and stability status of the patient in the fundamental postures.

For primary stability problems, mechanical support or other assistance must be provided. This can be done simply by partial or complete reduction of stress, which may include non–weight bearing or partial weight bearing of the spine and extremities or temporary bracing. If the stability problem is only in a particular range of movement, that movement must be managed. If an underlying mobility problem is present, it must be managed and temporarily taken out of the initial exercise movement. The alteration in posture can effectively limit complete or partial motion with little need for active control by the patient. The patient must be trained to deal with the stability problem independently of the mobility problem or be at a great mechanical advantage to avoid compensation. The secondary mobility problem, once managed, should be reintroduced in a nonstressful manner so that the previous compensatory pattern is not activated.

Manual articular and soft-tissue techniques, when appropriate, can be used for the primary mobility problem, followed by movement to integrate any improved range and benefit from more appropriate tone. If the limitation in mobility seems to be the result of weakness, one should make sure that the proximal structures have the requisite amount of stability before strengthening and then proceed with strengthening or endurance activities with a focus on recruitment, relaxation, timing, coordination, and reproducibility. Note that the word *resistance* was not used initially. Resistance is not synonymous with strengthening and is only 1 of many techniques used to improve functional movement in early movement reeducation. However, the later sections on position and pattern address resistance in greater detail. Posture should be used to mechanically block or restrict substitution of stronger segments and improve quality at the segment being exercised.

Posture for Recruitment and Facilitation The clinician must facilitate or stimulate the correct motor program, coordination, and sequence of movement. Although verbal and visual feedback is helpful through demonstration and cueing, kinesthetic feedback is paramount to motor learning.[56] Correct body position or posture will improve feedback. The posture and movement that occur early in the developmental sequence require a less complex motor task and activate a more basic motor program. This creates positive feedback and reinforcement and marks the point (posture) at which appropriate and inappropriate actions and reactions meet. From this point, the clinician can manipulate frequency, intensity, and duration, or advance to a more difficult posture in the appropriate sequence.

The clinician must also consider developmental biomechanics by dividing movement ability into 2 categories: internal forces and external forces. Internal forces include the center of gravity, base of support, and line of gravity. External forces include gravity, inertia of the body segment, and ground reaction forces. Accordingly, the clinician should evaluate the patient's abilities in the same manner by first observing management of the mass of the body over the particular base provided by the posture. The clinician then advances the patient toward more external stresses such as inertia, gravity, and ground reaction forces. This interaction requires various degrees of acceleration production, deceleration control, anticipatory weight shifting, and increased proprioception. Resistance and movement can stress static and dynamic postures, but the clinician should also understand that resistance and movement could be used to refine movement and stimulate appropriate reactions.[56] Postures must be chosen that reduce compensation and allow the patient to exercise below the level at which the impairment hinders movement or control. This is easily accomplished by creating "self-limited" exercises.[3] Such exercises require passive or active "locking" by limiting movement of the area that the patient will most likely use to substitute or "cheat" with during exercise.

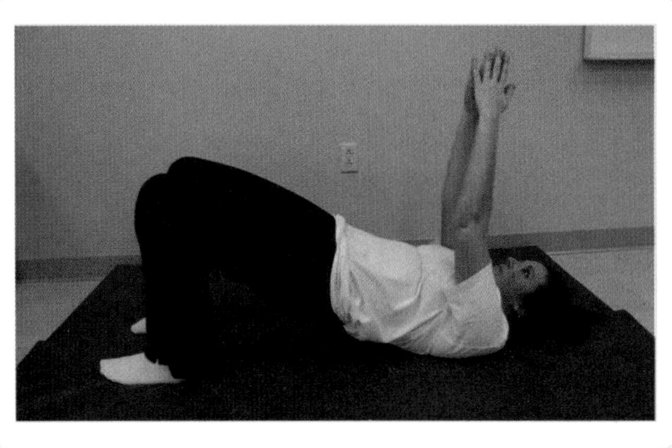

Figure 19-2 **Supine bridging movement**

To review, posture identifies the fundamental movements used in growth and development. These movements serve as steps toward the acquisition of skill and are also helpful in the presence of skill when quality is questionable. Figures 19-2 through 19-5 illustrate a few examples of these types of movements.

By following this natural sequence of movement, the clinician can observe the point at which a mobility or stability problem will first limit the quality of a whole movement pattern. The specific posture of the body is as important as the movement that is introduced onto that posture. Clinicians may already know the movement pattern that they want to train, but they also need to consider the posture of the body as the fundamental neuromuscular platform when making a corrective exercise choice. The posture is the soil and the movement is the seed. A chop pattern with the arms can be performed while supine, seated, half kneeling, tall kneeling, and standing. Each posture will require different levels of stability and motor control.

When stability and motor control are the primary problems, a posture must be selected to start the corrective exercise process. A patient with a mild knee sprain or even a total knee replacement may demonstrate segmental rolling to one side, but "logroll" to the other simply to avoid using a flexion-adduction-medial rotation movement pattern with the involved lower extremity. The clinician has now identified where success and failure meet in the developmental sequence. The knee problem creates a dynamic stability problem in the developmental sequence long before partial or full weight bearing is an issue. Consequently, it must be addressed at that level. The patient is provided with an example of how limited knee mobility can greatly affect movement patterns (such as rolling) that seem to require little of the knee. However, by restoring the bilateral segmental rolling function, measurable

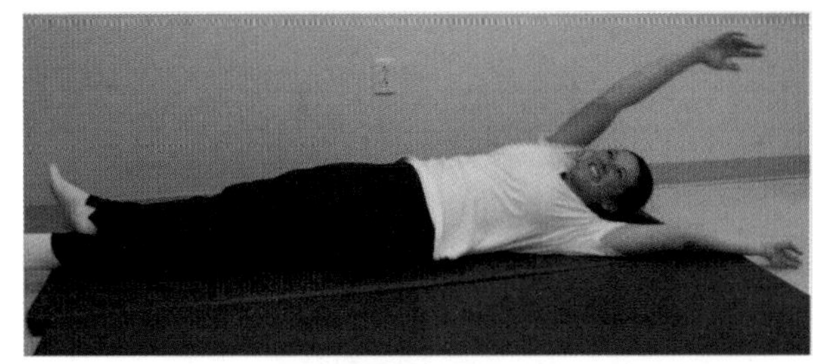

Figure 19-3 **Rolling to prone**

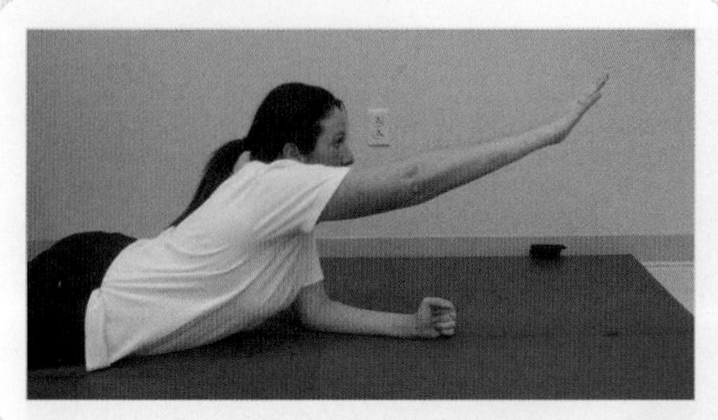

Figure 19-4 Prone on elbows with reaching

qualitative and quantitative improvements in many gait problems can be achieved. With use of postural progression, the earliest level of functional limitation can easily be identified and incorporated into the exercise program. Limitations can also be placed on the posture and movement (the self-limited concept) to control postural compensation and focus. If rolling from prone to supine does not present a problem, a more complex posture can be assumed. The obvious next choice would be to move to quadruped. From the all-fours position, alternate arms and legs can be lifted to an extended and flexed position. They can also be tucked into a flexed and extended position by bringing the alternate knee to the alternate elbow. This causes a significant motor control load by moving from 4 points of stability to 2. The load becomes even greater as movement of the extremities causes weight shifting, which must be managed continuously. If the movements are not compromised, the next progressive posture would be half kneeling with a narrow base. If this narrow-base half-kneeling posture demonstrates asymmetry and dysfunction, this is the posture for which the corrective exercise will be developed. Slightly widening the base improves control, and as control is developed, the base can be narrowed to challenge motor control.

Clinical Pearl

The clinician must define postural levels of success and failure to identify the postural level at which therapeutic exercise intervention should start. Otherwise, the clinician could potentially prescribe exercise at a postural level at which the patient makes significant amounts of inappropriate compensation and substitution during exercise.

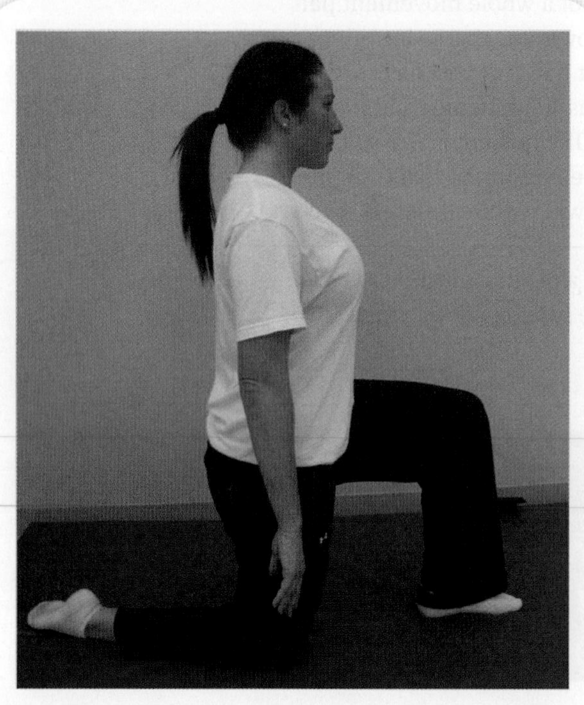

Figure 19-5 Half-kneeling position

Position

The word *position* describes not only the location of the anatomic structure (eg, joint, muscle group, or ligament) at which impairment has been identified but also the location (with respect to movement and load) at which the greatest and least limitations occur. The limitations can be either reduced strength and control or restricted movement. The primary questions to ask for this principle appear in Table 19-4. Orthopedic manual assessment of joints and muscles in various functional positions demonstrates the influence of the impairment and symptoms throughout the range of movement. The clinician will identify various deficits. Each will be qualified or quantified through assessment and objective testing, and then addressed through the appropriate dosage and positioning for exercise.

Purpose is the obvious reason for exercise intervention, whereas posture describes the orientation of the body in space. Position refers to the specific mobilizing or stabilizing segment. Attention should be paid to positions of body segments not directly involved in the posture or movement pattern. For the "single-leg bridge" (Figure 19-6), the hip is moving toward extension. If ROM were broken down into thirds, this exercise would involve only the extension third of movement. The flexion third and middle third of movement are not needed because no impairment was identified in those respective ranges. Not only was the hip in extension, but the knee was also in flexion. This is important because the hamstring muscle will try to assist hip extension in the end range of movement when gluteal strength is not optimal. However, the hamstrings cannot assist hip extension to any significant degree because of "active insufficiency." Likewise, the lumbar extensors cannot assist the extension pattern because of the passive stretch placed on them via maximal passive hip flexion. Hip extension proprioception is now void of any inappropriate patterning or compensation from the hamstrings or spinal erectors through the positional use of active and passive insufficiency.[57]

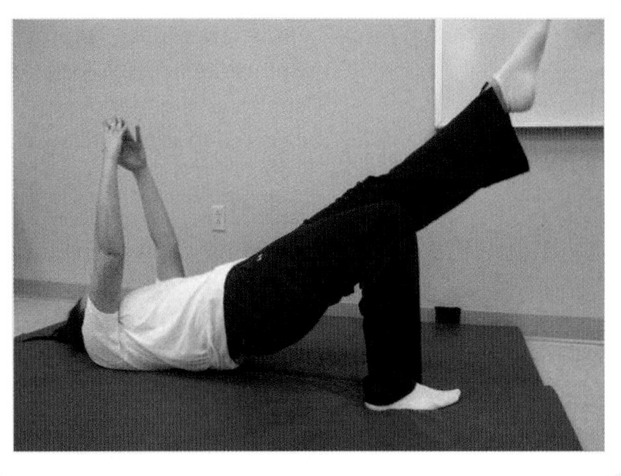

Figure 19-6 **Single-leg bridge**

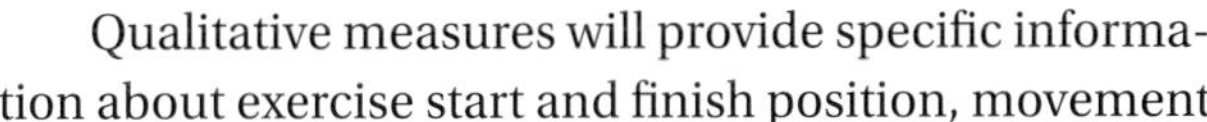

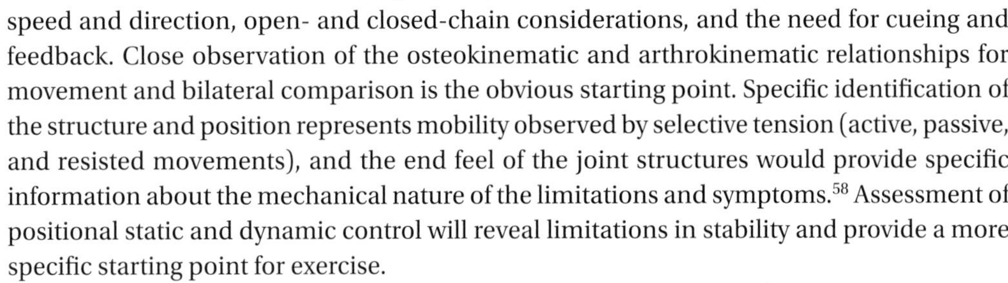

Qualitative measures will provide specific information about exercise start and finish position, movement speed and direction, open- and closed-chain considerations, and the need for cueing and feedback. Close observation of the osteokinematic and arthrokinematic relationships for movement and bilateral comparison is the obvious starting point. Specific identification of the structure and position represents mobility observed by selective tension (active, passive, and resisted movements), and the end feel of the joint structures would provide specific information about the mechanical nature of the limitations and symptoms.[58] Assessment of positional static and dynamic control will reveal limitations in stability and provide a more specific starting point for exercise.

Quantitative measures will reveal a degree of deficit, which can be recorded in the form of a percentage through bilateral comparison and compared with normative data when possible. ROM, strength, endurance, and recovery time should be considered, along with many other (quantitative) clinical parameters, to describe isolated or positional function. This will provide clear communication and specific documentation for goals, as well as be a tracking device for the effectiveness of treatment, information that will help define the baseline for initial exercise considerations. As stated earlier, any limitation in mobility or stability requires bilateral comparison, in addition to clearing of the joints above and below. The proximal and distal structures must also be compared with their contralateral counterparts. This central point of physical examination is often overlooked. Cyriax[58] noted, "Positive signs must always be balanced by corroborative negative signs. If a lesion appears to lie at or near one joint, this region must be examined for signs identifying its site. It is equally essential for the adjacent joints and the structures around them to be examined so that, by contrast, their normality can be established. These negative findings then reinforce the positive findings emanating elsewhere; then only can the diagnosis be regarded and established."

After position and movement options are established, a trial exercise session should be used to observe and quantify performance before prescription of exercise. Variables, including intensity and duration, can be used to establish strength or endurance baselines. Bilateral comparison should be used to document a deficit in performance, which is also recorded as a percentage. A maximum repetition test (with or without resistance) to fatigue, onset of symptoms, or loss of exercise quality is a common example. This will allow close tracking of home exercise compliance and help to establish a rate of improvement. If all other factors are addressed, the rate of improvement should be quite large. This is the benefit of correct dosage in prescription of exercise position and appropriate workload. Most of the significant improvement is not a result of training volume, tissue metabolism, or muscle hypertrophy, but of the efficient adaptive response of neural factors.[59] These factors can include motor recruitment efficiency, improved timing, increased proprioceptive awareness, improved agonist/antagonist coordination, appropriate phasic/tonic response to activity, task familiarity, and motor learning, as well as psychological factors. Usually, greater deficits are associated with more drastic improvement. Treatments should be geared to stimulate these changes whenever possible.

Pattern

The primary questions to ask for the pattern principle appear in Table 19-4. The word *pattern* serves as a cue to the clinician to continually consider the functional movements of the human body occurring in unified patterns that occupy 3-dimensional space and cross 3 planes (frontal, sagittal, and transverse).[3] Sometimes this is not easily ascertained by observing the design and use of fixed-axis exercise equipment and the movement patterns suggested in some rehabilitation protocols. The basic patterns of proprioceptive neuromuscular facilitation (PNF), for both the extremities and the spine, are excellent examples of how the brain groups movement. Muscles of the trunk and extremities are recruited in the most advantageous sequence (proprioception) to create movement (mobility) or control (stability) movement. Not only does this provide efficient and economical function, but it also effectively protects the respective joints and muscles from undue stress and strain. Voss et al[60] clearly and eloquently stated, "The mass movement patterns of facilitation are spiral and diagonal in character and closely resemble the movements used in sports and work activities. The spiral and diagonal character is in keeping with the spiral rotatory characteristics of the skeletal system of bones and joints and the ligamentous structures. This type of motion is also in harmony with the topographical alignment of the muscles from origin to insertion and with the structural characteristics of the individual muscles." When a structure within the sequence is limited by impairment, the entire pattern is limited in some way. The clinician should document the limited pattern, as well as the isolated segment causing the pattern to be limited. The isolated segment is usually identified in the evaluation process and outlined in the "position" considerations. The resultant effect on one or more movement patterns must also be investigated. A review of the basic PNF patterns can be beneficial to the rehabilitation specialist. Once a structure is evaluated, one should look at the basic PNF patterns involving that structure. Multiple patterns can be limited in some way, but usually one pattern in particular will demonstrate significantly reduced function. Obviously, poor function in a muscle group or joint can limit the strength, endurance, and ROM of an entire PNF pattern to some degree. However, the clinician must not simply view reduced function of a PNF pattern as an output problem. It should be equally viewed as an input problem. When muscle and joint functions are not optimal, mechanoreceptor and muscle spindle functions are not optimal. This can create an input or proprioceptive problem and greatly distort joint position and muscle tension information, which distorts the initial information (before movement is initiated), as well as feedback (once movement is in progress). Therefore, the clinician cannot consider only functional output. Altered proprioception, if not properly identified and outlined, can unintentionally become part of the recommended exercises and therefore be reinforced. The clinician must focus on synergistic and integrated function at all levels of rehabilitation. An orthopedic outpatient cannot afford to have a problem simply isolated 3 times a week for 30 minutes only to reintegrate the same problem at a subconscious level during necessary daily activities throughout the remaining week. PNF-style movement pattern exercise can often be taught as easily as an isolated movement and will produce a significantly greater benefit. Therapeutic exercise is no longer limited by sets as repetitions of the same activity. Successive intervals of increasing difficulty (although not physically stressful) that build on the accomplishment of an earlier task will reinforce one level of function and continually be a challenge for the next. A simple movement set focused on isolation of a problem can quickly be followed by a pattern that will improve integration. The integration can be followed by a familiar fundamental movement or functional activity that may reduce the amount of conscious and deliberate movement and give the clinician a chance to observe subcortical control of mobility and stability, as well as appropriate use of phasic and tonic responses.

Clinical Pearl

By continuously considering the pattern options, as well as pattern limitations, the clinician will be able to refine the exercise prescription and reduce unnecessary supplemental movements that could easily be incorporated into pattern-based exercise.

Direction, speed, and amount of resistance (or assistance) will be used to produce more refined patterns. Manual resistance, weighted cable or elastic resistance, weight-shifting activities, and even proprioceptive taping can improve recruitment and facilitate coordination. The clinician should refrain from initially discussing specific structural control such as "pelvic tilting" or "scapular retraction." Instead, the clinician should use posture and position to set the initial movement and design proprioceptive feedback to produce a more normal pattern whenever possible.

Reestablishing Proprioception and Neuromuscular Control

Although the concept and value of proprioceptive mechanoreceptors have been documented in the literature, treatment techniques focused on improving their function have not generally been incorporated into the overall rehabilitation program. The neurosensory function of the capsuloligamentous structures has taken a back seat to the mechanical structural role. This is mainly a result of lack of information about how mechanoreceptors contribute to the specific functional activities and how they can be specifically activated.[61,62]

Effects of Injury on the Proprioceptive System

After injury to the capsuloligamentous structures, it is thought that partial deafferentation of the joint occurs as the mechanoreceptors become disrupted. This partial deafferentation may be caused by either direct or indirect injury. Direct effects of trauma include disruption of the joint capsule or ligaments, whereas posttraumatic joint effusion or hemarthrosis[19] illustrate indirect effects.

Whether from a direct or indirect cause, the resultant partial deafferentation alters the afferent information received by the CNS and, therefore, the resulting reflex pathways to the dynamic stabilizing structures. These pathways are required by both the feed-forward and feedback motor control systems to dynamically stabilize the joint. A disruption in the proprioceptive pathway will result in an alteration in position and kinesthesia.[63,64] Barrett[65] showed that there is an increase in the threshold for detection of passive motion in a majority of patients with anterior cruciate ligament (ACL) rupture and functional instability. Corrigan et al,[66] who also found diminished proprioception after ACL rupture, confirmed this finding. Diminished proprioceptive sensitivity has likewise been shown to cause giving way or episodes of instability in the ACL-deficient knee.[67] Therefore, injury to the capsuloligamentous structures not only reduces the mechanical stability of the joint but also diminishes the capability of the dynamic neuromuscular restraint system. Consequently, any aberration in joint motion and position sense will affect both the feed-forward and feedback neuromuscular control systems. Without adequate anticipatory muscle activity, the static structures may be exposed to insult unless the reactive muscle activity can be initiated to contribute to dynamic restraint.

Restoration of Proprioception and Prevention of Reinjury

Although it has been demonstrated that a proprioceptive deficit occurs after knee injury, both kinesthetic awareness and reposition sense can be at least partially restored with surgery and rehabilitation. A number of studies examined proprioception after ACL reconstruction. Barrett[65] measured proprioception after autogenous graft repair and found that proprioception was better after repair than in an average patient with an ACL deficiency but still significantly worse than in a normal knee. He further noted that patients' satisfaction was more closely correlated with their proprioception than with their clinical score.[65] Harter et al[68] could not demonstrate a significant difference in the reproduction of passive positioning between the operative and nonoperative knee at an average of 3 years after ACL reconstruction. Kinesthesia has been reported to be restored after surgery, as detected by a threshold for detection of passive motion in the midrange of motion.[63] A longer threshold for detection of passive motion was observed in a knee with a reconstructed ACL than in the contralateral uninvolved knee when tested at the end ROM.[63] Lephart et al[69] found similar results in patients after arthroscopically assisted ACL reconstruction with a patellar-tendon autograft or allograft. The importance of incorporating a proprioceptive element in any comprehensive rehabilitation program is justified from the results of these studies.

Methods to enhance proprioception after injury or surgery could improve function and decrease the risk for reinjury. Ihara and Nakayama[70] demonstrated a reduction in neuromuscular lag time with dynamic joint control after a 3-week training period on an unstable board. Maintenance of equilibrium and an improvement in reaction to sudden perturbations on the unstable board improved neuromuscular coordination. This phenomenon was first reported by Freeman and Wyke, in 1967, when they stated that proprioceptive deficits could be reduced with training on an unstable surface.[51] They found that proprioceptive training through stabilometry, or training on an unstable surface, significantly reduced episodes of giving way after ankle sprains. Tropp et al[53] confirmed the work of Freeman and Wyke by demonstrating that the results of stabilometry could be improved with coordination training on an unstable board.

Relationship of Proprioception to Function

Barrett[65] demonstrated the relationship between proprioception and function. Their study suggested that limb function relied more on proprioceptive input than on strength during activity. Blackburn and Voight[33] also found high correlation between diminished kinesthesia and the single-leg hop test. The single-leg hop test was chosen for its integrative measure of neuromuscular control because a high degree of proprioceptive sensibility and functional ability is required to successfully propel the body forward and land safely on the limb. Giove et al[71] reported a higher success rate in returning athletes to competitive sports with adequate hamstring rehabilitation. Tibone et al[72] and Ihara and Nakayama[70] found that simple hamstring strengthening alone was not adequate; it was necessary to obtain voluntary or reflex-level control of knee instability for return to functional activities. Walla et al[73] found that 95% of patients were able to successfully avoid surgery after ACL injury when they could achieve "reflex-level" hamstring control. Ihara and Nakayama[70] found that the reflex arc between stressing the ACL and hamstring contraction could be shortened with training. With the use of unstable boards, the researchers were able to successfully decrease the reaction time. Because afferent input is altered after joint injury, proprioceptive sensitivity to retrain these altered afferent pathways is critical for shortening the time lag in muscular reaction to counteract the excessive strain on the passive structures and guard against injury.

Restoration of Efficient Motor Control

How do we modify afferent/efferent characteristics? The mechanoreceptors in and around the respective joints offer information about change in position, motion, and loading of the joint to the CNS, which, in turn, stimulates the muscles around the joint to function.[70] If a time lag exists in the neuromuscular reaction, injury may occur. The shorter the time lag, the less stress on the ligaments and other soft tissue structures around the joint. Therefore, the foundation of neuromuscular control is to facilitate the integration of peripheral sensations related to joint position and then process this information into an effective efferent motor response. The main objective of the rehabilitation program for neuromuscular control is to develop or reestablish the afferent and efferent characteristics around the joint that are essential for dynamic restraint.[21]

Several different afferent and efferent characteristics contribute to efficient regulation of motor control. As discussed earlier, these characteristics include the sensitivity of the mechanoreceptors and facilitation of the afferent neural pathways, enhancement of muscle stiffness, and production of reflex muscle activation. The specific rehabilitation techniques must also take into consideration the levels of CNS integration. For the rehabilitation program to be complete, each of the 3 levels must be addressed to produce dynamic stability. The plasticity of the neuromuscular system permits rapid adaptations during the rehabilitation program that enhance preparatory and reactive activity.[21,40,46,69,70,74]

Clinical Pearl

Specific rehabilitation techniques that produce adaptations to enhance the efficiency of neuromuscular techniques include balance training, biofeedback training, reflex facilitation through reactive training, and eccentric and high-repetition/low-load exercises.[21]

The 3-Phase Rehabilitation Model

The following is a 3-phase model designed to progressively retrain the neuromuscular system for complex functions of sports and ADL (Table 19-6). The model phases are successively more demanding and provide sequential training toward the objective of reestablishment of neuromuscular control. This 3-phase model has also been described as RNT. Ideally, the phases should be followed in order and should use the 4 rehabilitation considerations mentioned earlier (the 4 Ps) at each phase. Application of the 4 Ps at each phase is crucial to place successive demands on the athlete during rehabilitation. In addition, progression of exercise is guided by the 4 × 4 design. The 4 × 4 method of therapeutic exercise design refers to the 4 possible exercise positions combined with the 4 types of resistance used (Table 19-7).

The difficulty of any exercise can be increased by either changing the position (non-weight bearing being the easiest and standing being the toughest) or changing the resistance (unloaded with core activation being the easiest and loaded without core activation being the hardest). It is important to remember that exercises that present too much difficulty will force the patient to revert back to a compensation pattern. Therefore, the first set of exercises following a change in mobility will

Table 19-6 Three-Phase Rehabilitation Model

Phase	Description	Objective
1	Restore static stability through proprioception and kinesthesia	Restoration of proprioception
2	Restore dynamic stability	Encourage preparatory agonist-antagonist cocontraction
3	Restore reactive neuromuscular control	Initiate reflex muscular stabilization

Table 19-7 Four-by-Four Method for Design of Therapeutic Exercise

The 4 Positions	The 4 Types of Resistance
Non-weight bearing (supine or prone)	Unloaded with core activation
Quadruped	Unloaded without core activation
Kneeling (half kneeling or tall kneeling)	Loaded with core activation
Standing (lunge, split, squat, single leg)	Loaded without core activation

give all the information that one needs to know by producing 1 of 3 responses:

- **It is too easy.** The patient can perform the movement for more than 30 repetitions with good quality.
- **It is challenging, but possible.** The patient can perform the movement 8 to 15 times with good quality of movement and no signs of stress. Between 5 and 15 repetitions, however, there is a sharp decline in quality as demonstrated by a limited ability to maintain full ROM, balance, stabilization, and coordination, or the patient just becomes physically fatigued.
- **It is too difficult.** The patient has sloppy, stressful, poorly coordinated movement from the beginning, and it only gets worse.

Using this as a corrective exercise base, the clinician can observe the response and act accordingly. If the initial choice of exercise is too difficult, decrease the difficulty, observe the response to the next set, and repeat the process. If the initial exercise is too easy, increase the difficulty, observe the response to the next set, and repeat the process. Increasing difficulty rarely means increased resistance. A more advanced posture, a smaller base of support, or a more complex or involved movement pattern is usually indicated to increase the difficulty. A typical example is some form of activity with a rolling movement pattern moving to a quadruped exercise, then going to a half-kneeling activity, and finally progressing to movement with a single-leg stance.

Phase I: Restore Static Stability Through Proprioception and Kinesthesia

Functional neuromuscular rehabilitation activities are designed to both restore functional stability about the joint and enhance motor control skills. The RNT program is centered on stimulation of both the peripheral and central reflex pathways to the skeletal muscles. The first objective that should be addressed in the RNT program is restoration of proprioception. Reliable kinesthetic and proprioceptive information provides the foundation on which dynamic stability and motor control is based. It has already been established that altered afferent information received by the CNS can alter the feed-forward and feedback motor control systems. Therefore, the first objective of the RNT program is to restore the neurosensory properties of the damaged structures while at the same time enhancing the sensitivity of the secondary peripheral afferents.[69]

To facilitate appropriate kinesthetic and proprioceptive input into the CNS, joint reposition exercises should be used to provide maximal stimulation of the peripheral mechanoreceptors. The use of closed-kinetic-chain activities creates axial loads that maximally stimulate the articular mechanoreceptors via the increase in compressive force.[10,55] The use of closed-chain exercises not only enhances joint congruency and neurosensory feedback but also minimizes shearing stress about the joint.[75] At the same time, the muscle receptors are facilitated by the change in both length and tension.[10,55] The objective is to induce unanticipated perturbations and thereby stimulate reflex stabilization. Persistent use of these pathways will decrease the response time when an unanticipated joint load occurs.[76] In addition to weightbearing exercises, active and passive joint-repositioning exercises can be used to enhance the conscious appreciation of proprioception. Rhythmic stabilization exercises can

Table 19-8 Upper-Extremity Neuromuscular Exercises

Phase I: Proprioception and Kinesthesia	Phase II: Dynamic Stabilization	Phase III: Reactive Neuromuscular Control
Goals		
Normalize motion	Enhance dynamic functional stability	Improve reactive neuromuscular abilities
Restore proprioception and kinesthesia	Reestablish neuromuscular control	Enhance dynamic stability
Establish muscular balance	Restore muscular balance	Improve power and endurance
Diminish pain and inflammation	Maintain normalized motion	Gradual return to activities/throwing
Stability Exercises		
Joint repositioning	PNF D_2 Flex/Ext	PNF D2 Flex/Ext
Movement awareness	Supine	RS with T-band
RS	Side-lying	Perturbation RS
RI	Seated	Perturbation RS—eyes closed
SRH	Standing	90 degree/90 degree
PNF D_2 Flex/Ext	PNF D_2 Flex/Ext at end range	ER at end-range RS
PNF D_2 Flex/Ext RS, SRH, RI	90 degrees/90 ER at end range	ER Conc/Ecc
Side-lying RS, SRH, RI	Scapular strengthening	ER Conc/Ecc RS
Weight bearing (axial compression)	Scapular PNF—RS, SRH	ER/IR Conc/Ecc
Weightbearing RS, RI	ER/IR at 90 degree abduction—eyes closed	ER/IR Conc/Ecc RS
Standing while leaning on hands	PNF D_2 Flex/Ext—eyes closed	Eyes closed
Quadruped position	Balance beam	Standing on one leg
Tripod position	PNF D_2 Flex/Ext—balance beam	Reactive plyoballs
Biped position	Slide board—side to side	Pushups on unstable surface
Axial compression with ball on wall	Slide board pushups	UE plyometrics
OTIS	Axial compression—side to side	Two-handed overhead throw
	Axial compression—unstable surfaces	Side-to-side overhead throw
	Plyometrics—two handed (light and easy)	One-handed baseball throw
	Two-handed chest throw	Endurance
	Two-handed underhand throw	Wall dribble
		Wall baseball throw
		Axial compression circles
		Axial compression—side/side
		Sports specific
		Underweighted throwing
		Overweighted throwing
		Oscillating devices
		Boing
		Body blade

Conc, concentric; Ecc, eccentric; ER, external rotation; Ext, extension; Flex, flexion; IR, internal rotation; OTIS, oscillating techniques for isometric stabilization; PNF, proprioceptive neuromuscular facilitation; RI, reciprocal isometrics; RS, rhythmic stabilization; SRH, slow-reversal-hold; UE, upper extremity.

be included early in the RNT program to enhance neuromuscular coordination in response to unexpected joint translation. The intensity of the exercises can be manipulated by increasing either the weight loaded across the joint or the size of the perturbation (Tables 19-8 and 19-9). The addition of a compressive sleeve, wrap, or taping about the joint can also provide additional proprioceptive information by stimulating the cutaneous mechanoreceptors.[21,65,77,78] Figures 19-7 through 19-10 provide examples of exercises that can be begun in this phase.

Table 19-9 Lower-Extremity Neuromuscular Exercises

Phase I: Proprioception and Kinesthesia	Phase II: Dynamic Stabilization	Phase III: Reactive Neuromuscular Control
Goals		
Normalize motion Restore proprioception and kinesthesia Establish muscular balance Diminish pain and inflammation Develop static control and posture	Enhance dynamic functional stability Reestablish neuromuscular control Restore muscular balance Maintain normalized motion	Improve reactive neuromuscular abilities Enhance dynamic stability Improve power and endurance Gradual return to activities, running, jumping, cutting
Stability Exercises		

Bilateral to unilateral
Eyes open to eyes closed
Stable to unstable surfaces
  Level surfaces
  Foam pad
Controlled to uncontrolled
PNF
  Rhythmic stabilization
  Rhythmic isometrics
  Slow reversal hold
	OTIS
	  AWS
	  PWS
	  MWS
	  LWS
	  Chops/lifts
	ITIS
	PACE
	PNF
	  Rhythmic stabilization
	  Rhythmic isometrics
	  Slow-reversal-hold
	Stable to unstable surface
	  Rocker board
	  Wobble board
	  BAPS
	  Balance beam
	  Foam rollers
	  DynaDisc
		Squats
		Assisted
		  AWS
		  PWS
		  MWS
		  LWS
		Chops/lifts
		Lunges (front and lateral)
		  AWS
		  PWS
		  MWS
		  LWS
		Stationary walking with unidirectional WS
		Stationary running
		  PWS
		  MWS
		  LWS
		  AWS
		  Mountain climber
		CKC side to side
		  Fitter
		  Slide board
		Plyometrics
		  Jumps in place
		  Standing jumps
		  Bounding
		  Multiple hops and bounds
		  Hops with rotation
		  Bounds with rotation
		  Resisted lateral bounds
		  Box jumps
		  Depth jumps
		Multidirectional training
		  Lunges
		  Rock wall
		  Clock drill
		  Step-tos
		  Four-square
		Agility training

AWS, anterior weight shift; BAPS, biomechanical ankle platform system; CKC, closed-chain kinetic; ITIS, impulse techniques for isometric stabilization; LWS, lateral weight shift; MWS, medial weight shift; OTIS, oscillating techniques for isometric stabilization; PACE, partial-arc controlled exercise; PNF, proprioceptive neuromuscular facilitation; PWS, posterior weight shift; WS, weight shift.

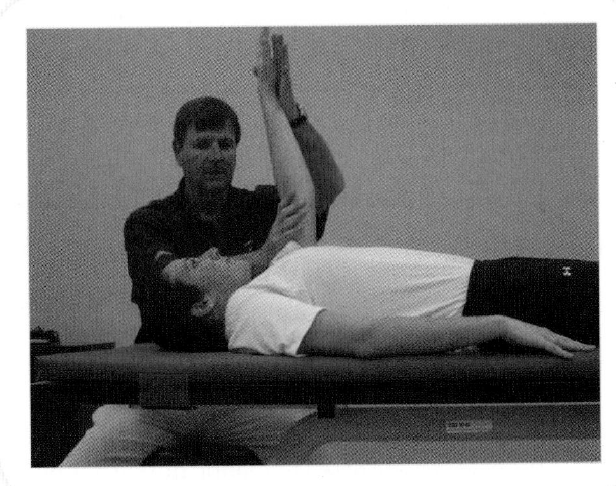

Figure 19-7 Rhythmic stabilization

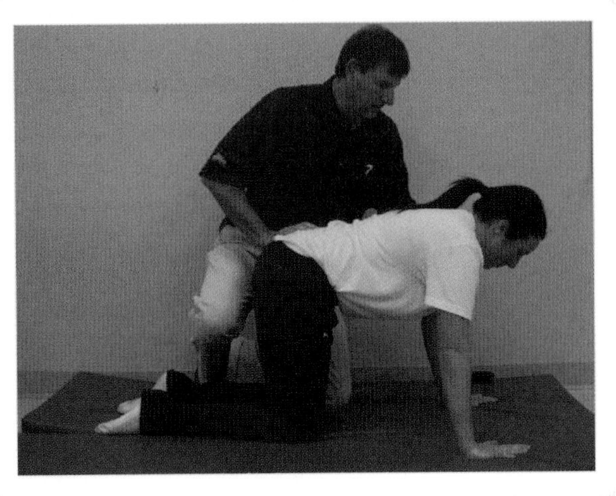

Figure 19-8 Quadruped position with manual perturbations

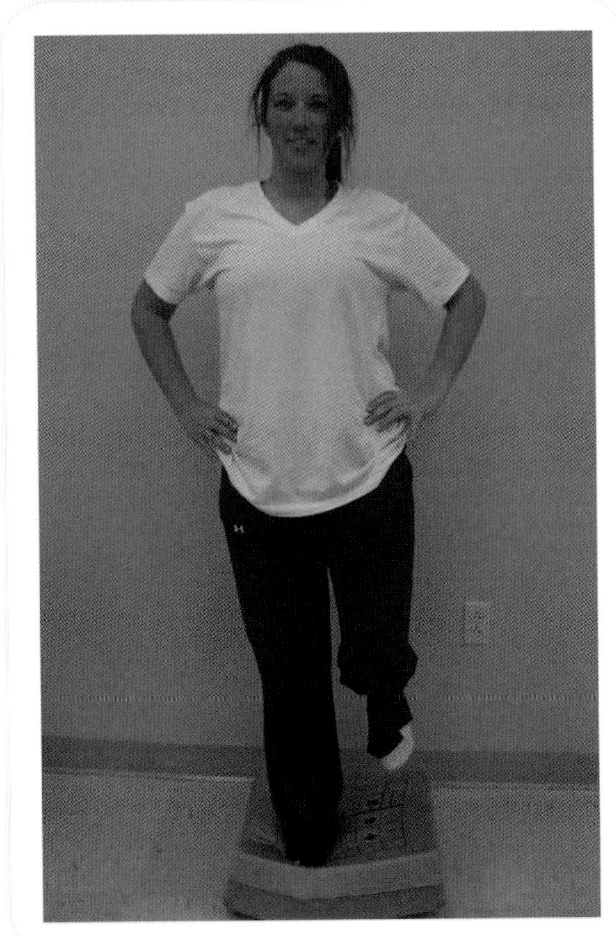

Figure 19-9 Single-limb balance on an unstable (foam) base

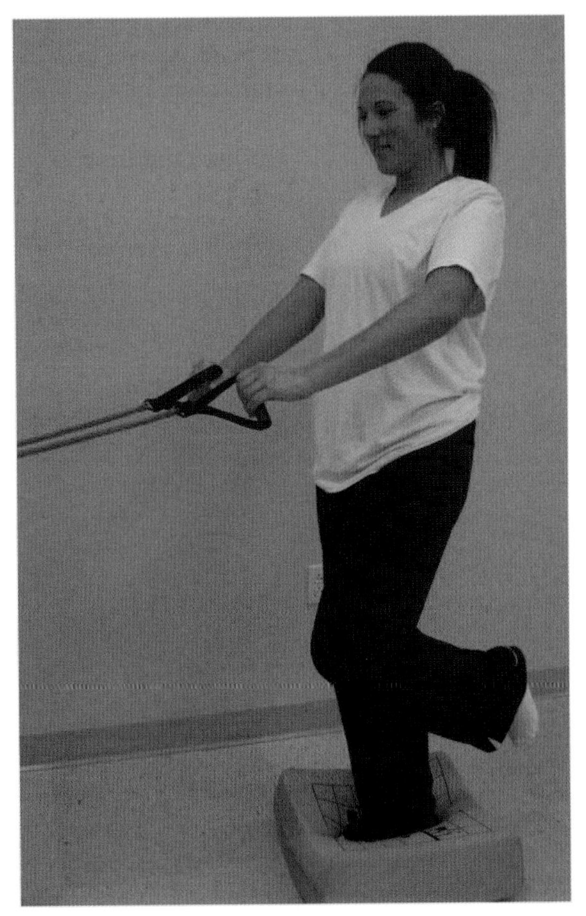

Figure 19-10 Single-limb balance with oscillating techniques for isometric stabilization

Box 19-6 Balance Variables That Can Be Manipulated in the Dynamic Stability Phase to Produce a Sensory Response

Bilateral to unilateral stance	Stable to unstable surfaces
Eyes open to eyes closed	

Phase II: Restore Dynamic Stability

The second objective of the RNT program is to encourage preparatory agonist-antagonist cocontraction. Efficient coactivation of the musculature restores the normal force couples that are necessary to balance joint forces, increase joint congruency, and thereby reduce the loads imparted onto the static structures.[21] The cornerstone of rehabilitation during this phase is postural stability training. Environmental conditions are manipulated to produce a sensory response (Box 19-6). The use of unstable surfaces allows the clinician to use positions of compromise to produce maximal afferent input into the spinal cord and thus produce a reflex response. Dynamic coactivation of the muscles about the joint to produce a stabilizing force requires both the feed-forward and feedback motor control systems. To facilitate these pathways, the joint must be placed in positions of compromise for the patient to develop reactive stabilizing strategies. Although it was once believed that the speed of the stretch reflexes could not be directly enhanced, efforts to do so have been successful in human and animal studies. This has significant implications for reestablishing the reactive capability of the dynamic restraint system. Reducing electromechanical delay between joint loading and protective muscle activation can increase dynamic stability. In the controlled clinical environment, positions of vulnerability can be used safely (see Tables 19-8 and 19-9). Figures 19-11 and 19-12 provide examples of exercises that can be implemented in this phase.

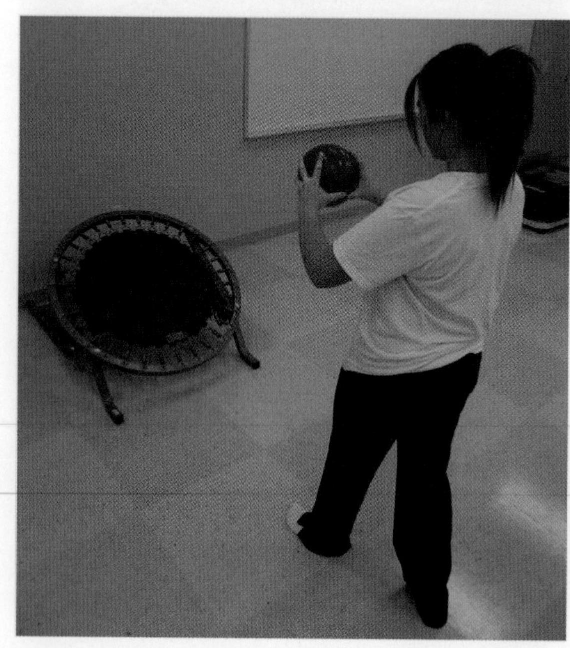

Figure 19-11 Plyoback, two-handed upper-extremity chest pass

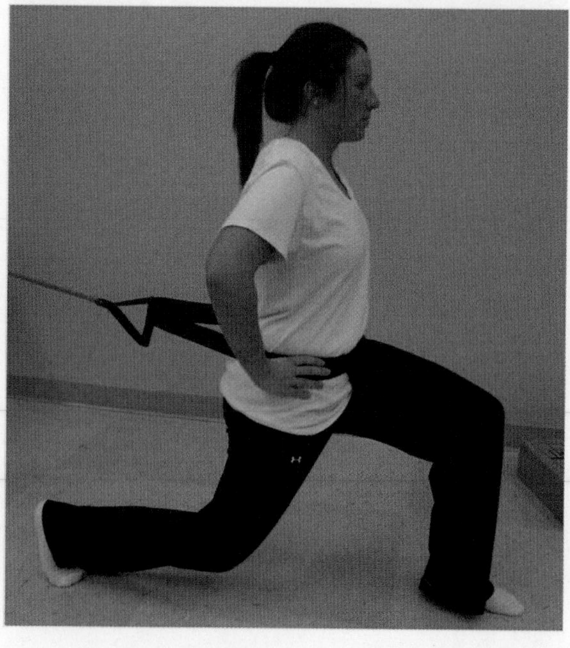

Figure 19-12 Lunging movement, forward with sport cord resistance

Proprioceptive training for functionally unstable joints after injury has been documented in the literature.[38,53,70,79] Tropp et al[53] and Wester et al[80] reported that ankle disk training significantly reduced the incidence of ankle sprains. Concerning the mechanism of the effects, Tropp et al[53] suggested that unstable surface training reduced the proprioceptive deficit. Sheth et al[79] demonstrated changes in healthy adults in patterns of contraction of the inversion and eversion musculature before and after training on an unstable surface. They concluded that the changes would be supported by the concept of reciprocal Ia inhibition via the mechanoreceptors in the muscles. Konradsen and Ravin[81] also suggested from their work that afferent input from the calf musculature was responsible for dynamic protection against sudden ankle inversion stress. Pinstaar et al[82] reported that postural sway was restored after 8 weeks of ankle disk training when performed 3 to 5 times a week. Tropp and Odenrick also showed that postural control improved after 6 weeks of training when performed 15 minutes per day.[39] Bernier and Perrin,[54] whose program consisted of balance exercises progressing from simple to complex sessions (3 times a week for 10 minutes each time), also found that postural sway was improved after 6 weeks of training. Although each of these training programs do have some differences, postural control improved after 6 to 8 weeks of proprioceptive training in subjects with functional instability of the ankle.

Phase III: Restore Reactive Neuromuscular Control

Dynamic reactive neuromuscular control activities should be initiated into the overall rehabilitation program after adequate healing and dynamic stability have been achieved. The key objective is to initiate reflex muscular stabilization.

Progression of these activities is predicated on the athlete satisfactorily completing the activities that are considered prerequisites for the activity being considered. With this in mind, progression of activities must be goal oriented and specific to the tasks that will be expected of the athlete.

The general progression of activities to develop dynamic reactive neuromuscular control is from slow-speed to fast-speed activities, from low-force to high-force activities, and from controlled to uncontrolled activities. Initially, these exercises should evoke a balance reaction or weight shift in the lower extremities and ultimately progress to a movement pattern. A sudden alteration in joint position induced by either the clinician or the athlete may decrease the response time and serve to develop reactive strategies to unexpected events. These reactions can be as simple as static control with little or no visible movement or as complex as a dynamic plyometric response requiring explosive acceleration, deceleration, or change in direction. The exercises will allow the clinician to challenge the patient by using visual or proprioceptive input, or both, via tubing (oscillating techniques for isometric stabilization) and other devices (eg, medicine balls, foam rolls, or visual obstacles). Although these exercises will improve physiologic parameters, they are specifically designed to facilitate neuromuscular reactions. Therefore, the clinician must be concerned with the kinesthetic input and quality of the movement patterns rather than the particular number of sets and repetitions. When fatigue occurs, motor control becomes poor and all training effects are lost. Therefore, during the exercise progression, all aspects of normal function should be observed, including isometric, concentric, and eccentric muscle control; articular loading and unloading; balance control during weight shifting and changes in direction; controlled acceleration and deceleration; and demonstration of both conscious and unconscious control (see Tables 19-7 and 19-8). Figures 19-13 through 19-15 are examples of exercises that can be implemented in this phase.

When dynamic stability and reflex stabilization have been achieved, the focus of the neuromuscular rehabilitation program is to restore ADL and sport-specific skills. It is

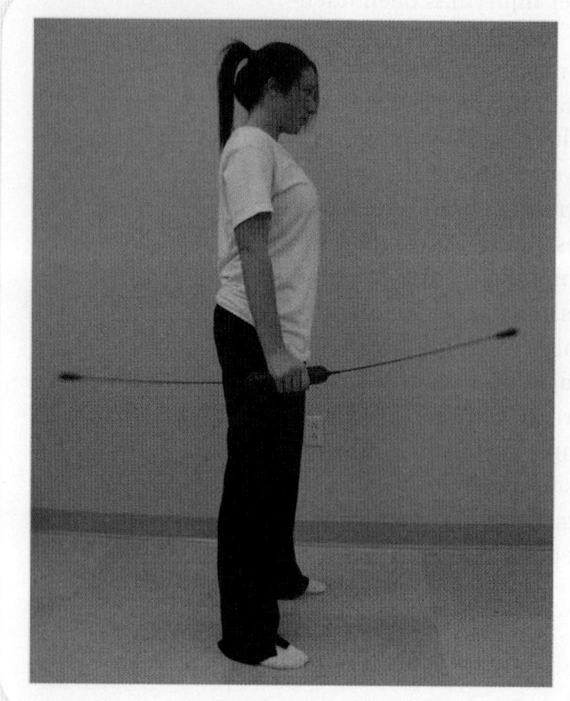

Figure 19-13 **Dynamic training; Body Blade, low position**

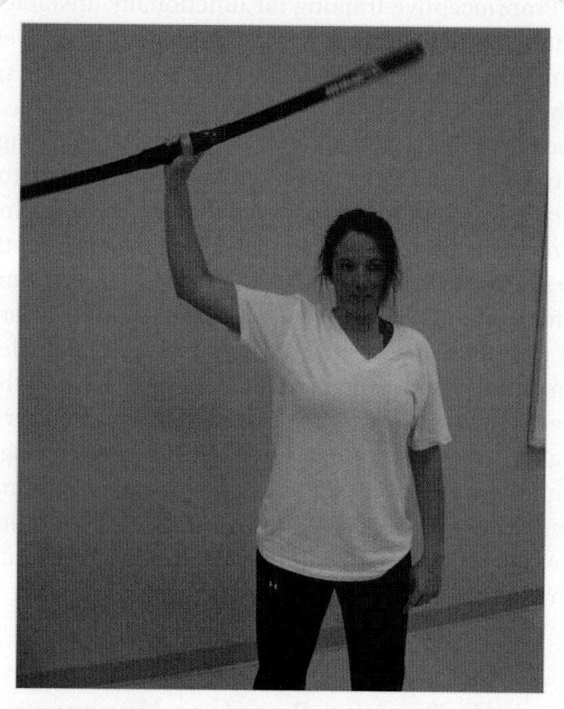

Figure 19-14 **Dynamic training; Body Blade, elevated position**

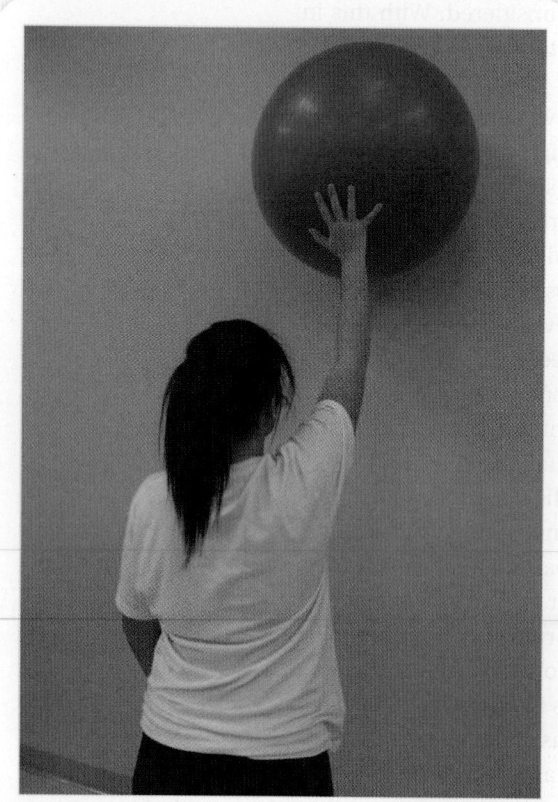

Figure 19-15 **Elevated wall dribble**

essential that the exercise program be specific to the patient's needs. The most important factor to consider during rehabilitation of patients is that they should be performing functional activities that simulate their ADL requirements. This rule applies not only to the specific joints involved but also to the speed and amplitude of movement required in ADL. Exercise and training drills that will refine the physiologic parameters required for return to preinjury levels of function should be incorporated into the program. The progression should be from straight plane to multiplane movement patterns. ADL movement does not occur along a single joint or plane of movement. Therefore, exercise for the kinetic chain must involve all 3 planes simultaneously. Emphasis in the RNT program must be placed on progression from simple to complex neuromotor patterns that are specific to the demands placed on the patient during function. The function progression breaks an activity down into its component parts so that they can be performed in a sequence that allows acquisition or reacquisition of the activity. Basic conditioning and skill acquisition must be achieved before advanced conditioning and skill acquisition. The training program should begin with simple activities, such as walking/running, and then progress to highly complex motor skills requiring refined neuromuscular mechanisms, including proprioceptive and kinesthetic awareness, which provides reflex joint stabilization. A significant amount of "controlled chaos" should be included in the program. Unexpected activities during ADL are by nature unstable. The more patients rehearse in this type of environment, the better they will react under unrehearsed conditions. The clinician needs to learn how to categorize, prioritize, and plan effectively because corrective exercises will evolve and equipment will change. The clinician's professional skill must be based in a systematic approach. Just being great at a technique is not good enough. Technical aspects of exercise will change. The clinician should not worry. This system is not based on exercise. It is based on human movement, not equipment, techniques, or trends. The final and most important consideration of this phase is to make the rehabilitation program fun. The first 3 letters of functional are FUN. If the program is not fun, compliance will suffer and so will the results.

SUMMARY

1. Increased attention has been devoted to the development of balance, proprioception, and neuromuscular control in the rehabilitation and reconditioning of athletes after injury.
2. It is believed that injury results in altered somatosensory input, which influences neuromuscular control.
3. If static and dynamic balance and neuromuscular control are not reestablished after injury, the patient will be susceptible to recurrent injury and performance may decline.
4. The 3-phase model for RNT may be an excellent method to assist athletes in regaining optimal neuromuscular performance and high-level function after injury or surgery.
5. The 3-phase model consists of restoring static stability through proprioception and kinesthesia, dynamic stability, and reactive neuromuscular control.
6. Current information has been synthesized to produce a new perspective for therapeutic exercise decisions. This new perspective was specifically designed to improve treatment efficiency and effectiveness and have a focus on function.
7. The 4 principles of purpose, posture, position, and pattern assist problem solving by providing a framework that categorizes clinical information in a hierarchy.
8. The 4 principles serve as quick reminders of the hierarchy, interaction, and application for each therapeutic exercise prescription principle. The questions of *what, when, where,* and *how* for functional movement assessment and exercise prescription are answered in the appropriate order.
   a. Functional evaluation and assessment = purpose.
   b. Identification of motor control = posture.
   c. Identification of osteokinematic and arthrokinematic limitations = position.
   d. Integration of synergistic movement patterns = pattern.
9. The clinician should always ask whether the program makes sense. If it does not make sense, it is probably not functional and therefore not optimally effective.
10. Clinical wisdom is the result of experience and applied knowledge. Intense familiarity and practical observation improve application. To be of benefit, the knowledge available must be organized and tempered by an objective and inclusive framework. It is hoped that this framework will provide a starting point to better organize and apply each clinician's knowledge and experience of functional exercise prescription.

REFERENCES

1. Barnett M, Ross D, Schmidt R, Todd B. Motor skills learning and the specificity of training principle. *Res Q.* 1973;44:440-447.
2. McNair PJ, Marshall RN. Landing characteristics in subjects with normal and anterior cruciate ligament deficient knee joints. *Arch Phys Med.* 1994;75:584-589.
3. Cook G. *The Four P's (Exercise Prescription): Functional Exercise Training Course Manual.* Greeley, CO: North American Sports Medicine Institute Advances in Clinical Education; 1997.
4. American College of Sports Medicine. *Exercise Management for Persons with Chronic Diseases and Disabilities.* Champaign, IL: Human Kinetics; 1997.
5. Barrack RL, Lund PJ, Skinner HB. Knee joint proprioception revisited. *J Sport Rehabil.* 1994;3:18-42.
6. Barrack RL, Skinner HB. The sensory function of knee ligaments. In: Daniel D, ed. *Knee Ligaments: Structure, Function, Injury, and Repair.* New York, NY: Raven Press; 1990;95-114.
7. Ciccotti MR, Kerlan R, Perry J, Pink M. An electromyographic analysis of the knee during functional activities: I. The normal profile. *Am J Sports Med.* 1994;22:645-650.
8. Cook G. *Functional Movement Service Manual.* Danville, VA: Athletic Testing Services; 1998.
9. Grigg P. Response of joint afferent neurons in cat medial articular nerve to active and passive movements of the knee. *Brain Res.* 1976;118:482-485.
10. Grigg P. Peripheral neural mechanisms in proprioception. *J Sport Rehabil.* 1994;3:1-17.
11. Grigg P, Finerman GA, Riley LH. Joint position sense after total hip replacement. *J Bone Joint Surg Am.* 1973;55:1016-1025.
12. Grigg P, Hoffman AH. Ruffini mechanoreceptors in isolated joint capsule. Reflexes correlated with strain energy density. *Somatosens Res.* 1984;2:149-162.
13. Grigg P, Hoffman AH. Properties of Ruffini afferents revealed by stress analysis of isolated sections of cat knee capsule. *J Neurophysiol.* 1982;47:41-54.
14. Guyton AC. *Textbook of Medical Physiology.* 6th ed. Philadelphia, PA: Saunders; 1991.
15. Skinner HB, Barrack RL, Cook SD, Haddad RJ. Joint position sense in total knee arthroplasty. *J Orthop Res.* 1984;1:276-283.
16. Cross MJ, McCloskey DI. Position sense following surgical removal of joints in man. *Brain Res.* 1973;55:443-445.
17. Freeman MAR, Wyke B. Articular reflexes of the ankle joint. An electromyographic study of normal and abnormal influences of ankle-joint mechanoreceptors upon reflex activity in leg muscles. *Br J Surg.* 1967;54:990-1001.
18. Sherrington CS. *The Interactive Action of the Nervous System.* New Haven, CT: Yale University Press; 1911.
19. Kennedy JC, Alexander IJ, Hayes KC. Nerve supply to the human knee and its functional importance. *Am J Sports Med.* 1982;10:329-335.
20. Clark FJ, Burgess PR. Slowly adapting receptors in cat knee joint: can they signal joint angle? *J Neurophysiol.* 1975;38:1448-1463.
21. Lephart S. Reestablishing proprioception, kinesthesia, joint position sense and neuromuscular control in rehab. In: Prentice WE, ed. *Rehabilitation Techniques in Sports Medicine.* 2nd ed. St. Louis, MO: Mosby; 1994;118-137.
22. Schulte MJ, Happel LT. Joint innervation in injury. *Clin Sports Med.* 1990;9:511-517.
23. Willis WD, Grossman RG. *Medical Neurobiology.* 3rd ed. St. Louis, MO: Mosby; 1981.
24. Voight ML, Blackburn TA, Hardin JA, et al. The effects of muscle fatigue on the relationship of arm dominance to shoulder proprioception. *J Orthop Sports Phys Ther.* 1996;23:348-352.
25. Voight ML, Cook G, Blackburn TA. Functional lower quarter exercise through reactive neuromuscular training. In: Bandy WE, ed. *Current Trends for the Rehabilitation of the Athlete.* Lacrosse, WI: SPTS Home Study Course; 1997.
26. Phillips CG, Powell TS, Wiesendanger M. Protection from low threshold muscle afferents of hand and forearm area 3A of Babson's cortex. *J Physiol.* 1971;217:419-446.
27. Borsa PA, Lephart SM, Kocher MS, Lephart SP. Functional assessment and rehabilitation of shoulder proprioception for glenohumeral instability. *J Sport Rehabil.* 1994;3:84-104.
28. Tippett S, Voight ML. *Functional Progressions for Sports Rehabilitation.* Champaign, IL: Human Kinetics; 1995.
29. Voight ML. *Functional Exercise Training.* Presented at the 1990 National Athletic Training Association Annual Conference, Indianapolis, IN; 1990.
30. Voight ML. Proprioceptive concerns in rehabilitation. In: *Proceedings of the XXVth FIMS World Congress of Sports Medicine,* Athens, Greece: The International Federation of Sports Medicine; 1994.
31. Voight ML, Draovitch P. Plyometric training. In: Albert M, ed. *Eccentric Muscle Training in Sports and Orthopaedics.* New York, NY: Churchill Livingstone; 1991;45-73.
32. Small C, Waters CL, Voight ML. Comparison of two methods for measuring hamstring reaction time using the Kin-Com isokinetic dynamometer. *J Orthop Sports Phys Ther.* 1994;19:335-340.
33. Blackburn TA, Voight ML. Single leg stance: development of a reliable testing procedure. In: *Proceedings of the 12th International Congress of the World Confederation for Physical Therapy.* Washington, DC: APTA; 1995.
34. Swanik CB, Lephart SM, Giannantonio FP, Fu F. Reestablishing proprioception and neuromuscular control in the ACL-injured athlete. *J Sport Rehabil.* 1997;6:183-206.

35. Rine RM, Voight ML, Laporta L, Mancini R. A paradigm to evaluate ankle instability using postural sway measures [abstract]. *Phys Ther.* 1994;74:S72.
36. Voight ML, Rine RM, Apfel P, et al. The effects of leg dominance and AFO on static and dynamic balance abilities [abstract]. *Phys Ther.* 1993;73:S51.
37. Voight ML, Rine RM, Briese K, Powell C. Comparison of sway in double versus single leg stance in unimpaired adults [abstract]. *Phys Ther.* 1993;73:S51.
38. Tropp H, Askling C, Gillquist J. Prevention of ankle sprains. *Am J Sports Med.* 1985;13:259-262.
39. Tropp H, Odenrick P. Postural control in single limb stance. *J Orthop Res.* 1988;6:833-839.
40. Beard DJ, Dodd CF, Trundle HR, et al. Proprioception after rupture of the ACL: an objective indication of the need for surgery? *J Bone Joint Surg Br.* 1993;75:311.
41. Pope MH, Johnson DW, Brown DW, Tighe C. The role of the musculature in injuries to the medial collateral ligament. *J Bone Joint Surg Am.* 1972;61:398-402.
42. Wojtys E, Huston L. Neuromuscular performance in normal and anterior cruciate ligament-deficient lower extremities. *Am J Sports Med.* 1994;22:89-104.
43. Dunn TG, Gillig SE, Ponser ES, Weil N. The learning process in biofeedback: is it feed-forward or feedback? *Biofeedback Self Regul.* 1986;11:143-155.
44. Belen'kii VY, Gurfinkle VS, Pal'tsev YI. Elements of control of voluntary movements. *Biofizika.* 1967;12: 135-141.
45. Lee WA. Anticipatory control of postural and task muscles during rapid arm flexion. *J Mot Behav.* 1980;12:185-196.
46. Hodgson JA, Roy RR, DeLeon R, et al. Can the mammalian lumbar spinal cord learn a motor task? *Med Sci Sports Exerc.* 1994;26:1491-1497.
47. Schmidt RA. *Motor Control and Learning.* Champaign, IL: Human Kinetics; 1988.
48. Scully R, Barnes M. *Physical Therapy.* Philadelphia, PA: Lippincott; 1989.
49. Cook G, Fields K. *Functional Training for the Torso.* Colorado Springs, CO: National Strength and Conditioning Association; 1997:14-19.
50. Sullivan PE, Markos PD, Minor MD. *An Integrated Approach to Therapeutic Exercise: Theory and Clinical Application.* Reston, VA: Reston Publishing; 1982.
51. Freeman MAR, Wyke B. Articular contributions to limb reflexes. *Br J Surg.* 1966;53:61-69.
52. Janda V. Muscles and motor control in low back pain: assessment and management. In: Twomey L, ed. *Physical Therapy of the Low Back.* New York, NY: Churchill Livingstone; 1987:253-278.
53. Tropp H, Ekstrand J, Gillquist J. Factors affecting stabilometry recordings of single leg stance. *Am J Sports Med.* 1984;12:185-188.
54. Bernier JN, Perrin DH. Effect of coordination training on proprioception of the functionally unstable ankle. *J Orthop Sports Phys Ther.* 1998;27:264-275.
55. Clark FJ, Burgess RC, Chapin JW, Lipscomb WT. Role of intramuscular receptors in the awareness of limb position. *J Neurophysiol.* 1985;54:1529-1540.
56. Voight ML, Cook G. Clinical application of closed kinetic chain exercise. *J Sport Rehabil.* 1996;5:25-44.
57. Kendall FP, McCreary KE, Provance PG. *Muscle Testing and Function.* 4th ed. Baltimore, MD: Williams & Wilkins; 1993.
58. Cyriax J. *Textbook of Orthopedic Medicine.* Vol. I. Diagnosis of Soft Tissue Lesions. 8th ed. London, UK: Bailliere Tindall; 1982.
59. Baechle TR. *Essentials of Strength Training and Conditioning.* Champaign, IL: Human Kinetics; 1994.
60. Voss DE, Ionta MK, Myers BJ. *Proprioceptive Neuromuscular Facilitation: Patterns and Techniques.* 3rd ed. Philadelphia, PA: Harper & Row; 1985.
61. Gandevia SC, McCloskey DI. Joint sense, muscle sense and their contribution as position sense, measured at the distal interphalangeal joint of the middle finger. *J Physiol.* 1976;260:387-407.
62. Glenncross D, Thornton E. Position sense following joint injury. *Am J Sports Med.* 1981;21:23-27.
63. Barrack RL, Skinner HB, Buckley SL. Proprioception in the anterior cruciate deficient knee. *Am J Sports Med.* 1989;17:1-6.
64. Skinner HB, Wyatt MP, Hodgdon JA, et al. Effect of fatigue on joint position sense of the knee. *J Orthop Res.* 1986;4:112-118.
65. Barrett DS. Proprioception and function after anterior cruciate reconstruction. *J Bone Joint Surg Br.* 1991;3:833-837.
66. Corrigan JP, Cashman WF, Brady MP. Proprioception in the cruciate deficient knee. *J Bone Joint Surg Br.* 1992;74:247-250.
67. Borsa PA, Lephart SM, Irrgang JJ, et al. The effects of joint position and direction of joint motion on proprioceptive sensibility in anterior cruciate ligament deficient athletes. *Am J Sports Med.* 1997;25:336-340.
68. Harter RA, Osternig LR, Singer SL, et al. Long-term evaluation of knee stability and function following surgical reconstruction for anterior cruciate ligament insufficiency. *Am J Sports Med.* 1988;16:434-442.
69. Lephart SM, Pincivero DM, Giraldo JL, Fu F. The role of proprioception in the management and rehabilitation of athletic injuries. *Am J Sports Med.* 1997;25:130-137.
70. Ihara H, Nakayama A. Dynamic joint control training for knee ligament injuries. *Am J Sports Med.* 1986;14:309-315.
71. Giove TP, Miller SJ, Kent BE, et al. Non-operative treatment of the torn anterior cruciate ligament. *J Bone Joint Surg Am.* 1983;65:184-192.
72. Tibone JE, Antich TJ, Funton GS, et al. Functional analysis of anterior cruciate ligament instability. *Am J Sports Med.* 1986;14:276-284.
73. Walla DJ, Albright JP, McAuley E, et al. Hamstring control and the unstable anterior cruciate ligament-deficient knee. *Am J Sports Med.* 1985;13:34-39.

74. Wojtys E, Huston LJ, Taylor PD, Bastian SD. Neuromuscular adaptations in isokinetic, isotonic, and agility training programs. *Am J Sports Med.* 1996;24:187-192.

75. Voight ML, Bell S, Rhodes D. Instrumented testing of tibial translation during a positive Lachman's test and selected closed-chain activities in anterior cruciate deficient knees. *J Orthop Sports Phys Ther.* 1992;15:49.

76. Ognibene J, McMahon K, Harris M, et al. Effects of unilateral proprioceptive perturbation training on postural sway and joint reaction times of healthy subjects. In: *Proceedings of the National Athletic Training Association Annual Meeting.* Champaign, IL: Human Kinetics; 2000.

77. Matsusaka N, Yokoyama S, Tsurusaki T, et al. Effect of ankle disk training combined with tactile stimulation to the leg and foot in functional instability of the ankle. *Am J Sports Med.* 2001;29:25-30.

78. Perlau RC, Frank C, Fick G. The effects of elastic bandages on human knee proprioception in the uninjured population. *Am J Sports Med.* 1995;23:251-255.

79. Sheth P, Yu B, Laskowski ER, et al. Ankle disk training influences reaction times of selected muscles in a simulated ankle sprain. *Am J Sports Med.* 1997;25:538-543.

80. Wester JU, Jespersen SM, Nielsen KD, et al. Wobble board training after partial sprains of the lateral ligaments of the ankle: a prospective randomized study. *J Orthop Sports Phys Ther.* 1996;23:332-336.

81. Konradsen L, Ravin JB. Prolonged peroneal reaction time in ankle instability. *Int J Sports Med.* 1991;12:290-292.

82. Pinstaar A, Brynhildsen J, Tropp H. Postural corrections after standardized perturbations of single limb stance: effect of training and orthotic devices in patients with ankle instability. *Br J Sports Med.* 1996;30:151-155.

20

Rehabilitation of Shoulder Injuries

Joseph B. Myers, Terri Jo Rucinski, William E. Prentice, and Rob Schneider

OBJECTIVES

After completion of this chapter, the physical therapist should be able to do the following:

- Review the functional anatomy and biomechanics associated with normal function of the shoulder joint complex.
- Differentiate the various rehabilitative strengthening techniques for the shoulder, including both open- and closed-kinetic-chain isotonic, plyometric, isokinetic, and proprioceptive neuromuscular facilitation exercises.
- Compare the various techniques for regaining range of motion, including stretching exercises and joint mobilization.
- Administer exercises that may be used to reestablish neuromuscular control.
- Relate biomechanical principles to the rehabilitation of various shoulder injuries/pathologies.
- Discuss criteria for progression of the rehabilitation program for different shoulder injuries/pathologies.
- Describe and explain the rationale for various treatment techniques in the management of shoulder injuries.

Functional Anatomy and Biomechanics

The anatomy of the shoulder joint complex allows for tremendous range of motion. This wide range of motion of the shoulder complex proximal permits precise positioning of the hand distally, to allow both gross and skilled movements. However, the high degree of mobility requires some compromise in stability, which, in turn, increases the vulnerability of the shoulder joint to injury, particularly in dynamic overhead athletic activities.[5]

The shoulder girdle complex is composed of 3 bones—the scapula, the clavicle, and the humerus—that are connected either to one another or to the axial skeleton or trunk via the glenohumeral joint, the acromioclavicular joint, the sternoclavicular joint, and the scapulothoracic joint (Figure 20-1). Dynamic movement and stabilization of the shoulder complex require integrated function of all four articulations if normal motion is to occur.

Sternoclavicular Joint

The clavicle articulates with the manubrium of the sternum to form the sternoclavicular joint, the only direct skeletal connection between the upper extremity and the trunk. The sternal articulating surface is larger than the sternum, causing the clavicle to rise much higher than the sternum. A fibrocartilaginous disk is interposed between the 2 articulating surfaces. It functions as a shock absorber against the medial forces and also helps to prevent any displacement upward. The articular disk is placed so that the clavicle moves on the disk, and the disk, in turn, moves separately on the sternum. The clavicle is permitted to move up and down, forward and backward, in combination, and in rotation.

The sternoclavicular joint is extremely weak because of its bony arrangement, but it is held securely by strong ligaments that tend to pull the sternal end of the clavicle downward and toward the sternum, in effect anchoring it. The main ligaments are the anterior sternoclavicular, which prevents upward displacement of the clavicle; the posterior sternoclavicular, which also prevents upward displacement of the clavicle; the interclavicular, which

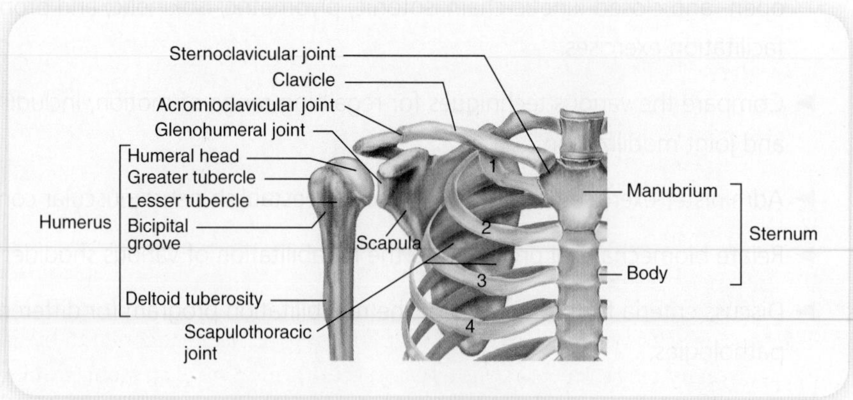

Figure 20-1 Skeletal anatomy of the shoulder complex

(Reproduced with permission from Prentice. *Principles of Athletic Training.* 14th ed. New York: McGraw-Hill; 2011.)

prevents lateral displacement of the clavicle; and the costoclavicular, which prevents lateral and upward displacement of the clavicle.[3]

It should also be noted that for the scapula to abduct and upward rotate throughout 180 degrees of humeral abduction, clavicular movement must occur at both the sternoclavicular and acromioclavicular joints. The clavicle must elevate approximately 40 degrees to allow upward scapular rotation.[93]

Acromioclavicular Joint

The acromioclavicular joint is a gliding articulation of the lateral end of the clavicle with the acromion process. This is a rather weak joint. A fibrocartilaginous disk separates the 2 articulating surfaces. A thin, fibrous capsule surrounds the joint.

The acromioclavicular ligament consists of anterior, posterior, superior, and inferior portions. In addition to the acromioclavicular ligament, the coracoclavicular ligament joins the coracoid process and the clavicle and helps to maintain the position of the clavicle relative to the acromion. The coracoclavicular ligament is further divided into the trapezoid ligament, which prevents overriding of the clavicle on the acromion, and the conoid ligament, which limits upward movement of the clavicle on the acromion. As the arm moves into an elevated position, there is a posterior rotation of the clavicle on its long axis that permits the scapula to continue rotating, thus allowing full elevation. The clavicle must rotate approximately 50 degrees for full elevation to occur; otherwise elevation would be limited to approximately 110 degrees.[93]

Coracoacromial Arch

The coracoacromial ligament connects the coracoid to the acromion. This ligament, along with the acromion and the coracoid, forms the coracoacromial arch over the glenohumeral joint. In the subacromial space between the coracoacromial arch superiorly and the humeral head inferiorly lies the supraspinatus tendon, the long head of the biceps tendon, and the subacromial bursa. Each of these structures is subject to irritation and inflammation resulting either from excessive humeral head translation or from impingement during repeated overhead activities. In asymptomatic individuals the optimal subacromial space appears to be about 9 to 10 mm.[94]

Glenohumeral Joint

The glenohumeral joint is an enarthrodial, or ball-and-socket, synovial joint in which the round head of the humerus articulates with the shallow glenoid cavity of the scapula. The cavity is deepened slightly by a fibrocartilaginous rim called the *glenoid labrum*. The humeral head is larger than the glenoid, and at any point during elevation, only 25% to 30% of the humeral head is in contact with the glenoid.[47] The glenohumeral joint is maintained by both static and dynamic restraints. Position is maintained statically by the glenoid labrum and the capsular ligaments, and dynamically by the deltoid and rotator cuff muscles.

Surrounding the articulation is a loose, articular capsule that is attached to the labrum. This capsule is strongly reinforced by the superior, middle, and inferior glenohumeral ligaments and by the tough coracohumeral ligament, which attaches to the coracoid process and to the greater tuberosity of the humerus.[87]

The long tendon of the biceps muscle passes superiorly across the head of the humerus and then through the bicipital groove. In the anatomical position the long head of the biceps moves in close relationship with the humerus. The transverse humeral ligament maintains the long head of the biceps tendon within the bicipital groove by passing over it from the lesser and the greater tuberosities, converting the bicipital groove into a canal.

Scapulothoracic Joint

The scapulothoracic joint is not a true joint, but the movement of the scapula on the wall of the thoracic cage is critical to shoulder joint motion.[92] The scapula is capable of 5 degrees of freedom movement, including 3 rotations (orientations) and 2 translations (positions).[54,76] Rotation of the scapula can occur around its 3 orthogonal axes, with upward/downward rotation occurring around an anteroposterior axis, internal/external rotation occurring around a superoinferior axis, and anterior/posterior tipping occurring around a mediolateral axis. In addition to rotating, the scapula can translate superoinferiorly (scapular elevation and depression), and anteroposteriorly on the thorax. Because anterior/posterior translation is limited by the rib cage, protraction/retraction results from the anterior/posterior translation (Figure 20-2). During humeral elevation (flexion, scaption, or abduction), the scapula and humerus must move in a synchronous fashion in order to maintain glenohumeral joint congruency, length-tension relationships for the numerous muscles attaching on the scapula, and adequate subacromial space clearance. Commonly termed *scapulohumeral rhythm*, as the humerus elevates, the scapula synchronously upwardly rotates, posteriorly tips, externally rotates, elevates, and translates posteriorly (retracts). Alterations in these scapular movement patterns have been identified in individuals with varying degrees of rotator tendinopathy (subacromial impingement and rotator cuff tears),[35,69,71,79,103,122] pathologic internal impingement,[61] glenohumeral instability,[88] frozen shoulder,[37,101] and osteoarthritis,[37] as well as highly influenced by fatigue,[33,34,108,119] upper-quarter posture and tightness,[11,12,13] and even history of participation in overhead athletics.[30,63,83,90]

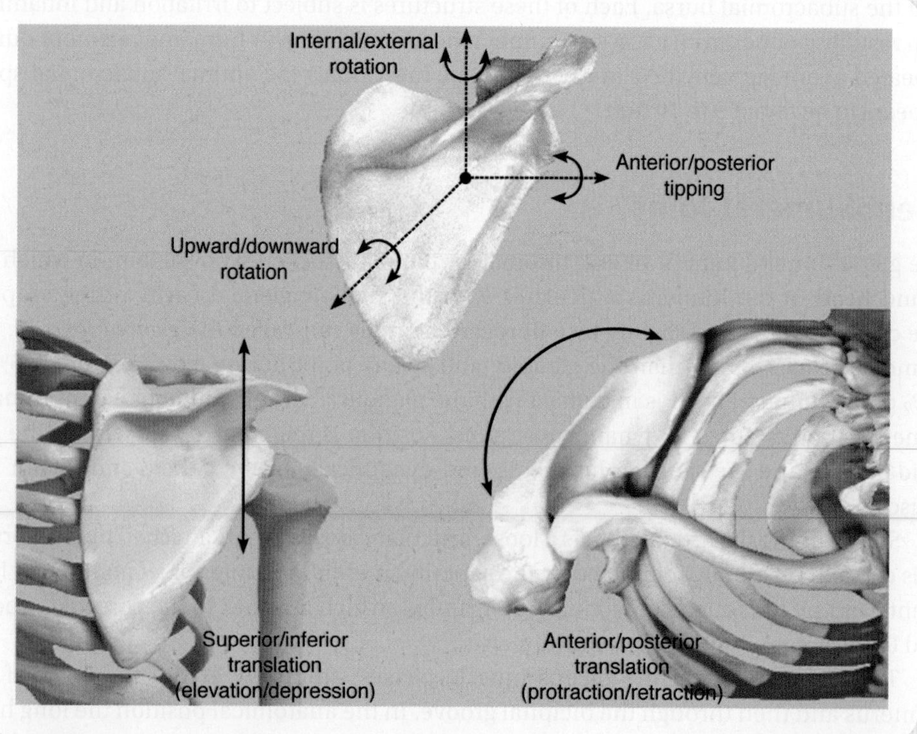

Figure 20-2 Scapular motions

Stability in the Shoulder Joint

Maintaining stability, while the 4 articulations of the shoulder complex collectively allow for a high degree of mobility, is critical in normal function of the shoulder joint. Instability is very often the cause of many of the specific injuries to the shoulder that are discussed later in this chapter. In the glenohumeral joint, the rounded humeral head articulates with a relatively flat glenoid on the scapula. During movement of the shoulder joint, it is essential to maintain the positioning of the humeral head relative to the glenoid. Likewise it is also critical for the glenoid to adjust its position relative to the moving humeral head while simultaneously maintaining a stable base. The glenohumeral joint is inherently unstable, and stability depends on the coordinated and synchronous function of both static and dynamic stabilizers.[74]

Static Stabilizers

The primary static stabilizers of the glenohumeral joint are the glenohumeral ligaments, the posterior capsule, and the glenoid labrum.

The glenohumeral ligaments appear to produce a major restraint in shoulder flexion, extension, and rotation. The anterior glenohumeral ligament is tight when the shoulder is in extension, abduction, and/or external rotation. The posterior glenohumeral ligament is tight in flexion and external rotation. The inferior glenohumeral ligament is tight when the shoulder is abducted, extended, and/or externally rotated. The middle glenohumeral ligament is tight when in flexion and external rotation. Additionally, the middle glenohumeral ligament and the subscapularis tendon limit lateral rotation from 45 to 75 degrees of abduction and are important anterior stabilizers of the glenohumeral joint.[3] The inferior glenohumeral ligament is a primary check against both anterior and posterior dislocation of the humeral head and is the most important stabilizing structure of the shoulder in the overhead patient.[3]

The tendons of the rotator cuff muscles blend into the glenohumeral joint capsule at their insertions about the humeral head (Figure 20-3). As these muscles contract, tension

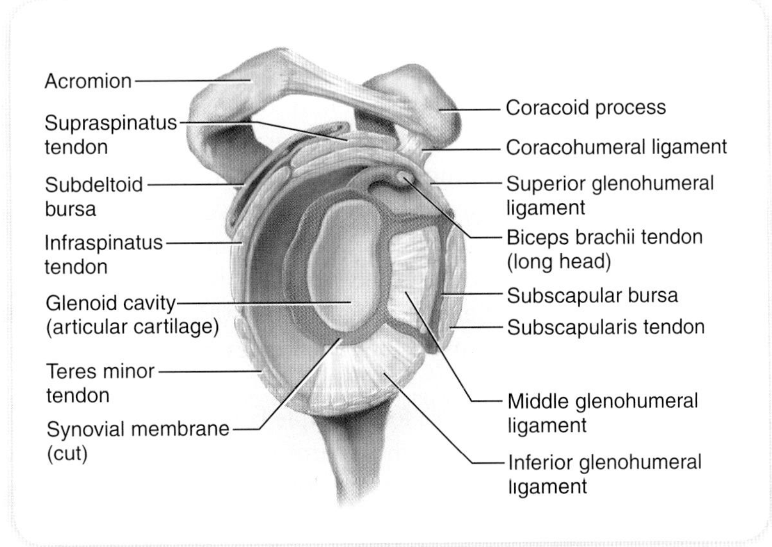

Figure 20-3 Rotator cuff tendons blend into the joint capsule, creating force couples in the frontal plane

(Reproduced with permission from Prentice. *Principles of Athletic Training*. 14th ed. New York: McGraw-Hill; 2011.)

is produced, dynamically tightening the capsule and helping to center the humeral head in the glenoid fossa. This creates both static and dynamic control of humeral head movement.

The posterior capsule is tight when the shoulder is in flexion, abduction, internal rotation, or any combination of these. The superior and middle segment of the posterior capsule has the greatest tension, while the shoulder is internally rotated.

The bones and articular surfaces within the shoulder are positioned to contribute to static stability. The glenoid labrum, which is tightly attached to the bottom half of the glenoid and loosely attached at the top, increases the glenoid depth approximately 2 times, enhancing glenohumeral stability.[66] The scapula faces 30 degrees anteriorly to the chest wall and is tilted upward 3 degrees to enable easier movement on the anterior frontal plane and movements above the shoulder.[4] The glenoid is tilted upward 5 degrees to help control inferior instability.[72]

The Dynamic Stabilizers of the Glenohumeral Joint

The muscles that cross the glenohumeral joint produce motion and function to establish dynamic stability to compensate for a bony and ligamentous arrangement that allows for a great deal of mobility. Movements at the glenohumeral joint include flexion, extension, abduction, adduction, horizontal adduction/abduction, circumduction, and humeral rotation.

The muscles acting on the glenohumeral joint may be classified into two groups. The first group consists of muscles that originate on the axial skeleton and attach to the humerus; these include the latissimus dorsi and the pectoralis major. The second group originates on the scapula and attaches to the humerus; these include the deltoid, the teres major, the coracobrachialis, the subscapularis, the supraspinatus, the infraspinatus, and the teres minor. These muscles constitute the short rotator muscles whose tendons insert into the articular capsule and serve as reinforcing structures. The biceps and triceps muscles attach on the glenoid and affect elbow motion.

The muscles of the rotator cuff, the subscapularis, infraspinatus, supraspinatus, and teres minor along with the long head of the biceps function to provide dynamic stability to control the position and prevent excessive displacement or translation of the humeral head relative to the position of the glenoid.[9,70,121]

Stabilization of the humeral head occurs through coactivation of the rotator cuff muscles. This creates a series of force couples that act to compress the humeral head into the glenoid, minimizing humeral head translation. A force couple involves the action of 2 opposing forces acting in opposite directions to impose rotation about an axis. These force couples can establish dynamic equilibrium of the glenohumeral joint regardless of the position of the humerus. If an imbalance exists between the muscular components that create these force couples, abnormal glenohumeral mechanics occur.

In the frontal plane a force couple exists between the subscapularis anteriorly and the infraspinatus and teres minor posteriorly (see Figure 20-3). Coactivation of the infraspinatus, teres minor, and subscapularis muscles both depresses and compresses the humeral head during overhead movements.

In the coronal plane, there is a critical force couple between the deltoid and the inferior rotator cuff muscles (Figure 20-4). With the arm fully adducted, contraction of the deltoid produces a vertical force in a superior direction causing an upward translation of the humeral head relative to the glenoid. Coactivation of the inferior rotator cuff muscles produces both a compressive force and a downward translation of the humerus that counterbalances the force of the deltoid, stabilizing the humeral head. The supraspinatus compresses the humeral head into the glenoid and, along with the deltoid, initiates abduction on this stable base. Dynamic stability is created by an increase in joint compression forces from contraction of the supraspinatus and by humeral head depression from contraction of the inferior rotator cuff muscles.[9,27,70,121]

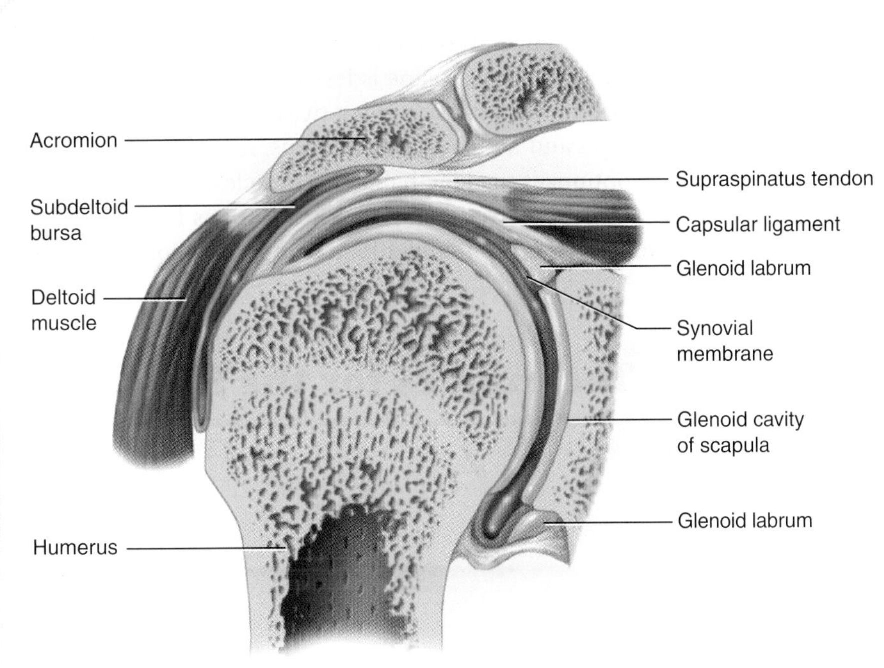

Figure 20-4 **Coronal plane force couples**

(Reproduced with permission from Prentice. *Principles of Athletic Training.* 14th ed. New York: McGraw-Hill; 2011.)

The long head of the biceps tendon also contributes to dynamic stability by limiting superior translation of the humerus during elbow flexion and supination.

Scapular Stability and Mobility

Like the glenohumeral muscles, the scapular muscles play a critical role in normal function of the shoulder. The scapular muscles produce movement of the scapula on the thorax and help to dynamically position the glenoid relative to the moving humerus. They include the levator scapula and upper trapezius, which elevate the scapula; the middle trapezius and rhomboids, which retract the scapula; the lower trapezius, which retracts, upwardly rotates, and depresses the scapula; the pectoralis minor, which depresses the scapula; and the serratus anterior, which protracts and upwardly rotates the scapula (in combination with the upper and lower trapezius). Collectively they function to maintain a consistent length-tension relationship with the glenohumeral muscles.[58,59,80]

The only attachment of the scapula to the thorax is through these muscles. The muscle stabilizers must fix the position of the scapula on the thorax, providing a stable base for the rotator cuff to perform its intended function on the humerus. It has been suggested that the serratus anterior moves the scapula while the other scapular muscles function to provide scapular stability.[58,59] The scapular muscles act isometrically, concentrically, or eccentrically, depending on the movement desired and whether the movement is speeding up or slowing down.[72]

Plane of the Scapula

The concept of the plane of the scapula refers to the angle of the scapula in its resting position, usually 35 to 45 degrees anterior to the frontal plane toward the sagittal plane. When the limb is positioned in the plane of the scapula, the mechanical axis of the glenohumeral joint is in line with the mechanical axis of the scapula. The glenohumeral joint capsule is lax, and the deltoid and supraspinatus muscles are optimally positioned to elevate the humerus. Movement of the humerus in this plane is less restricted than in the frontal or sagittal planes because the glenohumeral capsule is not twisted.[39] Because the rotator cuff muscles originate on the scapula and attach to the humerus, repositioning the humerus into the plane of the scapula optimizes the length of those muscles, improving the length–tension relationship. This is likely to increase muscle force.[39] It has been recommended that many strengthening exercises for the shoulder joint complex be done in the scapular plane.[39,128,129]

Rehabilitation Techniques for the Shoulder

Stretching Exercises

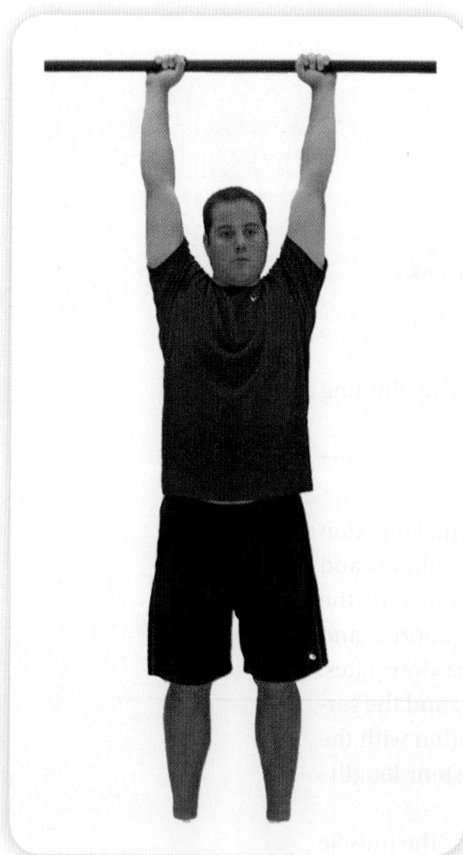

Figure 20-5 Static hanging

Hanging from a chinning bar is a good general stretch for the musculature in the shoulder complex.

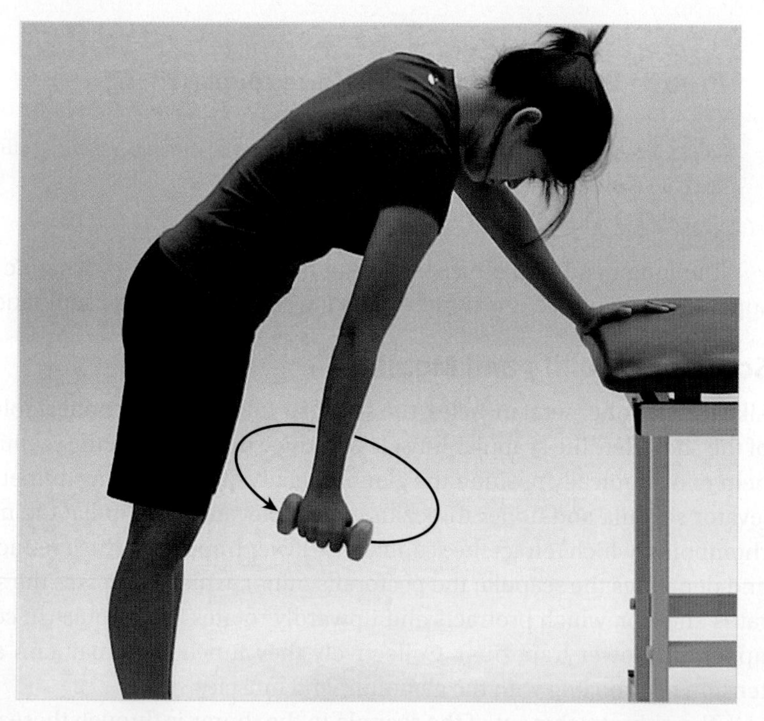

Figure 20-6 Codman's circumduction exercise

The patient holds a dumbbell in the hand and moves it in a circular pattern, reversing direction periodically. This technique is useful as a general stretch in the early stages of rehabilitation when motion above 90 degrees is restricted.

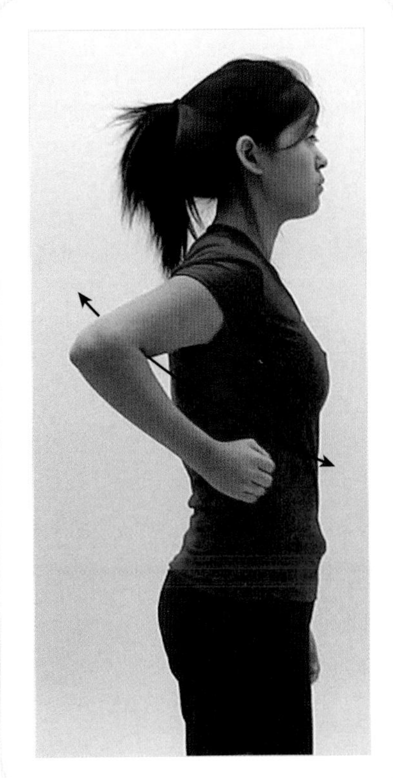

Figure 20-7 **Sawing**

The patient moves the arm forward and backward as if performing a sawing motion. This technique is useful as a general stretch in the early stages of rehabilitation when motion above 90 degrees is restricted.

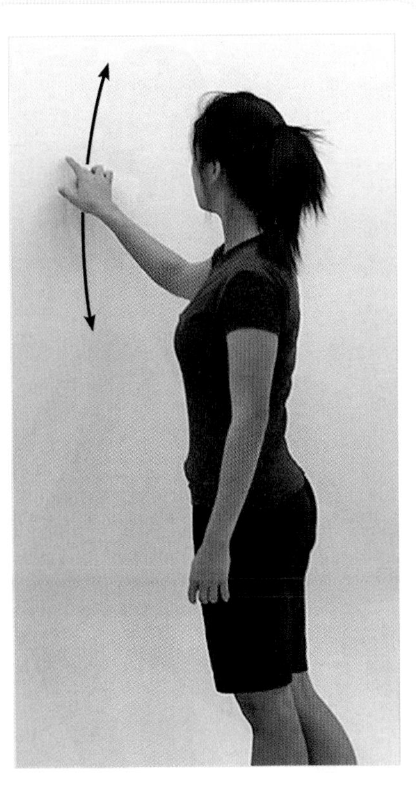

Figure 20-8 **Wall climbing**

The patient uses the fingers to "walk" the hand up a wall. This technique is useful when attempting to regain full-range elevation. ROM should be restricted to a pain-free arc.

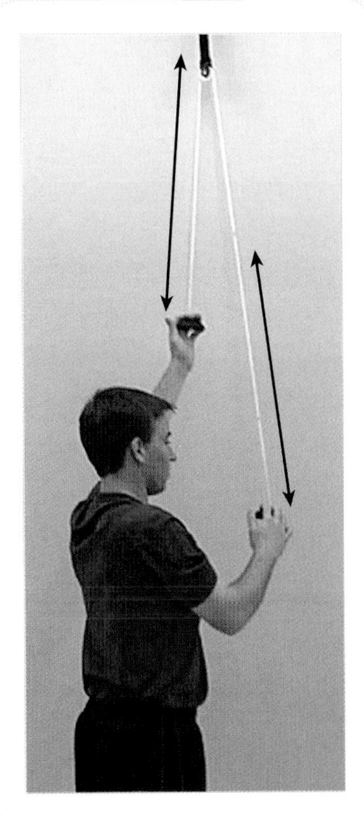

Figure 20-9 **Rope and pulley exercise**

This exercise may be used as an active-assistive exercise when trying to regain full overhead motion. ROM should be restricted to a pain-free arc.

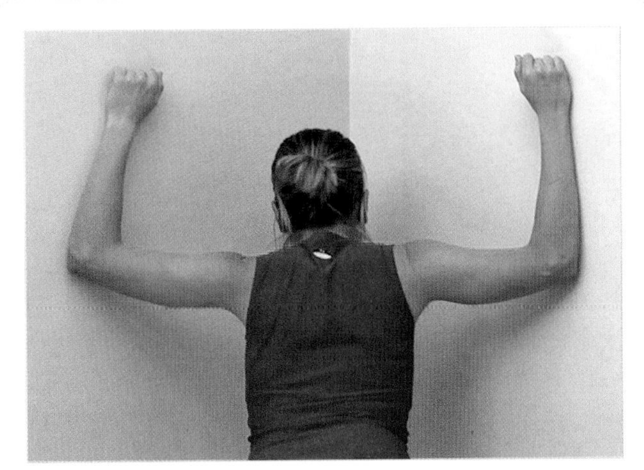

Figure 20-10 **Wall/corner stretch**

Used to stretch the pectoralis major and minor, anterior deltoid, and coracobrachialis, and the anterior joint capsule.

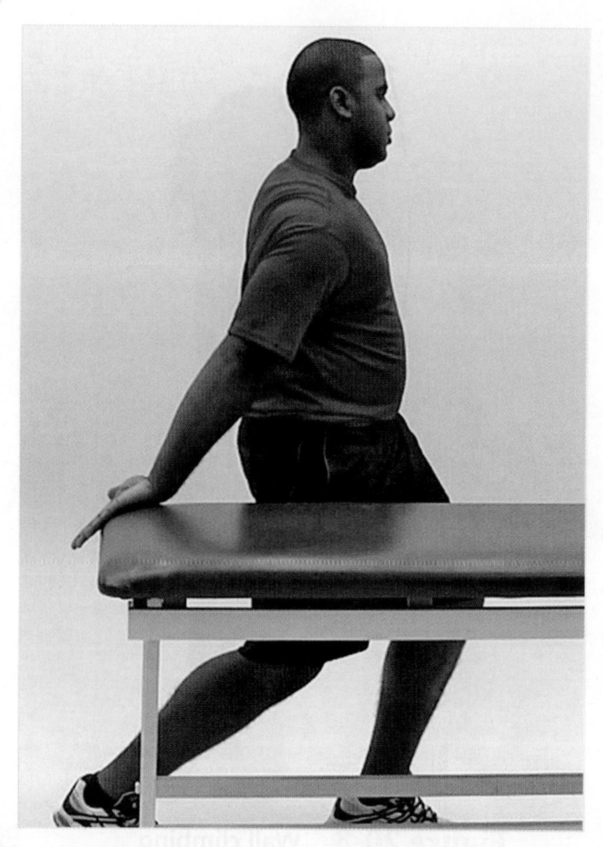

Figure 20-11 Shoulder flexors stretch standing

Used to stretch the anterior deltoid, coracobrachialis, pectoralis major, and biceps muscles, and the anterior joint capsule.

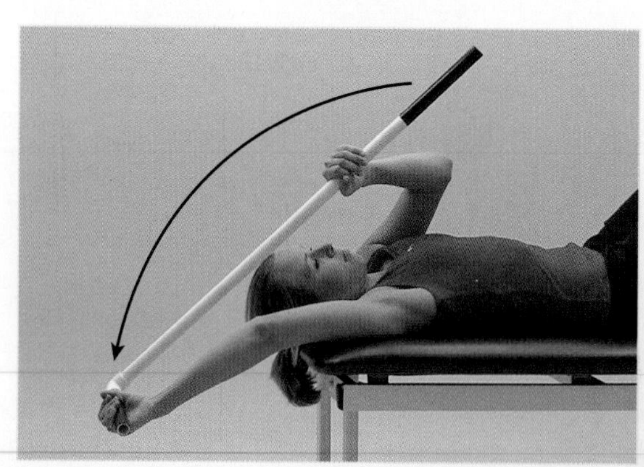

Figure 20-12 Shoulder extensor stretch using an L-bar

Used to stretch the latissimus dorsi, teres major and minor, posterior deltoid, and triceps muscles, and the inferior joint capsule.

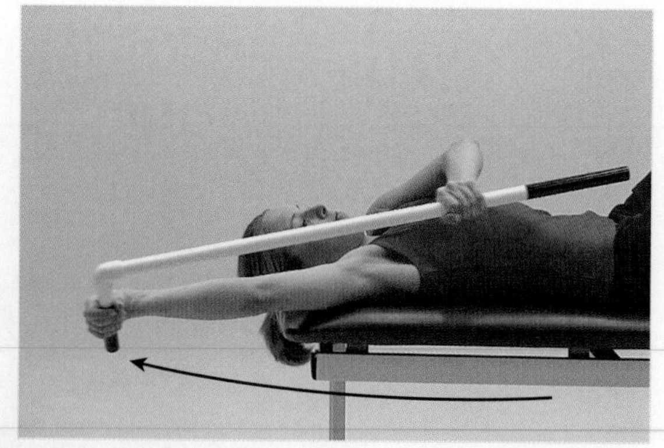

Figure 20-13 Shoulder adductors stretch using an L-bar

Used to stretch the latissimus dorsi, teres major and minor, pectoralis major and minor, posterior deltoid, and triceps muscles, and the inferior joint capsule.

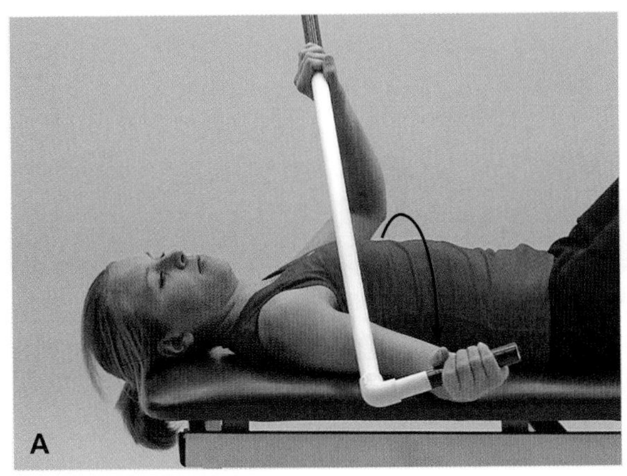

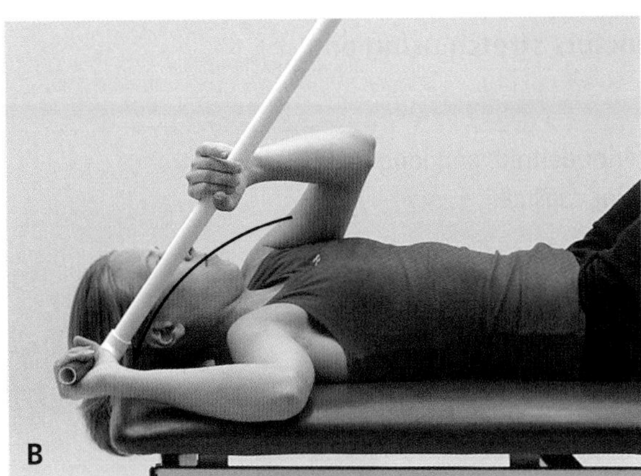

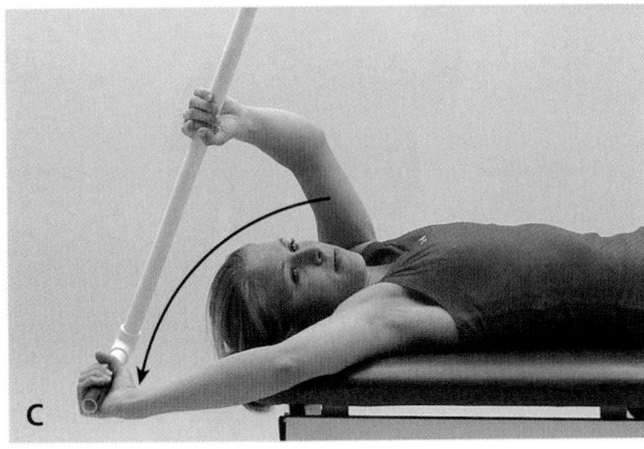

Figure 20-14 Shoulder medial rotators stretch using an L-bar

Used to stretch the subscapularis, pectoralis major, latissimus dorsi, teres major, and anterior deltoid muscles, and the anterior joint capsule. This stretch should be done at (**A**) 0 degrees, (**B**) 90 degrees, and (**C**) 135 degrees.

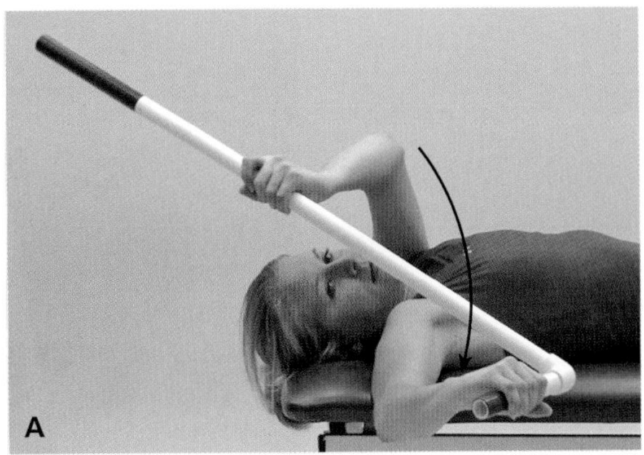

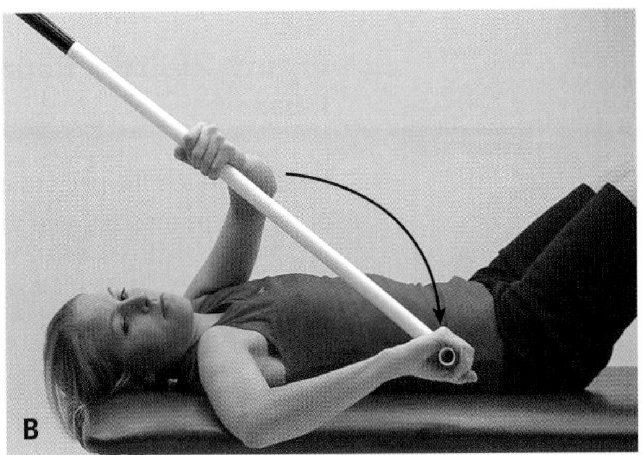

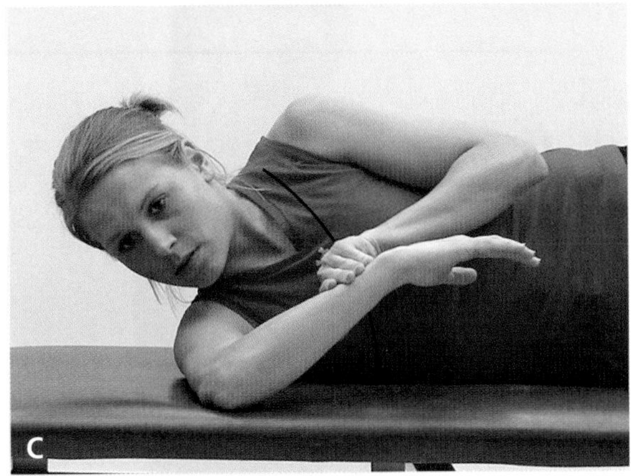

Figure 20-15 Shoulder external rotators stretch using an L-bar

Used to stretch the infraspinatus, teres minor, and posterior deltoid muscles, and the posterior joint capsule. This stretch should be done at (**A**) 90 degrees and (**B**) 135 degrees. **C.** The Sleeper Stretch can also be used to stretch the external rotators.

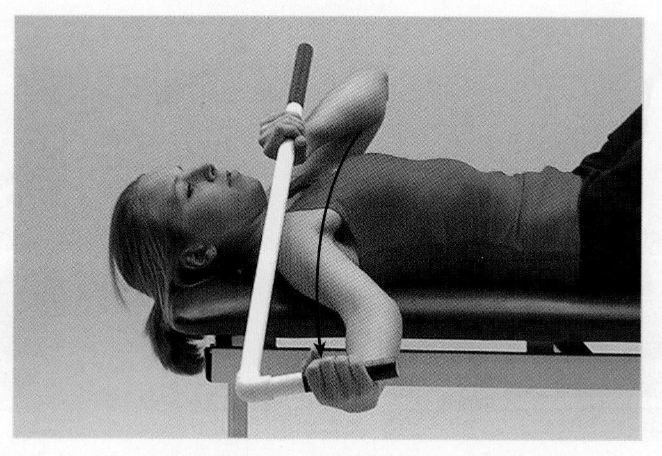

Figure 20-16 **Horizontal adductors stretch using an L-bar**

Used to stretch the pectoralis major, anterior deltoid, and long head of the biceps muscles, and the anterior joint capsule.

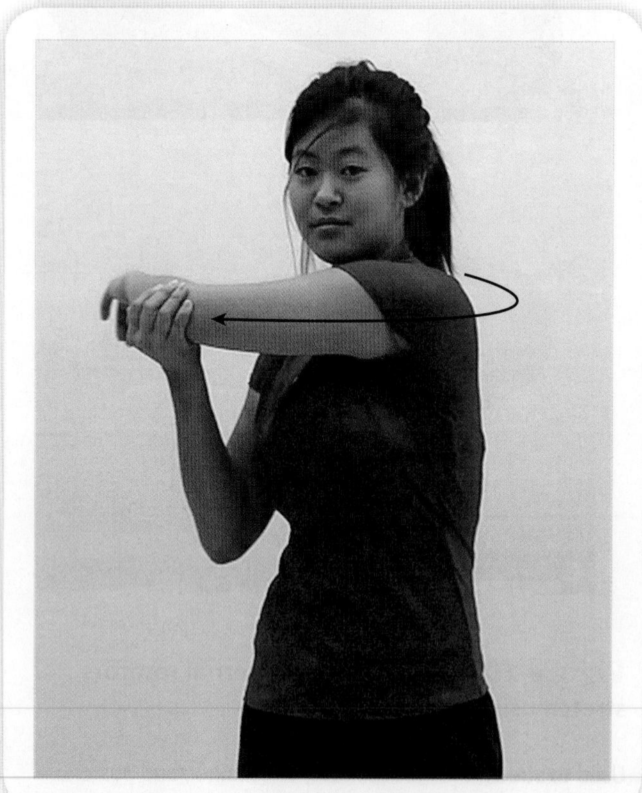

Figure 20-17 **Horizontal abductors stretch**

Used to stretch the posterior deltoid, infraspinatus, teres minor, rhomboids, and middle trapezius muscles, and the posterior capsule. This position might be uncomfortable for patients with shoulder impingement syndrome.

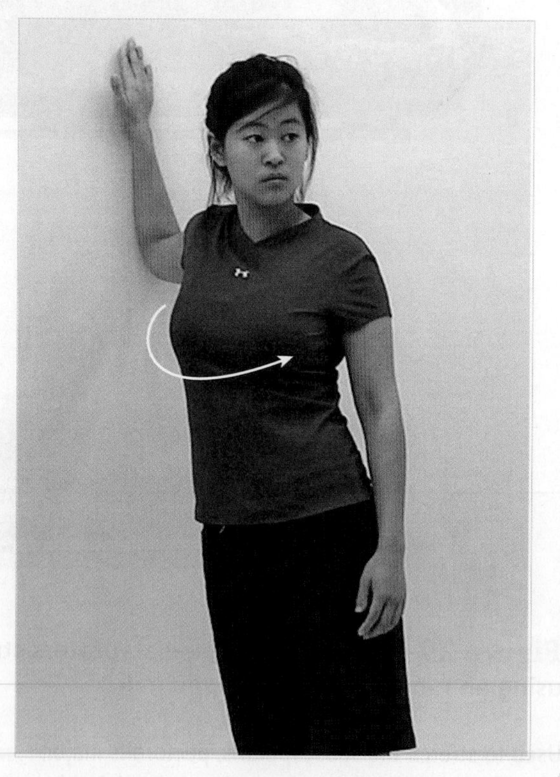

Figure 20-18 **Anterior capsule stretch**

Self-stretch using the wall.

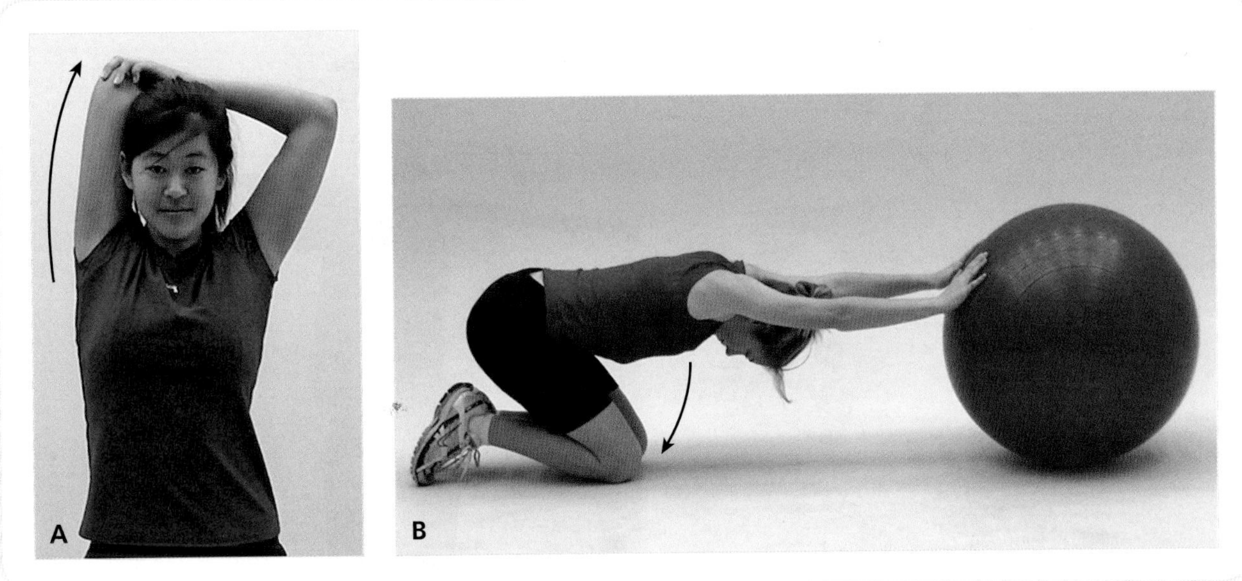

Figure 20-19 **Inferior capsule stretch**

A. Self-stretch done with the arm in the fully elevated overhead position. This position might be uncomfortable for patients with shoulder impingement syndrome. **B.** Inferior capsule stretch can also be done using a stability ball.

Strengthening Techniques

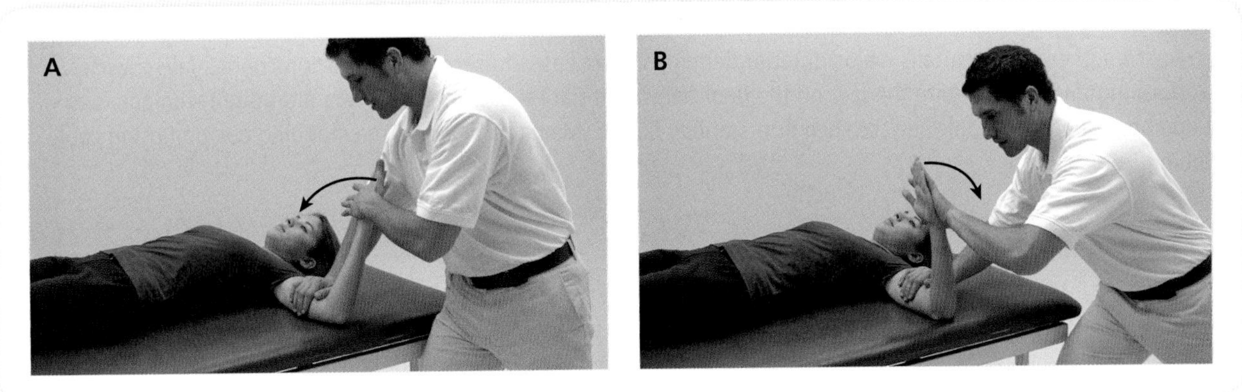

Figure 20-20

A. Isometric medial rotation, and (**B**) isometric lateral rotation, are useful in the early stages of a shoulder rehabilitation program when full ROM isotonic exercise is likely to exacerbate a problem.

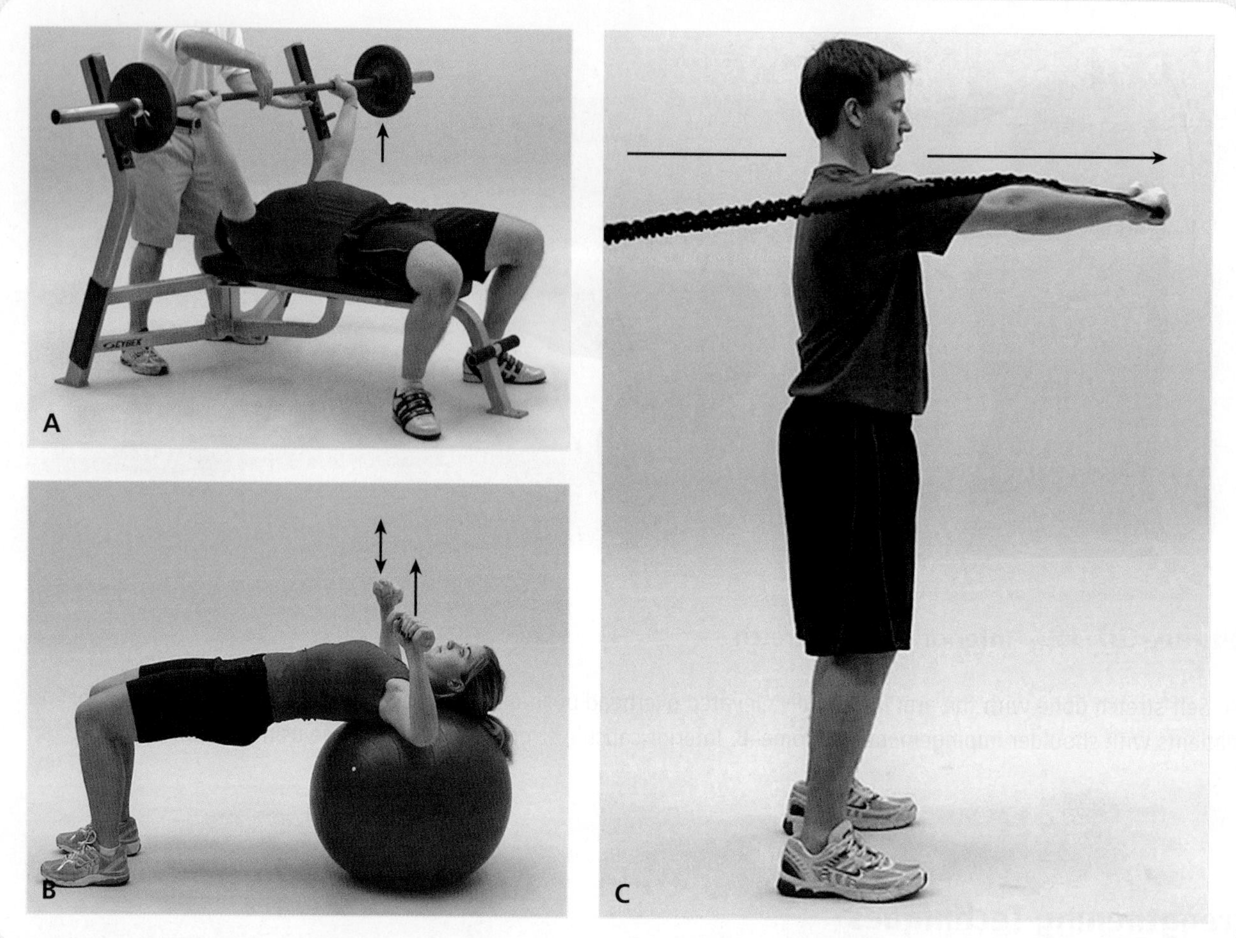

Figure 20-21 **Chest press**

Used to strengthen the pectoralis major, anterior deltoid, and triceps, and secondarily the coracobrachialis muscles. **A.** Performing this exercise with the feet on the floor helps to isolate these muscles. **B.** An alternate technique is to use dumbbells on an unstable surface such as a stability ball. **C.** May also be done in a standing position using cable or tubing.

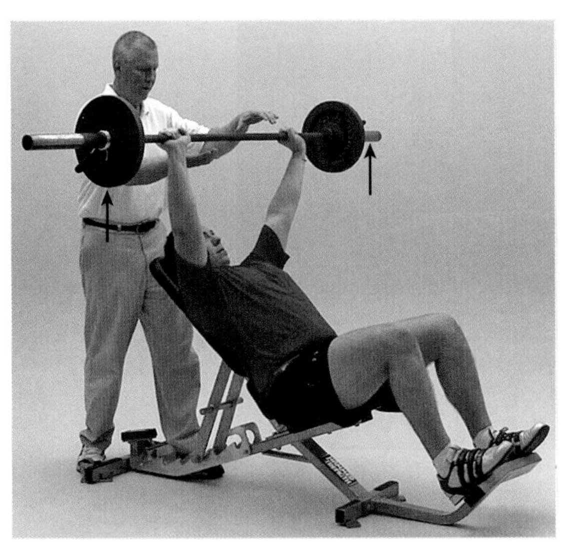

Figure 20-22 **Incline bench press**

Used to strengthen the pectoralis major (upper fibers), triceps, middle and anterior deltoid, and secondarily, the coracobrachialis, upper trapezius, and levator scapula muscles.

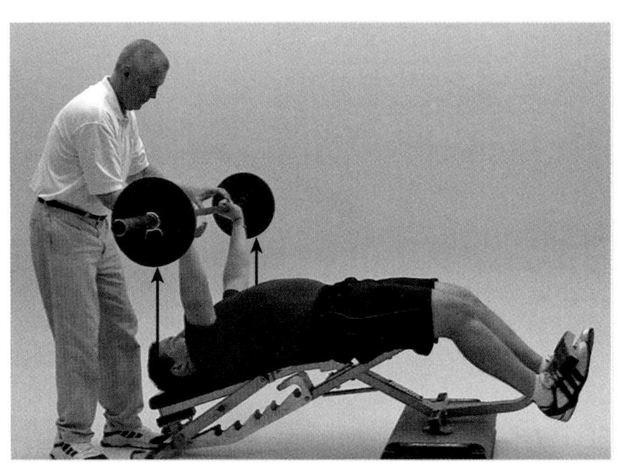

Figure 20-23 **Decline bench press**

Used to strengthen the pectoralis major (lower fibers), triceps, anterior deltoid, coracobrachialis, and latissimus dorsi muscles.

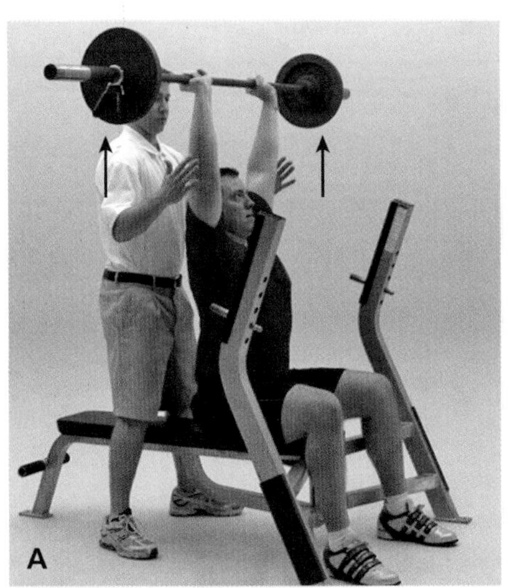

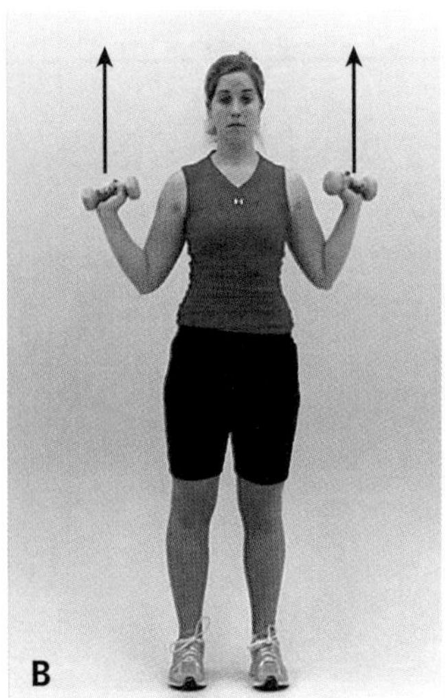

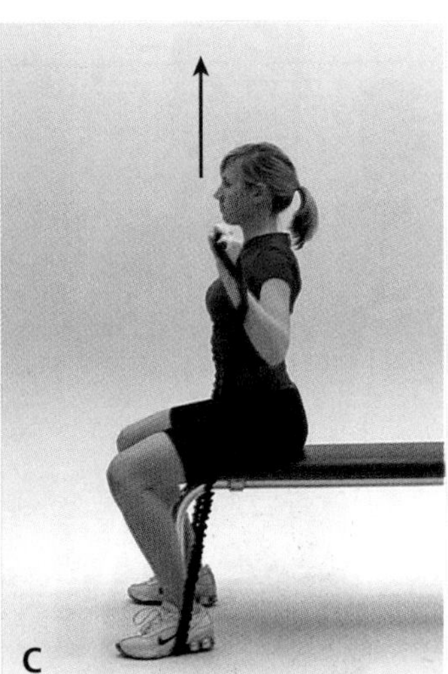

Figure 20-24 **Military press**

Used to strengthen the middle deltoid, upper trapezius, levator scapula, and triceps. **A.** Performed in a seated position on a bench. **B.** In a standing position using dumbbells. **C.** In a seated position using cable or tubing.

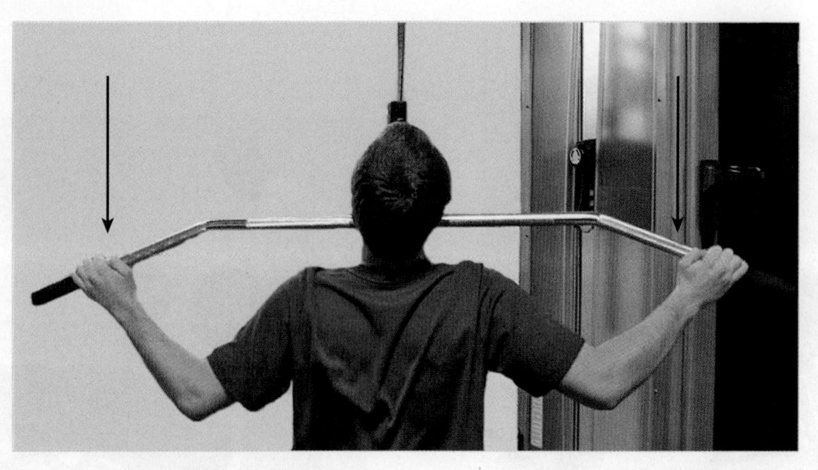

Figure 20-25 Lat pull-downs

Used to strengthen primarily the latissimus dorsi, teres major, and pectoralis minor, and secondarily the biceps muscles. This exercise should be done by pulling the bar down in front of the head. Pull-ups done on a chinning bar can also be used as an alternative strengthening technique.

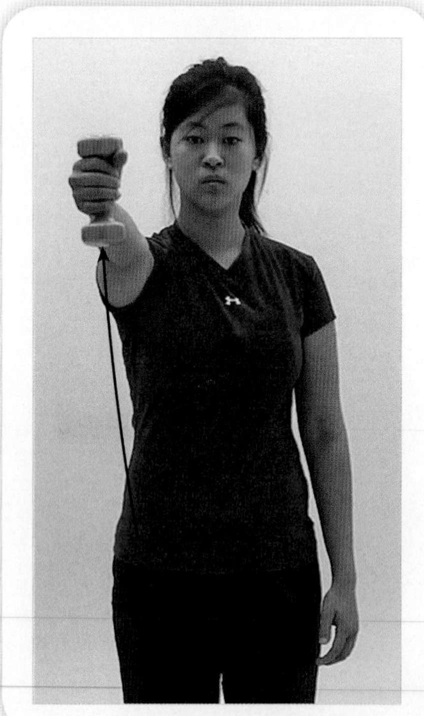

Figure 20-26 Shoulder flexion

Used to strengthen primarily the anterior deltoid and coracobrachialis, and secondarily the middle deltoid, pectoralis major, and biceps brachii muscles. Note that the thumb should point upward.

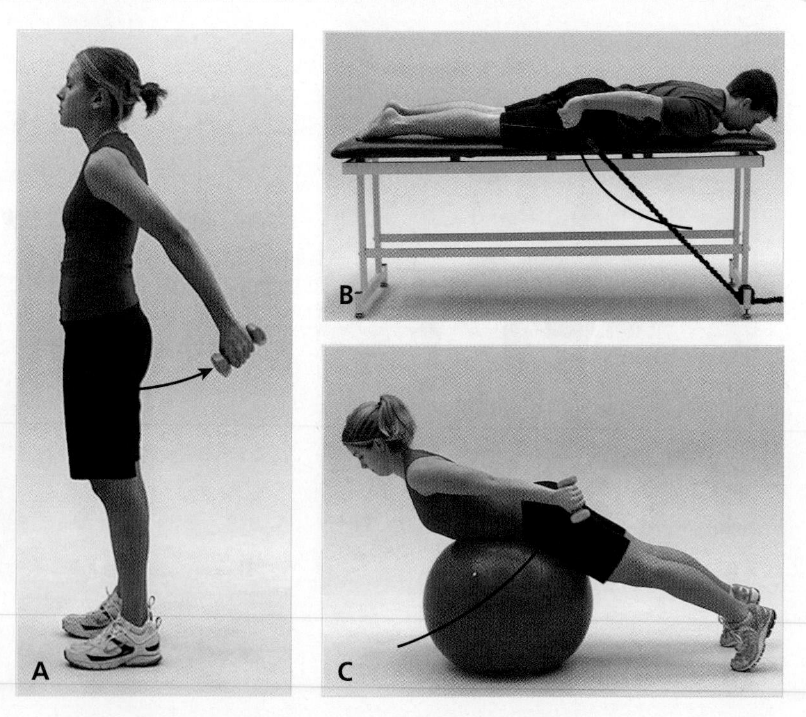

Figure 20-27 Shoulder extension

Used to strengthen primarily the latissimus dorsi, teres major, and posterior deltoid, and secondarily, the teres minor and the long head of the triceps muscles. Note that the thumb should point downward. May be done (**A**) standing using a dumbbell, (**B**) lying prone using cable or tubing, or (**C**) using dumbbells prone on a stability ball.

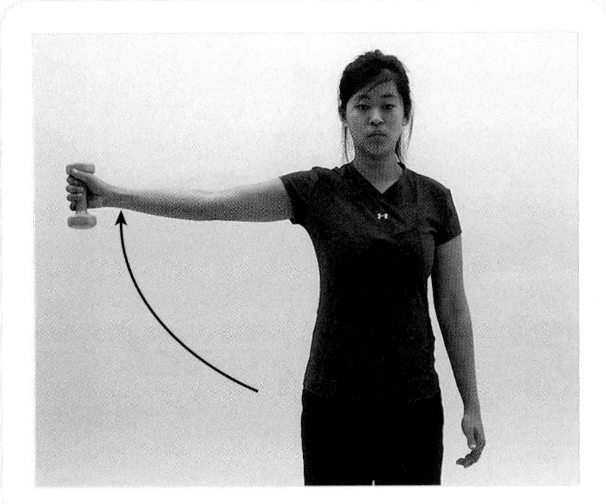

Figure 20-28 **Shoulder abduction to 90 degrees**

Used to strengthen primarily the middle deltoid and supraspinatus, and secondarily, the anterior and posterior deltoid and serratus anterior muscles.

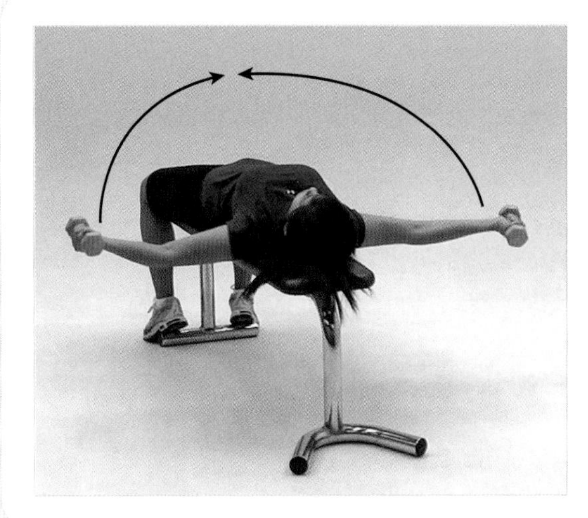

Figure 20-29 **Flys (shoulder horizontal adduction)**

Used to strengthen primarily the pectoralis major, and secondarily, the anterior deltoid. Note that the elbow may be slightly flexed. May be done in a supine position or standing with surgical tubing or wall pulleys behind.

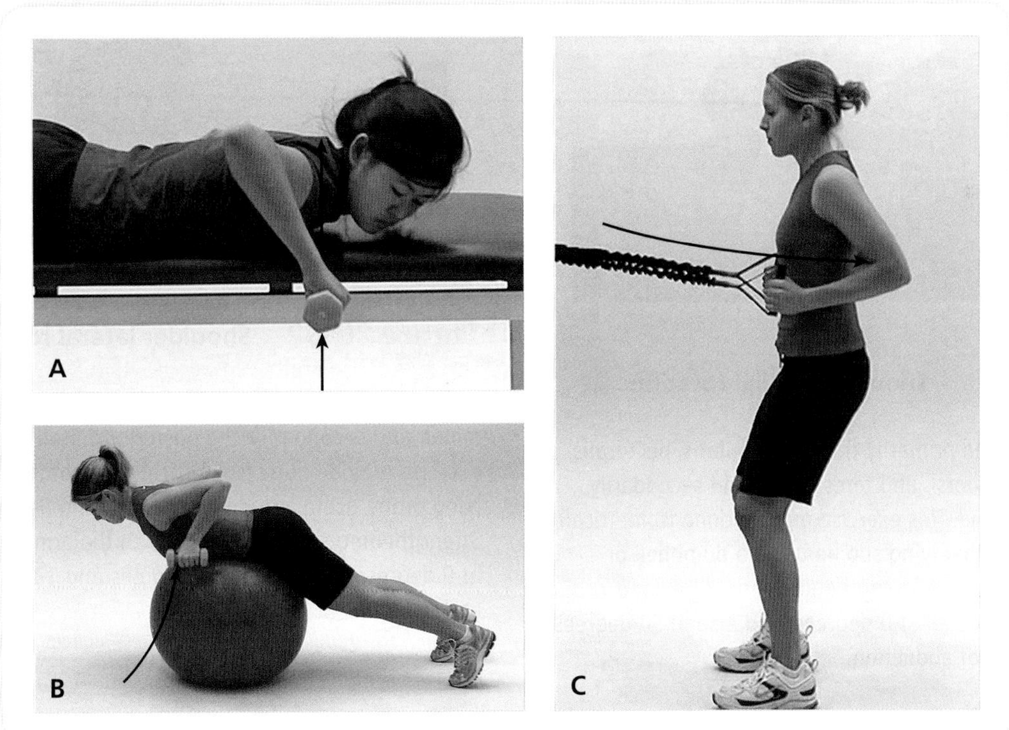

Figure 20-30 **Reverse flys (shoulder horizontal abduction)**

Used to strengthen primarily the posterior deltoid, and secondarily, the infraspinatus, teres minor, rhomboids, and middle trapezius muscles. **A.** May be done lying prone using dumbbells. **B.** Prone on a stability ball. **C.** Standing using cables or tubing. Note that with the thumb pointed upward the middle trapezius is more active, and with the thumb pointed downward the rhomboids are more active.

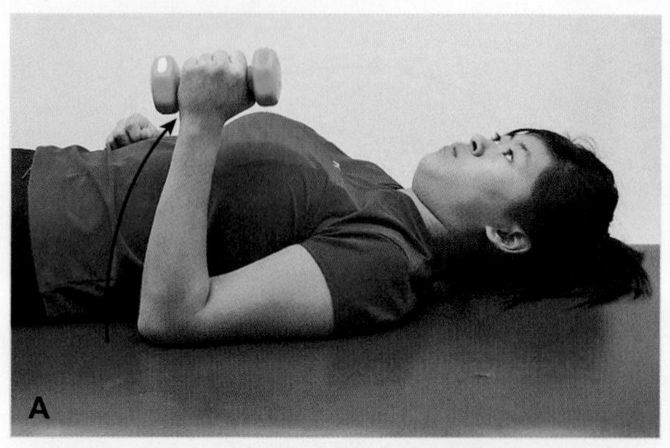
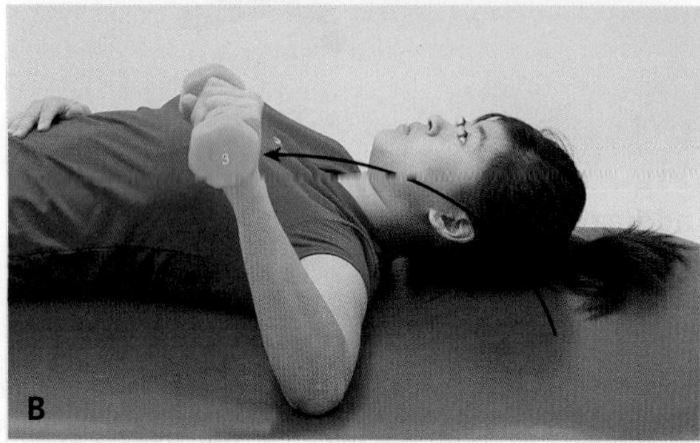
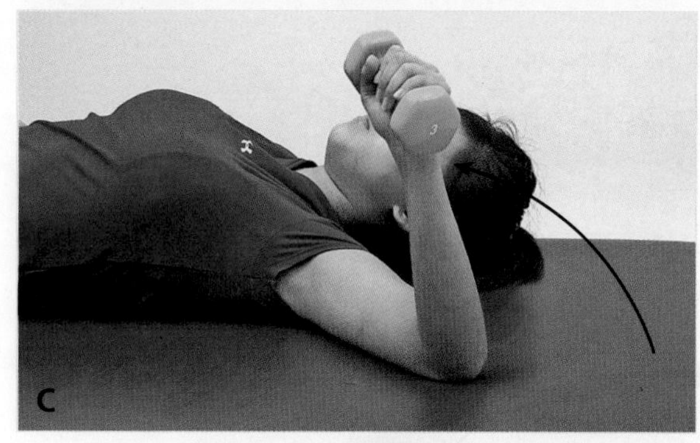

Figure 20-31 Shoulder medial rotation

Used to strengthen primarily the subscapularis, pectoralis major, latissimus dorsi, and teres major, and secondarily, the anterior deltoid. This exercise may be done isometrically or isotonically, either lying supine using a dumbbell or standing using tubing. Strengthening should be done with the arm fully adducted at 0 degrees, and also in 90 degrees and 135 degrees of abduction.

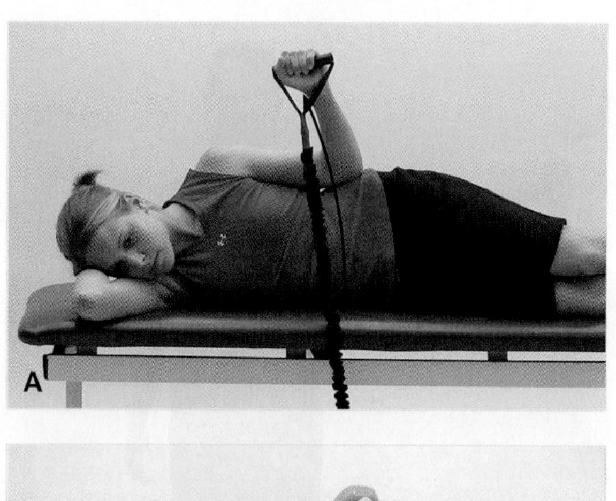
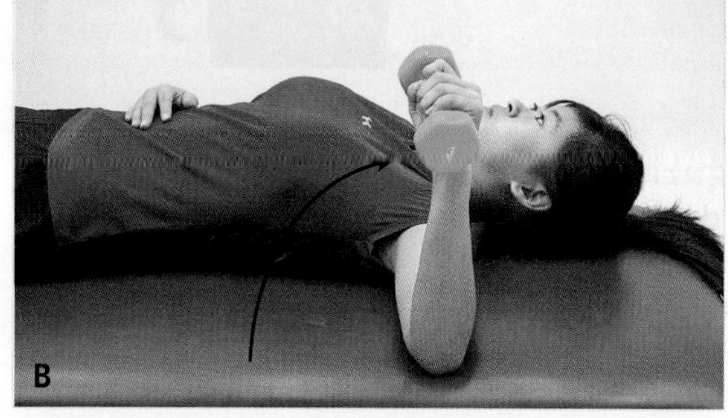
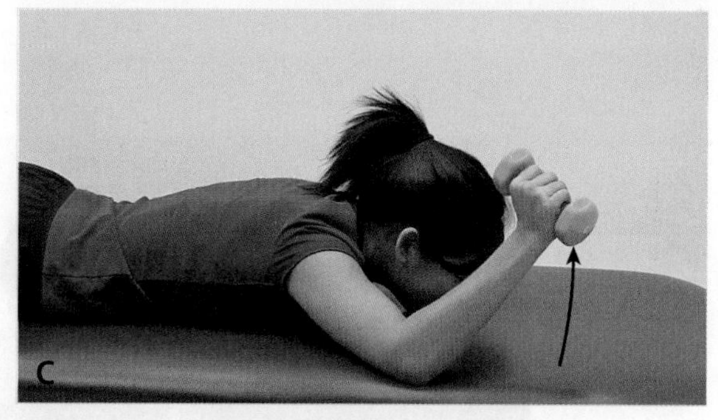

Figure 20-32 Shoulder lateral rotation

Used to strengthen primarily the infraspinatus and teres minor, and secondarily, the posterior deltoid muscles. This exercise may be done isometrically or isotonically, either lying prone using a dumbbell or standing using tubing. Strengthening should be done with the arm fully adducted at 0 degrees, and also in 90 degrees and 135 degrees of abduction.

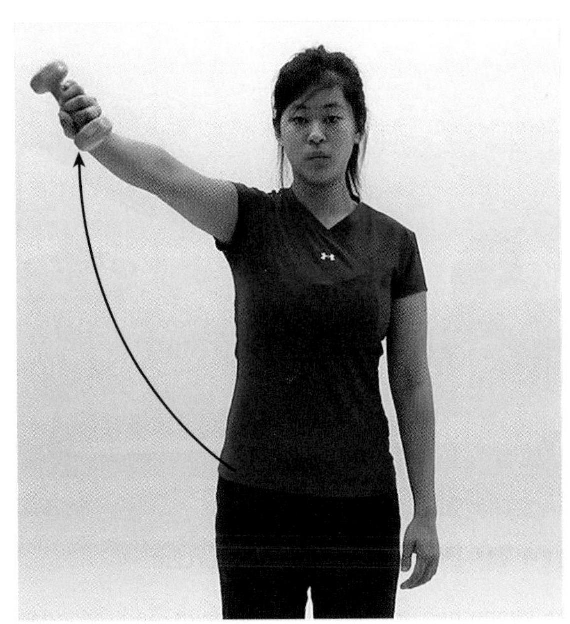

Figure 20-33 **Scaption**

Used to strengthen primarily the supraspinatus in the plane of the scapula, and secondarily, the anterior and middle deltoid muscles. This exercise should be done standing with the arm horizontally adducted to 45 degrees.

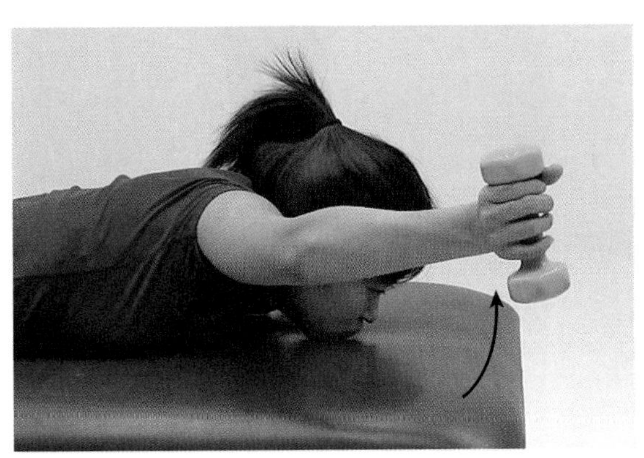

Figure 20-34 **Alternative supraspinatus exercise**

Used to strengthen primarily the supraspinatus, and secondarily, the posterior deltoid. In the prone position with the arm abducted to 100 degrees, the arm is horizontally abducted in extreme lateral rotation. Note that the thumb should point upward.

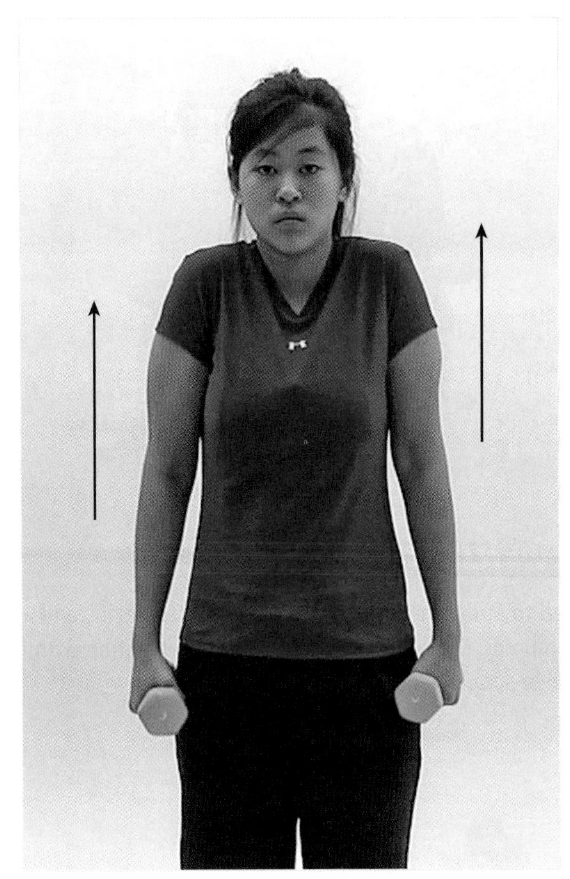

Figure 20-35 **Shoulder shrugs**

Used to strengthen primarily the upper trapezius and the levator scapula, and secondarily, the rhomboids.

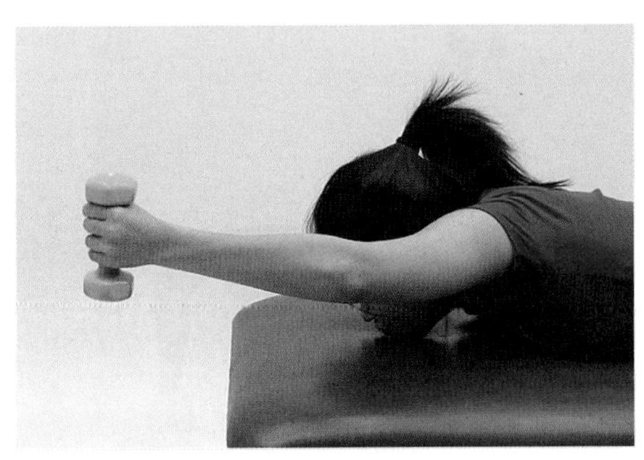

Figure 20-36 **Superman**

Used to strengthen primarily the inferior trapezius, and secondarily, the middle trapezius. May be done lying prone using either dumbbells or tubing.

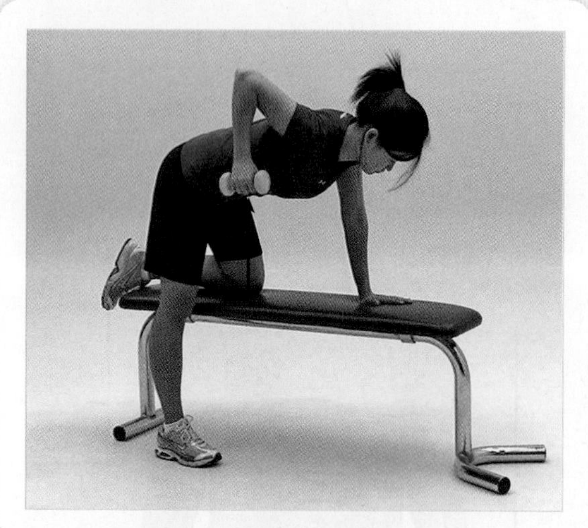

Figure 20-37 **Bent-over rows**

Used to strengthen primarily the middle trapezius and rhomboids. Done standing in a bent-over position with 1 knee supported on a bench.

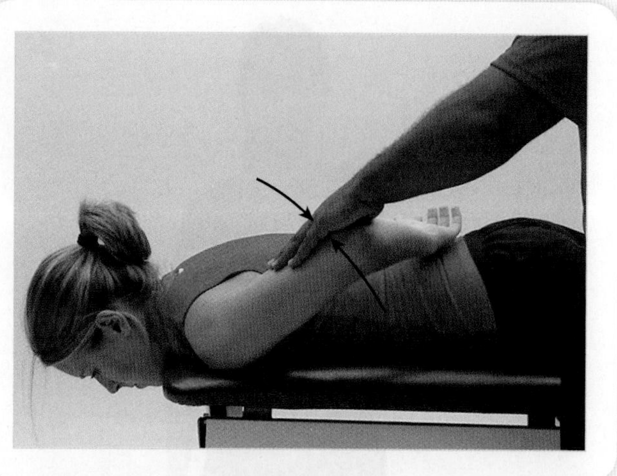

Figure 20-38 **Rhomboids exercise**

Used to strengthen primarily the rhomboids, and secondarily, the inferior trapezius. Should be done lying prone with manual resistance applied at the elbow.

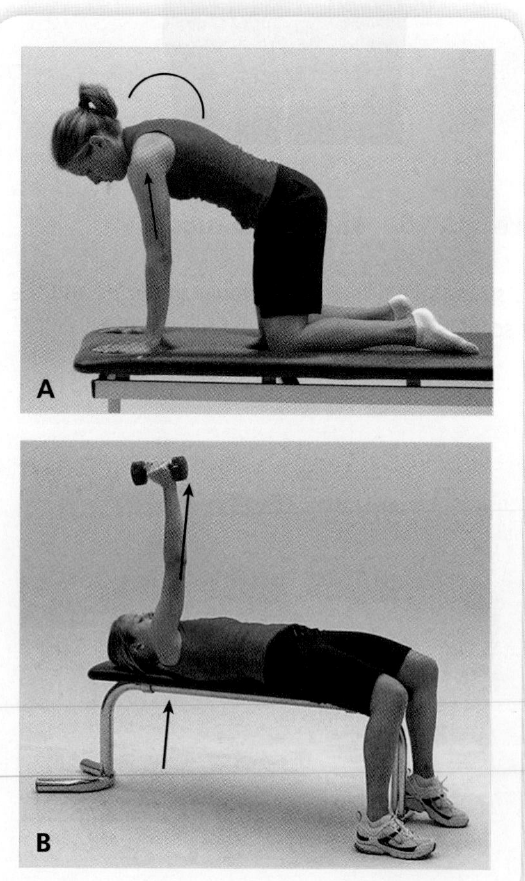

Figure 20-39 **Pushups with a plus**

Used to strengthen the serratus anterior. There are several variations to this exercise, including **(A)** regular pushups, and **(B)** weight-loaded pushups with a plus.

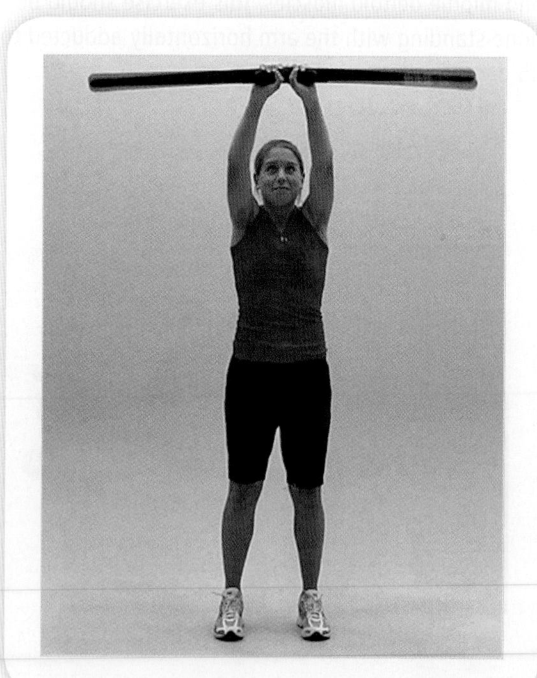

Figure 20-40 **Scapular strengthening using a Body Blade**

Holding an oscillating Body Blade with both hands, the patient moves from a fully adducted position in front of the body to a fully elevated overhead position.

Closed-Kinetic-Chain Exercises

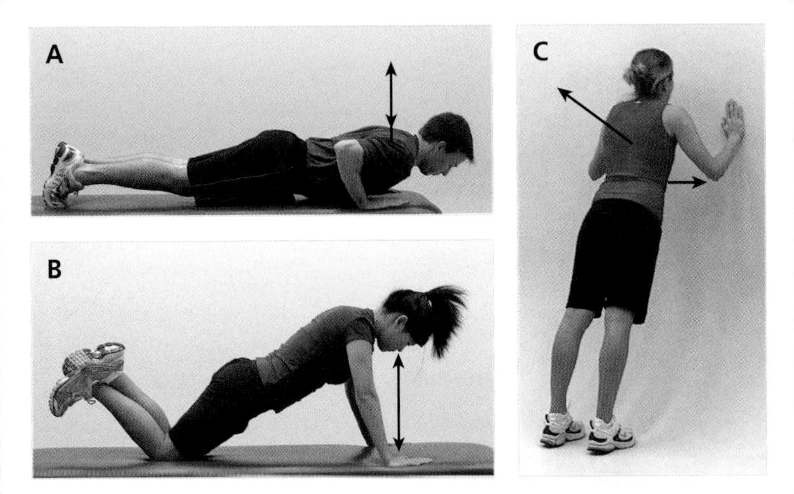

Figure 20-41 **Pushups**

May be done with (**A**) weight supported on feet, or (**B**) modified to support weight on the knees. **C.** Wall pushups.

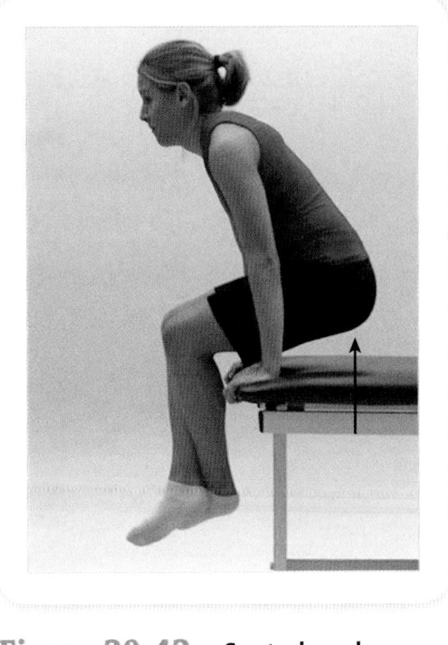

Figure 20-42 **Seated pushup**

Done sitting on the end of a table. Place hands on the tab le and lift weight upward off of the table isotonically.

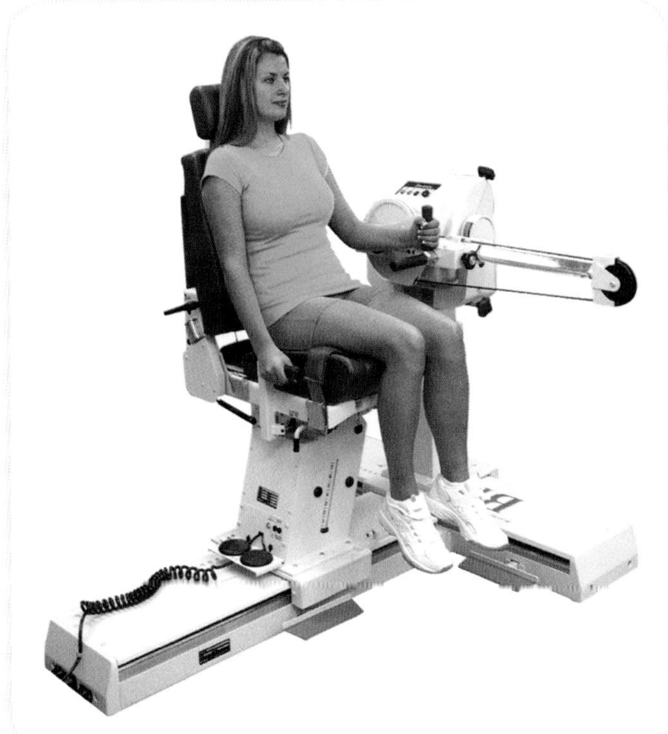

Figure 20-43 **Isokinetic upper-extremity closed-chain device**

One of the only isokinetic closed-kinetic-chain exercise devices currently available. (Photo courtesy Biodex Medical Systems, Inc.)

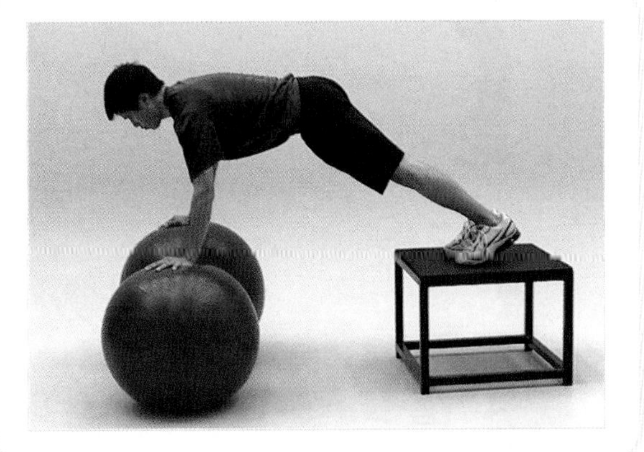

Figure 20-44 **Pushups on a stability ball**

An advanced closed chain strengthening exercise that requires substantial upper body strength.

Plyometric Exercises

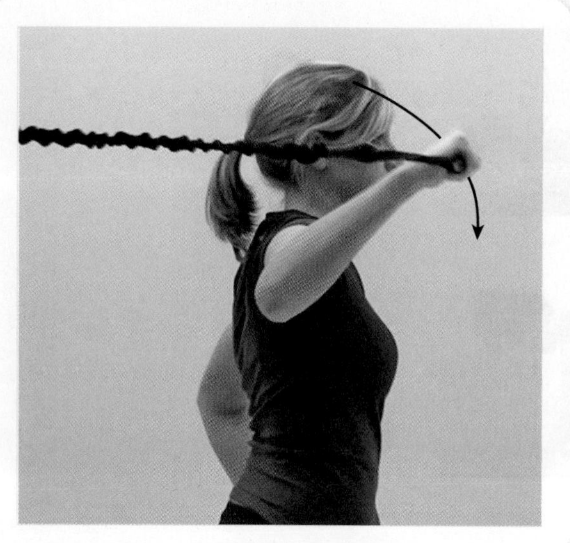

Figure 20-45 Cable or tubing

To strengthen the medial rotators, use a quick eccentric stretch of the medial rotators to facilitate a concentric contraction of those muscles.

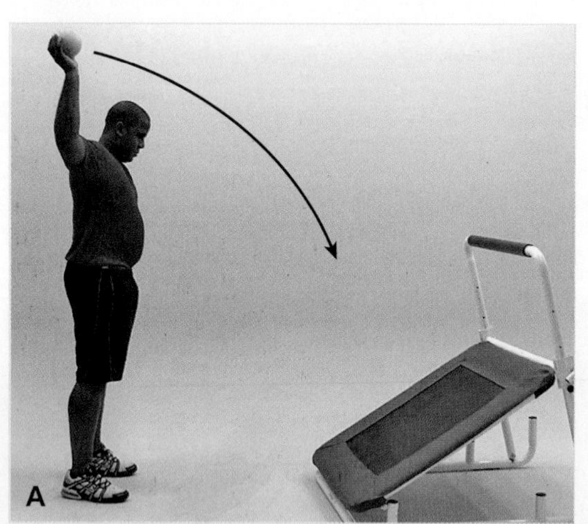

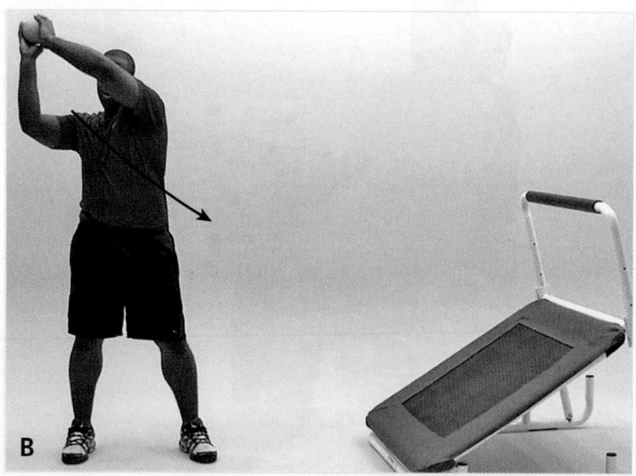

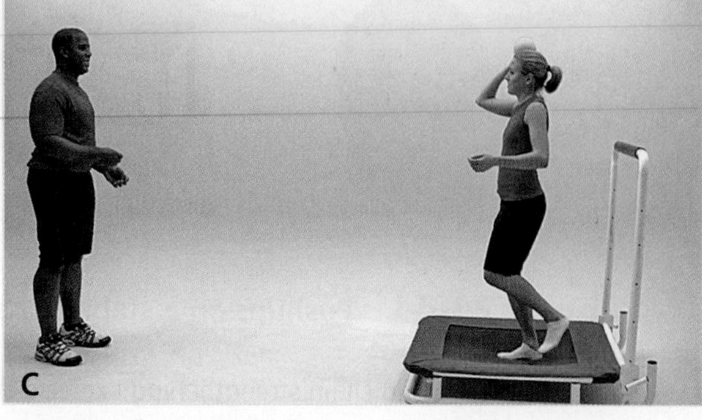

Figure 20-46 Plyoback

The patient should catch the ball, decelerate it, then immediately accelerate in the opposite direction. **A.** Single-arm toss. **B.** Two-arm toss with trunk rotation. **C.** Standing single-leg and single-arm toss on unstable surface.

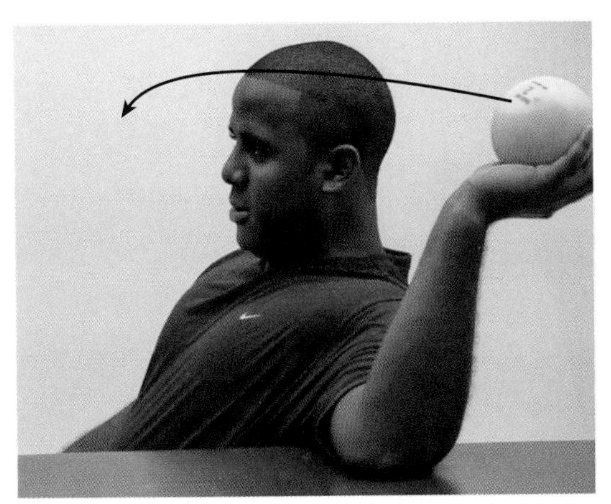

Figure 20-47 **Seated single-arm weighted-ball throw**

The patient should be seated with the arm abducted to 90 degrees and the elbow supported on a table. The therapist tosses the ball to the hand, creating an overload in lateral rotation that forces the patient to dynamically stabilize in that position.

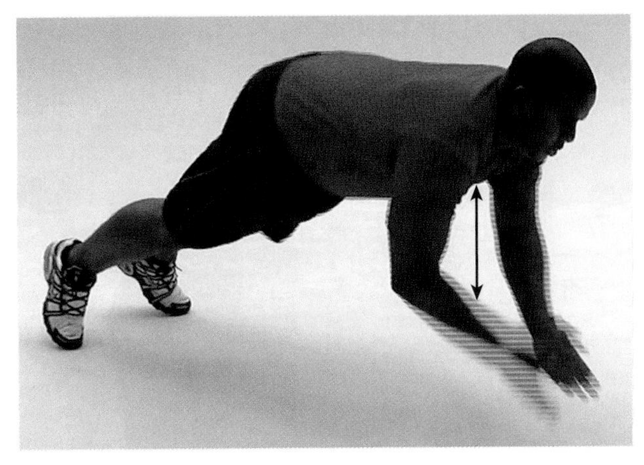

Figure 20-48 **Pushups with a clap**

The patient pushes off the ground, claps his hands, and catches his weight as he decelerates.

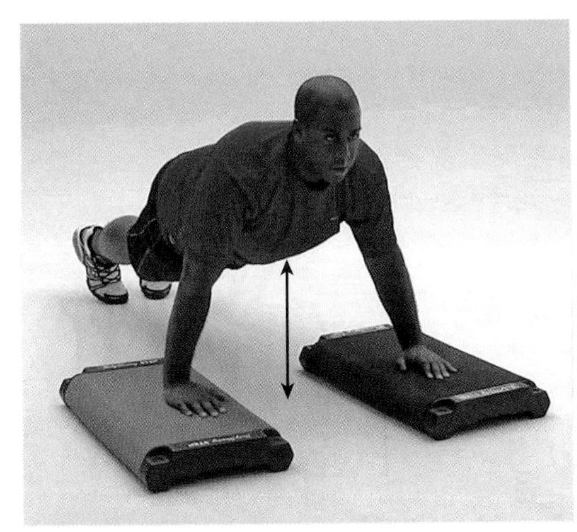

Figure 20-49 **Pushups on boxes**

When performing a plyometric pushup on boxes, the patient can stretch the anterior muscles, which facilitates a concentric contraction.

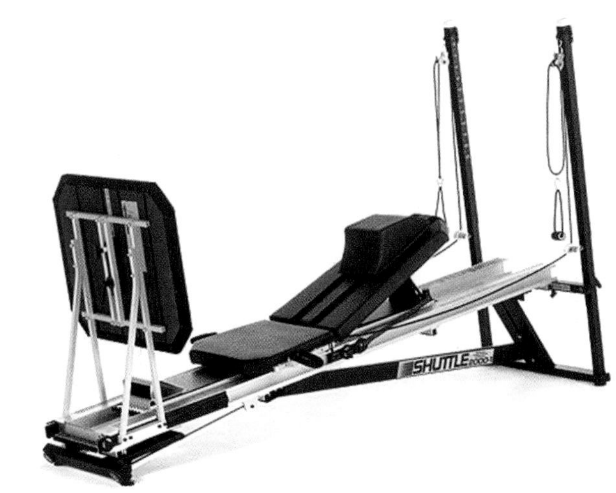

Figure 20-50 **Shuttle 2000-1**

The exercise machine can be used for plyometric exercises in either the upper or the lower extremity.

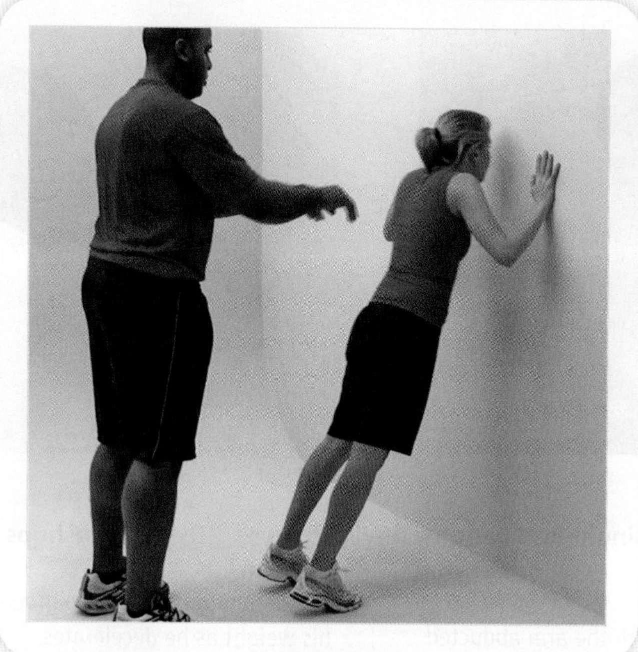

Figure 20-51 **Push into wall**

The therapist stands behind the patient and pushes her toward the wall. The patient decelerates the forces and then pushes off the wall immediately.

Isokinetic Exercises

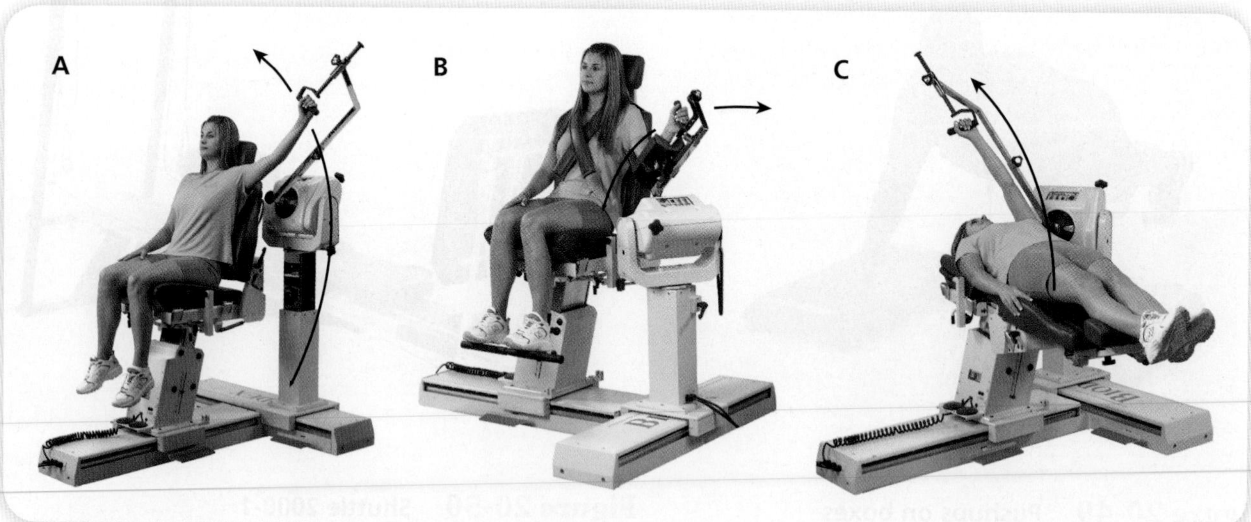

Figure 20-52

When using an isokinetic device for strengthening the shoulder, the patient should be set up such that strengthening can be done in a scapular plane. **A.** Shoulder abduction/adduction, (**B**) internal and external rotation, and (**C**) Diagonal 1 PNF pattern. (Courtesy Biodex Medical Systems.)

Proprioceptive Neuromuscular Facilitation Strengthening Techniques

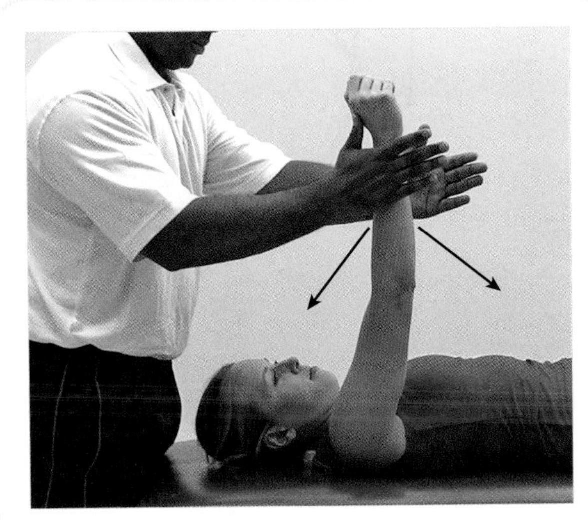

Figure 20-53 **Rhythmic contraction**

Using either a diagonal 1 (D1) or diagonal 2 (D2) pattern. The patient uses an isometric cocontraction to maintain a specific position within the ROM while the therapist repeatedly changes the direction of passive pressure.

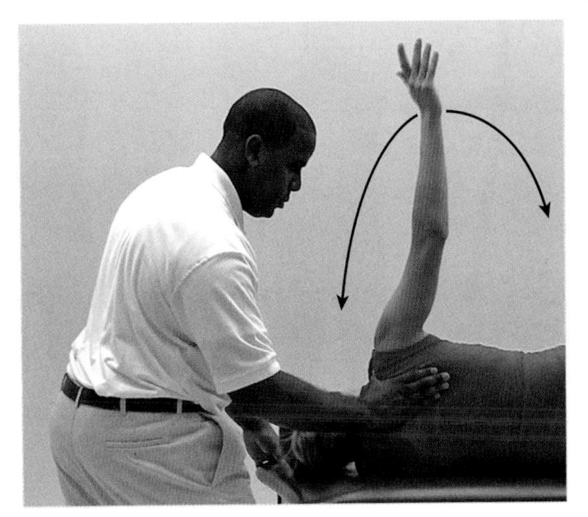

Figure 20-54 **PNF technique for scapula**

As the patient moves through either a D1 or a D2 pattern, the therapist applies resistance at the appropriate scapular border.

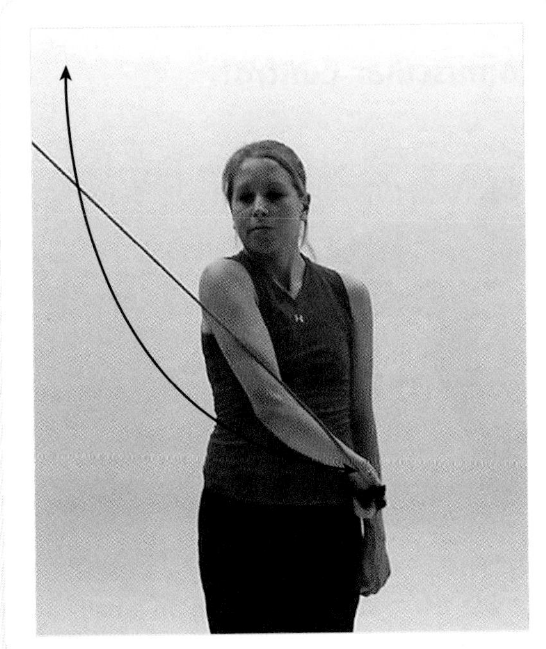

Figure 20-55

The patient can use resistance from tubing through a PNF movement pattern.

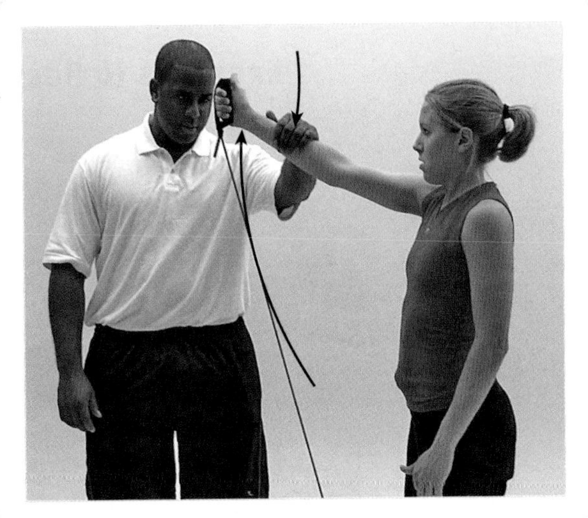

Figure 20-56 **PNF using both manual resistance and surgical tubing**

Rhythmic stabilization can be performed as the patient isometrically holds a specific position in the ROM with surgical tubing and force applied by the therapist.

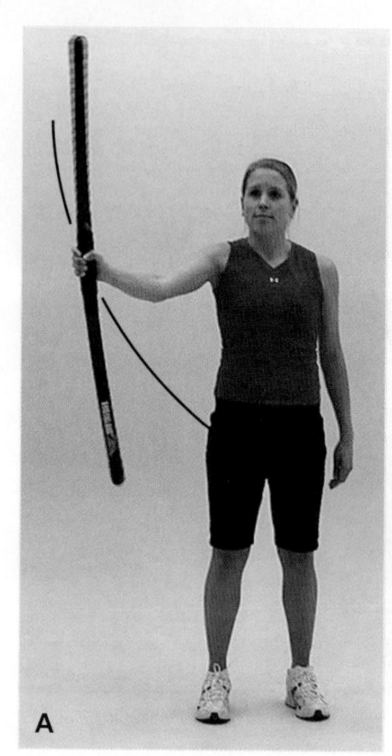

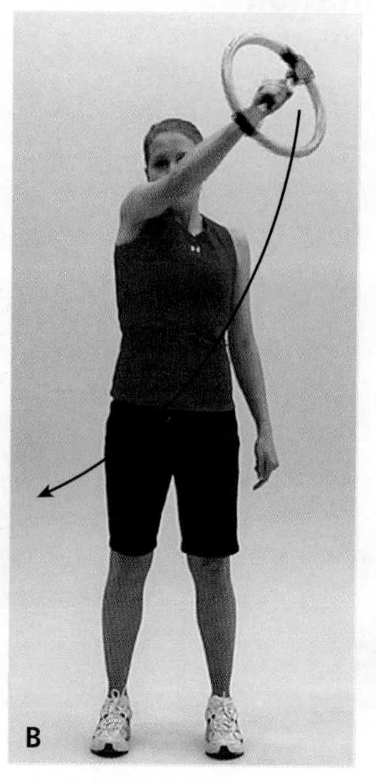

Figure 20-57

PNF using (**A**) Body Blade or (**B**) Centrifugal Ring Blade.

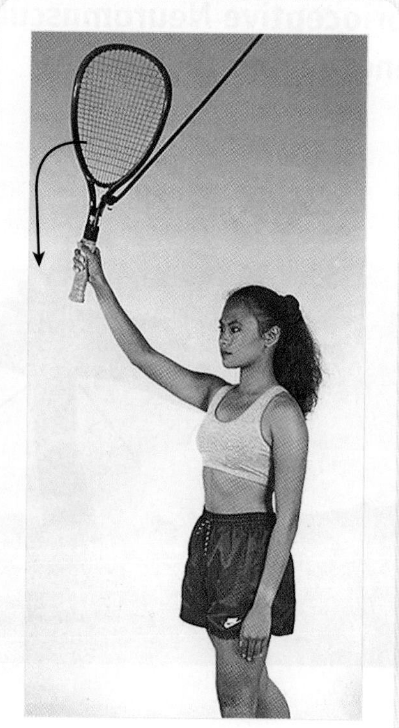

Figure 20-58

Surgical tubing may be attached to a tennis racket as the patient practices an overhead serve technique. This is useful as a functional progression technique.

Exercises to Reestablish Neuromuscular Control

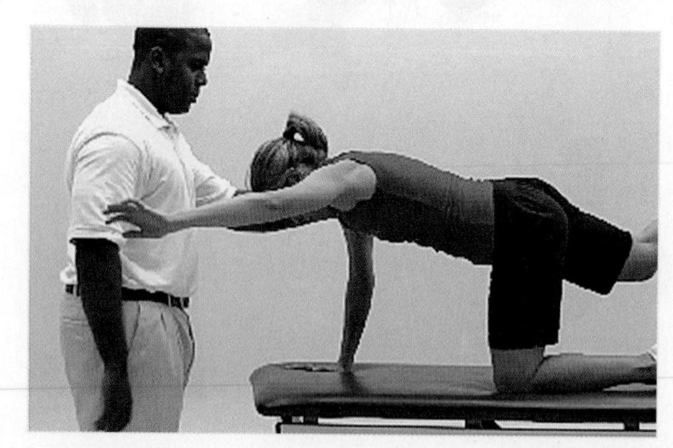

Figure 20-59

Weight shifting on a stable surface may be done kneeling in a 2-point position. The therapist can apply random directional pressure to which the patient must respond to maintain a static position. In the 2- and 3-point positions, the arm that is supported in a closed kinetic chain is using shoulder force couples to maintain neuromuscular control.

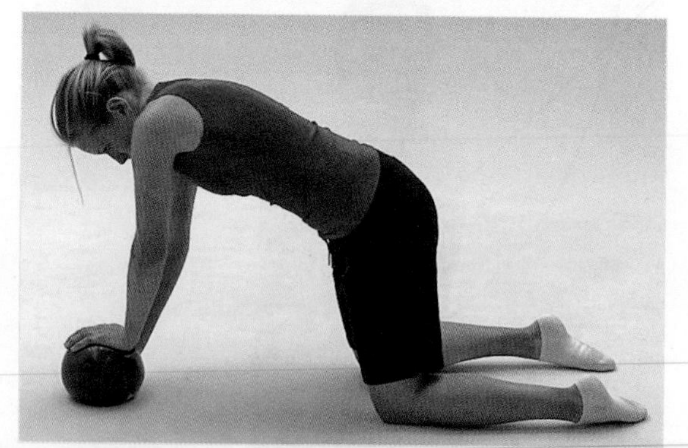

Figure 20-60 Weight shifting on a ball

In a pushup position with weight supported on a ball, the patient shifts weight from side to side and/or forward and backwards. Weight shifting on an unstable surface facilitates cocontraction of the muscles involved in the force couples that collectively maintain dynamic stability.

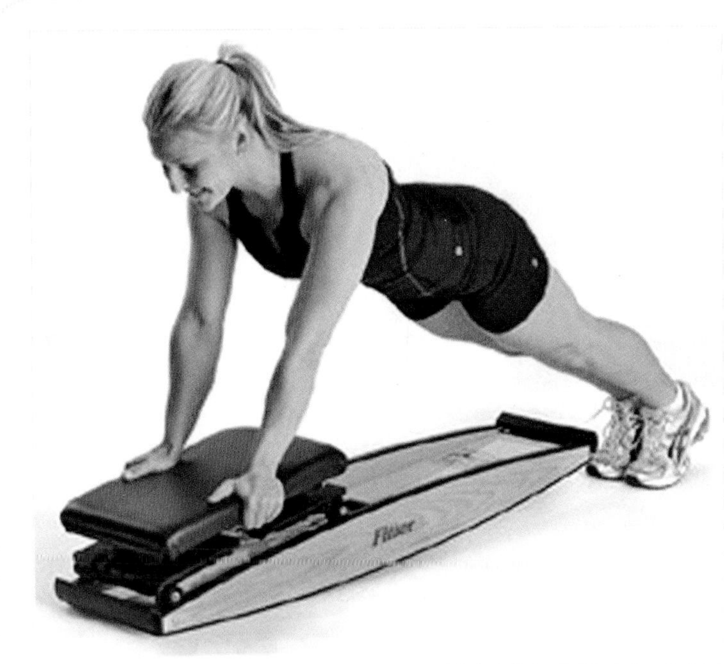

Figure 20-61 **Weight shifting on a Fitter**

In a kneeling position the patient shifts weight front to back using a Fitter. Weight shifting on an unstable surface facilitates cocontraction of the muscles involved in the force couples that collectively maintain dynamic stability. (Courtesy Fitter International, Inc.)

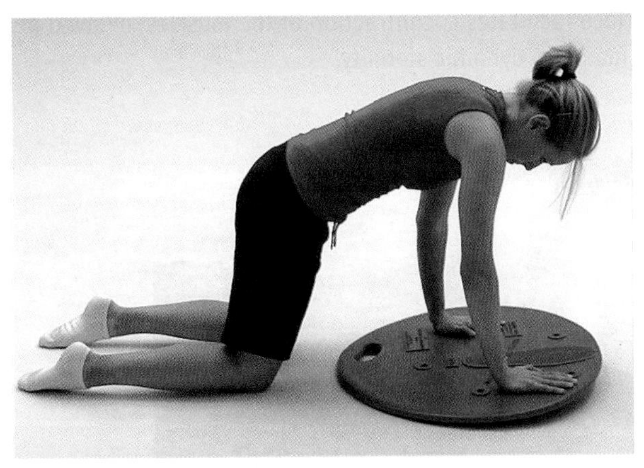

Figure 20-62 **Weight shifting on a biomechanical ankle platform system (BAPS) board**

In a kneeling position the patient shifts weight from side to side and/or backwards and forward using a BAPS board. Weight shifting on an unstable surface facilitates cocontraction of the muscles involved in the force couples that collectively maintain dynamic stability.

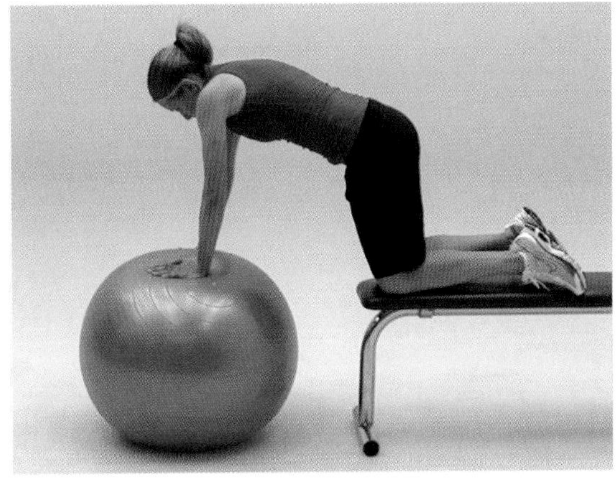

Figure 20-63 **Weight shifting on a stability ball**

With the feet supported on a bench, the patient shifts weight from side to side and/or backwards and forward using a stability ball. Weight shifting on an unstable surface facilitates cocontraction of the muscles involved in the force couples that collectively maintain dynamic stability.

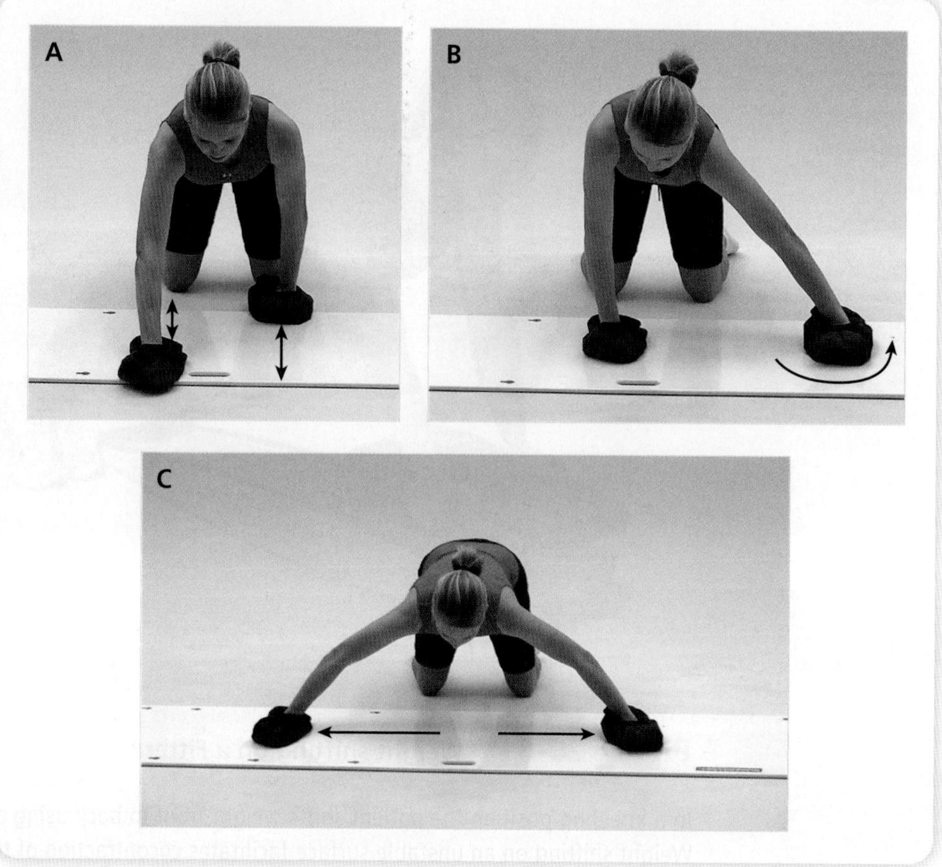

Figure 20-64 **Slide board exercises**

A. Forward and backwards motion. **B.** Wax-on/wax-off motion. **C.** Lateral motion. The patient shifts weight from side to side and/or backwards and forward using a slide board. Weight shifting on an unstable surface facilitates cocontraction of the muscles involved in the force couples that collectively maintain dynamic stability.

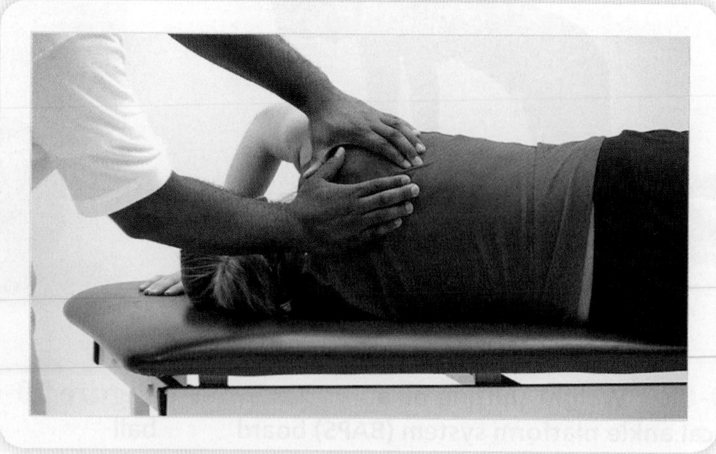

Figure 20-65 **Scapular neuromuscular control exercises**

The patient's hand is placed on the table, creating a closed kinetic chain, and the therapist applies pressure to the scapula in a random direction. The patient moves the scapula isotonically into the direction of resistance.

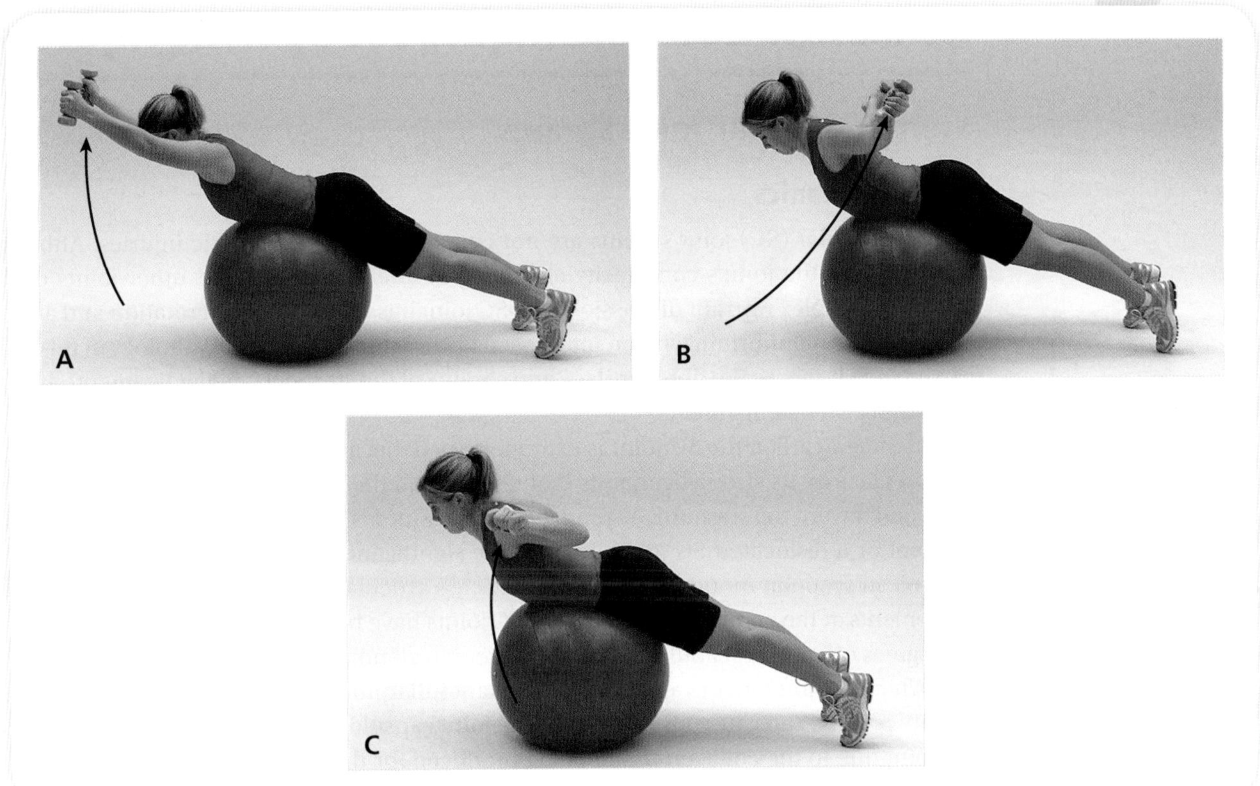

Figure 20-66 **Stability ball exercises**

The patient lies in a prone position on the stability ball and maintains a stable position and performs (**A**) Ys, (**B**) Ts, and (**C**) Ws.

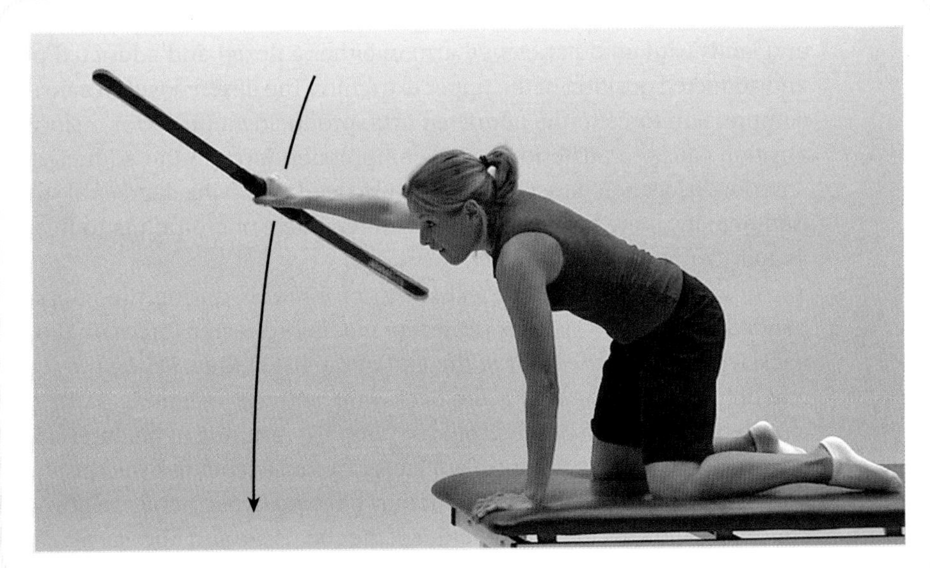

Figure 20-67 **Body Blade exercises**

The patient is in a 3-point kneeling position holding an oscillating Body Blade in 1 hand while working on neuromuscular control in the weightbearing shoulder.

Rehabilitation Techniques for Specific Injuries

Sternoclavicular Joint Sprains

Pathomechanics

Sternoclavicular (SC) joint sprains are not commonly seen as athletic injuries. Although they are rare, the joint's complexity and integral interaction with the other joints of the shoulder complex warrant discussion. The SC joint has multiple axis of rotation and articulates with the manubrium with an interposed fibrocartilaginous disc. Pathology of this joint can include injury to the fibrocartilage and sprains of the sternoclavicular ligaments and/or the costoclavicular ligaments.[49]

As stated earlier, the SC joint is extremely weak because of its bony arrangement. It is held in place by its strong ligaments that tend to pull the sternal end of the clavicle downward and toward the sternum. A sprain of these ligaments often results in either a subluxing SC joint or a dislocated SC joint. This can be significant because the joint plays an integral role in scapular motion through the clavicle's articulation with the scapula. Combined movements at the acromioclavicular and SC joints have been reported to account for up to 60 degrees of upward scapular rotation inherent in glenohumeral abduction.[3]

When this joint incurs an injury, a resultant inflammatory process occurs. The inflammatory process can cause an increase in the joint capsule pressure as well as a stiffening of the joint due to the collagen tissue being produced for the healing tissues. The pathogenesis of this inflammatory process can cause an altering of the joint mechanics as well as an increase in pain felt at the joint. This often results adversely on the shoulder complex.[106]

Injury Mechanism

After motor vehicle accidents, the most common source of injuries to the SC joint is sports participation.[89] The SC joint can be injured by direct or indirect forces, resulting in sprains, dislocations, or physical injuries.[49] Direct force injuries are usually the result of a blow to the anteromedial aspect of the clavicle and produce a posterior dislocation.[49] Indirect force injuries can occur in many different sporting events, usually when the patient falls and lands with an outstretched arm in either a flexed and adducted position or extended and adducted position of the upper extremity. The flexed position causes an anterior lateral compression force to the adducted arm, producing a posterior dislocation. The extended position causes a posterior lateral compression force to the adducted arm, leading to an anterior dislocation. Lesser forces can also lead to varying degrees of sprains to the SC joint. Additionally, there have been reports of repetitive microtrauma to this joint in sports such as golf, gymnastics, and rowing.[95,106]

In golf, an example of mechanism of injury is during the backswing.[74] For a right-handed golfer, the SC joint is subject to medially directed forces on the left at the top of the backswing and on the right at the end of the backswing. When the right arm is abducted and fully coiled at the end of the backswing and the beginning of the downswing, there is a posterior retraction of the shoulder complex, resulting in an anterior SC joint stress. As a result of the repetitive nature of golf, this can cause repetitive microtrauma leading to irritation of the joint. Over time the joint may become hypermobile relative to its normal stable condition, allowing for degeneration of the soft tissue and fibrocartilaginous disc. This often results in a painful syndrome affecting the mechanics of the joint and muscular control of the shoulder complex.[95] Similar examples are found in gymnastics and rowing.

Rehabilitation Concerns

In addressing the rehabilitation of a patient with a SC joint injury, it is important to address the function of the joint on shoulder complex movement. The SC joint acts as the sole passive attachment of the shoulder complex to the axial skeleton. As noted earlier in the chapter, the clavicle must elevate approximately 40 degrees to allow upward scapular rotation.[93]

In most cases the primary problem reported by the injured patient is discomfort associated with end-range movement of the shoulder complex. It is important to identify the cause of the pain (ie, ligamentous instability, disc degeneration, or ligamentous trauma).

In cases where there is ligamentous instability as well as disc degeneration, the rehabilitation should focus on strengthening the muscles attached to the clavicle in a range that does not put further stress on the joint. Muscles such as the pectoralis minor, sternal fibers of the pectoralis major, and upper trapezius are strengthened to help control the motion of the clavicle during motion of the shoulder complex. Exercises include incline bench, shoulder shrugs, and the seated press-up, in a limited ROM (see Figures 20-22, 20-35, and 20-42). In addition to addressing the dynamic supports of the SC joint, the therapist should employ the appropriate modalities necessary to control pain and the inflammatory process. It is also noteworthy, in cases where dislocation or subluxation has occurred, to consider the structures in close proximity to the SC joint. In the case of a posterior dislocation, signs of circulatory vessel compromise nerve tissue impingement, and difficulty swallowing may be seen. It is important to avoid these symptoms and communicate with the patient's physician regarding any lasting symptoms.[106]

When dealing with ligamentous trauma that lacks instability, the therapist should also address the associated pain with the appropriate modalities and utilize exercises that strengthen muscle with clavicular attachments. In all of the above scenarios, it is important to address the role of the SC joint on shoulder complex movement. A full evaluation of the shoulder complex should be performed to address issues related to scapular elevation. Exercises such as Superman, bent-over row, rhomboids, and pushups with a plus should be included to help control upward rotation of the scapula (see Figures 20-36 through 20-39). Appropriate progression should be followed while addressing the healing stages for the appropriate tissues.

Rehabilitation Progression

In the initial stages of rehabilitation, the primary goal is to minimize pain and inflammation associated with shoulder complex motion. The therapist should limit activities to midrange exercises and incorporate the use of therapeutic modalities along with the use of NSAID intervention from the physician. Ultrasound is often useful for increasing blood flow and facilitating the process of healing. Occasionally a shoulder sling or figure 8 strap can help minimize stress at the joint. During this phase of the rehabilitation progression, the therapist should identify the sport-specific needs of the patient so as to tailor the later phases of rehabilitation to the patient's demands. The patient should also continue to work on exercises that maintain cardiorespiratory fitness.

When the pain and inflammation have been controlled, the patient should gradually engage in a controlled increase of stress to the tissues of the joint. This is a good time to begin low-grade joint mobilizations resisted exercises for the muscles attaching to the clavicle. Exercises in this phase are best done in the midrange to minimize pain. As the patient's tolerance increases, the resistance and ROM can be increased. During this phase it is also important to address any limitations there might be in the patient's ROM. Emphasis should be placed on restoring the normal mechanics of the shoulder complex during shoulder movements.

As the patient begins to enter the pain-free stages of the progression, the therapist should gradually incorporate sport-specific demands into the exercise program. Examples of this are PNF with rubber tubing for the golfer (see Figures 20-55 and 20-56); Stair Climber with feet on chair for the gymnast (see Figure 20-44); and rowing machine for the rower.

Criteria for Returning to Full Activity

The patient may return to full activity when (a) the rehabilitation program has been progressed to the appropriate time and stress for the specific demands of the patient's sport; (b) the patient shows improved strength in the muscles used to protect the SC joint when compared to the uninjured side; and (c) the patient no longer has associated pain with movements of the shoulder complex that will inevitably occur with the demands of their sport.

Acromioclavicular Joint Sprains

Pathomechanics

The acromioclavicular (AC) joint is composed of a bony articulation between the clavicle and the scapula. The soft tissues included in the joint are the hyaline cartilage coating the ends of the bony articulations, a fibrocartilaginous disc between the 2 bones, the AC ligaments, and the costoclavicular ligaments. There have been 2 conflicting papers regarding the motion available at the joint. Codman reported little movement at the joint, whereas Inman reported exactly the opposite.[22,48] Multiple authors have reported degenerative changes at the AC joint by age 40 years in the average healthy adult.[29,102]

The AC joint provides the bridge between the clavicle and the scapula. When an injury occurs to the joint, all soft tissue should be considered in the rehabilitation process. An elaborate grading system has been reported to categorize injuries based on the soft tissue that is involved in the injury (Table 20-1).[99] Through evaluation by X-ray, the patient's injury should be categorized so as to provide the therapist with a guideline for rehabilitation.

Injury Mechanism

Type I or type II AC joint sprains are most commonly seen in athletics as a result of a direct fall on the point of the shoulder with the arm at the side in an adducted position or falling on an outstretched arm. The injury mechanism for type III and type IV sprains usually involves a direct impact that forces the acromion process downward, backward, and inward while the clavicle is pushed down against the rib cage. The impact can produce a number of injuries: (a) fracture of the clavicle; (b) AC joint sprain; (c) AC and coracoclavicular joint sprain; or (d) a combination of the previous injury with concomitant muscle tearing of the deltoid and trapezius at their clavicular attachments.[3] Another possible mechanism for injury to the AC joint is repetitive compression of the joint often seen in weight lifting.[106]

Rehabilitation Concerns

Management of AC injuries is dependent on the type of injury.[40] Age, level of play, and the demand on the patient can also factor into the management of this injury. Most physicians prefer to handle type I and type II injuries conservatively, but some authors suggest that type I and type II injuries can cause further problems to the patient later in life.[6,26] These injuries might require surgical excision of the distal 2 cm of the clavicle. The therapist should consider when developing a treatment plan (a) the stability of the AC joint; (b) the amount of time the patient was immobilized; (c) pain, as a guide for the type of exercises being used; and (d) the soft tissue that was involved in the injury. Rehabilitation of these injuries should focus on strengthening the deltoid and trapezius muscles. Additional strengthening of the clavicular fibers of the pectoralis major should also be done. Other muscles that help restore the proper mechanics to the shoulder complex should also be done.

Type I Treatment for the type I injury consists of ice to relieve pain and a sling to support the extremity for several days. The amount of time in the sling usually depends on the patient's ability to tolerate pain and begin carrying their involved extremity with the

Table 20-1 Acromioclavicular Sprain Classification

Type I
- Sprain of the AC ligaments
- AC ligament intact
- Coracoclavicular ligament, deltoid and trapezius muscles intact

Type II
- AC joint disrupted with tearing of the AC ligament
- Coracoclavicular ligament sprained
- Deltoid and trapezius muscles intact

Type III
- AC ligament disrupted
- AC joint displaced and the shoulder complex displaced inferiorly
- Coracoclavicular ligament disrupted with a coracoclavicular interspace 25% to 100% greater than the normal shoulder
- Deltoid and trapezius muscles usually detached from distal end of the clavicle

Type IV
- AC ligaments disrupted with the AC joint displaced and the clavicle anatomically displaced posteriorly through the trapezius muscle
- Coracoclavicular ligaments disrupted with wider interspace
- Deltoid and trapezius muscles detached

Type V
- AC and coracoclavicular ligaments disrupted
- AC joint dislocated and gross displacement between the clavicle and the scapula
- Deltoid and trapezius muscles detached from distal end of the clavicle

Type VI
- AC and coracoclavicular ligaments disrupted
- Distal clavicle inferior to the acromion or the coracoid process
- Deltoid and trapezius muscles detached from distal end of the clavicle

appropriate posture. The therapist can have the patient begin active assisted ROM immediately and then incorporate isometric exercises to the muscles with clavicular attachments. This will help restore the appropriate carrying posture for the involved upper extremity. When the patient is able to remove the sling, the therapist should increase the exercise program to incorporate PRE exercises for the muscles with clavicular attachments and add exercises to encourage appropriate scapular motion. This will help prevent related shoulder discomfort due to poor glenohumeral mechanics after return to activity.

Type II The treatment for type II injuries is also nonsurgical. Because this type of injury to the AC joint involves complete disruption of the AC ligaments, immobilization plays a greater role in the treatment of these patients. There is no consensus as to the duration of immobilization. Some authors recommend 7 to 14 days; others suggest using a sling that not only supports the upper extremity but depresses the clavicle.[1,106] This debate is fueled by disagreements regarding the time it takes the body to produce collagen and bridge the gap left from the injury. It has been reported that tissue mobilized too early shows a greater amount of type III collagen than the stronger type I collagen.[53] The time needed to heal the soft tissues involved in this injury must be considered prior to beginning exercises that stress the injury. Heavy lifting and contact sports should be avoided for 8 to 12 weeks.

Type III Many authors recommend a nonoperative approach for this type of injury, most agreeing that a sling is adequate for allowing the patient to rest comfortably.[3] Use of this nonoperative technique is reported to have limited success. Cox reported improved results without support of the arm in 62% of his patients, whereas only 25% had relief after 3 to 6 weeks of immobilization and a sling.[26]

Operative management of this type of injury can be summarized with the following options:

1. Stabilization of clavicle to coracoid with a screw.
2. Resection of distal clavicle.
3. Transarticular AC fixation with pins.
4. Use of coracoclavicular ligament as a substitute AC ligament.

Taft et al found superior results with coracoclavicular fixation. They found that patients with AC fixation had a higher rate of posttraumatic arthritis than those managed with a coracoclavicular screw.[112]

Type IV, V, and VI Types IV, V, and VI injuries require open reduction and internal fixation. Operative procedures are designed to attempt realignment of the clavicle to the scapula. The immobilization for this type of injury is longer and therefore the rehabilitation time is longer. After immobilization, the concerns are similar to those previously discussed.

Rehabilitation Progression

Early in the rehabilitation progression, the therapist should be concerned with application of cold therapy and pressure for the first 24 to 48 hours to control local hemorrhage. Fitting the patient for a sling is also important to control the patient's pain. Time in the sling depends on the severity of the injury. After the patient has been seen by a physician for differential diagnosis, the rehabilitation progression should be tailored to the type of sprain according to the diagnosis.

Types I, II, and III sprains should be handled similarly at first, with the time of progression accelerated with less-severe sprains. Exercises should begin with encouraging the patient to use the involved extremity for activities of daily living activities and gentle range-of-motion exercises. Return of normal ROM in the patient's shoulder is the first objective goal. The patient can also begin isometric exercises to maintain or restore muscle function in the shoulder. These exercises can be started while the patient is in the sling. Once the sling is removed, pendulum exercises can be started to encourage movement. In type III sprains, the therapist should hold off doing passive ROM exercises in the end ranges of shoulder elevation for the first 7 days. The patient should have full passive ROM by 2 to 3 weeks. Once the patient has full active ROM, a program of progressive resistive exercises should begin. Strengthening of the deltoid and upper trapezius muscles should be emphasized. The therapist should evaluate the patient's shoulder mechanics to identify problems with neuromuscular control and address specific deficiencies as noted. As the patient regains strength in the involved extremity, sport-specific exercises should be incorporated into the rehabilitation program. Gradual return to activity should be supervised by the patient's coach and therapist.

In the case of types IV, V, and VI AC sprains, a postsurgical progression should be followed. The therapist should design a program that is broken down into 4 phases of rehabilitation with the goal of returning the patient to the patient's activity as quickly as possible.[3] Contact with the physician is important to determine the time frame in which each phase may begin. Common surgeries for this injury include open reduction with pin or screw fixation and/or acromioplasty.

The early stage of rehabilitation should be designed with the goal of reestablishing pain-free ROM, preventing muscle atrophy, and decreasing pain and inflammation. Range-of-motion exercises may include Codman's exercises (see Figure 20-6), rope and pulley exercises (see Figure 20-9), L-bar exercises (see Figures 20-11 to 20-16), and self-capsular stretches (see Figures 20-17 and 20-19). Strengthening exercises in this phase may include isometrics in all of the cardinal planes and isometrics for medial and lateral rotation of the glenohumeral joint at 0 degrees of elevation (see Figure 20-20).

As rehabilitation progresses, the therapist has the goal of regaining and improving muscle strength, normalizing arthrokinematics, and improving neuromuscular control of the shoulder complex. Prior to advancing to this phase, the patient should have full ROM, minimal pain and tenderness, and a 4/5 manual muscle test for internal rotation, external rotation, and flexion. Initiation of isotonic PRE exercises should begin. Shoulder medial and lateral rotation (see Figures 20-31 and 20-32), shoulder flexion and abduction to 90 degrees (see Figures 20-26 and 20-28), scaption (see Figure 20-33), bicep curls, and triceps extensions should be included. Additionally, a program of scapular stabilizing exercises should begin. Exercises should include Superman exercises (see Figure 20-36), rhomboids exercises (see Figure 20-38), shoulder shrugs (see Figure 20-35), and seated pushups (see Figure 20-42). To help normalize arthrokinematics of the shoulder, complex joint mobilization techniques should be used for the glenohumeral, AC, SC, and scapulothoracic joints (see Figures 13-10 to 13-20). To complete this phase the patient should begin neuromuscular control exercises (see Figures 20-59 to 20-67), trunk exercises, and a low-impact aerobic exercise program.

During the advanced strengthening phase of rehabilitation, the goals should be to improve strength, power, and endurance of muscles as well as to improve neuromuscular control of the shoulder complex, and preparing the patient to return to sport-specific activities. Prior to advancing to this phase, the therapist should use the criteria of full pain-free ROM, no pain or tenderness, and strength of 70% compared to the uninvolved shoulder. The emphasis in this phase is on high-speed strengthening, eccentric exercises, and multiplanar motions. The patient should advance to surgical tubing exercises (see Figure 20-45), plyometric exercises (see Figures 20-46 to 20-51), PNF diagonal strengthening (see Figures 20-53 to 20-58), and isokinetic strengthening exercises (see Figure 20-52).

When the patient is ready to return to activity, the therapist should progressively increase activities that prepare the patient for a fully functional return. An interval program of sport-specific activities should be started. Exercises from stage III should be continued. The patient should progressively increase the time of participation in sport-specific activities as tolerated. For contact and collision sport patients, the AC joint should be protected.

Criteria for Returning to Full Activity

Prior to returning to full activity the patient should have full ROM and no pain or tenderness. Isokinetic strength testing should meet the demands of the patient's sport, and the patient should have successfully completed the final phase of the rehabilitation progression.

Clavicle Fractures

Pathomechanics

Clavicle fractures are one of the most common fractures in sports. The clavicle acts as a strut connecting the upper extremity to the trunk of the body.[31] Forces acting on the clavicle are most likely to cause a fracture of the bone medial to the attachment of the coracoclavicular ligaments.[4] Intact AC and coracoclavicular ligaments help keep fractures nondisplaced and stabilized.

Injury Mechanism

In athletics, the mechanism for injury often depends on the sport played. The mechanism can be direct or indirect. Fractures can result from a fall on an outstretched arm, a fall or blow to the point of the shoulder, or less commonly a direct blow as in stick sports like lacrosse and hockey.[95]

Rehabilitation Concerns

Early identification of the fracture is an important factor in rehabilitation. If stabilization occurs early, with minimal damage and irritation to the surrounding structures, the likelihood of an uncomplicated return to sports is increased. Other factors influencing the likelihood of complications are injuries to the AC, coracoclavicular, and SC ligaments. Treatment for clavicle fractures includes approximation of the fracture and immobilization for 6 to 8 weeks. Most commonly a figure-8 wrap is used, with the involved arm in a sling.

When designing a rehabilitation program for a patient who has sustained a clavicle fracture, the therapist should consider the function of the clavicle. The clavicle acts as a strut offering shoulder girdle stability and allowing the upper extremity to move more freely about the thorax by positioning the extremity away from the body axis.[42] Mobility of the clavicle is therefore very important to normal shoulder mechanics. Joint mobilization techniques are started immediately after the immobilization period in order to restore normal arthrokinematics. The clavicle also serves as an insertion point for the deltoid, upper trapezius, and pectoralis major muscles, providing stability and aiding in neuromuscular control of the shoulder complex. It is important to address these muscles with the appropriate exercises in order to restore normal shoulder mechanics.

Rehabilitation Progression

For the first 6 to 8 weeks, the patient is immobilized in the figure-8 brace and sling. If good approximation and healing of the fracture is occurring at 6 weeks, the patient may begin gentle isometric exercises for the upper extremity. Utilization of the involved extremity below 90 degrees of elevation should be encouraged to prevent muscle atrophy and excessive loss of glenohumeral ROM. After the immobilization period, the patient should begin a program to regain full active and passive ROM. Joint mobilization techniques are used to restore normal arthrokinematics (see Figures 13-10 to 13-12). The patient may continue to wear the sling for the next 3 to 4 weeks while regaining the ability to carry the arm in an appropriate posture without the figure-8 brace. The patient should begin a strengthening program utilizing progressive resistance as ROM improves. Once full ROM is achieved, the patient should begin resisted diagonal PNF exercises and continue to increase the strength of the shoulder complex muscle, including the periscapular muscles, to enable normal neuromuscular control of the shoulder.

Criteria for Return

The patient may return to activity when the fracture is clinically united, full active and passive ROM is achieved, and the patient has the strength and neuromuscular control to meet the demands of their sport.

Glenohumeral Dislocations/Instabilities (Surgical Versus Nonsurgical Rehabilitation)

Pathomechanics

Dislocations of the glenohumeral joint involve the temporary displacement of the humeral head from its normal position in the glenoid labral fossa. From a biomechanical perspective, the resultant force vector is directed outside the arc of contact in the glenoid fossa, creating a dislocating moment of the humeral head by pivoting about the labral rim.[32]

Shoulder dislocations account for up to 50% of all dislocations. The inherent instability of the shoulder joint necessary for the extreme mobility of this joint makes the glenohumeral joint susceptible to dislocation. The most common kind of dislocation is that occurring anteriorly. Posterior dislocations account for only 1% to 4.3% of all shoulder dislocations. Inferior dislocations are extremely rare. Of dislocations caused by direct trauma, 85% to 90% are recurring.[104]

In an anterior glenohumeral dislocation, the head of the humerus is forced out of its anterior capsule in an anterior direction past the glenoid labrum and then downward to rest under the coracoid process. The pathology that ensues is extensive, with torn capsular and ligamentous tissue, possibly tendinous avulsion of the rotator cuff muscles, and profuse hemorrhage. A tear or detachment of the glenoid labrum might also be present. Healing is usually slow, and the detached labrum and capsule can produce a permanent anterior defect on the glenoid labrum called a Bankart lesion. Another defect that can occur with anterior dislocation can be found on the posterior lateral aspect of the humeral head called a *Hill-Sachs lesion*. This is caused by compressive forces between the humeral head and the glenoid rim while the humeral head rests in the dislocated position. Additional complications can arise if the head of the humerus comes into contact with and injures the brachial nerves and vessels. Rotator cuff tears can also arise as a result of the dislocation. The bicipital tendon might also sublux from its canal as the result of a rupture of the transverse ligament.[104]

Posterior dislocations can also result in significant soft-tissue damage. Tears of the posterior glenoid labrum are common in posterior dislocation. A fracture of the lesser tubercle can occur if the subscapularis tendon avulses its attachment.

Glenohumeral dislocations are usually very disabling. The patient assumes an obvious disabled posture and the deformity itself is obvious. A positive sulcus sign is usually present at the time of the dislocation, and the deformity can be easily recognized on an X-ray. As detailed above, the damage can be extensive to the soft tissue.

Injury Mechanism

When discussing the mechanism of injury for dislocations of the glenohumeral joint, it is necessary to categorize the injury as traumatic or atraumatic, and anterior or posterior. An anterior dislocation of the glenohumeral joint can result from direct impact on the posterior or posterolateral aspect of the shoulder. The most common mechanism is forced abduction, external rotation, and extension that forces the humeral head out of the glenoid cavity.[73] An arm tackle in football or rugby or abnormal forces created in executing a throw can produce a sequence of events resulting in dislocation. The injury mechanism for a posterior glenohumeral dislocation is usually forced adduction and internal rotation of the shoulder or a fall on an extended and internally rotated arm.

The two mechanisms described for anterior dislocation can be categorized as traumatic or atraumatic. The following acronyms have been described to summarize the two mechanisms.[56]

Traumatic	**A**traumatic
Unidirectional	**M**ultidirectional
Bankart lesion	**B**ilateral involvement
Surgery required	**R**ehabilitation effective
	Inferior capsular shift recommended

The AMBRI group can be characterized by subluxation or dislocation episodes without trauma, resulting in a stretched capsuloligamentous complex that lacks end-range stabilizing ability. Several authors report a high rate of recurrence for dislocations, especially those in the TUBS category.[100]

Rehabilitation Concerns

Management of shoulder dislocation depends on a number of factors that need to be identified. Mechanism, chronology, and direction of instability all need to be considered in the development of a conservatively managed rehabilitation program. No single rehabilitation program is an absolute solution for success in the treatment of a shoulder dislocation. The therapist should thoroughly evaluate the injury and discuss those objective findings with the team physician. The initial concern in rehabilitation focuses on maintaining appropriate reduction of the glenohumeral joint. The patient is immobilized in a reduced position for a period of time, depending on the type of management used in the reduction (surgical versus nonsurgical). For the purpose of this section, the discussion will continue with conservative management in mind. The principles of rehabilitation, however, remain constant regardless of whether the physician's management is surgical or nonsurgical. Surgical rehabilitation should be based on the healing time of tissue affected by the surgery. The limitations of motion in the early stages of rehabilitation should also be based on surgical fixation. It is extremely important that the therapist and physician communicate prior to the start of rehabilitation. After the immobilization period, the rehabilitation program should be focused on restoring the appropriate axis of rotation for the glenohumeral joint, optimizing the stabilizing muscle's length-tension relationship, and restoring proper neuromuscular control to the shoulder complex. In the uninjured shoulder complex with intact capsuloligamentous structures, the glenohumeral joint maintains a tight axis of rotation within the glenoid fossa. This is accomplished dynamically with complex neuromuscular control of the periscapular muscles, rotator cuff muscles, and intact passive structures of the joint. Because the extent of damage in this type of injury is variable, the exercises employed to restore these normal mechanics should also vary.[99] As the therapist helps the patient regain full ROM, a safe zone of positioning should be followed. Starting in the plane of the scapula is safe because the axis of rotation for forces acting on the joint fall in the center of this plane. The least-provocative position is somewhere between 20 and 55 degrees of scapular plane abduction. Keeping the humerus below 55 degrees prevents subacromial impingement, while avoiding full adduction minimizes excessive tension across the supraspinatus/coracohumeral and/or capsuloligamentous complex. As ROM improves, the therapist should progress the exercise program into positions outside the safe zone, accommodating the demands that the patient will need to meet. Specific strengthening should be given to address the muscles of the shoulder complex responsible for maintaining the axis of rotation, such as the supraspinatus and rotator cuff muscles. The periscapular muscles should also be addressed in order to provide the rotator cuff muscles with their optimal length-tension relationship for more efficient usage. In the later stages of rehabilitation, neuromuscular control exercises are incorporated with sport-specific exercises to prepare the patient for return to activity.[56]

Rehabilitation Progression

The first step in a successful rehabilitation program is the removal of the patient from activities that may put the patient at risk for reinjury to the glenohumeral joint. A reasonable time frame for return to activity is approximately 12 weeks, with unrestricted activity coming closer to 20 weeks. This is variable, depending on the extent of soft-tissue damage and the type of intervention chosen by the patient and physician. Some exercises previously used by the patient might produce undesired forces on noncontractile tissues and need to be modified to be performed safely. Pushups, pull-downs, and the bench press are performed with the hands in close and avoiding the last 10 to 20 degrees of shoulder extension. Pull-downs

Table 20-2 Exercise Modification Per Direction of Instability

Direction of Instability	Position to Avoid	Exercises to Be Modified or Avoided
Anterior	Combined position of external rotation and abduction	Fly, pull-down, pushup, bench press, military press
Posterior	Combined position of internal rotation, horizontal adduction, and flexion	Fly, pushup bench press, weightbearing exercises
Inferior	Full elevation, dependent arm	Shrugs, elbow curls, military press

and military presses are performed with wide bars and machines are kept in front rather than behind the head. Supine fly exercises are limited to 30 degrees in the coronal plane while maintaining glenohumeral internal rotation. Table 20-2 provides further modifications dependent on directional instability.[3]

During phase 1 the patient is immobilized in a sling. This lasts for up to 3 weeks with first-time dislocations. The goal of this phase is to limit the inflammatory process, decrease pain, and retard muscle atrophy. Passive ROM exercises can be initiated along with low-grade joint mobilization techniques to encourage relaxation of the shoulder musculature. Isometric exercises are also started. The patient begins with submaximal contractions and increases to maximal contractions for as long as 8 seconds. The protective phase is a good time to initiate a scapulothoracic exercise program, avoiding elevated positions of the upper extremity that put stability at risk. Patients should begin an aerobic training regime with the lower extremity, such as stationary biking.

Phase 2 begins after the patient has been removed from the sling. This phase lasts from 3 to 8 weeks postinjury and focuses on full return of active ROM. The program begins with the use of an L-bar performing active assistive ROM (see Figures 20-11 to 20-16). Manual therapy techniques can also begin using PNF techniques to help reestablish neuromuscular control (see Figures 12-3 to 12-10). Exercises with the hands on the ground can help begin strengthening the scapular stabilizers more aggressively. These exercises should begin on a stable surface like a table, progressing the amount of weight bearing by advancing from the table to the ground (see Figure 20-59). Advancing to a less stable surface like a biomechanical ankle platform system (BAPS) board (see Figure 20-62) or stability ball (see Figure 20-63) will also help reestablish neuromuscular control.

At 6 to 12 weeks the therapist should gradually enter phase 3 of the rehabilitation progression. The goal of this phase is to restore normal strength and neuromuscular control. Prophylactic stretching is done, as full ROM should already be present. Scapular and rotator cuff exercises should focus on strength and endurance. Weightbearing exercises should be made more challenging by adding motion to the demands of the stabilization. Scapular exercises should be performed in the weight room with guidance from the therapist in order to meet the challenge of the patient's strength. Weight shifting on a Fitter (see Figure 20-61) and closed-kinetic-chain strengthening on a stair climber (see Figure 20-44) for endurance are started. Strengthening exercises progress from PRE to plyometric. Rotator cuff exercises using surgical tubing with emphasis on eccentrics are added.[2] Progression to multiangle exercises and sport-specific positioning is started. The Body Blade is a good rehabilitation tool for this phase (see Figure 20-67), progressing from static to dynamic stabilization and single-position to multiplanar dynamic exercises.

Phase 4 is the functional progression. Patients are gradually returned to their sport with interval training and progressive activity increasing the demands on endurance and stability. This can last as long as 20 weeks, depending on the patient's shoulder strength, lack of pain, and ability to protect the involved shoulder. The physician should be consulted prior to full return to activity.

Criteria for Return to Activity

At 20 to 26 weeks, the patient should be ready for return to activity. This decision should be based on (a) full pain-free ROM; (b) normal shoulder strength; (c) pain-free sport-specific activities; and (d) ability to protect the patient's shoulder from reinjury. Some therapist and physicians like the patient to use a protective shoulder harness during participation.

Multidirectional Instabilities of the Glenohumeral Joint

Pathomechanics

Multidirectional instabilities are an inherent risk of the glenohumeral joint. The shoulder has the greatest ROM of all the joints in the human body. The bony restraints are minimal, and the forces that can be generated in overhead motions of throwing and other athletic activities far exceed the strength of the static restraints of the joint. Attenuation of force is multifactorial, with time, distance, and speed determining forces applied to the joint. Thus, stability of the joint must be evaluated based on the patient's ability to dynamically control all of these factors in order to have a stable joint. In cases of multidirectional instability, there are 2 categories for pathology: atraumatic and traumatic. The atraumatic category includes patients who have congenitally loose joints or who have increased the demands on their shoulder prior to having developed the muscular maturity to meet these demands. When forces are generated at the glenohumeral joint that the stabilizing muscles are unable to handle (this occurs most commonly during the deceleration phase of throwing), the humeral head tends to translate anteriorly and inferiorly into the capsuloligamentous structures.[123] Over time, repetitive microtrauma causes these structures to stretch. Lephart et al described the essential importance of tension in the anterior capsule of the glenohumeral joint as a protective mechanism against excessive strain in these capsuloligamentous structures.[65] They theorized that the loss of this protective reflex joint stabilization can increase the potential for continuing shoulder injury. Proprioceptive deficits have been identified in individuals with multidirectional instability[4] and even generalized laxity.[10] Increased translation of the humeral head also increases the demand on the posterior structures of the glenohumeral joint, leading to repetitive microtrauma and breakdown of those soft tissues.[123] In this type of instability there will usually be some inferior laxity, leading to a positive sulcus sign. Although the anterior glenoid labrum is usually intact during the early stages of this instability, splitting and partial detachment can develop.[3] The patient usually has some pain and clicking when the arm is held by the side. Any symptoms and signs associated with anterior or posterior recurrent instability may be present.

Injury Mechanism

It is generally believed that the cause of multidirectional instability is excessive joint volume with laxity of the capsuloligamentous complex. In the patient, this laxity might be an inherent condition that becomes more pronounced with the superimposed trauma of sport. This type of instability might also occur as a result of extensive capsulolabral trauma in patients who do not appear to have laxity of other joints.[95]

Rehabilitation Concerns

The rehabilitation concerns for multidirectional instability are similar to those already discussed in relation to shoulder instabilities. The complexity of this program is increased because of the addition of inferior instability. The success of the program is often determined by the patient's tissue status and compliance.[109] Additionally, this program emphasizes the anterior and posterior musculature. These muscles working together are referred to as force couples and are believed to be essential stabilizers of the joint.[16] The rehabilitation program should also address the neuromuscular control of these muscles to promote dynamic stability.[43] Compliance is often an extremely important factor in maintaining good results with this type of instability. The patient must continue to do the exercise program even after symptoms have subsided. If the patient is not compliant, subluxation usually recurs. For cases where conservative treatment is not successful, Neer recommended an inferior capsular shift surgical procedure that has proven successful in restoring joint stability when used in conjunction with a rehabilitation program.[85]

Surgical management of multidirectional instability remains controversial.[36] Arthroscopic thermal capsulorrhaphy, when performed alone, has fallen out of favor as the surgery of choice as a result of high failure rates and complications.[25,45,96] The role that the rotator interval plays with regard to instability has come to the forefront. Although the integrity of the rotator interval and its relationship to shoulder stability is agreed upon,[18,25,96] the closure of the rotator interval in unstable shoulders remains an orthopedic dilemma. Although the dilemma is ongoing as to whether this closure is performed arthroscopically or via an open incision, or in combination with thermal techniques, there are several factors that can be agreed upon. The first is that the redundant capsule needs to be imbricated, the labrum, reverse Bankart, or reverse bony Bankart need to be repaired, and the rotator interval needs to be closed.[10,12] Wilk et al[131] suggest a postoperative rehabilitation program that is based on 6 factors: (a) type of instability; (b) patient's inflammatory response to surgery; (c) concomitant surgical procedures; (d) precautions following surgery; (e) gradual rate of progression; and (f) team approach to treatment. These factors determine the type and aggressiveness of the program. First, it must be determined whether the instability is congenital or acquired. Congenital instabilities should be treated more conservatively. Second, some patients respond to surgery with excessive scarring and proliferation of collagen ground tissue. Progression should be adjusted weekly based on assessing capsular end feel. The third factor takes into account any other procedures performed at the time of surgery. Precautions should be followed based on the tissue healing time of the other procedures. Surgical precautions also should be communicated to the therapist based on the tissues involved; passive range of motion (PROM) after surgery should be cautious. The authors suggest conservative PROM progression for the first 8 weeks postsurgery. The gradual progression (factor 5) contrasts to one that moves faster and then slows down. The speed of progression should be based on a weekly scheduled assessment of capsular end feel and progress. The sixth factor ensures a successful rehabilitation outcome by open and continuous communication between the patient, surgeon, and therapist.[131]

Rehabilitation Progression

The rehabilitation program should begin with reestablishing muscle tone and proper scapulothoracic posture. This helps provide a steady base with appropriate length-tension relationships for the anterior and posterior muscles of the shoulder complex acting as force couples. Strengthening of the rotator cuff muscles in the plane of the scapula should progress to higher resistance, starting at 0 degrees of shoulder elevation. As the patient becomes asymptomatic, the therapist should incorporate an emphasis on neuromuscular control exercises like PNF, rhythmic stabilization, and weightbearing activity to establish coactivation at the glenohumeral joint.[28] Sport-specific training can then be added, first in the rehabilitation setting and then in the competitive setting. For successful results, the patient might have to continue a program of maintenance for neuromuscular control for as long as they wish to be asymptomatic.

Shoulder Impingement

Pathomechanics

Shoulder impingement syndrome was first identified by Dr. Charles Neer,[85] who observed that impingement involves a mechanical compression of the supraspinatus tendon, the subacromial bursa, and the long head of the biceps tendon, all of which are located under the coracoacromial arch. This syndrome has been described as a continuum during which repetitive compression eventually leads to irritation and inflammation that progresses to fibrosis and eventually to rupture of the rotator cuff. Neer has identified 3 stages of shoulder impingement:

Stage I

- Seen in patients younger than 25 years of age with report of repetitive overhead activity
- Localized hemorrhage and edema with tenderness at supraspinatus insertion and anterior acromion
- Painful arc between 60 and 119 degrees; increased with resistance at 90 degrees
- Muscle tests revealing weakness secondary to pain
- Positive Neer or Hawkins-Kennedy impingement signs (Figures 20-68 and 20-69)
- Normal radiographs, typically
- Reversible; usually resolving with rest, activity modification, and rehabilitation program

Stage II

- Seen in patients 25 to 40 years of age with report of repetitive overhead activity
- Many of the same clinical findings as in stage I

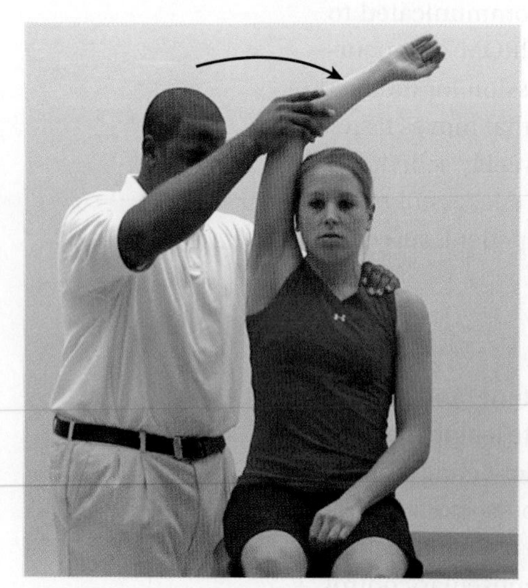

Figure 20-68 Neer impingement test

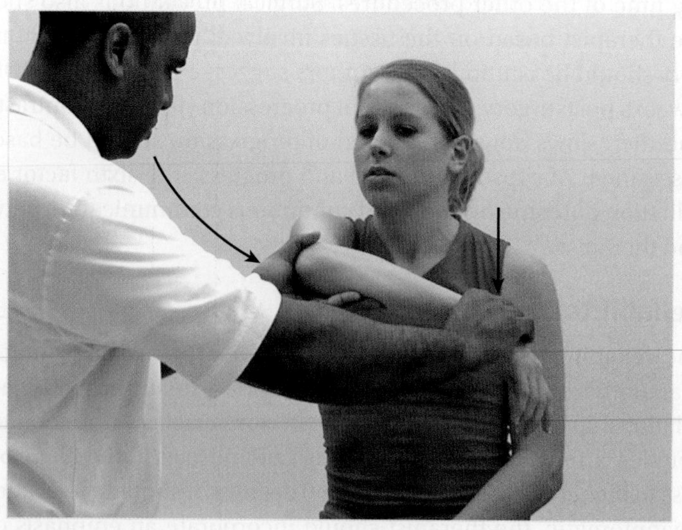

Figure 20-69 Hawkins-Kennedy impingement test

- Severity of symptoms worse than stage I, progressing to pain with activity and night pain
- More soft-tissue crepitus or catching at 100 degrees
- Restriction in passive ROM as a result of fibrosis
- Possibly radiographs showing osteophytes under acromion, degenerative AC joint changes
- No longer reversible with rest; possibly helped by a long-term rehabilitation program

Stage III

- Seen in patients older than 40 years of age with history of chronic tendinitis and prolonged pain
- Many of the same clinical findings as stage II
- Tear in rotator cuff usually less than 1 cm
- More limitation in active and passive ROM
- Possibly a prominent capsular laxity with multidirectional instability seen on radiograph
- Atrophy of infraspinatus and supraspinatus caused by disuse
- Treatment typically surgical following a failed conservative approach

Neer's impingement theory was based primarily on the treatment of older, nonathletic patients. The older population will likely exhibit what has been referred to as "outside" or "outlet" impingement.[8,85] In outside impingement there is contact of the rotator cuff with the coracoacromial ligament or the acromion with fraying, abrasion, inflammation, fibrosis, and degeneration of the superior surface of the cuff within the subacromial space. There might also be evidence of degenerative processes, including spurring, decreased joint space due to fibrotic changes, and decreased vascularity.

Internal or "nonoutlet" impingement is more likely to occur in the younger overhead patient. With internal impingement, the subacromial space appears relatively normal. With humeral elevation and internal rotation, the rotator cuff is compressed between the posterior superior glenoid labrum (or glenoid rim) and the humeral head. Although this compression is a normal biomechanical phenomenon, it can become pathologic in overhead patients because of the repetitive nature of overhead sports. The result is inflammation on the undersurface of the rotator cuff tendon, posterior superior tears in the glenoid labrum, and lesions in the posterior humeral head (Bankart lesion).

The mechanical impingement syndrome, as originally proposed by Neer, has been referred to as primary impingement. Jobe and Kvnite have proposed that an unstable shoulder permits excessive translation of the humeral head in an anterior and superior direction, resulting in what has been termed secondary impingement.[50] Based on the relationship of shoulder instability to shoulder impingement, Jobe and Kvnite have proposed an alternative system of classification:[50]

Group IA

- Found in recreational patients older than 35 years of age with pure mechanical impingement and no instability
- Positive impingement signs
- Lesions on the superior surface of the rotator cuff, possibly with subacromial spurring
- Possibly some arthritic changes in the glenohumeral joint

Group IB

- Found in recreational patients older than 35 years who demonstrate instability with impingement secondary to mechanical trauma
- Positive impingement signs
- Lesions found on the undersurface of the rotator cuff, superior glenoid, and humeral head

Group II

- Found in young overhead patients (younger than age 35 years) who demonstrate instability and impingement secondary to repetitive microtrauma
- Positive impingement signs with excessive anterior translation of humeral head
- Lesions on the posterior superior glenoid rim, posterior humeral head, or anterior inferior capsule
- Lesions on the undersurface of the rotator cuff

Group III

- Found in young overhead patients (younger than age 35 years)
- Positive impingement signs with atraumatic multidirectional, usually bilateral, humeral instabilities
- Demonstrated generalized laxity in all joints
- Humeral head lesions as in group II but less severe

Group IV

- Found in young overhead patients (younger than age 35 years) with anterior instability resulting from a traumatic event but without impingement
- Posterior defect in the humeral head
- Damage in the posterior glenoid labrum

It has also been proposed that wear of the rotator cuff is a result of intrinsic tendon pathology, including tendinopathy and partial or small complete tears with age-related thinning, degeneration, and weakening. This permits superior migration of the humeral head, leading to secondary impingement, thus creating a cycle that can ultimately lead to full-thickness tears.[120]

A "critical zone" of vascular insufficiency has been proposed to exist in the tendon of the supraspinatus, which is found at approximately 1 cm proximal to its distal insertion on the humerus. It has been hypothesized that when the humerus is adducted and internally rotated, a "wringing out" of the blood supply occurs in this tendon. Should this occur repetitively, such as in the recovery phase on a swimming stroke, ultimately irritation and inflammation may lead to partial or complete rotator cuff tears.[97]

It is likely that some as yet unidentified combination of mechanical, traumatic, degenerative, and vascular processes collectively lead to pathology in the rotator cuff.

Injury Mechanism

Shoulder impingement syndrome occurs when there is compromise of the subacromial space under the coracoacromial arch. When the dynamic and static stabilizers of the shoulder complex for one reason or another fail to maintain this subacromial space, the soft-tissue structures are compressed, leading to irritation and inflammation.[44] In athletes, impingement most often occurs in repetitive overhead activities such as throwing,

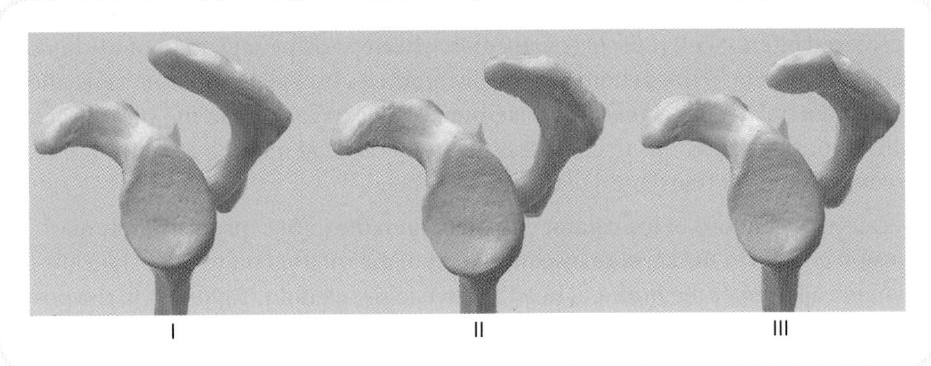

Figure 20-70 **Acromion shapes**

Type I, flat; type II, curved; and type III, hooked.

swimming, serving a tennis ball, spiking a volleyball, or during handstands in gymnastics. There is ongoing disagreement regarding the specific mechanisms that cause shoulder impingement syndrome. It has been proposed that mechanical impingement can result from either structural or functional causes. Structural causes can be attributed to existing congenital abnormalities or to degenerative changes under the coracoacromial arch and might include the following:

- An abnormally shaped acromion (Figure 20-70). Patients with a type III or hook-shaped acromion are approximately 70% more likely to exhibit signs of impingement than those with a flat or slightly curved acromion.[7]
- Inherent capsular laxity compromises the ability of the glenohumeral joint capsule to act as both a static and a dynamic stabilizer.[50]
- Ongoing or recurring tendinitis or subacromial bursitis causes a loss of space under the coracoacromial arch, which can potentially lead to irritation of other, uninflamed structures, setting up a vicious degenerative cycle.[106]
- Laxity in the anterior capsule due to recurrent subluxation or dislocation can allow an anterior migration of the humeral head, which can cause impingement under the coracoid process.[126]
- Postural malalignments, such as a forward head, round shoulders, and an increased kyphotic curve that cause the scapular glenoid to be positioned such that the space under the coracoacromial arch is decreased, can also contribute to impingement.

Functional causes include adaptive changes that occur with repetitive overhead activities, altering the normal biomechanical function of the shoulder complex. These include the following:

- Failure of the rotator cuff to dynamically stabilize the humeral head relative to the glenoid, producing excessive translation and instability. The inferior rotator cuff muscles (infraspinatus, teres minor, subscapularis) should act collectively to both depress and compress the humeral head. In the overhead or throwing patient, the internal rotators must be capable of producing humeral rotation on the order of 7000 degrees per second.[117] The subscapularis tends to be stronger than the infraspinatus and teres minor, creating a strength imbalance in the existing force couple in the transverse plane. This imbalance produces excessive anterior translation of the humeral head. Furthermore, weakness in the inferior rotator cuff muscles creates an imbalance in the existing force couple with the deltoid in the coronal plane.

Myers et al demonstrated that patients with subacromial impingement demonstrated decreased inferior cuff muscle coactivation while excessive activation of the middle deltoid is present.[82] The deltoid potentially produces excessive superior translation of the humeral head, decreasing subacromial space. Weakness in the supraspinatus, which normally functions to compress the humeral head into the glenoid, allows for excessive superior translation of the humeral head.[74]

- Because the tendons of the rotator cuff blend into the joint capsule, we rely on tension created in the capsule by contraction of the rotator cuff to both statically and dynamically center the humeral head relative to the glenoid. Tightness in the posterior and inferior portions of the glenohumeral joint capsule causes an anterosuperior migration of the humeral head, again decreasing the subacromial space. In the overhead patient, ROM in internal rotation is usually limited by tightness of both the muscles that externally rotate and the posterior capsule. There tends to be excessive external rotation, primarily due to laxity in the anterior joint capsule.[14]
- The scapular muscles function to dynamically position the glenoid relative to the humeral head, maintaining a normal length–tension relationship with the rotator cuff. As the humerus moves into elevation, the scapula should also move so that the glenoid is able to adjust regardless of the position of the elevating humerus. Weakness in the serratus anterior, which elevates, upward rotates, and abducts the scapula, or weakness in the levator scapula or upper trapezius, which elevate the scapula, will compromise positioning of the glenoid during humeral elevation, interfering with normal scapulohumeral rhythm.[23] Altered scapular movement patterns commonly identified in patients with subacromial impingement includes decreased upward rotation, external rotation, and posterior tipping, all of which have the potential to compromise subacromial space height, contributing to impingement.[23,35,69,71,122]
- It is critical for the scapula to maintain a stable base on which the highly mobile humerus can move. Weakness in the rhomboids and/or middle trapezius, which function eccentrically to decelerate the scapula in high-velocity throwing motions, can contribute to scapular hypermobility. Likewise, weakness in the inferior trapezius creates an imbalance in the force couple with the upper trapezius and levator scapula, contributing to scapular hypermobility.[23]
- An injury that affects normal arthrokinematic motion at either the SC joint or the AC joint can also contribute to shoulder impingement. Any limitation in posterior superior clavicular rotation and/or clavicular elevation will prevent normal upward rotation of the scapula during humeral elevation, compromising the subacromial space.

Rehabilitation Concerns

Management of shoulder impingement involves gradually restoring normal biomechanics to the shoulder joint in an effort to maintain space under the coracoacromial arch during overhead activities.[55,114] The therapist should address the pathomechanics and the adaptive changes that most often occur with overhead activities.

Overhead activities that involve humeral elevation (full abduction or forward flexion) or a position of humeral flexion, horizontal adduction, and internal rotation are likely to increase the pain.[68] The patient complains of diffuse pain around the acromion or glenohumeral joint. Palpation of the subacromial space increases the pain.

Exercises should concentrate on strengthening the dynamic stabilizers, the rotator cuff muscles that act to both compress and depress the humeral head relative to the glenoid (see Figures 20-31 and 20-32).[51,81,114] The inferior rotator cuff muscles in particular should be strengthened to recreate a balance in the force couple with the deltoid in the coronal plane. The supraspinatus should be strengthened to assist in compression of the humeral head into the glenoid (see Figures 20-33 and 20-34).[113] The external rotators, the infraspinatus and teres minor, are generally weaker concentrically but stronger eccentrically than the internal rotators and should be strengthened to recreate a balance in the force couple with the subscapularis in the transverse plane.

The external rotators and the posterior portion of the joint capsule are tight and tend to limit internal rotation and should be stretched (see Figures 20-15, 20-17, and 20-19). Both horizontal adduction and sleeper stretches have been demonstrated effective to stretch the posterior shoulder.[62,75] There is excessive external rotation because of laxity in the anterior portion of the joint capsule, and stretching should be avoided. There might be some tightness in both the inferior and the posterior portions of the joint capsule; this can be decreased by using posterior and inferior glenohumeral joint mobilizations (see Figures 13-13, 13-14, 13-16, and 13-17).

Strengthening of the muscles that abduct, elevate, and upwardly rotate the scapula (these include the serratus anterior, upper trapezius, and levator scapula) should also be incorporated (see Figures 20-35, 20-39, and 20-40). The middle trapezius and rhomboids should be strengthened eccentrically to help decelerate the scapula during throwing activities (see Figures 20-37 and 20-38). The inferior trapezius should also be strengthened to recreate a balance in the force couple with the upper trapezius, facilitating scapular upward rotation and stability (see Figure 20-36).

Anterior, posterior, inferior, and superior joint mobilizations at both the SC and the AC joint should be done to assure normal arthrokinematic motion at these joints (see Figures 13-10 to 13-12).

Strengthening of the lower-extremity and trunk muscles to provide core stability is essential for reducing the stresses and strains placed on the shoulder and arm, and this is also important for the overhead patient (see Figure 20-40).

Rehabilitation Progression

In the early stages of a rehabilitation program, the primary goal of the therapist is to minimize the pain associated with the impingement syndrome. This can be accomplished by utilizing some combination of activity modification, therapeutic modalities, and appropriate use of NSAIDs.

Initially, the therapist should have a coach evaluate the patient's technique in performing the overhead activity, to rule out faulty performance techniques. Once existing performance techniques have been corrected, the therapist must make some decision about limiting the activity that caused the problem in the first place. Activity limitation, however, does not mean immobilization. Instead, a baseline of tolerable activity should be established. The key is to initially control the frequency and the level of the load on the rotator cuff and then to gradually and systematically increase the level and the frequency of that activity. It might be necessary to initially restrict activity, avoiding any exercise that places the shoulder in the impingement position, to give the inflammation a chance to subside. During this period of restricted activity, the patient should continue to engage in exercises to maintain cardiorespiratory fitness. Working on an upper-extremity ergometer will help to improve both cardiorespiratory fitness and muscular endurance in the shoulder complex.

Therapeutic modalities such as electrical stimulating currents and/or heat and cold therapy may be used to modulate pain. Ultrasound and the diathermies are most useful for elevating tissue temperatures, increasing blood flow, and facilitating the process of healing. NSAIDs prescribed by the team physician are useful not only as analgesics, but also for their long-lasting antiinflammatory capabilities.

Once pain and inflammation have been controlled, exercises should concentrate on strengthening the dynamic stabilizers of the glenohumeral joint, stretching the inferior and posterior portions of the joint capsule and external rotators, strengthening the scapular muscles that collectively produce normal scapulohumeral rhythm, and maintaining normal arthrokinematic motions of the AC and SC joints.

REHABILITATION PLAN

ARTHROSCOPIC ANTERIOR CAPSULOLABRAL REPAIR OF THE SHOULDER COMPLEX

INJURY SITUATION A 27-year-old male baseball player returns to the throwing rotation of his baseball club after having elbow surgery 5 months earlier. Three weeks after returning, he starts complaining of posterior shoulder pain. After 3 months of using ice and nonsteroidal antiinflammatory drug (NSAID) therapy, he begins to have difficulty with his velocity and control of his pitches, and is now also having anterior shoulder pain near the bicipital groove. The patient is diagnosed by an orthopedist with posterior impingement secondary to multidirectional instability of the glenohumeral joint. An MRI revealed an additional lesion of the superior labral attachment, and some degenerative tearing of the rotator cuff.

SIGNS AND SYMPTOMS The patient complains of posterior cuff pain whenever he externally rotates. He has 165 degrees of external rotation and 35 degrees of internal rotation. Horizontal adduction of the humerus is only 15 degrees. Tenderness is present along the posterior glenohumeral joint line. He also has a positive O'Brien test for superior labral pathology (SLAP lesion), apprehension sign, and relocation test. The patient is evaluated for other factors that have stressed the throwing motion. Evaluation revealed an extremely tight hip flexibility pattern: bilateral hip flexion of 70 degrees, hip internal rotation of 15 degrees bilaterally, and hip external rotation of 50 degrees bilaterally.

MANAGEMENT PLAN The patient underwent arthroscopic anterior capsulolabral repair of the shoulder to address his instability and was rehabilitated with the goal of returning to play in 8 to 12 months.

PHASE ONE Protection Phase

GOALS: Allow soft-tissue healing, diminish pain and inflammation, initiate protected motion, retard muscle atrophy.

Estimated Length of Time (ELT): Day 1 to Week 6

For the first 2 to 3 weeks the patient uses a sling, full time for 7 to 10 days, sleeping with it for the full 2 weeks, and then gradual weaning of the sling. Exercises include hand and wrist range of motion and active cervical spine range of motion. During this phase, cryotherapy is used before and after treatments. Passive and active assisted range of motion for the glenohumeral joint is cautiously performed in a restricted range of motion. Shoulder rotation is done in 20 degrees of abduction; external rotation (ER) is to 30 degrees and internal rotation (IR) is allowed to 25 or 30 degrees for the first 3 weeks, advancing to 50 degrees by week 6. Passive forward elevation (PFE) is progressed to 90 degrees for the first 3 weeks, advancing to 135 degrees by 6 weeks. Active assisted forward elevation (AFE) can be progressed between weeks 3 and 6 to 115 degrees. Moist heat can be used prior to therapy after 10 days. Passive range of motion (ROM) is performed by the therapist and active-assisted ROM by the patient.

During this phase, ROM is progressed based on the end feel the therapist gets when evaluating the patient. With a hard end feel, the therapist may choose to be more aggressive, making sure not to surpass the ROM guidelines. A soft end feel dictates a slower progression. Range of motion is not the main focus of this phase; healing of the repaired tissue is the prime goal. The minimally invasive nature of arthroscopy leads to less pain and inflammation. Therefore, it is important to stress to the patient the importance of protection. Educating the patient to minimize load to less than 5 pounds and limiting repetitive activities is very important. ROM of the patient's hips is also addressed during this phase. Aggressive stretching and core stability exercises may be started to maintain an increased state of flexibility of the pitcher's total rotational capabilities.

Shoulder strengthening begins early in this phase with rhythmic stabilization, scapular stabilizing exercises, isometric exercises for the rotator cuff muscles, and proprioceptive neuromuscular facilitation (PNF) control exercises in a restricted range of motion. Although scapular stabilizing exercises are begun, protraction should not begin until the end of this phase. Protraction has been shown to stress the anterior and inferior portions of the joint capsule. Scapula elevation and retraction are allowed.[125] By the end of this phase, the patient should have met all ROM goals set and they should be pain free within these guidelines. Advancement to the second phase should not occur unless these goals are met.

PHASE TWO Intermediate Phase

GOALS: Restore full ROM, restore functional ROM, normalize arthrokinematics, improve dynamic stability, improve muscular strength.

Estimated Length of Time (ELT): Weeks 7 to 12

During this phase the patient's ROM will ultimately be progressed to fully functional by 12 weeks: at week 9, PFE to

155 degrees, 75 degrees of ER at 90 degrees of abduction, 50 to 65 degrees of ER at 20 degrees of abduction, and 60 to 65 degrees of IR. Active forward elevation should progress to 145 degrees. Aggressive stretching may be used during this phase if the goal is not met by 9 weeks. This may include joint mobilization and capsular stretching techniques. From week 9 to week 12, the therapist begins to gradually progress ROM exercises to a position functional for this pitcher.

In this phase, strengthening exercises include progressive resistive exercise (PRE) in all planes of shoulder motion and IR- and ER-resisted exercises. Exercises begin in the scapular plane and work their way to more functional planes. Incremental stresses are added to the anterior capsule working toward the 90/90 position. Resistance progresses from isotonic to gentle plyometrics. Gentle plyometrics are defined as two-handed, low-load activity like the pushup. Rhythmic stabilization drills continue to be progressed with increasing difficulty. Aggressive strengthening may be initiated if ROM goals are achieved. Strengthening should emphasize high repetitions (30 to 50 reps) and low resistance (1 to 3 pounds). Weight room activities, including pushups, dumbbell press (without allowing the arm to drop below the body), and latissimus pull-downs in front of body, bicep, and triceps exercises with arm at the side may begin. Exercises should be performed asymptomatically. If symptoms of pain or instability occur, a thorough evaluation of the patient should be performed and the program adjusted accordingly.

PHASE THREE Advanced Activity and Strengthening

GOALS: Improve strength, power, and endurance; enhance neuromuscular control; functional activities.

Estimated Length of Time (ELT): Weeks 12 to 24

The criteria for progression to this phase should be: Active range of motion (AROM) goals met without pain or substitution patterns, and appropriate scapular posture and dynamic control present during exercises. The patient should maintain established ROM and should continue stretching exercises. Throwing-specific exercises are initiated, including throwing a ball into the Plyoback.

During this phase, additional lifting exercises are added to begin building power and strength. Full dumbbell incline and bench press are added. Shoulder raises to 90 degrees in the sagittal and frontal planes, overhead dumbbell press, pectoralis major flys, and dead lifts can be worked in. Lifting exercises that put the bar behind the head and dips should still be avoided.

At week 16, the therapist will initiate a formal interval-throwing program. Each step is performed at least 2 times on separate days prior to advancing. Throwing should be performed without pain or any increasing symptoms. If symptoms appear, the patient will be regressed to the previous step and remain there until symptom-free.

PHASE FOUR Return to Full Activity

GOALS: Complete elimination of pain and full return to activity.

Estimated Length of Time (ELT): Weeks 24 to 36

Usually by week 24 the patient will begin throwing off the pitcher's mound. In this phase, the number of throws, intensity, and type of pitch are progressed gradually to increase the stress at the glenohumeral joint. By 6 to 7 months the patient will progress to game-type situations and return to competition. The patient will begin by limiting his pitch count and progressing if he can maintain his pain- and symptom-free status. Full return may take as long as 9 to 12 months.

Criteria for Returning to Competitive Pitching

1. Full functional ROM
2. No pain or tenderness
3. Satisfactory muscular strength
4. Satisfactory clinical exam

DISCUSSION QUESTIONS

1. What other factors may affect the pitcher's ability to generate velocity of the baseball when he throws the ball?
2. Can the therapist truly simulate the demands of pitching during the rehabilitation process?
3. Should the patient be allowed to take NSAIDs during the rehabilitation progression?
4. What muscles generate the greatest amounts of torque during the patient's throwing motion?
5. What other areas of the thrower's body should be targeted for strengthening, to ensure that he will recover his delivery speed and power?

Strengthening exercises are done to establish neuromuscular control of the humerus and the scapula (see Figures 20-59 through 20-67). Strengthening exercises should progress from isometric pain-free contractions to isotonic full-range pain-free contractions. Humeral control exercises should be used to strengthen the rotator cuff to restrict migration of the humeral head and to regain voluntary control of the humeral head positioning through rotator cuff stabilization.[127] Scapular control exercises should be used to maintain a normal relationship between the glenohumeral and scapulothoracic joints.[58,59,68]

Closed-kinetic-chain exercises for the shoulder should be primarily eccentric. They tend to compress the joint, providing stability, and are perhaps best used for establishing scapular stability and control.

Gradually, the duration and intensity of the exercise may be progressed within individual patient tolerance limitations, using increased pain or stiffness as a guide for progression, eventually progressing to full-range overhead activities.

Criteria for Returning to Full Activity

The patient may return to full activity when (a) the gradual program used to increase the duration and intensity of the workout has allowed the patient to complete a normal workout without pain; (b) the patient exhibits improved strength in the appropriate rotator cuff and the scapular muscles; (c) there is no longer a positive impingement sign, drop arm test, or empty can test; and (d) the patient can discontinue use of antiinflammatory medications without a return of pain. After return to play, or even as a prophylactic measure prior to injury athletes (especially those who participate in overhead sports) benefit from participation in an injury prevention program. Although the literature is currently void of scientifically validated injury prevention programs for the overhead patient, the literature and clinical experience do support the inclusion of overhead athletic specific resistance tubing exercises,[84,110,111] shoulder flexibility,[62,75] and upper quarter posture exercises[60] for purposes of injury prevention.

Rotator Cuff Tendinitis and Tears

Pathomechanics

Rotator cuff injury has often been described as a continuum starting with impingement of the tendon that, through repetitive compression, eventually leads to irritation and inflammation and eventually fibrosis of the rotator cuff tendon. This idea began with the work of Codman in 1934, when he identified a critical zone near the insertion of the supraspinatus tendon.[78] Since then many researchers in sports medicine have studied this area and expanded the information base, leading to the identification of other causative factors.[51,91] Neer is also credited with developing a system of classification for rotator cuff disease. This system seemed to be appropriate until sports medicine professionals began dealing with overhead patients as a separate entity due to the acceleration of repetitive stresses applied to the shoulder. Disease in the overhead patient usually results from failure from one or both of these chronic stresses: repetitive tension or compression of the tissue. We now regard rotator cuff injury in athletics as an accumulation of microtrauma to both the static and the dynamic stabilizers of the shoulder complex. Meister and Andrews classified these causative traumas based on the pathophysiology of events leading to rotator cuff failure. Their 5 categories of classification for modes of failure are primary compressive, secondary compressive, primary tensile overload, secondary tensile overload, and macrotraumatic.[78]

Injury Mechanism

Rotator cuff tendinopathy is a gradation of tendon failure, so it is important to identify the causative factors. The following classification system helps group injury mechanisms to better aid the therapist in developing a rehabilitation plan.

Primary compressive disease results from direct compression of the cuff tissue. This occurs when something interferes with the gliding of the cuff tendon in the already tight subacromial space. A predisposing factor in this category is a type III hooked acromion process, a common factor seen in younger patients with rotator cuff disease. Other factors in younger patients include a congenitally thick coracoacromial ligament and the presence of an os acromiale. In younger patients, a primary impingement without one of these associated factors is rare. In middle-aged athletes/patients, degenerative spurring on the undersurface of the acromion process can cause irritation of the tendon and eventually lead to complete tearing of the tendon. These individuals are often seen because they experience pain during such activities as tennis and golf.

Secondary compressive disease is a primary result of glenohumeral instability. The high forces generated by the overhead patient can cause chronic repetitive trauma to the glenoid labrum and capsuloligamentous structures, leading to subtle instability. Patients with inherent multidirectional instability, such as swimmers, are also at risk. The additional volume created in the glenohumeral capsule allows for extraneous movement of the humeral head, leading to compressive forces in the subacromial space.

Primary tensile overload can also cause tendon irritation and failure. The rotator cuff resists horizontal adduction, internal rotation, and anterior translation of the humeral head, as well as the distraction forces found in the deceleration phase of throwing and overhead sports. The repetitive high forces generated by eccentric activity in the rotator cuff while attempting to maintain a central axis of rotation can cause microtrauma to the tendon and eventually lead to tendon failure. This type of mechanism is not associated with previous instability of the joint. Causes for this mechanism often are found when evaluating the patient's mechanics and taking a complete history during the evaluation. The therapist might find that the throwing patient had a history of injury to another area of the body where the muscles are used in the deceleration phase of overhead motion (eg, the right-handed pitcher who sprained his left ankle).

Secondary tensile disease is often a result of primary tensile overload. In this case, the repetitive irritation and weakening of the rotator cuff allows for subtle instability. In contrast to secondary compressive disease of the tendon, the rotator cuff tendon experiences greater distractive and tensile forces because the humeral head is allowed to translate anteriorly. Over time, the increased tensile force causes failure of the tendon.

Macrotraumatic failure occurs as a direct result of one distinct traumatic event. The mechanism for this is often a fall on an outstretched arm. This is rarely seen in patients with normal, healthy rotator cuff tendons. For this to occur, forces generated by the fall must be greater than the tensile strength of the tendon. Because the tensile strength of bone is less than that of young healthy tendon, it is rare to see this in a patient. It is more common to see a longitudinal tear in the tendon with an avulsion of the greater tubercle.

Rehabilitation Concerns

When designing a rehabilitation program for rotator cuff tendinopathy, the basic concerns remain the same regardless of the extent to which the tendon is damaged. Instead, rehabilitation should be based on why and how the tendon has been damaged. Once the cause of the tendinopathy is identified and secondary factors are known, a comprehensive program can be designed. If a comprehensive rehabilitation program does not relieve the painful shoulder, surgical repair of the tendon and alteration of the glenohumeral joint are performed. Surgical rehabilitation is similar to the nonsurgical plan, with the time of progression altered based on tissue healing and tendon histology.

Conservative Management Stage I of the rehabilitation process is focused on reducing inflammation and removing the patient from the activity that caused pain. Pain should not be a part of the rehabilitation process. The therapist may employ therapeutic modalities to aid in patient comfort. A course of NSAIDs is usually followed during this stage of rehabilitation. ROM exercises begin, avoiding further irritation of the tendon. Attention is paid to restoring appropriate arthrokinematics to the shoulder complex. If the injury is a result of a compressive disease to the tendon, capsular stretching may be done (see Figures 20-17 and 20-19). Active strengthening of the glenohumeral joint should begin, concentrating on the force couples acting around the joint. Beginning with isometric exercises for the medial and lateral rotators of the joint (see Figure 20-20), and progressing to isotonic exercises if the patient does not experience pain (see Figures 20-31 and 20-32). A towel roll under the patient's arm can help initiate coactivation of the shoulder muscles, increasing joint stability. Exercises might need to be altered to limit translational forces of the humeral head. Strengthening of the supraspinatus may begin if 90 degrees of elevation in the scapular plane is available (see Figures 20-33 and 20-34). Aggressive pain-free strengthening of the periscapular muscles should also start, as the restoration of normal scapular control will be essential to removal of abnormal stresses of the rotator cuff tendon in later stages. The therapist might want to begin with manual resistance, progressing to free-weight exercises (see Figures 20-35 to 20-39).

In stage II, the healing process progresses and ROM will need to be restored. The therapist might need to be more aggressive in stretching techniques, addressing capsular tightness as it develops. The prone-on-elbows position is a good technique for self-mobilization. This position should be avoided if compressive disease was part of the irritation. If pain continues to be absent, strengthening gets increasingly aggressive. Isokinetic exercises at speeds greater than 200 degrees per second for shoulder medial and lateral rotation may begin (see Figure 20-52).[41]

Aggressive neuromuscular control exercises are started in this stage: quick reversals during PNF diagonal patterns, starting with manual resistance from the therapist and advancing to resistance applied by surgical tubing (see Figures 20-55 and 20-56). A Body Blade may also be used for rhythmic stabilization (see Figure 20-57). The exercise program should now progress to free weights, and eccentric exercises of the rotator cuff should be emphasized to meet the demands of the shoulder in overhead activities. Strengthening of the deltoid and upper trapezius muscles can begin above 90 degrees of elevation. Exercises include the military press (see Figure 20-24), shoulder flexion (see Figure 20-26), and reverse flys (see Figure 20-30). Pushups can also be added. It might be necessary to restrict ROM so the body does not go below the elbow, to prevent excessive translation of the glenohumeral joint. Combining this exercise with serratus anterior strengthening in a modified pushup with a plus is recommended (see Figure 20-39).

In the later part of this stage, exercises should progress to plyometric strengthening[132]. Surgical tubing is used to allow the patient to exercise in 90 degrees of elevation with the elbow bent to 90 degrees (see Figure 20-45). Plyoball exercises are initiated (see Figures 20-46 and 20-47). The weight and distance of the exercises can be altered to increase demands. The Shuttle 2000-1 is an excellent exercise to increase eccentric strength in a plyometric fashion (see Figure 20-50).

Stage III of the rehabilitation focuses on sport-specific activities. With throwing and overhead patients, an interval overhead program begins. Total body conditioning, return of strength, and increased endurance are the emphasis. The patient should remain pain-free as sport-specific activities are advanced and a gradual return to sport is achieved.

Postsurgical Management If conservative management is insufficient, surgical repair is often indicated. Postsurgical outcomes for patients having had a rotator cuff repair can be quite good.[15,19,21,24,46,77,98,105,116,130] The type of repair done depends on the classification of the injury. Subacromial decompression has been described by Neer as a method to stimulate tissue healing and increase the subacromial space.[85] Additional procedures may be done as open repairs of the tendon along with a capsular tightening procedure. One example

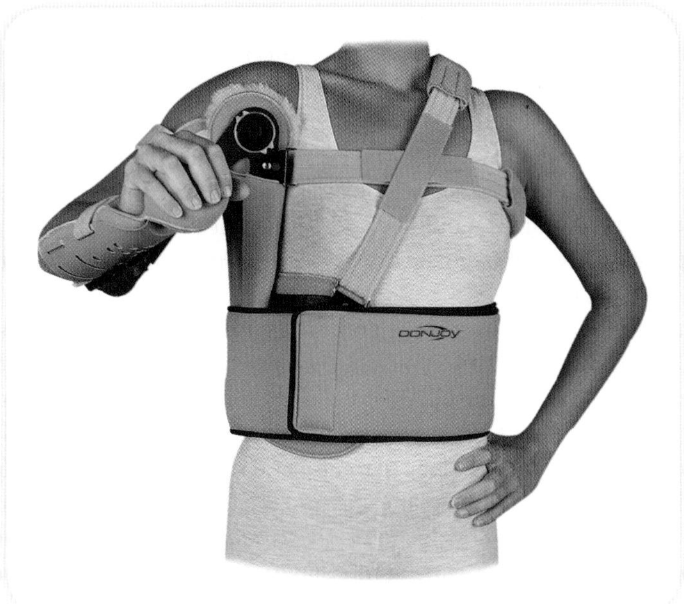

Figure 20-71 **Airplane splint**

(Courtesy DonJoy.)

is a modified Bankart procedure and capsulolabral reconstruction.[49] Surgical repairs can be done both open or closed. Closed arthroscopic rotator cuff repairs are becoming more common. The arthroscopic cuff repair addresses the deficiency of the rotator cuff by repairing the tear through the use of sutures and/or suture anchors. The arthroscopic technique spares the atrophy of the deltoid muscles and limits the presence of adhesions. Patients tend to show a much more rapid recovery of function with this repair.[38,67,115]

Stage I usually begins with some form of immobilization. This does not mean complete lack of movement. Instead it refers to restricting positions based on the surgical repair. In open repairs, flexion and abduction might be restricted for as long as 4 weeks. When the repair addresses the capsulolabral complex, the patient might spend up to 2 weeks in an airplane splint (Figure 20-71). Some surgeons have adopted a delayed start to mobilization and rehabilitation because of a few studies that have shown improved healing rates without associated stiffness.[57] During this phase, load across the repaired tendon should be minimized. ROM should be passive and in a safe range. During weeks 0 to 4 postoperation, the ROM in forward elevation should be kept below 125 degrees and external rotation should be at 20 degrees of abduction and less than 45 degrees. During weeks 4 to 6 postoperation, forward elevation can advance to 145 degrees and ER to 60 degrees. The patient may also advance to abduction at 90 degrees to begin external rotation ROM up to 45 degrees.

Pain control and prevention of muscle atrophy are addressed in this stage. Shoulder shrugs, isometrics, and joint mobilization for pain control can be done. Later in this stage, active assistive exercises with the L-bar and multiangle isometrics are done in the pain-free ROM, usually best done in supine position during this phase.

Stage II collagen and elastin components have begun to stabilize. Healing tissue should have a decreased level of elastin and an increased level of collagen by now.[106,131] Regaining full ROM and increasing the stress to healing tissue for better collagen alignment is important in this stage. Achieving full passive ROM during this phase is important. Normalizing the quality of AROM and beginning to work on strength and endurance are also important goals. This phase often is defined by weeks 6 to 10 postoperative.

Active, and active assisted ROM exercises are added, progressing from no resistance to resistance with light free weights. If a primary repair has been done to the tendon, resisted supraspinatus exercises should be avoided until 10 weeks. Internal rotation and external rotation stretches are introduced at 70 to 90 degrees of abduction. A full scapula strengthening program should be introduced. The restoration of normal arthrokinematics and scapulothoracic rhythm is addressed with exercises emphasizing neuromuscular control. Postural control and endurance should be addressed. The patient can use a mirror to judge progress. The patient may also begin a core exercise program and cardiovascular exercises at this time.

Stage III collagen and elastin components are nearing maturation.[99,131] By week 14, the tissue should be considered mature. Typically, this stage is defined as weeks 10 to 16 postoperation. Goals during this stage are full AROM, maintaining full PROM, gradual restoration of strength, power, and endurance, and optimal neuromuscular control. Closed-chain exercise progression may be progressed. A balanced rotator cuff strengthening program should be followed, advancing out of the scapular plane and into the functional position for the patient.

Stage IV is typically defined by postoperative weeks 14 to 26 and begins the preparation for return to sports training. During this stage, strength training will be advanced to plyometric loading.

Criteria for Return to Activity

Return to full activity should be based on these criteria: (a) the patient has full active ROM; (b) normal mechanics have been restored in the shoulder complex; (c) the patient has at least 90% strength in the involved shoulder as compared to the uninvolved side; and (d) there is no pain present during overhead activity.

Adhesive Capsulitis (Frozen Shoulder)

Pathomechanics

Adhesive capsulitis is characterized by the loss of motion at the glenohumeral joint. The cause of this arthrofibrosis is not well defined. One set of criteria used for diagnosis of a frozen shoulder was described by Jobe et al in 1996, and included: (a) decreased glenohumeral motion and loss of synchronous shoulder girdle motion; (b) restricted elevation (less than 135 degrees or 90 degrees, depending on the author); (c) external rotation 50% to 60% of normal; and (d) arthrogram findings of 5 to 10 mL volume with obliteration of the normal axillary fold.[52] Other authors have identified histologic changes in different areas surrounding the glenohumeral joint.[106] Travell and Simons explained that a reflex autonomic reaction could be the underlying cause, because of the presence of subscapularis trigger points.[118] The result is a chronic inflammation with fibrosis and rotator cuff muscles that are tight and inelastic.

Injury Mechanism

For the purposes of this chapter, we separate this diagnosis into 2 categories: primary versus secondary frozen shoulder. Adhesive capsulitis may be considered primary when it develops spontaneously; it is considered secondary when a known underlying condition (eg, a fractured humeral head) is present.

Primary frozen shoulder usually has an insidious onset. The patient often describes a sequence of painful restrictions in the patient's shoulder, followed by a gradual stiffness with less pain. Factors that have been found to predispose a patient to idiopathic capsulitis include diabetes, hypothyroidism, and underlying cardiopulmonary involvement.[106] These factors were identified through epidemiologic studies and might have more to do with characteristic personalities of these patients. It is rare to see this type of frozen shoulder in the athletic population.

Secondary frozen shoulder is more commonly seen in the athletic population. It is associated with many different underlying diagnoses. Rockwood and Matsen listed 8 categories of conditions that should be considered in the differential diagnosis of frozen shoulder: trauma, other soft-tissue disorders about the shoulder, joint disorders, bone disorders, cervical spine disorders, intrathoracic disorders, abdominal disorders, and psychogenic disorder (Table 20-3).[99]

Rehabilitation Concerns

The primary concern for rehabilitation is proper differential diagnosis. Attempting to progress the patient into the strength or functional activities portion of a rehabilitation program can lead to exacerbation of the motion restriction. The single best treatment for adhesive capsulitis is prevention.

Depending on the stage of pathology when intervention is started, the rehabilitation program time frame can be shortened. In all cases, the goals of rehabilitation are the same: first relieving the pain in the acute stages of the disorder, gradually restoring proper arthrokinematics, gradually restoring ROM, and strengthening the muscles of the shoulder complex.

Rehabilitation Progression

In the acute phase, Codman's exercises and low-grade joint mobilization techniques can be used to relieve pain. This may be accompanied by therapeutic modalities and passive stretching of the upper trapezius and levator scapulae muscles. The therapist may also want to suggest that the patient sleep with a pillow under the involved arm to prevent internal rotation during sleep.

In the subacute phase, ROM is more aggressively addressed. Incorporating PNF techniques such as hold-relax can be helpful. Progressive demands should be placed on the patient with rhythmic stabilization techniques. Wall climbing (see Figure 20-8) and wall/corner stretches (see Figure 20-10) are also good additions to the rehabilitation program. As ROM returns, the program should start to address strengthening. Isometric exercises for the shoulder are often the best way to begin. Progressive strengthening will continue in the next phase.

The final phase of rehabilitation is a progressive strengthening of the shoulder complex. Exercises for maintenance of ROM continue, and a series of strengthening exercises should be added. The rehabilitation program should be tailored to meet the needs of the patient based on the differential diagnosis.

Table 20-3 Differential Diagnosis of Frozen Shoulder

Trauma
Fractures of the shoulder region
Fractures anywhere in the upper extremity
Misdiagnosed posterior shoulder dislocation
Hemarthrosis of shoulder secondary to trauma
Other Soft-Tissue Disorders about the Shoulder
Tendinitis of the rotator cuff
Tendinitis of the long head of biceps
Subacromial bursitis
Impingement
Suprascapular nerve impingement
Thoracic outlet syndrome
Joint Disorders
Degenerative arthritis of the AC joint
Degenerative arthritis of the glenohumeral joint
Septic arthritis
Other painful forms of arthritis
Bone Disorders
Avascular necrosis of the humeral head
Metastatic cancer
Paget disease
Primary bone tumor
Hyperparathyroidism
Cervical Spine Disorders
Cervical spondylosis
Cervical disc herniation
Infection
Intrathoracic Disorder
Diaphragmatic irritation
Pancoast tumor
Myocardial infarction
Abdominal Disorder
Gastric ulcer
Cholecystitis
Subphrenic abscess
Psychogenic

Source: Rockwood CA, Matsen FA. *The Shoulder.* Philadelphia, PA: WB Saunders; 1990.

Criteria for Return to Activity

The patient may return to the patient's previous level of activity once the proper physiologic and arthrokinematic motion has been restored to the glenohumeral joint. How long the patient went untreated and undiagnosed affects how long it takes to reach this point.

Thoracic Outlet Syndrome

Pathomechanics

Thoracic outlet syndrome is the compression of neurovascular structures within the thoracic outlet. The thoracic outlet is a cone-shaped passage, with the greater circumferential opening proximal to the spine and the narrow end passing into the distal extremity. On the proximal end, the cone is bordered anteriorly by the anterior scalene muscles, and posteriorly by the middle and posterior scalene muscles. Structures traveling through the thoracic outlet are the brachial plexus, subclavian artery and vein, and axillary vessels. The neurovascular structures pass distally under the clavicle and subclavius muscle. Beneath the neurovascular bundle is the first rib. At the narrow end of the cone, the bundle passes under the coracoid process of the scapula and into the upper extremity through the axilla. The distal end is bordered anteriorly by the pectoralis minor and posteriorly by the scapula.

Based on the anatomy of the thoracic outlet, there are several areas where neurovascular compression can occur. Therefore, pathology of the thoracic outlet syndrome is dependent on the structures being compressed.

Injury Mechanism

In 60% of the population affected by thoracic outlet syndrome, there is no report from the patient of an inciting episode.[64] Some of the theories presented by authors regarding the etiology of thoracic outlet syndrome include trauma, postural components, shortening of the pectoralis minor, shortening of the scalenes, and muscle hypertrophy.

There are 4 areas of vulnerability to compressive forces: the superior thoracic outlet, where the brachial plexus passes over the first rib; the scalene triangle, at the proximal end of the thoracic outlet, where there might be overlapping insertions of the anterior and middle scalenes onto the first rib; the costoclavicular interval, which is the space between the first rib and clavicle where the neurovascular bundle passes (the space can be narrowed by poor posture, inferior laxity of the glenohumeral joint, or an exostosis from a fracture of the clavicle); and under the coracoid process where the brachial plexus passes and is bordered anteriorly by the pectoralis minor.[106]

Rehabilitation Concerns

As described, thoracic outlet syndrome is an anatomy-based problem involving compressive forces applied to the neurovascular bundle. Conservative management of thoracic outlet syndrome is moderately successful, resulting in decreased symptoms 50% to 90% of the time. As the first course of treatment, rehabilitation should be based on encouraging the least provocative posture. Leffert advocated a detailed history and evaluation of the patient's activities and lifestyle to help identify where and when postural deficiency is occurring.[64]

Through a detailed history and evaluation of an patient's activity, the therapist can identify the cause of compression in the thoracic outlet. The rehabilitation program should be tailored to encourage good posture throughout the patient's day. Therapeutic exercises should be used to strengthen postural muscles, such as the rhomboids (see Figure 20-38), middle trapezius (see Figure 20-37), and upper trapezius (see Figure 20-35). Flexibility exercises are also used to increase the space in the thoracic outlet. Scalene stretches and wall/corner stretches (see Figure 20-10) are used to decrease the incidence of muscle impinging on the neurovascular bundle. Proper breathing technique should also be reviewed with the patient. The scalene muscles act as accessory breathing muscles, and improper breathing technique can lead to tightening of these muscles.

Rehabilitation Progression

The rehabilitation process begins by detailed evaluation of the patient's activities and symptoms. First, the patient is removed from activities exacerbating the neurovascular symptoms until the patient can maintain a symptom-free posture. During this time an erect posture is encouraged using stretching and strengthening exercises. Gradually encourage the patient to return to the patient's sport, for short periods of time, while maintaining a pain-free posture. The time of participation is increased at regular intervals if the patient remains free of pain. This helps build endurance of the postural muscles. Exercising on an upper-body ergometer, by pedaling backwards, can help build endurance. As the patient returns to sports, it may be necessary to alter strength-training methods that place the patient in a flexed posture.

Criteria for Return to Activity

If the patient responds to the rehabilitation program and can maintain a pain-free posture during the patient's sport-specific activity, participation can be resumed. The patient should have no muscular weakness, neurovascular symptoms, or pain. If the patient fails to respond to therapy, and functionally significant pain and weakness persist, surgical intervention might be indicated. Surgical procedure depends on the anatomical basis for the patient's symptoms.

Brachial Plexus Injuries (Stinger or Burner)

Pathomechanics

The brachial plexus begins at cervical roots C5 through C8 and thoracic root T1. The ventral rami of these roots are formed from a dorsal (sensory) and ventral (motor) root. The ventral rami join to form the brachial plexus. The ventral rami lie between the anterior and middle scalene muscles, where they run adjacent to the subclavian artery. The plexus continues distally passing over the first rib. It is deep to the sternocleidomastoid muscle in the neck.[86] Just caudal to the clavicle and subclavius muscle, the 5 ventral rami unite to form the 3 trunks of the plexus: superior, middle, and inferior. The superior trunk is composed of the C5 and C6 ventral roots. The middle trunk is formed by the C7 root, and the inferior trunk is formed by C8 and T1 ventral roots. After passing under the clavicle, the 3 trunks divide into 3 divisions that eventually contribute to the 3 cords of the brachial plexus.

The typical picture of a brachial plexus injury in sports is that of a traction injury. This syndrome is commonly referred to as *burner* or *stinger syndrome*. These injuries usually involve the C5 to C6 nerve roots. The patient will complain of a sharp, burning pain in the shoulder that radiates down the arm into the hand. Weakness in the muscles supplied by C5 and C6 (deltoid, biceps, supraspinatus, and infraspinatus) accompany the pain. Burning and pain are often transient, but weakness might last a few minutes or indefinitely.

Clancy et al classified brachial plexus injuries into 3 categories.[20] A grade I injury results in a transient loss of motor and sensory function that usually resolves completely within minutes. A grade II injury results in significant motor weakness and sensory loss that might last from 6 weeks to 4 months. Electromyography evaluation after 2 weeks will demonstrate abnormalities. Grade III lesions are characterized by motor and sensory loss for at least 1 year in duration.

Injury Mechanism

The structure of the brachial plexus is such that it winds its way through the musculoskeletal anatomy of the upper extremity as described. Clancy et al identified neck rotation, neck lateral flexion, shoulder abduction, shoulder external rotation, and simultaneous scapular and clavicular depression as potential mechanisms of injury.[20]

During neck rotation and lateral flexion to one side, the brachial plexus and the subclavius muscle on the opposite side are put on stretch and the clavicle is slightly elevated about its anteroposterior axis. If the arm is not elevated, the superior trunk of the plexus will assume the greatest amount of tension. If the shoulder is abducted and externally rotated, the brachial plexus migrates superiorly toward the coracoid process and the scapula retracts, putting the pectoralis minor on stretch. As the shoulder is moved into full abduction, a condition similar to a movable pulley is formed, where the coracoid process of the scapula acts as the pulley. In full abduction, most stress falls on the lower cords of the brachial plexus.[107] The addition of clavicular and scapula depression to the above scenarios would produce a downward force on the pulley system, bringing the brachial plexus into contact with the clavicle and the coracoid process. The portion of the plexus that receives the greatest amount of tensile stress depends on the position of the upper extremity during a collision.

Rehabilitation Concerns

Management of brachial plexus injuries begins with the gradual restoration of the patient's cervical ROM. Muscle tightness caused by the direct trauma, and by reflexive guarding that occurs because of pain, needs to be addressed. Gentle passive ROM exercises and stretching for the upper trapezius, levator scapulae, and scalene muscles should be done. The therapist should be careful not to cause sensory symptoms.

Butler advocates using an early intervention with gentle mobilization of the neural tissues.[17] The goal of early mobilization is to prevent scarring between the nerve and the bed or within the connective tissue of the nerve itself as the nerve heals. He advocates low tensile loads to avoid the possibility of irritating a nerve lesion such as axonotmesis or neurotmesis. More chronic, repetitive injuries may use the neural tension test positions to do mobilizations with higher grades.

Strengthening of the involved muscles is also addressed in the rehabilitation program. Supraspinatus strengthening exercises, like scaption (see Figure 20-33) and alternative supraspinatus exercises (see Figure 20-34), should be done. Other exercises for involved musculature are shoulder lateral rotation (see Figure 20-32) for the infraspinatus, forward flexion and abduction to 90 degrees (see Figures 20-26 and 20-28) to strengthen the deltoid, and bicep curls for elbow flexion.

The therapist should also work closely with the patient's coach to evaluate the patient's technique and correct any alteration in form that might be putting the patient at risk for burners. Prior to return to activity, the patient's equipment should be inspected for proper fitting, and a cervical neck roll should be used to decrease the amount of lateral flexion that occurs during impact, as in tackling.

Rehabilitation Progression

The patient is removed from activity immediately after the injury. The rehabilitation progression should begin with the restoration of both active and PROM ROM at the neck and shoulder. Neural tissue mobilizations utilizing the upper limb tension testing positions should begin with the patient in the testing positions (see Figure 8-4*A* and *B*).[17] For the median nerve, the testing position consists of shoulder depression, abduction, external rotation, and wrist and finger extension. For the radial nerve, the elbow is extended, the forearm pronated, the glenohumeral joint internally rotated, and the wrist, finger, and thumb flexed. The position for stretching the ulnar nerve consists of shoulder depression, wrist and finger extension, supination or pronation of the forearm, and elbow flexion. Mobilizations of distal joints, like the elbow and wrist, in large-grade movements should initiate the treatment phase. Progression should include grade 4 and grade 5 mobilizations in later phases of recovery.

As the patient gets return of ROM, strengthening of the neck and shoulder is incorporated into the rehabilitation program. Strengthening should progress from PRE-type strengthening with free weights to exercises that emphasize power and endurance. Functional progression begins with teaching proper technique for sport-specific demands that mimic the position of injury. The progressive return and proper technique are important to the rehabilitation program, as they address the psychological component of preparing the patient for return to sport.

Criteria for Return to Activity

Patients are allowed to return to play when they have full, pain-free ROM, full strength, and no prior episodes in that contest.[124] Additionally, football players should use a cervical neck roll. The patient's psychological readiness should also be considered prior to return to sport. Patients who are too protective of their neck and shoulder can expose themselves to further injury.

Myofascial Trigger Points

Pathology

Clinically, a trigger point (TP) is defined as a hyperirritable foci in muscle or fascia that is tender to palpation and may, upon compression, result in referred pain or tenderness in a characteristic "zone." This zone is distinct from myotomes, dermatomes, sclerotomes, or peripheral nerve distribution. TPs are identified via palpation of taut bands of muscle or discrete nodules or adhesions. Snapping of a taut band will usually initiate a local twitch response.[106]

Physiologically, the definition of a TP is not as clear. Muscles with myofascial TPs reveal no diagnostic abnormalities upon electromyographic examination. Routine laboratory tests show no abnormalities or significant changes attributable to TPs. Normal serum enzyme concentrations have been reported with a shift in the distribution of lactate dehydrogenase-isoenzymes. Skin temperature over active TPs might be higher in a 5- to 10-cm diameter.[118]

Travell and Simons classify TPs as follows[118]:

1. Active TPs. Symptomatic at rest with referral pain and tenderness upon direct compression. Associated weakness and contracture are often present.
2. Latent TPs. Pain is not present unless direct compression is applied. These might show up on clinical exam as stiffness and/or weakness in the region of tenderness.
3. Primary TPs. Located in specific muscles.
4. Associated TPs. Located within the referral zone of a primary TP's muscle or in a muscle that is functionally overloaded in compensation for a primary TP.

Pathology of a myofascial TP is identified with (a) a history of sudden onset during or shortly after an acute overload stress or chronic overload of the affected muscle; (b) characteristic patterns of pain in a muscle's referral zone; (c) weakness and restriction in the end ROM of the affected muscle; (d) a taut, palpable band in the affected muscle; (e) focal tenderness to direct compression, in the band of taut muscle fibers; (f) a local twitch response elicited by snapping of the tender spot; and (g) reproduction of the patient's pain through pressure on the tender spot.

Injury Mechanism

The most common mechanism for myofascial TPs in the shoulder region is acute muscle strain (Table 20-4). The damaged muscle tissue causes tearing of the sarcoplasmic reticulum and release of its stored calcium, with loss of the ability of that portion of the muscle

Table 20-4 Trigger Points of the Shoulder

Posterior Shoulder Pain
Deltoid
Levator scapulae
Supraspinatus
Subscapularis
Teres minor
Teres major
Serratus posterior superior
Triceps
Trapezius
Anterior Shoulder Pain
Infraspinatus
Deltoid
Scalene
Supraspinatus
Pectoralis major
Pectoralis minor
Biceps
Coracobrachialis

Source: Data from Travell and Simons.[118]

to remove calcium ions. The chronic stress of sustained muscle contraction can cause continued muscle damage, repeating the above cycle of damage. The combined presence of the normal muscle adenosine triphosphate supplies and excessive calcium initiate and maintain a sustained muscle band contracture. This produces a region of the muscle with an uncontrolled metabolism, to which the body responds with local vasoconstriction. This region of increased metabolism and decreased local circulation, with muscle fibers passing through that area, causes muscle shortening independent of local motor unit action potentials. This taut band can be palpated in the muscle.

Rehabilitation Concerns

The principal mechanism of myofascial TPs is related to muscular overload and fatigue, so the primary concern is identification of the incriminating activity. The therapist should take a detailed history of the patient's daily activity demands, as well as the changing demands of the patient's sport activities.

The cyclic nature of TPs requires interruption of the cycle for successful treatment. Interrupting the shortening of the muscle fibers and prevention of further breakdown of the muscle tissue components should be attempted using modified hold-relax techniques and postisometric stretching. Travell and Simons advocate a spray-and-stretch method, where vapocoolant spray is applied and passive stretching follows. Theoretically, when the muscle is placed in a stretched position and the skin receptors are cooled, a reflexive inhibition of the contracted muscle is facilitated, allowing for increased passive stretching.[118]

After a treatment session where PROM has been achieved, the muscle must be activated to stimulate normal actin and myosin cross bridging. Gentle AROM exercises or active assistive exercises with the L-bar might be a good activity to use as posttreatment activity. Normal muscle activity and endurance must be encouraged after ROM is restored. A gradual progression of shoulder exercises with an endurance emphasis should be used.

Rehabilitation Progression

Treatment progression for TPs should begin with temporary removal from activities that overload the contracted tissue. The patient is then treated with myofascial stretching techniques to increase the length of the contracted tissue. Immediate use of the extended ROM should be emphasized. Strengthening exercises are added once the patient can maintain the normal muscle length without initiating the return of the contracted myofascial band. As strength and function of the involved muscles return, the patient may gradually return to the patient's sport.

Criteria for Return to Activity

The patient may return to activity in a relatively short period of time if the patient can demonstrate the ability to function without reinitiating the myofascial TPs and associated taut bands. Early return without meeting this criterion can lead to greater regionalization of the symptoms.

SUMMARY

1. The high degree of mobility in the shoulder complex requires some compromise in stability, which, in turn, increases the vulnerability of the shoulder joint to injury, particularly in dynamic overhead athletic activities.
2. In rehabilitation of the SC joint, effort should be directed toward regaining normal clavicular motion that will allow the scapula to abduct and upward rotate throughout 180 degrees of humeral abduction. The clavicle must elevate approximately 40 degrees to allow upward scapular rotation.
3. AC joint sprains are most commonly seen in patients who experienced a direct fall on the point of the shoulder with the arm at the side in an adducted position or falling on an outstretched arm.
4. Management of AC injuries depends on the type of injury. Types I and II injuries are usually handled conservatively, focusing on strengthening of the deltoid, trapezius, and the clavicular fibers of the pectoralis major. Occasionally AC injuries require surgical excision of the distal portion of the clavicle.
5. Treatment for clavicle fractures includes approximation of the fracture and immobilization for 6 to 8 weeks, using a figure-8 wrap with the involved arm in a sling. Because mobility of the clavicle is important for normal shoulder mechanics, rehabilitation should focus on joint mobilization and strengthening of the deltoid, upper trapezius, and pectoralis major muscles.
6. Following a short immobilization period, rehabilitation for a dislocated shoulder should focus on restoring the appropriate axis of rotation for the glenohumeral joint, optimizing the stabilizing muscle's length–tension relationship, and restoring proper neuromuscular control of the shoulder complex. Similar rehabilitation strategies are applied in cases of multidirectional instabilities, which can occur as a result of recurrent dislocation.
7. Management of shoulder impingement involves gradually restoring normal biomechanics to the shoulder joint in an effort to maintain space under the coracoacromial arch during overhead activities. Techniques include strengthening of the rotator cuff muscles, strengthening of the muscles that abduct, elevate, and upwardly rotate the scapula, and stretching both the inferior and the posterior portions of the joint capsule and posterior rotator cuff musculature.
8. The basic concerns of a rehabilitation program for rotator cuff tendinopathy are based on why and how the tendon has been damaged. If a comprehensive rehabilitation program does not relieve the painful shoulder, surgical repair of the tendon and alteration of the glenohumeral joint are performed. Surgical rehabilitation is similar to the nonsurgical plan, with the time of progression altered, based on tissue healing and tendon histology.
9. In cases of adhesive capsulitis, the goals of rehabilitation are relieving the pain in the acute stages of the disorder, gradually restoring proper arthrokinematics, gradual restoration of ROM, and strengthening the muscles of the shoulder complex.
10. Rehabilitation for thoracic outlet syndrome should be directed toward encouraging the least-provocative posture combined with exercises to strengthen postural muscles (rhomboids, middle trapezius, upper trapezius) and stretching exercises for the scalenes to increase the space in the thoracic outlet in order to reduce muscle impingement on the neurovascular bundle.
11. Management of brachial plexus injuries includes the gradual restoration of cervical ROM, and stretching for the upper trapezius, levator scapulae, and scalene muscles.

12. After identifying the cause of myofascial TPs, rehabilitation may include a spray- and-stretch method with passive stretching, gentle active ROM exercises or active assistive exercises, encouraging normal muscle activity and endurance, and gradual improvement of muscle endurance.

REFERENCES

1. Allman FL. Fractures and ligamentous injuries of the clavicle and its articulations. *J Bone Joint Surg Am.* 1967;49:774.
2. Anderson L, Rush R, Shearer L. The effects of a TheraBand exercise program on shoulder internal rotation strength. *Phys Ther Suppl.* 1992;72(6):540.
3. Andrews JR, Wilk EK, eds. *The Athlete's Shoulder.* New York, NY: Churchill Livingstone; 1994.
4. Barden JM, Balyk R, Raso VJ, Moreau M, Bagnall K. Dynamic upper limb proprioception in multidirectional shoulder instability. *Clin Orthop.* 2004;420:181-189.
5. Bateman JE. *The Shoulder and Neck.* Philadelphia, PA: WB Saunders; 1971.
6. Bergfeld JA, Andrish JT, Clancy GW. Evaluation of the acromioclavicular joint following first and second degree sprains. *Am J Sports Med.* 1978;6:153.
7. Bigliani L, Kimmel J, McCann P. Repair of rotator cuff tears in tennis players. *Am J Sports Med.* 1992;20(2):112-117.
8. Bigliani L, Morrison D, April E. The morphology of the acromion and its relation to rotator cuff tears. *Orthop Transcr.* 1986;10:216.
9. Blackburn T, McCloud W, White B. EMG analysis of posterior rotator cuff exercises. *Athl Train.* 1990;25(1):40-45.
10. Blasier RB, Carpenter JE, Huston LJ. Shoulder proprioception: effects of joint laxity, joint position, and direction of motion. *Orthop Rev.* 1994;23(1):45-50.
11. Borich MR, Bright JM, Lorello DJ, Cieminski CJ, Buisman T, Ludewig PM. Scapular angular positioning at end range internal rotation in cases of glenohumeral internal rotation deficit. *J Orthop Sports Phys Ther.* 2006;36(12):926-934.
12. Borstad JD. Resting position variables at the shoulder: evidence to support a posture-impairment association. *Phys Ther.* 2006;86(4):549-557.
13. Borstad JD, Ludewig MP. The effect of long versus short pectoralis minor resting length on scapular kinematics in healthy individuals. *J Orthop Sports Phys Ther.* 2005;35(4):227-238.
14. Brewster C, Moynes D. Rehabilitation of the shoulder following rotator cuff injury or surgery. *J Orthop Sports Phys Ther.* 1993;17(2):422-426.
15. Burkhart SS, Esch JC, Jolson RS. The rotator crescent and rotator cable: An anatomic description of the shoulder's "suspension bridge." *Arthroscopy.* 1993;9:611-616.
16. Burkhead W, Rockwood C. Treatment of instability of rotator cuff injuries in the overhead athlete. *J Bone Joint Surg Am.* 1992;74:890.
17. Butler D. *The Sensitive Nervous System.* Adelaide, Australia: Noigroup; 2000.
18. Caprise PA Jr, Sekiya JK. Open and arthroscopic treatment of multidirectional instability of the shoulder. *Arthroscopy.* 2006;22(10):1126-1131.
19. Carpenter JE, Thomopoulos S, Flanagan CL, DeBano CM, Soslowsky LJ. Rotator cuff defect healing: a biomechanical and histologic analysis in an animal model. *J Shoulder Elbow Surg.* 1998;7:599-605.
20. Clancy WG, Brand RI, Bergfeld AJ. Upper trunk brachial plexus injuries in contact sports. *Am J Sports Med.* 1977;5:209.
21. Clark JM, Harryman DT. Tendons, ligaments, and capsule of the rotator cuff: gross and microscopic anatomy. *J Bone Joint Surg Am.* 1992;74:713-725.
22. Codman EA. Ruptures of the supraspinatus tendon and other lesions in or about the subacromial bursa. In: Codman EA, ed. *The Shoulder.* Boston, MA: Thomas Todd; 1934.
23. Cools AM, Witvrouw EE, DeClercq GA, Voight LM. Scapular muscle recruitment pattern: EMG response of the trapezius muscle to the sudden shoulder movement before and after a fatiguing exercise. *J Orthop Sports Phys Ther.* 2002;32(5):221-229.
24. Cooper DE, O'Brien, SJ Warren RF. Supporting layers of the glenohumeral joint: an anatomic study. *Clin Orthop.* 1993;(289):144-155.
25. Covey, Bahu AM, Ahmad C. Arthroscopic posterior/multidirectional instability. *Oper Tech Orthop.* 2008;18:33-45.
26. Cox JS. The fate of the acromioclavicular joint in athletic injuries. *Am J Sports Med.* 1981;9:50.
27. Culham E, Malcolm P. Functional anatomy of the shoulder complex. *J Orthop Sports Phys Ther.* 1993;18(1):342-350.
28. Davies G, Dickoff-Hoffman S. Neuromuscular testing and rehabilitation of the shoulder complex. *J Orthop Sports Phys Ther.* 1993;18(2):449-458.
29. Depalma AF. *Surgery of the Shoulder.* 2nd ed. Philadelphia, PA: Lippincott; 1973.
30. Downar JM, Sauers EL. Clinical measures of shoulder mobility in the professional baseball player. *J Athl Train.* 2005;40(1):23-29.

31. Dvir Z, Berme N. The shoulder complex in elevation of the arm: a mechanism approach. *J Biomech.* 1978;11:219-225.
32. Duncan A. Personal communication to the author. August 1997.
33. Ebaugh DD, McClure PW, Karduna AR. Effects of shoulder muscle fatigue caused by repetitive overhead activities on scapulothoracic and glenohumeral kinematics. *J Electromyogr Kinesiol.* 2006;16(3):224-235.
34. Ebaugh DD, McClure PW, Karduna AR. Scapulothoracic and glenohumeral kinematics following an external rotation fatigue protocol. *J Orthop Sports Phys Ther.* 2006;36(8):557-571.
35. Endo K, Ikata T, Katoh S, Takeda Y. Radiographic assessment of scapular rotational tilt in chronic shoulder impingement syndrome. *J Orthop Sci.* 2001;6(1):3-10.
36. Favorito P, Langenderfer M, Colosimo A, Heidt R Jr, Carlonas R. Arthroscopic laser-assisted capsular shift in the treatment of patients with multidirectional shoulder instability. *Am J Sports Med.* 2002;30:322-328.
37. Fayad F, Roby-Brami A, Yazbeck C, et al. Three-dimensional scapular kinematics and scapulohumeral rhythm in patients with glenohumeral osteoarthritis or frozen shoulder. *J Biomech.* 2008;41(2):326-332.
38. Gerber C, Schneeberger AG, Beck M, Schlegel U. Mechanical strength of repairs of the rotator cuff. *J Bone Joint Surg Br.* 1994;76:371-380.
39. Greenfield B. Special considerations in shoulder exercises: plane of the scapula. In: Andrews J, Wilk K, eds. *The Athlete's Shoulder.* New York, NY: Churchill Livingstone; 1993.
40. Gryzlo SM. Bony disorders: clinical assessment and treatment. In: Jobe FW, ed. *Operative Techniques in Upper Extremity Sports Injuries.* St. Louis, MO: Mosby; 1996.
41. Hageman P, Mason D, Rydlund K. Effects of position and speed on concentric isokinetic testing of the shoulder rotators. *J Orthop Sports Phys Ther.* 1989;11:64-69.
42. Hart DL, Carmichael SW. Biomechanics of the shoulder. *J Orthop Sports Phys Ther.* 1985;6(4):229-234.
43. Hawkins R, Bell R. Dynamic EMG analysis of the shoulder muscles during rotational and scapular strengthening exercises. In: Post M, Morey B, Hawkins R, eds. *Surgery of the Shoulder.* St. Louis, MO: Mosby; 1990.
44. Hawkins R, Kennedy J. Impingement syndrome in athletes. *Am J Sports Med.* 1980;8:151.
45. Hawkins RJ, Krishnan SG, Karas SG, Noonan TJ, Horan MP. Electrothermal arthroscopic shoulder capsulorrhaphy: a minimum 2-year follow-up. *Am J Sports Med.* 2007;35(9):1484-1488.
46. Hirose K, Kondo S, Choi HR, Mishima S, Iwata H, Ishiguro N. Spontaneous healing process of a supra-spinatus tendon tear in rabbits. *Arch Orthop Trauma Surg.* 2004;124(9):647.
47. Howell S, Kraft T. The role of the supraspinatus and infraspinatus muscles in glenohumeral kinematics of anterior shoulder instability. *Clin Orthop.* 1991;263:128-134.
48. Inman VT, Saunders JB, Abbott CL. Observations on the function of the shoulder joint. *J Bone Joint Surg.* 1996;26:1.
49. Jobe FW, ed. *Operative Techniques in Upper Extremity Sports Injuries.* St. Louis, MO: Mosby; 1996.
50. Jobe FW, Kvitne RS, Giangarra CE. Shoulder pain in the overhand and throwing athletes. The relationship of anterior instability and rotator cuff impingement. *Orthop Rev.* 1989;18:963-975.
51. Jobe F, Moynes D. Delineation of diagnostic criteria and a rehabilitation program for rotator cuff injuries. *Am J Sports Med.* 1982;10(6):336-339.
52. Jobe FW, Schwab, Wilk KE, Andrews EJ. Rehabilitation of the shoulder. In: Brotzman SB, ed. *Clinical Orthopedics Rehabilitation.* St. Louis, MO: Mosby; 1996.
53. Kannus P, Josza L, Renstrom P, et al. The effects of training, immobilization and remobilization on musculoskeletal tissue: 2. Remobilization and prevention of immobilization atrophy. *Scand J Med Sci Sports.* 1992;2:164-176.
54. Karduna AR, McClure PW, Michener LA, Sennett B. Dynamic measurements of three-dimensional scapular kinematics: a validation study. *J Biomech Eng.* 2001;123(2):184-190.
55. Keirns M. Nonoperative treatment of shoulder impingement. In: Andrews J, Wilk K, eds. *The Athlete's Shoulder.* New York, NY: Churchill Livingstone; 2008:527-544.
56. Kelley MJ. Anatomic and biomechanical rationale for rehabilitation of the athlete's shoulder. *J Sport Rehabil.* 1995;4:122-154.
57. Kibler WB, McMullen J, Uhl T. Shoulder rehabilitation strategies, guidelines, and practice. *Orthop Clin North Am.* 2001;32:527-538.
58. Kibler WB. Role of the scapula in the overhead throwing motion. *Contemp Orthop.* 1998;22:525-532.
59. Kibler WB. The role of the scapula in athletic shoulder function. *Am J Sports Med.* 1998;26(2):325-337.
60. Kluemper M, Uhl TL, Hazelrigg H. Effect of stretching and strengthening shoulder muscles of forward shoulder posture in competitive swimmers. *J Sport Rehabil.* 2006;15:58-70.
61. Laudner KG, Myers JB, Pasquale MR, Bradley JP, Lephart SM. Scapular dysfunction in throwers with pathologic internal impingement. *J Orthop Sports Phys Ther.* 2006;36(7):485-494.
62. Laudner KG, Sipes RC, Wilson JT. The acute effects of sleeper stretches on shoulder range of motion. *J Athl Train.* 2008;43(4):359-363.
63. Laudner KG, Stanek JM, Meister K. Differences in scapular upward rotation between baseball pitchers and position players. *Am J Sports Med.* 2007;35(12):2091-2095.
64. Leffert RD. Neurological problems. In: Rockwood CA, Matsen FA, eds. *The Shoulder.* Philadelphia, PA: WB Saunders; 1990.
65. Lephart SM, Warner JP, Borsa PA, Fu HF. Proprioception of the shoulder joint in healthy, unstable, and surgically repaired shoulders. *J Shoulder Elbow Surg.* 1994;3(6):371-380.

66. Lew W, Lewis J, Craig E. Stabilization by capsule ligaments and labrum: stability at the extremes of motion. In: Masten F, Fu F, Hawkins R, eds. *The Shoulder: A Balance of Mobility and Stability*. Rosemont, IL: American Academy of Orthopedic Surgery; 1993.
67. Lewis CW, Schlegel TF, Hawkins RJ, James SP, Turner AS. The effect of immobilization on rotator cuff healing using modified Mason-Allen stitches: a biomechanical study in sheep. *Biomed Sci Instrum.* 2001;37:263-268.
68. Litchfield R, Hawkins R, Dillman C. Rehabilitation for the overhead athlete. *J Orthop Sports Phys Ther.* 1993;18(2):433-441.
69. Ludewig PM, Cook TM. Alterations in shoulder kinematics and associated muscle activity in people with symptoms of shoulder impingement. *Phys Ther.* 2000;80(3):276-291.
70. Ludewig PM, Cook MT. Translations of the humerus in persons with shoulder impingement syndromes. *J Orthop Sports Phys Ther.* 2002;32(6):248-259.
71. Lukasiewicz AC, McClure P, Michener L, Pratt N, Sennett B. Comparison of 3-dimensional scapular position and orientation between subjects with and without shoulder impingement. *J Orthop Sports Phys Ther.* 1999;29(10):574-583, discussion 584-576.
72. Magee D, Reid D. Shoulder injuries. In: Zachazewski J, Magee D, Quillen W, eds. *Athletic Injuries and Rehabilitation.* Philadelphia, PA: WB Saunders; 1995:509-542.
73. Matsen FA, Thomas SC, Rockwood AC. Glenohumeral instability. In: Rockwood CA, Matsen FA, eds. *The Shoulder.* Philadelphia, PA: WB Saunders; 1990.
74. McCarroll J. Golf. In: Pettrone FA, ed. *Athletic Injuries of the Shoulder*. New York, NY: McGraw-Hill; 1995.
75. McClure P, Balaicuis J, Heiland D, Broersma ME, Thorndike CK, Wood A. A randomized controlled comparison of stretching procedures for posterior shoulder tightness. *J Orthop Sports Phys Ther.* 2007;37(3):108-114.
76. McClure PW, Michener LA, Sennett BJ, Karduna AR. Direct 3-dimensional measurement of scapular kinematics during dynamic movements in vivo. *J Shoulder Elbow Surg.* 2001;10(3):269-277.
77. McGough RL, Debski RE, Taskiran E, Fu FH, Woo SL. Mechanical properties of the long head of the biceps tendon. *Knee Surg Sports Traumatol Arthrosc.* 1996;3:226-229.
78. Meister K, Andrews RJ. Classification and treatment of rotator cuff injuries in the overhead athlete. *J Orthop Sports Phys Ther.* 1993;18(2):413-421.
79. Mell AG, LaScalza S, Guffey P, et al. Effect of rotator cuff pathology on shoulder rhythm. *J Shoulder Elbow Surg.* 2005;14(1 Suppl S):58S-64S.
80. Moseley J, Jobe F, Pink M. EMG analysis of the scapular muscles during a shoulder rehabilitation program. *Am J Sports Med.* 1992;20:128-134.
81. Mulligan E. Conservative management of shoulder impingement syndrome. *Athl Train.* 1988;23(4):348-353.
82. Myers JB, Hwang JH, Pasquale MR, Blackburn JT, Lephart SM. Rotator cuff coactivation ratios in participants with subacromial impingement syndrome. *J Sci Med Sport.* 2009;12(6):603-608.
83. Myers JB, Laudner KG, Pasquale MR, Bradley JP, Lephart SM. Scapular position and orientation in throwing athletes. *Am J Sports Med.* 2005;33(2): 263-271.
84. Myers JB, Pasquale MR, Laudner KG, Sell TC, Bradley JP, Lephart SM. On-the-field resistance tubing exercises for throwers: an electromyographic analysis. *J Athl Train.* 2005;40(1):15-22.
85. Neer C. Anterior acromioplasty for the chronic impingement syndrome in the shoulder: a preliminary report. *J Bone Joint Surg Am.* 1972;54:41.
86. Nicholas JA, Hershmann BE, eds. *The Upper Extremity in Sports Medicine.* St. Louis, MO: Mosby; 1990.
87. O'Brien S, Neeves M, Arnoczky A. The anatomy and histology of the inferior glenohumeral ligament complex of the shoulder. *Am J Sports Educ.* 1990;18:451.
88. Ogston JB, Ludewig PM. Differences in 3-dimensional shoulder kinematics between persons with multidirectional instability and asymptomatic controls. *Am J Sports Med.* 2007;35(8):1361-1370.
89. Omer GE. Osteotomy of the clavicle in surgical reduction of anterior sternoclavicular dislocations. *J Trauma.* 1967;7(4):584-590.
90. Oyama S, Myers JB, Wassinger CA, Ricci RD, Lephart SM. Asymmetric resting scapular posture in healthy overhead athletes. *J Athl Train.* 2008;43(6):565-570.
91. Ozaki J, Fujimoto S, Nakagawa Y. Tears of the rotator cuff of the shoulder associated with pathological changes in the acromion: a study of cadavers. *J Bone Joint Surg Am.* 1988;70:1224.
92. Paine R, Voight M. The role of the scapula. *J Orthop Sports Phys Ther.* 1993;18(1):386-391.
93. Peat M, Culham E. Functional anatomy of the shoulder complex. In: Andrews J, Wilk K, eds. *The Athlete's Shoulder.* New York, NY: Churchill Livingstone; 1993.
94. Petersson C, Redlund-Johnell I. The subacromial space in normal shoulder radiographs. *Acta Orthop Scand.* 1984;55:57.
95. Pettrone FA, ed. *Athletic Injuries of the Shoulder.* New York, NY: McGraw-Hill; 1995.
96. Provencher M, Saldua N. The rotator interval of the shoulder: anatomy, biomechanics, and repair techniques. *Oper Tech Orthop.* 2008;18:9-22.
97. Rathburn J, McNab I. The microvascular pattern of the rotator cuff. *J Bone Joint Surg Br.* 1970;52:540.
98. Reilly P, Amis AA, Wallace AL, Emery RJ. Supraspinatus tears: propagation and strain alteration. *J Shoulder Elbow Surg.* 2003;12:134-138.
99. Rockwood C, Matsen F. *The Shoulder.* Philadelphia, PA: WB Saunders; 1990.
100. Rowe CR. Prognosis in dislocation of the shoulder. *J Bone Joint Surg Am.* 1956;38:957.

101. Rundquist PJ, Anderson DD, Guanche CA, Ludewig PM. Shoulder kinematics in subjects with frozen shoulder. *Arch Phys Med Rehabil.* 2003;84(10):1473-1479.

102. Salter EG, Shelley BS, Nasca R. A morphological study of the acromioclavicular joint in humans [abstract]. *Anat Rec.* 1985;211:353.

103. Scibek JS, Mell AG, Downie BK, Carpenter JE, Hughes RE. Shoulder kinematics in patients with full-thickness rotator cuff tears after a subacromial injection. *J Shoulder Elbow Surg.* 2007;17(1):172-181.

104. Skyhar M, Warren R, Altcheck D. Instability of the shoulder. In: Nicholas A, Hershmann BE, eds. *The Upper Extremity in Sports Medicine.* St. Louis, MO: Mosby; 1990.

105. Soslowsky LJ, Thomopoulos S, Esmail A, et al. Rotator cuff tendinosis in an animal model: role of extrinsic and overuse factors. *Ann Biomed Eng.* 2002;30: 1057-1063.

106. Souza TA. *Sports Injuries of the Shoulder: Conservative Management.* New York, NY: Churchill Livingstone; 1994.

107. Stevens JH. The classic brachial plexus paralysis. In: Codman EA, ed. *The Shoulder.* Boston, MA: Thomas Todd; 1934:344-350.

108. Su KP, Johnson MP, Gracely EJ, Karduna AR. Scapular rotation in swimmers with and without impingement syndrome: practice effects. *Med Sci Sports Exerc.* 2004;36(7):1121-1123.

109. Sutter JS. Conservative treatment of shoulder instability. In: Andrews J, Wilk EK, eds. *The Athlete's Shoulder.* New York, NY: Churchill Livingstone; 1994.

110. Swanik KA, Lephart SM, Swanik CB, Lephart SP, Stone DA, Fu FH. The effects of shoulder plyometric training on proprioception and selected muscle performance characteristics. *J Shoulder Elbow Surg.* 2002;11(6): 579-586.

111. Swanik KA, Swanik CB, Lephart SM, Huxel K. The effect of functional training on the incidence of shoulder pain and strength in intercollegiate swimmers. *J Sport Rehabil.* 2002;11(2):140-154.

112. Taft TN, Wilson FC, Ogelsby JW. Dislocation of the AC joint, an end result study. *J Bone Joint Surg Am.* 1987;69:1045.

113. Takeda Y, Kashiwguchi S, Endo K, Matsuura T, Sasa T. The most effective exercise for strengthening the supraspinatus muscle. *Am J Sports Med.* 2002;30:374-381.

114. Thein L. Impingement syndrome and its conservative management. *J Orthop Sports Phys Ther.* 1989;11(5):183-191.

115. Thomopoulos S, Williams GR, Soslowsky LJ. Tendon to bone healing: differences in biomechanical, structural, and compositional properties due to a range of activity levels. *J Biomech Eng.* 2003;125:106-113.

116. Thompson WO, Debski RE, Boardman ND, et al. A biomechanical analysis of rotator cuff deficiency in a cadaveric model. *Am J Sports Med.* 1996;24:286-292.

117. Townsend H, Jobe F, Pink M. EMG analysis of the glenohumeral muscles during a baseball rehabilitation program. *Am J Sports Med.* 1991;19(3):264-272.

118. Travell JG, Simons GD. *Myofascial Pain and Dysfunction: The Trigger Point Manual.* Baltimore, MD: Williams & Wilkins; 1983.

119. Tsai NT, McClure PW, Karduna AR. Effects of muscle fatigue on 3-dimensional scapular kinematics. *Arch Phys Med Rehabil.* 2003;84(7):1000-1005.

120. Uthoff H, Loeher J, Sarkar K. The pathogenesis of rotator cuff tears. In: Takagishi N, ed. *The Shoulder.* Philadelphia, PA: Professional Post Graduate Services; 1987.

121. Von Eisenhart-Rothe R, Jager A, Englmeier K, Vogl TJ, Graichen H. Relevance of arm position and muscle activity in three-dimensional glenohumeral translation in patients with traumatic and atraumatic shoulder instability. *Am J Sports Med.* 2002;30:514-522.

122. Warner JJ, Micheli LJ, Arslanian LE, Kennedy J, Kennedy R. Scapulothoracic motion in normal shoulders and shoulders with glenohumeral instability and impingement syndrome: a study using moire topographic analysis. *Clin Orthop.* 1992;(285):191-199.

123. Warner J, Michili L, Arslanin L. Patterns of flexibility, laxity, and strength in normal shoulders and shoulders with instability and impingement. *Am J Sports Med.* 1990;17(4):366-375.

124. Warren RF. Neurological injuries in football. In: Jordan BD, Tsiaris P, Warren FR, eds. *Sports Neurology.* Rockville, MD: Aspen; 1989.

125. Weiser WM, Lee TQ, McMaster WC, McMahon PJ. Effects of simulated scapular protraction on anterior glenohumeral stability. *Am J Sports Med.* 1999;27(6):801-805.

126. Wilk K, Andrews J. Rehabilitation following subacromial decompression. *Orthopedics.* 1993;16(3):349-358.

127. Wilk K, Arrigo C. An integrated approach to upper extremity exercises. *Orthop Phys Ther Clin N Am.* 1992;9(2):337-360.

128. Wilk K, Arrigo C. Current concepts in the rehabilitation of the athletic shoulder. *J Orthop Sports Phys Ther.* 1993;18(1):365-378.

129. Wilk K, Arrigo C. Current concepts in rehabilitation of the shoulder. In: Andrews J, Wilk K, eds. *The Athlete's Shoulder.* New York, NY: Churchill Livingstone; 1993.

130. Wilk KE, Arrigo CA, Andrews JR. Current concepts: the stabilizing structures of the glenohumeral joint. *J Orthop Sports Phys Ther.* 1997;25:364-379.

131. Wilk KE, Reinhold MM, Dugas JR, Andrews JR. Rehabilitation following thermal-assisted capsular shrinkage of the glenohumeral joint: current concepts. *J Orthop Sports Phys Ther.* 2002;32(6):268-287.

132. Wilk K, Voight M, Kearns M. Stretch shortening drills for the upper extremity: theory and application. *J Orthop Sports Phys Ther.* 1993;17(5):225-239.

Videos are available at www.accessphysiotherapy.com. Subscription is required.

21

Rehabilitation of the Elbow

Todd S. Ellenbecker, Tad E. Pieczynski, and David Carfagno

OBJECTIVES

After completion of this chapter, the physical therapist should be able to do the following:

- Discuss the functional anatomy and biomechanics associated with normal function of the elbow.
- Identify the various techniques for regaining range of motion including stretching exercises and joint mobilizations.
- Perform specific clinical tests to identify ligamentous laxity and tendon pathology in the injured elbow.
- Discuss criteria for progression of the rehabilitation program for different elbow injuries.
- Demonstrate the various rehabilitative strengthening techniques for the elbow, including open- and closed-kinetic chain isometric, isotonic, plyometric, isokinetic, and functional exercises.

Treatment of elbow injuries in active individuals requires an understanding of the mechanism of injury and the anatomy and biomechanics of the human elbow and upper-extremity kinetic chain, as well as a structured and detailed clinical examination to identify the structure or structures involved. Treatment of the injured elbow of both a younger adolescent patient and an older active patient requires this same approach. This approach consists of understanding the specific anatomical vulnerabilities present in the young athletes' elbow, as well as the effects of years of repetitive stress and the clinical ramifications these stresses produce in the aging elbow joint. An overview of the most common elbow injuries, as well as a review of the musculoskeletal adaptations of the elbow, will provide a platform for the discussion of examination and most specifically treatment concepts for patients with elbow injury. The important interplay between the elbow and shoulder joints in the upper-extremity kinetic chain is highlighted throughout this chapter in order to support comprehensive examination and intervention strategies, as well as the total-arm strength treatment concept.

Functional Anatomy and Biomechanics

Anatomically, the elbow joint comprises 3 joints. The humeroulnar joint, humeroradial joint, and the proximal radioulnar joint are the articulations that make up the elbow complex (Figure 21-1). The elbow allows for flexion, extension, pronation, and supination movement patterns about the joint complex. The bony limitations, ligamentous support, and muscular stability help to protect it from vulnerability of overuse and resultant injury.

The elbow complex comprises 3 bones: the distal humerus, proximal ulna, and proximal radius. The articulations among these 3 bones dictate elbow movement patterns.[125] It is also important to mention that the appropriate strength and function of the upper quarter (defined as the cervical spine to the hand, including the scapulothoracic joint) need to be addressed when evaluating the elbow specifically. The elbow complex has an intricate mechanical articulation between the 3 separate joints of the upper quarter in order to allow for function.

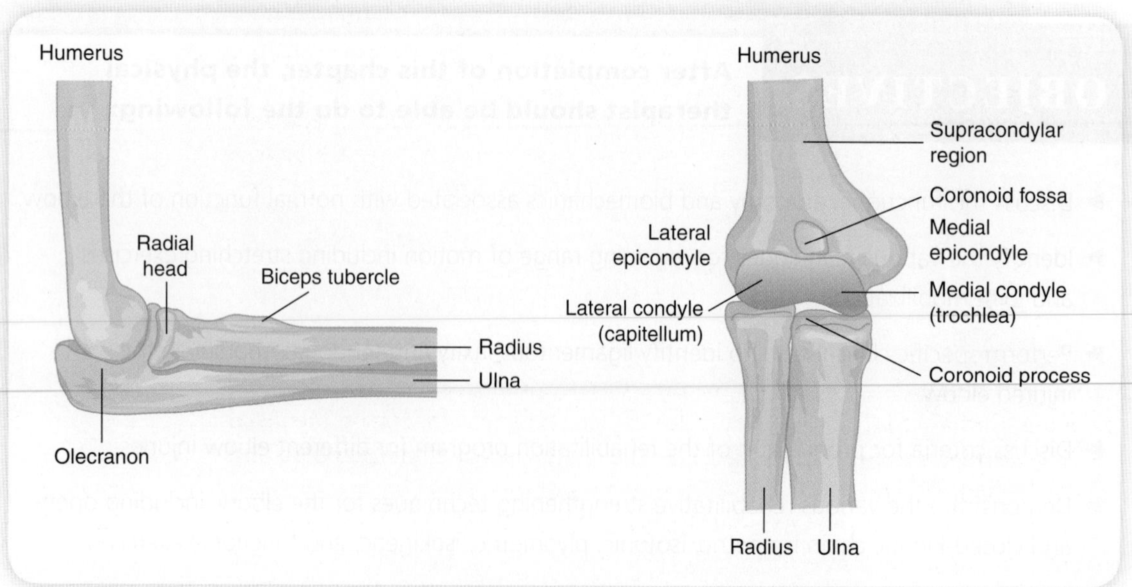

Figure 21-1 **Articulations of the elbow joint complex**

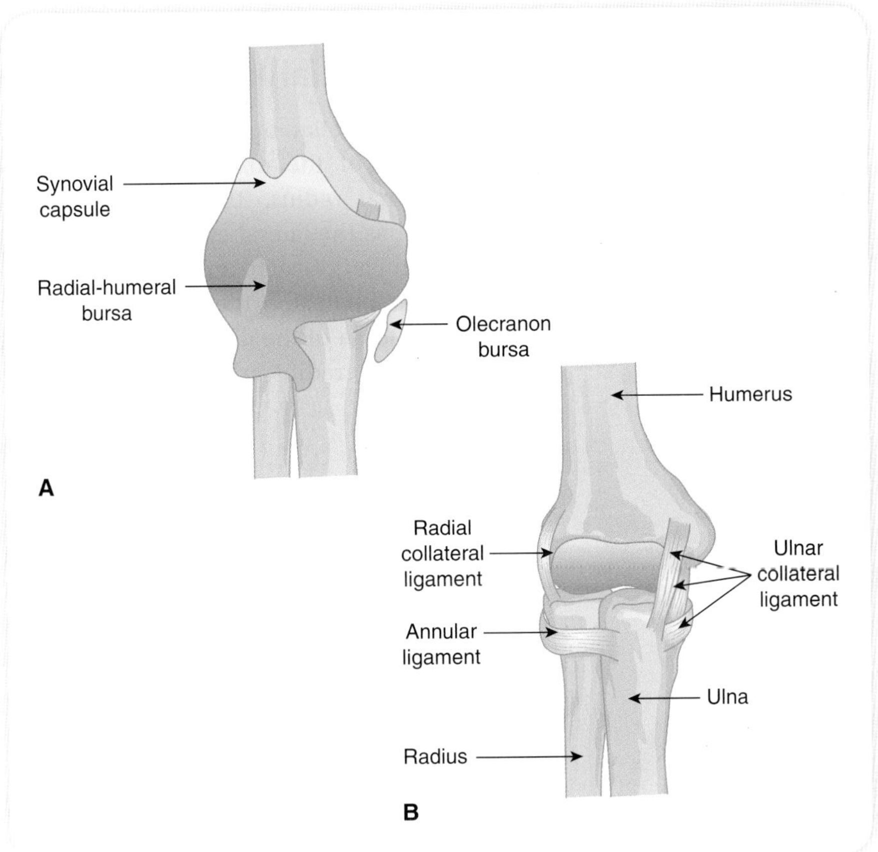

Figure 21-2

A. Elbow joint capsule. **B.** Medial ulnar collateral ligament complex.

In the elbow, the joint capsule plays an important role. The capsule is continuous (Figure 21-2*A*) among the 3 articulations and highly innervated.[87,92] This is important not only for support of the elbow joint complex but also for proprioception of the joint. The capsule of the elbow functions as a neurologic link between the shoulder and the hand within the upper-extremity kinetic chain. Therefore, function of the capsule has an effect on upper-quarter activity and is an obvious important consideration during the rehabilitation process, if injury does occur.

Humeroulnar Joint

The humeroulnar joint is the articulation between the distal humerus medially and the proximal ulna. The humerus has distinct features distally. The medial aspect has the medial epicondyle and an hourglass-shaped trochlea, located anteromedial on the distal humerus.[2,53] The trochlea extends more distal than the lateral aspect of the humerus. The trochlea articulates with the trochlear notch of the proximal ulna.

Because of the more distal projection of the humerus medially, the elbow complex demonstrates a carrying angle that is essentially an abducted position of the elbow in the anatomic position. The normal carrying angle (Figure 21-3) is 10 to 15 degrees in females and 5 degrees in males.[7]

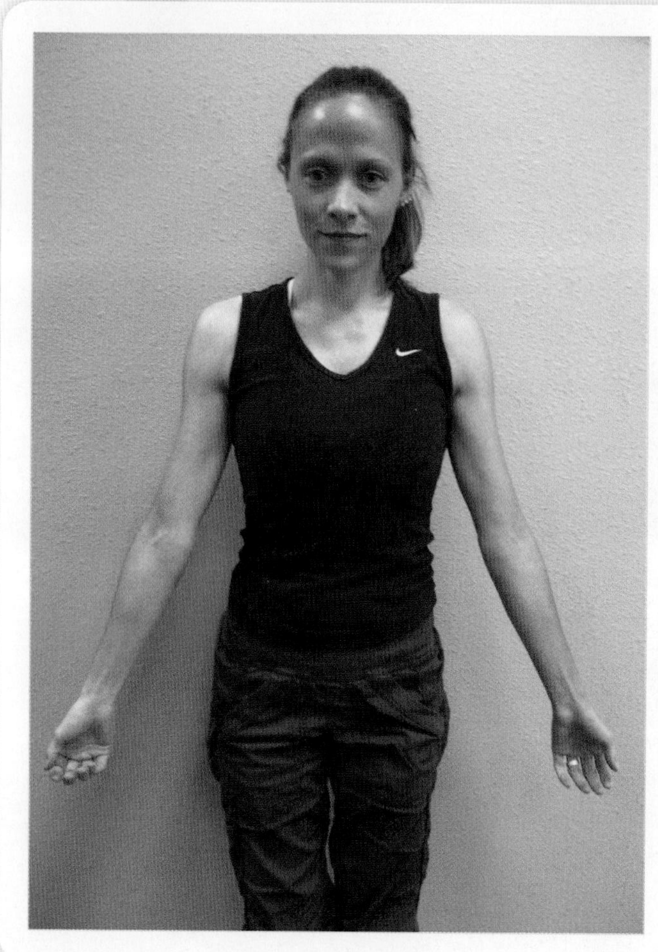

Figure 21-3 Carrying angle of the human elbow

Radiocapitellar Joint (Humeroradial Joint)

The radiocapitellar or humeroradial joint is the articulation of the distal lateral humerus and the proximal radius. The lateral aspect of the humerus has the lateral epicondyle and the capitellum, which is located anterolateral on the distal humerus. With flexion, the radius is in contact with the radial fossa of the distal humerus, whereas in extension, the radius and the humerus are not in contact.

Proximal Radioulnar Joint

The proximal radioulnar joint is the articulation between the radial notch of the proximal lateral aspect of the ulna, the radial head, and the capitellum of the distal humerus. The proximal and distal radioulnar joints are important for supination and pronation. Proximally, the radius articulates with the ulna by the support of the annular ligament, which attaches to the ulnar notch anteriorly and posteriorly. This ligament circles the radial head and adds support. The interosseous membrane is the connective tissue that functions to complete the interval between the 2 bones. When there is a fall on the outstretched arm, the interosseous membrane can shift forces off the radius—the main weightbearing bone of the forearm—to the ulna. This prevents the radial head from having forceful contact with the capitellum. Distally, the concave radius articulates with the convex ulna. With supination and pronation, the radius moves on the more stationary ulna.

Ligamentous Structures

The stability of the elbow starts with the joint capsule and excellent bony congruity inherent to the three articulations of the human elbow. The capsule is loose anteriorly and posteriorly to allow for movement in flexion and extension.[131] The joint capsule is taut medially and laterally as a result of the added support of the collateral ligaments.

The medial (ulnar) collateral ligament (MUCL) is fan shaped in nature and has 3 bands (see Figure 21-2*B*). The anterior band of the MUCL is the primary stabilizer of the elbow against valgus loads when the elbow is near extension.[131] The posterior band of the MUCL becomes taut after 60 degrees of elbow flexion and assists in stabilizing against valgus stress when the elbow is in a flexed position. The oblique band of the MUCL does not technically cross the elbow joint and this does not provide extensive stabilization to the medial elbow like the anterior and posterior bands.

The lateral elbow complex consists of 4 structures. The radial collateral ligament attachments are from the lateral epicondyle to the annular ligament. The lateral ulnar collateral ligament is the primary lateral stabilizer and passes over the annular ligament into the supinator tubercle. It reinforces the elbow laterally, as well as re-enforcing the humeroradial joint.[103,131] The accessory lateral collateral ligament passes from the supinator tubercle into the annular ligament. The annular ligament is the main support of the radial head in the radial notch of the ulna. The interosseous membrane is a syndesmotic tissue that connects the ulna and the radius in the forearm.

Dynamic Stabilizers of the Elbow Complex

The elbow flexors are the biceps brachii, brachialis, and brachioradialis muscles (Figure 21-4). The biceps brachii originates via 2 heads proximally at the shoulder: the long head from the supraglenoid tuberosity of the scapula, and the short head from the coracoid process of the scapula. The insertion is achieved by a common tendon at the radial tuberosity and lacertus fibrosis to origins of the forearm flexors. The functions of the biceps brachii are flexion of the elbow and supination the forearm.[136] The brachialis originates from the lower two-thirds of the anterior humerus and inserts on the coronoid process and tuberosity of the ulna. It functions to flex the elbow. The brachioradialis, which originates from the lower two-thirds of the lateral humerus and attaches to the lateral styloid process of the distal radius, functions as an elbow flexor as well as a weak pronator and supinator of the forearm.

The elbow extensors are the triceps brachii and the anconeus muscles. The triceps brachii has long, medial, and lateral heads. The long head originates at the infraglenoid tuberosity of the scapula, the lateral and medial heads to the posterior aspect of the humerus. The insertion is via the common tendon posteriorly at the olecranon. Through this insertion along with the anconeus muscle that assists the triceps, extension of the elbow complex is accomplished.

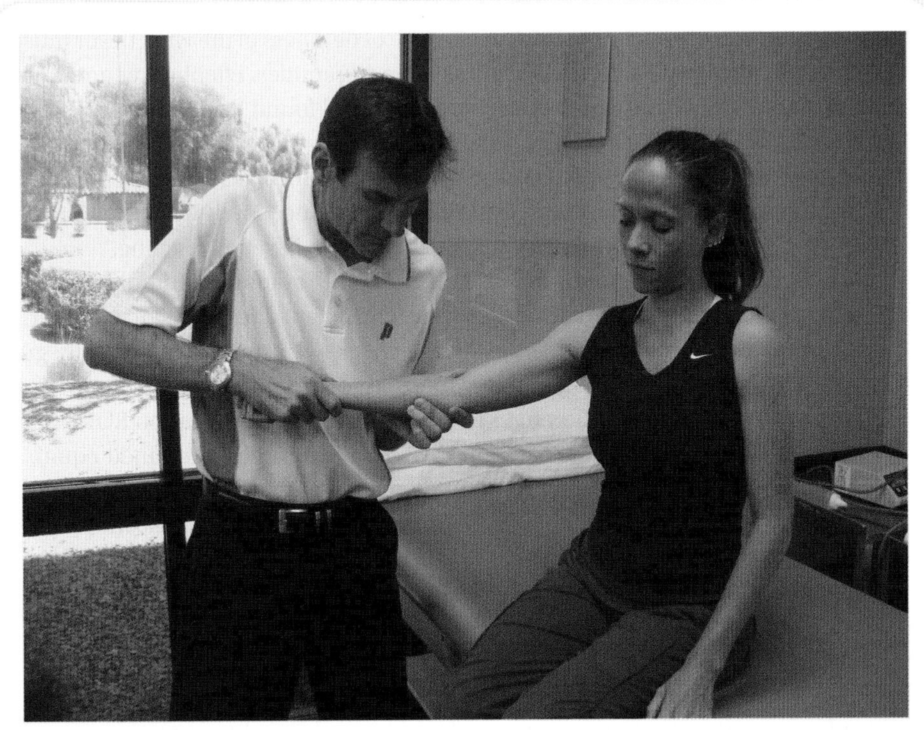

Figure 21-4 **Valgus stress test to evaluate the medial ulnar collateral ligament complex**

Clinical Examination of the Elbow

Although it is beyond the scope of this chapter to describe a complete elbow examination, several important components necessary in the comprehensive examination of the athletes elbow are discussed. Structural inspection of the athletes elbow must include a complete and thorough inspection of the entire upper extremity and trunk, because of the reliance of the entire upper-extremity kinetic chain on the core for power generation and force attenuation during functional activities.[37] Adaptive changes are commonly encountered during clinical examination of the athletic elbow, particularly in the unilaterally dominant upper-extremity athlete. In these athletes, use of the contralateral extremity as a baseline is particularly important to determine the degree of actual adaptation that may be a contributing factor in the patient's injury presentation.

Anatomical adaptation of the athlete's elbow can be categorized into 4 main categories for the purpose of this chapter. These include range of motion (ROM), osseous, ligamentous, and muscular. Each is presented in the context of the clinical examination of the patient with elbow dysfunction.

Range of Motion Adaptations

King et al[77] initially reported on elbow ROM in professional baseball pitchers. Fifty percent of the pitchers they examined were found to have a flexion contracture of the dominant elbow with 30% of subjects demonstrating a cubitus valgus deformity. Chinn et al[21] measured world-class professional adult tennis players and reported significant elbow flexion contractures on the dominant arm, but no presence of a cubitus valgus deformity.

More recently, Ellenbecker et al[38] measured elbow extension in a population of 40 healthy professional baseball pitchers and found flexion contractures averaging 5 degrees. Directly related to elbow function was wrist flexibility, which Ellenbecker et al[38] reported as significantly less in extension on the dominant arm because of tightness of the wrist flexor musculature, with no difference in wrist flexion ROM between extremities. Ellenbecker and Roetert[41] measured senior tennis players age 55 years and older and found flexion contractures averaging 10 degrees in the dominant elbow, as well as significantly less wrist flexion ROM. The higher utilization of the wrist extensor musculature is likely the cause of limited wrist flexor ROM among the senior tennis players, as opposed to the reduced wrist extension ROM seen from excessive overuse of the wrist flexor muscles inherent in baseball pitching.[47,112]

More proximally, measurement of ROM of humeral rotation in the older overhead athlete is also recommended. Several studies show consistent alterations of shoulder rotational ROM in the overhead athlete.[42,75,114] Ellenbecker et al[42] showed statistically greater dominant-shoulder external rotation and less internal rotation in a sample of professional baseball pitchers. Despite these differences in internal and external rotation ROM, the total rotation (internal rotation + external rotation) between extremities remained equal, such that any increases in external rotation ROM were matched by decreases in internal rotation ROM in this uninjured population. Elite level tennis players had significantly less internal rotation and no significant difference in external rotation on the dominant arm, and an overall decrease in total rotation ROM on the dominant arm of approximately 10 degrees. Careful monitoring of glenohumeral joint ROM is recommended for the athlete with an elbow injury.

Based on the findings of these descriptive profiles, the finding of an elbow flexion contracture and limited wrist flexion or extension ROM, as well as reduced glenohumeral joint internal rotation, can be expected during the examination of the older athlete who performs a unilateral upper-extremity sport. Careful measurement during the clinical examination is recommended to determine baseline levels of ROM loss in the distal upper extremity.

This careful measurement serves to determine if rehabilitative interventions are needed as well as to assess progress during rehabilitation.

Osseous Adaptation

In a study by Priest et al,[108] 84 world-ranked tennis players were studied using radiography, and an average of 6.5 bony changes were found on the dominant elbow of each player. Additionally, they reported twice as many bony adaptations, such as spurs, on the medial aspect of the elbow as compared to the lateral aspect. The coronoid process of the ulna was the number 1 site of osseous adaptation or spurring. An average of 44% increase in thickness of the anterior humeral cortex was found on the dominant arm of these players, with an 11% increase in cortical thickness reported in the radius of the dominant tennis playing extremity.

Additionally, in an MRI study, Waslewski et al[137] found osteophytes at the proximal or distal insertion of the ulnar collateral ligament in 5 of 20 asymptomatic professional baseball pitchers, as well as posterior osteophytes in 2 of 20 pitchers.

Ligamentous Laxity

Manual clinical examination of the human elbow to assess medial and lateral laxity can be challenging, given the presence of humeral rotation and small increases in joint opening that often present with ulnar collateral ligament injury. Ellenbecker et al[38] measured medial elbow joint laxity in 40 asymptomatic professional baseball pitchers to determine if bilateral differences in medial elbow laxity exist in healthy pitchers with a long history of repetitive overuse to the medial aspect of the elbow. A Telos stress radiography device was used to assess medial elbow joint opening, using a standardized valgus stress of 15 daN (kPa) with the elbow placed in 25 degrees of elbow flexion and the forearm supinated. The joint space between the medial epicondyle and coronoid process of the ulna was measured using anterior-posterior radiographs by a musculoskeletal radiologist and compared bilaterally, with and without the application of the valgus stress. Results showed significant differences between extremities with stress application, with the dominant elbow opening 1.20 mm, and the nondominant elbow opening 0.88 mm. This difference, although statistically significant, averaged 0.32 mm between the dominant and nondominant elbow and would be virtually unidentifiable with manual assessment. Previous research by Rijke et al[113] using stress radiography identified a critical level of 0.5-mm increase in medial elbow joint opening in elbows with ulnar collateral ligament injury. Thus, the results of the study by Ellenbecker et al[38] do support this 0.5-mm critical level, as asymptomatic professional pitchers in their study exhibited less than this 0.5 mm of medial elbow joint laxity.

Muscular Adaptations

Several methods can be used to measure upper-extremity strength in athletic populations. These can range from measuring grip strength with a grip strength dynamometer to the use of isokinetic dynamometers to measure specific joint motions and muscular parameters. Increased forearm circumference was measured on the dominant forearm in world-class tennis players,[21] as well as in the dominant forearm of senior tennis players.[80]

Isometric grip strength dynamometer measurements in elite adult and senior tennis players demonstrated unilateral increases in strength. Increases ranging from 10% to 30% have been reported using standardized measurement methods.[21,34,37,80]

Isokinetic dynamometers have been used to measure specific muscular performance parameters in elite-level tennis players and baseball pitchers.[34,37,39,40] Specific patterns of unilateral muscular development have been identified by reviewing the isokinetic literature from different populations of overhead athletes. Ellenbecker[34] measured isokinetic wrist and forearm strength in mature adult tennis players who were highly skilled, and found 10% to 25% greater wrist flexion and extension as well as forearm pronation strength on the dominant extremity as compared to the non-dominant extremity. Additionally, no significant difference between extremities in forearm supination strength was measured. No significant difference between extremities was found in elbow flexion strength in elite tennis players, but dominant arm elbow extension strength was significantly stronger than the non–tennis-playing extremity.[39]

Research on professional throwing athletes has identified significantly greater wrist flexion and forearm pronation strength on the dominant arm by as much as 15% to 35% when compared to the nondominant extremity,[37] with no difference in wrist extension strength or forearm supination strength between extremities. Wilk, Arrigo, and Andrews[139] reported 10% to 20% greater elbow flexion strength in professional baseball pitchers on the dominant arm, as well as 5% to 15% greater elbow extension strength as compared to the nondominant extremity.

These data help to portray the chronic muscular adaptations that can be present in the senior athlete who may present with elbow injury, as well as help to determine realistic and accurate discharge strength levels following rehabilitation. Failure to return the dominant extremity-stabilizing musculature to its preinjury status (10% to as much as 35% greater than the nondominant) in these athletes may represent an incomplete rehabilitation and prohibit the return to full activity.

Clinical Examination Methods

In addition to the examination methods outlined in the previous section, including accurate measurement of both distal and proximal joint ROM, radiographic screening, and muscular strength assessment, several other tests should be included in the comprehensive examination of the elbow of the older active patient. Although it is beyond the scope of this chapter to completely review all of the necessary tests, several are highlighted based on their overall importance. The reader is referred to Morrey[92] and Ellenbecker and Mattalino[37] for more complete chapters solely on examination of the elbow.

Clinical testing of the joints proximal and distal to the elbow allows the examiner to rule out referred symptoms and ensure that elbow pain is from a local musculoskeletal origin. Overpressure of the cervical spine in the motions of flexion/extension and lateral flexion/rotation, as well as quadrant or Spurling test combining extension with ipsilateral lateral flexion and rotation, are commonly used to clear the cervical spine and rule out radicular symptoms.[50]

Additionally, clearing the glenohumeral joint, and determining whether concomitant impingement or instability is present, is also highly recommended.[37] Use of the sulcus sign[88] to determine the presence of multidirectional instability of the glenohumeral joint, along with the subluxation/relocation sign[67] and load and shift test, can provide valuable insight into the status of the glenohumeral joint. The impingement signs of Neer[94] and Hawkins and Kennedy[57] are also helpful to rule out proximal tendon pathology.

In addition to the clearing tests for the glenohumeral joint, full inspection of the scapulothoracic joint is recommended. Removal of the patient's shirt or examination of the patient in a gown with full exposure of the upper back is highly recommended. Kibler et al[76] has recently presented a classification system for scapular pathology. Careful observation of the patient at rest and with the hands placed upon the hips, as well as during active overhead movements, is recommended to identify prominence of particular borders of the scapula, as well as a lack of close association with the thoracic wall during movement.[73,74] Bilateral comparison provides the primary basis for identifying scapular pathology; however, in many athletes, bilateral scapular pathology can be observed.

The presence of overuse injuries in the elbow occurring with proximal injury to the shoulder complex or with scapulothoracic dysfunction is widely reported,[33,37,92,95,96] and thus a thorough inspection of the proximal joint is extremely important in the comprehensive management of elbow pathology.

Elbow Joint: Special Tests

Several tests specific for the elbow should be performed to assist in the diagnosis of elbow dysfunction. These include the Tinel test, varus and valgus stress tests, the milking test, valgus extension overpressure test, bounce home test, and provocation tests. The Tinel test involves tapping of the ulnar nerve in the medial region of the elbow over the cubital tunnel retinaculum. Reproduction of paresthesia or tingling along the distal course of the ulnar nerve indicates irritability of the ulnar nerve.[92]

The valgus stress test (see Figure 21-4) is used to evaluate the integrity of the ulnar collateral ligament. The position used for testing the anterior band of the ulnar collateral ligament is characterized by 15 to 25 degrees of elbow flexion and forearm supination. The elbow flexion position is used to unlock the olecranon from the olecranon fossa and decreases the stability provided by the osseous congruity of the joint. This places a greater relative stress on the medial ulnar collateral ligament.[93] Reproduction of medial elbow pain, in addition to unilateral increases in ulnohumeral joint laxity, indicates a positive test. Grading the test is typically performed using the American Academy of Orthopedic Surgeons guidelines of 0 to 5 mm grade I, 5 to 10 mm grade II, and greater than 10 mm grade III.[38] Performing the test using a position of greater than 25 degrees of elbow flexion will increase the amount of humeral rotation during performance of the valgus stress test and lead to misleading information to the clinician's hands. The test is typically performed with the shoulder in the scapular plane, but can be performed with the shoulder in the coronal plane, to minimize compensatory movements at the shoulder during testing. The milking sign is a test the patient performs on himself, with the elbow held in approximately 90 degrees of flexion. By reaching under the involved elbow with the contralateral extremity, the patient grasps the thumb of their injured extremity and pulls in a lateral direction, thus imposing a valgus stress to the flexed elbow. Some patients may not have enough flexibility to perform this maneuver, and a valgus stress can be imparted by the examiner to mimic this movement, which stresses the posterior band of the ulnar collateral ligament.[93]

The varus stress test is performed using similar degrees of elbow flexion and shoulder and forearm positioning. This test assesses the integrity of the lateral ulnar collateral ligament, and should be performed along with the valgus stress test, to completely evaluate the medial/lateral stability of the ulnohumeral joint.

The valgus extension overpressure test has been reported by Andrews et al[7] to determine whether posterior elbow pain is caused by a posteromedial osteophyte abutting the medial margin of the trochlea and the olecranon fossa. This test is performed by passively extending the elbow while maintaining a valgus stress to it. This test is meant to simulate the stresses imparted to the posterior medial part of the elbow during the acceleration phase of the throwing or serving motion. Reproduction of pain in the posteromedial aspect of the elbow indicates a positive test.

Finally, the moving valgus test described by O'Driscoll et al[101] has been recommended to provide a stress to the ulnar collateral ligament and identify ulnar collateral ligament injury. This test is performed with the patient in a seated position with the shoulder abducted 90 degrees in the coronal plane to simulate the throwing motion. The elbow is then flexed to 120 degrees while an external rotation force is maintained by the examiner. This external rotation force creates a valgus load at the elbow. The elbow is then moved from 120 degrees of flexion to 70 degrees of elbow flexion. A positive test involves recreation of medial elbow pain in what has been termed the "shear zone" between 120 and 70 degrees.

This test has resulted in a specificity of 75% and sensitivity of 100% when tested against an arthroscopic evaluation the MUCL. This test can used to determine the integrity of the ulnar collateral ligament in the throwing athlete with medial elbow pain.

The use of provocation tests can be applied when screening the muscle tendon units of the elbow. Provocation tests consist of manual muscle tests to determine pain reproduction. The specific tests, used to screen the elbow joint of a patient with suspected elbow pathology, include wrist and finger flexion and extension as well as forearm pronation and supination.[33] These tests can be used to provoke the muscle tendon unit at the lateral or medial epicondyle. Testing of the elbow at or near full extension can often recreate localized lateral or medial elbow pain secondary to tendon degeneration.[79] Reproduction of lateral or medial elbow pain with resistive muscle testing (provocation testing) may indicate concomitant tendon injury at the elbow and directs the clinician to perform a more complete elbow examination.

Rehabilitation Techniques for Specific Injuries

Overuse injuries constitute the majority of elbow injuries sustained by the athletic elbow patient, with one of the most common being humeral epicondylitis.[37,98] Repetitive overuse is one of the primary etiologic factors evident in the history of most patients with elbow dysfunction. Epidemiologic research on adult tennis players reports incidences of humeral epicondylitis ranging from 35% to 50%.[20,55,71,78,109] The incidence reported in elite junior players is significantly less (11% to 12%).[143]

Pathomechanics

Etiology of Humeral Epicondylitis

Reported in the literature as early as 1873 by Runge,[117] humeral epicondylitis or "tennis elbow," as it is more popularly known, has been studied extensively by many authors. Cyriax, in 1936, listed 26 causes of tennis elbow,[25] while an extensive study of this overuse disorder by Goldie, in 1964, reported hypervascularization of the extensor aponeurosis and an increased quantity of free nerve endings in the subtendinous space.[48] More recently, Leadbetter[84] described humeral epicondylitis as a degenerative condition consisting of a time-dependent process that includes vascular, chemical, and cellular events that lead to a failure of the cell-matrix healing response in human tendon. This description of tendon injury differs from earlier theories where an inflammatory response was considered as a primary factor; hence Leadbetter[84] and Nirschl[96] used the term "tendinosis" as opposed to the original term of "tendonitis."

Nirschl[95,96] has defined humeral epicondylitis as an extraarticular tendinous injury characterized by excessive vascular granulation and an impaired healing response in the tendon, which he has termed "angiofibroblastic hyperplasia." In the most recent and thorough histopathologic analysis, Nirschl et al[79] studied specimens of injured tendon obtained from areas of chronic overuse and reported that these specimens did not contain large numbers of lymphocytes, macrophages, and neutrophils. Instead, tendinosis appears to be a degenerative process characterized by large populations of fibroblasts, disorganized collagen, and vascular hyperplasia.[79] It is not clear why tendinosis is painful, given the lack of inflammatory cells, and it is also unknown why the collagen does not mature or heal typically.

Structures Involved in Humeral Epicondylitis

Nirschl[96] described the primary structure involved in lateral humeral epicondylitis as the tendon of the extensor carpi radialis brevis. Approximately one-third of cases involve the tendon of the extensor digitorum communis.[79] Additionally, the extensor carpi radialis longus and extensor carpi ulnaris can be involved as well. The primary site of medial humeral epicondylitis is the flexor carpi radialis, followed by the pronator teres, and flexor carpi ulnaris tendons.[95,96]

Recent research describes in detail the anatomy of the lateral epicondylar region.[18,51] The specific location of the extensor carpi radialis brevis tendon lies inferior to the tendinous origin of the extensor carpi radialis longus, which can be palpated along the anterior surface of the supracondylar ridge just proximal or cephalad to the extensor carpi radialis brevis tendon on the lateral epicondyle.[18] Greenbaum et al[51] describe the pyramidal slope or shape of the lateral epicondyle and explain how both the extensor carpi radialis brevis and the extensor communis originate from the entire anterior surface of the lateral epicondyle. These specific relationships are important for the clinician to bear in mind when palpating for the region of maximal tenderness during the clinical examination process. Although detailed recent reports are not present in the literature regarding the medial epicondyle, careful palpation can be used to discriminate between the muscle tendon junctions of the pronator teres and flexor carpi radialis. Additionally, palpation of the MUCL, which originates from nearly the entire inferior surface of the medial epicondyle and inserts into the anterior medial aspect of the coronoid process of the ulna, should be performed. Understanding the involved structures, as well as a detailed knowledge of the exact locations where these structures can be palpated, can assist the clinician in better localizing the painful tendon or tendons involved.

Dijs et al[30] studied 70 patients with lateral epicondylitis. They reported the area of maximal involvement in these cases: the extensor carpi radialis longus in only 1% and the extensor carpi radialis brevis in 90%. The body of the extensor carpi radialis tendon was implicated in 1% of cases, and 8% were at the muscle tendon junction over the most proximal part of the muscle of the extensor carpi radialis brevis.

Epidemiology of Humeral Epicondylitis

Nirschl[95,96] reports that the incidence of lateral humeral epicondylitis is far greater than that of medial epicondylitis in recreational tennis players and in the leading arm of golfers (left arm in a right-handed golfer). Medial humeral epicondylitis is far more common in elite tennis players and throwing athletes, as a result of the powerful loading of the flexor and pronator muscle tendon units during the valgus extension overload inherent in the acceleration phase of those overhead movement patterns. Additionally, the trailing arm of the golfer (right arm in a right-handed golfer) is more likely to have medial symptoms than lateral.

Rehabilitation Progression: Humeral Epicondylitis

Following the detailed examination, a detailed rehabilitation program can commence. Three main stages of rehabilitation can conceptually be applied for the patient: protected function, total-arm strength, and the return to activity phase. Each is discussed in greater detail in this section of the chapter with specific highlights on the therapeutic exercises utilized during each stage of the rehabilitation process.

Protected Function Phase

During this first phase in the rehabilitation process, care is taken to protect the injured muscle tendon unit from stress, but not function. Nirschl[95,96] cautions against the use of an immobilizer or sling because of further atrophy of the musculature and negative effects on the upper-extremity kinetic chain. Protection of the patient from offending activities is recommended, with cessation of throwing and serving suggested for medial-based humeral symptoms. Allowing the patient to bat or hit 200 backhands allows for continued activity while minimizing stress to the injured area. Very often however, sport activity must cease entirely to allow the muscle tendon unit time to heal and to most importantly allow formal rehabilitation to progress. Continued work or sport performance can severely slow the progression of resistive exercise and other long-term treatments in physical therapy.

Use of modalities may be helpful during this time period; however, agreement on a clearly superior modality or sequence of modalities has not been substantiated in the literature.[18,82] A metaanalysis of 185 studies on treatment of humeral epicondylitis showed glaring deficits in the scientific quality of the investigations, with no significantly superior treatment approach identified. Although many modalities or sequences of modalities have anecdotally produced superior results, there is a great need for prospective, randomized, controlled clinical trials in order to identify optimal methods for intervention. Modalities such as ultrasound,[13,98] electrical stimulation and ice, cortisone injection,[71,98] nonsteroidal antiinflammatory drugs,[115] acupuncture,[19] transverse friction massage,[61] and dimethyl sulfoxide application[106] have all been reported to provide varying levels of relief in the literature. Boyer and Hastings,[18] in a comprehensive review of the treatment of humeral epicondylitis, reported no significant difference with the use of low-energy laser, acupuncture, extracorporeal shockwave therapy, or steroid injection.

The use of cortisone injection has been widely reported in the literature during the pain reduction phase of treatment of this often-recalcitrant condition. Dijs et al[30] compared the effects of traditional physical therapy and cortisone injection in 70 patients diagnosed with humeral epicondylitis. In their research, 91% of patients who received the cortisone injection received initial relief, as compared with 47% who reported relief from undergoing physical therapy. After only 3 months the recurrence rate (of primary symptoms) in their subjects, however, was 51% in the cortisone injection group, and only 5% in the physical therapy group. Similar findings were reported in a study by Verhaar et al[135] comparing physical therapy, consisting of Mills manipulation and cross-friction massage, with corticosteroid injection in a prospective, randomized, controlled clinical trial in 106 patients with humeral epicondylitis. At 6 weeks, 22 of 53 subjects reported complete relief from the cortisone injection, whereas only 3 subjects had complete relief from this type of physical therapy treatment. At 1 year, there were no differences between treatment groups regarding the course of treatment. These results show the short-term benefit from the corticosteroid injection, as well as the ineffectiveness of physical therapy using manipulation and cross-friction massage.

Several recent studies deserve further discussion as they also can be used to direct clinicians in the development of appropriate interventions. Nirschl et al[97] studied the effects of iontophoresis with dexamethasone in 199 patients with humeral epicondylitis. Results showed that 52% of the subjects in the treatment group reported overall improvement on the investigators' improvement index, with only 33% of the placebo group reporting improvement 2 days after the series of treatments with iontophoresis. One month following the treatment, there was no statistical difference in the overall improvement in the patients in the treatment group versus the control group. One additional finding from this study that has clinical relevance was the presence of greater pain relief in the group that underwent 6 treatments in a 10-day period, as opposed to subjects in the treatment group who underwent treatment over a longer period of time. Although this study does support the use of iontophoresis with dexamethasone, it does not report substantial benefits during follow-up.

Haake et al[54] studied the effects of extracorporeal shock wave therapy in 272 patients with humeral epicondylitis in a multicenter prospective randomized control study. They reported that extracorporeal shock wave therapy was ineffective in the treatment of humeral epicondylitis. Similarly, Basford et al[10] used low-intensity Nd:YAG laser irradiation at 7 points along the forearm 3 times a week for 4 weeks and reported it to be ineffective in the treatment of lateral humeral epicondylitis.

Based on this review of the literature, it appears that no standardized modality or modality sequence has been identified that is clearly statistically more effective than any other at the present time. Clinical reviews by Nirschl[95,96] and Ellenbecker and Mattalino[37] advocate the use of multiple modalities, such as electrical stimulation and ultrasound, as well as iontophoresis with dexamethasone, in order to assist in pain reduction and encourage local increases in blood flow. The copious use of ice or cryotherapy following increases in daily activity is also recommended. The use of therapeutic modalities with cortisone injection, if needed, can only be seen as one part of the treatment sequence, with increasing evidence being generated favoring progressive resistive exercise.

Exercise is one of the most powerful modalities used in rehabilitative medicine. Research shows increases in local blood flow following isometric contractions at levels as submaximal as 5% to 50% of maximum voluntary contraction both during the contraction and for periods of up to 1 minute postcontraction.[65] Two studies showed superior results in the treatment of humeral epicondylitis using progressive resistive exercise as compared with ultrasound.[46] In a study by Svernl and Adolffson,[127] 38 patients with lateral humeral epicondylitis were randomly assigned to a contract relax stretching or eccentric exercise treatment group. Result of this study showed a 71% report of full recovery in the eccentric exercise group, as compared to the group that performed contract-relax stretching, which only found 39% of the subjects rating themselves as fully recovered. These studies support the heavy reliance on the successful application of progressive resistive exercise, with an eccentric component, in the treatment of humeral epicondylitis.

Total-Arm Strength Rehabilitation

Early application of resistive exercise for the treatment of humeral epicondylitis focuses on the important principle that states that "proximal stability is needed to promote distal mobility."[126] The initial application of resistive exercise actually consists of specific exercises to strengthen the upper-extremity proximal force couples.[62] The rotator cuff (deltoid and rotator cuff musculature) and lower trapezius force couples are targeted to enhance proximal stabilization using a low-resistance, high-repetition exercise format (ie, 3 sets of 15, <60 repetition maximum loading). Specific exercises such as side-lying external rotation, prone horizontal abduction, and prone extension, both with externally rotated humeral positions and prone external rotation, all have been shown to elicit high levels of posterior rotator cuff activation during electromyogram research (Figure 21-5).[9,15,130] Additionally, exercises such as the serratus press (Figure 21-6) and manual scapular protraction and retraction resistance (Figure 21-7) can be safely applied without stress to the distal aspect of the upper extremity during this important phase of rehabilitation. The use of cuff weights allows some of the rotator cuff and scapular exercises to be

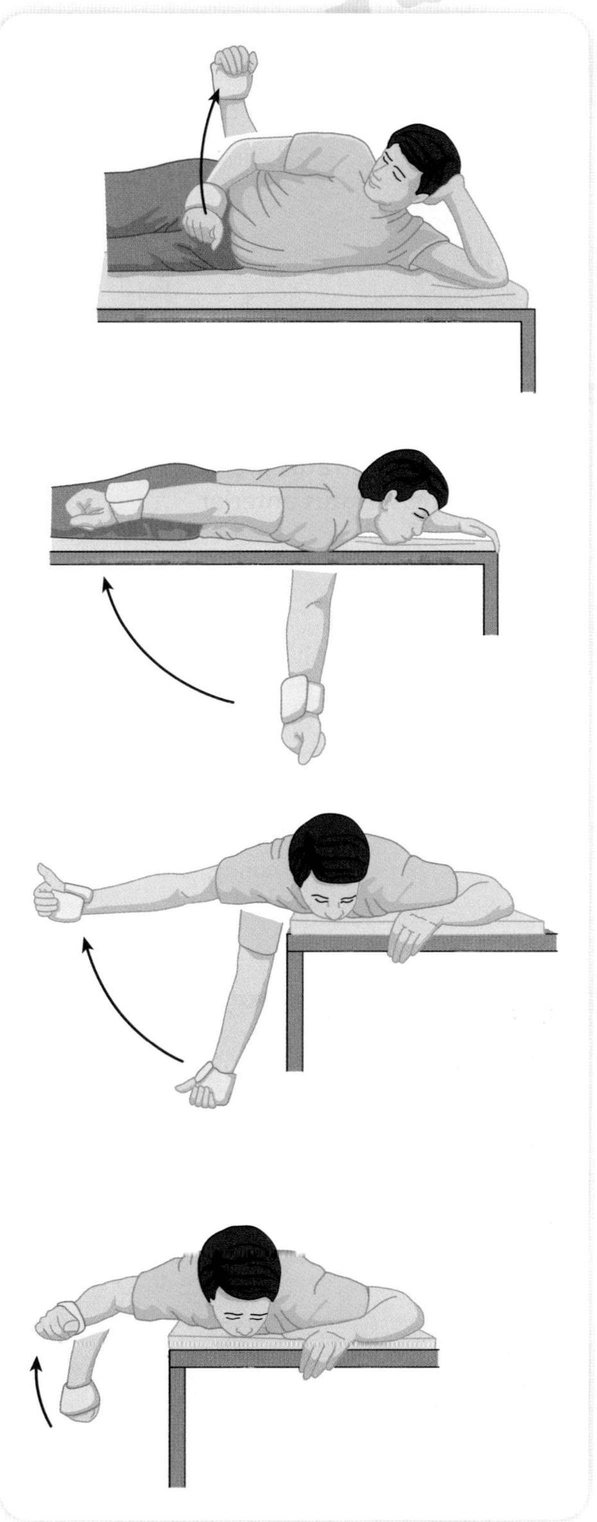

Figure 21-5 Rotator cuff exercises used during rehabilitation of elbow injuries

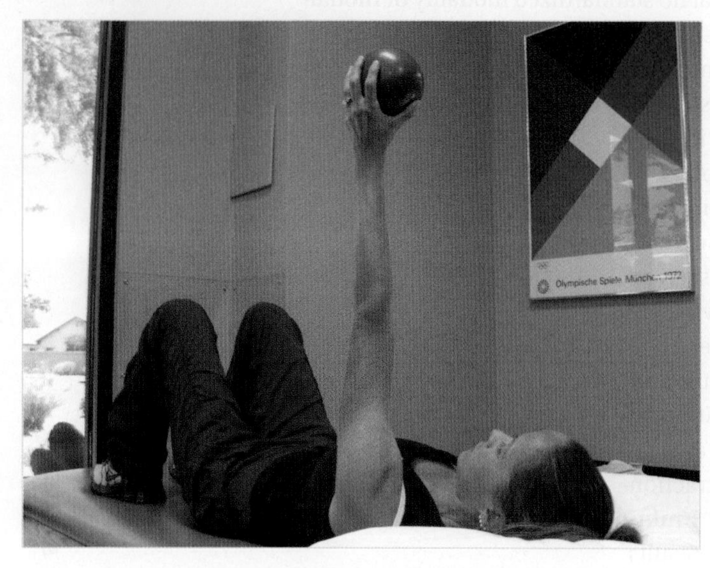

Figure 21-6 **Serratus press exercise used to recruit and strengthen the serratus anterior**

performed with the weight attached proximal to the elbow, to further minimize overload to the elbow and forearm during the earliest phases of rehabilitation if needed for some patients.

The initial application of exercise to the distal aspect of the extremity follows a pattern that stresses the injured muscle-tendon unit last. For example, the initial distal exercise sequence for the patient with lateral humeral epicondylitis would include wrist flexion and forearm pronation, which provides most of the tensile stress to the medially inserting tendons which are not directly involved in lateral humeral epicondylitis (Figure 21-8). Gradual addition of wrist extension and forearm supination, as well as radial and ulnar deviation exercises are added as signs and symptoms allow. Additional progression is based on the elbow position utilized during distal exercises. Initially, most patients tolerate the exercises in a more pain-free fashion with the elbow placed in slight flexion, with a progression to more extended and functional elbow positions, as signs and symptoms allow. These exercises are performed with light weights, often as little as 1 lb or 0.5 kg, as well as tan or yellow Thera-Band, emphasizing both the concentric and eccentric portions of the exercise movement. According to the research by Svernl and Adolffson,[127] the eccentric portion of the exercise may actually have a greater benefit than the concentric portion; however, more research is needed before a greater and clearer understanding of the role isolated eccentric exercise plays in the rehabilitation of degenerative tendon conditions is achieved. Multiple sets of 15 to 20 repetitions are recommended to promote muscular endurance. Several studies show superior results in the treatment of humeral epicondylitis using progressive resistive exercise. [24,82,107,127,132]

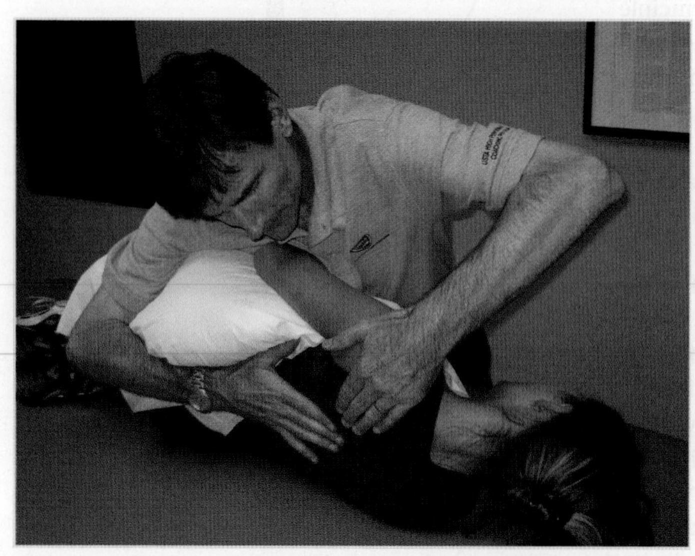

Figure 21-7 **Manual scapular retraction exercise**

Once the patient can tolerate the most basic series of distal exercises (wrist flexion/extension, forearm pronation/supination, and wrist radial/ulnar deviation), exercises are progressed to include activities that involve simultaneous contraction of the wrist and forearm musculature with elbow flexion/extension ROM. These include exercises such as exercise ball dribbling (Figure 21-9), the Body Blade (Hymanson, TX), the B.O.I.N.G. arm exerciser device (OPTP, Minneapolis, MN) (Figures 21-10 and 21-11), Thera-Band (Hygenic Corp, Akron, OH), resistance bar external oscillations (Figure 21-12) (which combine wrist and forearm stabilization with posterior rotator cuff and scapular exercise), and seated rowing (Figure 21-13). Additionally, the use of closed-kinetic-chain exercise for the upper extremity is added to promote cocontraction and mimic functional positions with joint approximation (Figures 21-14 to 21-16).[35]

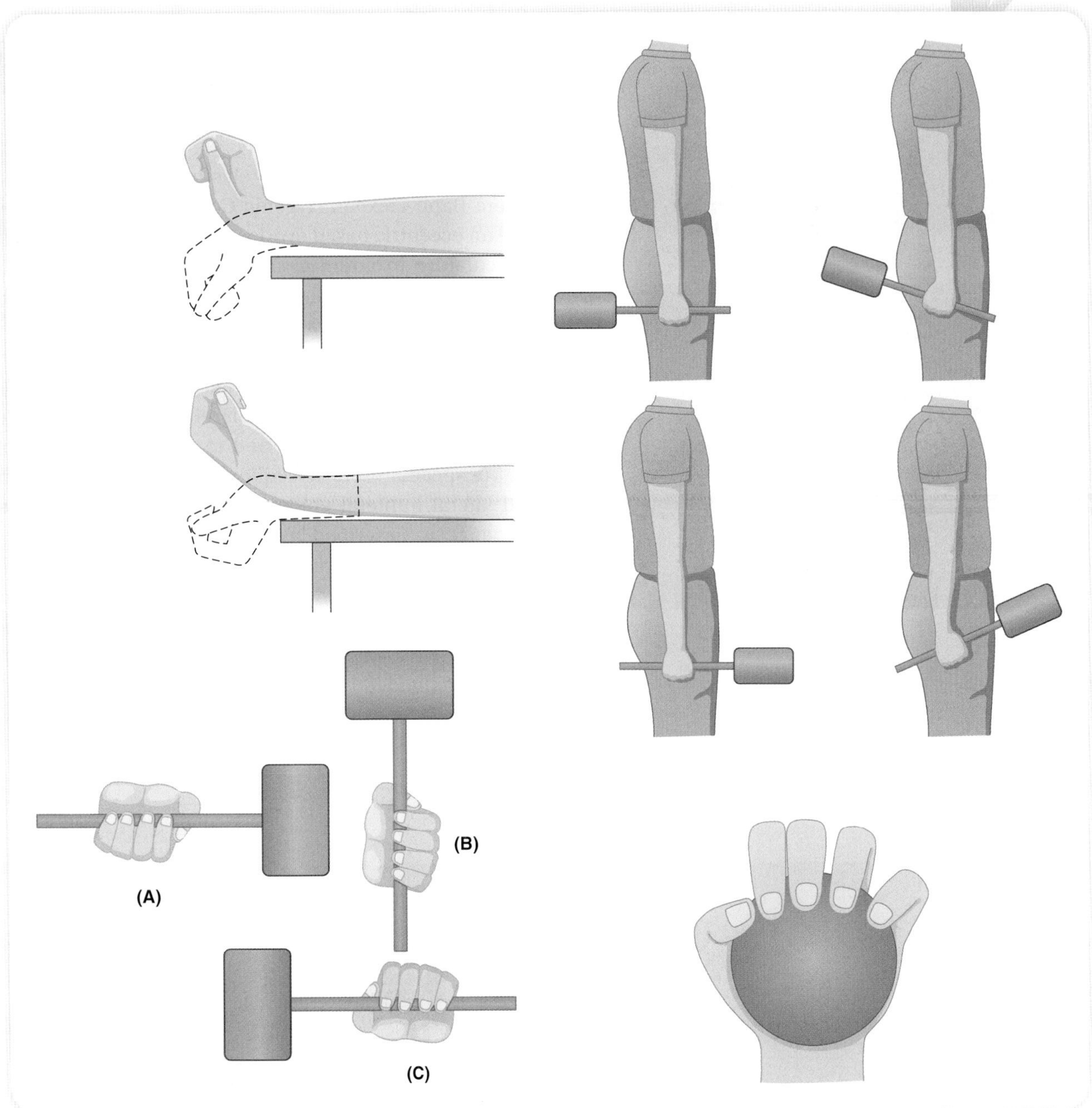

Figure 21-8

Distal upper extremity isotonic exercise patterns, including wrist flexion and extension, radial and ulnar deviation, and forearm pronation and supination.

Svernl & Adolffson[127] followed 38 patients with lateral humeral epicondylitis who were randomly assigned to a contract-relax stretching or eccentric exercise treatment group. Results of their study showed that 71% of the eccentric exercise group reported full recovery, as compared to 39% of the subjects who performed contract-relax stretching and rated themselves as fully recovered. Croisior et al[24] compared the effectiveness of a passive standardized treatment in patients diagnosed with chronic humeral epicondylitis (nonexercise control) to a program that included eccentric isokinetic exercise. After training the

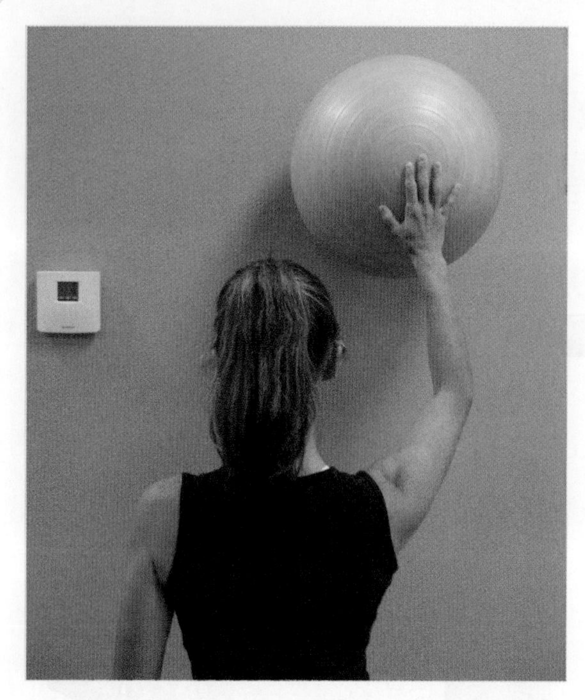

Figure 21-9

Ball dribbling using an exercise ball to promote rapid contraction of the musculature in an endurance-oriented fashion.

patients in the eccentric exercise group had a significant reduction in pain intensity, an absence of bilateral strength deficit in the wrist extensors and forearm supinators, improved tendon imaging and improved disability status with rating scales.

Tyler et al[132] used an elastic based flexible bar (Thera-Band Flexbar, Hygenic Corp, Akron, OH) to provide an eccentric based overload to the wrist and forearm musculature in addition to a traditional rehabilitation program. Results of their research, performed initially on patients with lateral humeral epicondylitis using a twisting type exercise to eccentrically load the extensor musculature in an elbow-extended position, showed superior results to traditional rehabilitation exercises alone.[132] The reader is referred to the Tyler et al article for the specific exercise sequence used for both medial and lateral humeral epicondylitis. The Flexbar exercise sequence is described as beginning with preparatory prelading the wrist and hand musculature (concentrically), followed by a slow eccentric release of the same muscles. This sequence can be performed for either wrist flexion or wrist extension. Multiple sets of 15 repetitions are recommended by the researchers,[132] with slight levels

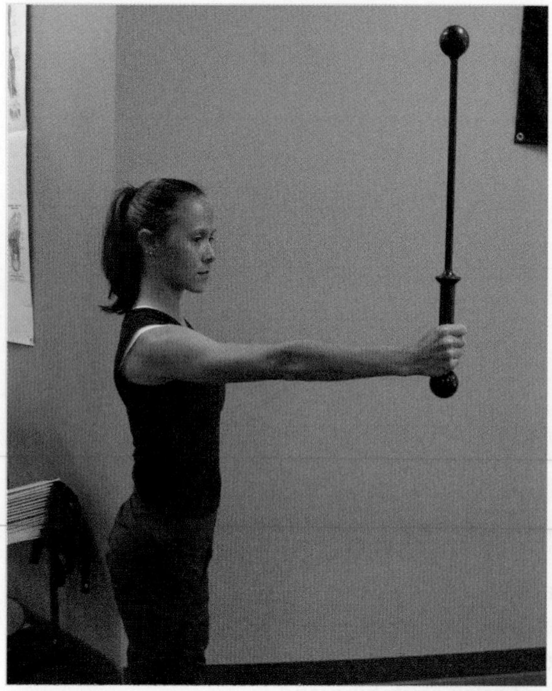

Figure 21-10 **Oscillatory exercise using the B.O.I.N.G. (Biomechanical Oscillation Integrates Neuromuscular Gain), device**

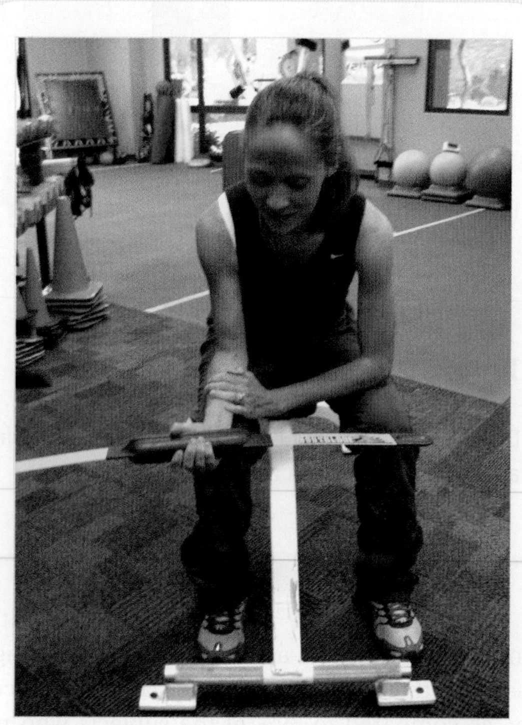

Figure 21-11 **Oscillatory exercise using the Body Blade device**

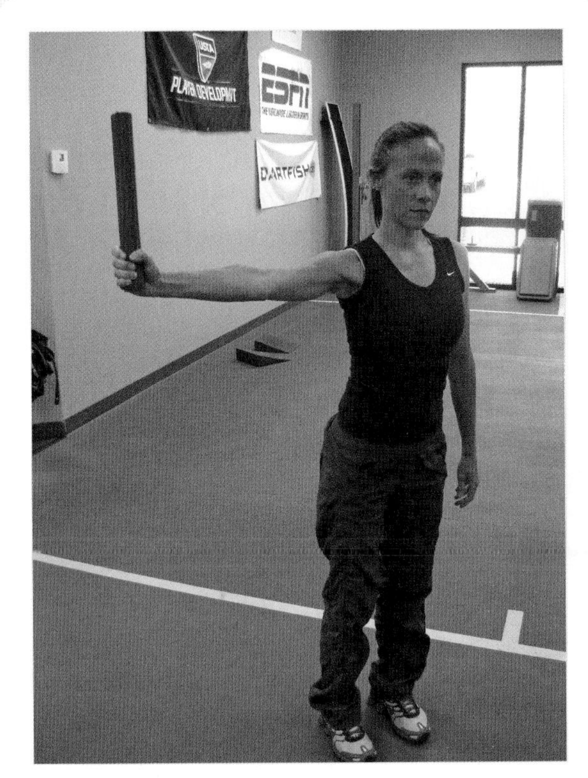

Figure 21-12 Oscillatory exercise using the Thera-Band flex bar

Oscillations can be performed in a sagittal and frontal plane direction to target specific muscle group activation.

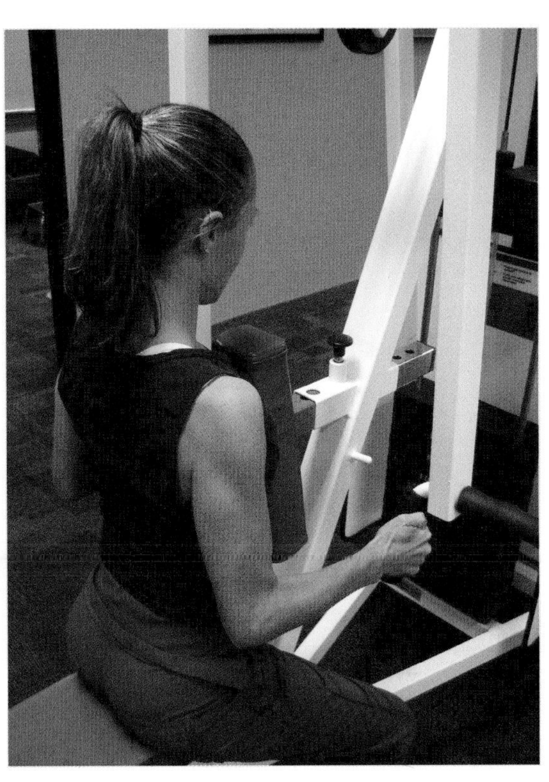

Figure 21-13 Seated rowing exercise used for proximal stabilization and total-arm strength

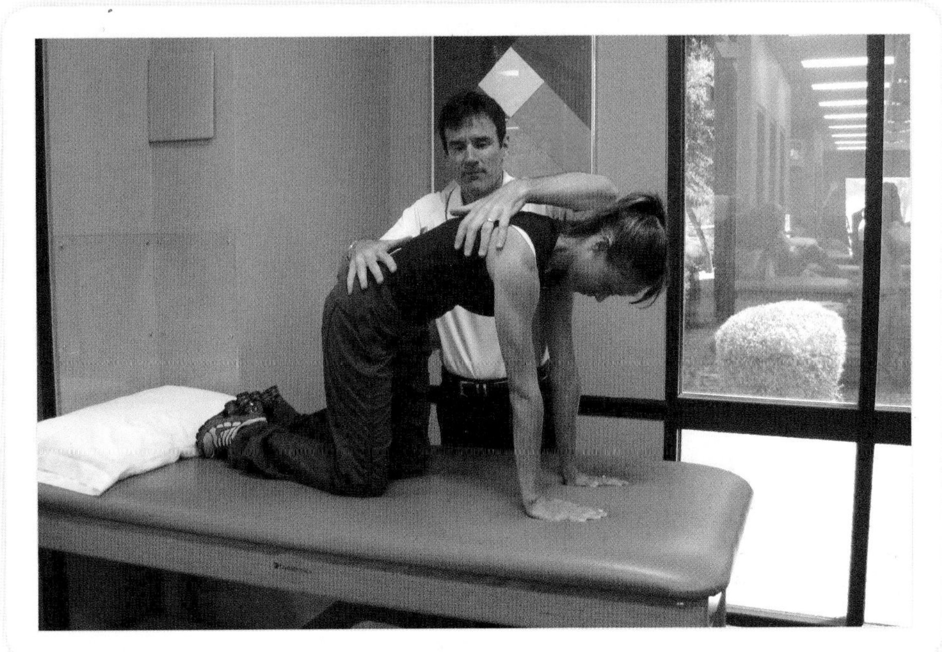

Figure 21-14 Quadruped rhythmic stabilization exercise

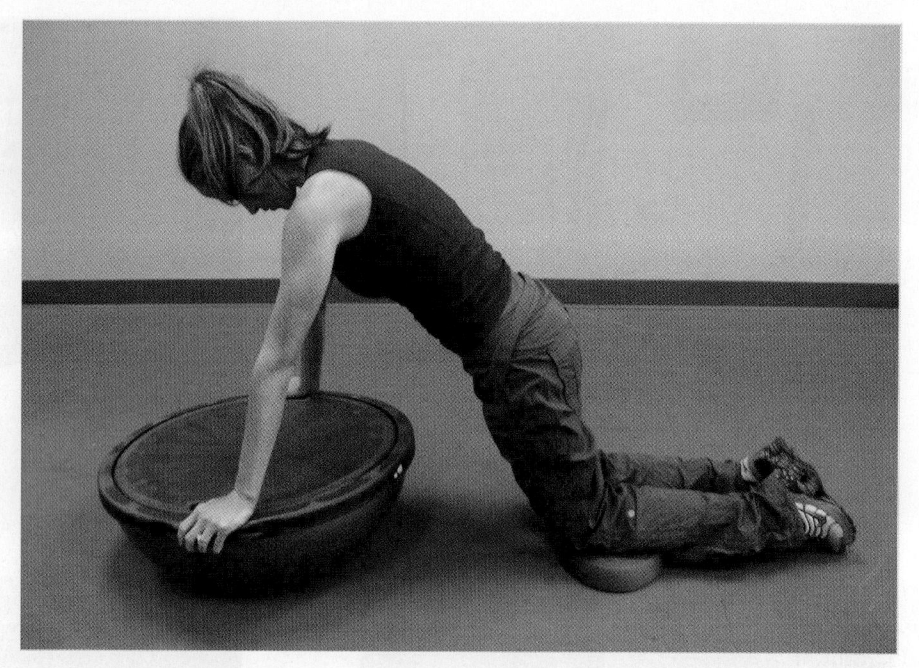

Figure 21-15 Closed-chain upper-extremity exercise using the BOSU platform

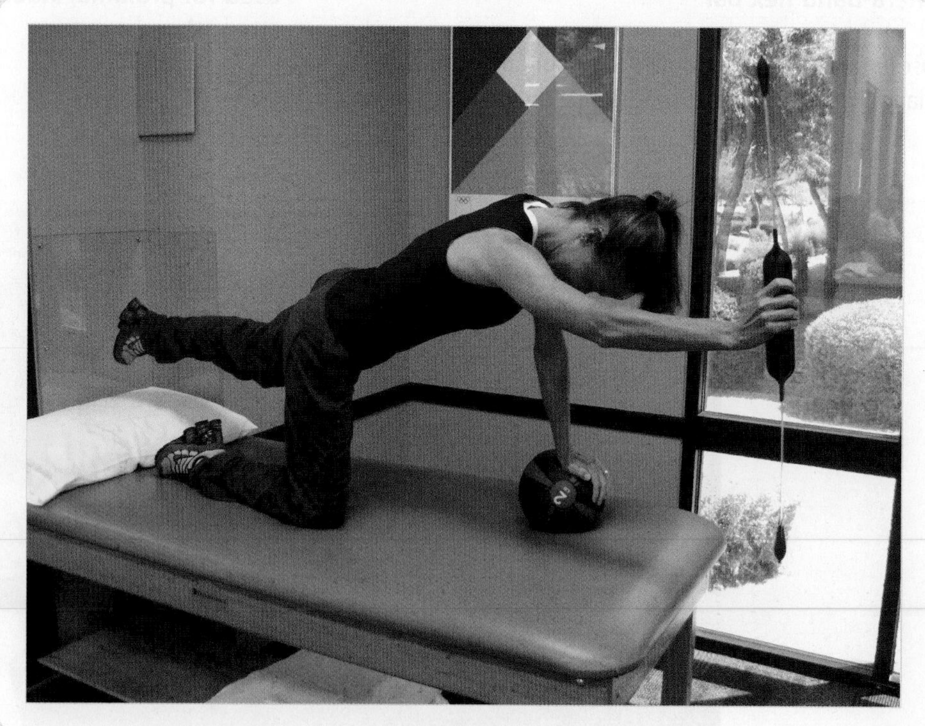

Figure 21-16 Pointer closed-chain upper extremity exercise using the Body Blade to promote instability in the open-chain limb and a medicine ball under the closed-chain limb

of discomfort (Visual Analog Scale [VAS] levels 3 to 4) during the exercise being allowed, which is similar to other types of eccentric training programs.[82] The addition of this exercise, coupled with eccentric wrist flexion exercises with elastic tubing or bands for multiple sets, is used to provide a controlled overload to the wrist, forearm, and finger musculature in this stage of the rehabilitation program. These site-specific exercises are integrated with total extremity focus as described above, including the scapular stabilizers and rotator cuff, to complete the comprehensive rehabilitation program.

Most recently, Peterson et al[107] studied a group of 81 patients with a 3-month history (mean duration: 107 weeks) of chronic lateral elbow pain. Patients were randomly allocated to an exercise group or a control group for a 3-month period of either concentric and eccentric exercise (exercise group) or a "wait-and-see" control group. Exercises consisted of controlled wrist flexion and extension starting with a 1 kg (women) or 2 kg (men) water container that was increased by one-tenth (1 dL of water) into the container with subjects performing 45 repetitions (3 sets of 15 repetitions). After 3 months of training, subjects in the exercise group had a greater relief of pain with a maximal muscle test provocation and elongation provocation test. Specifically, 72% of the subjects in the exercise group had a 30% diminution in pain during the maximal voluntary muscle provocation test as compared with 44% in the control group. This study demonstrates the continued support of an exercise-based approach to elbow tendon pathology.

In addition to the resistive exercise, the use of gentle passive stretching to optimize the muscle tendon unit length is indicated. Combined stretches with the patient in the supine position are indicated to elongate the biarticular muscle tendon units of the elbow, forearm and wrist using a combination of elbow, and wrist and forearm positions (Figure 21-17). Additionally, stretching the distal aspect of the extremity in varying positions of glenohumeral joint elevation is also indicated.[37] Mobilization of the ulnohumeral joint can also be effective in cases where significant flexion contractures exist. Use of ulnohumeral distraction with the elbow near full extension will selectively tension the anterior joint capsule (Figure 21-18).[17]

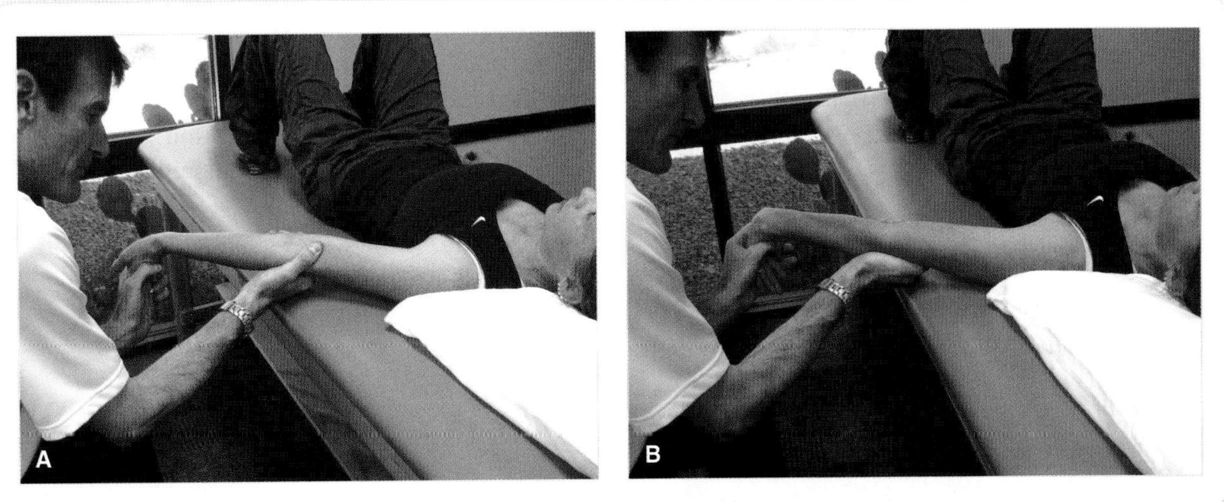

Figure 21-17 Passive stretching of the wrist and forearm musculature

A. Wrist flexion and pronation to stretch the wrist extensors, and (**B**) wrist extension and supination to stretch the flexors and pronators of the distal upper extremity.

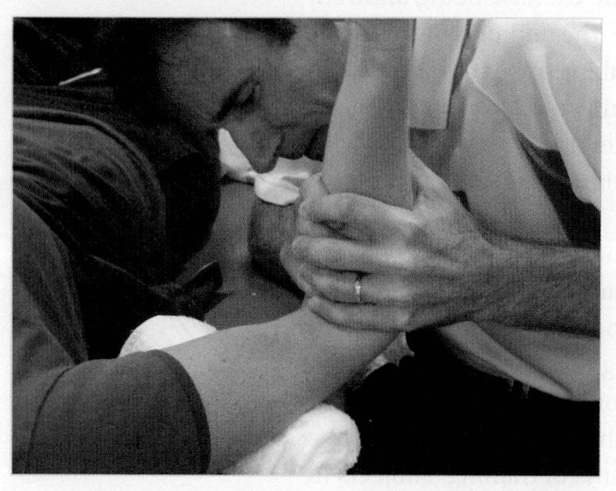

Figure 21-18 **Ulnohumeral joint distraction mobilization**

Altering the position of elbow flexion and extension selectively stresses portions of the anterior and posterior capsule.

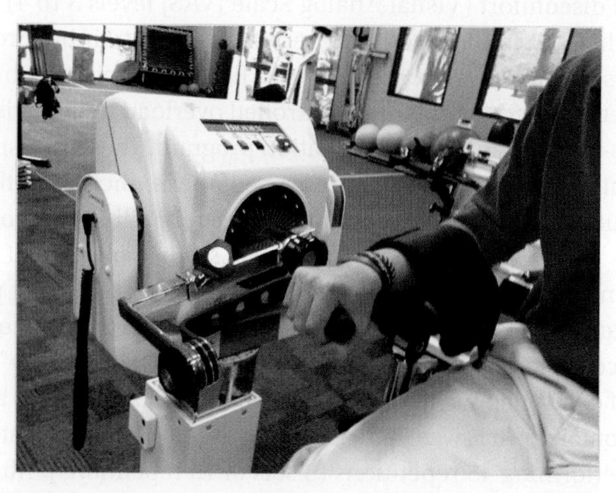

Figure 21-19 **Isokinetic wrist flexion/extension exercise on the Biodex™ isokinetic dynamometer**

As the patients tolerate the distal isotonic exercise progression pain-free at a level of 3 to 5 pounds or medium-level elastic tubing or bands, as well as demonstrate a tolerance to the oscillatory type exercises in this phase of rehabilitation, they are progressed to the isokinetic form of exercise. Advantages of isokinetic exercise are the inherent accommodative resistance and utilization of faster, more functional contractile velocities, in addition to providing isolated patterns to elicit high levels of muscular activation. The initial pattern of exercise used anecdotally has been wrist flexion/extension (Figure 21-19), with forearm pronation/supination (Figure 21-20) added after successful tolerance of a trial treatment of wrist flexion/extension. Contractile velocities ranging between 180 and 300 degrees per second, with 6 to 8 sets of 15 to 20 repetitions, are used to foster local muscular endurance.[45] In addition to isokinetic exercise, plyometric wrist snaps (Figure 21-21) and wrist flips (Figure 21-22), as well as upper-extremity patterns, are utilized to begin to train the elbow for functional and sport specific demands.

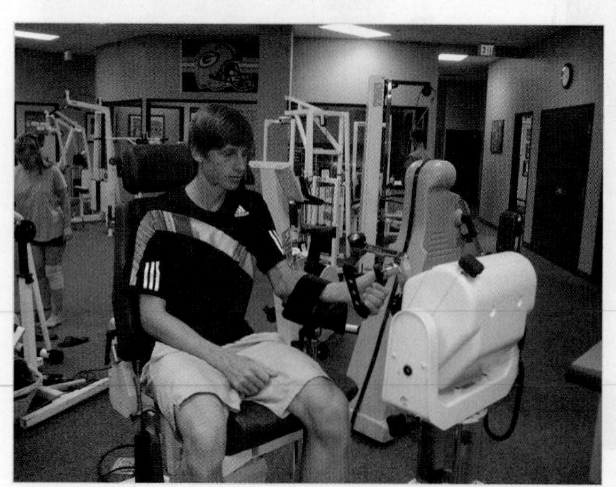

Figure 21-20 **Isokinetic forearm pronation/supination exercise on the Biodex™ isokinetic dynamometer**

Return to Activity Phase

Of the 3 phases in the rehabilitation process for humeral epicondylitis, return to activity is the one that is most frequently ignored or cut short, resulting in serious potential for reinjury and the development of a "chronic" status of this injury. Objective criterion for entry into this stage are tolerance of the previously stated resistive

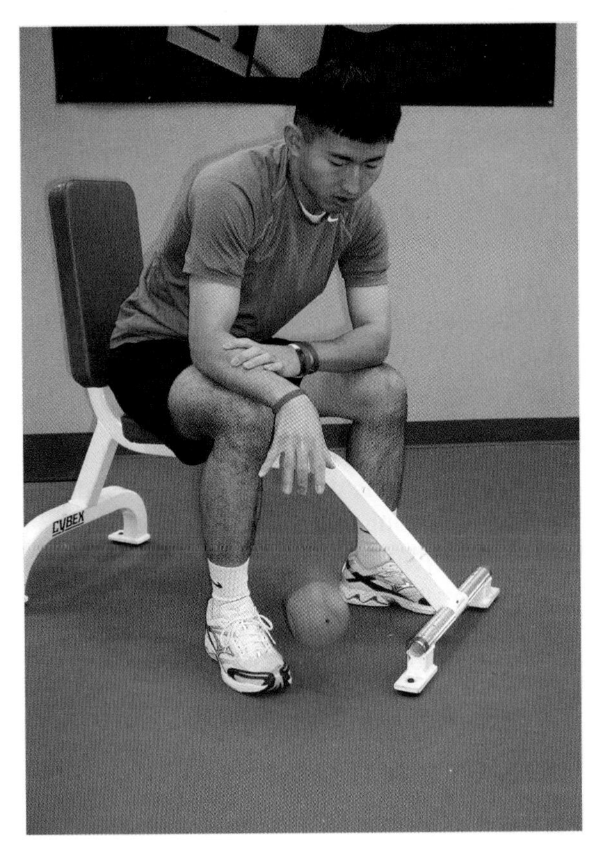

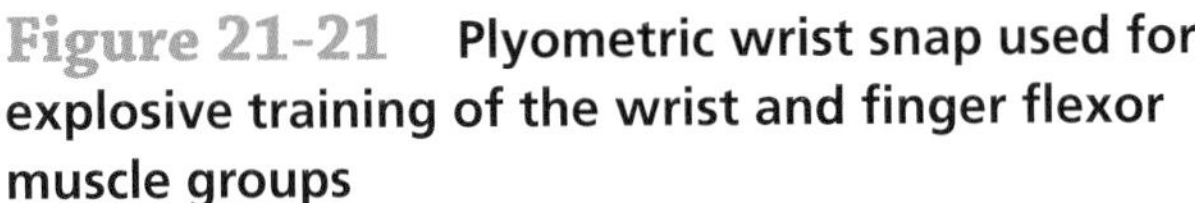

Figure 21-21 Plyometric wrist snap used for explosive training of the wrist and finger flexor muscle groups

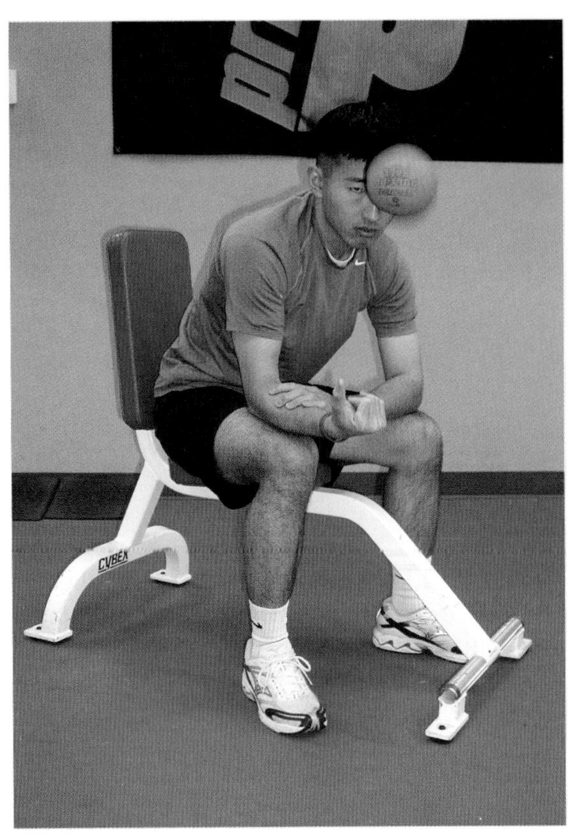

Figure 21-22 Plyometric wrist flip used for explosive training of the wrist and finger flexor muscle groups

exercise series, objectively documented strength equal to the contralateral extremity with either manual muscle testing or, preferably, isokinetic testing distal grip strength measured with a dynamometer, and functional ROM. It is important to note that often in the elite athlete, chronic musculoskeletal adaptations exist that prevent attainment of full elbow ROM. Recall that this is often secondary to the osseous and capsular adaptations discussed earlier in this chapter.

Characteristics of interval sport return programs include alternate day performance, as well as gradual progressions of intensity and repetitions of sport activities. For example, utilizing low-compression tennis balls such as the Pro-Penn Star Ball (Penn Racquet Sports, Phoenix, AZ) or Wilson Gator Ball (Wilson Sporting Goods, Chicago, IL) during the initial contact phase of the return to tennis decreases impact stress and increases tolerance to the activity. Performing the interval program under supervision, either during therapy or with a knowledgeable teaching professional or coach, allows for the biomechanical evaluation of technique and guards against overzealous intensity levels, which can be a common mistake in well-intentioned, motivated patients. Using the return program on alternate days, with rest between sessions, allows for recovery and decreases the potential for reinjury.

Two other important aspects of the return to sport activity are the continued application of resistive exercise and the modification or evaluation of the patient's equipment.

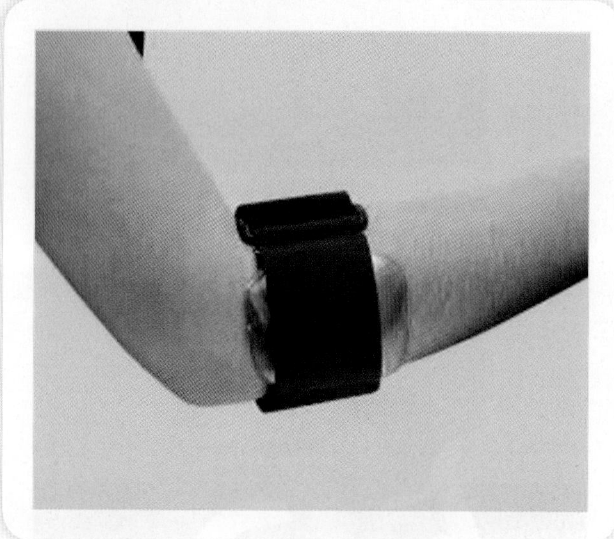

Figure 21-23 **Counterforce brace applied the elbow for a patient with lateral humeral epicondylitis**

Continuation of the total-arm strength rehabilitation exercises using elastic resistance, medicine balls, and isotonic or isokinetic resistance is important to continue to enhance not only strength but also muscular endurance. Inspection and modification of the patient's tennis racquet or golf clubs is also important. For example, lowering the string tension several pounds and ensuring that the player uses a more resilient or softer string, such as a coreless multifilament synthetic string or gut, is widely recommended for tennis players with upper-extremity injury histories.[95,96,98] Grip size is also very important with research showing changes in muscular activity with alteration of handle or grip size.[1] Measurement of proper grip size has been described by Nirschl as corresponding to the distance between the distal tip of the ring finger along the radial border of the finger to the proximal palmar crease.[95] Nirschl has also recommended the use of a counterforce brace (Figure 21-23) in order to decrease stress on the insertion of the flexor and extensor tendons during work or sport activity.[52]

Additional Treatments Presently Used for Tendon Injury

Platelet-Rich Plasma

Platelet-rich plasma (PRP) is a treatment modality that can be utilized in many orthopedic injuries involving tendon and ligament. Such treatment involves localized injections of PRP at various concentrations into the injured tissues, which has been theorized to improve healing by delivering a high concentration of platelets to the injured region.[8] Research demonstrates that platelets are involved in healing through clot formation and the release of growth factors and cytokines, although which specific factors and how they are regulated is still not completely understood. Growth factors in the PRP concentrate include, but are not limited to, transforming growth factor β_1, platelet-derived growth factor, vascular endothelial growth factor, epithelial growth factor, hepatocyte growth factor, and insulin-like growth factor 1.[44] No classification system currently exists to regulate PRP preparation, including regulation of methods of platelet concentration, activation, and the presence of white blood cell concentration. As a result, much of the literature that relates to the use of PRP is difficult to cross-reference and compare despite, recent attempts to unify a system.[29]

The literature supporting the use of PRP treatment for tendon injuries demonstrates mixed results with variable success related to the location of the injured tendons and ligaments. Various cell culture and animal studies demonstrate the efficacy of PRP. In one animal study, PRP used in posttendon repair not only increased healing strength and load-to-failure, it did so without increasing adhesion formation or inflammation 2 weeks following surgery. Although many of the animal studies are encouraging, the results in human studies have been limited.[120,129] During 1 large, stratified, block-randomized, double-blind, placebo-controlled trial by deVos, it was concluded that PRP injection therapy did not improve pain and activity when compared to saline injections used with controls. Although this study was performed on patients with chronic Achilles tendinopathy, it illustrates the equivocal nature of PRP treatment.[28]

Since the deVos study was released in 2006 there have been numerous other PRP studies exhibiting variable success which is often dependent upon the anatomical area of administration. One such area in which treatment with PRP has been encouraging and has almost become an established treatment based on level I data is lateral and medial epicondylar tendinopathies. A 2006 level II cohort study comparing PRP and bupivacaine injection for elbow epicondylitis resulted in statistically significant improvement in patients' VAS for pain score and Mayo elbow score. Of note, the study excluded patients taking nonsteroidal antiinflammatory drugs, a common treatment currently utilized for such diagnoses.[91] Further evidence supporting PRP has emerged in a level 1 double-blinded randomized control trial of patients with lateral epicondylitis. This study included patients that had failed nonsteroidal antiinflammatory drug therapy, physical therapy, bracing, and other conservative therapies commonly used. Patients were randomized and received either a PRP injection or corticosteroid injection and were then followed for 1 and eventually 2 years. The PRP group had better improvement with fewer interventions and operations, with concurrent reductions in the disabilities of the arm, shoulder, and hand and VAS scores even after 2 years. Furthermore, there were no reported complications with the PRP treatment.[49,105] In a similar randomized control study that included lateral epicondylitis and plantar fasciitis, PRP outperformed corticosteroid injections with significant improvement in function and pain.[104]

More recent studies have compared PRP with autologous whole blood in the treatment of lateral epicondylitis. While the patients receiving PRP consistently performed better in a level 1 randomized, controlled study, only one time point at 6 weeks showed any statistically significant difference.[128] A second study utilizing a similar model demonstrated no difference between the 2 groups at 6 months.[23] These results, however, are not straightforward because of confounding factors of red blood cells and white blood cells possibly playing a role in the healing process. More research is needed to decipher the appropriate concentrations of PRP and whether other blood components should be included in order to positively impact healing.

Postoperative Rehabilitation Progression

In a study of more than 3000 cases of humeral epicondylitis, Nirschl[96] has reported that 92% respond to nonoperative treatment. Characteristics of patients who often require surgical correction for this condition are failure of nonoperative rehabilitation programs, minimal relief with corticosteroid injection, and intense pain in the injured elbow even at rest. Surgical treatment for lateral humeral epicondylitis, as reported by Nirschl,[96] involves a small incision from the radial head to 1 inch proximal to the lateral epicondyle. Through this incision, Nirschl removes the pathologic tissue he termed *angiofibroblastic hyperplasia*, without disturbing the attachment of the extensor aponeurosis, in order to preserve stability of the elbow.[96] Vascular enhancement is afforded by drilling holes into the cortical bone in the anterior lateral epicondyle to cancellous bone level. Postoperative immobilization is brief (48 hours), with early motion of the wrist and fingers on postoperative day 1, progressing to elbow active assistive ROM during the first 2 to 3 weeks. Resistive exercise is gradually applied after the third postoperative week, with a return to normal daily activities expected at 8 weeks postoperatively and a return to sport activity several months thereafter.[95,96]

Rehabilitation Following Elbow Arthroscopy

Repetitive stresses to the athletic elbow often result in loose body formation and osteochondral injury, in addition to the more commonly reported tendon injury resulting in humeral epicondylitis. Andrews and Soffer[4] report that the most common indications for elbow arthroscopy are loose body removal and removal of osteophytes. Posteromedial decompression includes the excision of osteophytes, with or without resection of additional posteromedial bone from the proximal olecranon.[3] Early emphasis on regaining full-extension ROM is possible because of the minimally invasive arthroscopic procedure. The senior author's postoperative protocol following arthroscopic procedures of the elbow is presented in Appendix 1. Progressive application of resistive exercise to increase both strength and local muscle endurance forms the bulk of the rehabilitation protocol. Use of early shoulder and scapular stabilization is also recommended in these patients in preparation to the return to overhead activities and aggressive functional activity following discharge.

Outcomes following elbow arthroscopy for posteromedial osteophyte and loose body removal were reported by Oglive-Harris et al,[102] where 21 patients were followed for an average of 35 months postoperatively, rendering good and excellent results in 7 and 14 patients, respectively. O'Driscoll and Morrey[100] reported that arthroscopic removal of loose bodies was of benefit in 75% of all patients; however, when loose bodies were not secondary to some other intraarticular condition, 100% of patients rated the procedure as beneficial. Andrews and Timmerman[5] reviewed the results of 73 cases of arthroscopic elbow surgery in professional baseball pitchers. Eighty percent of players were able to return to full activity, returning to pitching at their preinjury level for at least 1 season. Further review of these patients found that 25% returned for additional surgery, often requiring stabilization and reconstruction of the ulnar collateral ligament as a result of valgus instability. This important study shows the close association between medial elbow laxity and posterior medial osteochondral injury and highlights the importance of identifying subtle instability in the athletic elbow.

Reddy et al[110] retrospectively reviewed a sample of 172 patients who underwent elbow arthroscopy and had a mean follow-up of 42 months. Fifty-six percent of these patients had an excellent result, which allowed them a full return to activity, with 36% having a good result. A 1.6% complication rate was reported, with an overall conclusion that this procedure is both safe and efficacious for the treatment of osteochondral injury of the elbow.

Ellenbecker and Mattalino[37] measured muscular strength at a mean of 8 weeks postoperatively in 8 professional baseball pitchers following arthroscopic removal of loose bodies and posteromedial olecranon spur resection. Results showed a complete return of wrist flexion/extension strength and forearm pronation/supination strength at 8 weeks following arthroscopy. This allows for a gradual progression to interval sport return programs between 8 and 12 weeks postoperatively.

Valgus Extension Overload Injuries

Repeated activities, such as overhead throwing, tennis serving, or throwing the javelin, can lead to characteristic patterns of osseous and osteochondral injury in both the older active patient, as well as the adolescent elbow. These injuries are commonly referred to as valgus extension overload injuries.[142]

Pathomechanics

As a result of the valgus stress incurred during throwing or the serving motion, traction placed via the medial aspect of the elbow can create bony spurs or osteophytes at the medial epicondyle or coronoid process of the elbow.[11,60,123] Additionally, the valgus stress during elbow extension creates impingement, which leads to the development of osteophyte formation at the posterior and posteromedial aspects of the olecranon tip, causing chondromalacia and loose body formation.[142] The combined motion of valgus pressure with the powerful extension of the elbow leads to posterior osteophyte formation, because of impingement of the posterior medial aspect of the ulna against the trochlea and olecranon fossa. Joyce[70] has reported the presence of chondromalacia in the medial groove of the trochlea, which often precedes osteophyte formation. Erosion to subchondral bone is often witnessed when olecranon osteophytes are initially developing. Injury to the ulnar collateral ligament and medial muscle-tendon units of the flexor-pronator group can also occur with this type of repetitive loading.[60,144]

During the valgus stress that occurs to the human elbow during the acceleration phase of both the throwing and serving motions, lateral compressive forces occur in the lateral aspect of the elbow, specifically at the radio-capitellar joint. Of great concern in the immature pediatric throwing athlete is osteochondritis dissecans and Panner disease.[37,70] Both of these injuries are covered in Chapter 30. In the older adult elbow, the radiocapitellar joint can be the site of joint degeneration and osteochondral injury from the compressive loading.[60] This lateral compressive loading is increased in the elbow with MUCL laxity or ligament injury.[37]

Ulnar Collateral Ligament Injury

Pathomechanics and Mechanism of Injury

Attenuation of the ulnar collateral ligament can produce valgus instability of the elbow, which can lead to medial joint pain, ulnar nerve compromise, and lateral radiocapitellar and posterolateral osseous dysfunction, which results in severe dysfunction in the throwing or racquet sport athlete. The repetitive valgus loading that occurs in the elbow during the acceleration phase of the throwing or serving motion can attenuate this structure. Sprains and partial thickness tears of the MUCL can occur and progress to complete tears and avulsions of the ligament from its bony attachments.[31]

Rehabilitation Concerns

Nonoperative rehabilitation of the athlete with an ulnar collateral ligament sprain also involves the primary stages outlined in the rehabilitation of humeral epicondylitis. During the initial stage of rehabilitation, immobilization of the elbow is often a characteristic part of the process to decrease pain and enhance healing. Either an immobilizer or hinged brace is used to limit end ranges of elbow extension and flexion. Modalities are again used to assist in the healing process, as are gentle ROM, submaximal isometrics, and manual resistance of both wrist and forearm midrange movements.

Rehabilitation Progression

Use of a total-arm strength rehabilitation protocol is indicated to facilitate both muscular strength and endurance to the elbow, forearm, and wrist. In addition to previously mentioned exercises, particular attention is given to eccentric muscle work of the wrist flexors and forearm supinators to attempt to dynamically support the attenuated ulnar collateral ligament. Because of the intimate association between the flexor carpi ulnaris and the ulnar collateral ligament, early strengthening in the pattern of wrist flexion and ulnar deviation may provoke symptoms; however, later in rehabilitation, the repeated use of exercises to strengthen the muscles directly overlying the injured ligament to provide dynamic stabilization is highly recommended.[26]

In addition to distal strengthening, significant emphasis is placed on strengthening of the rotator cuff and scapular stabilizers of the throwing athlete with ulnar collateral ligament injury. In addition to increasing strength and endurance of the scapular stabilizers and rotator cuff musculature, attention is also directed toward the evaluation of shoulder ROM and specifically to the range of rotational ROM. Dines et al[31] has identified increased glenohumeral internal rotation ROM deficits in throwing athletes with ulnar collateral ligament injury as compared to cohorts of throwing athletes without medial elbow injury. This finding highlights the importance of evaluation and treatment of the entire upper extremity kinetic chain in the throwing athlete with ulnar collateral ligament injury. The application of specific interventions directed to stretch the posterior shoulder [64] to improve internal rotation ROM is recommended based on this new finding. Wilk et al[141] and Shanley et al[121] both have shown increases in shoulder injury risk with losses of approximately 12 degrees of internal rotation or more on the throwing arm, as well as losses of only 5 degrees or more of total rotation ROM[141] in baseball pitchers.

Progression to plyometric exercises, which impart a submaximal, controlled valgus stress to the medial aspect of the elbow such as a 90/90 shoulder and elbow medicine ball toss in later stages of rehabilitation, attempts to simulate loads placed on the medial elbow (Figure 21-24). Use of the isokinetic dynamometer for distal strengthening is also recommended, with additional training focused on the shoulder for internal/external rotation with the arm abducted 90 degrees and elbow flexed 90 degrees (Figure 21-25). Use of this position imparts a controlled valgus stress to the elbow in addition to strengthening the rotator cuff.[36]

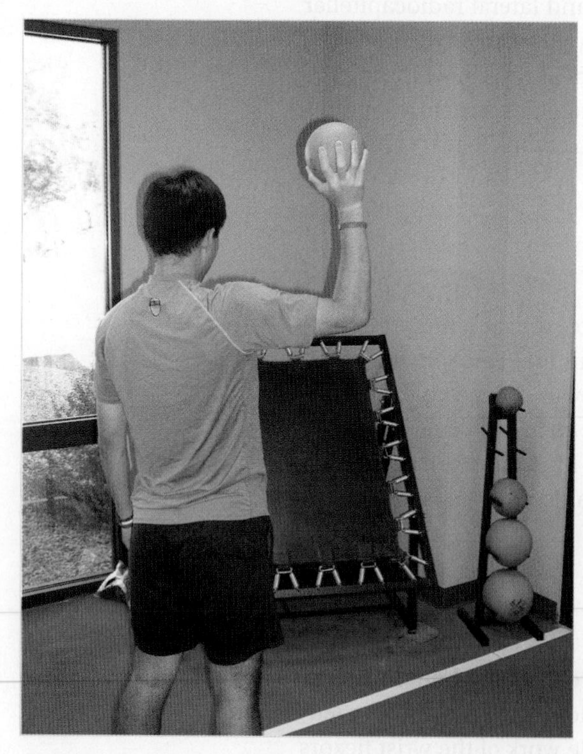

Figure 21-24

Plyometric 90/90 medicine ball toss to simulate loads placed to the medial elbow in the later stages of rehabilitation only to prepare the overhead athlete for a return to throwing.

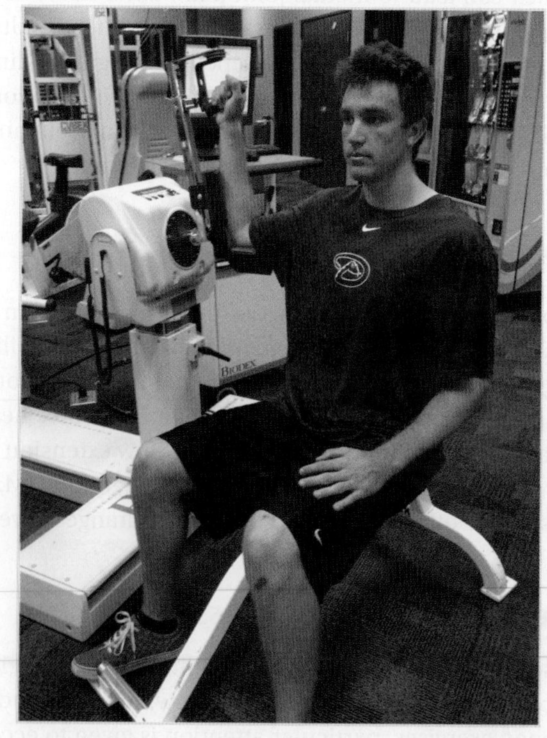

Figure 21-25 **Isokinetic 90/90 internal/external rotation training position on the Biodex™ isokinetic dynamometer**

A complete return of ROM and isokinetically documented appropriate elbow, forearm, and wrist strength are required before an interval program is initiated. Reoccurrence of pain, feelings of instability, or neural irritation with throwing or functional activity identify the patient as a potential candidate for an ulnar collateral ligament repair or reconstruction. It should be noted that many patients who undergo nonoperative rehabilitation may progress to the need for operative intervention.

Postoperative Rehabilitation Following Ulnar Collateral Ligament Reconstruction

Operative procedures for the athlete with valgus instability of the elbow have focused on direct primary repair of the ligament[81] as well as utilization of an autogenous graft for reconstruction of the medial elbow. Conway et al,[22] Jobe et al,[68] and Regan et al[111] reported that the palmaris tendon used as the autogenous graft, harvested from the ipsilateral forearm, fails at higher loads (357 N) and is 4 times stronger than the native anterior band of the ulnar collateral ligament, which fails at 260 N.

In a retrospective study by Conway et al[22] of 71 throwing athletes who underwent either surgical repair or reconstruction of the ulnar collateral ligament, 87% were found to have a midsubstance tear of the ulnar collateral ligament, 10% had a distal ulnar avulsion, and only 3% avulsed from the medial epicondyle. Thirty-nine percent of these elbows had calcification and scar formation in the ulnar collateral ligament with 16% demonstrating an osteophyte to the posteromedial olecranon most likely from the increased valgus extension overload secondary to ulnar collateral ligament attenuation.

The clinical evaluation of these patients preoperatively resulted in a positive valgus stress test in 8 of the 14 patients who underwent an ulnar collateral ligament repair, and 33 of 56 patients who underwent autogenous reconstruction. Valgus stress radiographs were also used in the preoperative evaluation with greater emphasis placed upon the subjective and clinical evaluation.[22] Fifty percent of these athletes demonstrated a flexion contracture that limited full elbow extension.

Surgical Technique for Ulnar Collateral Ligament Reconstruction

The surgical technique used to reconstruct the ulnar collateral ligament is described extensively by Conway et al,[22] Jobe et al,[68] and Jobe and Elattrache.[66] A 10-cm medial incision over the medial epicondyle is used to provide exposure with careful dissection and protection of the ulnar nerve carried out before the ulnar collateral ligament is addressed. If a primary repair is performed, adequate normal-appearing ligamentous tissue is required to allow for direct repair. If inadequate ligamentous tissue is present, a reconstruction is performed. Additional exposure is required to perform the reconstruction, which is obtained by transection of the flexor/pronator tendinous origin.

This has important ramifications with respect to rehabilitation. The removal of this tendinous origin results in a greater amount of time required for healing, and a longer time period before resistive exercise of the flexor/pronator muscles and forearm supination and wrist extension ROM can be performed.

Calcification within the ligament and surrounding soft tissues is also removed with relocation of the ulnar nerve performed by removing it from the cubital tunnel. The ulnar nerve is mobilized from the level of the arcade of Struthers to the interval between the two heads of the flexor carpi ulnaris. The attachment sites of the anterior band of the ulnar collateral ligament are identified and tunnels are drilled in the medial epicondyle and proximal ulna to approximate the anatomical location of the original ligament. The graft taken from the ipsilateral palmaris longus (if available) is then placed in a figure-of-8 fashion through the tunnels. The ulnar nerve is carefully transposed so that no impingement or tethering occurs. Reattachment of the flexor pronator origin is then performed. The elbow is immobilized in a position of 90 degrees of flexion, neutral forearm rotation, with the wrist left free to move.

Rehabilitation Concerns

The elbow remains immobilized for the first 10 days postoperatively, with gentle gripping exercises allowed in order to prevent further disuse atrophy. Active and passive ROM of the elbow, wrist, and shoulder are performed at 10 days postoperatively. Close monitoring of the ulnar nerve distribution in the distal upper extremity is recommended because of the transposition of the nerve that frequently accompanies surgical reconstruction of the MUCL. As discussed in the previous section entitled "Surgical Technique for UCL Reconstruction", care is taken to protect the graft by gradually progressing elbow extension ROM to 30 degrees by week 2 and finally to terminal ranges by 4 to 6 weeks postoperatively. Protection of the graft from large stresses is recommended, even though loss of extension ROM is an undesirable postoperative result. Therefore, progressive increases in elbow extension ROM and the use of gentle joint mobilization and contract-relax stretching techniques are warranted to achieve timely, optimal elbow extension. Because of the reattachment of the flexor-pronator tendinous insertion, limited ROM into wrist extension and forearm supination is performed for the first 6 weeks until healing of the flexor-pronator insertion takes place.

Rehabilitation of the postoperative elbow should also include activities to restore proprioceptive function to the injured joint. Kinesthesia is the perceived sensation of the position and movement of joints and muscles and an important part in the coordination of movement patterns in the peripheral joints. Simple use of exercises such as angular replication and end-range reproduction can be used early in rehabilitation, without visual assistance, to stimulate mechanoreceptors in the postoperative joint. These procedures are utilized early in the rehabilitation process concomitant with ROM and joint mobilization. Loss of kinesthetic awareness in the upper extremity following injury has been objectively identified by Smith and Brunolli.[124]

Rehabilitation Progression (Appendix 2)

The progression of resistive exercise follows previously discussed exercises, beginning with multiple-angle isometrics at week 2 and submaximal isotonics during the fourth postoperation week. Utilization of the total-arm strength concept is followed, with proximal weight attachment for glenohumeral exercises to prevent stresses placed across the elbow. No glenohumeral joint, internal or external rotation strengthening, is allowed for at least 6 weeks to as many as 16 weeks postoperation, because of the valgus stress placed upon the elbow with this movement pattern. During weeks 8 to 12 following surgery, both concentric and eccentric exercises are performed in the elbow extensors and flexors, as well as a continued total-arm strengthening emphasis, with all distal movement patterns described in nonoperative rehabilitation of humeral epicondylitis being applied. Plyometric exercises, ball dribbling, and closed-chain exercises are also introduced during this time frame.

Isokinetic training is introduced at 4 months postoperation, with isokinetic testing applied to identify areas needing specific emphasis.[139,140] Progression of isokinetic training patterns by these authors again follows from wrist extension/flexion to forearm pronation/supination, and, finally, to elbow extension/flexion. The isokinetic dynamometer is also used at 4 to 6 months postoperatively for shoulder internal/external rotation strengthening with 90 degrees of abduction and 90 degrees of elbow flexion to impart a gentle, controlled valgus stress to the elbow. At 4 months postoperation, throwing athletes begin an interval-throwing program to prepare the elbow for the stresses of functional activity.

The duration of rehabilitation postoperatively is often 6 months to a year. A slow revascularization of the graft through a sheath of granulation tissue that grows from the tissue adjacent to the site of implantation encircles the graft is the rationale provided by Jobe et al[68] for their time-based rehabilitation program. They are convinced that at least 1 year is required for the tendon graft and its surrounding tissues to develop sufficient strength and endurance to function as a ligament in the medial elbow.

Outcomes Following Ulnar Collateral Ligament Reconstruction

In their series of 56 reconstructed elbows, Conway et al[22] reported baseball players return to throwing 15 feet by 4.5 months, with competition at 12.5 months postoperation. The athlete with a repaired ulnar collateral ligament performed throwing activities of 15 feet at 3 months and competed at 9 months. Overall, an excellent result was achieved in 64% of the operative elbows of elite athletes. An excellent result was defined as achieving a level of activity equal to or greater than preinjury level. Bennett et al[12] reported improved stability in 13 of 14 cases of ulnar collateral ligament reconstruction in an active adult and working population, with improved stability reported in all cases of direct repair by Kuroda and Sakamaki.[81] A flexion contracture was reported in as many as 50% of the athletes at a mean of six years following an autogenous ulnar collateral ligament reconstruction.[22] Conway et al[22] did not feel that this finding limits performance, since elbow ROM during throwing ranges from 120 degrees to 20 degrees, although conscious effort during rehabilitation is given to regain as much extension as possible during the time-based rehabilitation program.

Elbow Dislocations

Failure of the normally stable osseous, ligamentous, capsular, and muscular constraints at the elbow ultimately can lead to dislocation in response to a macrotrauma.

Pathomechanics

The elbow is the second most commonly dislocated large joint behind the shoulder in the adult population and the most commonly dislocated joint in children younger than the age of 10 years.[86] It is reported that 7 of every 100,000 people suffer an elbow dislocation.[69] Inherent in any elbow dislocation is a degree of instability present at the joint. Rehabilitation and treatment are predicated upon regaining full functional mobility while maintaining elbow joint stability.

Mechanism of Injury

Elbow dislocations are typically the result of trauma as the person falls onto an outstretched arm. Two specific mechanisms of injury have been reported. Hyperextension along with an axially directed force causes the olecranon to act as a fulcrum, levering the trochlea over the coronoid process.[86] A posterolateral rotary-directed force can produce a rotational displacement of the ulna on the humerus leading to dislocation.[99] A combination of axial compression, elbow flexion, valgus stress, and forearm supination produces this type of displacement. Concomitant injuries associated with elbow dislocations include fractures, soft tissue tear or rupture of ligaments, muscles, and joint capsule, vascular and neural compromise, as well as articular cartilage defects. Following the dislocation event, the elbow typically presents with significant swelling, severe pain, and structural deformity with the forearm appearing shortened upon observation.

Classification

Traditionally, elbow dislocations are classified according to the direction of ulnar displacement relative to the humerus. The overwhelming majority of cases involve a posterior dislocation versus the rare incidence of both anterior and lateral dislocation. Posterior dislocations are further subdivided into posterior, posteromedial, and posterolateral groups. Approximately 90% of all elbow dislocations are posterior and posterolateral.[6] Other classifications include simple versus complete dislocations. Simple dislocations involve minimal disruption of the congruity of bony and soft-tissue restraints, which usually allow for early initiated motion and rehabilitation. Complete dislocations involve the destruction of the bony restraints and soft tissue, particularly the ulnar collateral ligament. The ulnar collateral ligament and bony articulation provide the majority of stability at the elbow absorbing 54% and 33% of the valgus forces at 90 degrees of elbow flexion and 31% each at 0 degrees of elbow flexion.[93] Complete dislocations generally require a longer immobilization and recovery period to allow for healing of the primary restraints. Further classification is used to describe posterolateral instability as it progresses to dislocation. This classification is divided into 3 stages and based upon a circular disruption of bone and soft tissue that starts laterally and progresses toward the medial side of the elbow.[99] Stage 1 involves a partial or complete rupture of the lateral collateral ligament resulting in subluxation. In stage 2, the entire lateral collateral ligament is ruptured along with part of the anterior and posterior capsule leading to a *perched* dislocation. Perched refers to the position of the coronoid process as it sits "perched" on the posterior aspect of the trochlea. Stage 3 posterolateral dislocations are considered complete dislocations. Stage 3A involves all soft tissues around the elbow including the posterior band of the ulnar collateral ligament with the exception of the anterior band. In stage 3B, complete disruption of both lateral and ulnar collateral ligament complexes results in gross multidirectional instability.

Rehabilitation Concerns

Immediate care of elbow dislocations initially involves reduction, evaluation of the neurovascular triad for compromise, and further assessment of ligamentous stability. Radiographs and MRI are obtained to determine the extent of bony and soft-tissue damage. The elbow is typically placed in a posterior splint at 90 degrees flexion and immobilized until cleared to begin ROM activities. Severe damage to bony and soft-tissue restraints may require surgical intervention.

Rehabilitation Progression

Elbow rehabilitation guidelines following dislocation comprise 3 distinct phases, as proposed by Harrelson and Leaver-Dunn.[56] Phase 1 is the immediate motion phase and generally starts anywhere from 1 to 10 days postinjury. Early active ROM (all planes) within a protected and pain-free range is initiated to prevent adhesion formation and flexion contracture, which causes subsequent loss of motion and pain. For simple dislocations, immediate motion protocols have been shown to produce favorable results including return of full motion, early return to athletic and competitive activities, and low incidence of recurrent instability.[116,133,134] Passive ROM is not indicated early because of the possibility of heterotopic ossification. Management of pain and inflammation is conducted with ice, compression, and use of modalities. Strengthening activities can include gripping, shoulder and wrist isotonics, and gentle multiangle submax-to-max isometrics for both elbow flexion and extension. All exercises should be completed in a pain-free ROM. Care should be taken to avoid valgus stresses at the elbow. The posterior splint is usually discharged; however, a hinged elbow brace may be utilized to protect ROM within the limits of stability.

Phase 2 consists of the intermediate phase from days 10 to 14. During this period chief concern is achieving full elbow ROM particularly extension. Strength, endurance, and power exercise are progressed to include elbow isotonics in all planes. Progressive resistive exercises are to be incorporated for the shoulder, wrist, and elbow. Inclusion of proprioceptive activities, rhythmic stabilization, plyometrics, and eccentric isotonics during the latter parts of this phase helps retrain the dynamic elbow stabilizers. Phase 3 is the advanced strengthening phase beginning from week 2 to 6. During this phase preparation is made for a gradual return to sport or activity. Exercise progression is to include sport specific activities and drills along with continued progressive resistive exercise. At this time, an interval-throwing program may be initiated for those returning to overhand throwing activities. Wilk and Arrigo[138] also include a return to activity phase as part of a general rehabilitation protocol. Sport-specific exercise and tests are conducted to determine appropriate stability requirements on the elbow. Upon clinical examination by the physician, ROM should be full and no pain present. Medical doctor clearance is ultimately required for return to activity. Bracing or taping may continue to be used to ensure stability and joint protection.

Elbow Fractures

Pathomechanics and Mechanism of Injury

Fractures that affect function at the elbow joint may occur at the distal humerus, capitellum, coronoid, olecranon, radial head and neck, supracondylar region, lateral condyle, and medial epicondyle. These fractures occur in both children and adults as the result of an acute traumatic injury, such as a direct collision or a fall on an outstretched hand. A thorough clinical examination and radiographs are important for obtaining a correct diagnosis so that appropriate treatment can be given. Clinical signs and symptoms of a fracture include history of traumatic onset, pain, swelling, tenderness, and ecchymosis. Elbow stability and neurovascular status should also be assessed immediately following injury. The presence of the posterior fat pad sign on radiographs has been suggested as a sign of an intracapsular elbow fracture in pediatric patients even if no fracture is seen on the radiograph. Effusion within the elbow joint elevates the posterior fat pad, making it visible on radiographs. In a prospective study, the presence of a posterior fat pad on radiographs was indicative of a fracture in 76% of the children evaluated. These results suggest that the children with an elevated posterior fat pad sign should be treated as though a nondisplaced elbow fracture is present, even if the fracture is not evident on radiographs.[122]

Types of Elbow Fractures

Supracondylar Fractures

Supracondylar fractures are the most common elbow fractures that occur in children and account for 60% of all elbow fractures.[32,89] They often occur in children who are around 7 years old.[27] The mechanism of injury is a fall on a hyperextended arm with pronation.[27,32] Because the supracondylar ridge is only 2 to 3 mm thick in children,[32] it has a high risk for injury with a hyperextension mechanism. The Gartland classification system is used to divide supracondylar fractures into 3 types.[32,89] Type I fractures are nondisplaced and usually treated with 3 weeks of immobilization. Type II fractures are moderately displaced, but there is contact between the fragments as the posterior periosteal hinge is intact. A complete displacement is classified as type III. Posteromedial displacement is associated with radial nerve injuries, and posterolateral displacement is associated with brachial artery or median nerve injury. Reduction and surgical stabilization is required for type III, and possibly for type II fractures.[32,89] Three to 4 weeks of immobilization is recommended following surgery.[27] Complications following supracondylar injury may include cubitus varus, transient nerve injury, and compartment syndrome.[32]

Full elbow ROM can be difficult to regain after supracondylar fractures and rehabilitation may last several months.[27] Loss of ROM will vary based on patient age, injury severity, and concomitant injuries. Keppler et al[72] investigated the effectiveness of physiotherapy in regaining elbow ROM after uncomplicated, operative treatment supracondylar humeral fractures without neurovascular injury in children between the ages of 5 and 12 years. At 12 and 18 weeks following surgery, results showed a significant improvement in elbow ROM in those children receiving physiotherapy compared to those not receiving treatment. However, at a 1-year follow-up, there was no significant difference between the children who had received physical therapy and those who did not.

Lateral Condyle Fractures

Lateral condyle fractures account for 12% to 20% of elbow fractures in children,[14,32,83,89] and are the second most common elbow fracture.[83] These fractures result from a fall on an outstretched hand with forearm supination.[89,90] A varus force may cause the extensor muscles and collateral ligament to avulse the lateral condyle.[32,90] Lateral condyle fractures are classified by the Milch system into 2 types based on the location of the fracture line.[32,89,90] Milch type I fractures occur when the fracture line is lateral to the trochlear groove or in the trochlear groove. Milch type II fractures extend medial to the trochlea, allowing lateral subluxation of the ulna and elbow instability. Proper classification in children may be difficult to assess because the trochlea is not ossified until the child is approximately 10 years old.[90]

Lateral condyle fractures with less than a 2-mm displacement may be treated nonoperatively with immobilization, if fracture healing is monitored.[32,83] For fractures displaced more than 2 mm, surgery is recommended.[83,89] Surgical treatment may involve open reduction and internal fixation[14,89] or intraoperative arthrography followed by closed reduction and percutaneous pinning, with no consensus for the optimal technique in the literature.[14] Complications following lateral condyle fractures may include delayed union, nonunion, avascular necrosis of the lateral condyle, and stiffness.[32,89]

Medial Epicondyle Fractures

Medial epicondyle fractures account for 8% to 10% of pediatric elbow fractures[89] and are most common in children between the ages of 9 and 15 years.[32] They are caused by a fall on an outstretched hand with forced wrist hyperextension and valgus stress at the elbow.[89] Associated elbow dislocation occurs in 50% of cases.[89] Possible complications to be aware of after medial epicondyle fractures include ulnar nerve irritation, elbow instability, nonunion, and stiffness.

Fractures with displacement up to 2 mm can be treated with immobilization. Surgery is a consideration for fractures displaced greater than 2 mm.[32] Farsetti et al[43] performed a long-term follow-up comparison of medial epicondyle fractures displaced greater than 5 mm treated surgically versus nonsurgically. Subjects were divided into 3 treatment groups: (a) nonsurgical treatment consisting of immobilization, (b) open reduction and internal fixation of the fragment, and (c) excision of the osteocartilaginous fragment.

Outcome measures included ROM, forearm muscle atrophy, elbow stability, grip strength, radiographs to assess epicondylar nonunion and posttraumatic arthritis, and electromyography if symptoms of nerve impairment were present. At an average follow-up of 34 years (range: 18 to 48 years), results showed patients treated with cast immobilization and patients treated with open reduction and internal fixation had similar functional outcomes, despite a high incidence of nonunion of the medial epicondyle in patients treated with cast immobilization only. A good functional outcome was defined as full or minimally restricted pain-free elbow motion, stable manual valgus stress testing, normal ipsilateral grip strength, minimal-to-no forearm muscle atrophy, and no radiographic signs of osteoarthritis. Good results were found in 16 of 19 patients in the immobilization group and in 15 of 17 patients following open reduction internal fixation. No good results were found in patients treated with excision of the epicondylar fragment. Because of poor long-term outcomes, surgical excision of the medial epicondyle should be avoided. Nonunion did not have negative effects on function. A study by Lee et al[85] also showed good to excellent results in subjects ages 7 to 17 years who had sustained medial epicondyle fractures (with greater than 5 mm displacement) that were treated operatively.

Radial Head and Neck Fractures

Radial head and neck fractures occur secondary to a fall on an outstretched hand with valgus stress.[32,89] Treatment is determined by the amount of displacement and angulation between the radial head and shaft. Nondisplaced fractures usually have no residual deficits despite minimal treatment. It has also been shown that displaced Mason type I radial head or neck fractures have good long-term outcomes with conservative treatment.[58] Sanchez-Sotelo[119] recommends nonoperative treatment for radial head fractures in adults with less than 2 mm displacement, less than 30% involvement of the articular surface, angulation of less than 30 degrees, and no instability. An angulation of 30 degrees or greater may be an indication for surgical consideration.[89] When treating displaced or comminuted radial head fractures, the clinician should be aware of possible associated injuries, including osteochondral and ligamentous injury.[63] Following radial fractures, complications may include malunion, radial head overgrowth, avascular necrosis, and nonunion.[89]

Rehabilitation Concerns

Strategies to Regain Elbow Range of Motion Following Immobilization

The amount and rate of progression of rehabilitation following an elbow fracture is determined by several factors, including severity of injury, length of immobilization, concomitant injuries, age of patient, and level of sport activities. The primary focus of rehabilitation is on optimizing the return of elbow ROM and strength, with progression to functional daily and sport activities as needed.

Elbow ROM may not be completely regained following traumatic injury. Decreased ROM may be because of osseous structures, but is usually a result of the joint capsule or soft-tissue structures (muscles, tendons, ligaments). The viscoelastic properties of soft tissue must be considered during treatment to regain elbow ROM. These properties include strain rate dependency, creep, stress relaxation, elastic deformation, and plastic deformation. Strain rate is the dependence of material properties on the rate or speed in which a load is applied. Rapidly applied forces will cause stiffness and elastic deformation whereas gradually applied forces will result in plastic deformation.

Creep is defined as the continued deformation of soft tissue with the application of a fixed load (eg, traction and dynamic splinting). Stress relaxation is the reduction of forces, over time, in a material that is stretched and held at a constant length (eg, serial casting and static splinting). Elastic deformation is the elongation produced by loading that is recovered

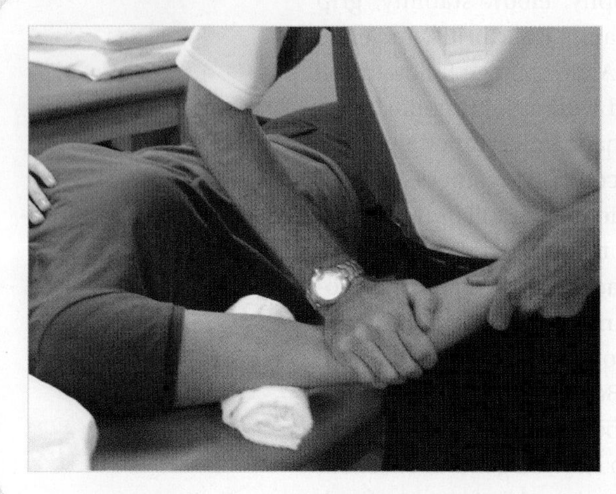

Figure 21-26 **Posterior glide of the ulnohumeral joint**

after the load is removed. There is no long-term effect on tissues. Plastic deformation is the elongation produced under loading that will remain after the removal of a load, resulting in a permanent increase in length.[16]

A study by Bonutti et al[16] evaluated the effectiveness of a patient-directed static progressive stretching program in the treatment of elbow contractures. Subjects had elbow contractures for 1 month to 42 years that did not respond to previous treatment consisting of physical therapy, dynamic splinting, serial casting, surgery, or a combination of these treatments. The orthosis providing a static progressive stretch was worn for 30 minutes with the patient increasing the amount of stretch every 5 minutes as tolerated. Separate 30-minute sessions were used in patients requiring flexion and extension improvement. Results showed an average improvement of 17 degrees extension and 14 degrees flexion. Improved results were seen in 4 to 6 weeks, with continued improvement in patients using the orthotic 3 months or more. There was no change in ROM in patients 1 year after discontinuation of the orthosis, suggesting that the plastic deformation of soft tissue occurred and the elongation of tissue was maintained over time.

Manual rehabilitation techniques for improving elbow ROM include passive ROM and joint mobilizations. Passive range is performed in elbow flexion, extension, supination, and pronation. Care should be taken with passive ROM into extension, as end range stretching of the flexors can potentially contribute to heterotrophic ossification, as discussed previously. Elbow joint mobilizations may be used to restore joint arthrokinematics. Joint distraction (see Figure 21-18), posterior glides of the ulna (Figure 21-26), medial and lateral ulna glides (Figure 21-27), radial distraction (Figure 21-28), and dorsal and ventral glides of the proximal radioulnar (Figure 21-29) joint are used to increase elbow ROM.[37] Shoulder passive ROM should also be performed early in the rehabilitation process to prevent glenohumeral capsular hypomobility, especially if the injury required prolonged immobilization.

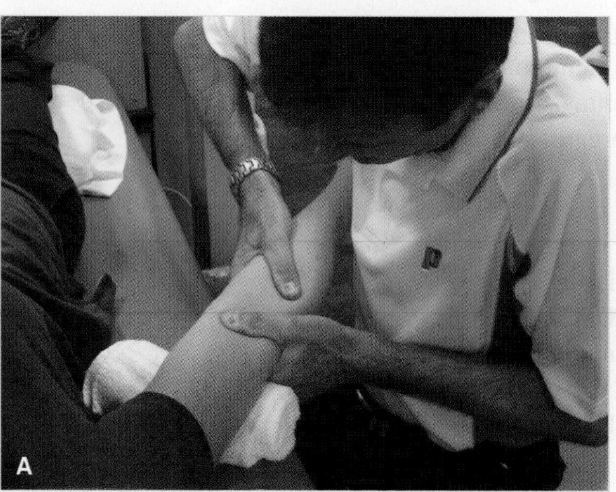

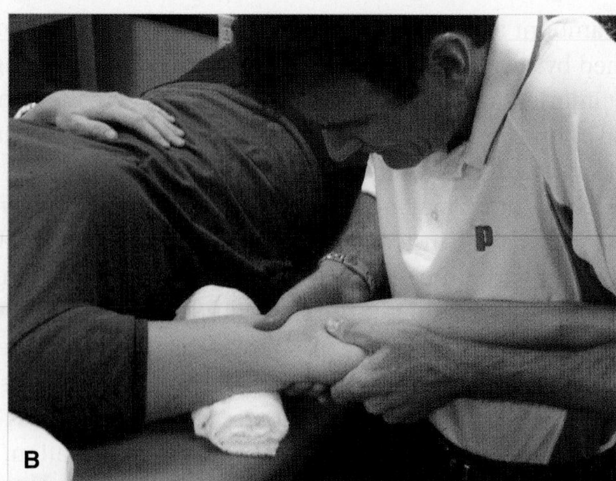

Figure 21-27 **Lateral and medial glides of the ulnohumeral joint**

A. Lateral glide. **B.** Medial glide.

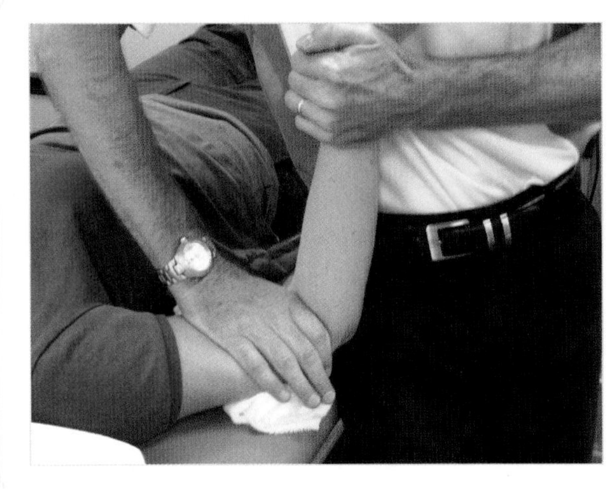

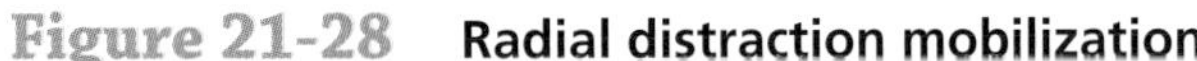

Figure 21-28 Radial distraction mobilization

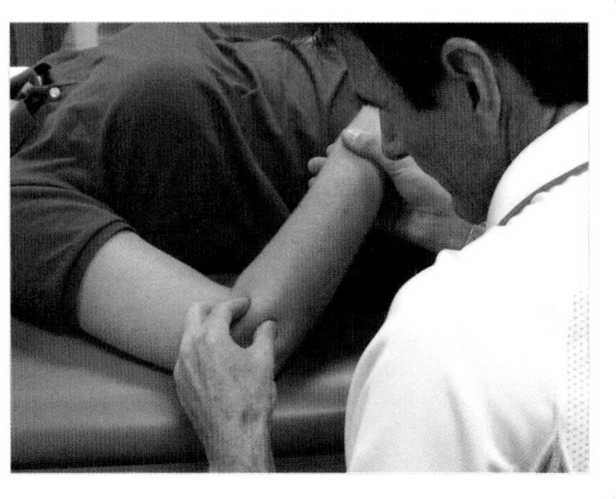

Figure 21-29 Dorsal and ventral glides of the proximal radioulnar joint

Pediatric Considerations

When diagnosing and treating pediatric elbow injuries, consideration must be given to bone maturation and growth. In young children, the elbow joint is cartilaginous with the appearance of apophyseal ossification centers between the ages of 2 and 10 years. It is important to be aware of the apophyseal ossification centers at the elbow so that they are not misinterpreted as fractures on a radiograph. The ossification centers with the date of appearance in parentheses include the capitellum (2 years), radial head (4 years), medial epicondyle (5 years), trochlea (7 years), olecranon (9 years), and lateral epicondyle (10 years).[32] Because the soft tissues surrounding the apophyses are stronger than the cartilage present at the apophyses, injurious forces causing a sprain or strain in an adult may cause an avulsion fracture in children. The most common site for an avulsion fracture is the medial epicondyle. Medial epicondyle avulsion fractures occur in young throwing athletes due to an acute valgus stress and flexor-pronator muscle contraction.[59] There is an acute onset of medial elbow pain after forceful contraction such as during a baseball pitch. The avulsion commonly occurs during late cocking or early acceleration phase of throwing. A "pop" may be heard at time of injury. If a medial epicondyle avulsion fracture is suspected, it is important to assess the ulnar nerve, point tenderness of the medial epicondyle, swelling, ecchymosis, and valgus instability.

The Salter-Harris classification system[118] is commonly used to describe acute physeal injuries (Figure 21-30). There are 5 types of fractures in this classification, with type II fractures being the most common. Type I fractures occur when the epiphysis separates completely from the metaphysis. The mechanism of injury involves shear, torsion, and avulsion forces. Treatment consists of casting with excellent prognosis unless vascular damage is present. In a type II fracture, the fracture line extends along the growth plate and into the metaphysis. The triangular-shaped metaphyseal fragment is referred to as the Thurston-Holland sign. Type III fractures are intraarticular and extend from the joint surface to the weak zone of the growth plate and reaches the periphery of the plate. There is good prognosis with proper reduction and intact vascular supply. Surgery may be needed for type III fractures. Type IV fractures are characterized by the fracture extending from the joint surface through the epiphysis, across the full thickness of the growth plate, and through a portion of the metaphysis. Surgery is required for this type of fracture, and there is usually a poor prognosis unless the growth plate is completely and accurately aligned. A type V fracture is rare and involves crushing of the growth plate, which inhibits further growth.

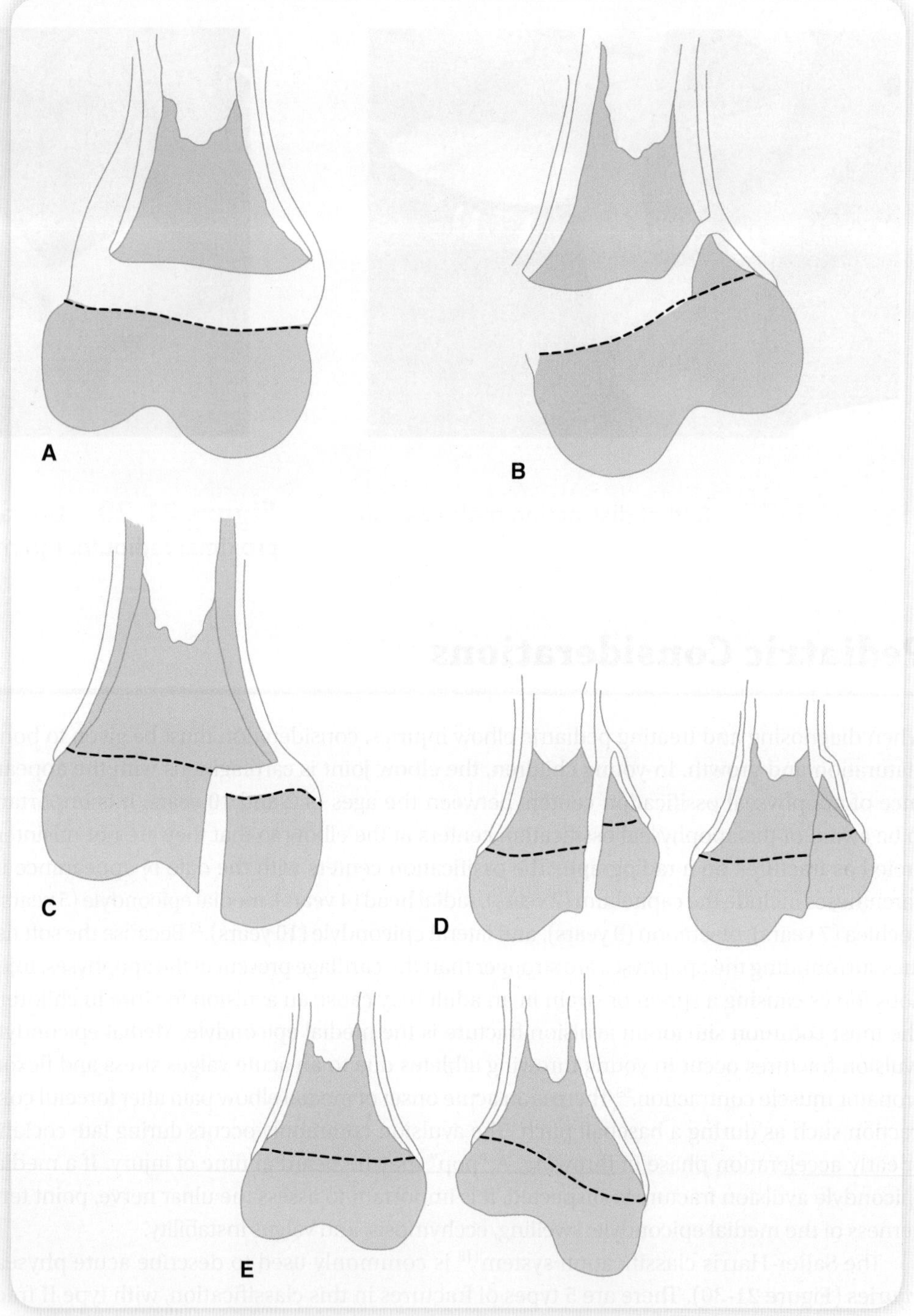

Figure 21-30 **Salter-Harris fracture classification**

A. Type I. B. Type II. C. Type III. D. Type IV. E. Type V.

Similar to elbow fractures in adults, treatment of pediatric elbow fractures varies based on location and type of fracture. Protection of the open growth plates is an important consideration to optimize long-term outcomes. Prolonged immobilization following injury can be more conservative in children than adults, as children do not develop the amount of stiffness and soft-tissue contractures as adults. Pediatric injuries may require less rehabilitation as a result of decreased ROM restriction when compared to adults.

Appendix 1: Postoperative Protocol for Elbow Arthroscopy and Removal of Loose Bodies

Acute Phase

Primary goals

1. Reduce pain and postoperative edema
2. Regain joint ROM and muscle length
3. Initiate submaximal resistive exercise as tolerated

Postoperative Days 1 and 2

1. Removal of bulky postoperative dressing and replacement with Ace wrap.
2. Electric stimulation and ice to decrease pain/inflammation.
3. Initiation of ROM exercise for the glenohumeral joint, elbow, forearm, and wrist.
4. Initiation of submaximal strengthening exercises including:
   a. putty
   b. isometric elbow and wrist flexion/extension
   c. isometric forearm pronation/supination

Postoperative Days 2 to 7

1. ROM and joint mobilization to terminal ranges for the elbow, forearm, and wrist (avoid overaggressive elbow extension passive ROM)
2. Begin progressive resistance exercise program with 0 to 1 lb weight and 3 sets of 15 repetitions
   a. wrist flexion curls
   b. wrist extension curls
   c. radial deviation
   d. ulnar deviation
   e. forearm pronation
   f. forearm supination
3. Upper body ergometer

Intermediate Phase

Primary goals

1. Begin total-arm strength-training program
2. Emphasize full elbow ROM

Postoperative 1 to 3 Weeks

1. Continue progressive resistance exercise program adding:
   a. elbow extension
   b. elbow flexion
   c. isolated rotator cuff program (Jobe exercises)

d. seated row
e. manual and isotonic scapular program
f. closed-chain, upper-extremity program

Advanced/Return to Activity Phase

Primary goals

1. Advance strengthening progression of distal upper extremity
2. Prepare patient for return to functional activity with simulation of joint angles and muscular demands inherent in intended sport activity

Postoperative 4 to 8 Weeks

1. Isokinetic exercise introduction using wrist flexion/extension and forearm pronation/supination movement patterns
2. Upper-extremity plyometrics with medicine balls
3. Isokinetic test to formally assess distal strength
4. Interval sport return program
   a. criterion for advancement:
      i. full, pain-free ROM
      ii. 85% to 100% return of muscle strength
      iii. no provocation of pain on clinical exam
5. Upper-extremity strength and flexibility maintenance program

Appendix 2: Postoperative Rehabilitation Following Ulnar Collateral Ligament Reconstruction Using Autogenous Graft

Postoperative Week 1

Brace

- Posterior splint applied immediately postoperatively with elbow placed in 90 degrees of flexion. Progression to hinged ROM brace dependent on patient tolerance. ROM brace to remain locked at 90 degrees for week 1.

Rehab

- Modalities to decrease elbow swelling and control pain.
- ROM forearm pronation/supination and wrist flexion/extension.
- ROM glenohumeral joint and scapulothoracic joint mobilization.
- Shoulder isometrics (no internal rotation or external rotation as a result of valgus stress on elbow).
- Gripping exercises with balls or putty.

Postoperative Week 2

Brace

- ROM set in hinged elbow brace from 30-100 degrees.

Rehab

- Continue with above exercises and ROM.
- Initiate isometric muscular work of wrist flexion/extension, radial/ulnar deviation, and elbow flexion/extension within ROM available at ulnohumeral joint.
- Initiate closed-chain exercise over Swiss balls (wax-on/off) with limited weight bearing over extremity.
- Begin scapular protraction/retraction manual resistance in side-lying with the elbow in 90 degrees of elbow flexion.

Postoperative Week 3

Brace

- Hinged elbow brace is opened to 15 to 110 degrees. (ROM in brace is gradually increased 5 degrees in extension and 10 degrees in flexion each week unless otherwise specified by physician.)

Rehab

- No changes in exercises during this time period.

Postoperative Weeks 4 to 5

Brace

- Hinged elbow brace set at 10 degrees-120 degrees.

Rehab

- Begin submaximal isotonic exercise for wrist flexion/extension, radial/ulnar deviation and forearm pronation/supination with light 1-lb weight or Thera tubing (yellow or red).
- Begin shoulder isotonic exercise program with prone extension, prone horizontal abduction and standing scaption to 80 degrees elevation as tolerated. Continue to avoid rotational strengthening patterns, due to valgus stress at ulnohumeral joint. Weight attachment proximal to elbow with cuff weights recommended for introduction.
- Initiate seated rowing using Thera tube or machine/cables.

Postoperative Week 6

*Brace**

- Hinged elbow brace set at 0 to 130 degrees.

Rehab

- Begin elbow flexion/extension isotonics using available ranges and avoiding a "bounce home" type movement at end range extension.
- Initiate shoulder internal rotation and external rotation patterns using both isotonic machine or cables (submax), Thera tube (yellow or red to start), and initiation of side-lying external rotation pattern.
- Begin ball dribbling off ground using Swiss balls, Body Blade, Thera-Band resistance bar oscillation, and B.O.I.N.G. using patterns of radial/ulnar deviation and pronation/supination with varied shoulder positions less than 90 degrees of elevation.

---

*Discontinuation of hinged elbow brace occurs between 6 and 10 weeks postoperative, as designated by referring physician.

Postoperative Weeks 10 to 12

Rehab

- Plyometric program initiated using Swiss ball, progressing to medicine ball. Patterns consisting of initially a 2-hand chest pass and progressing to side throws, wood chops, and eventually eccentric arm deceleration with contralateral arm throwing.
- Continuation of shoulder, elbow, forearm, and wrist isotonics.
- Rhythmic stabilization techniques using both open- and closed-chain environments.
- Closed-chain step-up progression.

Postoperative Week 12

Rehab

- Initiation of isokinetic training using the pattern of wrist flexion/extension at speeds ranging from 180 to 300 degrees per second. ROM stops used at 0 to 35 degrees wrist extension and 0 to 55 degrees wrist flexion. Upon successful completion of wrist flexion/extension during several trial treatments, isokinetic forearm pronation and supination is initiated using ROM stops of 0 to 50 degrees of pronation and supination.
- Shoulder isokinetic internal rotation/external rotation is initiated submaximally using speeds between 210 degrees and 300 degrees per second in the modified base position.

Postoperative Week 14 (Return to Activity Phase)

Rehab

- Initiation of elbow extension/flexion isokinetics using speeds between 180 degrees and 300 degrees per second and ROM stops at 10 degrees extension and 125 degrees flexion.
- Initiation of interval sport return programs.
- Continuation of upper-extremity strengthening programs and maintenance of particularly elbow extension ROM.
- A return to competitive levels of throwing or racquet sports is not expected until at least 6 months following surgery.

SUMMARY

1. The elbow joint is composed of the humeroulnar joint, humeroradial joint, and the proximal radioulnar joint. Motions in the elbow complex include flexion, extension, pronation, and supination.
2. Fractures in the elbow may occur from a direct blow or falling on an outstretched hand. They may be treated by casting or in some cases by surgical reduction and fixation. Following surgical fixation, the patient may require 12 weeks for rehabilitation.
3. Valgus extension overload injuries occur during the acceleration phase of the throwing motion and can result in the development of posterior medical osteophytes and loose bodies in the athletic elbow. Treatment via arthroscopy is followed by early immediate ROM and a progression of strength and functional training to restore full function to the elbow.

4. The ulnar collateral ligament is injured as a result of a repetitive valgus force. Reconstruction is vital to competitive throwing patients.
5. Elbow dislocations result from elbow hyperextension from a fall on an extended arm, with the radius and ulna dislocating posteriorly. The degree of stability present determines the course of rehabilitation. If the elbow is stable, a brief period of immobilization is followed by rehabilitation. An unstable dislocation requires surgical repair and thus a longer period of immobilization.
6. Medial epicondylitis results from repetitive microtrauma to the common flexor and pronator tendons during pronation and flexion of the forearm and wrist.
7. Lateral epicondylitis (tennis elbow) occurs with concentric or eccentric overload of the wrist extensors and supinators, most commonly the extensor carpi radialis brevis tendon.

REFERENCES

1. Adelsberg S. An EMG analysis of selected muscles with rackets of increasing grip size. *Am J Sports Med.* 1986;14:139-142.
2. An KN, Morrey BF. Biomechanics of the elbow. In: Morrey BF, ed. *The Elbow and Its Disorders.* Philadelphia, PA: Saunders; 1993:53-72.
3. Andrews JR, Heggland EJH, Fleisig GS, Zheng N. Relationship of ulnar collateral ligament strain to amount of medial olecranon osteotomy. *Am J Sports Med.* 2001;29(6):716-721.
4. Andrews JR, Soffer SR. *Elbow Arthroscopy.* St. Louis, MO: Mosby-Yearbook; 1994.
5. Andrews JR, Timmerman LA. Outcome of elbow surgery in professional baseball players. *Am J Sports Med.* 1995;23:407-4134.
6. Andrews JR, Wilk KE, Groh G. Elbow rehabilitation. In: Brotzman SB, ed. *Clinical Orthopaedic Rehabilitation.* Philadelphia, PA: Mosby-Yearbook; 1996:67-71.
7. Andrews JR, Wilk KE, Satterwhite YE, Tedder JL. Physical examination of the thrower's elbow. *J Orthop Sports Phys Ther.* 1993;6:296-304.
8. Arnoczky SP, Delos D, Rodeo SA. What is platelet-rich plasma? *Oper Tech Sports Med.* 2011;19:142-148.
9. Ballentyne BT, O'Hare SJ, Paschall JL, et al. Electromyographic activity of selected shoulder muscles in commonly used therapeutic exercises. *Phys Ther.* 1993;73:668-682.
10. Basford JR, Sheffield CG, Cieslak KR. Laser therapy: a randomized, controlled trial of the effects of low intensity Nd:YAG laser irradiation on lateral epicondylitis. *Arch Phys Med Rehabil.* 2000;81:1504-1510.
11. Bennett GE. Elbow and shoulder lesions of baseball players. *Am J Surg.* 1959;98:484-492.
12. Bennett JB, Green MS, Tullos HS. Surgical management of chronic medial elbow instability. *Clin Orthop Relat Res.* 1992;278:62-68.
13. Bernhang AM, Dehner W, Fogarty C. Tennis elbow: a biomechanical approach. *Am J Sports Med.* 1974;2:235-260.
14. Bhandari M, Tornetta P, Swiontkowski MF. Displaced lateral condyle fractures of the distal humerus. *J Orthop Trauma.* 2003;17:306-308.
15. Blackburn TA, McLeod WD, White B, et al. EMG analysis of posterior rotator cuff exercises. *Athl Train.* 1990;25:40-45.
16. Bonutti PM, Windau JE, Ables BA, Miller BG. Static progressive stretch to reestablish elbow range of motion. *Clin Orthop Relat Res.* 1994;303:128-134.
17. Bowling RW, Rockar PA. The elbow complex. In: Davies GJ, Gould JA, eds. *Orthopaedic and Sports Physical Therapy.* St. Louis, MO: Mosby; 1985:476-496.
18. Boyer MI, Hastings H. Lateral tennis elbow: is there any science out there? *J Shoulder Elbow Surg.* 1999;8:481-491.
19. Brattberg G. Acupuncture therapy for tennis elbow. *Pain.* 1983;16:285-288.
20. Carroll R. Tennis elbow: incidence in local league players. *Br J Sports Med.* 1981;15:250-255.
21. Chinn CJ, Priest JD, Kent BE. Upper extremity range of motion, grip strength, and girth in highly skilled tennis players. *Phys Ther.* 1974;54:474-482.
22. Conway JE, Jobe FW, Glousman RE, Pink M. Medial instability of the elbow in throwing athletes. *J Bone Joint Surg Am.* 1992;74(1):67-83.
23. Creaney L, Wallace A, Curtis M, Connell D: Growth factor-based therapies provide additional benefit beyond physical therapy in resistant elbow tendinopathy: a prospective, single-blind, randomised trial of autologous blood injections versus platelet-rich plasma injections. *Br J Sports Med.* 2011;45:966-971.
24. Croisier JL, Foidart-Dessalle, M, Tinant, F, et.al. An isokinetic eccentric programme for the management of chronic lateral epicondylar tendinopathy. *Br J Sports Med.* 2007;41:269-275.

25. Cyriax JH, Cyriax PJ. *Illustrated Manual of Orthopaedic Medicine.* London, UK: Butterworths; 1983.
26. Davidson PA, Pink M, Perry J, Jobe FW. Functional anatomy of the flexor pronator muscle group in relation to the medial collateral ligament of the elbow. *Am J Sports Med.* 1995;23(2):245-250.
27. de las Heras J, Duran D, de la Cerdo J, Romanillos O, Martinez-Miranda J, Rodriguez-Merchain EC. Supracondylar fractures of the humerus in children. *Clin Orthop Relat Res.* 2005;432:57-64.
28. De Vos RJ, Weir A, Van Schie HTM, Bierma-Zeinstra R, Verhaar J Weinans H, Tol JL. Platelet-rich plasma injection for chronic Achilles tendinopathy. *JAMA.* 2010;303:144-149.
29. DeLong JM, Russell RP, Mazzocca AD: Platelet-rich plasma: the PAW classification system. *Arthroscopy.* 2012;28:998-1009.
30. Dijs H, Mortier G, Driessens M, DeRidder A, Willems J, Devroey TA. Retrospective study of the conservative treatment of tennis elbow. *Acta Belg Med Phys.* 1990;13:73-77.
31. Dines JS, Frank JB, Akerman M, et al: Glenohumeral internal rotation deficits in baseball players with ulnar collateral ligament deficiency. *Am J Sports Med.* 2009;37(3):566-70.
32. Do T, Herrara-Soto J. Elbow injuries in children. *Curr Opin Pediatr.* 2003;15:68-73.
33. Ellenbecker TS. Rehabilitation of shoulder and elbow injuries in tennis players. *Clin Sports Med.* 1995;14:87-110.
34. Ellenbecker TS. A total arm strength isokinetic profile of highly skilled tennis players. *Isokinet Exerc Sci.* 1991;1:9-21.
35. Ellenbecker TS, Davies GJ. *Closed Kinetic Chain Exercise.* Champaign, IL: Human Kinetics; 2001.
36. Ellenbecker TS, Davies GJ, Rowinski MJ. Concentric versus eccentric isokinetic strengthening of the rotator cuff: objective testing versus functional test. *Am J Sports Med.* 1988;16(1):64-69.
37. Ellenbecker TS, Mattalino AJ. *The Elbow in Sport.* Champaign, IL: Human Kinetics; 1997.
38. Ellenbecker TS, Mattalino AJ, Elam EA, Caplinger RA. Medial elbow laxity in professional baseball pitchers: a bilateral comparison using stress radiography. *Am J Sports Med.* 1998;26(3):420-424.
39. Ellenbecker TS, Roetert EP. Isokinetic profile of elbow flexion and extension strength in elite junior tennis players. *J Orthop Sports Phys Ther.* 2003;33(2):79-84.
40. Ellenbecker TS, Roetert EP. *Isokinetic Profile of Wrist and Forearm Strength in Female Elite Junior Tennis Players.* Platform presentation presented at the APTA Annual Conference and Exposition, Washington DC, June, 2003.
41. Ellenbecker TS, Roetert EP. Unpublished data from the USTA on range of motion of the elbow and wrist in senior tennis players; 1994.
42. Ellenbecker TS, Roetert EP, Bailie DS, Davies GJ, Brown SW. Glenohumeral joint total rotation range of motion in elite tennis players and baseball pitchers. *Med Sci Sports Exerc.* 2002;34(12):2052-2056.
43. Farsetti P, Potenza V, Caterini R, Ippolito E. Long-term results of treatment of fractures of the medial humeral epicondyle in children. *J Bone Joint Surg Am.* 2001;83(9):1299-1305.
44. Ficek K, Kamiński T, Wach E, Cholewiński J. Application of platelet rich plasma in sports medicine. *J Hum Kinet.* 2011;30:85- 97.
45. Fleck SJ, Kraemer WJ. *Designing Resistance Training Programs.* Champaign, IL: Human Kinetics; 1987.
46. Gam AN, Warming S, Larsen LH, et al. Treatment of myofascial trigger points with ultrasound combined with massage and exercise. A randomized controlled trial. *Pain.* 1998;77(1):73-79.
47. Glousman RE, Barron J, Jobe FW, et al. An electromyographic analysis of the elbow in normal and injured pitchers with medial collateral ligament insufficiency. *Am J Sports Med.* 1992;20:311-317.
48. Goldie I. Epicondylitis lateralis humeri. *Acta Chir Scand Suppl.* 1964;339:1-114.
49. Gosens T, Peerbooms JC, Van Laar W, Den Oudsten B. A double-blind randomized controlled trial with 2-year follow-up: ongoing positive effect of platelet-rich plasma versus corticosteroid injection in lateral epicondylitis. *Am J Sports Med.* 2011;39:1200-1208.
50. Gould JA, Davies GJ. Orthopaedic and sports rehabilitation concepts. In: Gould JA, Davies GJ, eds. *Orthopaedic and Sports Physical Therapy.* St. Louis, MO: Mosby, 1985:181-198.
51. Greenbaum B, Itamura J, Vangsness CT, Tibone J, Atkinson R. Extensor carpi radialis brevis. *J Bone Joint Surg Br.* 1999;81(5):926-929.
52. Groppel JL, Nirschl RP. A biomechanical and electromyographical analysis of the effects of counter force braces on the tennis player. *Am J Sports Med.* 1986;14:195-200.
53. Guerra JJ, Timmerman LA. Clinical anatomy, histology, and pathomechanics of the elbow in sports. *Oper Tech Sports Med.* 1996;4:69-76.
54. Haake M, Konig IR, Decker T, et al. Extracorporeal shock wave therapy in the treatment of lateral epicondylitis: a randomized multicenter trial. *J Bone Joint Surg Am.* 2002;84:1982-1991.
55. Hang YS, Peng SM. An epidemiological study of upper extremity injury in tennis players with particular reference to tennis elbow. *J Formos Med Assoc.* 1984;83:307-316.
56. Harrelson GL, Leaver-Dunn D. Elbow rehabilitation. In: Andrews JR, Harrelson GL, Wilk KE, eds. *Physical Rehabilitation of the Injured Athlete.* 2nd ed. Philadelphia, PA: Saunders, 1998:554-588.
57. Hawkins RJ, Kennedy JC. Impingement syndrome in athletes. *Am J Sports Med.* 1980;8:151-158.

58. Herbertson P, Josefsson PO, Hasserius R, Karlsson C, Besjakov J, Karlsson MK. Displaced mason type I fractures of the radial head and neck in adults: a fifteen-to thirty-three-year follow-up study. *J Shoulder Elbow Surg.* 2005;14:73-77.
59. Hughes PE, Paletta GA. Little leaguer's elbow, medial epicondyle injury, and osteochondritis dissecans. *Sports Med Arthroscopy Rev.* 2003;11:30-39.
60. Indelicato PA, Jobe FW, Kerlan RK, Carter VS, Shields CL, Lombardo SJ. Correctable elbow lesions in professional baseball players: a review of 25 cases. *Am J Sports Med.* 1979;7:72-75.
61. Ingham K. Transverse cross friction massage. *Phys Sportsmed.* 1981;9(10):116.
62. Inman VT, Saunders JB de CM, Abbot LC. Observations on the function of the shoulder joint. *J Bone Joint Surg Am.* 1944;26:1-30.
63. Itamura J, Roidis N, Mirzayan R, Vaishnzv S, Learch T, Shean C. Radial head fractures: MRI evaluation of associated injuries. *J Shoulder Elbow Surg.* 2005;14:421-424.
64. Izumi T, Aoki M, Muraki T, Hidaka E. Stretching positions of the posterior capsule of the glenohumeral joint. *Am J Sports Med.* 2008;36(10):2014-2022.
65. Jensen BR, Sjogaard G, Bornmyr S, Arborelius M, Jorgensen K. Intramuscular laser-Doppler flowmetry in the supraspinatus muscle during isometric contractions. *Eur J Appl Physiol Occup Physiol.* 1995;71(4):373-378.
66. Jobe FW, Elattrache NS. Diagnosis and treatment of ulnar collateral ligament injuries in athletes. In: Morrey BF, ed. *The Elbow and its Disorders.* 2nd ed. Philadelphia, PA: Saunders, 1993:566-572.
67. Jobe FW, Kvitne RS. Shoulder pain in the overhand or throwing athlete: the relationship of anterior instability and rotator cuff impingement. *Orthop Rev.* 1989;28(9):963-975.
68. Jobe FW, Stark H, Lombardo SJ. Reconstruction of the ulnar collateral ligament in athletes. *J Bone Joint Surg Am.* 1986;68:1158-1163.
69. Josefsson PO, Nilsson BE. Incidence of elbow dislocations. *Acta Orthop Scand.* 1986;57:537-538.
70. Joyce ME, Jelsma RD, Andrews JR. Throwing injuries to the elbow. *Sports Med Arthroscopy Rev.* 1995;3:224-236.
71. Kamien M. A rational management of tennis elbow. *Sports Med.* 1990;9:173-191.
72. Keppler P, Salem K, Schwarting B, Kintzl L. The effectiveness of physiotherapy after operative treatment of supracondylar humeral fractures in children. *J Pediatr Orthop.* 2005;25:314-316.
73. Kibler WB. The role of the scapula in athletic shoulder function. *Am J Sports Med.* 1998;26(2):325-337.
74. Kibler WB. Role of the scapula in the overhead throwing motion. *Contemp Orthop.* 1991;22(5):525-532.
75. Kibler WB, Chandler TJ, Livingston BP, Roetert EP. Shoulder range of motion in elite tennis players. *Am J Sports Med.* 1996;24(3):279-285.
76. Kibler WB, Uhl TL, Maddux JWQ, Brooks PV, Zeller B, McMullen J. Qualitative clinical evaluation of scapular dysfunction: a reliability study. *J Shoulder Elbow Surg.* 2002;11:550-556.
77. King JW, Brelsford HJ, Tullos HS. Analysis of the pitching arm of the professional baseball pitcher. *Clin Orthop.* 1969;67:116-123.
78. Kitai E, Itay S, Ruder A, et al. Ann epidemiological study of lateral epicondylitis in amateur male players. *Ann Chir Main.* 1986;5:113-121.
79. Kraushaar BS, Nirschl RP. Tendinosis of the elbow (tennis elbow). Clinical features and findings of histopathological, immunohistochemical and electron microscopy studies. *J Bone Joint Surgery Am.* 1999;81:259-278.
80. Kulund DN, Rockwell DA, Brubaker CE. The long term effects of playing tennis. *Phys Sportsmed.* 1979;7:87-92.
81. Kuroda S, Sakamaki K. Ulnar collateral ligament tears of the elbow joint. *Clin Orthop Relat Res.* 1986;208: 266-271.
82. Labelle H, Guibert R, Joncas J, Newman N, Fallaha M, Rivard CH. Lack of scientific evidence for the treatment of lateral epicondylitis of the elbow. *J Bone Joint Surg Br.* 1992;74:646-651.
83. Launay F, Leet A, Jacopin S, Jouve J, Bollini G, Sponseller PD. Lateral humeral condyle fractures in children: a comparison to two approaches in treatment. *J Pediatr Orthop.* 2004;24:385-391.
84. Leadbetter WB. Cell matrix response in tendon injury. *Clin Sports Med.* 1992;11:533-579.
85. Lee H, Shen H, Chang J, Lee C, Wu S. Operative treatment of displaced medial epicondyle fractures in children and adolescents. *J Shoulder Elbow Surg.* 2005;14:178-185.
86. Linscheid RL, O'Driscoll SW. Elbow dislocation. In: Morrey BF, ed. *The Elbow and Its Disorders.* 2nd ed. Philadelphia, PA: Saunders, 1993:441-452.
87. Magee DJ. Elbow. In: Magee DJ, ed. *Orthopedic Physical Assessment.* Philadelphia, PA: Saunders; 1997:247-274.
88. McFarland EG, Torpey BM, Carl LA. Evaluation of shoulder laxity. *Sports Med.* 1996;22:264-272.
89. Milbrandt TA, Copley LA. Common elbow injuries in children: evaluation, treatment, and clinical outcomes. *Curr Opin Orthop.* 2004;15:286-294.
90. Mirsky EC, Karas EH, Weiner L. Lateral condyle fractures in children: evaluation of classification and treatment. *J Orthop Trauma.* 1997;11(2):117-120.
91. Mishra A, Pavelko T. Treatment of chronic elbow tendinosis with buffered platelet-rich plasma. *Am J Sports Med.* 2006;34:1774-1778.
92. Morrey BF. *The Elbow and its Disorders.* 2nd ed. Philadelphia, PA: Saunders; 1993.
93. Morrey BF, An KN. Articular and ligamentous contributions to the stability of the elbow joint. *Am J Sports Med.* 1983;11:315.
94. Neer CS. Impingement lesions. *Clin Orthop.* 1973;173:70-77.

95. Nirschl RP. Muscle and tendon trauma: tennis elbow. In: Morrey BF, ed. *The Elbow and its Disorders*. 2nd ed. Philadelphia, PA: Saunders; 1993:537-552.
96. Nirschl RP. Elbow tendinosis/tennis elbow. *Clin Sports Med.* 1992;11:851-870.
97. Nirschl RP, Rodin DM, Ochiai DH, Maartmann-Moe C. Iontophoretic administration of dexamethasone sodium phosphate for acute epicondylitis: a randomized, double-blinded, placebo controlled study. *Am J Sports Med.* 2003;31(2):189-195.
98. Nirschl R, Sobel J. Conservative treatment of tennis elbow. *Phys Sportsmed.* 1981;9:43-54.
99. O'Driscoll SW. Elbow instability. *Hand Clin.* 1994;10: 405-415.
100. O'Driscoll SW, Morrey BF. Arthroscopy of the elbow. *J Bone Joint Surg Am.* 1992;74:84-94.
101. O'Driscoll SW, Lawton RL, Smith AM. The moving valgus stress test for medial ulnar collateral ligament tears of the elbow. *Am J Sports Med.* 2005;33(2):231-239.
102. Oglive-Harris DJ, Gordon R, MacKay M. Arthroscopic treatment for posterior impingement in degenerative arthritis of the elbow. *Arthroscopy.* 1995;11(4):437-443.
103. Olsen BS, Sojbjerg JO, Dalstra M, Sneppen O. Kinematics of the lateral ligamentous constraints of the elbow joint. *J Shoulder Elbow Surg.* 1996;5:333-341.
104. Omar AS, Ibrahim ME, Ahmed AS, Said M. Local injection of autologous platelet rich plasma and corticosteroid in treatment of lateral epicondylitis and plantar fasciitis: randomized clinical trial. *Egyptian Rheumatologist.* 2012;34:43-49.
105. Peerbooms JC, Sluimer J, Bruijn DJ, Gosens T. Positive effect of an autologous platelet concentrate in lateral epicondylitis in a double-blind randomized controlled trial: platelet-rich plasma versus corticosteroid injection with a 1-year follow-up. *Am J Sports Med.* 2010;38:255-262.
106. Percy EC, Carson JD. The use of DMSO in tennis elbow and rotator cuff tendinitis. A double blind study. *Med Sci Sports Exerc.* 1981;13:215-219.
107. Peterson M, Butler S, Eriksson M, Svardsudd K. A randomized controlled trial of exercise versus wait-list in chronic tennis elbow (lateral epicondylosis). *Ups J Med Sci.* 2011;116(4):269-279.
108. Priest JD, Jones HH, Nagel DA. Elbow injuries in highly skilled tennis players. *J Sports Med.* 1974;2(3): 137-149.
109. Priest JD, Jones HH, Tichenor CJC, et al. Arm and elbow changes in expert tennis players. *Minn Med.* 1977;60:399-404.
110. Reddy AS, Kvitne RS, Yocum LA, Elattrache NS, Glousman RE, Jobe FW. Arthroscopy of the elbow: A long term clinical review. *Arthroscopy.* 2000;16(6): 588-594.
111. Regan WD, Korinek SL, Morrey BF, An KN. Biomechanical study of ligaments around the elbow joint. *Clin Orthop.* 1991;271:170-179.
112. Rhu KN, McCormick J, Jobe FW, et al. An electromyographic analysis of shoulder function in tennis players. *Am J Sports Med.* 1988;16:481-485.
113. Rijke AM, Goitz HT, McCue FC. Stress radiography of the medial elbow ligaments. *Radiology.* 1994;191:213-216.
114. Roetert EP, Ellenbecker TS, Brown SW. Shoulder internal and external rotation range of motion in nationally ranked junior tennis players: a longitudinal analysis. *J Strength Cond Res.* 2000;14(2):140-143.
115. Rosenthal M. The efficacy of flurbiprofen versus piroxicam in the treatment of acute soft tissue rheumatism. *Curr Med Res Opin.* 1984;9:304-309.
116. Ross G, McDevitt ER, Chronister R, et al. Treatment of simple elbow dislocation using an immediate motion protocol. *Am J Sports Med.* 1999;27(3):308-311.
117. Runge F. Zur genese unt behand lung bes schreibekramp fes. *Berl Kun Woschenschr.* 1873;10:245-248.
118. Salter RB, Harris WR. Injuries involving the epiphyseal plate. *J Bone Joint Surg Am.* 1963;45:587-632.
119. Sanchez-Sotelo J, Barwood SA, Blaine TA. Current concepts in elbow fracture care. *Curr Opin Orthop.* 2004;15:300-310.
120. Sato D, Takahara M, Narita A, et al. Effect of platelet-rich plasma with fibrin matrix on healing of intrasynovial flexor tendons. *J Hand Surg Am.* 2012;37:1356-1363.
121. Shanley E, Rauh MJ, Michener LA, Ellenbecker TS, Garrison JC, Thigpen CA. Shoulder range of motion measures as risk factors for shoulder and elbow injuries in high school softball and baseball players. *Am J Sports Med.* 2011;39:1997-2006.
122. Skaggs DL, Mirzayan R. The posterior fat pad sign in association with occult fracture of the elbow in children. *J Bone Joint Surg Am.* 1999;10:1429-1433.
123. Slocum DB. Classification of the elbow injuries from baseball pitching. *Am J Sports Med.* 1978;6:62.
124. Smith R, Brunulli J. Shoulder kinesthesia after anterior glenohumeral dislocation. *Phys Ther.* 1989;69(2):106-112.
125. Stroyan M, Wilk KE. The functional anatomy of the elbow complex. *J Orthop Sports Phys Ther.* 1993;17:279-288.
126. Sullivan PE, Markos PD, Minor MD. *An Integrated Approach to Therapeutic Exercise: Theory and Clinical Application.* Reston, VA: Reston Publishing; 1982.
127. Svernl AB, Adolfsson L. Non-operative treatment regime including eccentric training for lateral humeral epicondylalgia. *Scand J Med Sci Sports.* 2001;11(6):328-334.
128. Thanasas C, Papadimitriou G, Charalambidis C, Paraskevopoulos I, Papanikolaou A. Platelet-rich plasma versus autologous whole blood for the treatment of chronic lateral elbow epicondylitis: a randomized controlled clinical trial. *Am J Sports Med.* 2011;39:2130-2134.
129. Tinsley BA, Ferreira JV, Dukas AG, Mazzocca AD. Platelet-rich plasma nonoperative injection therapy—a review of indications and evidence. *Oper Tech Sports Med.* 2012;20:192-200.

130. Townsend H, Jobe FW, Pink M, et al. Electromyographic analysis of the glenohumeral muscles during a baseball rehabilitation program. *Am J Sports Med.* 1991;19:264-272.

131. Tullos HS, Ryan WJ. Functional anatomy of the elbow. In: Zarins B, Andres JR, Carson WD, eds. *Injuries to the Throwing Arm.* Philadelphia, PA: Saunders; 1985.

132. Tyler TF, Thomas GC, Nicholas SJ, McHugh MP. Addition of isolated wrist extensor eccentric exercise to standard treatment for chronic lateral epicondylosis: a prospective randomized trial. *J Shoulder Elbow Surg.* 2010;19(6):917-922.

133. Uhl TL. Uncomplicated elbow dislocation rehabilitation. *Athl Ther Today.* 2000;5(3):31-35.

134. Uhl TL, Gould M, Gieck JH. Rehabilitation after posterolateral dislocation of the elbow in a collegiate football player: a case report. *J Athl Train.* 2000;35(1):108-110.

135. Verhaar JAN, Walenkamp GHIM, Kester ADM, Linden AJVD. Local corticosteroid injection versus Cyriax-type physiotherapy for tennis elbow. *J Bone Joint Surg Br.* 1995;77:128-132.

136. Warfel JH. *Muscles of the Arm. The Extremities, Muscles, and Motor Points.* Philadelphia, PA: Lea & Febinger; 1993.

137. Waslewski GL, Lund P, Chilvers M, Taljanovic M, Krupinski E. *MRI Evaluation of the Ulnar Collateral Ligament of the Elbow in Asymptomatic, Professional Baseball Players.* Presented at the AOSSM Meeting, San Diego, CA; 2002.

138. Wilk KE, Arrigo CA. Rehabilitation of elbow injuries. In: Andrews JR, Harrelson GL, Wilk KE, eds. *Physical Rehabilitation of the Injured Athlete.* 3rd ed. Philadelphia, PA: Saunders, 2004:590-618.

139. Wilk KE, Arrigo CA, Andrews JR. Rehabilitation of the elbow in the throwing athlete. *J Orthop Sports Phys Ther.* 1993;17:305-317.

140. Wilk KE, Azar FM, Andrews JR. Conservative and operative rehabilitation of the elbow in sports. *Sports Med Arthroscopy Rev.* 1995;3:237-258.

141. Wilk KE, Macrina LC, Fleisig GS, et al. Correlation of glenohumeral internal rotation deficit and total rotational motion to shoulder injuries in professional baseball pitchers. *Am J Sports Med.* 2011;39:329-335.

142. Wilson FD, Andrews JR, Blackburn TA, McCluskey G. Valgus extension overload in the pitching elbow. *Am J Sports Med.* 1983;11(2):83-88.

143. Winge S, Jorgensen U, Nielsen AL. Epidemiology of injuries in Danish championship tennis. *Int J Sports Med.* 1989;10:368-371.

144. Wolf BR, Altchek DW. Elbow problems in elite tennis players. *Tech Shoulder Elbow Surg.* 2003;4(2):55-68.

22

Rehabilitation of the Wrist, Hand, and Digits

Jeanine Beasley and Dianna Lunsford

OBJECTIVES

After completion of this chapter, the physical therapist should be able to do the following:

- Discuss key concepts of functional anatomy and biomechanics involved in the normal wrist and hand.
- Relate biomechanics and tissue healing principles to the rehabilitation of various wrist and hand conditions.
- Discuss criteria for progression of the rehabilitation program for specific hand and wrist conditions.
- Describe the rationale for specific orthotic techniques in the management of selected wrist and hand conditions.

Functional Anatomy and Biomechanics

The hand is an intricate balance of muscles, tendons, and joints working in unison. This balance combines mobility, stability, and dexterity allowing the hand to perform a multitude of activities. Any disruption of this balance as a result of an injury or condition can greatly alter the ability of the hand to perform activities of daily living (ADL). At work, the hand is the most frequently injured part of the body.[79] Hand conditions can occur as a single injury, over time as in cumulative trauma, or because of a disease process.

Treatment of hand conditions requires a complete history and evaluation. These evaluations can include subjective and objective assessments that assist the physician and therapist in determining the specific hand dysfunction. A diagnosis of "hand pain" or "wrist pain" does the client a disservice and may lend itself to treatment that is not specific to the condition. The reader is referred to the text, *Rehabilitation of the Hand and Upper Extremity* (6th ed.),[72] for a complete discussion of evaluations and assessments.

Treatment of the hand is based on the phases of wound healing. Initially, the inflammatory phase usually lasts 3 to 5 days. It is typically a time of vascular dilation and edema.[62,89] The extremity is often immobilized during this phase. For example, following a surgery, a bulky dressing can provide immobilization during this phase. This phase can be prolonged in cases of overactive patients or aggressive therapy. Diabetes or specific medications can prolong this and other phases of wound healing. The second phase is the fibroplasia phase, which typically lasts from 5 to 21 days.[62,89] During this phase, the fibroblasts lay down collagen in a random network. Depending on the specific diagnosis, special protected motion exercises may be allowed during this phase. An example of this is treatment of a newly repaired flexor tendon, which generally begins with passive range of motion (PROM) in a protective orthosis during this phase to avoid stress on or rupture of the repair.[62]

The third phase is the maturation phase that usually begins at 3 weeks. It continues for several months. Here the randomly oriented collagen matures and develops strength with intermolecular crosslinking.[62,89] Adhesions also form during this phase. Some treatment protocols are often progressed during this phase. Care should be taken to use caution during the application of stress to the area in order to protect the healing tissues.

The Wrist

The wrist is the connecting link between the hand and forearm.[97] The wrist joints are comprised of 8 carpal bones that are arranged in 2 rows. The proximal row articulates with the distal radius and the triangular fibrocartilage complex (TFCC) of the ulna proximally. The distal row articulates with the metacarpals distally. There is an intricate relationship between the carpal bones. Ligaments interconnect the carpal bones, as well as connect the carpal bones to the radius and ulna.[8,16] During range of motion (ROM) the carpal bones demonstrate complex kinematics.[8] Flexion and extension occur through synchronous movement of proximal and distal carpal rows. Some authors have debated these kinematic theories noting that the scaphoid sometimes acts as part of the proximal row and other times acts as a link between the proximal and distal carpal row.[46,49,58] Palmer et al[58] demonstrated that many ADL involve a wrist arc from radial deviation and wrist extension to ulnar deviation and wrist flexion also called the "dart throwers arc" (Figure 22-1). The scaphoid and lunate are stable and have minimal intercarpal movements during the dart throwers motion as noted during kinematic studies.[70] An example of an application of this concept would be initiating a gentle active motion exercise program for a carpal ligament repair to the scaphoid and lunate using the "dart throwers arc" in order to protect these repairs.

Functional movement of the wrist, or the amount of wrist movement needed to do most ADL was found by Ryu et al[69] to be 40 degrees of flexion, 40 degrees of extension, and a

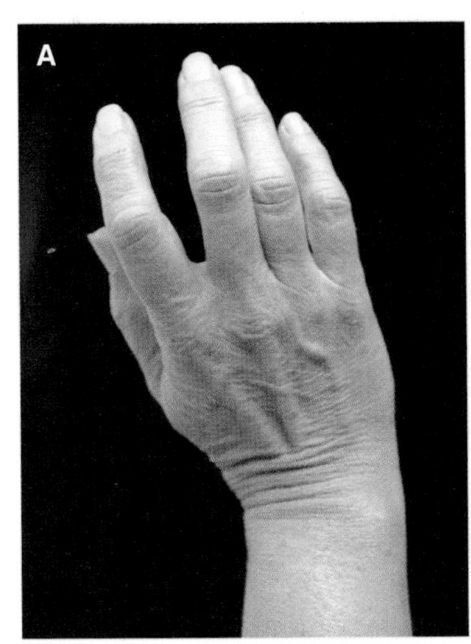

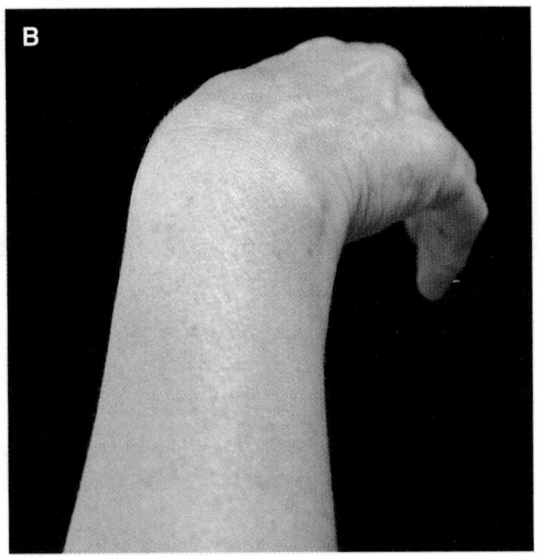

Figure 22-1 **Dart throwers arc**

(**A**) The scaphoid and lunate are most stable and have minimal intercarpal movements during the dart throwers motion as noted by kinematic studies.[11] This movement involves a wrist arc from radial deviation and wrist extension to (**B**) ulnar deviation and wrist flexion. Palmer et al[10] demonstrated that many ADL involve this motion. Initiating a gentle active motion exercise program for a carpal ligament repair to the scaphoid and lunate may be best done using the dart throwers arc to protect these repairs.

combined arc of 40 degrees of radial and ulnar deviation. It is important for the therapist to remember to not sacrifice joint stability or increase joint pain when attempting to increase ROM. A pain-free stable joint with adequate functional motion, as discussed above, serves the client's functional activities better than a joint with greater ROM, greater pain, and less stability.

Stability of the ulnar side of the wrist is provided by the TFCC.[97] This ligament arises from the radius and inserts into the base of the ulnar styloid, the ulnar carpals, and the base of the fifth metacarpal.[97] This ligament complex is the major stabilizer of the distal radioulnar joint (DRUJ) and is a load-bearing column between the distal ulna and ulnar carpals.[97] Injury to the TFCC can result in pain with pronation and supination of the forearm and with ulnar deviation. Diagnostically, this pain may be reduced when the examiner provides support to the ulna during pronation and supination (Figure 22-2). Treatment for this condition is discussed in the section entitled "Injuries to the Distal Radioulnar Joint".

The flexor carpi ulnaris (FCU) with its insertion into the pisiform, a sesamoid bone, is unique in that it is the only muscle with a tendinous insertion into the wrist. The proximity of this easily palpated bone to the ulnar nerve can sometimes be troublesome in cases of blows to the area or a pisiform fracture. In cases of ulnar nerve compression, symptoms should be differentiated to determine if the problem arises from the Guyon canal (located under the pisiform) or at the cubital tunnel of the elbow. Compression of the ulnar nerve at the cubital tunnel is a more common condition.

The dorsal wrist has an extensor retinaculum (fascia) with 6 extensor compartments that are separated by septa.[68] The purpose of the retinaculum is to prevent bowstringing or subluxation of the tendons during wrist movement. The fibro-osseous tunnels or

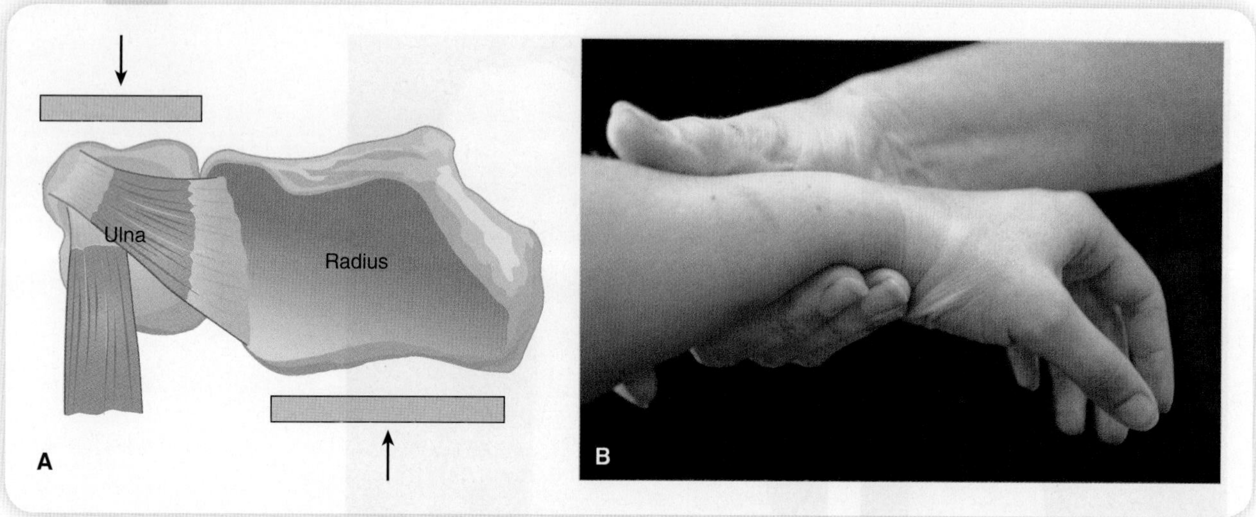

Figure 22-2

A. Injury to the TFCC can result in forearm pain with pronation and supination, as well as with wrist ulnar deviation. Support to the distal ulna may provide support and decrease pain (see Figure 22-11 for an example of an orthosis to support the distal ulna). **B.** This pain may be reduced when the instability of the DRUJ is supported by the examiner. This is completed by providing compression of the distal ulna dorsally and a counterforce to the distal radius in volar direction.

compartments position and maintain the extensor tendons in their synovial sheaths.[68] The first compartment comprises extensor pollicis brevis and abductor pollicis longus. One of the most common wrist conditions that affects the tendons in this first compartment is known as de Quervain disease. The second compartment contains extensor carpi radialis longus and extensor carpi radialis brevis. The third contains extensor pollicis longus. This tendon is often injured in distal radius fractures. In the fourth compartment lies the extensor digitorum communis and extensor indices proprius. The fifth compartment contains extensor digiti minimi. In the final, sixth compartment is the extensor carpi ulnaris.

Volarly, the long finger flexors, long thumb flexor, median nerve, and radial artery pass through the carpal tunnel. The carpal tunnel consists of a concave arch of carpal bones. The roof of this arch includes the transverse carpal ligament, forearm fascia, and the distal aponeurosis of the thenar and hypothenar muscles.[68] The carpal tunnel is the site of one of the most common hand pathologies, carpal tunnel syndrome (CTS). Any condition that increases pressure in the tunnel can lead to compression of the median nerve. This can result in pain and paresthesia in the median nerve distribution.

The Hand

The metacarpophalangeal (MCP) joints allow for several planes of motion, including flexion, extension, abduction, adduction, and a slight degree of pronation and supination. The metacarpal head has a convex shape, which fits with a shallow concave proximal phalanx. The stability of the MCP joint is provided by its capsule, collateral ligaments, accessory collateral ligaments, volar plate, and musculotendinous units. The collateral ligaments are laterally positioned and are dorsal to the axis of rotation. In extension, the collateral ligament is lax; in flexion, it is taut.[41] If the MCP joint is immobilized in extension, the lax collateral ligament can shorten. Flexion of the MCP is considered the "safe position" in order to prevent tightening of the collateral ligaments; however, care should be taken to

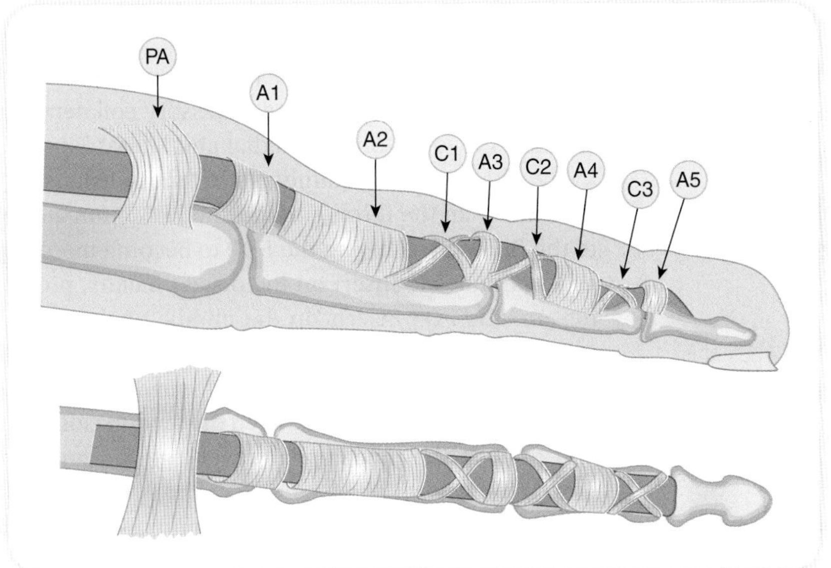

Figure 22-3 **The pulleys of the flexor tendons**

(Reprinted, with permission, from Strickland JW. Development of flexor tendon surgery: twenty-five years of progress. *J Hand Surg*. 2000;25:214-235.)

consider the specific condition when immobilizing the MCP joint. Several tendons cross the MCP joints. On the flexor surface, the flexor digitorum superficialis (FDS) and flexor digitorum profundus (FDP) are held closely to the bones by pulleys. The A1 pulley (Figure 22-3) is the site of tendon drag or locking in the case of a trigger finger. The FDS flexes the proximal interphalangeal (PIP) joint, and the FDP flexes the distal interphalangeal (DIP) joint. Injuries to the flexor tendons are categorized by zones (Figure 22-4). Zone 1 is distal to the insertion of FDS whereas zone 2 is located from the A1 pulley to the insertion of FDS. Zone 3 includes the distal border of the carpal tunnel to the A1 pulley. Zone 4 consists of the area covered by the transverse carpal ligament. Zone 5 spans from the proximal border of the transverse carpal ligament to the flexor musculocutaneous junction (Figure 22-4). The interosseous muscles are lateral to the MCP joints and are responsible for abduction and adduction of the MCP joints. The lumbrical muscles, volar to the axis of rotation of the MCP joint, insert into the lateral bands, dorsal to the PIP and DIP joints. Their function is MCP joint flexion and interphalangeal (IP) joint extension. (This is why it is possible to have active IP extension with radial nerve palsy.) The extensor mechanism crosses the MCP joint dorsally. Sagittal bands hold the extensor digitorum communis tendons centrally. Injuries and treatment to the extensor tendons are also categorized by zones (Figure 22-5). One way to remember this system is to locate the odd-numbered zones over the joints.

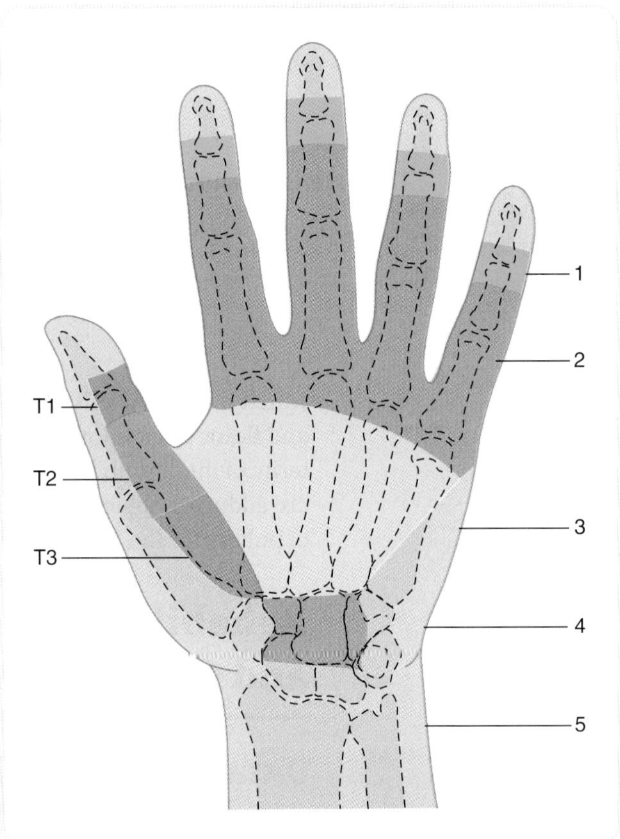

Figure 22-4 **The flexor tendon zones**

(Reprinted, with permission, from Kleinert HE, Schepel S, Gill T. Flexor tendon injuries. *Surg Clin North Am*. 1981;61:267-286.)

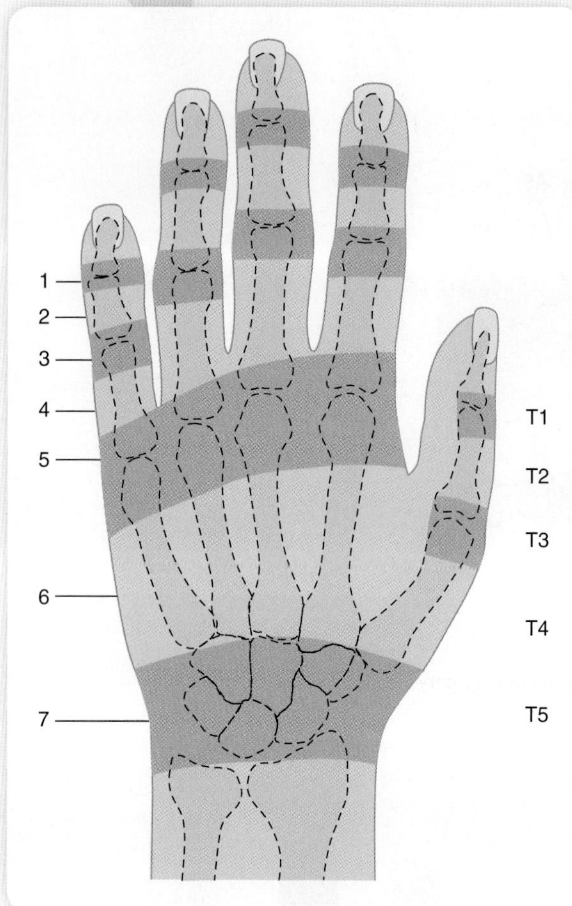

Figure 22-5 The extensor tendon zones

(Reprinted, with permission, from Kleinert HE, Schepel S, Gill T. Flexor tendon injuries. *Surg Clin North Am.* 1981;61:267-286.)

The Fingers

The IP joints are bicondylar hinge joints that allow flexion and extension. Collateral and accessory collateral ligaments stabilize the joints on the medial and lateral aspects, respectively. The collateral ligaments are taut in extension and lax in flexion. On the flexor surface, the FDS bifurcates proximal to the PIP joint, allowing the FDP to become more superficial as it continues to insert on the distal phalanx, providing DIP flexion. The FDS inserts on the middle phalanx for PIP flexion. Five annular pulleys and 3 cruciate ligaments between the MCP and DIP joints prevent bowstringing of the tendons. These pulleys and ligaments keep the tendon close to the bone and provide the mechanical advantage for composite digit flexion (see Figure 22-3).

On the extensor surface, the common extensor tendons cross the MCP joints and then divide into 3 slips. The central slip inserts on the dorsal middle phalanx, allowing for PIP extension. The 2 lateral slips, called the *lateral bands*, receive attachments from the lumbricals, travel dorsal and lateral to the PIP joint, rejoin after the PIP joint, and insert as the terminal extensor into the DIP joint. This delicately balanced system serves to extend the IP joints.

The Thumb

The thumb is responsible for 40% to 50% of the function of the hand.[87] The thumb's ability to oppose the digits, grasp, and pinch occurs as a consequence of the thumb's unique ability to balance mobility with joint stability. The thumb carpal metacarpal joint is a biconcave saddle joint that allows for ROM in a wide variety of planes. This necessary motion is controlled with joint stability provided by the strong joint capsule and supporting ligaments. There are 4 extrinsic thumb muscles, which include extensor pollicis longus, extensor pollicis brevis, abductor pollicis longus, and flexor pollicis longus. The 5 intrinsic muscles that add to the unique mobility and dexterity of the thumb include the abductor pollicis brevis, opponens pollicis, abductor pollicis, adductor pollicis, and flexor pollicis brevis. The thumb, like the other digits, has a series of pulleys for the flexor tendons.

Rehabilitation Techniques for Specific Injuries and Conditions

Distal Radius Fractures

Pathomechanics

Fractures of the distal radius can be described by several classification systems. It is important that the therapist has an understanding of the type of fracture and how different types of fractures need to be treated. Some of the questions the therapist may ask are: Is the fracture intraarticular or extraarticular, displaced or nondisplaced? If displaced, in which direction? Is the fracture simple or comminuted, open or closed? Is the radius shortened? and Is the ulna also fractured? Answers to these questions will help the therapist select interventions and determine expected outcomes.

It is important to consider the normal anatomy when evaluating wrist fractures. The normal radius is tilted volarly. If in a fracture the volar tilt becomes dorsal, motion will be affected, which can ultimately lead to midcarpal instability, decreased strength, increased ulnar loading, and a dysfunctional DRUJ.[52] Another complicating factor is the length of the radius. The normal radius is longer than the ulna. If the radius is shortened in a comminuted fracture, there is a high potential for disability.[12,34,52] Radial shortening may lead to DRUJ pain, especially with pronation and supination activities. This can result in reduced grip strength because of pain and limited use of the hand. The DRUJ is discussed in greater detail later in the section entitled "Injuries to the Distal Radioulnar Joint".

The type of fracture, size of the fragments, and displacement determine the initial treatment. Stable fractures may require casting; however, more complex fractures may require internal or external fixation by a surgeon.

Injury Mechanism

As is true of most wrist injuries, many distal radius fractures occur from a fall on an outstretched hand (otherwise known as a FOOSH injury). The presence of this condition in the middle-aged population may indicate a need for a bone density test to rule out osteoporosis, especially when it occurs with a low-impact event.

Rehabilitation Concerns

Rehabilitation may be initiated while the wrist is immobilized. Rehabilitation following a distal radius fracture is similar regardless of the method of fixation. While immobilized, ROM and edema control of noninvolved joints is essential, so that when immobilization is discontinued, rehabilitation can be concentrated on the wrist and forearm. This should include shoulder ROM in all planes, elbow flexion and extension, and finger flexion and extension. Finger exercises should include isolated MCP flexion, composite flexion (full fist), and intrinsic minus fisting (MCP extension with IP flexion) (Exercise 22-1). Coban or an Isotoner glove may be used for edema control if necessary. This helps prevent muscle atrophy, aids in muscle pumping to decrease edema, and, most importantly, prevents edema-related hypomobility. Shoulder slings are not usually recommended as they can contribute to shoulder and elbow stiffness. Other concerns include complications of CTS or complex regional pain syndrome.[42] Both conditions are best managed by early detection and intervention. Another complication is an extensor pollicis longus rupture.[42] It is thought that this occurs from the extensor pollicis longus rubbing through bone around the fracture site near the Lister tubercle. In such a condition, the patient would be unable to actively extend the thumb IP joint, and surgical intervention is required. If the fracture is stabilized with a fixator or if pins are present, pin site care may be performed depending on the physician's preference.

Rehabilitation Progression

Once immobilization is discontinued per the physician, ROM of the wrist can be initiated. This includes active wrist flexion, extension, radial and ulnar deviation, and forearm pronation and supination. The patient should be instructed on wrist extension with full composite digital flexion (Exercise 22-2). This isolates the wrist extensors rather than using the extensor digitorum communis so as to prevent extrinsic extensor tendon tightness. This tightness is most commonly seen with plate fixation or prolonged immobilization. Active ROM to decrease extrinsic extensor tightness requires simultaneous wrist and digital motion. Active ROM to decrease flexor tendon tightness would include simultaneous wrist and digital extension. Exercises should also include forearm rotation (supination and pronation).

Instruction should be provided to perform these exercises with the elbow at 90 degrees and held close to the side of the body to avoid compensation from the shoulder (Exercise 22-3).

The initiation of PROM is dependent upon the stability of the fracture. A lightweight hammer or mallet in the hand during pronation and supination exercises is a helpful tool to gently stretch and increase this motion (Exercise 22-4). Gentle joint mobilizations to the radius and ulna are also helpful in increasing motion. When providing forearm rotation passively, gentle pressure should be applied at the distal radius, proximal to the wrist, not at the hand. This will avoid placing unnecessary torque across the carpals. Gentle wrist distraction combined with flexion and extension may be effective in increasing ROM in a pain-free range. Contract and relax techniques may also be helpful in obtaining the desired ROM. Orthotics can be effective tools in increasing ROM in patients who are not progressing. Wrist extension limitations can be treated effectively with a serial night orthosis (Figure 22-6). The wrist is held in comfortable maximum extension during the fabrication process. The night orthosis gently and progressively stretches the wrist into greater extension. The orthosis is remolded at each therapy visit as gains in extension are made. It is very effective in patients that are having difficulty obtaining a functional range (40 degrees). Caution should be noted not to apply undue pressure on the median nerve. A static progressive orthosis can be also used periodically during the day to increase wrist PROM. Daytime use of this orthosis may help to achieve greater wrist flexion and/or extension (Figure 22-7). The orthosis is usually worn for 20 to 30 minutes, 2 to 3 times daily. The patient adjusts this orthosis as gains are made. This type of

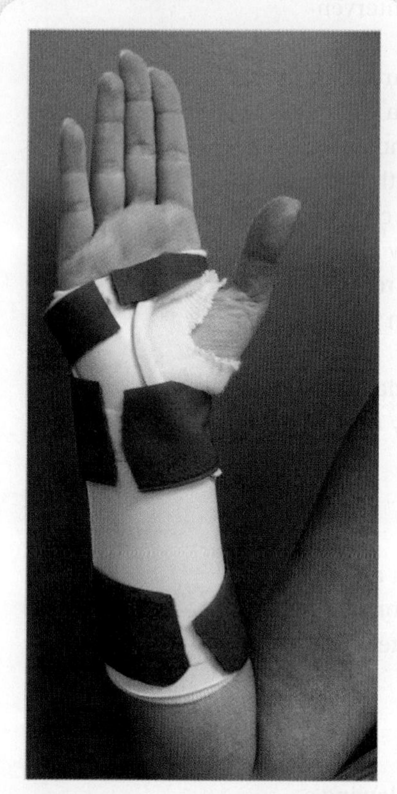

Figure 22-6 **A wrist orthosis is used for a variety of conditions**

With conservative management of CTS it can be beneficial to keep the wrist in a neutral position at night. After a healed wrist fracture, wrist extension limitations can be treated effectively with a serial night orthosis. In the clinic, the orthosis is molded while the wrist is held in comfortable maximum extension. The night orthosis gently stretches the wrist into progressively more extension. The orthosis is remolded at each therapy visit as gains in extension are made.

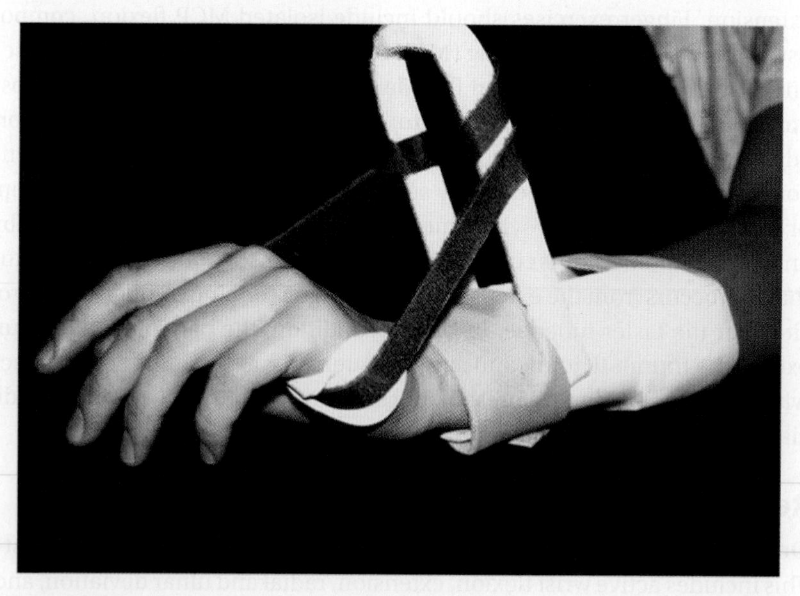

Figure 22-7

A static progressive orthosis can be utilized periodically during the day to increase wrist ROM. Daytime static progressive orthosis for wrist flexion and/or extension is usually worn for 20 to 30 minutes, 2 to 3 times daily. The patient adjusts this orthosis as gains are made. This orthosis demonstrates static progressive extension.

orthosis is also available commercially. Static progressive or dynamic pronation and supination orthotic management may be utilized 2 to 3 times a day so as to not interfere with functional use of the hand (Figure 22-8).[21]

Active motion can be progressed to strengthening after adequate ROM is achieved, typically occurring at approximately 8 weeks after injury or surgery, when the fracture is healed and stable. Strengthening a wrist with limited motion too soon may result in developing strength in less-than-ideal ROM. All strengthening exercises should be pain free and can include light weights, Thera-Band, or tubing, and can be graded for wrist and forearm motions. This can be in conjunction with comfortable progressive weightbearing exercises such as wall pushups that progress to the countertop, stairs, and then to a floor mat (Exercise 22-5). Weight bearing on a ball and gentle ball rolling can be the next progression (Exercise 22-6).

Mass grasp or grip strength is often decreased after wrist fracture. Therapy putty is one tool used to address strengthening of mass grasp. Putty is available in a variety of grades, from soft to hard, to provide different levels of resistance. The type of putty used for grip strengthening should be soft enough to provide a pain-free level of resistance. If the patients aggravate pain in an attempt to increase strength, the pain will limit their function during ADL, and may increase edema. Patient needs and preferences with regards to level of strengthening should be taken into consideration to ensure best practice.

Athletes, particularly those in contact sports, can require additional protection as they resume athletic activity. Many referees will not allow a rigid orthosis or cast to be used as a possible weapon on the field of play. A soft cast or various padding materials may be used. The best care for both the patient and the other team players should be considered. Families may want their children in high-school sports to return to play too quickly. The patient and family should be cautioned to avoid the possibility of additional injury or chronic conditions that may result from premature return to the field of play.

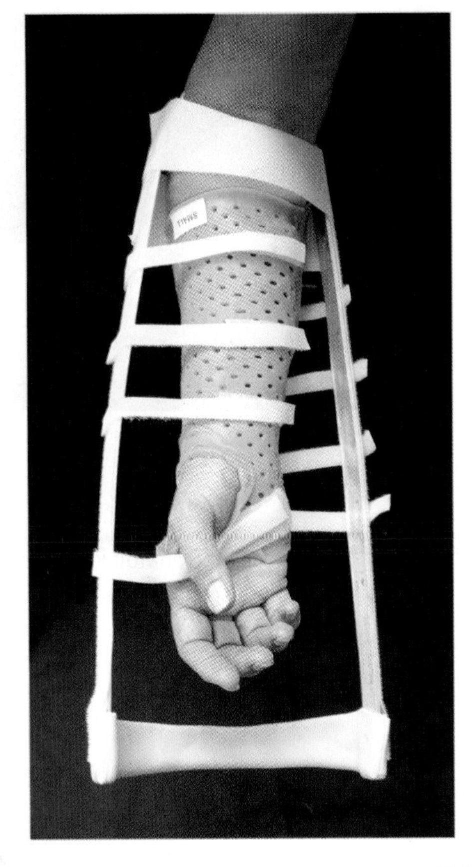

Figure 22-8 A static progressive orthosis to increase pronation and supination of the forearm

It is used when stiffness occurs following a healed distal radius fracture and worn 2 to 3 times a day for 20 to 30 minutes. This orthosis is based on a concept by Kay Collelo Abram.[21]

Scaphoid Fracture

Pathomechanics

Fractures of the scaphoid account for 60% of all carpal injuries.[12,50,90] The prognosis is related to the site of the fracture, obliquity, displacement, and promptness of diagnosis and treatment. The blood supply of the scaphoid occurs distal to proximal. A fracture through the proximal one-third of the scaphoid may result in delayed union or avascular necrosis secondary to the limited blood supply. It can take 20 weeks or longer for a proximal fracture to heal.[50] Surgical intervention is necessary if the fracture is displaced or results in a nonunion. Not treating the fracture can lead to carpal instability and periscaphoid arthritis.[59,88]

Injury Mechanism

Scaphoid fractures result from a fall on an outstretched hand (FOOSH injury) placing the wrist in hyperextension and radial deviation.[90] A proper diagnosis is a primary concern. Diagnosis is often difficult and not easily confirmed with a standard radiograph and many go undiagnosed or misdiagnosed as wrist sprains. A bone scan and/or MRI may be needed for definitive diagnosis. Patients usually have wrist pain with this fracture, especially when palpated in the anatomic snuffbox (Figure 22-9).

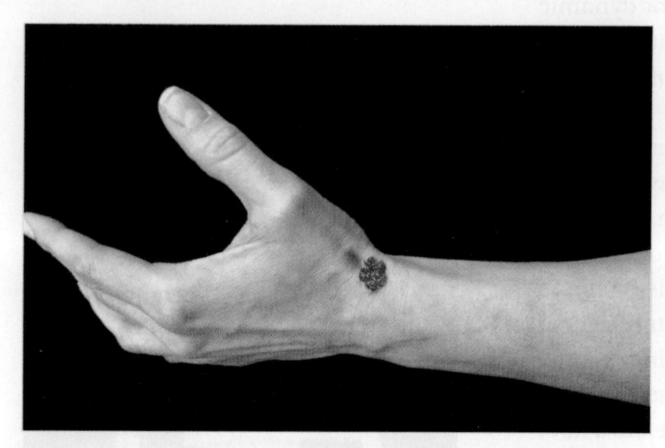

Figure 22-9

The asterisk (*) indicates the anatomic snuffbox, which can be painful to palpation in a scaphoid fracture.

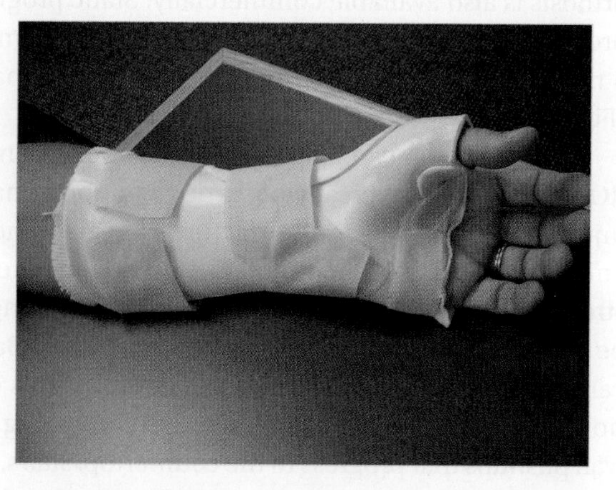

Figure 22-10

A forearm-based thumb spica orthosis includes the thumb and wrist. It is most commonly used for a scaphoid fracture, thumb metacarpal fracture, or de Quervain tendonitis.

Rehabilitation Concerns

Nonunions can result in cases that are misdiagnosed as a wrist sprain.[24] Greater concern about nonunion exists when the fracture is at the proximal pole because of the limited or absent blood supply in that region. Scaphoid nonunion may lead to carpal instability or periscaphoid arthritis. A client who is not progressing in therapy and has persistent complaints of wrist pain may need to be further evaluated by the physician for a possible scaphoid fracture.

Rehabilitation Progression

Once the diagnosis has been made, the initial treatment of the nondisplaced scaphoid fracture is casting. As a result of the limited blood supply, healing is slow to occur. Casting usually continues for at least 8 to 10 weeks with distal scaphoid fractures followed by fabrication of a custom thumb spica orthosis (Figure 22-10) for continued protection. Fractures of the middle portion of the scaphoid require 6 weeks in a long arm cast followed by 6 weeks in a short arm cast.[24] Fractures of the proximal pole of the scaphoid may require an additional 3 to 6 months of casting or orthotic wear.[50,90] The initiation of wrist active range of motion (AROM) is determined by the surgeon, based on evidence of fracture healing. The "dart throwers arc" may be the preferred AROM exercise to prevent overstretching of nearby carpal ligaments (see Figure 22-1).[70] The thumb spica orthosis is worn between exercises and at night as the patient progresses. Active ROM exercises including wrist flexion, extension (see Exercise 22-2), and radial and ulnar deviation are completed in a pain-free range. Thumb flexion and extension, abduction and adduction, and opposition to each finger are also initiated (Exercise 22-7*A* to *C*). Some patients may be overly aggressive with their home exercise programs, possibly as a result of the long period of immobilization. This aggression may overstretch the healing carpal ligaments compromising wrist stability. It is typical to have ligament injuries associated with the scaphoid fracture. Progressing wrist PROM to the point of pain can compromise long-term function. Grip strength measurements are often diminished in the presence of pain. Strengthening exercises are delayed until healing is complete, adequate AROM has been achieved, and pain is under control. It is important to note that joint stability should not be sacrificed for an increase in ROM. Care should be taken not to return an athlete to a sport too quickly.

Rehabilitation after an open reduction and internal fixation of the scaphoid follows the same progression as outlined above. The period of immobilization may be less because of the repair of the scaphoid with rigid fixation.[24,50,90]

Injuries to the Distal Radioulnar Joint

Pathomechanics

The DRUJ is a complex system (see Figure 22-2*A*). The design of the structures at the DRUJ allows for forearm pronation and supination while providing the necessary stability to the ulnar side of the wrist. The TFCC at the distal ulna provides support and stability to the DRUJ. Pain in this area can be caused by fractures of the ulna, arthritis, synovitis, dislocation, DRUJ instability, tendonitis, and/or tears of the TFCC.[71] A complete evaluation by an experienced hand surgeon is often needed to make an accurate diagnosis. Some of these conditions can be evaluated by radiography, but others are difficult to diagnose, largely because of the soft-tissue involvement. The distal ulna is more prominent in pronation and less prominent in supination when palpated. When the DRUJ loses stability as a result of a disruption of the TFCC, the ulna can displace during ROM, making a popping or clicking noise. Patients can have significant pain, limiting ADL. Injuries are often overlooked and patients often become frustrated when there is a delay in diagnosis and treatment.

Injury Mechanism

A fracture to the distal radius commonly includes an injury to the DRUJ. This may include a fracture to the ulnar styloid or an injury to the TFCC. Arthritis at the DRUJ can result in pain with pronation and supination. Injuries and tears to the TFCC can be a result of excessive load in wrist ulnar deviation and forearm rotation activities.

Rehabilitation Concerns

Patients with persistent pain at the distal ulna should be tested to determine if depression and support of the ulna during pronation and supination relieves their symptoms (see Figure 22-2*B*). Manually depressing the ulna can reduce pain by providing support to weakened ligaments. A simple wristband that provides padding at the dorsal ulna and volar radius can be very helpful in decreasing pain and providing support to the TFCC (Figure 22-11).

Surgical intervention can include arthroscopy, ulnar resection, ulnar shortening, hemiresection interposition arthroplasty, fusion with proximal pseudoarthrodesis, repair to the TFCC, and tethering of the distal ulna.[6,23,71,83] Each procedure has an individualized and specific period of immobilization with specific casting and/or orthotic positioning (specified by the surgeon), followed by gentle and gradual return of ROM. The therapist should contact the surgeon to determine the point at which gentle AROM can be initiated. It is important to avoid aggressive ROM that can stretch out ligaments that provide the necessary stability to the DRUJ. All ROM should be kept pain free, as stability was a major area of concern prior to surgery.

Rehabilitation Progression

The key to successful management of injuries to the DRUJ is gradual progression in a pain-free range. Motions that need to be addressed for AROM are flexion, extension, radial deviation, ulnar deviation, supination, and pronation. Strengthening exercises are delayed until healing is complete, adequate ROM has been achieved, and pain is under control. Joint stability should not be sacrificed for an increase in ROM. Care should be taken not to return

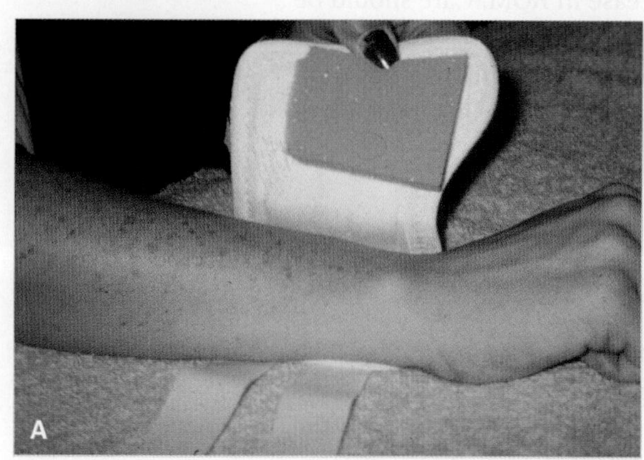

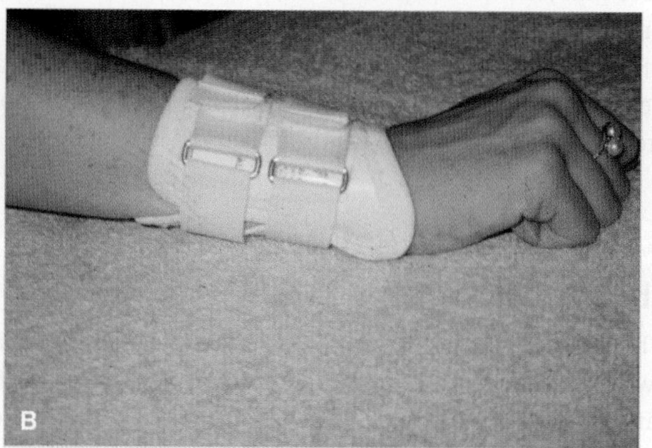

Figure 22-11

A. A prefabricated wrist wrap orthosis (Count'R-force) with padding at the dorsal ulna and the volar wrist is very helpful in managing painful pronation and supination caused by disruption of the triangular fibrocartilage. **B.** The wrist wrap orthosis allows partial wrist movement while supporting the distal ulna.

this patient to work, sport, or other activities too quickly. The wristband (see Figure 22-11) can be helpful in returning a patient to activities by decreasing any persistent pain with forearm rotation.

Carpal Tunnel Syndrome

Pathomechanics

CTS occurs as a result of compression of the median nerve at the level of the wrist. The carpal tunnel is made up of the carpal bones dorsally and transverse carpal ligament volarly. Located in the carpal tunnel are the FDS and FDP to all digits, flexor pollicis longus, median nerve, and median artery.[14] If the space within the carpal tunnel is decreased as a result of inflammation, cyst, tumor, scar tissue, fracture, edema, or other conditions, the median nerve can be compressed. Research has shown when intratunnel pressure of the wrist was measured, even a small change in wrist position increased this pressure. Studies by Burke et al[14] and Weiss et al[92] found that the lowest intratunnel pressure is with the wrist in a near-neutral position. This information should influence the night orthosis design. Many prefabricated orthoses place the wrist in far too much wrist extension, potentially aggravating symptoms. Symptoms of classic CTS are numbness and tingling in the median nerve distribution, pain or waking at night, and clumsiness or weakness in the hand. Symptoms may increase with static positioning (eg, driving or reading a newspaper),[2] vibration, activation of the lumbricals,[37] and changes in joint position.[92] Diagnosis is made by history, the Phalen test (Figure 22-12), the Tinel sign, nerve conduction studies, direct pressure over the carpal tunnel (Figure 22-13), and electromyography. It is important to note that negative nerve conduction studies are not always conclusive. A study by Grundberg showed that 11.3% of the patients with negative tests had positive clinical and surgical findings.[36]

Injury Mechanism

There are many conditions and injuries that contribute to median nerve compression caused by elevated carpal pressures. These include tenosynovitis, fracture, carpal

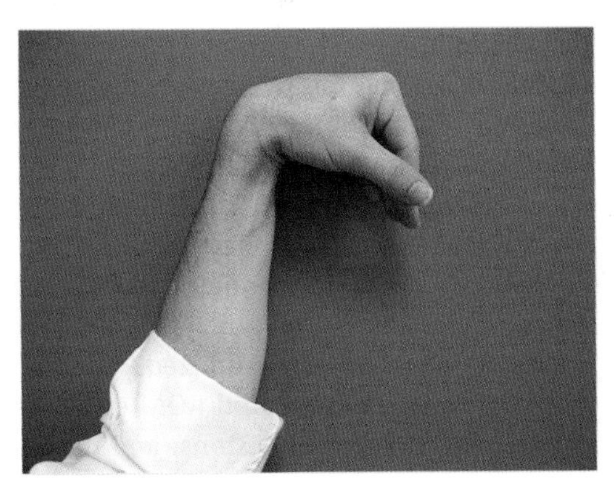

Figure 22-12

The Phalen test for CTS is full wrist flexion, which increases the pressure in the carpal canal. The test is positive if there is numbness and tingling in the median nerve distribution within 60 seconds.

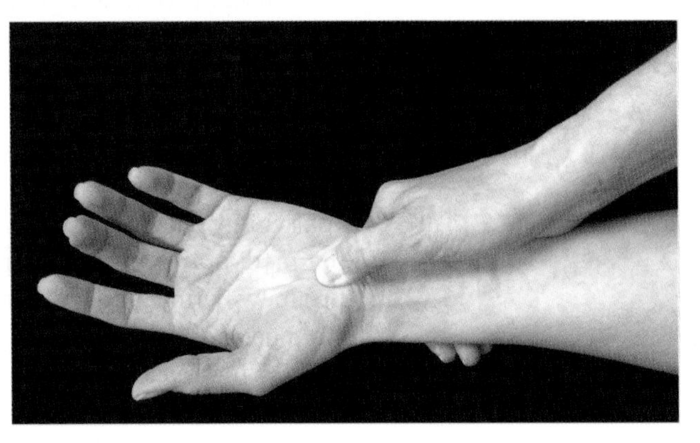

Figure 22-13

Pressure over the carpal tunnel may produce the symptoms of numbness and tingling in the median nerve distribution. Positive findings should be correlated with other clinical symptoms and assessments.

dislocation, cysts, tumor, diabetes, alcoholism, pregnancy, menopause, thyroid disorders, obesity, vibration, external forces, tendon load, and changes in joint position.[37,44,91]

Rehabilitation Concerns

Research suggests that there are several effective interventions for conservative management of CTS, including orthotic intervention.[55,63] Conservative treatment is the first-line intervention and consists of a night orthosis with the wrist in a neutral position (see Figure 22-6) and relative rest from aggravating sources. Occasionally, physicians will recommend a full-time wrist orthosis. Prefabricated orthoses may need to be adapted as they often place the wrist in extension as opposed to a near-neutral position. In some cases of CTS, it is also necessary to limit movement of digits 2 to 5 because of the action of the lumbricals moving into the carpal tunnel with digit flexion.[37] Including the MCP joints in extension within the splint has been reported to be effective in decreasing symptoms (Figure 22-14).[3,29] Nerve gliding exercises described by Butler[15] should only be used with extreme caution so as not to increase symptoms. It is difficult for many patients to keep nerve gliding techniques symptom free. Forced nerve gliding may result in increased inflammation, fibrosis, and edema[82] to the nerve, which will worsen instead of improve symptoms. Activity analysis to determine activities that increase symptoms should be done to see if changes in technique would help to decrease or avoid symptoms. Grip strengthening, conservatively, has been found to be contraindicated by several authors because of the action of the lumbricals increasing pressure in the carpal tunnel.[29]

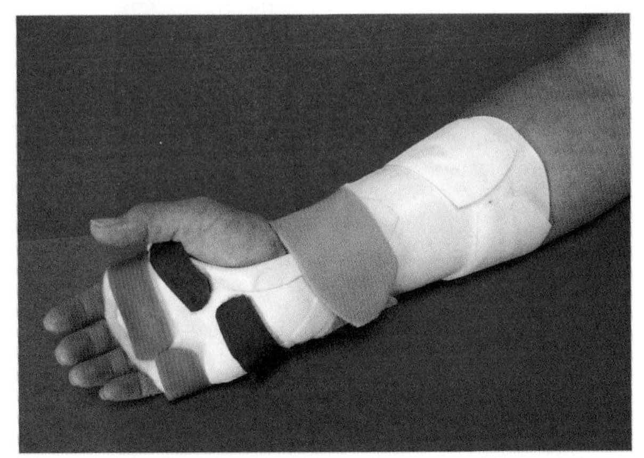

Figure 22-14

In some cases of CTS, it is necessary to limit movement of digits 2 to 5 because of the action of the lumbricals moving into the carpal tunnel with digit flexion.[34] Including the MCP joints in extension within the splint has been reported to be effective in decreasing symptoms.[40]

If conservative treatment fails, a carpal tunnel release may be performed. There are 2 standard approaches to this release. The open technique exposes and releases the transverse carpal ligament and the endoscopic technique uses portals to view and then release the transverse carpal ligament. Surgeon preference determines the type of procedure selected, with reports of advantages and disadvantages to each procedure.[13,19,39,56,86] The lack of visualization of the nerve has been a critique of the endoscopic technique, with the possibility of complications such as an incomplete release[86] or the possibility of injury to the median nerve and other structures.[56] Critics of the open technique report longer return to work time and greater scar tenderness.[13,29] Rehabilitation is dictated by the individual needs of each patient rather than by the surgical technique utilized. Rehabilitation following release consists of wound care, scar management, and ROM exercises.[29] Tendon gliding exercises are used to improve ROM, prevent adhesions, and decrease edema. Tendon glides begin with full finger extension, and then hook fist to maximize FDP pull-through in relation to FDS. The digits are also placed into a straight fist to maximize FDS pull-through, as well as a composite (full) fist to use all of the finger flexors. Full extension should be performed between each position and should be kept pain free (see Exercise 22-1). The FDS is also isolated by holding all but 1 digit in MCP extension and flexing each digit at the PIP joint individually (Exercise 22-8). Wrist AROM should also be performed in a pain-free range.

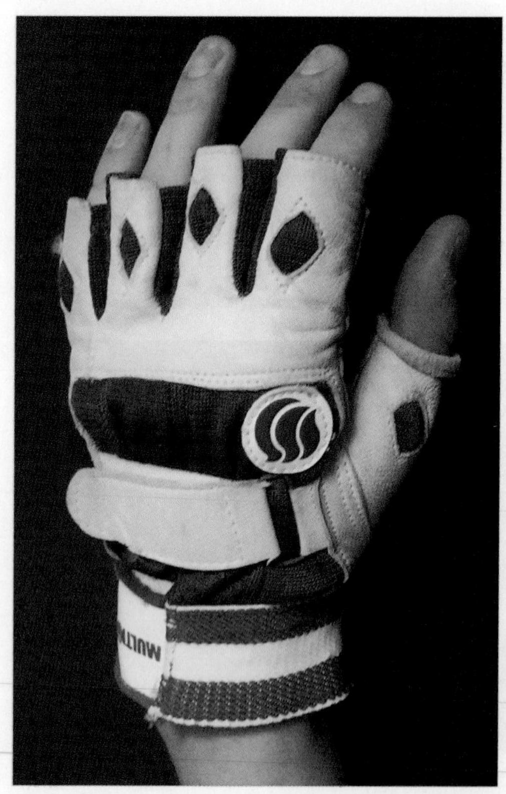

Figure 22-15

Patients that have persistent pain may benefit from padded bicycle gloves as they return to their sports. This glove protects the sensitive area while allowing a gradual return to such activities as golf or tennis.

Rehabilitation Progression

The postoperative progression after carpal tunnel release involves a gradual return to normal use. Grip strengthening and repetitive activities should be initiated gradually in order to prevent inflammation and aggravation of the preoperative symptoms.[29] Returning to work will require an evaluation of the conditions that may have aggravated the symptoms. Padded work gloves can be helpful in decreasing vibration and protecting sensitive incision sites (Figure 22-15). Workstation evaluation and adaptations may be needed to avoid awkward and repetitive movements whenever possible.

Boxer's Fracture

Pathomechanics

A boxer's fracture is a fracture of the fifth metacarpal neck, which is the most commonly fractured metacarpal.[39] On impact with a solid object, the metacarpal will frequently shorten and angulate. Because of the large degree of mobility of the fifth metacarpal, less-than-perfect anatomic reduction is acceptable, allowing adequate hand function.[7]

Injury Mechanism

This injury occurs most frequently from contact against an object with a closed fist. It can also be the result of a fall. Many patients who sustain this fracture because of a hostile encounter are reluctant to admit the true cause of the injury.

Rehabilitation Concerns

If the injury is open, the risk of infection is serious. This is especially true when a closed fist has struck another's mouth and come in contact with the opponent's teeth and/or saliva. If the injury is closed, treatment consists of proper immobilization, edema control, and ROM of noninvolved joints. Proximal IP joint extension can be problematic especially of the fifth digit. In some cases, open reduction and internal fixation is required. Postoperatively, proper orthotic management, edema control, and AROM of uninvolved joints are important.[26,39]

Treatment is immobilization in a plaster gutter support, or in a thermoplastic orthosis (Figure 22-16). The latter is often preferred, as it allows removal of the orthosis for ROM of the wrist and digits, as well as skin hygiene. The orthosis immobilizes the ring and small finger metacarpals and MCP joints. The MCP joints are placed in comfortable flexion and the wrist is usually left free. The orthosis should be adjusted and remolded as edema decreases. Immobilization with the orthosis is continued for approximately 4 to 6 weeks. If there is an open wound present, it should be monitored for infection and the physician should be contacted immediately. The physician may place the patient on a course of antibiotics when an open wound is present.

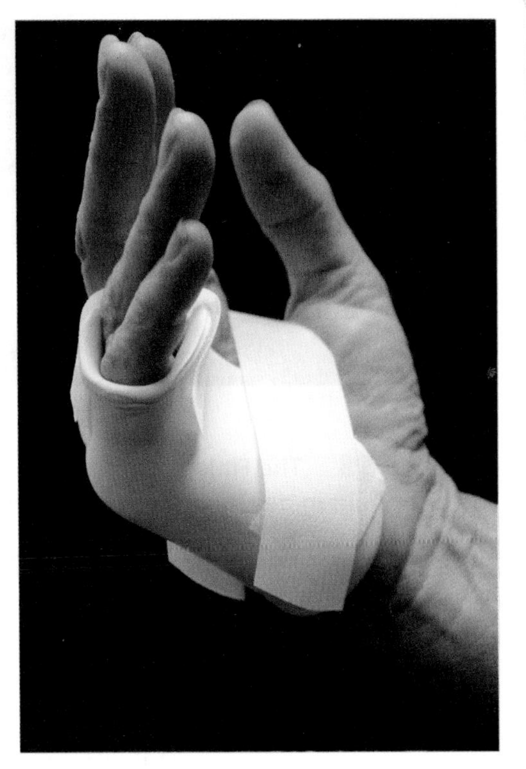

Figure 22-16

A boxer's fracture orthosis often protects the ring and small finger proximal phalanxes and the MCP joint.

Rehabilitation Progression

During the time of immobilization, AROM to noninvolved joints is maintained. The surgeon, based on the stability of the fracture or surgical fixation, should determine the initiation of MCP AROM to the involved digits. At approximately 6 weeks, the orthosis is often discontinued if there is evidence of radiographic healing, but may be used as needed for protection during heavier activities. A buddy tape (Figure 22-17) may be used when MCP AROM is allowed to promote proper digital alignment. A patient may gradually resume normal activity without the orthosis when there is evidence of radiographic healing. Gentle grip strengthening exercises with putty can be initiated with a healed fracture usually at 6 to 8 weeks after injury or surgical intervention.

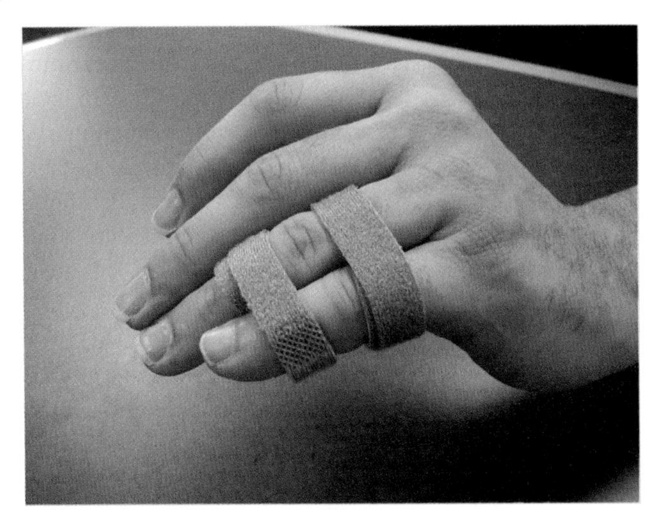

Figure 22-17

Buddy taping may be utilized to encourage or maintain proper digit alignment when adequate healing allows MCP AROM following a boxer's fracture.

de Quervain Tenosynovitis

Pathomechanics

de Quervain tenosynovitis is an inflammation in the first dorsal compartment affecting abductor pollicis longus and extensor pollicis brevis.[4,48] The Finkelstein test,[33] which involves thumb flexion into the palm with passive wrist ulnar deviation, can assist with making the diagnosis (Figure 22-18). It may be helpful to compare the level of pain elicited to the noninjured side. This test alone cannot confirm the diagnosis, as it can be uncomfortable in the normal population. The results of the Finkelstein test must be considered in conjunction with other clinical findings.

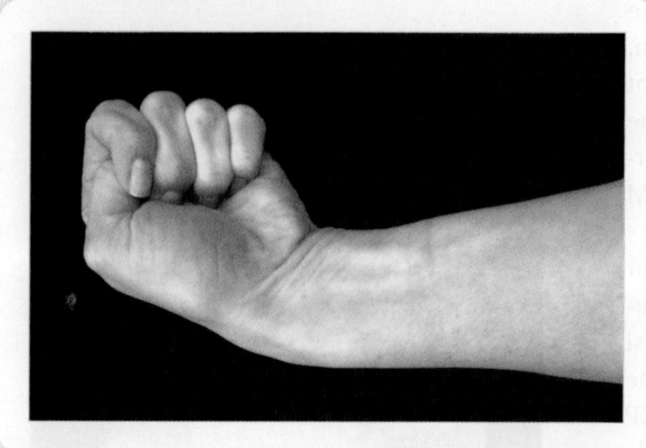

Figure 22-18 The Finkelstein test will be positive for pain in de Quervain tenosynovitis

Passive flexion of the thumb with wrist ulnar deviation is the provocative position.[51,52] Always compare to the noninvolved side, as this test can be uncomfortable with a normal hand.

Injury Mechanism

Repeated wrist movements may cause de Quervain tenosynovitis. Less-frequent causes include a direct blow to the radial styloid, acute strain as in lifting, or a ganglion cyst in the first dorsal compartment.[4,48]

Rehabilitation Concerns

Initial treatment is rest from aggravating activities. Modalities for edema reduction and pain control such as ultrasound and ice are widely utilized by clinicians for this condition. Ice is used for its ability to manage inflammation and pain.[4,31] Michlovitz[54] reports that ultrasound at lower intensities most likely produces its therapeutic effects by the phenomenon known as *microstreaming*. This is reported to cause changes in cell permeability and may help to promote healing. Michlovitz[54] discusses that low-dose pulsed ultrasound may be effective in acute and subacute rehabilitation of tendonitis, but stresses that further study is needed. In addition, an analysis of activities should be performed to determine aggravating activities. These activities should then be avoided or adapted as necessary.

Orthotic management for de Quervain tenosynovitis includes immobilization of the thumb at the MCP and carpometacarpal (CMC) joints as well as the wrist (see Figure 22-10).[96] Immobilization is usually full time with removal of the orthosis for hygiene for the first 4 to 6 weeks. Many patients need to be reminded not to "fight" their orthosis, but to relax and let it support them. Resisting the orthosis can aggravate symptoms. Some patients may have a combined condition that includes irritation to the radial sensory nerve. This nerve irritation can include hypersensitivity that makes the area painful to touch. These patients may also be unable to tolerate ice. Clinical use of a transcutaneous electrical nerve stimulation may be effective for pain control for these patients until the nerve symptoms subside. As the pain from the tendon is reduced after 4 to 6 weeks, the patient slowly decreases the wear time of the orthosis. Activity is resumed gradually, while avoiding irritating activities. If pain is persistent, immobilization is continued. Patients who do not respond to conservative management may be candidates for surgical intervention of the first dorsal compartment.

Various surgical techniques are used to treat this condition. Some surgeons hope to prevent the complication of a tendon subluxation with an internal tendon sling to help stabilize the release. This surgery will require a thumb spica orthosis for approximately 6 weeks postoperatively, with the initiation of gentle thumb and wrist AROM usually at the 4-week point.[4,48] AROM consists of gentle thumb opposition, flexion, and extension (see Exercise 22-7), as well as wrist flexion and extension (see Exercise 22-2). If the release to the first dorsal compartment does not include an internal sling, then gentle AROM as described above can begin after the sutures are removed. This is usually 10 to 14 days after surgery. After a simple release (no internal sling), some physicians prefer a thumb spica orthosis for a few weeks. The patient gradually resumes normal activity around the sixth week after surgery.[48] It is important that the therapist consult with the physician to implement the preferred postoperative protocol.

Complications from surgery include hypersensitivity, complex regional pain syndrome, incomplete release, tendon subluxation, and injury to the radial sensory nerve.[48] A radial sensory nerve injury will present itself as a very different type of pain than the patient had before surgery. The patient may complain of numbness, or pain that is burning, shooting, or electrical in nature. Care should be taken to avoid any pressure from the orthosis in the area of the radial sensory nerve at the wrist during the preoperative or postoperative programs.

Rehabilitation Progression

Early strengthening exercises should be avoided or symptoms could be exacerbated. Increased symptoms are likely to limit return to normal activity. Patients should have pain-free ROM in the affected area as the primary goal. Aggravating activities should be addressed and adapted as appropriate. Some patients may benefit from the support and protection of a soft neoprene orthosis as they return to activities (Figure 22-19).[5] This soft orthosis allows ROM, but provides gentle support and padding to an area that can be hypersensitive. It also allows more activity because it is more flexible than a custom thermoplastic/ridged orthosis and the hand is protected during ADL.

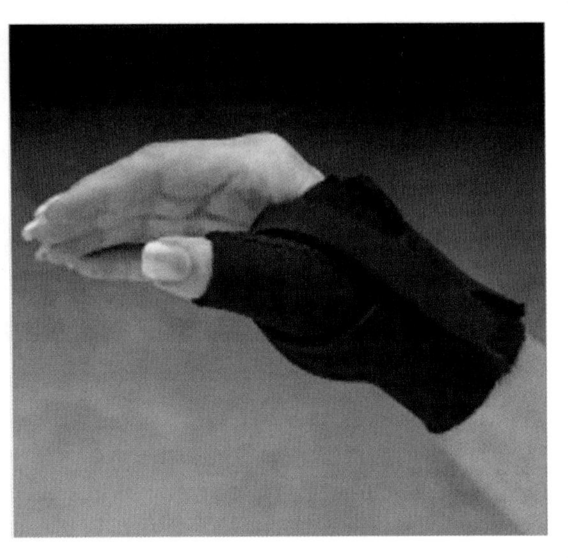

Figure 22-19

Some patients, who have difficulty returning to activities because of nerve pain, appreciate the support and protection of a soft neoprene orthosis. This Comfort Cool soft orthosis allows good ROM, but provides gentle support and padding to an area that can be hypersensitive. This orthosis will then allow more activity as the patient is not fearful of bumping or hitting the hand accidentally during daily living activities.[56] (Photo and splint courtesy of North Coast Medical, Inc., Gilroy, CA.)

Trigger Finger

Pathomechanics

Trigger finger or stenosing flexor tenosynovitis can be described as a discrepancy between the flexor tendon and the A1 pulley, which is located at the level of the metacarpal head. This disproportionate size does not allow for smooth gliding of the flexor tendon within the sheath. This may cause pain, "catching," or even locking of the digit in flexion. Occasionally pain is identified by the patient to be in the dorsal PIP joint, the DIP joint, or the entire finger. This pain, is, however, referred pain[18] from the flexor tendon and/or the A1 pulley. In addition, a nodule may also be present and may be palpated. Patel and Bassini described 6 stages of trigger finger (Table 22-1).[60]

Table 22-1 Patel and Bassini's Stages of Stenosing Tenosynovitis[58]

Stages	Description
1	Normal
2	Uneven
3	Triggering = Clicking = Catching
4	Locking of finger in flexion on extension, unlocked by active finger motion
5	Locking of finger in flexion on extension, unlocked by passive finger motion
6	Locked finger in flexion or extension

Injury Mechanism

Triggering may be the result of flexor tendon inflammation or thickening of the tissues for a variety of reasons. This may be caused by overuse of the flexors, thereby causing a larger inflamed or even bulbous tendon. Also, diseases such as arthritis and diabetes can cause changes in the soft tissues. Because use of the regular use of the hand for daily tasks, a perpetual cycle may occur causing a constant irritation of the tendon, limiting a smooth glide.

Rehabilitation Concerns

Often, patients are not referred immediately from the physician for therapeutic intervention. In many cases, a patient is provided with a cortisone injection to the flexor tendon at the site of the A1 pulley. This has been reported to have

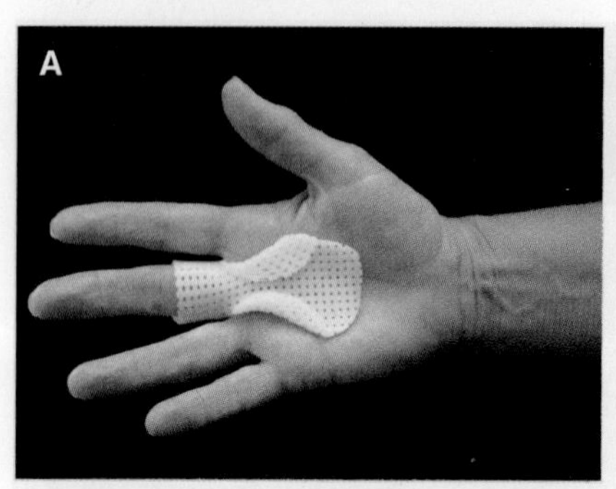

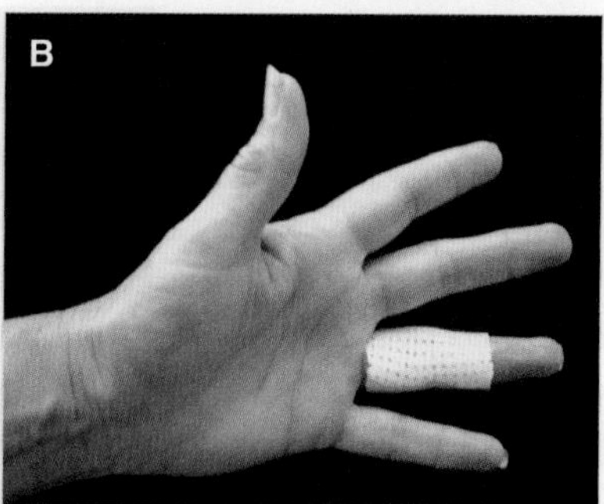

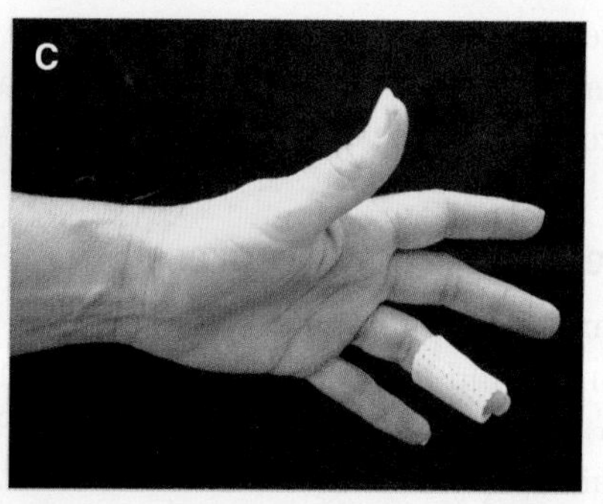

Figure 22-20

A. The literature notes many types of orthosis that effectively limit the amount of tendon glide excursion in the treatment of trigger finger. This orthosis limits MCP flexion. **B.** This orthosis limits PIP flexion. **C.** This orthosis limits DIP flexion.

varying levels of success.[61] A patient may be referred to a therapist for an orthosis, modalities, and possible PROM.[30] Modalities may provide some benefit to the inflamed tendons and for pain control.

Orthotic use in all stages, with the exception of the last stage, has been effective for many patients.[20,30,80,81,85,95] The literature discusses the many types of orthoses that are recommended to limit the amount of tendon glide/excursion (Figure 22-20). This immobilization may decrease pain and inflammation as well as decrease the active "catching" of the thumb or digit. Immobilization with an orthosis is done full-time for 3 to 6 weeks, with removal of the orthotic for hygiene purposes, avoiding active motion.[20] Patients who do not respond to immobilization may require a surgical release of the A1 pulley.

Therapy considerations for a postsurgical trigger-finger release include active motion as early as the same day. The focus of therapy includes wound care as needed, ROM, edema control techniques, and eventual scar management.

Rehabilitation Progression

Patients are usually seen in therapy for only a few postoperative visits. Many patients are discharged prior to beginning a strengthening program. Strengthening can be initiated, if needed, at approximately 3 weeks postsurgery. This can be done with Theraputty and should be gradual without irritation or pain. Occasionally, hypersensitivity of the scar is noted and will need to be addressed with desensitization techniques. If overuse was a primary cause of the initial trigger finger, patient education should be provided. This would include avoiding sustained gross grasp and repetitive digital flexion activities. Analysis of activities with modifications and adaptations to the environment should be performed and provided as needed.

Osteoarthritis of the Carpometacarpal Joint

Pathomechanics

Osteoarthritis (OA) can affect all of the joints of the thumb. A swan-neck deformity is common, involving 21% of patients with OA.[95] This deformity is often characterized by metacarpal adduction, CMC subluxation from the trapezium, MCP joint hyperextension, and IP joint flexion (Figure 22-21*A*). Pinch is often painful because the CMC subluxation becomes more pronounced during heavy pinch activities. The thumb IP joint sometimes assumes a

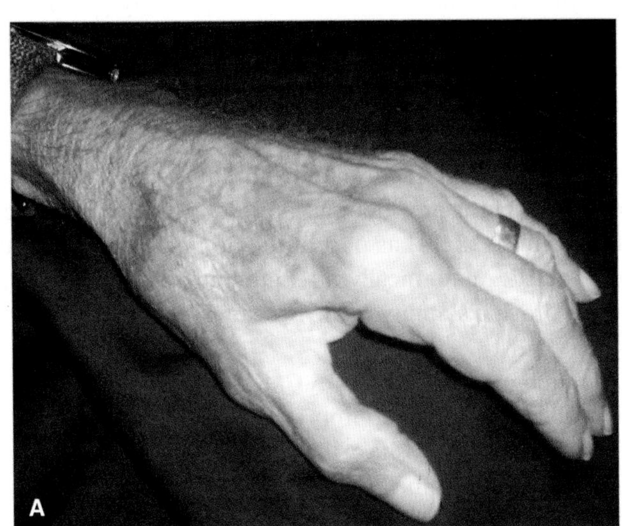

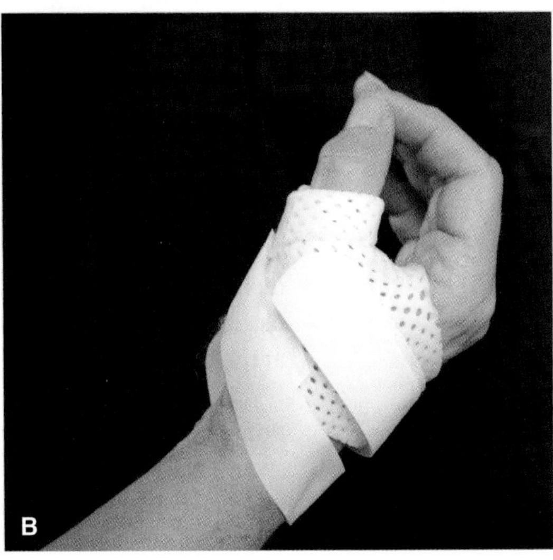

Figure 22-21

A. OA can affect all of the joints of the thumb. A swan-neck deformity is often characterized by metacarpal adduction, CMC subluxation from the trapezium, MCP joint hyperextension, and IP joint flexion. **B.** Designing and fabricating a thumb orthosis for the OA CMC joint requires careful positioning during fabrication to immobilize the CMC appropriately. A gentle correction of the swan-neck deformity would place the thumb (opposite of the deformity) in metacarpal abduction, align the metacarpal on the trapezium, flex the MCP joint, and extend the IP joint in joints that are passively correctable.

flexed position. The Eaton classification has been widely used to define severity and guide treatment of this deformity through radiographs.[28] When evaluating the thumb, determine the specific pattern of deformity so that treatment can be more specific in terms of orthotic support and therapeutic management.

Injury Mechanism

Osteoarthritis is often called the wear-and-tear disease, but research demonstrates that the breakdown in the articular cartilage is caused by both mechanical and chemical factors.[9] Complex biomechanical factors appear to activate the chondrocytes to produce degradative enzymes.[40,96] Mechanical factors, such as abnormal loading of the joint from trauma, heavy labor, joint instability, aging, and obesity, can increase the risk of OA.[40] Affected persons have a genetic susceptibility, and OA occurs more frequently in women older than age 50 years than in men of the same age.[47,96]

Rehabilitation Concerns

General principles of exercise include avoiding painful AROM and PROM by working within the client's comfort level. General AROM exercises for the hand include wrist flexion and extension, gentle digit flexion and extension, and thumb opposition. Encouraging CMC motion in flexion and abduction with the thumb MCP and IP joints flexed can assist the patient in relearning CMC movement instead of overusing the MCP and IP joints during ADL (see Exercise 22-7*D* and *E*). There is moderate evidence to support hand exercises in OA for increasing grip strength, improving function, improving ROM, and pain reduction.[84] Combining joint protection and painfree hand home exercises were found to be an effective means to increase hand function, as measured by grip strength and self-reported global functioning in persons with hand OA.[27] Exercise programs that utilize AROM as opposed to pinch strengthening[66,76,84] were found to be more effective. Even light putty-pinching exercises impart large forces[22] to an unstable CMC joint and may aggravate a potential deformity. Stability must not be sacrificed for a possible increase in strength. A stable pain-free thumb provides a post against which the digits can grip and pinch effectively. Stretching and massaging the first web space at the adductor pollicis brevis may help reduce muscle tightness that can promote the adduction contracture and subsequent MCP hyperextension deformity.[1] Thumb web space stretching or widening can be done by having the client grasp a 1-inch wooden dowel[11] (Exercise 22-9*A*) as part of the home program, as well as techniques to relax the adductor pollicis. Anatomically, strengthening the first dorsal interosseous (Exercise 22-9*B*) may help provide stability to the base of the CMC as it originates at the base of the first metacarpal.[1]

Designing and fabricating a thumb orthosis for the OA CMC joint requires careful positioning during fabrication to immobilize the CMC appropriately. A gentle correction of the swan-neck deformity would place the thumb (opposite of the deformity) in metacarpal abduction, align the metacarpal on the trapezium, flex the MCP joint, and extend the IP joint.[11] Stabilizing the CMC joint with an appropriate orthosis can decrease pain and increase function in patients that are passively correctable (see Figure 22-21*B*).[84,93] Research indicates that specific orthoses were preferred by patients. Weiss et al[93,94] found that a hand-based thumb orthosis and a short, flexible, neoprene orthosis were preferred. Night CMC orthoses were found to decrease pain and disability after 12 months of wear.[94] Use of an orthosis also is effective in reducing the need for surgery. One study reported after wearing the orthoses for 7 months, only 30% of the patients reported wanting to have surgery.[65] A systematic review published by Valdes and Marik[84] found that orthotic provision had a positive impact on decreasing hand pain and increasing hand strength and function in patients with OA. The therapist has several choices when selecting the proper orthosis for the client. The orthosis can be custom fabricated of lightweight thermoplastics, or in some cases a soft material (eg, Neoprene) can be used if the strapping is applied properly, to counteract the deforming forces. There are also several prefabricated options available. The authors of this chapter have had good patient acceptance and reported pain reduction with both the neoprene Comfort Cool Thumb CMC Restriction Splint (see Figure 22-19) (available from North Coast Medical) and The Push MetaGrip (Figure 22-22) (available from HandLab). This client acceptance is attributable to decreased pain and increased joint stability when using the properly fit orthoses during pinching activities. Clients often misinterpret this as an increase in strength. A stable, pain-free thumb is important to hand function and provides a post that the digits can grip and pinch effectively.

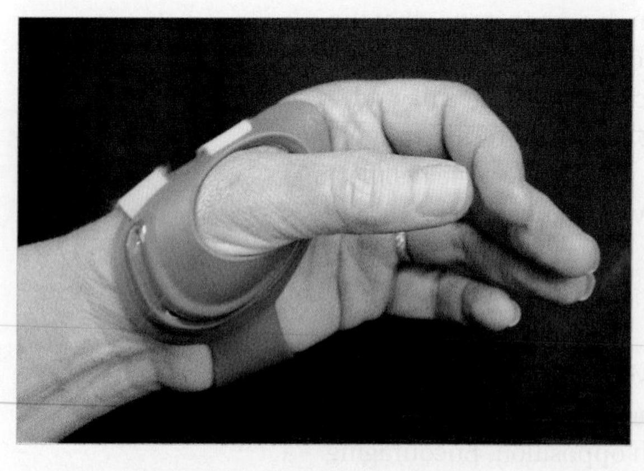

Figure 22-22

The Push MetaGrip is a prefabricated option that has high patient acceptance. This acceptance is often attributable to decreased pain and increased joint stability when using the properly fitted orthoses during pinching activities.

Rehabilitation Progression

OA is a chronic condition with remissions and exacerbations. The principles above will continue as the client progresses through the disease process. It is important to avoid pain during daily activities and during treatment so as to avoid joint deformities. CMC surgery may be indicated as the disease progresses.

Ulnar Collateral Ligament Sprain (Gamekeeper's or Skier's Thumb)

Pathomechanics

Injury to the ulnar collateral ligament (UCL) of the thumb MCP joint is one of the most common ligament injuries.[10,17,38,51,73,78] The injury is classified as grade I when there is pain but minimal damage to the ligament; grade II is a partial tear with some joint instability; and grade III is a complete disruption of the UCL with more than 30 degrees of lateral instability. It is most often the distal attachment of the ligament where the rupture occurs.[38,51]

The patient will complain of pain or tenderness on the ulnar side of the MCP joint, as well as inflammation, in all classifications. If the ligament is completely torn, one must also be concerned about a Stener lesion. A Stener lesion is where the torn UCL protrudes beneath the adductor aponeurosis. This places the aponeurosis between the ligament and its insertion. If this occurs, reattachment will not occur and surgery is needed.[78]

Injury Mechanism

UCL injuries occur when a torsional load is applied to the thumb.[16] It frequently occurs in pole sports as a result of a fall on an outstretched hand when landing with a pole on an abducted thumb.[10,17,38,51,73,78] This injury is referred to as gamekeeper's injury as well as skier's thumb. Gamekeeper's injury occurs most frequently from chronic repeated stress on the UCL[78] whereas skier's thumb occurs most commonly as an acute injury.[38] Football players also may sustain this injury while abducting the thumb before making a tackle.[51]

Rehabilitation Concerns

Early diagnosis and treatment are important. An unstable thumb MCP joint or a Stener lesion, if not treated, can become chronically painful and unstable possibly resulting in arthritic changes and reduced pinch strength.[10,17,78] Treatment for incomplete (grade I or II) tears and some grade III avulsions is often immobilization in a thumb spica cast or orthosis (Figure 22-23). This is often utilized for 6 to 8 weeks, depending on the preferences of the physician. Care should be taken to avoid MCP radial deviation during the immobilization phase so as to prevent stretching of the healing UCL. There is some support for using an orthosis rather than a cast for immobilization.[32,43] In addition to treatment with an orthosis, there is some support for early initiation of AROM.[43,45] There has also been some support for utilization of a hinged orthosis. This orthosis allows for motion in flexion and extension but prevents MCP ulnar and radial deviation.[35,53,74]

Treatment for Stener lesions or displaced bony avulsion injuries is a surgical repair. Early operative intervention is recommended because delayed reconstruction is less successful.[17] Postoperatively, a thumb spica orthosis is usually worn for 6 to 8 weeks with initiation of thumb AROM based on physician preferences.

Rehabilitation Progression

Some patients, as they return to sports or specific activities, prefer to continue to wear a thin hand-based thumb spica orthosis (see Figure 22-23) for protection. This orthosis can be fabricated with light (1/16 in) orthotic materials that can fit under a ski or other sport's glove. A simple Velcro thumb sling described by Fillon may be preferred by patients who require a softer option.[35] The orthosis secures the thumb to the index digit avoiding ulnar deviation. These patients will gradually wean from the orthosis as they progress.

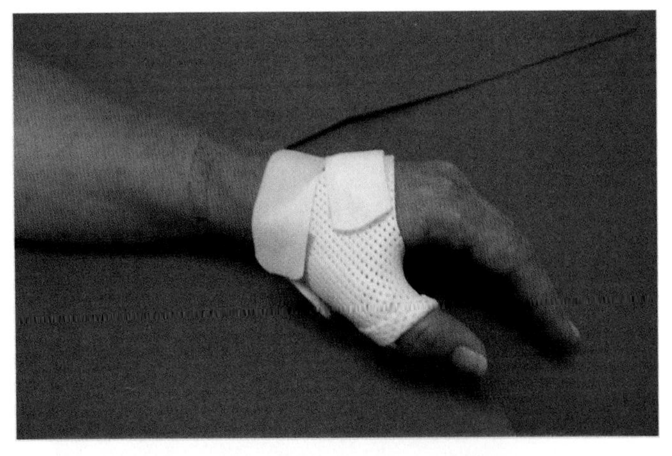

Figure 22-23

A hand-based thumb spica orthosis is utilized for protection of the UCL. This condition is often referred to as gamekeeper's thumb or skier's thumb.

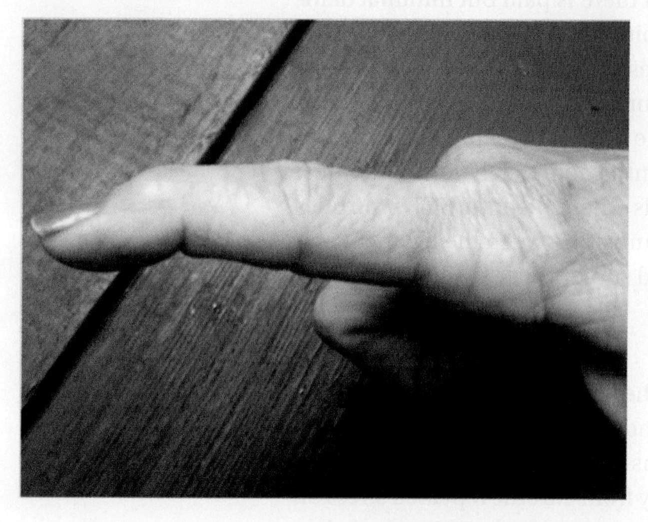

Figure 22-24 A mallet finger deformity with DIP flexion

Mallet Finger

Pathomechanics

A mallet finger is the avulsion of the terminal extensor tendon, which is responsible for extension of the DIP joint.[70] The patient will be unable to extend the DIP joint actively upon examination (Figure 22-24). It may occur with or without fracture of bone. If there is a large fracture fragment where the fracture fragment is displaced greater than 2 mm, or the DIP joint has volar subluxation on radiograph, the injury will require open reduction and internal fixation.

Injury Mechanism

The injury mechanism is forced flexion of the DIP joint while it is held in full extension.[77] It frequently happens when a ball or some other object strikes the fully extended digit. It also may occur when tucking in bedding or when the tendon is weakened by the arthritic process.

Rehabilitation Concerns

Rehabilitation of the mallet finger requires excellent orthotic/casting skills and good patient compliance. There is a tendency to minimize this condition and many patients are noncompliant. Treatment includes an orthosis that places the DIP joint in slight hyperextension (Figure 22-25) for 6 to 8 weeks with no flexion of the DIP joint.[25,57,77] If the DIP joint is flexed even once during the immobilization period, the 6-week immobilization period begins again at that time. An orthosis or cast should be custom made,[64] comfortable to the patient, and designed not to cause skin breakdown. If the splint is removable, the patient should be able to reapply it with the DIP held in hyperextension. Skin integrity needs to be monitored

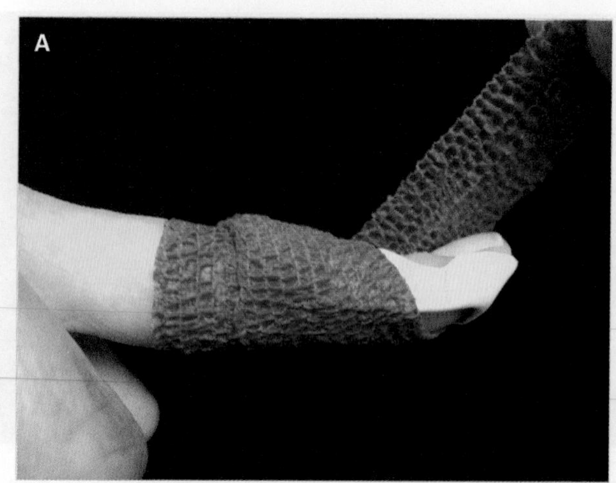

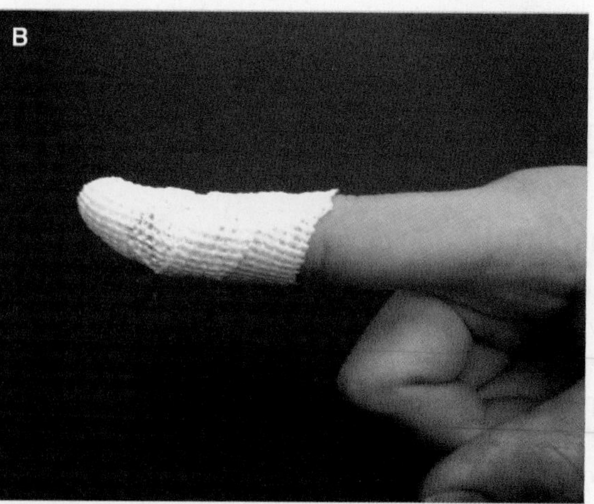

Figure 22-25

A. A mallet finger orthosis must hold the DIP in slight hyperextension. Skin integrity needs to be monitored with the orthosis being modified or redesigned if irritation occurs. B. Waterproof QuickCast II material allows full-time wear even while bathing.

and the orthosis be modified or redesigned if irritation occurs. Because of this challenge, many clinicians utilize a waterproof QuickCast II material that allows full-time wear even while bathing. The QuickCast II material is heated with a hair dryer and quickly applied to the digit held in slight DIP hyperextension (Figure 22-26*A–E*). Patients return weekly for cast changes. If the cast becomes loose between cast changes, it can be held snug by an overwrap of Coban. Range of motion of noninvolved fingers and joints should be maintained. Athletes may require cast changes with each game or practice as a consequence of perspiration. The therapist can instruct the team's athletic trainer in the QuickCast II technique so as to reduce the number of visits the athlete has to make to the clinic.

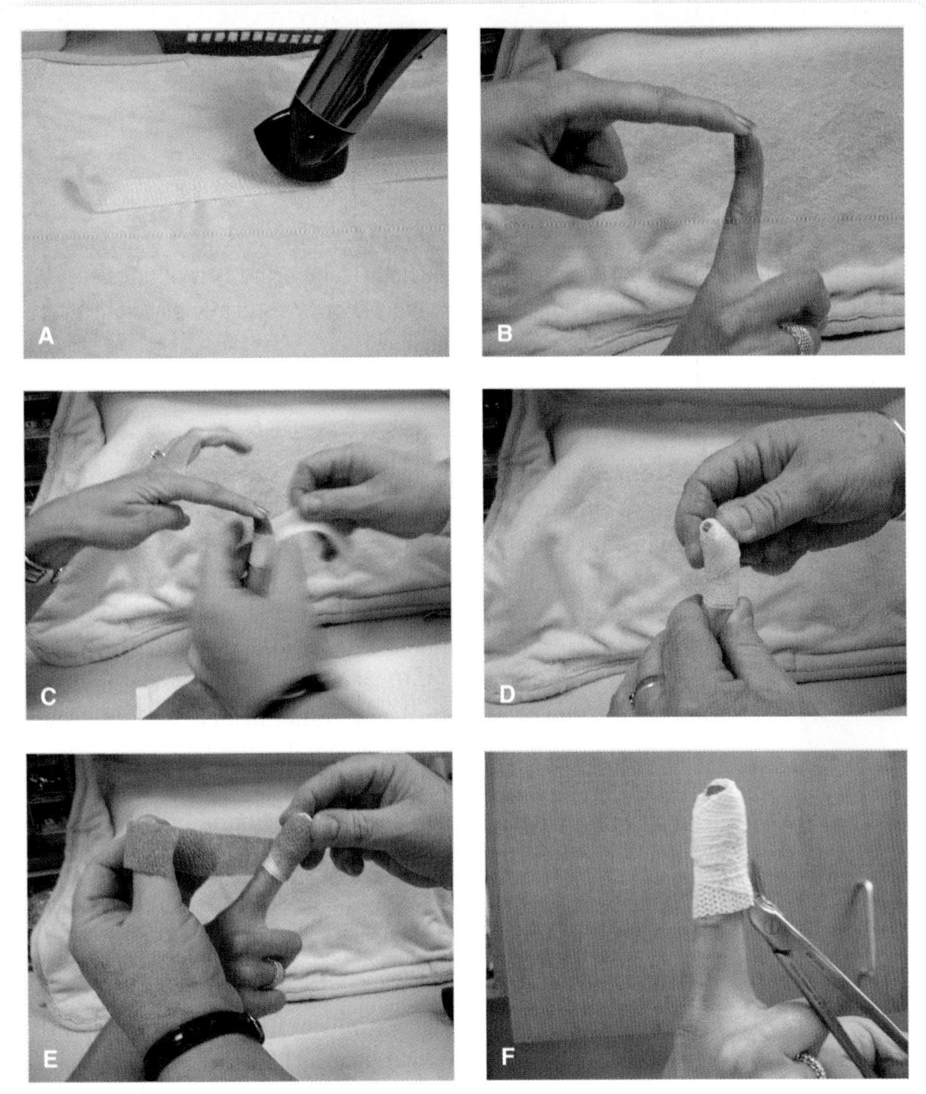

Figure 22-26

A. The QuickCast II material can be heated up with a hair dryer. **B.** The digit held in slight DIP hyperextension at all times. **C** and **D.** The cast is quickly applied and the position of slight hyperextension maintained as the orthosis cools. Patients return weekly for cast changes. **E.** If the cast becomes loose between cast changes, it can be held snug by an overwrap of Coban. ROM of noninvolved fingers and joints should be maintained. PIP flexion with the DIP cast will not put tension on the injury and should be encouraged. **F.** The cast is removed with a special short scissors.

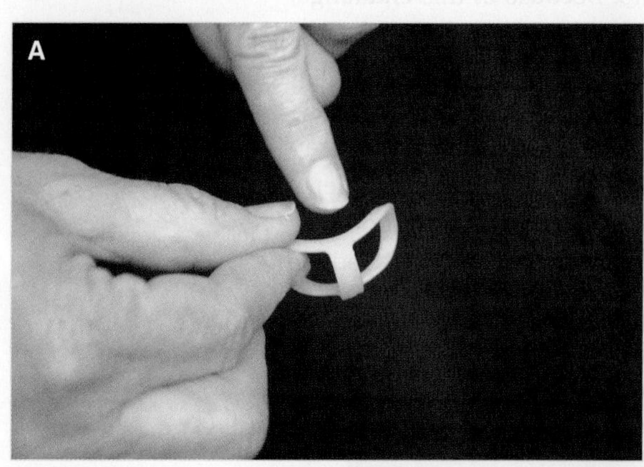

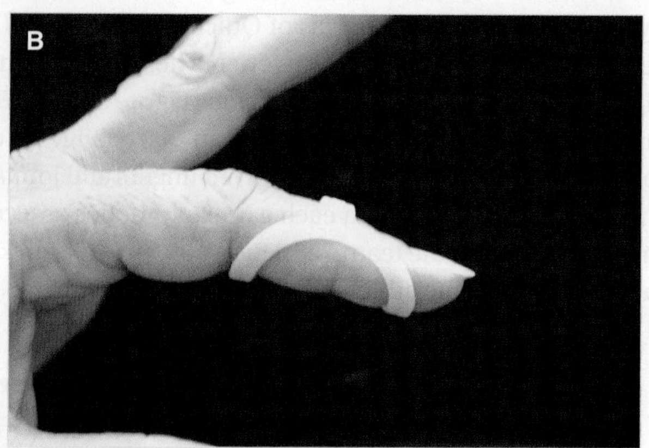

Figure 22-27

A. Once the tendon is healed, often at approximately 6 to 8 weeks,[94] orthotic weaning is initiated with a schedule of 2 hours on, 2 hours off, and at least 1 month of night orthotic wear.[96] An adjusted Oval 8 orthosis facilitates easy donning and doffing during this phase. The Oval 8 is heated up at this junction and the orthosis gently placed in slight hyperextension. **B.** The Oval 8 holding the digit in place and in slight hyperextension.

Rehabilitation Progression

Once the tendon is healed, often at approximately 6 to 8 weeks,[57] orthotic weaning is initiated. If an extensor lag is present, use of the orthosis either continues or the physician evaluates for the possibility of surgery. Orthotic weaning is initiated with a schedule of 2 hours on, 2 hours off, and at least 1 month of night splinting.[57] If no extension lag develops, then the time out of the orthosis is gradually increased. An adjusted Oval 8 orthosis facilitates easy donning and doffing during this phase (Figure 22-27). Gentle DIP joint AROM consists of initiating light use of the hand. No attempt should be made to passively flex the DIP joint or to stretch out the tendon with DIP joint blocking (Exercise 22-10). Full ROM is usually gained through regular functional hand use. Athletes should wear a DIP joint orthosis for no less than 8 weeks.

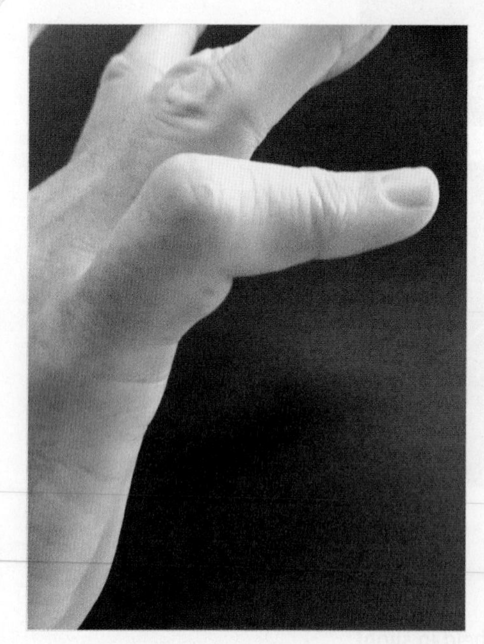

Figure 22-28

A boutonnière deformity may start as a PIP contracture. It can in time result in hyperextension of the DIP joint.

Boutonnière Deformity

Pathomechanics

The posture of a finger with a boutonnière deformity is PIP joint flexion and DIP joint hyperextension (Figure 22-28). It is caused by interruption of the central slip. Normally, the central slip will initiate extension of flexed PIP joints. When the central slip is disrupted, the extensor muscle displaces proximally and shifts the lateral bands shift volarly. The FDS is then unopposed without an intact central slip and will flex the PIP joint. The lateral bands displace volarly and may become fixed as the deformity progresses. This then makes passive correction very difficult. The DIP joint hyperextends because all the force to extend the PIP is transmitted to the DIP joint.[68]

Once a fixed deformity is present, treatment can be challenging. Treatment within 6 weeks of the initial injury is associated with better outcomes.[75] Many patients do not seek immediate medical attention, mistakenly feeling that the finger was "just jammed" and that it will resolve quickly. Treatment for the acute injury is uninterrupted immobilization, with an orthosis or QuickCast II, of the PIP joint in full extension for 6 to 8 weeks[67] (Figure 22-29). The DIP joint is left free or blocked in slight flexion without strapping to encourage DIP flexion. This will synergistically relax the extrinsic and intrinsic extensor tendon muscles and exercises the oblique retinacular ligament.[49]

Injury Mechanism

Injury occurs when the extended finger is forcibly flexed, such as when being hit by a ball or because of a fall when striking the finger on another object.[67,73] Trauma to the dorsal aspect of the PIP joint can also be a mechanism of injury.[67]

Rehabilitation Concerns

Of primary concern is early and proper diagnosis and treatment. Radiographs can help to rule out a fracture or a PIP joint dislocation. It is also very important to immobilize the PIP in full extension. As edema decreases, frequent orthotic modifications are needed to assure full PIP joint extension. If diagnosis is made late and there is a fixed PIP flexion contracture, serial casting may be the best conservative measure to restore extension. Serial casting with QuickCast II is preferred by many patients as it is waterproof and more easily tolerated. Following return of full extension (usually after 6 to 8 weeks), the digit is then placed in a removable orthosis for the weaning program (see Figure 22-27*A*). Weaning occurs gradually with a return to the immobilization orthosis if an extension lag develops at the PIP joint.

Rehabilitation Progression

Weaning from the orthosis after 6 to 8 weeks may be initiated with a 2 hours on and 2 hours off daytime schedule and with night immobilization continuing for several weeks. Gentle

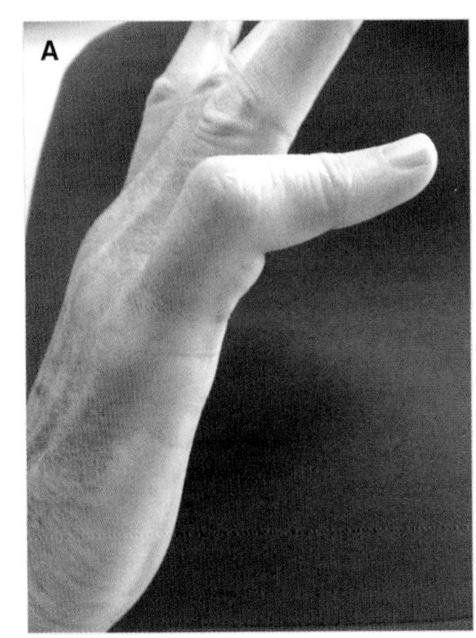

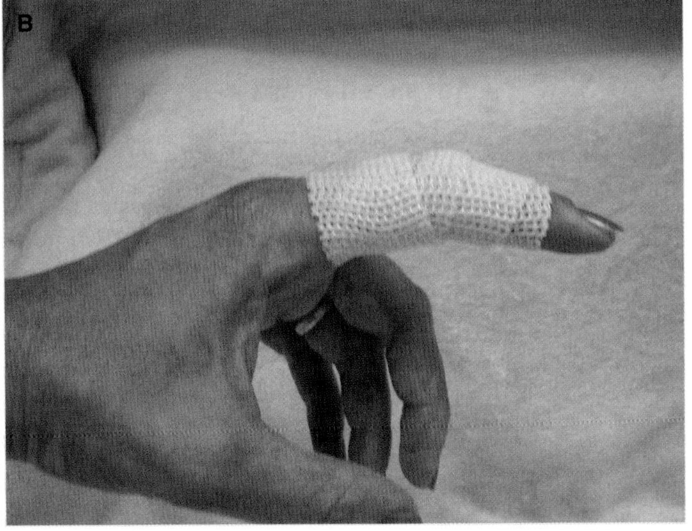

Figure 22-29

A. Treatment for the acute boutonnière injury is uninterrupted immobilization of the PIP joint in full extension for 6 to 8 weeks. The DIP joint is left free or blocked in slight flexion without strapping to encourage DIP flexion. This will synergistically relax the extrinsic and intrinsic extensor tendon muscles and exercise the oblique retinacular ligament.[13] **B.** Chronic injures usually require serial casting to gradually obtain full PIP extension.

PIP joint AROM begins gradually, observing for the development of PIP joint extension lag. If an extension lag develops, the patient is returned to the orthosis. If the extension lag is persistent, the patient should be referred to the surgeon for evaluation. Orthosis weaning programs that progress without an extension lag can gradually return to using the hand for light activities. Night immobilization may continue for 12 weeks and beyond.

Protocols

de Quervain Tendonitis Conservative Management Protocol

Acute Phase

The initial treatment is rest from aggravating activities. This includes full-time wear of the orthosis for 4 to 6 weeks (see Figure 22-10) with removal of the orthosis for bathing and skin care. The forearm-based orthosis includes the wrist, thumb (CMC), and MCP joints. Modalities to decrease inflammation may be utilized by the clinician during this phase as well. Goals for the acute phase include the following:

1. The patient will report reduced pain while wearing the orthosis.
2. The patient will be independent with the orthotic program.

Intermediate Phase

After wearing the orthosis for 4 to 6 weeks, weaning of the orthosis is initiated if the patient reports a decrease in pain (with a pain analog scale). This begins with a schedule of 2 hours on and 2 hours off during the day. Painful activities are avoided, and night immobilization continues. The time out of the orthosis gradually increases, as dictated by reduced pain levels. If the symptoms return during the weaning program, the physician should be contacted to determine if full-time immobilization with the orthosis should be resumed, or if surgery is an option. The goals of the intermediate phase are to wean from the orthosis during the day and to gradually return to ADL without an increase in pain.

Advanced Phase

The patient gradually weans from the night orthosis. Some activities including work activities may need to be avoided, modified or adapted as necessary to prevent recurrence of the condition. The goal of the advanced phase is to gradually wean from the night orthosis and return to full participation in ADL without an increase in pain.

Return to Function

Strengthening exercises should be avoided to prevent irritation to the involved tendons. Once the patient returns to pain-free ADL, formal strengthening programs are usually not needed. Work as well as all activities should be carefully analyzed and adapted as possible to avoid recurrence of painful symptoms. The goal of the return-to-function phase is to return to ADL and work activities without a recurrence of symptoms.

Mallet Finger Conservative Management Protocol

Acute Phase

Rehabilitation for a mallet finger requires precise fabrication of an orthosis or a cast. The orthosis or QuickCast II must be applied in slight DIP hyperextension and worn full-time for 6 to 8 weeks. The hyperextension position must be maintained at each weekly orthosis/cast change or the immobilization period must be initiated again from the beginning. When patients are wearing an orthosis, the patient should perform skin care checks and hygiene at least once a day. It is important that the patient is independent with the home orthosis/casting program including proper use and duration of wear, and avoids any unsupported DIP motion when removed for short time periods during skin care. If the patient is wearing a QuickCast II, it will need to be changed by the therapist at least once a week. Many patients are unable to obtain the position of slight DIP hyperextension at the initial therapy visit. This requires serial casting or a serial extension orthosis until the position is obtained (see Figure 22-26). The goals of the acute phase include achieving slight DIP hyperextension. Once this is obtained, a 6- to 8-week immobilization period begins. If the cast or orthosis becomes loose, Coban or tape should be used to secure it. The patient should be able to complete PIP AROM exercises in the DIP orthosis/cast.

Intermediate Phase

The cast/orthotic program continues for 6 to 8 weeks until full active DIP extension is achieved.[95,97] At the 6-week point, the DIP active extension position is carefully tested by having the digit supported in hyperextension by the examiner. The support is then briefly removed by the examiner to observe for full active DIP extension. If full active DIP extension is achieved, the patient moves on to the intermediate phase. If the DIP flexes slightly, support is immediately reapplied by the examiner and the orthosis/cast is reapplied. At this point, the immobilization may continue or the patient may consult with the physician regarding surgical intervention. The goal of the intermediate phase is full active DIP extension.

Advanced Phase

After full active DIP extension has been achieved by means of the continuous DIP orthosis/cast extension program, weaning from the orthosis is initiated. Weaning proceeds by gradually decreasing the amount of time in the orthosis and observing for DIP extension lags. This weaning usually involves a change in the wearing schedule to include 2 hours on and 2 hours off with continued night wear. An easily removable orthosis for this weaning period is the Oval 8 orthosis from 3-point products (see Figure 22-27). This orthosis is adjusted to place the DIP in slight hyperextension. The ease of donning and removal of this "ring style" orthosis may improve patient compliance. After 3 to 4 days, if full DIP extension is maintained, the wearing schedule or time out of the orthosis is increased to 4 hours on and 4 hours off and continues at night. This weaning procedure continues until the daytime orthosis is gradually discontinued, but wearing a night orthosis continues for at least 1 month.[96]

If at any point during the weaning program, the DIP demonstrates an extension lag, the orthosis is reapplied and the physician contacted. The patient may be a candidate for surgery if the orthosis program has been unsuccessful. Some physicians and/or patients may prefer another trial month of the full-time orthosis program as opposed to surgery. The goal of the advanced phase is successfully weaning from the orthosis during the day while maintaining full active DIP extension of the involved digit. It is important to note that if the patient has an extension lag, it will only increase after the orthosis is discontinued.[95,97]

Return to Function

The advanced phase ends with successful weaning from the daytime DIP orthosis. During the return-to-function phase the patient gradually weans from the night orthosis. One option is to wear the night orthosis every other night and gradually increase the number of nights out of the orthosis. This continues until night orthotic wear is eliminated and full active DIP extension is maintained. Blocking (Exercise 22-10) to the DIP, as well as PROM, are prohibited to avoid stress to the newly healed tendon. The patient gradually returns to using the digit for progressively more involved ADL. Once again (as stated previously), any return of the DIP extension lag is reported to the surgeon.

Exercises

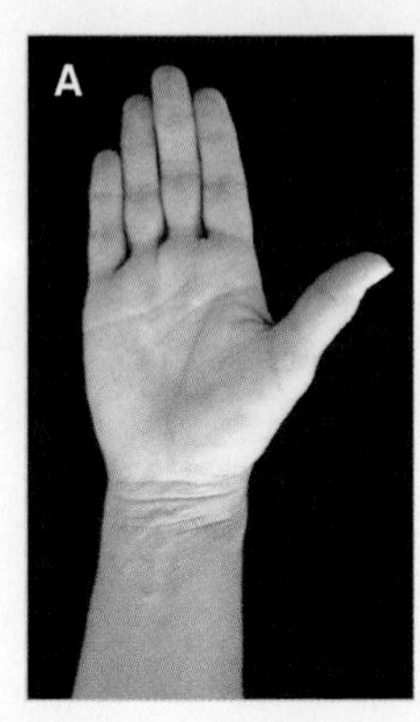
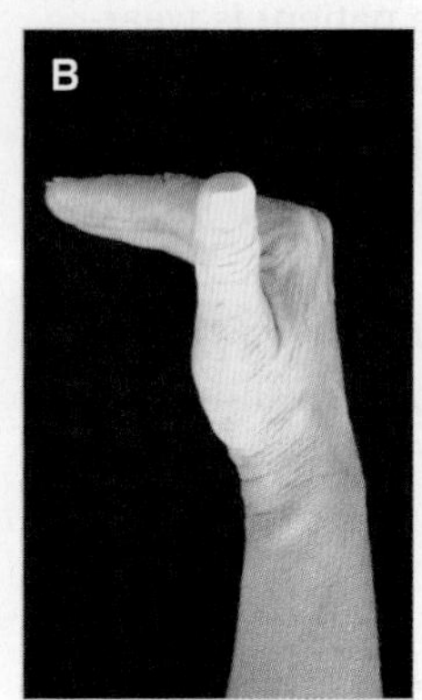
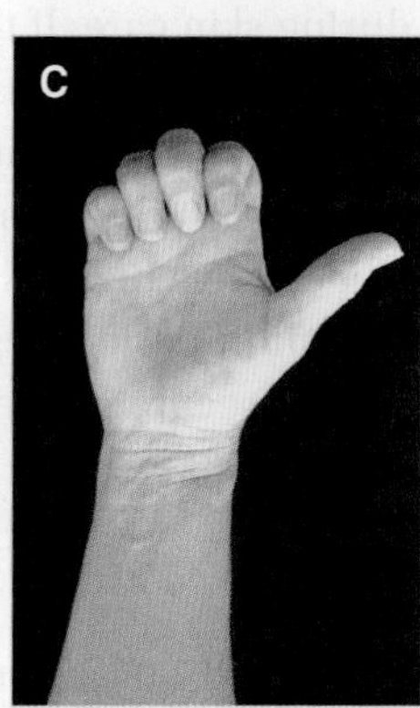
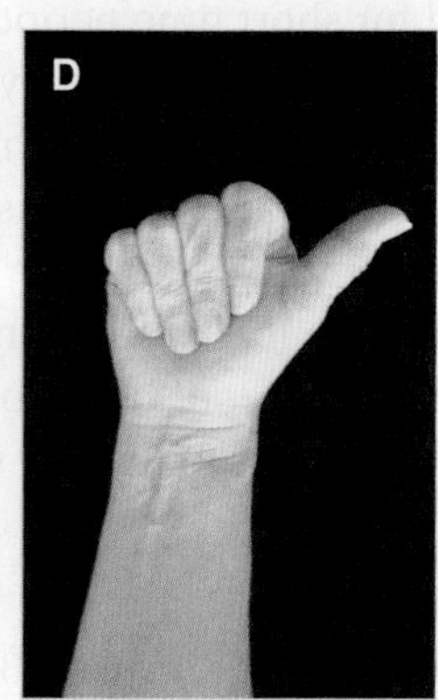
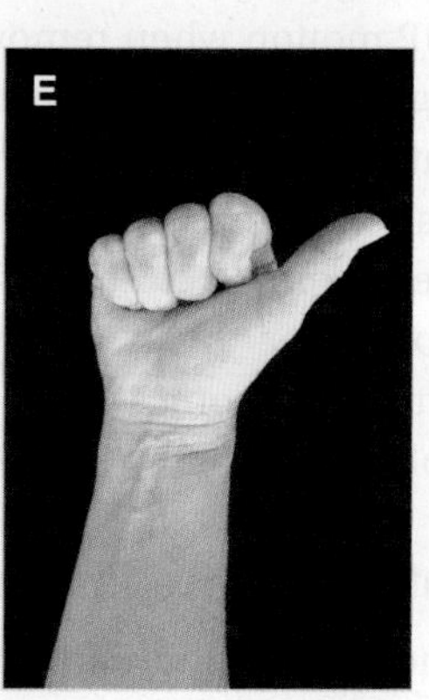

Exercise 22-1

Tendon gliding exercises allow for maximum gliding of the FDS and FDP. **A.** Start with full composite finger extension. **B.** Move to MCP flexion with IP extension activating the intrinsics and then return to extension. **C.** Move to hook fisting, which gives maximum differential tendon gliding between FDS and FDP and return to extension. **D.** Move to long fisting with MCP and PIP flexion and DIP extension for maximum FDS tendon glide and return to extension. **E.** Finally, move to composite flexion with full fisting, which gives the maximum glide of the FDP tendon.

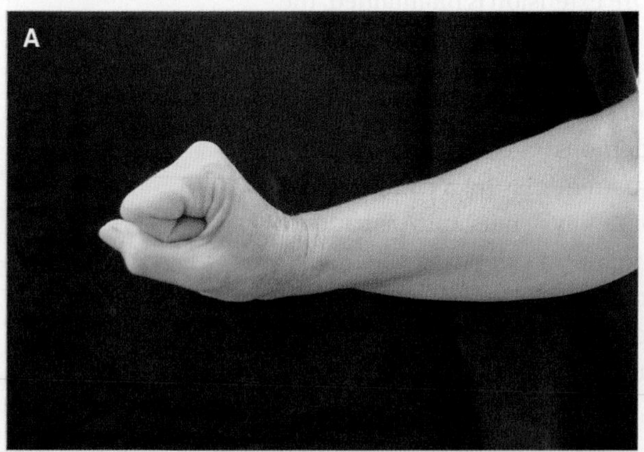
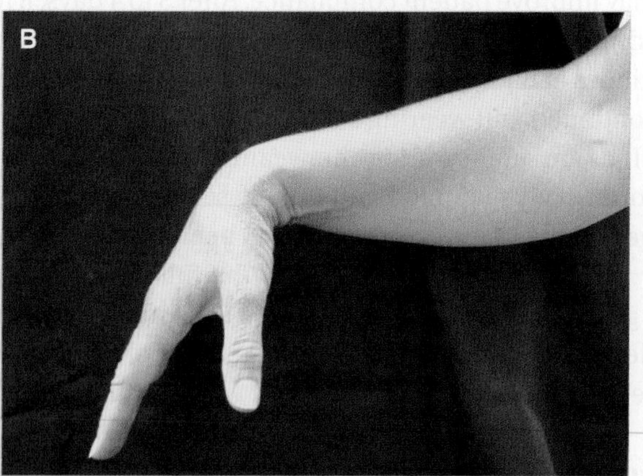

Exercise 22-2

A. Wrist extension encourages exercise of the common wrist extensor tendons (extensor carpi radialis longus, extensor carpi radialis brevis, and extensor carpi ulnaris). Digit flexion should be maintained to eliminate extensor digitorum communis contribution and to isolate the wrist musculature. **B.** Wrist flexion encourages exercise of the common wrist flexors (flexor carpi ulnaris, flexor carpi radialis). Digit extension should be maintained to avoid FDS and FDP contributions and to isolate the wrist musculature.

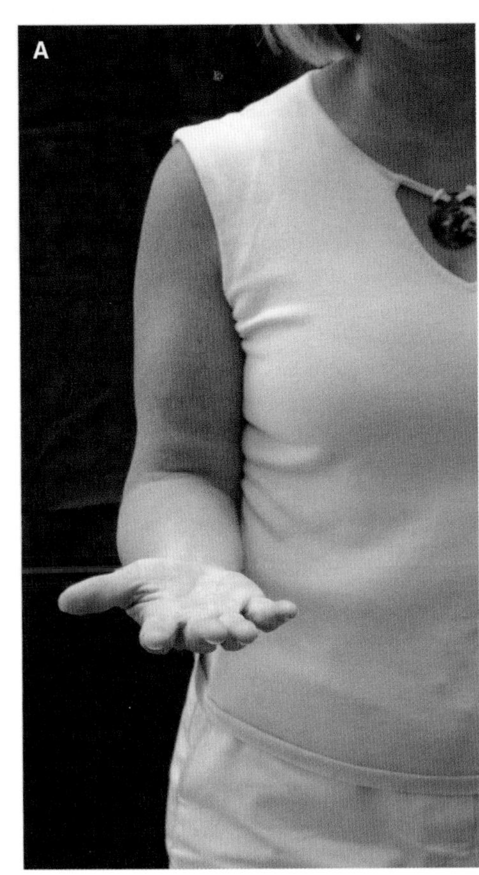

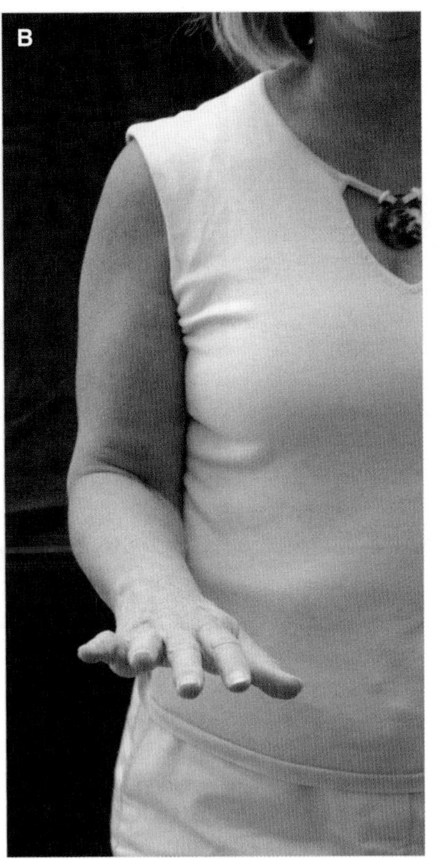

Exercise 22-3

A. Active supination exercises the supinator and the biceps. It should be done with elbow at 90 degrees of flexion with the humerus by the side. This eliminates shoulder rotation. **B.** Active pronation exercises should also be done in the same position.

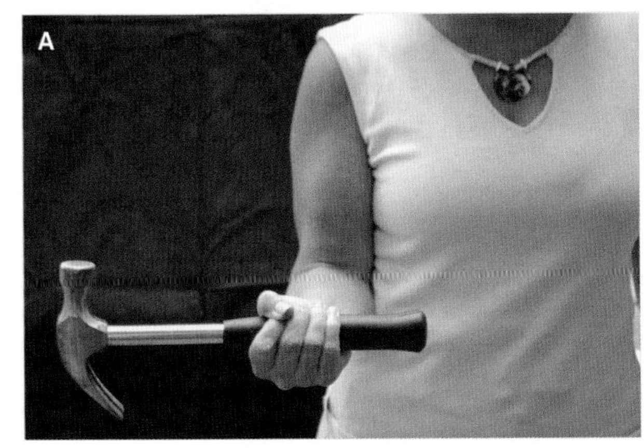

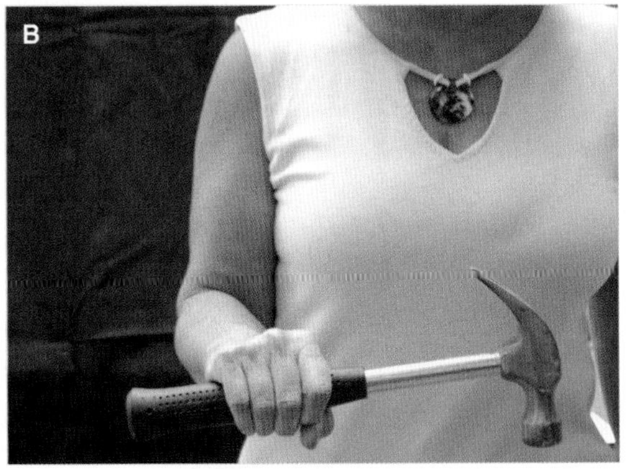

Exercise 22-4

A. Passive supination can be done with a hammer. The lever action of the hammer assists with the passive motion. **B.** Passive pronation is also done with the hammer.

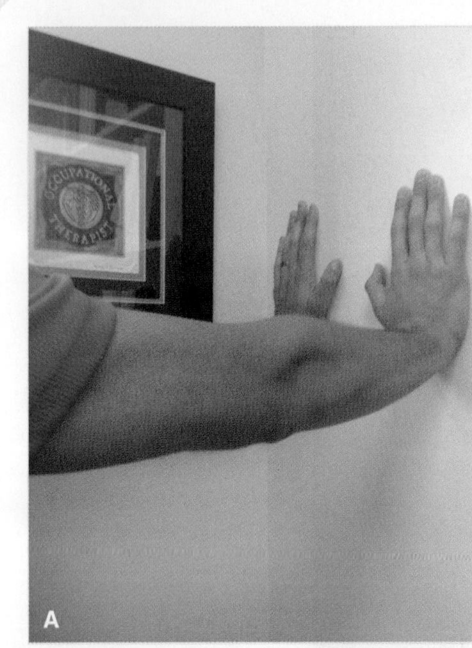

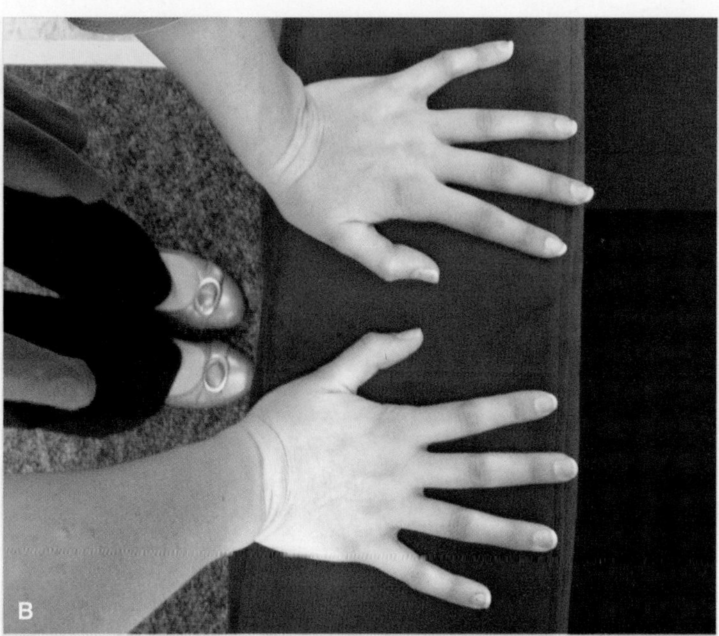

Exercise 22-5

A. Wall pushups encourage wrist motion and general upper-body strengthening. They also encourage weight bearing and closed-chain activities. **B.** Pushups can be progressed from the wall to a table or countertop. This encourages gradual progression of increased weight bearing to the extremity.

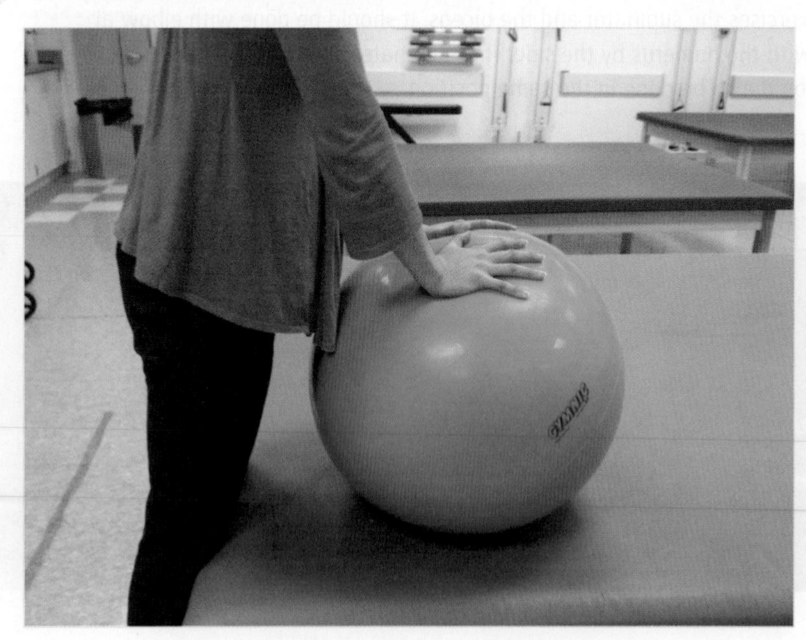

Exercise 22-6

Pushups on a ball encourage upper-extremity control.

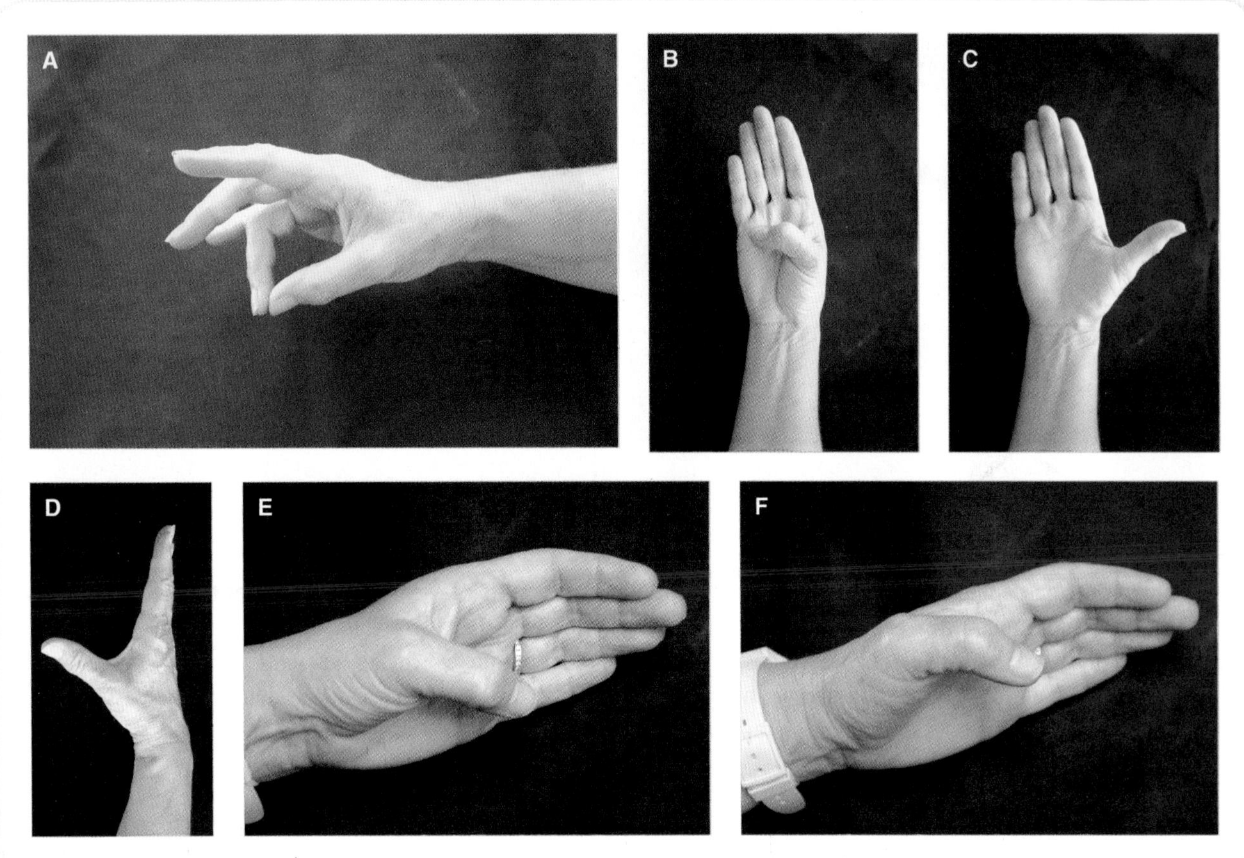

Exercise 22-7

Some of the more common AROM exercises to the thumb include (**A**) opposition, (**B**) flexion, (**C**) extension, and (**D**) palmar abduction. (**E**) Carpometacarpal (CMC) flexion with MCP and IP flexion is used in cases of CMC osteoarthritis. This encourages the patient to relearn how to move the CMC instead of over using the MCP and IP joints during ADL. (**F**) CMC abduction with MCP and IP flexion.

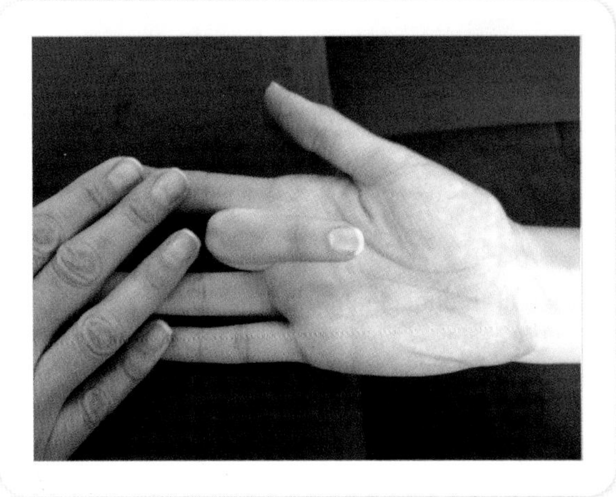

Exercise 22-8

To isolate active movement of the FDS, the noninvolved fingers are held in full extension, allowing only the involved finger to flex.

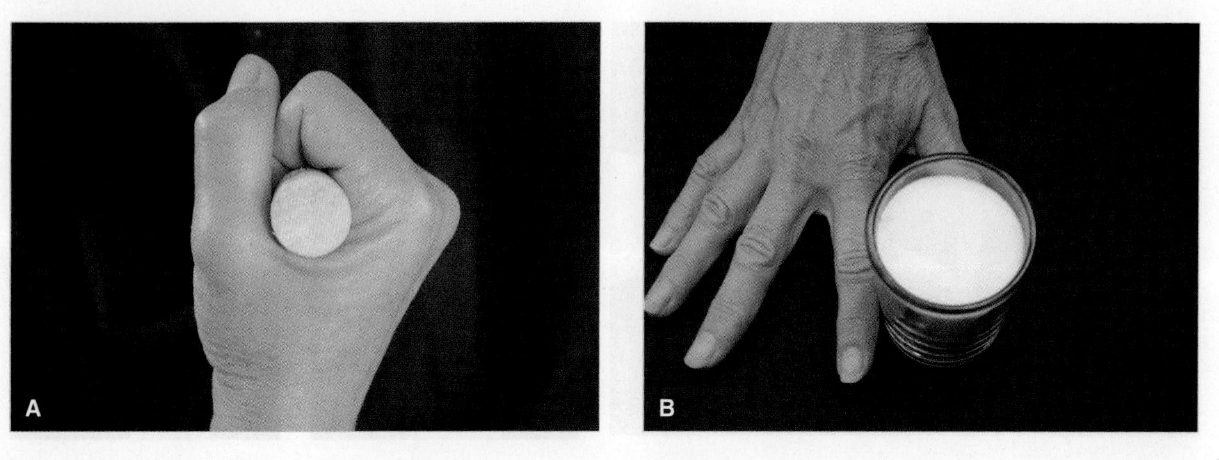

Exercise 22-9

A. Stretching and massaging the first web space to a tight adductor pollicis brevis may help prevent the adduction contracture and subsequent MCP hyperextension deformity.[76] Thumb web space stretching or widening can be done by having the client grasp a 1-inch wooden dowel as part of the home program, as well as techniques to relax the adductor pollicis (AP).[76,77] **B.** Anatomically, strengthening the first dorsal interossius may help provide stability to the base of the CMC as it originates at the base of the first metacarpal.[76]

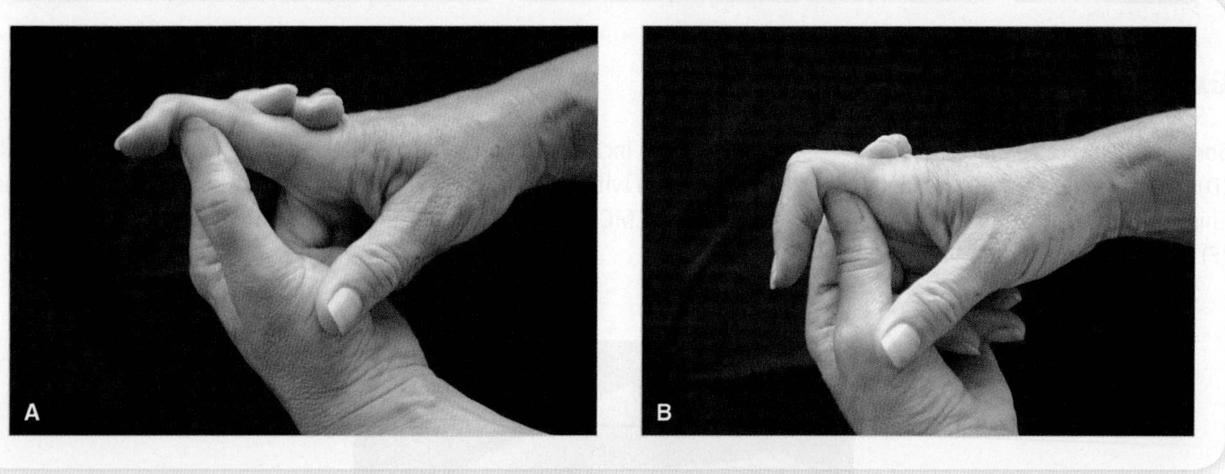

Exercise 22-10

A. Blocked DIP exercises encourage FDP pull-through. Stabilizing the middle phalanx allows the flexion force to concentrate at the DIP joint. **B.** Blocked PIP exercises encourage FDS pull-through. Stabilizing the proximal phalanx then allows the flexion force to act at the PIP joint.

SUMMARY

1. Scaphoid fractures may not be obvious on an initial radiograph. Some scaphoid fractures are misdiagnosed as wrist sprains. Proper immobilization is important in the long-term outcome.
2. CTS is usually treated by rest and with a night orthoses that place the wrist in a neutral wrist position.
3. Orthotic provision in patients with CMC OA has been demonstrated to decrease hand pain and increase hand strength and function. The therapist has several choices when selecting the proper orthosis for the client.
4. Boxer's fractures with an open wound have a high incidence of infection.
5. de Quervain tenosynovitis should be immobilized for 4 to 6 weeks in a thumb spica orthosis.
6. Trigger finger may be managed conservatively with the use of several types of orthoses for a minimum of 3 to 6 weeks of immobilization.
7. The goal in the treatment of UCL injuries (gamekeeper's thumb and skier's thumb) is stability of the MCP joint. Care should be taken to avoid any thumb MCP radial deviation.
8. Conservative management of a mallet finger requires a cooperative compliant patient. DIP flexion is not allowed at any time during the 6- to 8-week orthotic or casting program.
9. Early treatment of the boutonnière deformity is essential, as is a proper orthotic position. The PIP joint should be fully extended with the DIP joint free or in slight flexion. Serial casting can be effective in increasing extension in chronic boutonnière deformities.

REFERENCES

1. Albrecht J. *Caring for the Painful Thumb, More Than a Splint.* Christchurch, New Zealand: New Zealand Association of Hand Therapists; 2008.
2. Amadio PC. Carpal tunnel syndrome: surgeon's management. In: Skirven TM, Osterman AL, Fedorczyk JM, Amadio PC, eds. *Rehabilitation of the Hand and Upper Extremity.* 6th ed. Philadelphia, PA: Elsevier; 2011:657-665.
3. Baker N, Moehling K, Rubinstein E, Wollstein R, GustafsonN, Baratz M. The comparative effectiveness of combined lumbrical muscle splints and stretches on symptoms and function in carpal tunnel syndrome. *Arch Phys Med Rehabil.* 2012;93:1-10.
4. Baxter-Petralia P, Penney V. Cumulative trauma. In: Stanley BG, Tribuzi SM, eds. *Concepts in Hand Rehabilitation.* Philadelphia, PA: FA Davis; 1992:434-445.
5. Beasley J. Soft orthoses: indications and techniques. In: Skirven TM, Osterman AL, Fedorczyk JM, Amadio PC, eds. *Rehabilitation of the Hand and Upper Extremity.* 6th ed. Philadelphia, PA: Elsevier; 2011:1610-1619.
6. Bednar JM. The distal radioulnar joint: acute injuries and chronic injuries In: Skirven TM, Osterman AL, Fedorczyk JM, Amadio PC, eds. *Rehabilitation of the Hand and Upper Extremity.* 6th ed. Philadelphia, PA: Elsevier; 2011: 948-963.
7. Belsky MR, Leibman M. Extra-articular hand fractures, part I: surgeon's management—a practical approach. In: Skirven TM, Osterman AL, Fedorczyk JM, Amadio PC, eds. *Rehabilitation of the Hand and Upper Extremity.* 6th ed. Philadelphia, PA: Elsevier; 2011:377-385.
8. Berger AB. Anatomy and kinesiology of the wrist. In: Skirven TM, Osterman AL, Fedorczyk JM, Amadio PC, eds. *Rehabilitation of the Hand and Upper Extremity.* 6th ed. Philadelphia, PA: Elsevier; 2011:18-27.
9. Berenbaum, F. Osteoarthritis: B. Pathology and pathogenesis. In: Klippel JH, ed. *Primer on the Rheumatic Diseases.* 13th ed. New York, NY: Springer; 2008:229-234.
10. Bertini TH, Laidig TJ, Pettit NM, et al. Treatment of the injured athlete. In: Skirven TM, Osterman AL, Fedorczyk JM, Amadio PC, eds. *Rehabilitation of the Hand and*

Upper Extremity. 6th ed. Philadelphia, PA: Elsevier; 2011:1706-1713.

11. Biese (Beasley) J. Arthritis. In: Cooper C. *Fundamentals of Hand Therapy: Clinical Reasoning and Treatment Guidelines for Common Diagnoses of the Upper Extremity*. St. Louis, MO: Elsevier; 2007:348-375.
12. Bohler L. *The Treatment of Fractures*. 4th ed. Baltimore, MD: William Wood; 1942.
13. Brown RA, Gelberman RH, Seiler JG, et al. Carpal tunnel release: a prospective, randomized assessment of open and endoscopic methods. *J Bone Joint Surg Am*. 1993;75A:1265.
14. Burke DT, Burke MM, Stewart GW, Cambre A. Splinting for carpal tunnel syndrome: in search of the optimal angle. *Arch Phys Med Rehabil*. 1994;75:1241.
15. Butler DS. *Mobilization of the Nervous System*. Melbourne, Australia: Churchill Livingstone; 1991.
16. Cahalan TD, Cooney WP. Biomechanics. In: Jobe FW, Pink MM, Glousman RE, et al, eds. *Operative Techniques in Upper Extremity Sports Injuries*. St. Louis, MO: Mosby; 1996:109-123.
17. Campbell CS. Gamekeeper's thumb. *J Bone Joint Surg Br*. 1955;37:148-149.
18. Chin D, Jones N. Repetitive motion hand disorders. *J Calif Dent Assoc*. 2002;30:149-160.
19. Cobb TK, Dalley BK, Posteraro RH, Lewis RC. Anatomy of the flexor retinaculum. *Hand Surg*. 1993;18A:91.
20. Colbourn J, Heath N, Manary S, Pacifico D. Effectiveness of splinting for the treatment of trigger finger. *J Hand Ther*. 2008;21(4):336-43.
21. Colello-Abraham, K. Dynamic pronation-supination splinting. In: Hunter JM et al, eds. *Rehabilitation of the Hand*. 3rd ed. St. Louis, MO: Mosby; 1990:1134-1139.
22. Cooney WP, Chao EY. Biomechanical analysis of static forces in the thumb during hand function. *J Bone Joint Surg Am*. 1977;59(1):27-36.
23. Cooney WP, Linschied RI, Dobyns JH. Triangular fibro-cartilage tears. *J Hand Surg*. 1994;19(1):143-154.
24. Dell PC, Dell RB, Griggs R. Management of carpal fractures and dislocations. In: Skirven TM, Osterman AL, Fedorcyzk JM, Armadio PC, eds. *Rehabilitation of the Hand and Upper Extremity*. 6th ed. Philadelphia, PA: Elsevier; 2011:988-1001.
25. Doyle JR. Extensor tendons—acute injuries. In: Green DP, ed. *Operative Hand Surgery*. 2nd ed. New York, NY: Churchill Livingstone; 1988:55-71.
26. Dray GJ, Eaton RG. Dislocations and ligament injuries in the digits. In: Green DP, ed. *Operative Hand Surgery*. Vol. 1. 3rd ed. New York, NY: Churchill Livingstone; 1993:101-122.
27. Dunlop DD, Semanik P, Song J, Manheim LM, Shih V, Chang RW. Risk factors for functional decline in older adults with arthritis. *Arthritis Rheum*. 2005;52:1274-1282.
28. Eaton RG, Glickel SZ. Trapeziometacarpal osteoarthritis. Staging as a rationale for treatment. *Hand Clin*. 1987;3:455-471.
29. Evans RB. Therapist's management of carpal tunnel syndrome: a practical approach. In: Skirven TM, Osterman AL, Fedorczyk JM, Amadio PC, eds. *Rehabilitation of the Hand and Upper Extremity*. 6th ed. Philadelphia, PA: Elsevier; 2011:666-677.
30. Evans RB, Hunter JM, Burkhalter WE. Conservative management of the trigger finger: a new approach. *J Hand Ther*. 1988;1:59-68.
31. Fedorczyk JM. The use of physical agents in hand rehabilitation. In: Skirven TM, Osterman AL, Fedorczyk JM, Amadio PC, eds. *Rehabilitation of the Hand and Upper Extremity*. 6th ed. Philadelphia, PA: Elsevier; 2011:1495-1511.
32. Fillion PL. Ulnar collateral ligament thumb sling. *J Hand Ther*. 2004;17(1):69-70.
33. Finklestein H. Stenosing tendovaginitis at the radial styloid process. *J Bone Joint Surg*. 1930;12:509.
34. Gartland JJ, Werley CW. Evaluation of healed Colles' fractures. *J Bone Joint Surg Br*. 1961;43:245.
35. Gomez MA,Woo SLY, Amiel D, Harwood F, Kitabayashi L, Matyas JR. The effects of increased tension on healing medial collateral ligaments. *Am J Sports Med*. 1991;19:347-354.
36. Grundberg AB. Carpal tunnel decompression in spite of normal electromyography. *J Hand Surg*. 1983; 8A:348.
37. Ham SJ, Kolkman WF, Heeres J, den Boer JA. Changes in the carpal tunnel due to action of the flexor tendons: visualization with magnetic resonance imaging. *J Hand Surg*. 1996;21A:977.
38. Husband JB, McPherson SA. Bony skier's thumb injuries. *Clin Orthop Relat Res*. 1996;327:79-84.
39. Jupiter JB, Belsky MR. Fractures and dislocations of the hand. In: Browner BD, Jupiter JB, Levine AM, Trafton PG, eds. *Skeletal Trauma*. Philadelphia, PA: Saunders; 1992: 1153-1266.
40. Kalichman L, Hernández-Molina G. Hand osteoarthritis: an epidemiological perspective. Semin Arthritis Rheum. 2010;39:6:465-476.
41. Kaplan EM. *Joints and Ligaments in Functional and Surgical Anatomy of the Hand*. Philadelphia, PA: Lippincott; 1965.
42. Kozin SH, Wood MB. Early soft tissue complications after fractures of the distal part of the radius. *J Bone Joint Surg Am*. 1993;75:144.
43. Kuz JE, Husband JB, Tokar NT, McPherson SA. Outcome of avulsion fractures of the ulnar base of the proximal phalanx of the thumb treated nonsurgically. *J Hand Surg*. 1999;24A:275-282.
44. Lam N, Thurston A. Association of obesity, gender, age, and occupation with carpal tunnel syndrome. *Aust N Z J Surg*. 1998;68:190.
45. Landsman JC, Seitz WH Jr, Froimson AI, Leb RB, Bachner EJ. Splint immobilization of gamekeeper's thumb. *Orthopedics*. 1995;18(12):1161-1165.
46. Landsmeer JMF. Studies in the anatomy of articulation. 1. The equilibrium of the "intercalated" bone. *Acta Morphol Neerl Scand*. 1961;3:287-303.

47. Lawrence RC, Felson DT, Helmick CG, et al. Estimates of the prevalence of arthritis and other rheumatic conditions in the United States. Part II. *Arthritis Rheum.* 2008;58:26-35.
48. Lee MP, Biafora SJ, Selouf DS. Management of hand and wrist tendinopathies. In: Skirven TM, Osterman AL, Fedorczyk JM, Amadio PC, eds. *Rehabilitation of the Hand and Upper Extremity.* 6th ed. Philadelphia, PA: Elsevier; 2011:569-590.
49. Linscheid RL, Dobyns JH, Beabout JW, Bryan RS. Traumatic instability of the wrist. *J Bone Joint Surg Am.* 1972;54A:1262-1267.
50. Mazet R, Hohl M. Fractures of the carpal navicular: analysis of 91 cases and review of the literature. *J Bone Joint Surg Am.* 1967;45:82.
51. McCue FC, Nelson WE. Ulnar collateral ligament injuries of the thumb. *Phys Sportsmed.* 1993;21:67-80.
52. Medoff, RJ. Distal radius fractures: classification and management In: Skirven TM, Osterman AL, Fedorczyk JM, Amadio PC, eds. *Rehabilitation of the Hand and Upper Extremity.* 6th ed. Philadelphia, PA: Elsevier; 2011:941-948.
53. Michaud EJ, Flinn S, Seitz WH Jr. Treatment of grade III thumb metacarpophalangeal ulnar collateral ligament injuries with early controlled motion using a hinged splint. *J Hand Ther.* 2010;23:77-81.
54. Michlovitz S. Is there a role for ultrasound and electrical stimulation following injury to tendon and nerve? *J Hand Ther.* 2005;18:2.
55. Muller M, Tsui D, Schnur R, Biddulph-Deisroth L, Hard J, MacDermid JC. Effectiveness of hand therapy interventions in primary management of carpal tunnel syndrome: a systematic review. *J Hand Ther.* 2004;17: 210-228.
56. Murphy RX Jr, Jennings JF, Wukich DK. Major neurovascular complications of endoscopic carpal tunnel release. *J Hand Surg.* 1994;19A:114.
57. Oetgen ME, Dodds SD. Non-operative treatment of common finger injuries. *Curr Rev Musculoskelet Med.* 2008;1(2):97-102.
58. Palmer AK, Werner FW, Murphy D, Glisson R. Functional wrist motion: a biomechanical study. *J Hand Surg.* 1985;10A:39-46.
59. Palmer AK, Dobyns JH, Linscheid RL. Management of post-traumatic instability of the wrist secondary to ligament rupture. *J Hand Surg.* 1978;3:507.
60. Patel MR, Bassini L. Trigger fingers and thumb: when to splint, inject or operate. *J Hand Surg.* 1992;17:110-113.
61. Peters-Veluthamaningal C, van der Windt DA, Winters JC, Meyboom-de Jong B. Corticosteroid injection for trigger finger in adults. *Cochrane Database Syst Rev.* 2009;(1):CD005617.
62. Pettengil KM, Van Strien G. Postoperative management of flexor tendon injuries. In: Skirven TM, Osterman AL, Fedorczyk JM, Amadio PC, eds. *Rehabilitation of the Hand and Upper Extremity.* 6th ed. Philadelphia, PA: Elsevier; 2011:457-478.
63. Piazzini DB, Aprile I, Ferrara PE, et al. A systematic review of conservative treatment of carpal tunnel syndrome. *Clin Rehabil.* 2007;21:299-314.
64. Pike J, Mulpuri K, Metzger M, Ng G, Wells N, Goetz T. Blinded, prospective, randomized clinical trial comparing volar, dorsal, and custom thermoplastic splinting in treatment of acute mallet finger. *J Hand Surg Am.* 2010;35(4)580-588.
65. Rannou F, Dimet J, Boutron I, et al. Splint for base-of-thumb osteoarthritis: a randomized trial. *Ann Intern Med.* 2009;150:(10):661-669.
66. Rogers MW, Wilder FV. Exercise and hand osteoarthritis symptomatology: a controlled crossover trial. *J Hand Ther.* 2009;22:10-18.
67. Rosenthal EA, Elhassan BT. The extensor tendons: evaluation and treatment: part 5—tendon injuries and tendinopathies. In: Skirven TM, Osterman AL, Fedorcsyk JM, Amadio PC, eds. *Rehabilitation of the Hand and Upper Extremity.* 6th ed. Philadelphia, PA: Elsevier; 2011:513-520.
68. Rosenthal EA, Elhassan, BT. The extensor tendons: evaluation and surgical management. In: Skirven TM, Osterman AL, Fedorczyk JM, Amadi PC, eds. *Rehabilitation of the Hand and Upper Extremity.* 6th ed. Philadelphia, PA: Elsevier; 2011:487-513.
69. Ryu JY, Cooney WP, Askew LJ, An KN, Chao EY. Functional ranges of motion of the wrist joint. *J Hand Surg.* 1991;16A:409.
70. Saffar P, Semaan I. The study of the biomechanics of wrist motion in an oblique plane—a preliminary report. In: Schuind F, An KN, Cooney WP III, Garcia-Elias M, eds. *Advances in the Biomechanics of the Hand and Wrist.* New York, NY: Plenum Press; 1994:305-311.
71. Sam Dalal, S. Raj Murali The distal radio-ulnar joint. *Orthop Trauma.* 2012;26(1):44-52.
72. Skirven TM, Osterman AL, Fedorczyk JM, Amadio PC, eds. *Rehabilitation of the Hand and Upper Extremity.* 6th ed. Philadelphia, PA: Elsevier; 2011.
73. Smith RJ. Post-traumatic instability of the metacarpophalangeal joint of the thumb. *J Bone Joint Surg Am.* 1977;59:14-21.
74. Sollerman C, Abrahamsson SO, Lundborg G, Adalbert K. Functional splinting versus plaster cast for ruptures of the ulnar collateral ligament of the thumb. *Acta Orthop Scand.* 1991;62(6):524-526.
75. Souter WA. The boutonniere deformity. *J Bone Joint Surg.* 1967;49-B:710-721.
76. Stamm TA, Machold K, Smelen JS, et al. Join protection and home hand exercises improve hand function in patients with osteoarthritis: a randomized control trial. *Arthritis Rheum.* 2002;47:44-49.
77. Stark HH, Boyes JH, Wilson JN. Mallet finger. *J Bone Joint Surg Am.* 1962;44-A:1061-1068.
78. Stener B. Displacement of the ruptured ulnar collateral ligament of the metacarpophalangeal joint of the thumb. *J Bone Joint Surg Br.* 1962;44:869-879.

79. Sorock GS, Lombardi DA, Hauser RB, Eisen EA, Herrick RF, Mittleman MA. Acute traumatic occupational hand injuries: type location and severity. *J Occup Environ Med.* 2002;44(4):345-351.
80. Swezey RL. Trigger finger splinting. *Orthopedics.* 1999;22:180.
81. Tarbhai K, Hannah S, von Schroeder HP. Trigger finger treatment: a comparison of 2 splint designs. *J Hand Surg Am.* 2012;37(2):243-249.
82. Totten PA, Hunter JM. Therapeutic techniques to enhance nerve gliding in thoracic outlet syndrome and carpal tunnel syndrome. *Hand Clin.* 1991;7:505.
83. Trumble TE, Gilbert M, Vedder N. Ulnar shortening combined with arthroscopic repairs in the delayed management of triangular fibrocartilage complex tears. *J Hand Surg.* 1997;22A:807-813.
84. Valdes K, Marik T. A systemic review of conservative interventions for osteoarthritis of the hand. *J Hand Ther.* 2010;23(4):334-349
85. Valdes K. A retrospective review to determine the long-term efficacy of orthotic devices for trigger finger. *J Hand Ther.* 2012;25(1):89-96.
86. Van Heest A, Waters P, Simmons D, Schwartz JT. A cadaveric study of the single-portal endoscopic carpal tunnel release. *J Hand Surg.* 1995;20A:363.
87. Verdan C. The reconstruction of the thumb. *Surg Clin North Am.* 1968;48:1033.
88. Volz RG, Lieb M, Benjamin J. Biomechanics of the wrist. *Clin Orthop Relat Res.* 1980;149:112-117.
89. Von der Heyde RL, Evans RB. Wound classification and management. In: Skirven TM, Osterman AL, Fedorczyk JM, Amadio PC, eds. *Rehabilitation of the Hand and Upper Extremity.* 6th ed. Philadelphia, PA: Elsevier; 2011:219-232.
90. Weber ER, Chap EY. An experimental approach to the mechanism of scaphoid waist fractures. *J Hand Surg.* 1978;3A:142.
91. Weinstein SM, Herring SA. Nerve problems and compartment syndromes in the hand, wrist, and forearm. *Clin Sports Med.* 1992;11(1):161-188.
92. Weiss ND, Gordon L, Bloom T, So Y, Rempel DM. Position of the wrist associated with the lowest carpal tunnel pressure: implication for splint design. *J Bone Joint Surg Am.* 1995;77:1695-1699.
93. Weiss S, LaStayo PL, Mills A, Bramlet D. Splinting the degenerative basal joint: custom-made or prefabricated neoprene? *J Hand Ther.* 2004;17:401-406.
94. Weiss S, LaStayo PL, Mills A, Bramlet D. Prospective analysis of splinting the first carpometacarpal joint: an objective, subjective, and radiographic assessment. *J Hand Ther.* 2000;13:218-226.
95. Wilder FV, Barrett JP, Farina EJ. Joint-specific prevalence of osteoarthritis of the hand. *Osteoarthritis Cartilage.* 2006;14:953-957.
96. Witt J, Pess G, Gelberman RH. Treatment of de Quervain tenosynovitis: a prospective study of the results of injection of steroid and immobilization in a splint. *J Bone Joint Surg Am.* 1991;73:219-222.
97. Zemel NP. Fractures and ligament injuries of the wrist. In: Jobe FW, Pink MM, Glousman RE, eds. *Operative Techniques in Upper Extremity Sports Injuries.* St. Louis, MO: Mosby; 1996:652-698.

23

Rehabilitation of the Groin, Hip, and Thigh

Timothy F. Tyler, Stephanie M. Squitieri, and Gregory C. Thomas

OBJECTIVES

After completion of this chapter, the physical therapist should be able to do the following:

- Discuss the functional anatomy and biomechanics of the groin, hip, and thigh.
- Discuss injuries to the groin, hip, and thigh and describe the biomechanical changes that occur during and after injury.
- Discuss and describe the functional injury evaluation of the groin, thigh, and hip.
- Articulate the role previous injury may play in subsequent injuries in the athlete.
- Describe the at-risk populations and the mechanism of injury for muscle strains, muscle contusions, and acetabular labral injuries.
- Demonstrate application of various intervention strategies for a wide variety of hip pathologies including muscle strains and contusions and acetabular labral injuries.
- Apply principles of prevention and wellness using screening for imbalances and preseason-strengthening programs for susceptible populations.
- Apply principles of stretching, strengthening, open- and closed kinetic-chain exercises, plyometrics, isokinetics, and proprioceptive neuromuscular facilitation exercises to the hip complex as a part of comprehensive rehabilitation.

The occurrence of injuries to the hip, pelvis, and thigh are relatively small when compared to the other lower-extremity regions.[1-5] Although statistically less prevalent, a hip pathology can cause immediate gait abnormalities, lead to chronic pain, and give rise to premature degeneration in the hip joint itself. These injuries can vary significantly depending on the specific sporting activity involved.[6] Contact sports will have a high incidence of traumatic injuries, such as fractures, contusions, and dislocations, whereas endurance sports, like running, swimming, and biking, can lead to stress and overuse injuries. No matter what the injury, proper diagnosis and intervention is key to returning the athlete back to the athlete's sport(s) of choice. This chapter identifies common hip pathologies and directs an appropriate and concise rehabilitation program to optimize a patient's recovery time.

Anatomy and Biomechanics

The primary function of the hip joint is to support the weight of the head, arm, and trunk, while also serving as the connection between the lower extremities and the pelvic girdle. The anatomical design of the hip is well suited to handle this task as well as the increased loads that can be transmitted during athletic competition.[7] Joint impact forces such as running produces loads up to 3 to 5 times body weight.

The joint itself is the articulation between the acetabulum of the pelvis and the head of the femur. These 2 segments form a diarthrodial ball-and-socket joint with 3 degrees of freedom: flexion/extension in the sagittal plane, abduction/adduction in the frontal plane, and medial/lateral rotation in the transverse plane.

The cuplike concavity of the acetabulum is formed by the fusion of 3 bones: ilium, ischium, and pubis. These bones typically unite by the late teenage years.[8] The resulting socket is located on the lateral aspect of the pelvic bone and has an angular orientation of inferior and anterior. The femoral component of the joint has an angular orientation of superior and anterior. These orientations represent the angles of inclination and torsion respectfully. The angle of inclination is measured in the frontal plane between the axis of the head/neck and the axis of the shaft. Normal angles range between 125 and 135 degrees. A pathological increase in inclination is called *coxa valga*, and a decrease is referred to as *coxa vara*. The angle of torsion is measured in the transverse plane between the axis of the head/neck of the femur and the axis through the femoral condyles. It can best be viewed by looking down the length of the femur from top to bottom. Normal angles of torsion are between 10 and 15 degrees with an increase termed *anteversion* and a decrease called *retroversion*.[7] Both normal and abnormal angles are properties of the femur and independent of the hip joint.

The femoral and acetabular surfaces correspond well to each other, but given the increased need for stability at this joint, an accessory structure is needed. The entire periphery of the acetabulum is rimmed by a ring of wedge-shaped fibrocartilage called the *acetabular labrum*. This labrum not only deepens the socket but also increases the concavity of the socket through its triangular shape. This structural stability is reinforced by the hip joint capsule and its ligaments.

The capsule is attached proximally to the entire periphery of the acetabulum beyond the labrum. The distal end covers the head and neck like a sleeve and attaches to the base of the femoral neck. This capsule is considered to have 3 reinforcing ligaments: 2 anteriorly and 1 posteriorly. The 2 anterior ligaments are the iliofemoral ligament and pubofemoral ligament. These are often referred to as the *Y ligament of Bigelow*. The ischiofemoral ligament is the posterior capsular ligament.[7] Femoroacetabular anomalies may occur at the hip joint. These morphological variances include an abnormal femoral head interacting with a normal acetabulum, or, conversely, a normal femoral head acting on an abnormally formed acetabulum.[9]

Movements at the hip joint consist of arthrokinematic and osteokinematic actions. The arthrokinematics that occur within the joint can best be visualized as the movement of the convex head of the femur within the concavity of the acetabulum. Thus the convex on concave rule states that arthrokinematic motions are opposite of the osteokinematic movements. Hip flexion created by primary movers such as the iliopsoas, rectus femoris, tensor fascia lata, and sartorius occurs in the anterior direction around the coronal axis. During hip flexion there is a posterior glide of the humeral head. Full range through flexion is approximately 125 degrees.

The hip extensors are made up of the gluteus maximus and hamstrings, which consist of the biceps femoris, semimembranosus, and semitendinosus. Extension occurs posteriorly around the coronal axis causing an anterior glide of the femoral head. Normal range for extension is 10 degrees.

Abduction of the hip is brought about by the primary actions of the gluteus medius and gluteus minimus. This movement occurs away from the midsagittal plane in the lateral direction. Normal range is approximately 45 degrees, with inferior movement of the humeral head.

The gracilis, adductor magnus, longus, and brevis produce osteokinematic adduction toward the midsagittal plane. This results in a superior arthrokinematic femoral head glide within the acetabulum. Adduction range on average is 10 degrees.[7,10,11]

The final motion of the hip is hip rotation that occurs in the transverse plane of motion and is often overlooked. More importance has been given to the patients' ability to control hip rotation during function movements. In patients with patellofemoral pain syndrome, it has been suggested that a theoretical mechanism for pathology may be weak femoral external rotators that allow the femur to be in relative internal rotation and influence patellar alignment and kinematics. In fact, the role of the hip rotator muscles is frequently overlooked when addressing prevention and rehabilitation of lumbar spine injuries. Weak and/or shortened hip rotators may contribute to abnormal lumbopelvic posture and cause compensatory motion in the lumbar spine during daily activities. The detrimental effects of inadequately conditioned and prepared hip rotators may predispose the athlete to lumbar spine injuries. The small external rotators of the hip (piriformis, obturator internus, obturator externus, gemellus superior, gemellus inferior, and quadratus femoris) sometimes get fatigued or overpowered by the large internal rotators of the hip (gluteus maximus, gluteus medius, and gluteus minimus) creating muscle imbalance.

Hip Muscular Strains

A muscle strain, also called a *pull* or *tear*, is a common injury, particularly among people who participate in sports. The thigh has 3 sets of strong muscles: the hamstring muscles posteriorly, the quadriceps muscles anteriorly, and the adductor muscles medially. The hamstring and quadriceps muscle groups are particularly at risk for muscle strains because they cross both the hip and knee joints. They are also used for high-speed activities, such as track and field events, football, basketball, ice hockey, and soccer.

Most commonly, the mechanism of injury for muscle strains in the hip area is when a stretched muscle is forced to contract suddenly. A fall or direct blow to the muscle, overstretching, and overuse can tear muscle fibers resulting in a strain. The risk of muscle strain increases if the patient had a prior injury in the area, performs inadequate warm-up before exercising or attempts to do too much too quickly. Strains may be mild, moderate, or severe depending on the extent of the injury. Signs and symptoms may include pain over the injured muscle (the most common symptom of a hip strain), increased pain level with muscular contraction, swelling and discoloration (depending on the severity of the strain), and a loss of strength in the muscle.

Evaluation of hip muscle strains can be challenging when overlapping conditions exist. A muscle that is painful on contraction and painful when stretched may be strained. Certain exercises or stretches in specific ways, which stress the involved muscle, can help determine which muscle is injured. A radiograph or other diagnostic test may be used to rule out the possibility of a stress fracture of the hip, which has similar symptoms, including pain in the groin area, with weight bearing. In most cases, no additional tests are needed to confirm the diagnosis.

In general, interventions are chosen and rehabilitation programs designed to relieve pain, restore range of motion (ROM), and restore strength, in that order. Rest, ice, compression, and elevation is standard protocol for mild-to-moderate muscle strains. Gently massaging the area with ice may also help decrease swelling. Nonsteroidal anti-inflammatory drugs (NSAIDs) can be taken to reduce swelling and ease pain. Compression shorts/sleeve or a compression bandage may also be helpful to decrease swelling and provide support. If walking causes pain, consider limiting weight bearing and using crutches for the first day or two after the injury.

Adductor Muscle Strains

Adductor muscle strains can result in missed playing time for athletes in many sports. Adductor muscle strains are encountered most frequently in ice hockey and soccer.[12-14] These sports require a strong eccentric contraction of the adductor musculature during competition.[15,16] Recently, adductor muscle strength has been linked to the incidence of adductor muscle strains. Specifically, the strength ratio of the adduction–abduction muscles groups has been identified as a risk factor in professional ice hockey players.[17] Intervention programs can lower the incidence of adductor muscle strains, but cannot avoid them altogether. Therefore, proper injury treatment and rehabilitation must be implemented to limit the amount of missed playing time and avoid surgical intervention.[18]

Adductor Musculature

The group of muscles along the inner thigh is referred to as the adductor muscle group. This group of 6 muscles includes the pectineus, adductor longus, adductor brevis, adductor magnus, gracilis, and obturator externus. All of the adductor muscles are innervated by the obturator nerve except for the pectineus, which gets its motor intervention from the femoral nerve. These muscles originate in the inguinal region at various points on the pubis. They travel inferior to insert along the medial femur. The main action of this muscle group is to adduct the thigh in the open kinetic chain and stabilize the lower extremity to perturbations in the closed kinetic chain. Each individual muscle can also provide assistance in femoral flexion and rotation.[8,19] The adductor longus is thought to be the most frequently injured adductor muscle.[20] Its lack of mechanical advantage may make it more susceptible to strain.

Adductor Muscle Injury

A groin strain is defined as pain on palpation of the adductor tendons or the insertion on the pubic bone, or both, and groin pain during adduction against resistance.[18,21,22] Groin strains and muscle strains in general are graded as a first-degree strain if there is pain but minimal loss of strength and minimal restriction of motion. A second-degree strain is defined as tissue damage that compromises the strength of the muscle, but not including complete loss of strength and function. A third-degree strain denotes complete disruption of the muscle tendon unit. It includes complete loss of function of the muscle.[23] A thorough history and a physical examination is needed to differentiate groin strains from athletic pubalgia, osteitis pubis, hernia, hip-joint osteoarthrosis, rectal or testicular referred pain, piriformis syndrome, or presence of a coexisting fracture of the pelvis or the lower extremities.[20-23] Imaging studies can sometimes be useful to rule out other possible causes of inguinal pain.[24]

Adductor Muscle Strain Incidence

The exact incidence of adductor muscle strains in sport is unknown. This is partly a result of athletes playing through minor groin pain and the injury going unreported. In addition, overlapping diagnosis can also skew the exact incidence. Groin strains are among the most common injuries seen in ice hockey players.[25-27] It has been documented that groin strains accounted for 10% of all injuries in elite Swedish ice hockey players.[28] Furthermore, Molsa[29] reported that groin strains accounted for 43% of all muscles strains in elite Finish ice hockey players. Tyler et al[17] published the incidence of groin strains in a single National Hockey League (NHL) team of 3.2 strains per 1000 player-game exposures. In a larger study of 26 NHL teams, Emery et al[13] reported, the incidence of adductor strains in the NHL has increased over the last 6 years. The rate of injury was greatest during the preseason compared to regular and postseason play. Prospective soccer studies in Scandinavia report a groin strain incidence between 10 and 18 injuries per 100 soccer players.[30] Ekstrand and Gillquist[14] documented 32 groin strains in 180 male soccer players representing 13% of all injuries over the course of 1 year. Adductor muscle strains, certainly, are not isolated to these 2 sports.

Risk Factors

Previous studies have shown an association between strength and/or flexibility and musculoskeletal strains in various athletic populations.[14,31,32] Ekstrand and Gillquist[14] found that preseason hip abduction ROM was decreased in soccer players who subsequently sustained groin strains compared with uninjured players. This is in contrast to the data published on professional ice hockey players that found no relationship between passive or active abduction ROM (adductor flexibility) and adductor muscle strains.[17,33]

Adductor muscle strength has been associated with a subsequent muscle strain. Tyler et al[17] found that preseason hip adduction strength was 18% lower in NHL players who subsequently sustained groin strains, as compared to those who remained uninjured. The hip adduction to abduction strength ratio was also significantly different between the 2 groups. Adduction strength was 95% of abduction strength in the uninjured players but only 78% of abduction strength in the injured players. Additionally, in the players who sustained a groin strain, preseason adduction to abduction strength ratio was lower on the side that subsequently sustained a groin strain compared with the uninjured side. Adduction strength was 86% of abduction strength on the uninjured side, but only 70% of abduction strength on the injured side. Conversely, another study on adductor strains on ice hockey players found no relationship between peak isometric adductor torque and the incidence of adductor strains.[33] Unlike the previous study this study had multiple testers using a handheld dynamometer, which would increase the variability and decrease the likelihood of finding strength differences. However, the results of Emery et al[33] did demonstrate that players who practiced during the off season were less likely to sustain a groin injury as were rookies in the NHL. The final risk factor was the presence of a previous adductor strain. Tyler et al[17] also linked preexisting injury as a risk factor, as in their study, 4 of the 9 groin strains (44%) were recurrent injuries. This is consistent with the results of Seward et al[34] who reported a 32% recurrence rate for groin strains in athletes participating in Australian Rules Football.

Prevention

Now that researchers have identified players at risk for a future adductor strain, the next step is to design an intervention program to address all risk factors. Tyler et al[25] were able to demonstrate that a therapeutic intervention of strengthening the adductor muscle group could be an effective method for preventing adductor strains in professional ice hockey players. Prior to the 2000 and 2001 seasons, professional ice hockey players were strength tested. Thirty-three of these 58 players were classified as being "at risk," which was defined as having an adduction–abduction strength ratio of less than 80%, and placed on an intervention program. The intervention program consisted of strengthening and functional exercises aimed at increasing adductor strength (Table 23-1). The injuries were tracked over the course of the 2 seasons. In the present study, there were 3 adductor strains, which all occurred in game situations. This gives an incidence of 0.71 adductor strains per 1000 player-game exposures. Adductor strains accounted for approximately 2% of all injuries. In contrast, there were 11 adductor strains and an incidence of 3.2 adductor strains per 1000 player-game exposures in the 2 seasons prior to the intervention. In those prior 2 seasons, adductor strains accounted for approximately 8% of all injuries. This was also significantly lower than the incidence reported by Lorentzon et al[28] who found adductor strains to be 10% of all injuries. Of the 3 players who sustained adductor strains, none of the players had sustained a previous adductor strain on the same side. One player had bilateral adductor strains at different times during the first season. This study demonstrated that a therapeutic intervention of strengthening the adductor muscle group can be an effective method for preventing adductor strains in professional ice hockey players.

Rehabilitation

Despite the identification of risk factors and strengthening intervention for ice hockey players, adductor strains continue to occur in all sports.[24] The high incidence of recurrent strains could be a result of incomplete rehabilitation or inadequate time for complete tissue repair. Hömlich et al[18] demonstrated that a passive physical therapy program of massage,

Table 23-1 Adductor Strain Injury Prevention Program

Warm-up	Bike Adductor stretching Sumo squats Side lunges Kneeling pelvic tilts
Strengthening program	Ball squeezes (legs bent to legs straight) Different ball sizes Concentric adduction with weight against gravity Adduction in standing on cable column or elastic resistance Seated adduction machine Standing with involved foot on sliding board moving in sagittal plane Bilateral adduction on sliding board moving in frontal plane (ie, bilateral adduction simultaneously) Unilateral lunges with reciprocal arm movements
Sports-specific training	On ice, kneeling, adductor pulls together Standing resisted stride lengths on cable column to simulate skating Slide skating Cable column crossover pulls
Clinical goal	Adduction strength at least 80% of the abduction strength

stretching, and modalities were ineffective in treating chronic groin strains. By contrast, an 8- to 12-week active strengthening program consisting of progressive resistive adduction and abduction exercises, balance training, abdominal strengthening, and skating movements on a slide board proved more effective in treating chronic groin strains. An increased emphasis on strengthening exercises may reduce the recurrence rate of groin strains. An adductor muscle strain injury program progressing the athlete through the phases of healing was developed by Tyler et al[25] and anecdotally seems to be effective (Table 23-2). This

Table 23-2 Adductor Strain Postinjury Program

Phase I (acute)	RICE for first approximately 48 hours after injury NSAIDs Massage Transcutaneous electrical nerve stimulation (TENS) Ultrasound Submaximal isometric adduction with knees bent→with knees straight progressing to maximal isometric adduction, pain-free hip PROM in pain-free range Non-weightbearing hip progressive resistive exercises without weight in antigravity position (all except abduction), pain-free, low-load, high-repetition exercise Upper body and trunk strengthening Contralateral lower extremity (LE) strengthening Flexibility program for noninvolved muscles Bilateral balance board
Clinical milestone	Concentric adduction against gravity without pain
Phase II (subacute)	Bicycling/swimming Sumo squats Single-limb stance Concentric adduction with weight against gravity Standing with involved foot on sliding board moving in frontal plane Adduction in standing on cable column or Thera-Band Seated adduction machine Bilateral adduction on sliding board moving in frontal plane (ie, bilateral adduction simultaneously) Unilateral lunges (sagittal) with reciprocal arm movements Multiplane trunk tilting Balance board squats with throwbacks General flexibility program
Clinical milestone	Involved lower-extremity PROM equal to that of the uninvolved side and involved adductor strength at least 75% that of the ipsilateral abductors
Phase III (sports-specific training)	Phase II exercises with increase in load, intensity, speed, and volume Standing resisted stride lengths on cable column to simulate skating Slide board On ice, kneeling, adductor pulls together Lunges (in all planes) Correct or modify ice-skating technique
Clinical milestone	Adduction strength at least 90% to 100% of the abduction strength and involved muscle strength equal to that of the contralateral side

PROM, passive range of motion; RICE, rest, ice, compression, elevation.

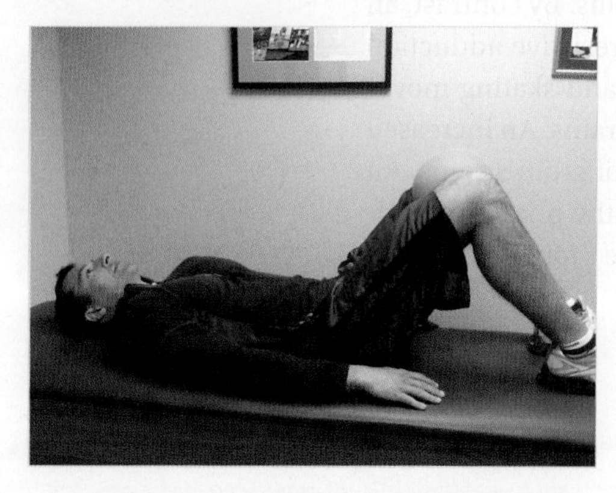

Figure 23-1 Ball squeeze

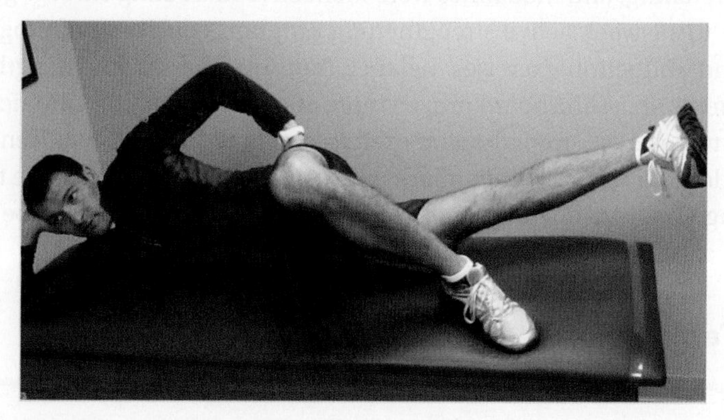

Figure 23-2 Side-lying hip adduction

type of treatment regime combines modalities and passive treatment immediately, followed by an active training program emphasizing eccentric resistive exercise. This method of rehabilitation program has been supported throughout the literature.[22,24] Exercises for this injury are shown in Figures 23-1 to 23-4. An adductor stretch is shown in Figure 23-5.

Hamstring Musculature

The Hamstrings actually comprise 3 separate muscles: the biceps femoris, semitendinosus, and semimembranosus. These muscles originate just underneath the gluteus maximus on the pelvic bone and attach on the tibia and fibula. The hamstrings are primarily fast-twitch muscles, responding to low repetitions and powerful movements. The primary functions of the hamstrings are knee flexion and hip extension.

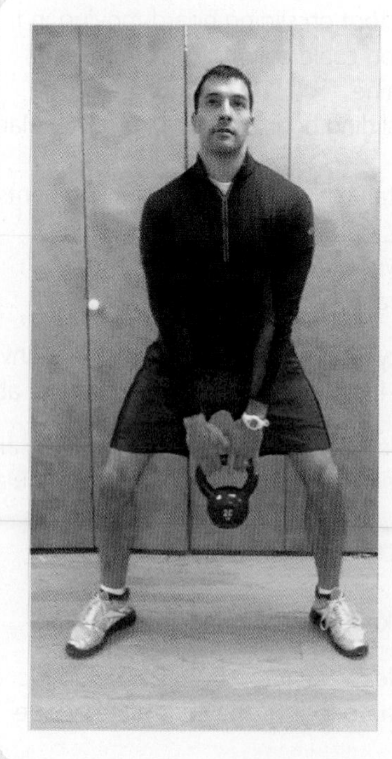

Figure 23-3 Sumo squats

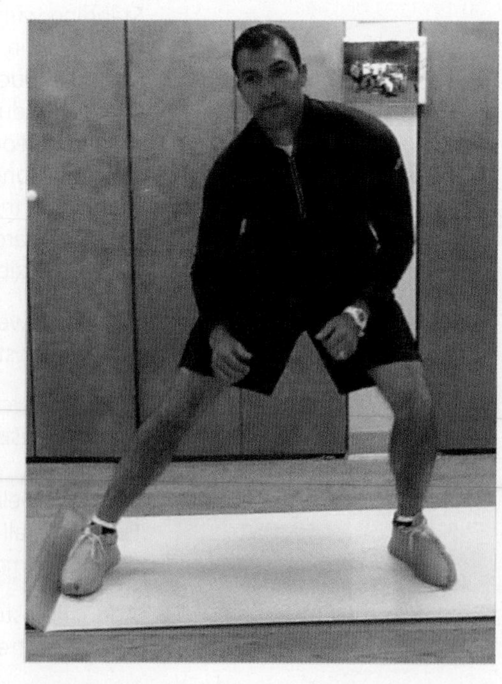

Figure 23-4 Slide board

Hamstring Muscle Injury

Hamstring muscle strains commonly result from a wide variety of sporting activities, particularly those requiring rapid acceleration and deceleration. An eccentric load to the muscle causes the majority of these injuries. Garrett et al[23,35] demonstrated that, in young athletes, hamstring muscle strains typically involve myotendinous disruption of the proximal biceps femoris muscle. Other authors also have shown experimentally that the weak link of the muscle complex is the myotendinous junction.[23,36] Although apophyseal fractures of the ischial tuberosity have been reported in young athletes, the majority of hamstring muscle strains are first- and second-degree strains.[37]

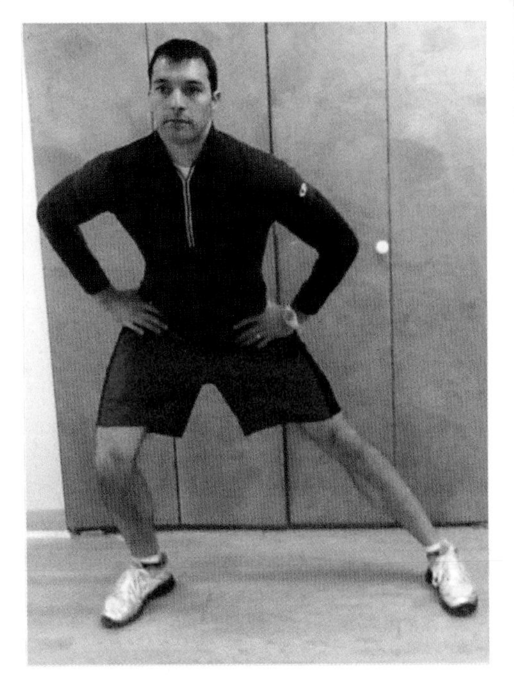

Figure 23-5 Adductor stretch

Hamstring Muscle Strain Incidence

Hamstring muscle strains are among the most common injuries in sports involving high-speed movement and physical contact. They can account for 12% to 16% of all injuries in athletes,[38-42] with a recurrence rate as high as 22% to 34%.[42-44] Hamstring strains are by far the most commonly seen muscle strains in Australian Rules Football, with an incidence of 8.05 injuries per 1000 player-game-hours. Soccer players are also susceptible to hamstring strains with an incidence of 3.0 per 1000 player-game-hours for hamstring strains. Overall, any athlete who sprints as part of their sport may contribute to the incidence of hamstring strains.

Risk Factors

Factors causing hamstring muscle injury have been studied for many years. It has been suggested that, strength deficits,[32] lack of flexibility,[45-46] muscle fatigue,[47] poor core stability,[48] inadequate proper warm-up,[49] poor lumbar posture,[50] and prior hamstring injury[51-53] may predispose an athlete to a hamstring strain.

Croisier et al[54] suggest that the persistence of muscle weakness and imbalance may give rise to recurrent hamstring muscle injuries and pain. These authors believe that when there is insufficient eccentric braking capacity of the hamstring muscles compared with the concentric motor action of the quadriceps muscles, the muscle may be at risk for injury.

Ekstrand and Gillquist[55] prospectively studied male Swedish soccer players and found hamstrings to be the muscle group most often injured. They noted that minor injuries increased the risk of having a more severe injury within 2 months. Likewise, Engebretsen et al examined more than 500 amateur soccer players and found that among all the risk factors, a previous hamstring strain was the greatest risk factor for a recurrent strain.[51] Others have noted a recurrence rate of 25% for hamstring injuries in intercollegiate football players.[56]

Prevention

It has been well established in the literature that eccentric training works in preventing hamstring strains.[1,32,57,58] Arnason et al[57] prospectively studied elite soccer teams in Iceland and Norway and found eccentric training combined with warm up stretching appeared to reduce the risk of hamstring strains; although no effect was found from flexibility training alone. Peterson et al[58] found that the addition of eccentric hamstring training decreased the rate of overall, new and recurrent acute hamstring injuries.

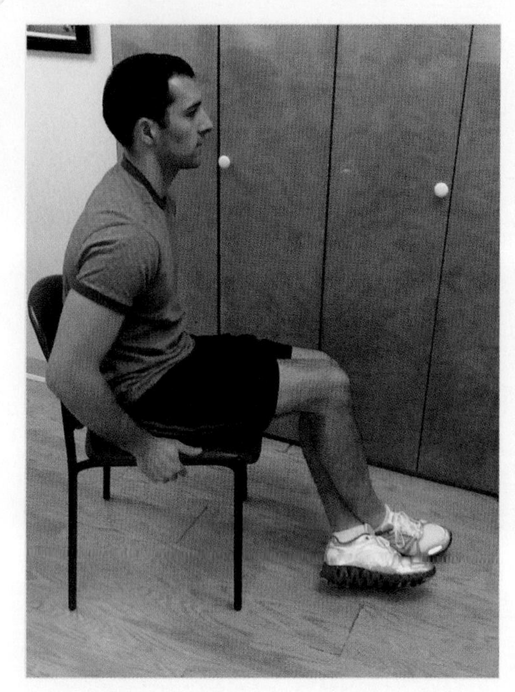

Figure 23-6 **Seated multiangle isometrics at 30, 60, 90 degrees of knee flexion**

Rehabilitation

There is no consensus for rehabilitation of the hamstring muscles after strain. However, a rehabilitation program consisting of progressive agility and trunk stabilization exercises has been shown to be more effective than a program emphasizing isolated hamstring stretching and strengthening in promoting return to sports and preventing injury recurrence in athletes suffering an acute hamstring strain.[48] The aim of the physical therapy is to restore full pain-free ROM and strength throughout the ROM. In addition, as a complement to the usual restoration of function, we emphasize restoring eccentric muscle strength and correction of agonist–antagonist imbalances in the rehabilitation process. We recommend the inclusion of eccentric exercises at a lengthened state of the hamstring muscles, submaximally, as soon as the patient can tolerate it. Our rationale is based on basic science animal research[59] and imaging studies of human muscle tissue[22] that have indicated incomplete healing following muscle strains. Fibrosis at the injury site is thought to be related to the risk of reinjury. Based on these observations, interventions aimed at remodeling the muscle tissue may be effective in reducing the risk associated with having had a prior muscle strain. Eccentric muscle contractions have been shown to result in muscle–tendon junction remodeling in an animal model,[60] and more recently have been shown to cause intramuscular collagen remodeling in humans.[61] Brockett et al[62] examined the angle torque curves of previously injured hamstring subjects and compared them to the noninvolved side, and uninjured controls. The authors found that peak hamstring torque occurred at a significantly shorter muscle length in the injured hamstring when compared to controls, implying a possible shift in the length–tension curve. It is possible that when an athlete sustains a hamstring strain the athlete may return to play with weakness at longer muscle lengths which can predispose them for another strain. It is our belief that training specifically in the lengthened state will allow the hamstring to achieve optimal strength at a longer operating length. Schmitt et al[63] developed a protocol for rehabilitating hamstring strains with an emphasis on lengthened state eccentric training in the latter stages. Rehabilitation during the acute stage would start with relative rest and protection of the injured muscle lasting from 1 to 3 days. Returning to exercise in this stage can lead to reinjury and disruption of the healing tissue. Multiangle isometrics, as shown in Figure 23-6, should be initiated to properly align the regenerating muscle fibers and limit the extent of connective tissue fibrosis. Static stretching is not recommended particularly during this stage because you want to prevent disruption of the healing fibers. Rest, ice, compression, and elevation, along with anti-inflammatory medication, are helpful during the immediate stages of treatment. Heat, ice, electrical stimulation, laser and ultrasound are modalities that can also be used in conjunction with each other during the rehabilitation program to facilitate a return to competition. The goals of this stage are to normalize gait, and obtain knee flexion strength at greater than 50% of the uninjured length upon manual muscle testing at 90 degrees of knee flexion.[63]

During the second phase of rehabilitation, an effective strengthening program should focus on concentric and eccentric contractions. The goals of this second phase are to progressively increase strength throughout the ROM and to improve neuromuscular control.[63] During this phase, end range lengthening should be avoided if painful. However, eccentric exercises can be achieved using an isokinetic dynamometer, if available, or by performing

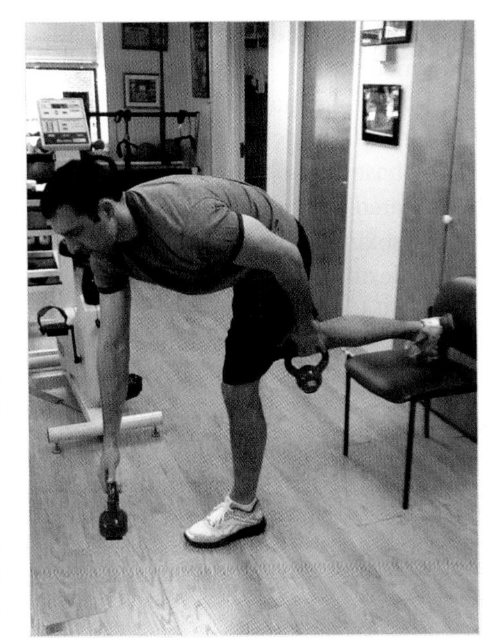

Figure 23-7 **Single-leg windmills**

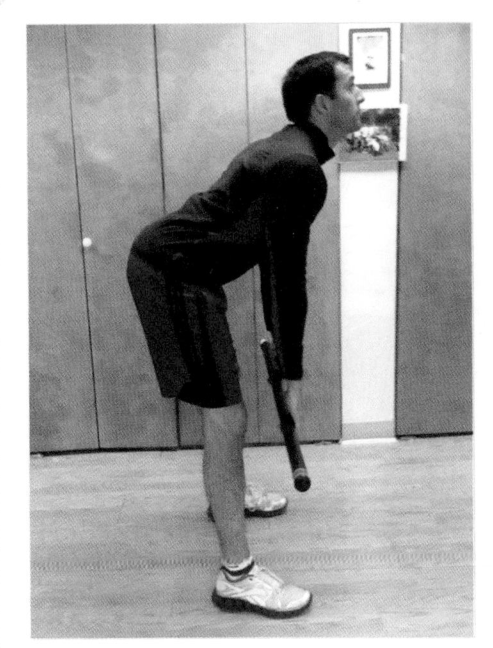

Figure 23-8 **Stiff-legged deadlift**

exercises such as straight-leg deadlift, single-leg windmills, and Nordic hamstring exercise.[63] Exercises are shown in Figures 23-7 to 23-9. Prior to athletic competition, a general warm-up (jogging, cycling) to increase tissue temperature followed by dynamic stretching that includes sports-specific movements is recommended. Examples of dynamic stretches for the legs include forward or backward lunges, high-knee marching, and straight-leg kicks (Figure 23-10). In order to complete this phase and progress to the next phase, there should

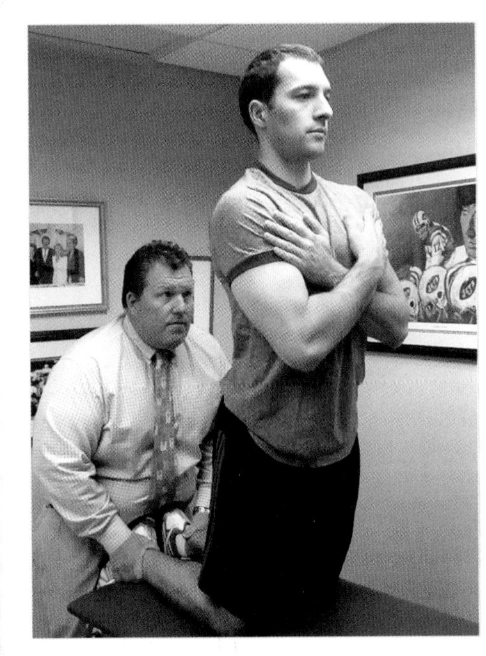

Figure 23-9 **Nordic hamstring exercise**

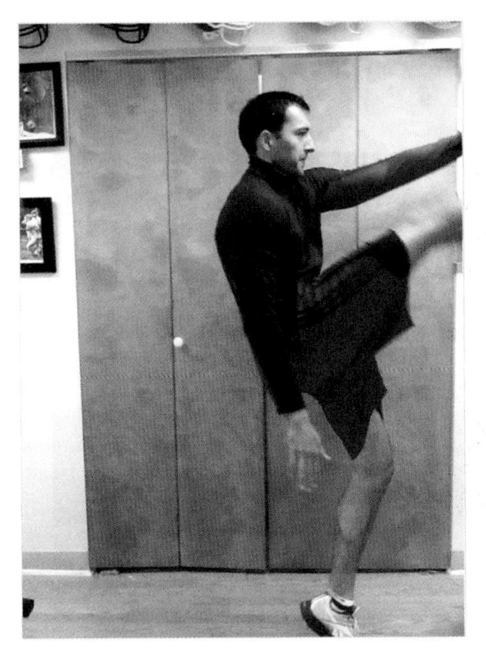

Figure 23-10 **Straight-leg kicks**

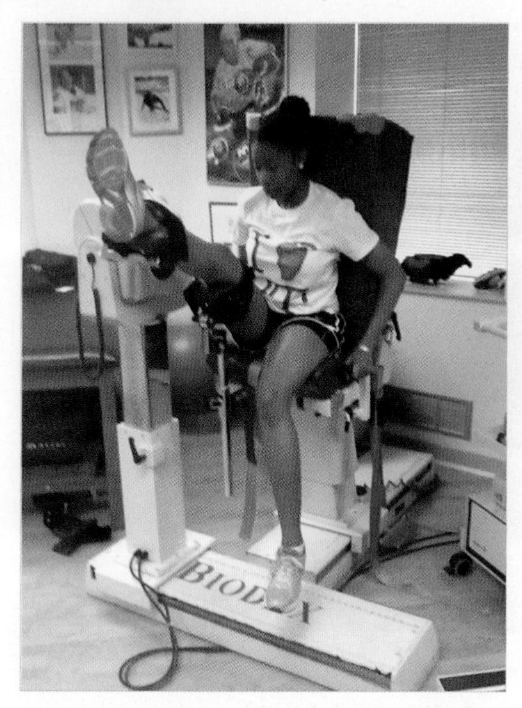

Figure 23-11 Lengthened-state eccentrics on isokinetic dynamometer

be full strength (5/5 on manual muscle test) or be within 20% of the uninjured leg in the zero to 90-degree range when measured with hand held dynamometer.[63]

During the third phase of rehabilitation, the focus is on functional movements and eccentric strengthening in a lengthened state. It is in this phase that plyometrics and sports specific activity may be initiated. Lengthened-state eccentrics can be performed using an isokinetic dynamometer (Biodex). The patient should be in hip flexion and then passively extends and flexes the knee into end ROM. The patient is told to resist passive motion as the knee extends. It is important to assure the hip is flexed as the knee extends to ensure the hamstring is truly at a lengthened state (Figure 23-11). An alternative to using the dynamometer for lengthened state eccentric training is by using a Thera-Band, cable column, or manual resistance, which is shown in Figure 23-12. Table 23-3 provides a hamstring protocol in an eccentric lengthened state.

Quadriceps Strain

The quadriceps is a group of 4 muscles that sit on the anterior aspect of the thigh. They are the vastus medialis, intermedius, lateralis, and, finally, the rectus femoris. The quadriceps attach to the front of the tibia via the patella tendon and originate at the top of the femur. The exception is the rectus femoris, which actually crosses the hip joint and originates on the pelvis. The function of the quadriceps as a whole is to extend the knee. The rectus femoris not only functions to extend the knee, but also acts as a hip flexor because it crosses the hip joint. Any of these muscles can strain (or tear) but probably the most common is the rectus femoris. The grading system is the same as the adductor strains. A grade III tear is felt as an abrupt, sudden, acute pain that occurs during activity (often while sprinting). It may be accompanied by swelling or bruises on the thigh. The rehabilitation of quadriceps strains follows the same

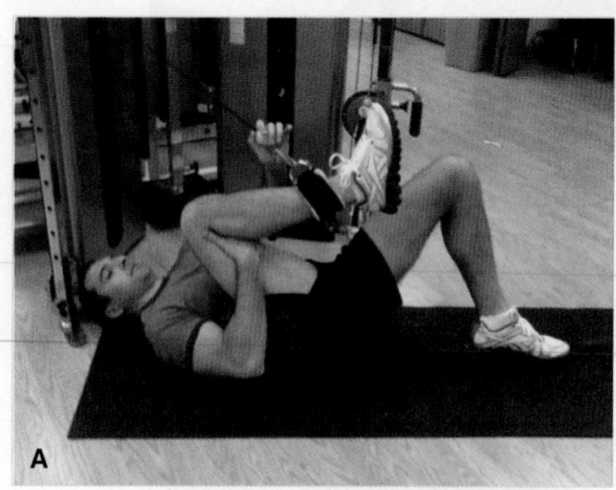

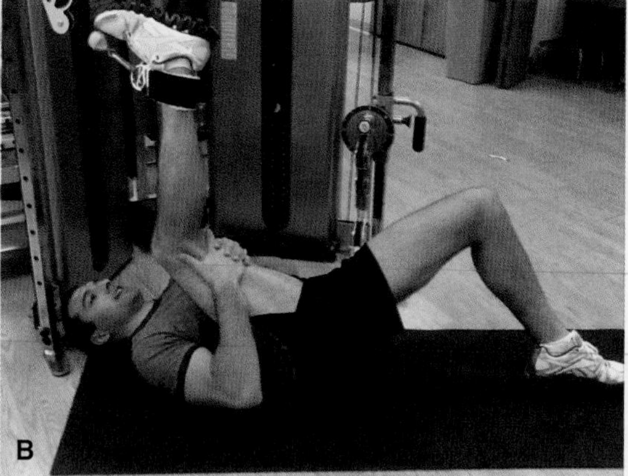

Figure 23-12

A, B. Lengthened-state eccentric training on cable column.

Table 23-3 Hamstring Strain Protocol in an Eccentric Lengthened State

Phase I (acute)	RICE (rest, ice, compression, elevation) for first approximately 48 hours after injury NSAIDs Soft-tissue mobilization (STM)/instrument-assisted soft-tissue mobilization (IASTM) Transcutaneous electrical nerve stimulation (TENS) Ultrasound Submaximal multiangle isometrics performed at 30, 60, and 90 degrees of knee flexion (see Figure 23-7) Progressive hip strengthening Stationary bicycle Single-leg balance Pain-free isotonic knee flexion (see Figure 23-9) Bilateral balance board
Clinical milestone	Pain-free isometric contraction against submaximal (50% to 75%) resistance during prone knee flexion manual muscle test Avoid excessive active or passive lengthening of the hamstrings
Phase II (subacute)	Bicycling Treadmill at moderate to high intensity Isokinetic eccentrics in a nonlengthened state Single-leg windmills (see Figure 23-8) Single-leg stance with perturbation (ball toss/reaches) Supine hamstring hurls on Swiss ball Seated adduction machine STM/IASTM Nordic hamstring exercise (see Figure 23-10) Shuttle jumps Prone leg drops Lateral/retro band walks
Clinical milestone	Full strength 5/5 without pain during prone knee flexion, pain-free forward and backward jogging, pain-free max eccentric contraction in a nonlengthened state, strength deficits less than 20% compared to the noninjured limb
Phase III (lengthened state training)	Treadmill moderate to high intensity as tolerated Hamstring dynamic stretching Isokinetic eccentric training at a lengthened state (Figures 23-14 to 23-16) STM/IASTM Plyometric training Sport-specific drills
Clinical milestone	Full strength without pain in the lengthened state, full ROM without pain, bilateral symmetry in knee flexion angle of peak torque, sport-specific movements without pain or symptoms

principles as the rehabilitation process of adductors and hamstring strains. Exercises for this type of injury initially are shown in Figures 23-13 and 23-14. Advanced exercises can be as given in Figures 23-15 and 23-16. Stretches are shown in Figures 23-17 through 23-19.

Avulsion Fractures

Avulsion fractures are the result of a sudden, forceful, eccentric or unbalanced contraction of a musculotendinous unit at its attachment at an apophysis. Traction epiphyses, or

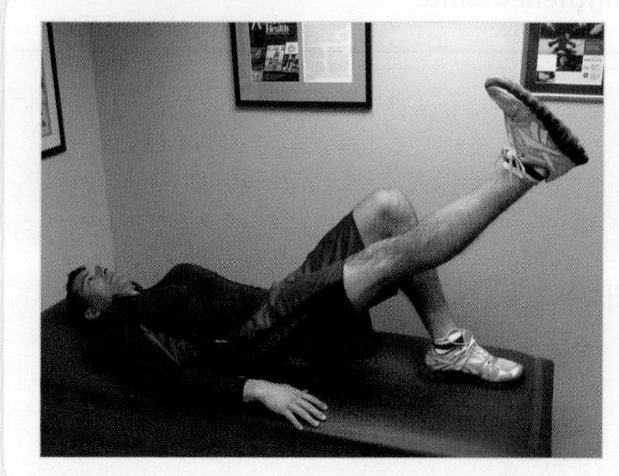

Figure 23-13 Straight-leg raises

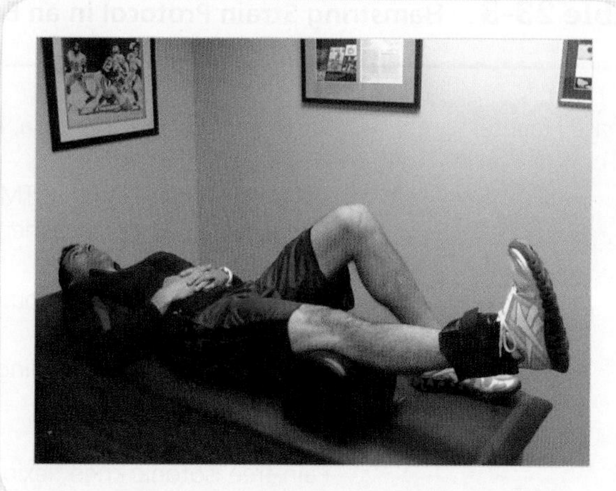

Figure 23-14 Short arc quads

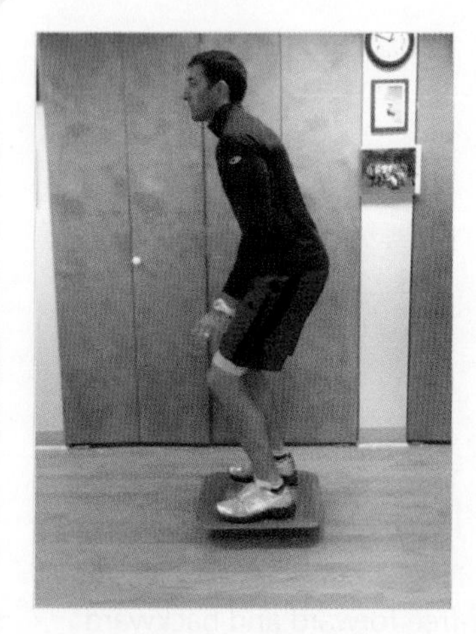

Figure 23-15 Balance board squats

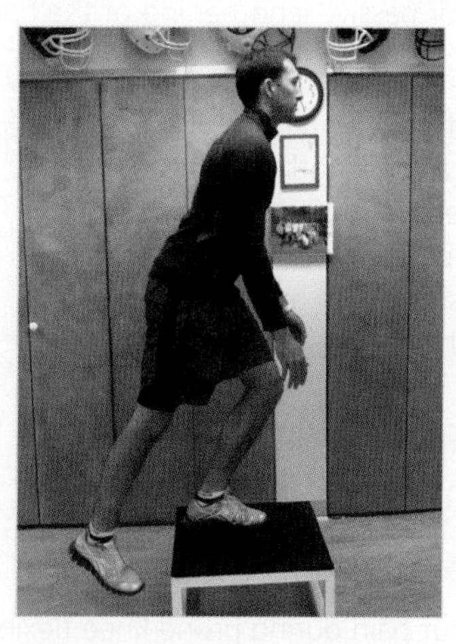

Figure 23-16 Step up

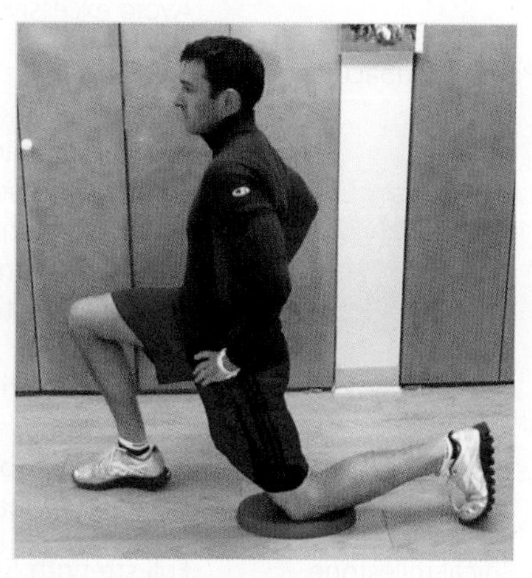

Figure 23-17 Kneeling hip flexor stretch

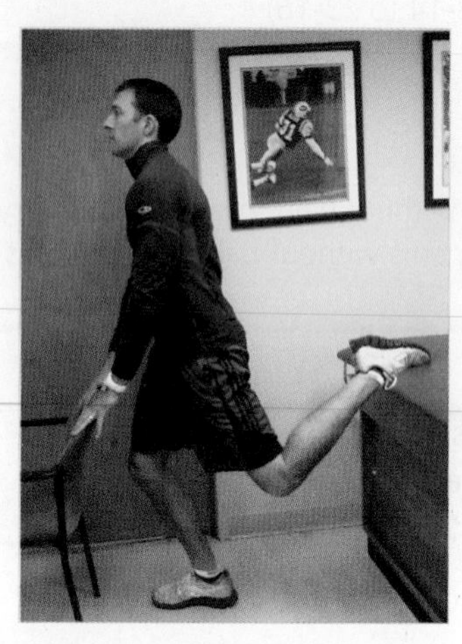

Figure 23-18 Standing hip flexor/quad stretch

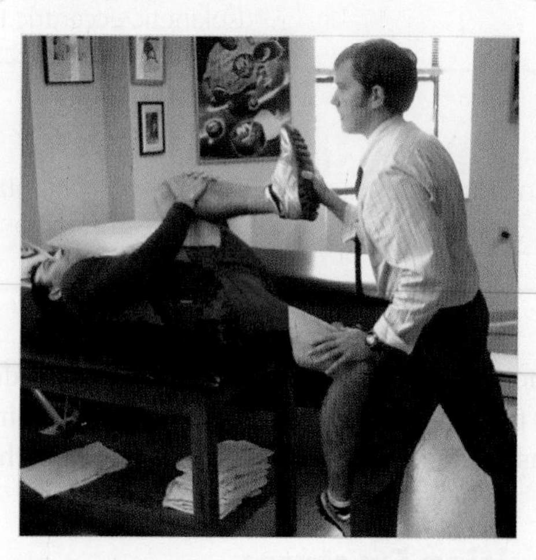

Figure 23-19 Thomas stretch

apophyses, are bony projections of forming bone that do not contribute to longitudinal growth of the bone. These epiphyseal plates are weaker than their associated ligaments; for this reason, injuries that would result in torn ligaments or tendons in adults may produce traumatic separation of the apophyses in adolescents. These injuries account for up to 15% of children's fractures.[64]

The ischial apophysis is the site of hamstring and adductor magnus origin and is the last apophysis to unite.[65] An avulsion here is the result of a violent or forceful hip flexion while the knee is extended. This injury is commonly seen in hurdlers, sprinters, cheerleaders, and dancers.

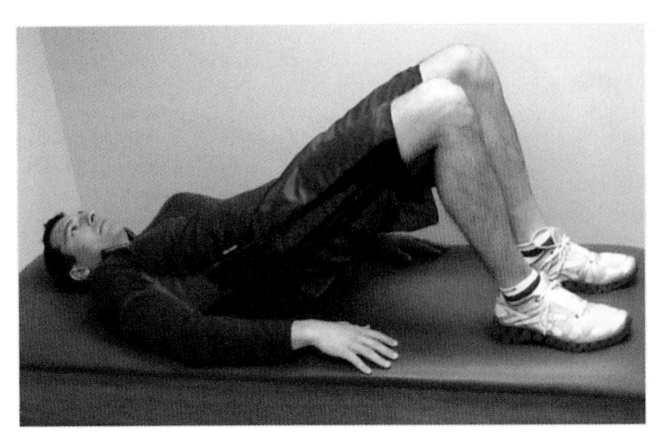

Figure 23-20 Bridges

The athlete will give a history report of a traumatic event that caused an acute onset of pain. They present with tenderness over the ischial tuberosity and pain with a straight-leg raise. An antalgic gait may be evident as well as statements of pain with sitting. Definitive diagnosis is performed radiographically. In older adults with no history of traumatic incident, a systemic or pathologic cause needs to be reviewed.[66]

Treatment for this injury begins with rest along with pain-free active range of motion (AROM) and passive ROM and protected weight bearing with crutches if needed.[67] With a reduction of pain, initiation of light strengthening and gentle stretching can be prescribed. Exercises shown in Figures 23-2 and 23-20 to 23-22 illustrate such interventions. Normalization of gait cycle is progressed throughout healing time. Progressive resistant exercises are introduced with return of ROM and cessation of pain. A steady advancement to sport-specific activities should concentrate on strengthening, proprioceptive training, and, finally, plyometrics (exercises shown in Figures 23-3, 23-15, 23-16, 23-27, and 23-30). Patients should not return to competition until full ROM and strength is restored.[24]

Another avulsion fracture in the pelvis involves the anterior inferior iliac spine. This injury cost commonly occurs in kicking sports. The anterior inferior iliac spine is the origin of the reflected head of rectus femoris. The tension load occurs in the kicking mechanics with a sudden contraction of the rectus while the hip is extended and the knee is flexed. Examination may reveal an antalgic gait pattern along with local tenderness and pain with resisted hip flexion.

Avulsion of the anterior superior iliac spine involves the same mechanics of hip extension with flexed knee, but involves a forceful contraction of the sartorius muscle. This is

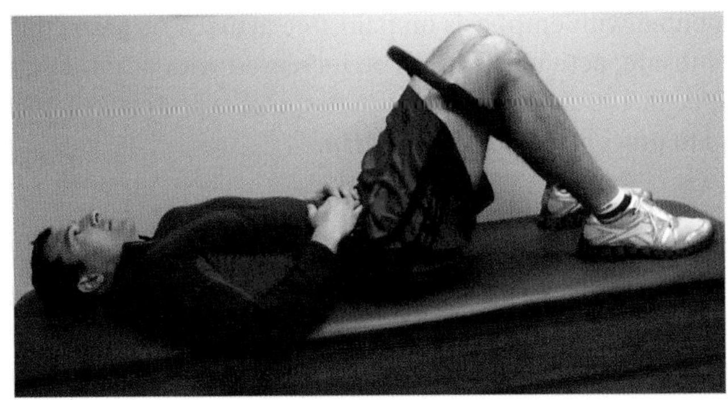

Figure 23-21 Ring squeezes

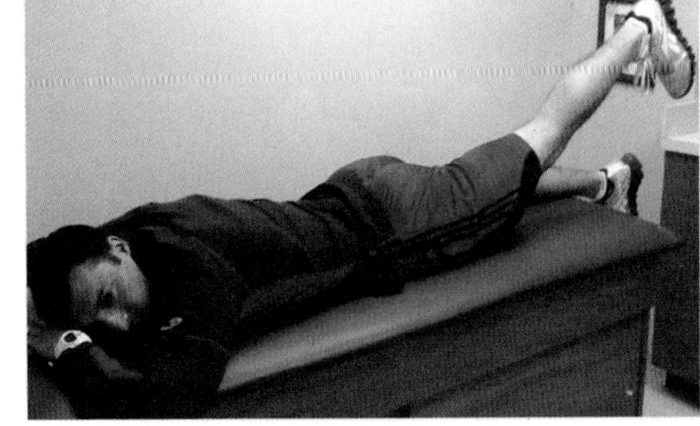

Figure 23-22 Prone hip extension

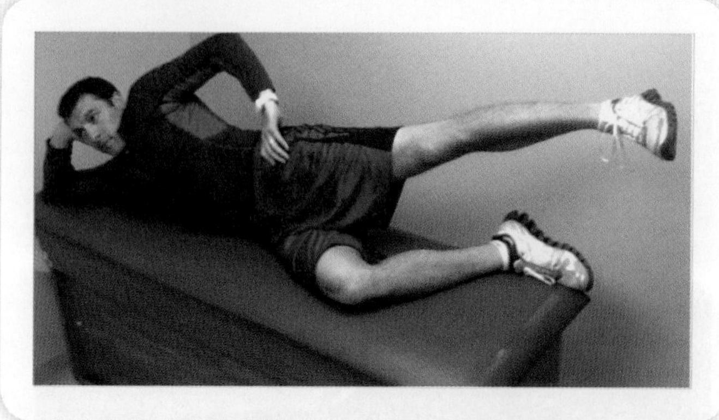

Figure 23-23 Hip abduction stretch

found in sprinters during high-speed hip extension. The athlete will present with palpable tenderness over the anatomical landmark.

Both injuries respond well to conservative treatment that involves initial rest and cessation of injuring activity. Rehabilitation is similar to that of the ischial avulsion fracture with emphasis on pain-free progression (exercises shown in Figures 23-13, 23-14, and 23-22 to 23-24).

Hip Pointer

A hip pointer occurs from a traumatic blow or fall to the iliac crest. It is also referred to as a contusion of the iliac crest. The impact causes bleeding from ruptured capillaries and infiltration of blood into muscles, tendons, and other soft tissues; that is, subperiosteal and subcutaneous regions.[8] The iliac crest has a minimal amount of overlying fatty or muscular tissue, which makes it more susceptible to injury than other more protected areas of the body. Hip pointers occur most commonly in contact sports such as football, rugby, and hockey, but also occur in noncontact sports, such as volleyball, as a result of a fall or dig onto the hip or side.

The signs and symptoms include a sudden onset of pain after a traumatic hit or fall onto that side. Pain is often localized (point tender) and may present with swelling and ecchymosis at the injury site. The athlete may present physically with guarding, decreased strength, pain with resistance, and gait abnormalities.[68]

Three grades of contusion can be distinguished based on physical findings. A grade I hip pointer presents with a normal gait and posture, but with complaints of pain, palpable tenderness, and minimal swelling. Grade II injuries are more painful with noticeable swelling and abnormal gait patterns. ROM is limited and trunk movement is painful. The posture may be flexed to the injured side. Finally, a grade III presents with severe pain, increased swelling, ecchymosis, limited ROM, and a slow and shortened stride length during gait.

Initial rehabilitation should consist of ice, compression, NSAIDs, and rest in a position of comfort. An assistive device may be utilized if gait is too painful. As pain decreases, interventions should focus on return of full ROM and stretching of all adjacent musculature (see Figures 23-17, 23-18, 23-25, and 23-26). Modalities may be utilized as needed to aid in pain reduction and tissue healing.[69,70] Progression to strength and aerobic training should be implemented with emphasis on pain-free activity. As pain continues to subside, activities should be increased with a transition to sport-specific training. With a return to sports, a protective pad will be worn to prevent reinjury to the area.

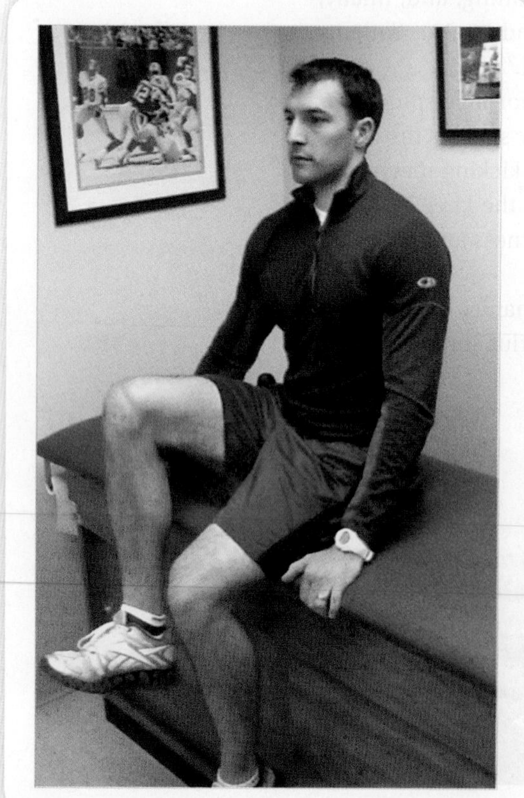

Figure 23-24 Seated hip flexion

Quadriceps Contusion

Pathomechanics

Because the quadriceps muscle is in the front of the thigh, a direct blow to the area that causes the muscle to compress against the femur can be very disabling.[1,31] A direct blow to the anterior portion of the muscle is usually more serious and disabling than a

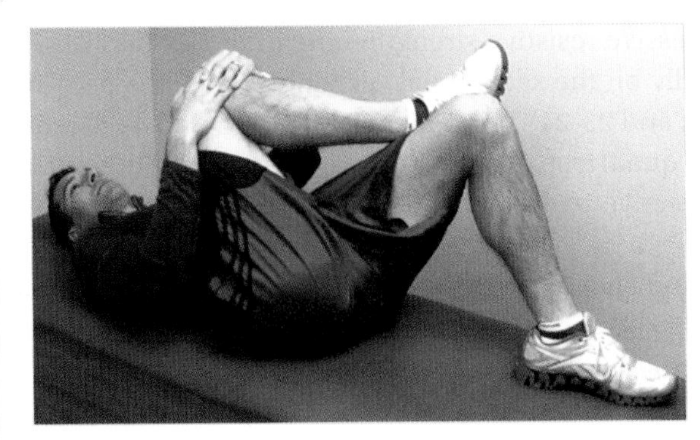

Figure 23-25 **Modified piriformis stretch**

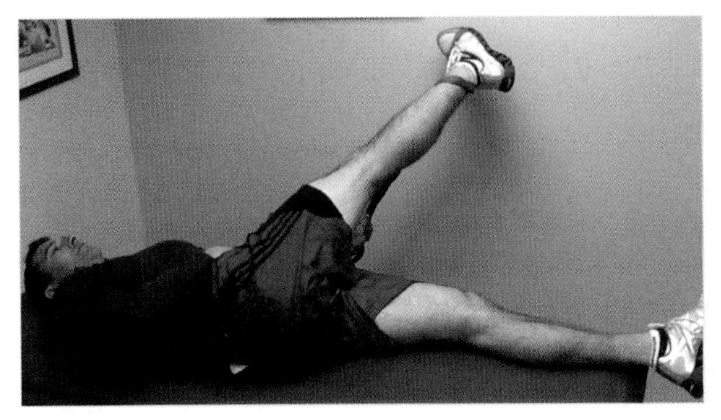

Figure 23-26 **Supine ITB stretch with strap**

direct blow to the lateral quadriceps area because of the differences in muscle mass present in the 2 areas. Blood vessels that break cause bleeding in the area where muscle tissue has been damaged.[3] If not treated correctly, or if treated too aggressively, a quadriceps contusion can lead to the formation of myositis ossificans (see "Myositis Ossificans" below). Ice hockey players are especially susceptible to this injury because of the velocity of the puck and players causing high impact.

At the time of injury, the patient may develop pain, loss of function to the quadriceps mechanism, and loss of knee flexion ROM. How forceful the blow was at the time of injury determines the grade of injury.

Injury Mechanism

A patient with a grade I contusion may present a normal gait cycle, negative swelling, and only mild discomfort on palpation. The patient's active knee flexion ROM while lying prone should be within normal limits. Resistive knee extension while sitting and lying supine with the knee bent over the end of a table may not cause discomfort.

A patient with a grade II contusion may have a normal gait cycle. Attempting to continue activity will likely cause the injury to become progressively disabling. If the gait cycle is abnormal, the patient will splint the knee in extension and avoid knee flexion while bearing weight because the knee feels like it will give out. This patient may also externally rotate the extremity to use the hip adductors to pull the leg through during the swing-through phase. This move may be accompanied by hiking the hip at push-off, which causes tilting of the pelvis in the frontal plane. Swelling may be moderate to severe, with a noticeable defect and pain on palpation. While the patient is lying prone, AROM in the knee may be limited, with possibly only 90 degrees of motion. Resistive knee extension while sitting and lying supine with the knee bent over the end of a table may be painful, and a noticeable weakness in the quadriceps mechanism may be evident.

A patient with a grade III contusion may herniate the muscle through the fascia to cause a marked defect, severe bleeding, and disability. The patient may not be able to ambulate without crutches. Pain, severe swelling, and a bulge of muscle tissue may be present on palpation. When the patient is lying prone, knee flexion AROM may be severely limited. Active resistive knee extension while the patient is sitting and lying supine with the knee bent over the end of a table may not be tolerated, and severe weakness may be present. If a grade III quadriceps contusion is diagnosed, a possible fracture should be ruled out.[71]

Rehabilitation Concerns and Progression

A patient with a grade I quadriceps contusion should begin ice and 24-hour compression immediately. Twenty-four–hour compression should be continued until all signs and symptoms are absent. Gentle, pain-free quadriceps exercises, such as quad sets, may be performed on the first day. Progressive resistive strengthening exercises may also be performed as soon as possible, usually on the second day, as long as they are pain-free (see exercises in Figures 23-13, 23-14, and 23-24) This patient's AROM should be carefully monitored. A patient with a grade I quadriceps contusion may try to continue normal activities, but compression and protective padding should be worn until the patient is symptom free.

A patient with a grade II contusion should be treated very conservatively. Crutches should be used until a normal gait can be accomplished free of pain. Ice, 24-hour compression, and electrical muscle stimulation modalities may be started immediately to decrease swelling, inflammation, pain, and to promote ROM.[29] Compression should be applied at all times to minimize bleeding into the area. Pain-free quadriceps isometric exercises may be performed as soon as possible, usually within the first 3 days. Between days 3 and 5, ice is continued with pain-free AROM while the patient is sitting and lying prone. AROM lying supine with the knee bent over the end of a table can be added. Passive stretching is contraindicated at this time and not used until the later phases of rehabilitation. Massage and heat modalities are also contraindicated in the early phases because of the possibility of promoting bleeding and eventually myositis ossificans. At approximately day 5, the patient may perform straight-leg raises without weights and then progress to weights, pain free (see exercise in Figure 23-13). As AROM increases and approaches 95 to 100 degrees of knee flexion, swimming, aquatic therapy, and biking may be performed, if the seat height is adjusted to the patient's available ROM. Between days 7 and 10, heat in the form of hot packs, ultrasound, or whirlpool, may be used, as long as swelling is absent and the patient is approaching full AROM while lying prone. Pain-free quadriceps progressive resistive strengthening exercises may be performed in the order given (see exercises in Figures 23-13 and 23-14), flexion with knee both extended and flexed (see exercises in Figures 23-3, 23-15, and 23-16), and isokinetics may be added. Ice or heat modalities, with AROM, should be continued before all exercises as a warm-up. Pain-free quadriceps stretching exercises should not be rushed and can be started between 10 and 14 days as needed (see exercises in Figure 23-18). A patient with a grade II quadriceps contusion may require 3 to 21 days for rehabilitation, depending upon the severity of the injury. Jogging, slide board (see exercise in Figure 23-4), plyometrics, and functional activities may be used after the fourteenth day. Compression and protective padding should be worn during physical activity until the patient is symptom free.

A patient with a grade III quadriceps contusion should use crutches, rest, ice, 24-hour compression, and electrical muscle stimulation modalities immediately to decrease pain, bleeding, and swelling and to counteract atrophy.[29] The patient may begin pain-free isometric quadriceps exercises between days 5 and 7. Ice and 24-hour compression should be continued from the very first day through day 7, with pain-free AROM exercises, while the patient is sitting and lying prone, added about day 7. AROM lying supine with the knee bent over the end of a table can also be added. At approximately day 10, the patient may perform straight-leg raises without weights and then progress to weights by day 14 (see exercise in Figure 23-13). Electrical muscle stimulation may be very helpful in this phase to counteract muscle atrophy and reeducate muscle contraction. Again, as AROM increases and approaches 95 to 100 degrees of knee flexion, swimming, aquatic therapy, and biking may be performed if the seat height is adjusted to the patient's available ROM. After day 14, the patient may use heat in the form of hot packs or whirlpool, as long as the swelling has decreased and the patient has gained AROM. At approximately the third week of rehabilitation, pain-free quadriceps progressive resistive strengthening exercises may be performed in the order presented (see exercises in Figures 23-13 to 23-16), and isokinetics. Pain-free quadriceps stretching may also be performed (see exercises in Figures 23-17 and 23-18) if the patient is careful not to overstretch the quadriceps muscles. A patient with a grade III quadriceps contusion may require 3 weeks to 3 months for rehabilitation. In general, at approximately week 3, the patient may begin jogging, slide board, plyometrics, and functional activities. Again, compression and protective padding should be worn during all competition until the patient is symptom free.[72]

Myositis Ossificans

Pathomechanics and Injury Mechanism

With a severe direct blow or repetitive direct blows to the quadriceps muscles that cause muscle tissue damage, bleeding, and injury to the periosteum of the femur, ectopic bone production may occur.[1,21] In 3 to 6 weeks, calcium formation may be seen on X-ray films. If the trauma was to the quadriceps muscles only, and not to the femur, a smaller bony mass may be seen on radiographs.[1]

If quadriceps contusion and strain are properly treated and rehabilitated, myositis ossificans can be prevented. Myositis ossificans can be caused by trying to "play through" a grade II or III quadriceps contusion or strain and by early use of stretching exercises into pain, ultrasound, and other heat modalities.[73]

Rehabilitation Concerns and Progression

After 1 year, surgical removal of the bony mass may be helpful. If the bony mass is removed too early, the trauma caused by the surgery may actually enhance the condition.

After radiographic diagnosis, intervention should follow that for a grade II or III quadriceps contusion or quadriceps strain (see treatment and rehabilitation for grade II and III quadriceps contusions and strains).[72] The bony mass usually stabilizes after the sixth month.[18] If the mass does not cause disability, the patient should be closely monitored and follow the treatment and rehabilitation programs outlined in grade II and III quadriceps contusions and strains. It has also been recommended that myositis can be treated using acetic acid with iontophoresis.[53]

Hip Dislocation

The capsule and ligaments of the hip joint permit little or no distraction even upon strong traction forces. The joint is also very difficult to traumatically dislocate (unlike the glenohumeral joint). Under circumstances where the joint surfaces are neither maximally congruent nor in a closed-pack position, the hip joint is at risk for traumatic dislocation. This position of particular vulnerability occurs when the hip joint is flexed, internally rotated and adducted.[7] In this position, a strong force up the femoral shaft toward the joint may push the femoral head out of the acetabulum. This is found predominantly in motor vehicle accidents as a consequence of the seated position of an individual within the car. Upon a head on collision the dashboard provides the load down the femoral shaft dislocating the hip joint.

Although rare in athletes, 2 general categories of hip dislocation exist: anterior and posterior.[74] Anterior dislocations compose only 10% of cases and occur in contact sports as a result of a violent force that send the hip into extension, abduction, and lateral rotation.[24,75] The more prevalent posterior dislocation occurs with excessive loads applied to a flexed, adducted, and internally rotated joint. This mechanism is found also in contact sports where the athlete has a high-speed uncontrolled fall onto a flexed knee such as in a gang tackle.

When a posterior dislocation is sustained, the athlete presents with severe pain in the hip region with inability to walk or move the involved leg. The affected limb will appear shortened, flexed, adducted, and internally rotated. Of great concern with this injury is the compromise of hip vascularity and the close relationship of the sciatic nerve. These 2 components make hip dislocations a medical emergency. The dislocated hip can occlude the lateral circumflex artery, which is the primary provider of circulation to the femoral head. This reduced flow can lead to avascular necrosis of the femoral head. Adults whose hips are reduced within 8 hours from the time of injury have a low incidence of avascular necrosis. Those whose reduction occurred more than 8 hours earlier have up to approximately a 40% chance of this complication.[64] Stretching or compression of the sciatic nerve as a result of this injury may lead to paralysis of hamstrings and muscularity distal to the knee that is innervated by the nerve.[76]

Medical treatment includes rapid reduction and hospitalization along with possible traction or immobilization in a hip spica cast until the joint is pain free, which is approximately 1 to 3 weeks. Following this initial time line, rehabilitation will begin with simple assisted ROM to maintain normal flexibility. Pain-free use of isometrics or muscular stimulation can be utilized to prevent excessive atrophy and aid in muscular reeducation acutely [69,70] Crutch ambulation with progressive weight bearing is implemented with advancement to gait normalization. Progressive resistance exercises can begin with return of painless ROM and concentration focused on proximal hip musculature (see exercises in Figures 23-2, 23-13, and 23-22 to 23-24). Advancement of exercise can progress as tolerated and with pain-free motions.

Labral Tears

Pathomechanics and Injury Mechanism

The acetabular labrum is a fibrocartilage ring around the rim of the acetabulum, located in the socket of the hip joint. It has the job of increasing the congruency of the hip joint, acting as a shock absorber during weight bearing.[77] The acetabular labrum can be torn if there is a twisting movement while the hip joint is bearing weight, and it frequently occurs during soccer activity. Golfers and ice hockey players are also susceptible to labral tears that can result in arthritis if not treated, according to a study reported at the annual meeting of the Radiological Society of North America in Chicago.

The onset of pain is immediate and usually located at the front of the hip joint. As with all hip problems, the pain may become diffuse and difficult to pinpoint. If the front of the hip joint is affected, there may be a pinching sensation when the patient flexes the hip by bringing the knee up to the chest. A mechanical catching or giving way sensation in the hip may also occur. Symptoms usually occur when the hip is changing position. The pain may be reproduced in sport during activities that require concomitant weight bearing and twisting; for example, driving a golf ball.[78]

Labrum tears can be the result of an underlying anatomic abnormality of the hip. Because a torn labrum not only causes pain and instability but also disturbs the mechanical function of the hip in its own right and predisposes to arthritis, a symptomatic labral tear is an indication for treatment both to prevent arthritis and improve symptoms. Nonoperative treatment of labral tears can be successful if the tear is small and stable. If nonoperative means are not successful, the results of hip arthroscopy have to be reported to be good.[79] A return to sports is usually possible between 2 and 3 months after the operation.

Although hip arthroscopy usually can allow symptom-relieving trimming of the torn labrum in a minimally invasive way, if the torn labrum occurred because of an underlying anatomic abnormality in the hip, it is usually advisable to correct the underlying anatomic hip abnormality first.[80]

Rehabilitation Concerns and Progression

An emerging surgical trend hip arthroscopy is becoming more common, especially among athletes. The application of this minimally invasive technique, combined with advances in MRI, is considered a significant advancement in treating many forms of chronic hip injuries. Although the surgery is new and emerging, the rehabilitation progression should take into consideration the basic science principles of soft-tissue healing (Table 23-4).

Following surgery, the patient is instructed to use bilateral crutches with partial weight bearing as tolerated for the first 2 weeks. Then, they are progressed to one crutch for 1 week, until they regain normal gait. Gait training to restore normal gait is paramount at this point in the rehabilitation. Some surgeons utilize a hip brace to restrict hip flexion ROM. During the second week, the patient may also begin some easy pool walking and stationary biking without resistance.

Table 23-4 Arthroscopic Hip Labral Repair Rehabilitation Guidelines

Weightbearing (WB) status	Foot flat with 20 lb of pressure Duration 2 to 4 weeks
Continuous passive motion (CPM)	Start 30 to 70 degrees Increase as tolerated 0 to 90 degrees Duration 2 weeks
Sleeping	Ace wrap feet when sleeping for 2 weeks
Brace	Daytime use Set at 0 to 90 degrees of hip flexion
Stationary bicycle	Immediate postoperatively 1 to 2 times/day × 15 to 20 minutes Avoid pinching in front of hip by setting seat high
Pool exercises	Begin postoperative day 14 or as soon as sutures are removed and wound is healed
Range of motion	Examine stool internal rotation—day 3 (may push early internal rotation within pain limits) Examine stool external rotation—day 7 (limit to 30 degrees internal rotation) 2 to 3 sets × 12 to 15 repetitions Quadriceps rocking—day 7 AROM—within limits of brace or as tolerated if no brace is worn PROM (passive range of motion)—within available pain-free limits after brace is removed
Strength	Quad sets/ankle pumps—day 1 Isometrics in neutral day 7 (within painful limits) Bridges—days 7 to 10 Isotonic weight equipment day 14 Except for leg press begin at 6 weeks Shuttle/Pilates begin at 3 to 4 weeks dependent on WB Trunk strength Transverse abdominis Side supports Trunk and low-back stabilization as tolerated

(continued)

Table 23-4 Arthroscopic Hip Labral Repair Rehabilitation Guidelines *(Continued)*

Function	No straight-leg raises for 4 weeks May begin pool walking in chest-high water Avoid antalgic gait Be aware of weakness of gluteus medius, side supports, and transverse abdominis strength in sagittal, coronal, and transverse planes
Balance	As soon as WB is permitted begin working on both double- and single-leg balance with eyes open and eyes closed 10 repetitions × 5 seconds is a good place to start
General considerations • Typically requires 3 months of supervised therapy • **Month 1: tissue healing phase (1 to 2 × per week)**	
Goals:	Pain control Decrease tissue inflammation Decrease swelling Maintenance of motion (flexion 0 to 90 degrees internal rotation as tolerated; internal rotation 0 to 30 degrees)
• **Month 2: early functional recovery (2 to 3 × per week)**	
Goals:	Full PROM Progress to full AROM Early strength gains Avoid flexor tendonitis and abductor tendonitis
• **Month 3: late functional recovery (2 to 3 × per week)**	
Goals:	Advance strength gains—focus on abductor and hip flexor strength Balance and proprioception Continue to monitor for development of tendonitis Progress to sport-specific activity in months 3 and 4 depending on strength Do not progress to running until abductor strength is equal to contralateral side Progression to sport-specific activities requires full strength return and muscle coordination
Precautions	• Avoid anything that causes either anterior or lateral impingement • Be aware of low-back sacroiliac joint dysfunction • Pay close attention for the onset of flexor tendonitis and abductor tendonitis • Patients with preoperative weakness in proximal hip musculature are at increased risk for postoperative tendonitis • Modification of activity with focus on decreasing inflammation takes precedent if tendonitis occurs

Independent ambulation is encouraged at the 3-week mark. Aerobic activity is increased to 30 minutes along with the activation of active assistive hip ROM exercises. Any explosive movements or rotational hip torque could potentially damage the hip capsule and labrum and are therefore to be avoided. During the first 4 to 6 weeks, pain-free exercise is recommended to avoid a synovitis, tendonitis, or overstretching.

At 2 weeks postoperation, light hip isotonics and more weightbearing exercises such as bridges and single-leg bridges are initiated (see exercises in Figures 23-1 and 23-20). Strengthening of the hip extensors, abductors, and external rotators are emphasized, along with light stretching for hamstrings, hip flexors, quadriceps, and the iliotibial band (ITB).

The straight-leg exercise is avoided until the fourth week following surgery, because of the potential for high compressive loading. ROM is pushed for internal rotation, but progressed more slowly for external rotation. Trunk strengthening is begun at this time with emphasis on the transverse abdominals and the back extensors.

At 6 weeks, the patient begins light internal-external hip-rotation stretching, which marks the first time stretches are introduced to the postoperative hip beyond the AROM. Eight weeks following surgery, lower-extremity strength work, which includes squats, Romanian dead lifts, four-way hip exercises, lunges, and lateral step work, is initiated (see exercises in Figures 23-8, 23-15, 23-16, 23-27, 23-28, and 23-30). The lifting program emphasizes lighter weights and higher repetitions and is designed to build endurance and avoid positions that could potentially aggravate the hip. Avoid anything that causes either anterior or lateral impingement. The physical therapist should be aware of overlapping condition such as low-back pain and sacroiliac dysfunction. In addition, monitoring for the onset of flexor tendonitis and abductor tendonitis can help prevent failures. Keep in mind that patients with preoperative weakness in proximal hip musculature are at increased risk for postoperative tendonitis.[80]

Following hip arthroscopy, patients should avoid weightbearing twists and turns on the hip for up to 3 months after surgery. Although not evidence based, similar to a healing meniscus, this compression with rotation is likely not beneficial to a healing labrum of patients in all age groups and of all occupations. It is recommended that patients attempt to keep their movements within the midline, certainly for a 6-week period. They can then gradually introduce rotational movements to the hip, but such movements must be under their own control. Rotational therapeutic exercises should start with non-weightbearing exercises and progress cautiously to full weight bearing. At the 3- to 4-month point, assuming no setbacks, patients are allowed to return to unprotected, full activities provided full strength and coordination have returned.

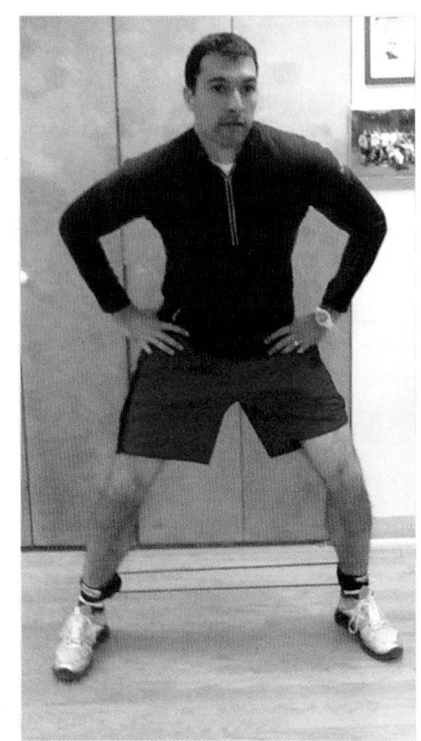

Figure 23-27 Lateral walks

Insidious Injuries

Bursitis

Bursae are lined with synovium and are synovial fluid filled sacs that exist normally at sites of friction between tendons and bone as well as between these structures and the overlying skin.[64] It is analogous to filling a balloon with oil and rubbing it between your fingers. The purpose of the bursae is to dissipate friction caused by 2 or more structures moving against one another.[8] The development of a bursitis is the product of 1 of 2 mechanisms, the most common being inflammation secondary to excessive friction or shear forces as a result of overuse. Posttraumatic bursitis is the other mechanism, and stems from direct blows and contusions that cause bleeding in the bursae with resultant inflammation.

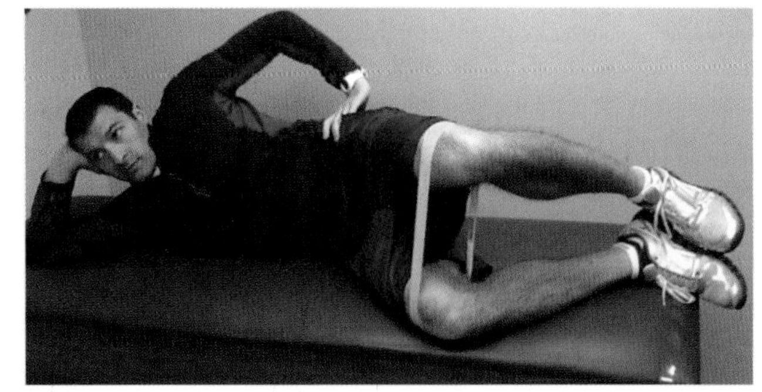

Figure 23-28 Clam shells

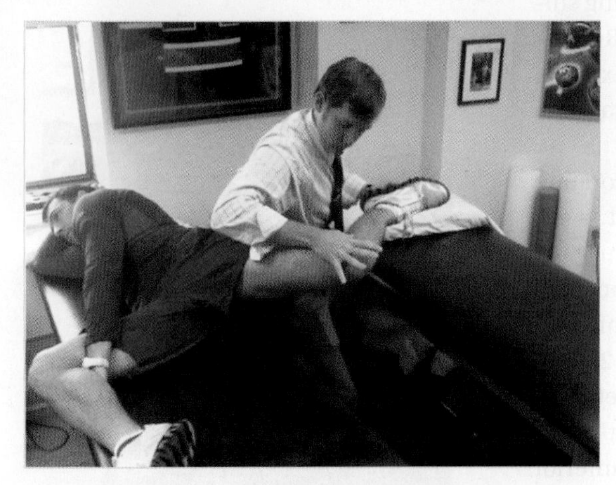

Figure 23-29 Passive Ober's stretch

The 3 major bursae around the hip joint that are susceptible to bursitis are the iliopsoas bursa, ischial bursa, and the greater trochanteric bursa.

Trochanteric Bursitis

The greater trochanteric bursa lies between the gluteus maximus, tensor fasciae latae, and the surface of the greater trochanter. Its location on the lateral aspect of the hip exposes it to contact injuries in sports such as football, soccer, and ice hockey. More commonly though, it is seen in the clinic as an overuse injury found in runners, bikers, and cross-country skiers. It may also be found in individuals with an increased Q angle, prominent trochanters, or a leg-length discrepancy. It is the repetitive motion of hip flexion and extension on an excessively compressed bursa that gives rise to irritation and inflammation. This can occur with tightness in tissues around the hip, for example, the ITB pulling across the hip, or hip adductors bringing the thigh into a more midline position. Poor running mechanics or continuous running on banked surfaces that brings the lower extremity into an increased adducted position can also cause undue strain at the hip.

Signs and symptoms of trochanteric bursitis include warmth and reported pain at the greater trochanter region of the hip. Pain with hip abduction resistance, palpable tenderness at lateral hip, pain with gait and possible swelling or ecchymosis at the surface of the greater trochanter, as well as pain with lying on affected side may be present.[81,82]

Intervention begins by taking a thorough history from the patient to determine activity level, length of onset, or mechanism of possible traumatic incident. Examination is then performed to check for ROM, tenderness, tightness, and weakness in surrounding soft-tissue structures. It is necessary to analyze gait and stair patterns as well as possibly analyzing running mechanics if subjective complaints warrant.

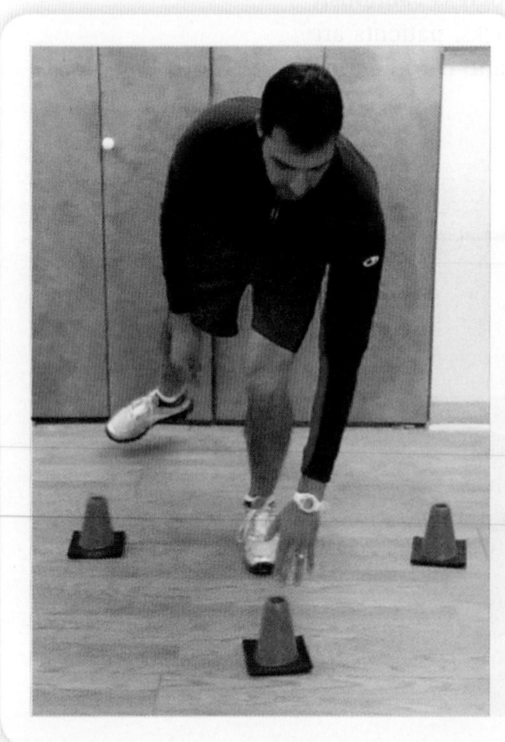

Figure 23-30 Cone touches

Initial home rehabilitation for the individual will consist of rest, ice, and nonsteroidal antiinflammatories. Clinical treatment emphasizes modalities for inflammation, for example, ultrasound, stretching of appropriate structures such as the ITB and adductors (see exercises in Figures 23-25, 23-26, and 23-29), as well as slow integration into progressive resistive exercises for encompassing hip musculature (see exercises in Figures 23-2, 23-13, 23-22 to 23-24, and 23-28).[70,83] If the underlying cause is a leg-length discrepancy, it should be corrected with the appropriate device. Upon normalization of ROM and flexibility, a gradual return to sport-specific activities should be implemented. Full return to sports should emphasize prevention with a regular stretching program or appropriate padding for traumatic injuries.

Ischial Bursitis

Although uncommon, ischial bursitis may occur as a complication of an injury to the hamstring insertion into the ischial tuberosity or as a direct trauma to a fall or hit. The symptoms include pain while sitting and localized tenderness. It is important to distinguish this bursitis from a hamstring tear at the origin. Initial treatment consists of rest, ice, and NSAIDs. Sitting cushion may be utilized as needed. General stretching of the hamstrings and progressive resistant exercises are implemented as pain subsides (see stretching in Figures 23-25 and 23-26, as well as exercises in Figures 23-2, 23-22 to 23-24, and 23-28).

Iliopsoas (Iliopectineal) Bursitis

Iliopsoas (*iliopectineal*) bursitis is most often caused by excessive activity. It is thought to be irritated by the iliopsoas muscle passing over the iliopectineal eminence. This rubbing may also be associated with a snapping hip. Pain is reported in the inguinal area and can radiate into femoral triangle. Associated palpable tenderness can be present by placing the hip in flexion and external rotation. This position can also help relieve symptoms. Treatment includes the rest, NSAIDs, and stretching of the iliopsoas (see stretches in Figures 23-17 and 23-18). Strengthening of any muscle imbalances can be initiated in pain-free arcs (see exercises in Figures 23-2, 23-13, and 23-22 to 23-24).

Snapping Hip Syndrome

Snapping hip syndrome (*coxa saltans*) can arise from 2 different sources: intraarticular and extraarticular. Intraarticular causes include loose bodies, osteocartilaginous exostosis, labral tears, synovial chondromatosis, and subluxation of the hip. More common, though, is the extraarticular causes of a "snapping hip." This occurs primarily, but not exclusively, when the ITB snapping is over the greater trochanter during hip flexion and extension. Hip adduction and knee extension will tighten the ITB and accentuate the snapping sensation. This continuous pathomechanical movement can lead directly to trochanteric bursitis. A second extraarticular source comes from the iliopsoas tendon as it passes just in front of the hip joint. This tendon can catch on the pelvic brim (iliopectineal eminence) and cause a snap when the hip is flexed.[84]

This syndrome is common in ballet dancers where 44% of reported hip pain involved a snapping or clicking. Most complaints concerned the sensation, with only one-third reporting pain.[85] The condition can present itself with specific flexion movements of the thigh such as situps. Both have signs and symptoms of an audible snap or click either laterally or anterior deep in the groin which may or may not be painful. They may also present with an associated bursitis.

Treatment for a patient with snapping hip syndrome begins with a thorough examination. During the subjective evaluation, the clinician must question the patient to determine which actions exacerbate symptoms during daily activities and athletics. The objective examination is designed to determine the severity of pathology and to perform a biomechanical assessment. The information gathered in this portion of the examination can be used to guide specific elements of the treatment program. Muscle-tendon length and strength, joint mobility testing, and palpation of the injured area are key to a proper examination. Biomechanical assessment of the patient includes both static (posture) and dynamic (gait/functional movement) elements. Perform static inspection of the entire lower extremity. Particular areas of attention during this portion of the examination include observation of genu recurvatum, knee flexion contracture, biomechanical abnormalities of the foot, hip flexion contracture, and the amount of internal or external rotation present in the lower extremity during static stance. Also take note of leg length. Gait analysis allows the clinician to confirm the findings of static examination and observe if a movement dysfunction is present. Functional movements (eg, squatting, stair accent/descent) may further demonstrate to the clinician the severity of the movement dysfunction.[85]

Once identification of contributing factors has been completed, treatment can be directed toward those factors. Intervention during the acute phase consists of standard antiinflammatory care and the elimination of activities that exacerbate symptoms.

Physical therapy modalities (eg, ice, ultrasound, electrical stimulation, iontophoresis) may be used during this time.[69,70] Activity modification depends on the severity of the pathology. Crutches may be used in severe cases, while simply decreasing the time and intensity of the aggravating activity is commonly used in less severe cases. Muscle weakness and/or tightness in the thigh or pelvis is addressed with a strengthening and stretching program (see exercises in Figures 23-2, 23-13, 23-22 to 23-24, and 23-28, and stretches in Figures 23-25, 23-26, and 23-29). Biomechanical abnormalities of the foot may require an orthotic to assist with foot stabilization or control (refer to Chapter 26). Leg-length deformities commonly require a lift in the shoe to assist with balancing the entire lower extremity. For those patients with a symptomatic snapping hip and trochanteric bursitis unresponsive to conservative therapy, a surgical procedure has been described as an effective method of treatment in this specific population.[86]

Osteitis Pubis

The anterior connection between the 2 pubic bones of the pelvis creates the pubic symphysis. This along with the sacroiliac joint completes the closure of the pelvic ring. Generally, there is little motion at this joint. Excessive forces, however, may occur to produce injury or dislocation. Osteitis pubis is the result of inflammation at the pubic symphysis. It is most often encountered in postoperative patient who have undergone invasive procedures around the pelvic region. In athletes, this pathology may present as a type of overuse injury or stress fracture. It is seen mainly in distance runners, soccer players, and in other sports requiring pivoting and kicking. The constant repetitive force at the symphysis can be the cause of inflammation and pain. The stress may also be caused by traction on muscles whose origins arise from the pubis symphysis region.[24]

Patients report pain in the groin region that may radiate down the medial thigh and is exacerbated with sporting activities. There is palpable tenderness over the pubic symphysis and statements of clicking or popping with various movements. Pain may also be present during normal gait, stair climbing, or lying on one's side. The examination should focus on subjective and objective findings as well as the effects that occur on other *activities of daily living*.[87]

Early treatment involves rest and the use of NSAIDs.[88] As pain subsides, intervention should concentrate on the deficits found and pelvic stabilization. Closed-chain exercises may be started for stabilization prior to moving to open-chain motions (see exercises in Figures 23-1, 23-15, 23-20, 23-28, and 23-31). Because the inflammation may be caused by traction at muscular origins, exercises should be modified based off subjective complaints of discomfort. Corticosteroid injection may be used if symptoms do not resolve with noninvasive treatment.[89]

Apophysitis

Apophysitis is an inflammatory response to overuse and chronic traction at an apophysis in athletic children (see "Avulsion Fractures" above). The injury is characterized with an insidious onset and palpable tenderness at the bony landmark. There may or may not be accompanying swelling present. Treatment consists of relative rest from high-intensity activity with management of inflammation and pain. Graded progression of flexibility with open- and closed-chain strengthening activities implemented (see exercises in Figures 23-2, 23-13, 23-20, 23-22 to 23-24, 23-27, and 23-28). With a cessation of pain, a return to sports program begins. Training is tailored for specific sports and monitored for the return of pain and irritation. If this is encountered, training is reduced to pain-free levels.

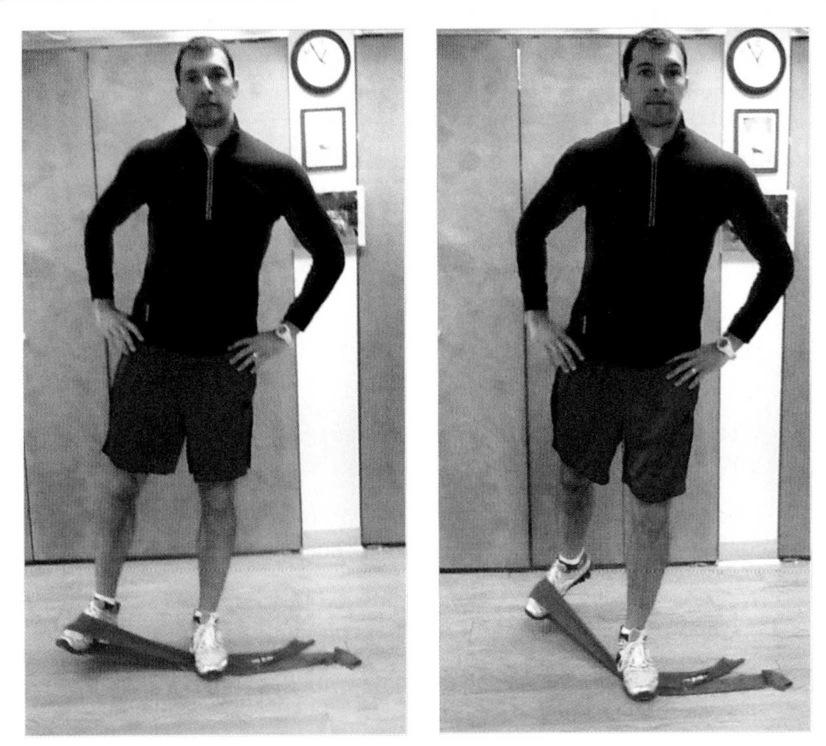

Figure 23-31

A, B. Standing hip abduction with Thera-Band at 2 angles.

Femoral Neck Stress Fracture

Bone is a specialized type of connective tissue that is capable of only a limited number of reactions to a large number of abnormal conditions. The basic nature of these reactions is best considered at a microscopic or cellular level. There are just 4 basic ways in which bone can react to abnormal conditions: (a) local death, (b) an alteration in bone deposition, (c) alteration in bone reabsorption, and (d) mechanical failure (fracture). The Wolf law states that intermittent stresses applied to bone result in architectural remodeling to allow adaptation to the new mechanical environment.[51] Thus bone is in a constant state of change with bone deposition being completed by osteoblasts while at the same time allowing for bone reabsorption by osteoclasts. This dynamic remodeling is based on applied stresses that occur in response to weight bearing and muscle contractions. Thus maintenance of healthy bone mass and structure relies on a balance between osteoclastic and osteoblastic activity.[90]

A stress fracture is a metabolic event in which an overuse repetitive injury exceeds the intrinsic ability of the bone to repair itself.[91,92] It is this stage where osteoclastic activity exceeds osteoblastic activity and leads to a stress fracture.[93-95] Although femoral neck stress fractures are rare, representing only 5% of all stress fractures, they do commonly occur in endurance athletes.[96,97] It is often associated with participation in sports involving running, jumping, or other lower-extremity repetitive stress.

Two types of stress fractures can occur in the femoral neck. They are described as transverse, which presents on the tension side of the neck, or compression fractures, which occur on the medial side of the femoral neck.[98] The tension fractures have a poor prognosis

Table 23-5 Protocol for Return to Running After a Hip or Pelvis Injury

Running Time Missed (Week)	Modification of Running Program
<1	No modification of preinjury training
1 to 2	Decrease 25% from preinjury mileage
2 to 3	Decrease 50% from preinjury mileage first week, 25% second week
≥4	Week 1: Walk 1 to 2 miles, alternating 1 minute fast and 1 minute normal pace
	Week 2: Walk 2 to 3 miles, alternating a 1.5-minute jog with a 1.5-minute walk
	Week 3: If no pain occurs, substitute a 10-minute jog every other day for walk/jog; incorporate rest days as needed
	Week 4: Same as week 3, but increase jog to 15 minutes every other day in lieu of walk/jog
	Week 5: Jog 15 minutes and alternate with 25 minutes every other day; incorporate rest days as needed
	Week 6: Jog 20 minutes and alternate with 30 minutes every other day; incorporate rest days as needed
	Week 7: Jog 20 minutes and alternate with 35 minutes every other day; incorporate rest days as needed
	Week 8: Jog 20 minutes and alternate with 40 minutes every other day; incorporate rest days as needed
	Week 9: Resume training at preinjury level if training errors have been corrected

Data from James SL. Running injuries of the knee. *Instr Course Lect.* 1998;47:407-417.

and are treated aggressively with open reduction and internal fixation. The fractures on the compression side heal well and respond favorably to noninvasive treatment.[98]

This section discusses rehabilitation of compression femoral neck stress fractures. An athlete with a possible stress fracture will present with reports of pain in groin and thigh, which is exacerbated with activities. It is important to obtain a detailed history to pinpoint any increased training regimes or changes in gear or equipment used in the training program. The patient may have an antalgic gait pattern or possible lurch and a decrease in available ROM secondary to pain. Table 23-5 is a protocol for return to running after a hip or pelvis injury.

Initial treatment of a diagnosed fracture includes rest, ice, NSAIDs, and cessation of painful activity. ROM and progressive resistant exercises are carried out within pain-free limits (see exercises in Figures 23-2, 23-13, and 23-22 to 23-24). Crutches with non-weightbearing ambulation can be prescribed until relief of pain in gait cycle. As pain reduces, a gradual increase from non-weightbearing to touchdown weight bearing to partial weight bearing to discontinuation of crutches is implemented. Utilization of cross training, or active rest, can be accomplished by activities such as water running, stationary bike riding, and upper-body ergometer training. Activity resumption requires recovery periods that allow for tissue healing and adaptation (see exercise in Figures 23-15, 23-16, and 23-27). A return to running should be initiated and monitored toward the end of rehabilitation. Training and rest days are key components in returning the athlete based off this injury etiology. See Table 28-4 for a return-to-running protocol. Increasing training volume by no more than 10% per week allows adaptation to mechanical stress as speed and intensity are gradually reintroduced.[24]

SUMMARY

1. Soft-tissue injuries to the hip, thigh, and groin can be extremely disabling and often require a substantial amount of time for full rehabilitation.
2. Early return after soft-tissue injury to the thigh often exacerbates the problem.
3. Previous injury to the soft tissues about the hip and thigh predispose athletes to additional injury, especially if not rehabilitated fully.
4. Pathologies of the acetabular labrum are more common than once thought and often treated with arthroscopic surgery and subsequent rehabilitation.
5. Snapping or clicking hip syndrome occurs most commonly when the ITB snaps over the greater trochanter causing trochanteric bursitis.
6. Hip dislocations are rare, but require careful rehabilitation in order to return the patient/client to full function.
7. The femur is subject to stress fractures (uncommon) and avulsion fractures.
8. Different patterns of injury exist in the skeletally mature (adult) patient than in the skeletally immature patient (children and adolescents).
9. Protection after soft-tissue injury is important to prevent further injury (padding, wrapping, compression shorts/sleeves).

REFERENCES

1. Berend KR, Vail TP. Hip arthroscopy in the adolescent and pediatric athlete. *Clin Sports Med.* 2001;20(4):763-778.
2. Byrd JW, Jones KS. Hip arthroscopy in athletes. *Clin Sports Med.* 2001;20(4):749-761.
3. Culpepper MI, Niemann KM. High school football injuries in Birmingham, Alabama. *South Med J.* 1983;76(7):873-875, 878.
4. Gomez E, DeLee JC, Farney WC. Incidence of injury in Texas girls' high school basketball. *Am J Sports Med.* 1996;24:684-687.
5. DeLee JC, Farney WC. Incidence of injury in texas high school football. *Am J Sports Med.* 1992;20:575-580.
6. Anderson K, Strickland SM, Warren R. Hip and groin injuries in athletes. *Am J Sports Med.* 2001;29(4): 521-533.
7. Norkin CC, Levangie PK. *Joint Structure and Function.* 2nd ed. Philadelphia, PA: FA Davis; 1992.
8. Moore KL. *Clinically Oriented Anatomy.* 3rd ed. Baltimore, MD: Lippincott Williams & Wilkins; 1992.
9. Ganz R, Parvizi J, Beck M, Leunig M, Notzli H, Siebenrock K. Femoroacetabular impingement: A cause for osteoarthritis of the hip. *Clin Orthop Relat Res.* 2003;417(12):112-120.
10. Sahrmann, SA. *Diagnosis and Treatment of Movement Impairment Syndromes.* St. Louis, MO: Mosby; 2002.
11. Smith ZK, Weiss EL, Lehmkuhl DL. *Brunstrom's Clinical Kinesiology.* 5th ed. 1996.
12. Lynch SA, Renstrom PA. Groin injuries in sport: treatment strategies. *Sports Med.* 1999;28(2):137-144.
13. Emery CA, Meeuwisse WH, Powell JW. 1. Groin and abdominal strain injuries in the National Hockey League. *Clin J Sport Med.* 1999;9:151-156.
14. Ekstrand J, Gillquist J. The avoidability of soccer injuries. *Int J Sports Med.* 1983;4:124-128.
15. Sim FH, Chao EY. Injury potential in modern ice hockey. *Am J Sports Med.* 1978;6(6):378-384.
16. Tegner Y, Lorentzon R. Ice hockey injuries: Incidence, nature and causes. *Br J Sports Med.* 1991;25(2):87-89.

17. Tyler TF, Nicholas SJ, Campbell RJ, McHugh MP. The association of hip strength and flexibility on the incidence of groin strains in professional ice hockey players. *Am J Sports Med.* 2001;29(2):124-128.
18. Holmich P, Uhrskou P, Ulnits L, et al. Effectiveness of active physical training as treatment for long-standing adductor-related groin pain in athletes: Randomized trial. *Lancet.* 1999;353:339-443.
19. Kendall FP, McCreary EK. *Muscles: Testing and Function.* Baltimore, MD: Williams and Wilkins; 3:1983.
20. Renstrom P, Peterson L. Groin injuries in athletes. *Br J Sports Med.* 1980;14:30-36.
21. Lynch SA, Renstrom PA. Groin injuries in sport: treatment strategies. *Sports Med.* 1999;28(2):137-144.
22. Meyers WC, Ricciardi R, Busconi BD, et al. *Groin Pain in Athletes.* 1999:281-289.
23. Speer KP, Lohnes J, Garrett WE. Radiographic imaging of muscle strain injury. *Am J Sports Med.* 1993;21(1):89-96.
24. Anderson K, Strickland SM, Warren R. Hip and groin injuries in athletes. *Am J Sports Med.* 2001;29(4):521-533.
25. Tyler TF, Campbell R, Nicholas SJ, Donellan S, McHugh MP. The effectiveness of a preseason exercise program on the prevention of groin strains in professional ice hockey players. *Am J Sports Med.* 2002;30(5):680-683.
26. Jorgenson U, Schmidt-Olsen S. The epidemiology of ice hockey injuries. *Br J Sports Med.* 1986;20(1):7-9.
27. Sim FH, Simonet WT, Malton JM, Lehn T. Ice hockey injuries. *Am J Sports Med.* 1987;15(1):30-40.
28. Lorentzon R, Wedren H, Pietila T. Incidences, nature, and causes of ice hockey injuries: a three year prospective study of a Swedish elite ice hockey team. *Am J Sports Med.* 1988;16:392-396.
29. Molsa J, Airaksinen O, Nasman O, Torstila I. Ice hockey injuries in Finland. A prospective epidemiologic study. *Am J Sports Med.* 1997;25(4):495-499.
30. Nielsen A, Yde J. Epidemiology and traumatology of injuries in soccer. *Am J Sports Med.* 1989;17:803-807.
31. Knapik JJ, Bauman CL, Jones BH, Harris JM, Vaughan L. Preseason strength and flexibility imbalances associated with athletic injuries in female athletes collegiate athletes. *Am J Sports Med.* 1991;19(1):76-81.
32. Orchard J, Marsden J, Lord S, Garlick D. Preseason hamstring muscle weakness associated with hamstring muscle injury in Australian footballers. *Am J Sports Med.* 1997;25(1):495-499.
33. Emery CA, Meeuwisse WH. Risk factors for groin injuries in hockey. *Med Sci Sports Exerc.* 2001;33(9): 1423-1433.
34. Seward H, Orchard J, Hazard H. Collinson: Football injuries in Australia at the elite level. *Med J Aust.* 1993;159:298-301.
35. Garrett WE Jr. Muscle strain injuries: clinical and basic aspects. *Med Sci Sports Exerc.* 1990;(22):436-443.
36. De Smet AA, Best TM. MR imaging of the distribution and location of acute hamstring injuries in athletes. *AJR Am J Roentgenol.* 2000;(174):393-399.
37. Wootton JR, Cross MJ, Holt KW. Avulsion of the ischial apophysis. The case for open reduction and internal fixation. *J Bone Joint Surg Br.* 1990;72:625-627.
38. Brooks JH, Fuller CW, Kemp SP, et al. Incidence, risk and prevention of hamstring muscle injuries in professional rugby union. *Am J Sports Med.* 2006;34: 1297-1306.
39. Woods C, Hawkins RD, Maltby S, et al. The Football Association Medical Research Programme: an audit of injuries in professional football—analysis of hamstring injuries. *Br J Sports Med.* 2004;38:36-41.
40. Ekstrand J, Hagglund M, Walden M. Epidemiology of muscle injuries in professional football (soccer). *Am J Sports Med.* 2011;29:1226-1232.
41. Elliot MC, Zarins B, Powell JW, et al. Hamstring strains in professional football players: a 10 year review. *Am J Sports Med.* 2011;39:1621-1628.
42. Orchard J, Seward H. Epidemiology of injuries in the Australian Football League, seasons 1997-2000. *Br J Sports Med.* 2002;36:39-44.
43. Malliaropoulos N, Isinkaye T, Tsitas K, et al. Reinjury after acute posterior thigh muscle strains in elite track and field athletes. *Am J Sports Med.* 2011;39:304-310.
44. Marcus C, Elliot CW, Zarins B, et al. Hamstring muscle strains in professional football players: 10 Year review. *Am J Sports Med.* 2011;39:843-850.
45. Fousekis K, Tsepis E, Poulmedis P. Intrinsic risk factors of noncontact quadriceps and hamstring strains in soccer: a prospective study of 100 professional players. *Br J Sports Med.* 2011;45:709-714.
46. Watsford ML, Murphy AJ, McLachlan KA, et al. A prospective study of the relationship between lower body stiffness and hamstring injury in professional Australian rules footballers. *Am J Sports Med.* 2010;38(10):2058-2064.
47. Small K, McNaughton LR, Greig M, et al. Soccer fatigue, sprinting, and hamstring injury risk. *Int J Sports Med.* 2009;8:587.
48. Sherry MA, Best TM. A comparison of 2 rehabilitation programs in the treatment of acute hamstring strains. *J Orthop Sports Phys Ther.* 2004;34(3):116-125.
49. Worrell TW. Factors associated with Hamstring injuries. An approach to treatment and preventative measures. *Sports Med.* 1994;17:338-345.
50. Hennessey L, Watson AW. Flexibility and posture assessment in relation to hamstring injury. *Br J Sports Med.* 1993;27:243-246.
51. Engebretsen AH, Myklebust G, Holme I, et al. Intrinsic risk factors for hamstring injuries among male soccer players: a prospective cohort study. *Am J Sports Med.* 2010;38(6):1147-1153.
52. Hägglund M, Waldén M, Ekstrand J. Previous injury as a risk factor for injury in elite football: a prospective study over two consecutive seasons. *Br J Sports Med.* 2006;40(9):767-772.
53. Verral GM, Slavotinek JP, Barnes PG, et al. Clinical risk factors for hamstring muscle strain injury: a prospective

study with correlation of injury by magnetic resonance imaging. *Br J Sports Med.* 2001;35(6):435-439.

54. Croisier JL. Factors associated with recurrent hamstring injuries. *Sports Med.* 2004;34(10):681-695.
55. Ekstrand J, Gillquist J. Soccer injuries and their mechanisms: a prospective study. *Med Sci Sports Exerc.* 1983;15(3): 267-270.
56. Heiser TM, Weber J, Sullivan G, et al. Prophylaxis and management of hamstring muscle injuries in intercollegiate football players. *Am J Sports Med.* 1984;12(5):368-370.
57. Arnason A, Andersen TE, Holme I, Engebretsen L, Bahr R. Prevention of hamstring strains in elite soccer: an intervention study. *Scand J Med Sci Sports.* 2008;18:40-48.
58. Petersen J, Thorborg K, Bachmann M, et al. preventive effect of eccentric training on acute hamstring injuries in men's soccer: a cluster randomized control trial. *Am J Sports Med.* 2011;39:2296-2303.
59. Nikolau P, Macdonald B, Glisson R, Seaber A, Garrett W. Biomechanical and histological evaluation of muscle after controlled strain injury. *Am J Sports Med.* 1987;15(1):9-14.
60. Frenette J, Cote CH. Modulation of structural protein content of the myotendinous junction following eccentric contractions. *Int J Sports Med.* 2000;21(5):313-320.
61. Mackey A, Donnelly A, Turpeenniemi-Hujanen T, Roper H. Skeletal muscle collagen content in humans following high force eccentric contractions. *J Appl Physiol.* 2004;97(1):197-203.
62. Brockett CL, Morgan DL, Proske U. Predicting hamstring strain injury in elite soccer: an intervention study. *Med Sci Sports Exerc.* 2004;44: 647-658.
63. Schmitt B, Tyler T, McHugh M. Clinical commentary: hamstring injury rehabilitation and prevention of reinjury using lengthened state eccentric training: a new concept. *Int J Sports Med.* 2012;7(3):1-9.
64. Salter RB. *Textbook of Disorders and Injuries of the Musculoskeletal System.* 3rd ed. Baltimore, MD: Williams and Wilkins; 1999.
65. Kujala UM, Orava S, Karpakka J, et al. Ischial tuberosity apophysitis and avulsion among athletes. *Int J Sports Med.* 1997;18(2):149-155.
66. Ly JQ, Bui-Mansfield LT, Taylor, DC. Radiologic demonstration of temporal development of bizarre parosteal osteochondromatous proliferation. *Clin Imaging.* 2004;28(3):216-218.
67. McBryne AM Jr. Stress fractured in runners. *Clin Sports Med.* 1985;4:737-752.
68. O'Kane JW. Anterior hip pain. *Am Fam Physician.* 1999;60(6):1687-1696.
69. Hecox B, Mehreteab TA, Weisberg J. *Physical Agents: A Comprehensive Text for Physical Therapists.* Upper Saddle River, NJ: Prentice Hall; 1994.
70. Cameron MH. *Physical Agents in Rehabilitation: From Research to Practice.* Philadelphia, PA: WB Saunders; 1999.
71. Vanden Bossche L, Vanderstraeten G. Heterotopic ossification: a review. *J Rehabil Med.* 2005;37(3):129-136.
72. Berg E. Deep muscle contusion complicated by myositis ossificans (a.k.a. heterotopic bone). *Orthop Nurs.* 2000;19(6):66-67.
73. Cetin C, Sekir U, Yildiz Y, Aydin T, Ors F, Kalyon TA. Chronic groin pain in an amateur soccer player. *Br J Sports Med.* 2004;38(2):223-224.
74. Chudick S, Answorth A, Lopez V, et al. Hip dislocations in athletes. *Sports Med Arthroscopic Rev.* 2002;10:123-133.
75. Scudese VA. Traumatic anterior hip redislocation. A case report. *Clin Orthop.* 1972;88:60-63.
76. Tennent TD, Chambler AF, Rossouw DJ. Posterior dislocation of the hip while playing basketball. *Br J Sports Med.* 1998;32(4):342-343.
77. Keene GS, Villar RN. Arthroscopic anatomy of the hip: an in vivo study. *Arthroscopy.* 1994;10(4):392-399.
78. Byrd JW, Jones KS. Diagnostic accuracy of clinical assessment, magnetic resonance imaging, magnetic resonance arthrography, and intra-articular injection in hip arthroscopy patients. *Am J Sports Med.* 2004;32(7): 1668-1674.
79. Byrd JW. Hip arthroscopy in athletes. *Instr Course Lect.* 2003;52:701-709.
80. Byrd JW, Jones KS. Prospective analysis of hip arthroscopy with 2-year follow-up. *Arthroscopy.* 2000;16(6):578-587.
81. Shbeeb MI, Matteson EL. Trochanteric bursitis (greater trochanter pain syndrome). *Mayo Clin Proc.* 1996;71(6):565-569.
82. Shbeeb MI, O'Duffy JD, Michet CJ Jr, O'Fallon WM, Matteson EL. Evaluation of glucocorticosteroid injection for the treatment of trochanteric bursitis. *J Rheumatol.* 1996;23(12):2104-2106.
83. Gerber JM, Herrin SO. Conservative treatment of calcific trochanteric bursitis. *J Manipulative Physiol Ther.* 1994;17(4):250-252.
84. Schaberg JE, Harper MC, Allen WC. The snapping hip syndrome. *Am J Sports Med.* 1984;12(5):361-365.
85. Reid DC. Prevention of hip and knee injuries in ballet dancers. *Sports Med.* 1988;6(5):295-307.
86. Zoltan DJ, Clancy WG Jr, Keene JS. A new operative approach to snapping hip and refractory trochanteric bursitis in athletes. *Am J Sports Med.* 1986;14(3):201-204.
87. Fricker PA, Taunton JE, Ammann W. Osteitis pubis in athletes. Infection, inflammation or injury? *Sports Med.* 1991;12(4):266-279.
88. Batt ME, McShane JM, Dillingham MF. Osteitis pubis in collegiate football players. *Med Sci Sports Exerc.* 1995;27(5):629-633.
89. Holt MA, Keene JS, Graf BK, Helwig DC. Treatment of osteitis pubis in athletes. Results of corticosteroid infections. *Am J Sports Med.* 1995;23(5):601-606.
90. Junqueira LC, Carneiro J, Kelly RO. *Basic Histology.* 9th ed. New York, NY: Long; 1998.
91. Monteleone GP Jr. Stress fractures in the athletes. *Orthop Clin North Am.* 1995;26:423-432.
92. Haverstock BD. Stress fractures of the foot and ankle. *Clin Podiatr Med Surg.* 2001;18:273-284.

93. Maitria RS, Johnson DL. Stress fractures. Clinical history and physical examination. *Clin Sports Med.* 1997;16(2):259-274.

94. Knapp ME. Late treatment of fractures and complications. 2. *Postgrad Med* 1966;40(2):A113-A118.

95. Shin AY, Gillingham BL. Fatigue fractures of the femoral neck in athletes. *J Am Acad Orthop Surg.* 1997;5(6):293-302.

96. Volpin G, Hoerer D, Groisman G, Zaltsman S, Stein H. Stress fractures of the femoral neck following strenuous activity. *J Orthop Trauma*. 1990;4:394-398.

97. Benell KL, Malcolm SA, Thomas SA, et al. Risk factors for stress fractures in track and field athletes. Twelve month prospective study. *Am J Sports Med.* 1996;24:810-818.

98. Fullerton LR, Snoway HA. Femoral neck stress fractures. *Am J Sports Med.* 1998;16:365-377.

24

Rehabilitation of the Knee

Robert C. Manske, B.J. Lehecka, Mark De Carlo, and Ryan McDivitt

OBJECTIVES

After completion of this chapter, the physical therapist should be able to do the following:

- Understand the functional biomechanics associated with normal function of the knee.
- Utilize a general rehabilitation progression when treating knee injuries.
- Integrate a comprehensive understanding of pathomechanics and mechanism of injury into the rehabilitation of ligamentous and meniscal injuries.
- Integrate a comprehensive understanding of pathomechanics and mechanism of injury into the rehabilitation of patellofemoral and extensor mechanism injuries.
- Justify the use of external supports to augment the rehabilitation process.
- Implement a functional progression to ensure safe return to activity.

Functional Biomechanics of the Knee

The study of biomechanics, along with functional anatomy, is a cornerstone to knee rehabilitation. A complete understanding of joint articulations, arthrokinematics, and the structures responsible for controlling movement is essential for the clinician to make sound decisions in the diagnosis and treatment of musculoskeletal disorders. Despite the relative simplicity of a hinge-type joint, the knee provides an interesting biomechanical study because of the intricacies required to maintain stability without good bony support along with attenuating forces greater than 4 times the weight of the body. The patellofemoral joint and the pain syndromes often associated with the knee also present an interesting study. A solid knowledge of the supporting structures and stress placed on the patellofemoral joint provides the framework for rehabilitation program design.

Tibiofemoral Joint

Tibiofemoral Articulation: Menisci-Femoral Condyles

The condyles of the distal femur articulate with the shallow, concave tibial plateau, resulting in significant tibiofemoral joint incongruence. Tibiofemoral stability would be insufficient if left solely to the skeletal structure. The medial and lateral menisci provide additional congruency to the joint through their semicircular shape and peripheral thickness, thus forming a wedge surrounding the femoral condyles.

The contact area of the menisci varies significantly during knee range of motion (ROM). In weight bearing, the total contact area of the menisci decreases with knee flexion. Although mean surface area increases in non-weightbearing conditions, total menisci contact area also decreases during knee flexion. Following a meniscectomy, surface contact area decreases, resulting in a greater amount of stress upon the contact surface.

Axial Forces

The ability of the tibiofemoral joint to withstand forces imposed by the superincumbent weight of the body combined with the ground reaction force transmitted through the distal extremity requires interaction of multiple structural factors. The longitudinal axis of the femur extends laterally to medially to the tibiofemoral articulation, resulting in an oblique angle formed 5 to 10 degrees away from vertical. It would seem that this alignment would produce a greater load on the lateral femoral condyle; however, a close look at the mechanical axis that connects the head of the femur with the superior surface of the talus contradicts this. The mechanical axis, which is the true line of weight bearing and determines the angle of force distribution, produces approximately equal weight bearing on the lateral and medial compartments of the tibiofemoral joints during bilateral stance.

Arthrokinematics

Arthrokinematics is a description of the accessory motion that occurs between articulating surfaces. The accessory motions of rolling and gliding of the joint surfaces occur in combination during the osteokinematic motion at the knee. This combination allows the articulating surfaces to stay in contact and permit maximal osteokinematic motion.

Arthrokinematic motion plays a prominent role in sagittal plane movements of the tibiofemoral joint. During knee flexion in the closed kinetic chain (CKC), the convex femur moves on a fixed, concave tibia. When a convex surface is moving on a concave surface, rolling and gliding occur in opposite directions. Because of this relationship, the femur must glide anteriorly to counteract the posteriorly directed roll that is occurring (Figure 24-1).

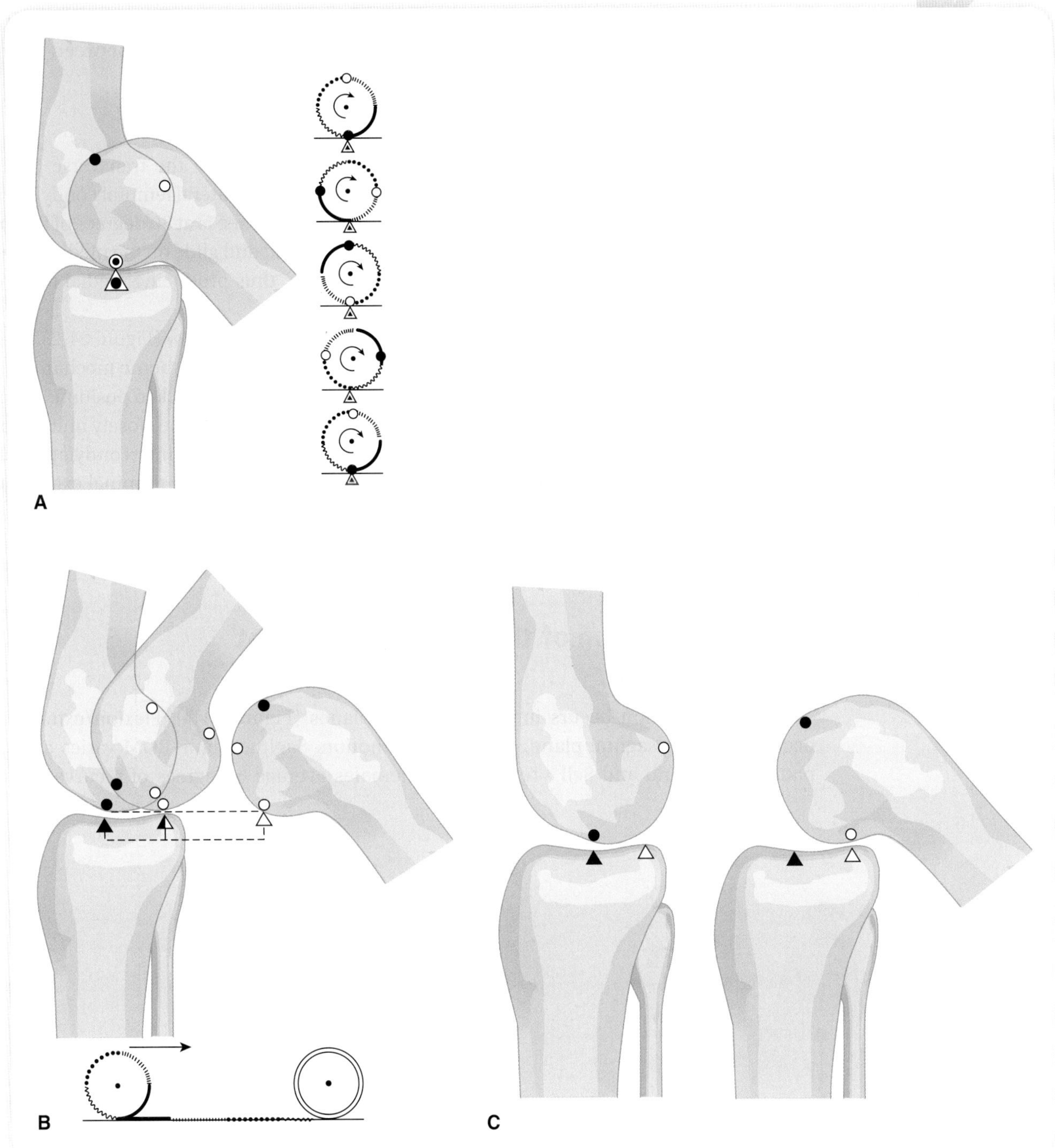

Figure 24-1 Arthrokinematic motion

A. Anterior gliding of the femur on the tibia. **B.** Posterior rolling of the femur on the tibia. **C.** Both gliding and rolling. (Reproduced from Scott WN. *The Knee*. St. Louis, MO: Mosby; 1994:77, with permission from Elsevier.)

Without the anterior glide of the femur, tibiofemoral flexion would be limited, as the femur would roll off the posterior tibia. During CKC knee extension, the femur rolls anteriorly and glides posteriorly. In the open kinetic chain (OKC), the concave tibia moves on the convex femur as rolling and gliding occur anteriorly with extension and posteriorly with flexion.

Although rolling and gliding must both occur to keep the tibia and femur in contact, the rolling and gliding do not happen simultaneously as the knee flexes. At the initiation of flexion, pure rolling occurs between the joint surfaces, with gliding becoming more prominent to terminal flexion. Once the gliding starts in early flexion, the ratio between rolling and gliding is 1:2, progressing to a 1:4 ratio at terminal flexion.

Screw-Home Mechanism

Near terminal knee extension, arthrokinematic motion occurs in the transverse plane. Because the medial femoral condyle is 1 to 2 cm longer than the lateral femoral condyle, the lateral femoral condyle completes all of its motion when the knee is at 30 degrees of flexion in a weight-bearing position. As the knee continues to extend and glide on the medial femoral condyle, it pivots on the fixed lateral femoral condyle, thus producing medial femoral rotation on the fixed tibia.

Rotation at terminal extension, called the *screw-home mechanism* (Figure 24-2), is an involuntary motion that occurs because of bony geometry. The screw-home mechanism is crucial for knee stability, locking the tibiofemoral joint into a close-packed position. As the femur internally rotates on the fixed tibia, the femoral condyles become closely united and congruent with the menisci, the tibial tubercles becomes lodged in the intercondylar notch, and the ligaments become taut. For the tibiofemoral joint to flex from terminal extension, the joint must first unlock. While this is also an automatic motion caused by the bony structure of the femoral condyles, the popliteus can initiate the lateral rotation of the femur on a fixed tibia to begin the unlocking of the tibiofemoral joint.

Kinematic Motion of the Tibiofemoral Joint

Flexion/extension

Tibiofemoral motion occurs in the 3 cardinal planes (Figure 24-3). Flexion/extension, occurring in the sagittal plane, is the largest motion. Sagittal plane ROM varies among patients. De Carlo and Sell[32] reported that females average 6 degrees of recurvatum to

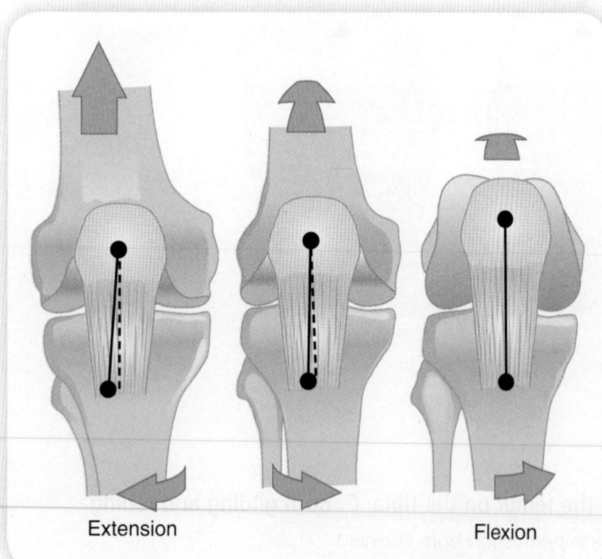

Figure 24-2 **The tibia externally rotates as the knee moves into terminal extension, creating a "screw-home" mechanism**

(Reproduced from Scott WN. *The Knee*. St. Louis, MO: Mosby; 1994:22, with permission from Elsevier.)

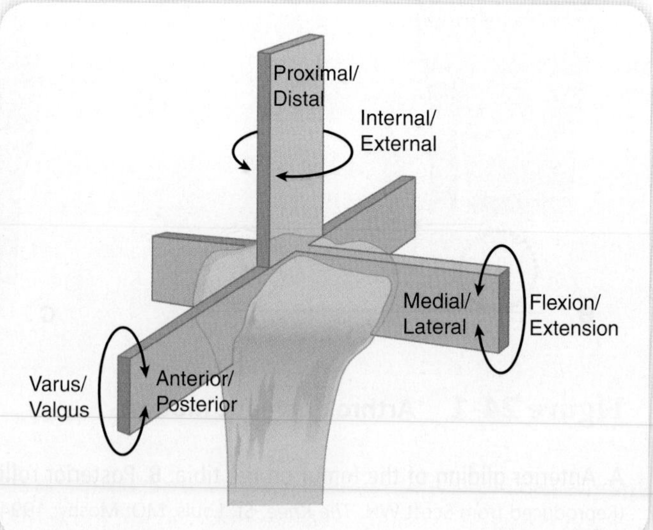

Figure 24-3 **Knee motion in each plane occurs around an axis**

(Reproduced from Scott WN. *The Knee*. St. Louis, MO: Mosby; 1994:17, with permission from Elsevier.)

143 degrees of flexion, whereas males average 5 degrees of recurvatum to 140 degrees of flexion. During sagittal plane motion, the instantaneous axis of rotation of the knee also varies. A study of a series of roentgenograms illustrated that the instantaneous axis of rotation forms a semicircle (Figure 24-4).[85] An abnormal instantaneous axis of rotation can result from internal derangement in the tibiofemoral joint, causing a compensatory attenuation of static supporting structures of the knee. These abnormal stresses on the articulating surfaces can result in early degenerative changes.

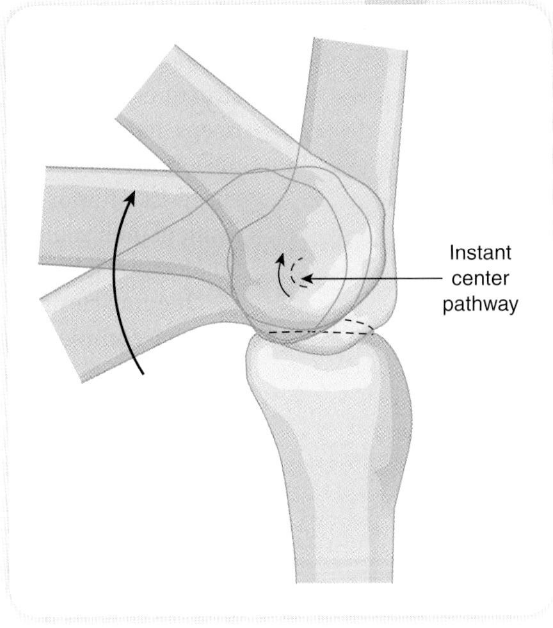

Figure 24-4 Normal instantaneous axis of rotation forms a semicircle

(Reproduced from Scott WN. *The Knee*. St. Louis, MO: Mosby; 1994:76, with permission from Elsevier.)

Rotation

Motion in the transverse plane is influenced by the position of the knee in the sagittal plane. In the close-packed position (terminal extension), motion in the transverse plane cannot occur. Rotation is greatest at 90 degrees of knee flexion. In this position, lateral rotation averages 45 degrees and medial rotation averages 30 degrees.[85] The axis for tibiofemoral rotation runs longitudinally through the medial tibial intercondylar tubercle.

Abduction/Adduction

Only a small amount of tibiofemoral motion occurs in the frontal plane. Similar to rotation, this motion is dictated by the position of the knee in the sagittal plane. Abduction and adduction, primarily limited by ligaments, reach a maximum at 30 degrees of knee flexion. The muscles do not contribute motion to the frontal plane.

Knee Stability

Stability of the tibiofemoral joint is of primary concern in the orthopedic setting. Although the bony structures of the knee contribute to stability in terminal extension, the knee must rely on soft tissues for stability during most of the degrees of movement. Injury to these structures (the menisci, muscles, and ligaments) often results in debilitating instability.

A review of the literature related to knee stability reveals varied and often contradictory information on the roles of different support structures.[68] The differences in results are because studies often test knee stability in a static scenario and in varied positions. Although describing the stabilizers individually provides a "clean and neat" presentation, one must remember that most of the structures work together to provide knee stability in all motions.

Menisci

The menisci contribute mainly to force distribution and dissipation, although they can provide a degree of stability to the tibiofemoral joint. Johnson et al[77] have made clinical observations that joint laxity can result after meniscectomy. The belief that the medial and lateral menisci act as anterior and posterior wedges to prevent anteroposterior movement is supported by several studies that found that resection of the medial meniscus resulted in more instability than resection of the lateral meniscus.[90,91,92,150] The studies often found that resection of the anterior cruciate ligament (ACL) exposed a greater reliance on the menisci for stability, but that the medial supporting structures must be intact for more effective stability.

Muscular Contributions

As the tibiofemoral joint becomes loaded, stability can be gained from multiple dynamic structures. The main muscular contributors to anteroposterior stabilization are the quadriceps, hamstring, gastrocnemius, and popliteus muscles. The quadriceps complex resists posteriorly directed forces on the tibia, while the hamstrings, gastrocnemius, and popliteus resist anterior displacement of the tibia. The popliteus and the semimembranosus, as a result of their multiple connections, are particularly crucial in the stability of the posterior tibiofemoral joint.

The muscles that contribute to medial stability as the knee flexes are part of the pes anserine complex (Figure 24-5). The iliotibial tract, popliteus, and biceps femoris provide lateral stability (Figure 24-6), but the popliteus is the main contributor, particularly in the posterolateral direction. It is uncertain what effect the dynamic structures have on rotational stabilization, but the position and action of the popliteus and hamstring muscles would suggest a minor contribution to rotational stability.

Ligaments and Stability

The role of ligaments in knee stability has been widely substantiated in the scientific literature as well as by practical clinical observations of ligament disruption. Ligaments enhance

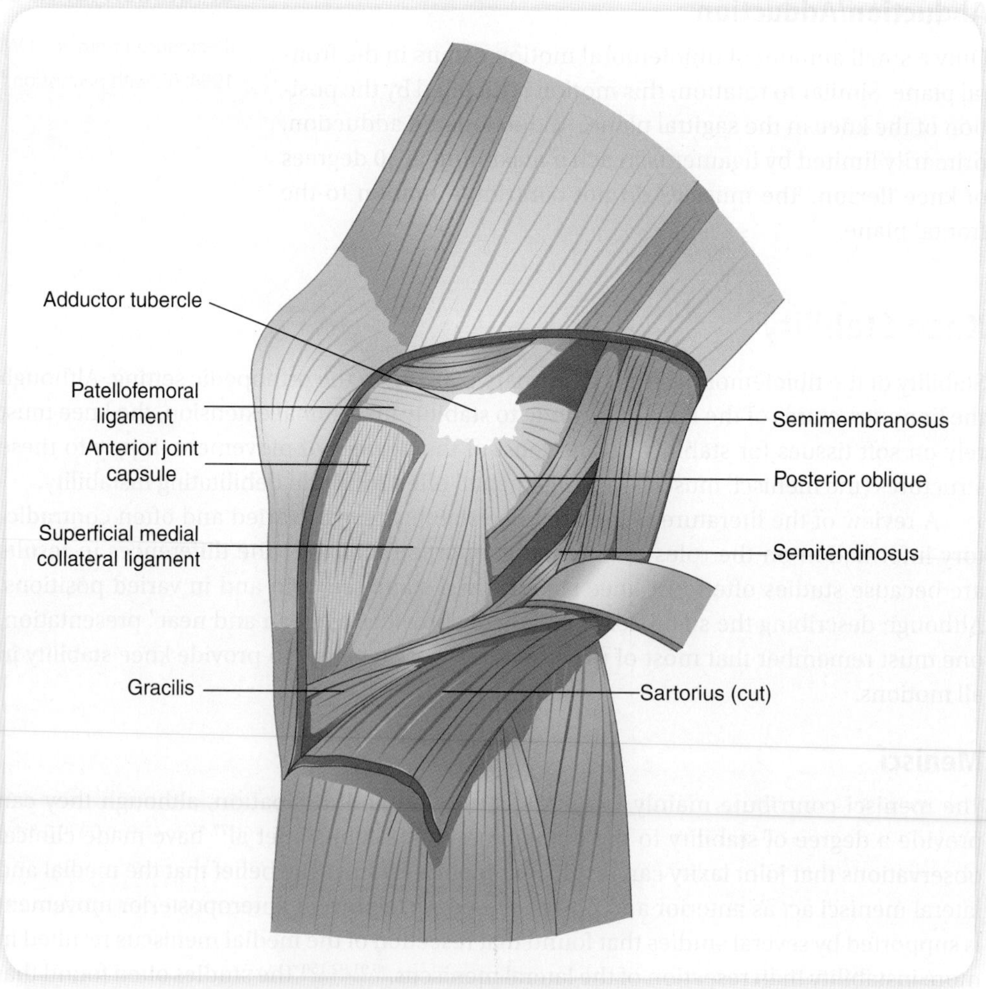

Figure 24-5 Medial static and dynamic stabilizers of the knee

(Reproduced from Scott WN. *The Knee*. St. Louis, MO: Mosby; 1994:36, with permission from Elsevier.)

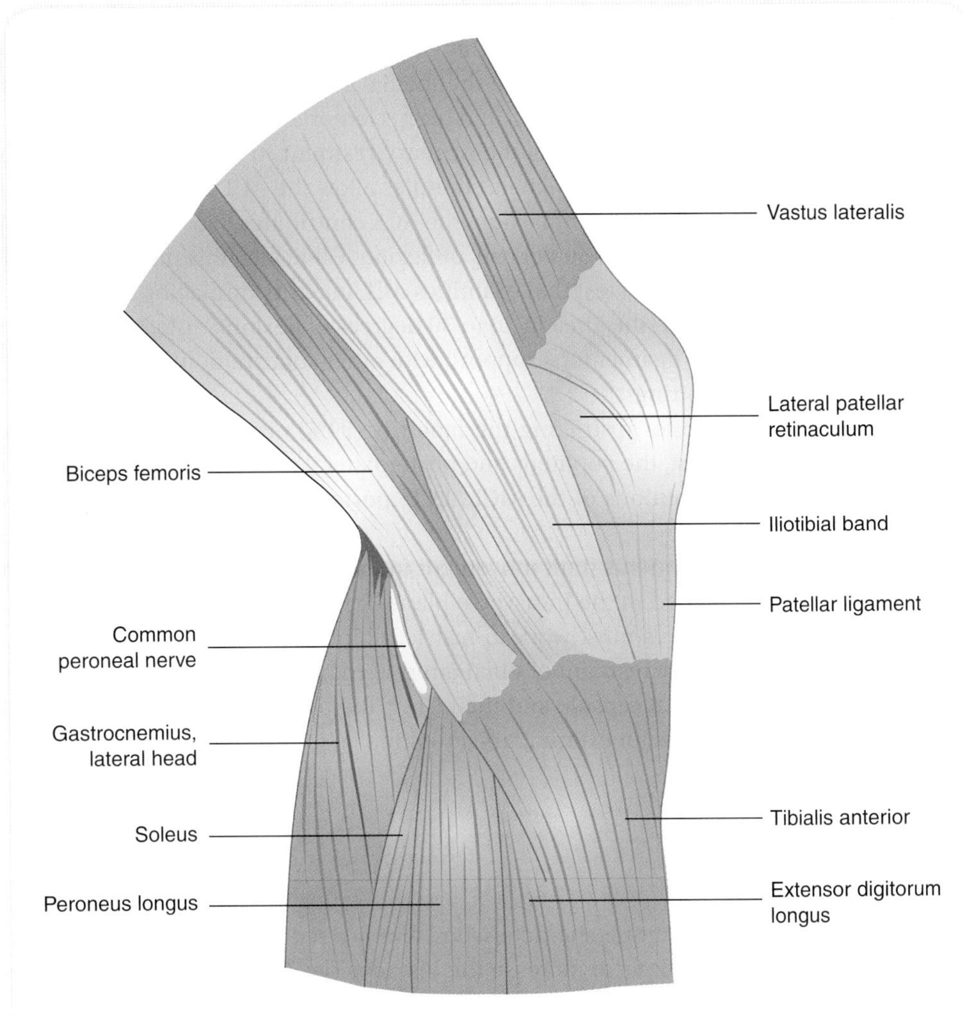

Figure 24-6 Lateral dynamic stabilizers of the knee

(Reproduced from Scott WN. *The Knee*. St. Louis, MO: Mosby; 1994:40, with permission from Elsevier.)

knee stability by their ability to restrict tensile forces along the orientation of their fibers. Knee stability is reliant on multiple ligamentous, meniscal, muscular, or bony structures. This is an important factor to consider when studying the biomechanics of ligaments, because no ligament acts alone in limiting knee motion, nor does 1 ligament limit 1 plane of movement.

The medial collateral ligament (MCL) is the primary stabilizer against valgus stress. Studies in which the superficial fibers of the MCL were disrupted showed an increase in knee valgus following an externally directed force. The superficial fibers also limited external rotation of the tibia, whereas sectioning the deeper fibers of the MCL did not significantly increase valgus movement or external rotation.[60] Secondary restraints include the ACL, posterior cruciate ligament (PCL) (especially at terminal extension), and the lateral compartment because of the increased compressive forces.[139]

The lateral collateral ligament (LCL) is the primary restraint to varus forces. The restraining effect of the LCL increases as the knee flexes. The LCL's maximal contribution in limiting lateral joint opening is 69% at 25 degrees of knee flexion. The ACL and PCL contribute as secondary stabilizers and provide maximal protection against varus forces at 8 degrees of flexion, but then decrease as the knee flexes. The lateral joint capsule, particularly the posterior portion, contributes to stability, but this effect also decreases with increased knee flexion.[55] Other secondary restraints include the medial compartment through compression and the popliteus, iliotibial band (ITB), and biceps femoris.

It is well established that the ACL is the primary restraint to anterior translation of the tibia. The anteromedial and posterolateral bundles allow the ACL to be taut during all ranges of knee motion. At 90 degrees of flexion, the ACL contributes 85% of the restraining force and this force increases up to 30 degrees of flexion. Clinically, this property is demonstrated by the classic Lachman test that examines ACL integrity by placing an anteriorly directed force to the tibia with the knee in 20 to 30 degrees of flexion.[21] The MCL and LCL provide minimal secondary ligamentous support, with other contributions from the posterior capsule, ITB, and hamstrings.

The PCL is responsible for restricting the majority (94%) or posterior tibial translation. If the PCL is not present, the popliteus and posterolateral capsule provide most of the support, with minor contributions of the MCL, LCL, posteromedial capsule, and medial capsule.

As noted previously, ligaments limit movement in the direction of the fibers. Because there is not a ligament aligned in the transverse plane, it is evident that a combination of ligaments and other structures must work to restrict tibiofemoral rotation. The ACL has been shown to be the primary restraint of tibial internal rotation, with secondary restraint provided by the posteromedial capsule and the LCL.[93] The posterolateral capsule and the MCL are the primary restraints for external tibial rotation.

Patellofemoral Joint

Functions of the Patella

The patella possesses very unique characteristics that are required for normal function of the knee. The patella functions to increase the distance (lever arm) from the joint axis, increase leverage of the quadriceps through gliding in the trochlear, provide a smooth articular surface, and provide a bony shield to the trochlea and condyles of the distal femur during knee flexion.[79]

The length of the lever arm changes from knee flexion to extension, modulating the force production that the patella provides. In full flexion, there is little anterior displacement of the quadriceps tendon. Thus, the patella contributes only 10% to the length of the lever arm in this position. As the knee extends, the patella migrates superiorly and anteriorly in the trochlear groove, leading to a greater mechanical advantage. The mechanical advantage reaches its peak at 45 degrees of knee flexion, where the patella contributes 30% to the lever arm. As the knee nears terminal extension, the effect of the patella on quadriceps force (Fq) decreases to the point where the quadriceps muscles must generate 60% more force to perform the last 15 degrees of knee extension. The inability of weakened quadriceps to perform this motion is demonstrated by a quadriceps lag during a straight-leg raise.

Patellofemoral Contact Areas

As the knee goes through a ROM, various portions of the patella articulate with the trochlea (Figure 24-7). Goodfellow et al[56] described the contact surfaces of the patellofemoral joint at different points of knee flexion during weightbearing conditions. At terminal extension, the patella lies slightly lateral and proximal to the trochlea without contact. The patella engages with the bony groove between 10 to 20 degrees of flexion. The area of contact is initiated at the inferior pole of the patella and moves superiorly on the retropatellar surface until 90 degrees of flexion, where the major contact point is on the superior pole. The contact of the patella from lateral to medial also varies with knee motion. During the first 90 degrees of flexion, the contact is exclusively lateral. After 90 degrees, the contact moves medially to the odd facet.

Patellofemoral Joint Reaction Force and Joint Stress

The amount of force that the posterior surface of the patella encounters with various activities is well documented. Clinically, understanding the ROM and load optimal for patellofemoral joint contact forces is very useful in treating patellofemoral disorders that result from abnormal force on the posterior surface of the patella. Patellofemoral joint reaction force[149] (Fpf) is determined by the following equation:

$$Fpf = kXFq$$

At a specific point of knee ROM, the amount of *Fq* multiplied by the angle of knee flexion (*X*) equals *Fpf*, or Fpf = kXFq, where *k* is a constant that is predetermined for each angle of knee flexion.

The amount of force that the patella encounters does not fully reveal the amount of stress placed on the patella. *Joint surface stress* is determined by the amount of force placed on a given area of joint surface. This relationship is expressed by the equation force/area = stress. Thus, the less area to which a force is applied, the greater amount of stress is applied to the joint. The amount of stress that is on a given point of the patella has important clinical implications. It is the amount of stress, not simply the joint reaction force, that can inflict abnormal wear or pain on the posterior surface of the patella.[59]

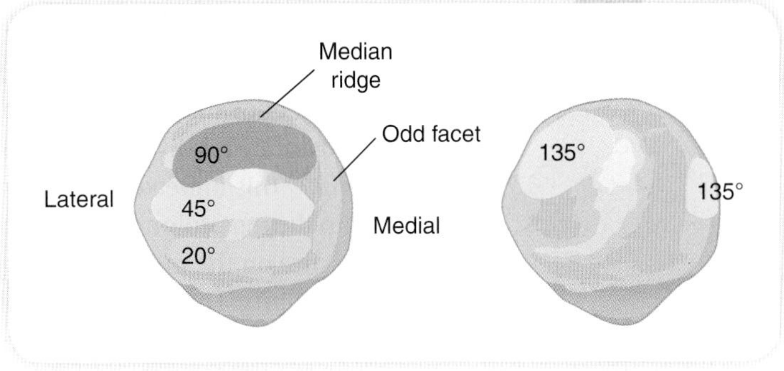

Figure 24-7 **Patellofemoral contact areas during varying degrees of flexion**

(Reproduced from Scott WN. *The Knee*. St. Louis, MO: Mosby; 1994:22, with permission from Elsevier.)

OKC Joint Reaction Force During OKC function, Fpf increases as the knee extends from 90 degrees of knee flexion. At 90 degrees of flexion, the patellar tendon and quadriceps muscles are perpendicular to each other and Fq tends to result in a low Fpf. As the knee extends from 90 to 60 degrees of knee flexion, Fq must increase, resulting in increased Fpf. After 60 degrees of knee flexion, Fq levels off and Fpf is relatively unchanged to end range.

OKC Joint Stress As a result of decreased joint surface area contact during knee extension, joint stress increases from 90 degrees of flexion to approximately 20 degrees of extension. Typically, there is little to no patellar contact area past 20 degrees of flexion to terminal extension; thus, joint stress often does not occur during this range. For the patients who do maintain some contact in this ROM, joint stress will be very high owing to the small contact area.

CKC Joint Reaction Force Investigation of joint reaction force in the CKC shows that in contrast to the OKC, Fpf decreases as the knee extends. This decrease in force is greatest between 30 and 90 degrees of flexion. Fpf decreases at a lesser rate past 30 degrees of flexion, particularly because there is relatively no contact between the articulating surfaces of the patellofemoral joint past 20 degrees.[149]

CKC Joint Stress As in the OKC, joint surface contact area increases as the knee extends from 90 degrees of flexion. However, the Fq required for knee extension decreases faster than the contact area decreases, resulting in a decrease of joint stress. Realizing when the patellofemoral joint is subjected to stress is crucial for exercise prescription to minimize the amount of injury to patellofemoral articular cartilage.

Functional Implications of Joint Reaction Force and Stress

Understanding the amount of Fpf and joint stress that are encountered with daily tasks can be useful in educating patients who have anterior knee pain. As a result of the elastic pull of the proximal and distal tendon units, there is a substantial amount of force present during sitting.[69] This increased stress accounts for a patient's subjective complaint of anterior knee pain during prolonged sitting. Although sitting can impose a low load with long duration pressure on the patellofemoral joint, dynamic movements frequently cause abnormal stress and injury. During gait, the joint reaction force is typically 50% of the body weight as the knee flexes to 10 to 15 degrees during initial contact.[69] Stair ambulation, which requires increased Fq and knee flexion, can produce far greater Fpf. As the knee reaches 60 degrees of flexion during stair ambulation, joint reaction force can be as much as 3.3 times the body weight.[30,69] As the knee approaches 130 degrees of flexion in deep-squatting activities, joint reaction force may reach 7.8 times the body weight.[30,69]

Force Dissipation

The patellofemoral joint is subjected to varying extremes of joint reaction force over small areas. Fortunately, the trochlea and articulating surface of the patella possess multiple properties responsible for dissipating patellofemoral joint stress. When compressed, articular cartilage allows fluid to flow freely within the matrix and permits the cartilage to expand laterally. The patella benefits from thickened articular cartilage that easily expands laterally during compression. As knee flexion increases, the patella will seat more deeply into the trochlea and contact more surface area, which reduces the stress at a given point. This property also contributes to greater patellofemoral joint stability. Because of the large amount of permeability and compressibility of the articular cartilage, there is greater stress on the matrix that composes the cartilage. Unfortunately, chronic wear to the matrix can lead to degeneration and eventual patellar lesions.

Patellar Stability

Static Stabilization The articulation of the patella with the trochlea represents the greatest contribution to patellar stability. The trochlea acts as a trough for the patella to glide within. There is a greater degree of dynamic muscle pull from the proximal–lateral direction, necessitating increased support to prevent excessive lateral movement. This support is provided in part by the large anterior extension of the lateral femoral condyle. A lack of lateral femoral condyle height can contribute to chronic patella subluxation or dislocation.

The lack of bony contact between the patella and trochlea from 20 degrees of flexion to terminal extension results in a dependence on soft-tissue restraints. Investigators have described the medial and lateral extensor retinacula as the primary restraints to excessive patellar movement in the frontal plane.[156] The added support of medial and lateral patellofemoral ligaments present in a portion of the population will reinforce the retinacula.[30,125]

Dynamic Stabilization The dynamic musculotendinous stabilizers are oriented in a longitudinal fashion proximal and distal to the patella. The single distal stabilizer, the patellar tendon, contains the patella inferiorly. Proximally, the quadriceps generate a superior pull through the quadriceps tendon.[30,48] The combination of these longitudinal forces provides stability during knee flexion by seating the patella into the trochlear groove. However, the longitudinal pull may decrease stability by pulling the patella out of the trochlear groove during knee hyperextension.

Based on the pull of the quadriceps muscle, an imbalance of the vastus lateralis and vastus medialis oblique can result in abnormal tracking of the patellofemoral joint and disrupt stability as the knee approaches terminal extension. There is controversy in recent literature regarding the role of this mechanism in aiding the stability of the patellofemoral joint and decreasing anterior knee pain, as well as optimal treatment techniques.[14,96,148]

Influence of Proximal and Distal Joint Position on the Patellofemoral Joint

Hip and Femur Changes in the position of the femur at the hip joint can alter the orientation of the trochlea. The osteokinematics of the femur in the frontal and transverse planes can affect the directional force of the quadriceps on the patella. Clinically, the most common abnormal movement pattern is hip adduction and internal rotation, causing an inward collapse of the knee and medial displacement of the trochlea. The insertion of the quadriceps at the tibial tubercle remains fixed, resulting in a more laterally aligned patella.

Kendall et al[80] cited dominance of the hip internal rotators and adductors as possible sources of this faulty movement pattern. In addition, positional weakness or increased length of the hip abductors and external rotators, particularly the posterior fibers of the gluteus medius, contributes to the inward collapse knee.

Tibia and Foot Rotation of the tibia can also influence the alignment of the patellofemoral joint. As the tibia rotates either medially or laterally against a fixed femur, the patella can either glide or rotate in the direction of the tibial tubercle. Whether glide or rotation occurs depends upon the proximal fixation of the patella.

Rotation of the tibia has several influences. The proximal tibia will laterally rotate with a dominance of muscle action of the biceps femoris or tensor fasciae latae–ITB. Medial rotation can be caused by the predominance of the semitendinosus and semimembranosus. Distally, tibial rotation is influenced by the position of the subtalar joint. Pronation will lead to medial rotation of the tibia, thus positioning the patella medially relative to the trochlea.

Quadriceps Angle

The quadriceps angle (Q angle) is the angle formed between a line connecting the anterior superior iliac spine to the midpoint of the patella and a line that connects the tibial tubercle with the midpoint of the patella (Figure 24-8). A 15-degree angle between these 2 lines is considered normal.[2,30] A Q angle greater than 20 degrees can contribute to pathology in the patellofemoral joint. A large Q angle can cause displacement of the patella laterally, resulting in a bowstringing effect against the lateral femoral condyle during quadriceps contraction.[73,89]

There are several concerns when using the Q angle as a diagnostic tool. A large Q angle has not been shown to predispose a knee to patellofemoral pain, nor do all patients with patellofemoral pain have a large Q angle. Also, the measure assumes that the patella is centered in the trochlea; however, a laterally subluxed patella can result in a false-positive finding.[57]

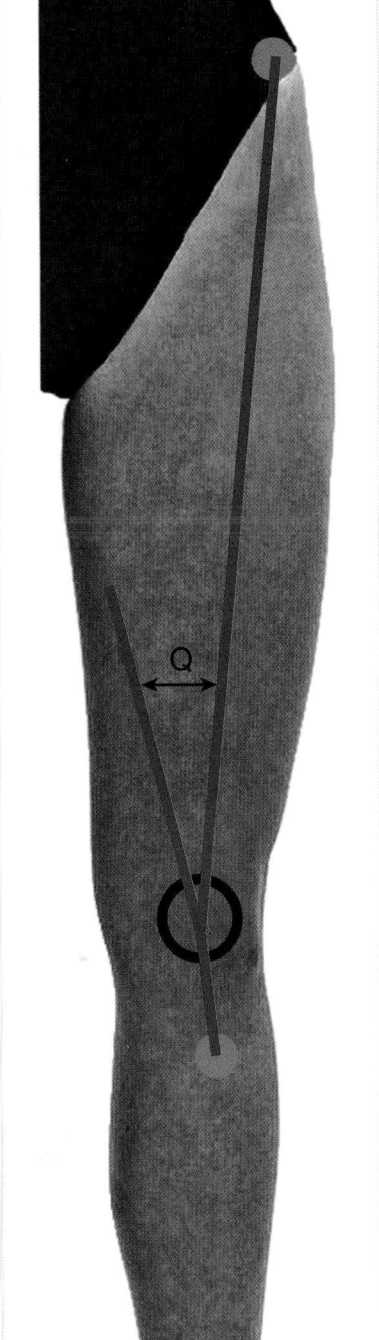

Figure 24-8 The Q angle

Overview of General Rehabilitation Progression Following Knee Injury

When treating knee injuries, the clinician should utilize a progression that considers the physiologic effects of the rehabilitation. This general progression should be understood so that guidelines and principles can be used to develop protocols for more specific knee pathologies or for surgical procedures.[102] When following any rehabilitation progression there are several general principles that should be considered: (a) awareness of joint inflammation or joint irritability; (b) the amount of motor control and muscular strength of the knee and lower extremity; (c) the ROM available at the joint; (d) the progression of weight bearing; and (e) the patients' present functional status compared to their ultimate desired outcome.[163]

Pain and inflammatory control, ROM, gait training, strengthening exercises, agility drills, and sport-specific exercises must all be implemented in a sequence that adheres to a criterion-based rehabilitation protocol. If the rehabilitation deviates from a criterion-based approach, the body will respond with adverse effects such as inflammation, swelling, pain, and further injury.

For purposes of this section, the general treatment plan has been divided into 4 phases. Many rehabilitation protocols set a time line to determine when it is appropriate to advance to the next phase. However, movement between phases should be criterion-based, requiring the patient to meet the goals outlined in each phase and not on a prespecified period of time. Advancing a patient into a later stage without full ROM or controlled swelling has a high probability of delaying the entire rehabilitation process. A skilled clinician knows when to advance a patient, delay a patient who has plateaued or regressed, or provide some overlap between phases.

Phase I

In the past, the majority of acute injuries requiring surgery were often repaired within days of the initial insult. As a result, patients were undergoing surgery with acute swelling and inflammation, ROM deficits, antalgic gait patterns, and muscular weakness. Immediate surgery following an ACL tear often led to a severe arthrofibrosis.[144] As with most injuries that require surgery, delaying surgery until the knee has passed the acute inflammatory stage and regained near-normal ROM and strength can contribute to a more optimal outcome.

Preoperative rehabilitation involves both mental and physical preparation. The patient must be given time to experience the psychological responses to injury as well as become emotionally prepared for the challenges of surgery and postoperative rehabilitation. Patient education about the surgical and rehabilitative procedures is of utmost importance. Using anatomical models or other resources, the clinician should explain the injury as well as the surgical technique. Detailed understanding of the postoperative rehabilitation program and goals is helpful. The patient must exhibit a positive attitude and have a sense of control over his/her situation. The clinician should also establish a good rapport with the patient during this time.

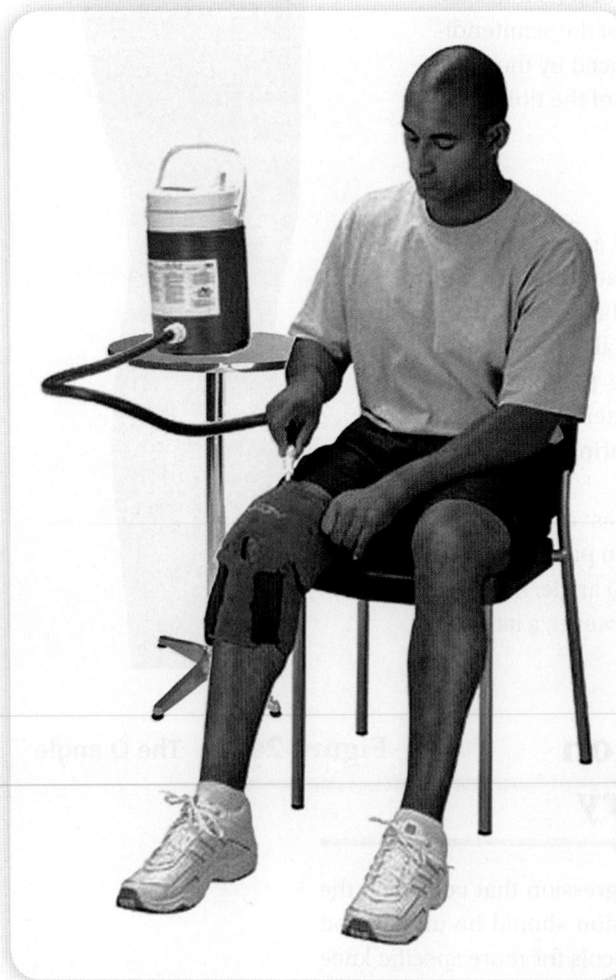

Figure 24-9 Cryo Cuff application provides cold and compression

After acute injury from either trauma or surgery the initial focus is placed on the elimination of pain and swelling, and restoration of ROM. In the early stages of rehabilitation, a knee Cryo Cuff (Aircast Inc., Summit, NJ) is an easy and effective way to control pain and swelling by means of cold and compression (Figure 24-9). Compression garments and ice bags can also be used. These early forms of treatment may minimize strength and motion losses following injury. Pain is often the main deterrent to motion and can lead to muscular and neurogenic inhibition, weakness and atrophy, and altered neuromuscular patterns. As the knee is acutely irritated at this time, care should be taken to not further irritate the tissues by rushing weightbearing status, progressing exercises too quickly, or forcing ROM.

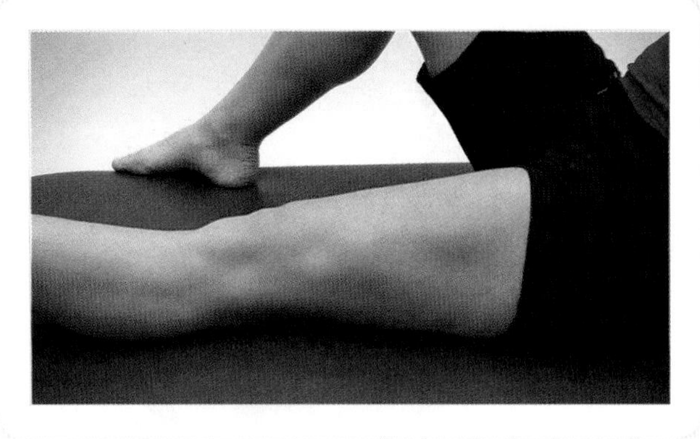

Figure 24-10 **Quadriceps setting is isometric quadriceps contraction performed in full extension for early strengthening and recruitment**

Early controlled knee ROM exercises are important to prevent joint fibrosis, and provide nutrition to the articular cartilage of the joint surfaces.[95] Motion exercises will help align collagen fibers providing a more flexible, strong scar that will help promote the full return of normal joint mechanics.[62] ROM exercises should begin almost immediately after the injury, with a greater emphasis placed on regaining extension. Among the many exercises to improve passive extension are heel props and prone hangs. Typically, flexion can be improved through exercises such as heel slides. However, because an active contraction of the rectus femoris is needed to perform a supine heel slide, a wall slide may be more useful early in rehabilitation. Alternatively, use of a towel under the foot to pull into flexion may also allow relaxation of the anterior musculature enough for the exercise to be tolerated. ROM should be the focus of treatment until both legs are symmetrical. Once the knee has achieved near 110 degrees of flexion, using a stationary bike with minimal tension can be an adjunct to gaining further flexion ROM. It has been shown that returning full ROM prior to surgery decreases postoperative complications.[135,143]

Once full ROM is restored and swelling and pain are minimal, basic level strengthening can begin. A resistive exercise continuum should be utilized, beginning with low-level isometric strengthening. Isometric quadriceps contraction from a long-sitting position, or quad sets, is an exercise often employed after a major knee injury (Figure 24-10). As strength and weightbearing improve, the patient can begin selective CKC exercises, such as minisquats, step-downs, and calf raises. Gait training can also begin during this period. As weight bearing becomes tolerable, gait should be practiced in a normal heel-to-toe pattern, with emphasis on obtaining full extension at heel strike and knee flexion at the swing through phase. Low-impact aerobics, such as stationary bicycle and stair machines, are also appropriate at this time.

The preoperative phase also includes measurement and testing of both extremities. Strength testing is achieved typically through an isokinetic strength assessment. Single-leg hop test is another functional measure that can be utilized. Other measurements that should be taken include ligament arthrometry, ROM, and subjective knee questionnaire.

Phase II

Phase II follows many of the same principles of the preoperative phase but also includes those patients whose injuries do not require surgery or who choose a nonoperative treatment. Immediate postinjury status is often thought of as the protection phase. Phase II is characterized by pain modulation, restoration of normal ROM, basic strengthening, and restoration of normal gait.

Pain modulation can take place through a number of modalities. Ice, compression, and elevation are staples during this period to control pain and swelling. Limiting ROM and weightbearing status through an immobilizer, brace, or crutches can appropriately protect and rest the joint, depending on the type of injury. The effects of pain and swelling and the effectiveness of a Cryo Cuff were discussed earlier in the preoperative section.

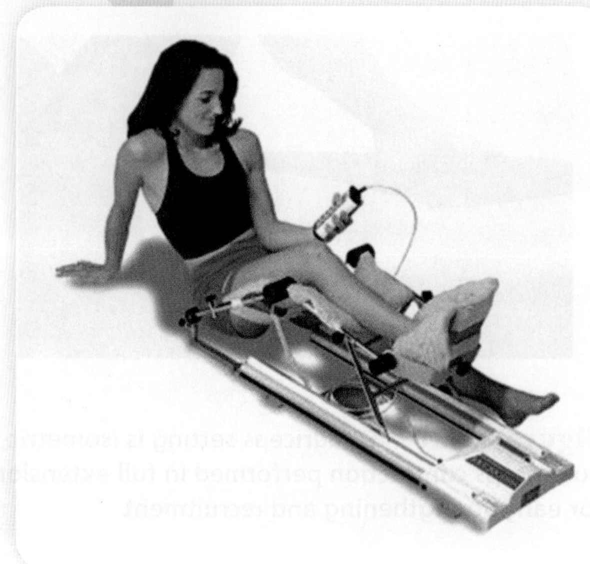

Figure 24-11 CPM device permits early motion

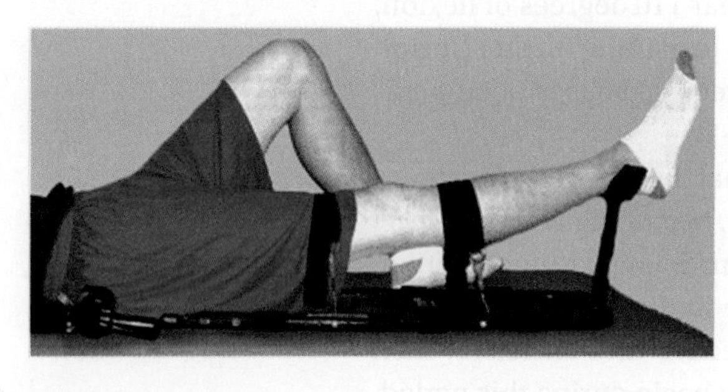

Figure 24-12 Extension board used to gain full hyperextension

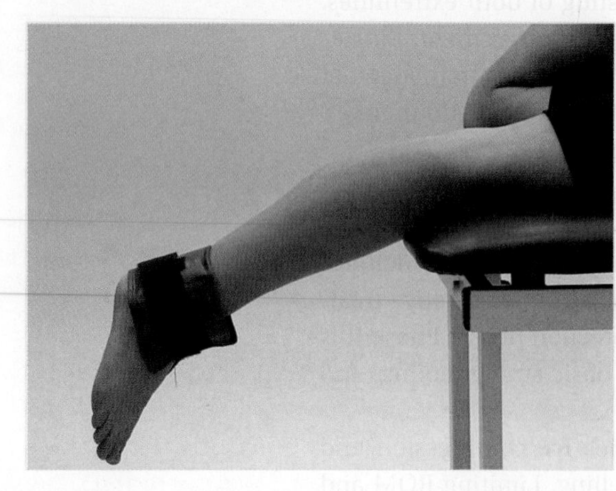

Figure 24-13 The prone hang is performed with the patient's distal thighs at the edge of the table

The importance of early ROM, when indicated, cannot be overstated. Motion is often the key to recovery. Often after surgery, a continuous passive motion (CPM) device is applied to the knee to begin early motion through a small arc (Figure 24-11). Especially with surgical patients with knee injuries an immediate emphasis is placed on regaining terminal knee extension. Terminal knee extension facilitates a normal gait pattern and also prevents scar tissue from forming in the femoral notch becoming a permanent block to knee extension.[51] Lack of full extension has been linked to quadriceps weakness, anterior knee pain, and crepitus.[136] This has led to a market of extension boards and devices aimed at achieving the motion (Figure 24-12). Exercise instruction for gaining knee extension includes prone hangs and heel props. Prone hangs allow passive knee extension with the involved knee and lower leg off the end of the table (Figure 24-13). Gravity-assistance from the prone position allows the weight of the extremity in gaining extension. An ankle cuff weight can be added for additional assistance. Heel props are performed in supine with the heel of the extremity propped onto a bolster, lifting the gastrocnemius and distal thigh from the table (Figure 24-14). This position allows the knee to relax into full extension with gravity assistance also. A weight or strap can be affixed superior to the patella for an increase in assistance.

Although not as urgent a concern, obtaining knee flexion is also important. Knee flexion can be improved through heel slides, wall slides, and active-assistive knee flexion in sitting. Heel slides are performed from a long-sitting position with knees starting in a position of extension then moving into knee flexion. Heel slides are typically more comfortable and tolerated better when done passively. The patient can grasp the lower leg and passively pulls it into further flexion (Figure 24-15). This can also be performed with a towel either under the foot or wrapped around the ankle. Wall slides involve the patient in a supine position with legs extended up a wall. The injured leg slowly slides down the wall with the assistance of gravity and the uninjured leg (Figure 24-16). If needed, an additional outside force from the patient's uninvolved leg, can be used to push the knee into deeper flexion. Active-assistive knee flexion is performed in a short-sitting position. From this position, the noninjured leg can pull the injured leg into even more flexion. A stationary bicycle also can be used as a mechanical means of attaining flexion. With both feet strapped into the pedals, the patient can use the contralateral leg to propel the knee into flexion. The clinician should adjust the seat to a position that is challenging to the patient. As this position becomes easy, the seat can be lowered, increasing the amount of flexion required at the knee to complete a revolution. If a full revolution cannot be completed, a rocking strategy can be employed. An alternating forward and backward pedaling motion is used until the knee gets "over the top" of the first revolution. A final strategy for increasing knee flexion is the use of the total gym (Engineering Fitness International, San Diego, CA). The amount of flexion and force used to gain it will be determined via the angle of the equipment and the use of the range-limiting protection strap.

Along with ROM, a few associated concepts to consider are flexibility and joint mobility. Improving flexibility means increasing the ability of soft-tissue structures to elongate through a range of joint motion. A lack of soft-tissue elongation may or may not be a result of the injury; however, balancing the available ROM is critical for normal biomechanics to occur at the knee. Mobilization of the patellofemoral and tibiofemoral joints may also be necessary for restoration of accessory motion, especially after a period of immobilization. Grades I and II mobilizations are oscillations applied at less-than-full joint mobility and can be useful in pain control and preventing restrictions of joint motion during the early phases of rehabilitation. Grades III and IV mobilizations are taken to the end of physiologic joint motion and are used to correct restrictions to joint motion. Inferior glides of the patellofemoral joint along with posterior glides of the tibiofemoral joint will help aid in increasing physiologic knee flexion. Superior patellofemoral glides and anterior tibiofemoral glides will help achieve full physiologic knee extension. The importance of the screw-home mechanism in knee extension should not be forgotten. In the patient struggling to achieve full extension, passive joint motion to external tibial rotation may need to be evaluated and mobilizations to external tibial passive mobility may need to be instituted. If present, 90 degrees of knee flexion is the best position to assess for this motion restriction.

Basic strengthening to regain leg control and improve quadriceps tone is also important during the early rehabilitation period. Exercises to improve leg control include quad sets, straight-leg raises, and active knee flexion and extension. Straight-leg raises are performed with the patient in a long-sitting position and the knee in full extension. The patient contracts the quadriceps muscle, much like performing a quad set, and then raises the leg 6 to 12 inches off the table (Figure 24-17). The straight-leg raise should be performed slowly in a controlled manner. Partial to full knee extension and flexion exercises are to be completed during this time, with ROM depending on the status of the articular cartilage and menisci. Sitting knee extensions are performed in a pain-free ROM off the edge of the table. With both flexion and extension, active assistance

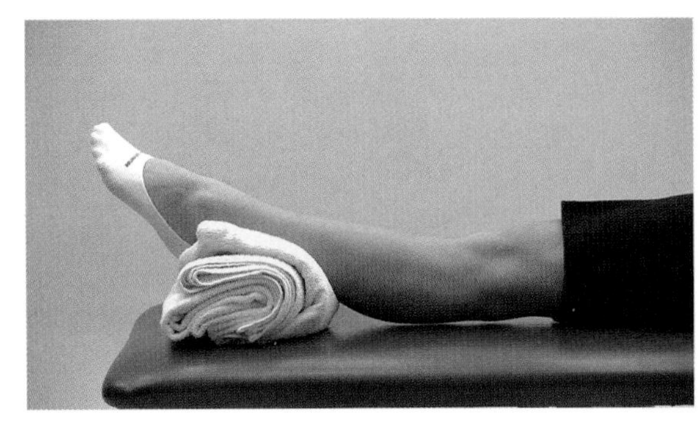

Figure 24-14 The heel prop is an early extension exercise

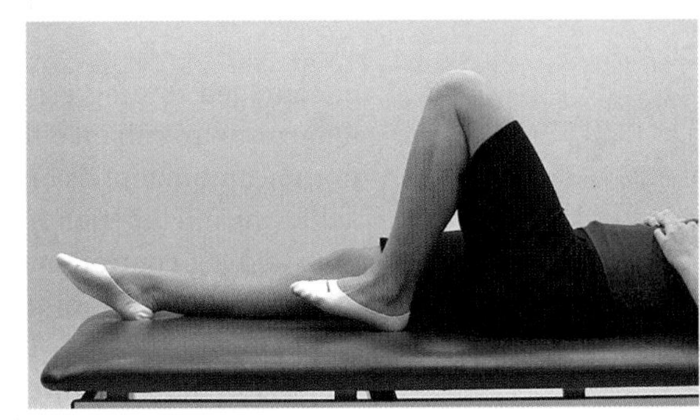

Figure 24-15 Heel slides are an effective means of obtaining knee flexion

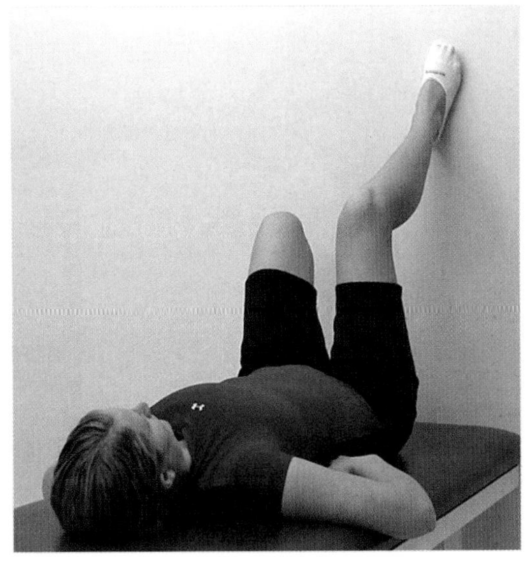

Figure 24-16 Wall slides are performed by slowly sliding the foot down the wall

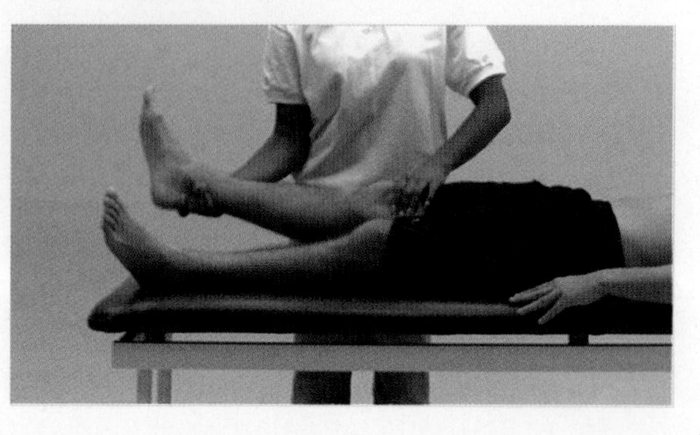

Figure 24-17 Straight-leg raise performed by initiating a quad set and maintaining knee extension while raising the leg off the table. This should progress from active-assisted to active

can be provided from the contralateral extremity. Additional resistance for these exercises should not be added until the patient is able to obtain full knee motion and at appropriate time frames dependent upon pathology.

Gait restoration is critical in affecting many aspects of early rehabilitation. Early postinjury the patient should ambulate with crutches until gait is normalized. Facilitation of quadriceps function is encouraged through full knee extension at heel strike and full weight bearing as tolerated during the stance phase of gait. Backward walking can be a means of obtaining active knee extension in those having difficulty obtaining full extension at heel strike. Early weight bearing also allows for joint compression and physiologic motion at the knee joint, which are conducive to cartilage nutrition and normal physiologic stresses to osseous and soft-tissue structures about the knee.

Toward the end of phase I, the patient should be encouraged to progress to full weight bearing without crutches. Practicing in front of a mirror may enhance the patient's ability to ambulate normally. Stance phase during normal ambulation is one of the most basic forms of CKC quadriceps strengthening. By achieving full independent weight bearing, the patient is able to regain good quadriceps tone and leg control, making it possible to implement more challenging strengthening exercises. Bilateral minisquats are performed with the feet shoulder-width apart and toes pointing forward. The patient slowly bends the hip and knees to one-quarter of a typical full squat, maintaining the knees in a position posterior to the toes (Figure 24-18). This minisquatting activity can be performed near a stable object at arm level for balance. The bilateral leg press is similar to the bilateral one-quarter knee bend in muscular activity. Bilateral calf raises are appropriate for strengthening the triceps surae musculature. The patient can begin this exercise from a flat surface and advance to standing on a stable object with heels hanging off the edge for a greater ROM. The patient should elevate as high as possible, contracting tightly at the top. Unilateral stance of the involved extremity, if tolerable, can be used to begin improving balance and proprioception.

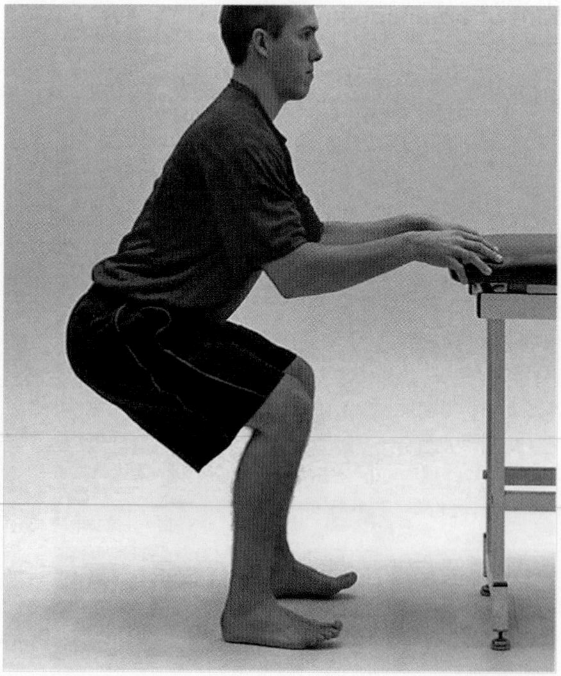

Working toward leg control and normal gait is aimed at improving the patient's function. Depending on the injury, a knee brace or taping of the patella may be appropriate to assist in returning function to the patient. Cross-training activities, such as swimming, biking, or stair machine, may be appropriate to initiate muscular endurance and aerobic capacity. Swimming is contraindicated in surgical patients with unhealed wounds.

Figure 24-18 Bilateral one-quarter squats permit early CKC strengthening of the quadriceps

Phase III

Once goals of phase II are achieved, the patient can move forward to phase III. If full terminal knee extension or flexion are still lacking, ROM must be placed at a priority. Full ROM must be achieved prior to more strenuous strengthening activities. If this criterion is not followed, the body may respond adversely. The main focus of phase III is advanced strengthening.

Strengthening activities of phase II are continued with either increased repetitions and or resistance. The patient should be encouraged to place more resistance on the involved side as tolerated, in a progression toward unilateral strengthening. Once the patient has sufficient leg control to perform a unilateral knee bend without difficulty, weight room activities may commence. A combination of both OKC and CKC activities, as well as concentric and eccentric muscular strengthening, should be utilized with most knee conditions. Chapter 11 provides an introductory discussion of OKC and CKC exercises.

OKC exercises for the knee are an excellent way to facilitate isolated quadriceps muscle strengthening. However, caution must be exercised, as patellofemoral compressive forces are distributed over a smaller contact area with progressive knee extension.[131] For patients with patellofemoral compressive issues a range of knee extension from 90 to 50 degrees may be tolerated more favorably. OKC extension exercises also produce an anterior shear force that significantly loads the ACL, particularly in the last 30 degrees of extension. Thus, a safer ROM for postoperative ACL patients may be between approximately 45 and 90 degrees of flexion. In any patient respective of pathology, performance of full terminal extension should be performed only if there is sufficient quadriceps strength and proper alignment to complete the exercise without pain.

CKC exercise is thought by some to be preferred for a more functional rehabilitation of the lower extremity. During CKC exercises, patellofemoral compressive forces become larger as flexion increases.[131] However, CKC exercises produce reduced shear forces across the tibiofemoral joint through cocontraction and axial loading.[12] Thus, a safe general range for patients to begin CKC exercise is from 0 degrees to approximately 45 degrees. A more advanced patient may go beyond 45 to 90 degrees of knee flexion if the exercise can be completed without pain.

Frequently, emphasis in rehabilitation is placed solely on concentric activity. However, eccentric activity is dominant in most athletic activities such as running, tennis, and throwing. Eccentric lower-extremity control is needed when landing from a jump in activities such as basketball, track and field, volleyball, and gymnastics. Additionally, eccentric control is recognized as important for efficient gait. In fact, many activities of daily living require eccentric activity, such as bending over to pick up an object or descending stairs.

The potential force of eccentric muscle activity can be described as part of the stretch-shortening cycle.[24] Muscle eccentric stretching loads potential energy into elastic elements that is transferred into kinetic energy during the concentric phase of a muscle contraction, thereby raising the peak potential force.[24] This is the premise behind plyometric activity. For example, consider a standing vertical leap. During the knee and hip flexion phase, stored potential energy occurs as the muscles lengthen eccentrically. This allows the athlete to jump higher than if jump from a static position of knee and hip flexion without eccentric loading.

Advanced strengthening in phase III should emphasize unilateral exercises, including leg press, step-downs, calf raises, and leg extensions. When starting unilateral extremity exercises a patient can performing leg press and leg extensions by using the uninvolved leg through the concentric phase followed by only the involved in the eccentric portion of the lift. Step-downs are performed by having the patient stand on a step with the affected extremity. The patient slowly lowers the contralateral leg to the floor while maintaining good biomechanical alignment of the lower extremity, then returning to the starting position (Figure 24-19). Initially, the height of the step should be small (2 to 4 in) and should increase as the exercise becomes easier. Difficulty of the exercise can be increased by performing the step-down to the front or back of the step. At this time more advanced exercises, such as light squats and lunges, can commence.

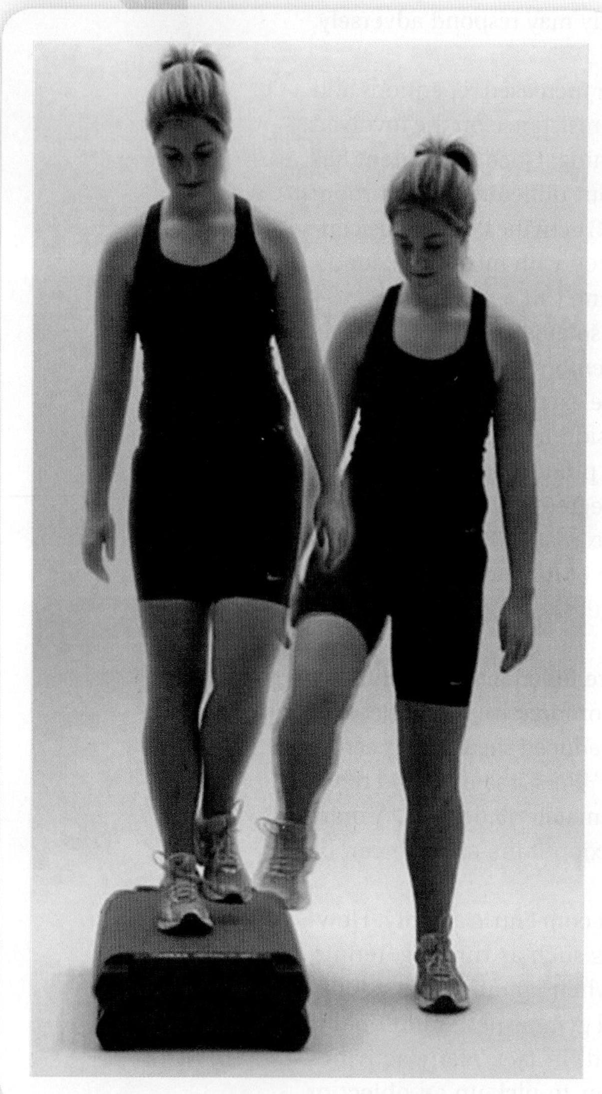

Figure 24-19 Step-downs can be made more challenging by increasing the height of the step

Aerobic exercise is always important and can be initiated with a stair machine, elliptical runner, or stationary bicycle. If aerobic exercise is already being done it can be progressed to greater intensity levels. If wounds have healed, the patient can also begin swimming and performing other hydrotherapy activity.

Toward the end of phase III, early agility drills can begin. Jumping rope, straight-ahead jogging, or easy position drills for athletes are appropriate. During this period, ROM should be maintained, pain and swelling should not occur, and a normal gait pattern should be achieved.

Phase IV

A functional return to prior activity status is the goal of the final phase. The patient can progress, once meeting the goals of phase III and maintaining the objectives, from the previous phase. Phase IV is characterized by a functional progression that includes activity- or sport-specific exercises, agility drills, and balance and proprioceptive training.

The patient continues advanced strengthening throughout the entire phase. Once 65% to 70% strength is attained in the involved leg (usually tested with an isokinetic strength assessment), agility activities and sports specific drills can be advanced safely. Weight-room activities and home strengthening exercises should progress from high repetition/low weight to low repetition/high weight. Moderate speed strengthening and cardiovascular conditioning should be continued during this period.

Activities and exercises during this phase should be functional, specific, and progressive. Whether a mail carrier or a football linebacker, the rehabilitation needs to focus on tasks required for that individual to return to his/her prior activity status. A mail carrier may be required to lift moderately heavy objects and walk long distances, while a linebacker requires explosive power and high-speed change of direction. Solo sport activities, such as shooting a basketball or hitting a tennis ball, are appropriate during this time.

Advanced agility drills can include lateral shuffles, cariocas, crossover drills, and backward running. By focusing on agility activities rather than on jogging, the patient is more apt to improve areas of confidence, moderate speed strength, quickness, and sport-specific skills. By avoiding the repetition and redundancy of jogging and making the activity purposeful and specific, the patient is often able to better absorb joint compressive forces and become more engaged in rehabilitation sessions.

As the patient progresses, agility training becomes more vigorous. Figure-of-eights and half-to-full-speed running should be included at this time. Typically, a functional progression will follow a scheme that gradually increases speed increments from half to three-quarter, to full-speed activity. Chapter 18 provides additional suggestions for functional progressions. Making certain activities are performed with proper technique is paramount. To begin, jumping movements should be performed straight up and down with no lateral moments at the knee. The patient should maintain the trunk over knees and knees over feet while keeping the hips, knees, and ankles in a straight line. Landing on the balls of the feet instead of flat-footed and assuming a position of slight flexion in the hips and knees is helpful.

During return to activity, the clinician should challenge the patient's balance through perturbation activities performed on a wobble board, foam, or trampoline. Performing the exercise unilaterally or with eyes closed increases the difficulty. These exercises improve joint stabilization patterns through cocontractions of the quadriceps and hamstrings. The patient also improves body awareness through an enhancement in proprioceptive information. Chapter 9 provides additional information regarding neuromuscular training.

Before a full return to prior activity level, the patient's involved extremity should be reevaluated. ROM, isokinetic strength assessment, ligament arthrometry, and a combination of subjective knee questionnaire and functional tests should all be compared to preoperative or preinjury status. The patient should have full ROM, acceptable ligament stability, and 80% strength bilaterally before returning to competitive athletic or recreational activities. The patient should complete a sport- or occupation-specific functional progression prior to full return.

Specific Rehabilitation Techniques for Ligamentous and Meniscal Injury

Medial Collateral Ligament Sprain

Pathomechanics

Although current research on knee ligament injuries appears to focus more on ACL injuries, the MCL remains the most commonly injured ligament of the knee.[173] In young, active patients, approximately 90% of all knee ligament injuries are to ACL, MCL, or a combination of the two.[112] Successful management of MCL injuries often depends on establishing the existence of an isolated lesion, with no associated damage to other knee structures, particularly the ACL. Isolated MCL injuries can heal spontaneously, without the need for surgical correction, even in complete ligament ruptures when the fragmented ends of the damaged tissue are not in close approximation.[174]

A clear understanding of the anatomy of the medial knee is important in understanding injury biomechanics and developing a treatment strategy. Warren and Marshall used the three-layer concept to describe the medial structures of the knee.[162] The first, most superficial layer is composed of the fascia surrounding the sartorius muscle. The intermediate second layer contains the superficial MCL, the medial patellofemoral ligament, and the ligaments of the posteromedial corner of the knee. The third and deepest layer of knee structures includes the capsule and the deep MCL. The MCL can tear midsubstance or at either the femoral or tibial attachment sites. Approximately 65% of MCL sprains occur at the proximal insertion site on the femur. On the basis of location of the injury, rehabilitation can vary substantially. MCL injuries occurring midsubstance or near femoral origin tend to develop more stiffness and readily incur ROM loss.[52] Restoration of full motion should be monitored closely within the first few weeks following injury. In contrast, injuries at the tibial attachment tend to heal with residual laxity and thus have easier return of ROM. As a result, additional protection may be required to allow the MCL to heal.

The grade of ligament injury is determined by the amount of joint laxity. A grade I MCL sprain presents with tenderness caused by microtears, no increased laxity, and a firm end point. A grade II sprain involves an incomplete tear with some increased laxity with valgus stress at 30 degrees of flexion and minimal laxity in full extension, and a firm end point. There is tenderness to palpation, hemorrhage, and pain on valgus stress test. A grade III sprain is a complete tear with significant laxity on valgus stress in full extension. No end point is evident, and as a result of not having opposing ends, pain is less than that experienced with grade I or II sprains. Significant laxity with valgus stress testing in full extension likely indicates injury to the medial joint capsule and the cruciate ligaments.

Mechanism of Injury

Injury to the MCL occurs as a result of valgus stress to the knee from a contact or noncontact force. The most common mechanism of injury for an isolated MCL injury is by a direct lateral contact, which is frequent during contact sports such as football. A direct force to the outside of the knee can result in a valgus stress to the medial aspect of the knee that exceeds the strength of the ligament. The patient will usually explain that the knee was hit on the lateral side with the foot planted and that there was immediate pain on the medial side of the knee that felt more like a "pulling" or "tearing" than a "pop." A true "popping" sensation may be more indicative of an MCL sprain with concomitant ACL rupture.

Less commonly, the MCL is injured through a noncontact mechanism that occurs when the foot is planted and an indirect rotational force is coupled with an increased valgus stress at the knee. This mechanism is common in sports that involve cutting maneuvers such as soccer, basketball, and football. This mechanism may be more likely to incur damage to other anatomical structures such as meniscus and ACL.

Rehabilitation Concerns

Historically, the standard of care for MCL injuries was surgical management.[118-121] Since the early 1980s, the treatment of MCL sprains has changed considerably.[71] The current approach is nonsurgical and includes limited immobilization with early ROM and strengthening exercises. Shelbourne and Patel[142] found the best approach for management of a combined MCL–ACL injury is achieved by treating the MCL injury nonsurgically and performing a delayed reconstruction of the ACL.

Patient advancement varies according to the location of the tear, degree of ligamentous instability, concomitant injuries involved, age, and activity demands. A patient with a grade III tear at the femoral attachment site typically will have more difficulty restoring motion, whereas patients with tears at the tibial insertion tend to have more instability.

Grade I injuries may be progressed as tolerated with or without the use of a hinged knee brace. Grade II injuries can be progressed as tolerated, depending on the patient's signs and symptoms. These injuries will display increased valgus laxity but retain a firm end point. A hinged knee brace can be used early in the rehabilitation, although an immobilizer may be used for patient comfort. Grade III injuries may be progressed as tolerated with a hinged brace or may be immobilized in 30 degrees of flexion for 1 to 3 weeks if a more conservative approach is used. This protection provides a stable environment for proper healing and tightening of the injured ligamentous complex. The physician and clinician should collaborate on patient progression at each clinical visit, as overlapping of the 3 phases is very common and has been built into this progression. There are several instances when operative management may be warranted: (a) a large bony avulsion exists; (b) there is a concomitant tibial plateau fracture; (c) there is a concomitant ACL injury; and (d) there is intraarticular entrapment of the end of the torn MCL. Surgery can be performed using primary reconstruction or via surgical repair. Kovachevich et al recently reported that no studies have compared the 2 forms of surgical treatment.[84] Therefore, at this time, no clear evidence-based recommendations can be made for either procedure.

Rehabilitation Progression

Phase I: 0 to 3 Weeks Phase I is characterized by protection, early healing, and restoring ROM. The clinical goals are to minimize pain and swelling and to attain full-weightbearing and normal gait with or without a brace or immobilizer.

A Cryo Cuff is to be used as tolerated throughout the day for control of pain and swelling. A stockinette can be worn to assist in swelling control. Antiinflammatory medications can be taken as prescribed by the physician. Immobilization is dependent on the patient's instability and pain. For patients with a grade I MCL injury, bracing is used as needed. Patients with a grade II injury use a brace and possibly an immobilizer. Grade III injuries are managed with a hinged brace, cast, or immobilizer. Immobilization times will vary depending on the severity of instability and physician's preference.

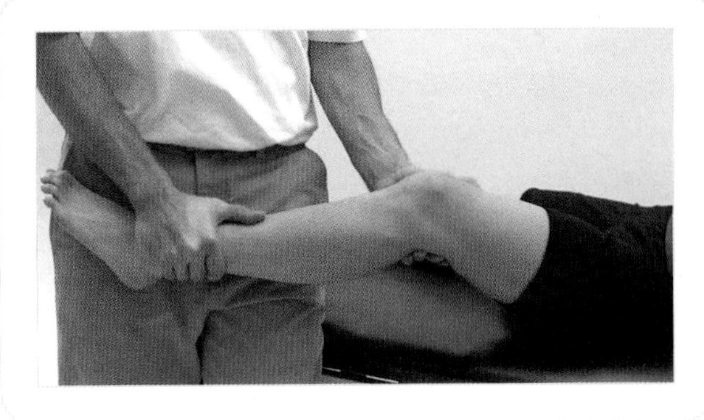

Figure 24-20 Stress shielding the MCL by applying a varus force to the knee while performing passive knee flexion range of motion

The patient may be allowed to weight bear as tolerated with or without protective devices, depending on pain status. ROM exercises are performed 3 times daily (prone hangs, heel props, wall slides, and heel slides). If an immobilization period is required, ROM exercise may be delayed.

Phase II: 1 to 5 Weeks Phase II rehabilitation focuses on restoring full ROM and beginning a strengthening program that utilizes both OKC and CKC exercises. Clinical goals include no swelling, full ROM, normal gait, pain-free activities of daily living, and initiation of strengthening and proprioception activities. ROM exercises are continued during this period. During attempts to gain passive flexion ROM the clinician can stress shield the healing MCL by applying a varus force (Figure 24-20) The patient should begin to exhibit a normal gait pattern without assistance from a hinged brace, or assistive devices. A brace can be worn as needed for comfort. Strengthening exercises begin bilaterally and are progressed to a unilateral exercise. The regimen consists of minisquats, step-downs, toe raises, leg presses, and leg extensions. Proprioceptive activities and nonimpact aerobic training, such as stationary bicycle, stair machine, and elliptical trainers, are initiated at this time.

By the end of phase II, the patient should possess full ROM, including terminal extension. Stockinette use can be discontinued at the end of this phase if no swelling is present. Use of the Cryo Cuff after exercise and for pain control can be continued as needed.

Phase III: 2 to 8 Weeks The final phase consists of a progressive return to functional activities. The goals of phase III include pain-free activities of daily living without a brace, weight-room strengthening, completing a functional progression with a brace, and return to sport or work with a brace. The clinician administers the functional progression and isokinetic strength assessment. For a return to full competitive activity, the patient should meet the following criteria:

1. Minimal to no pain
2. Full ROM
3. Quadriceps and hamstring strength equal to 90% of the uninvolved limb
4. Completion of a running progression program.

The average time for return to play varies with sport and injury extent. A grade I injury requires approximately 10 days for return to full activity, a grade II injury takes approximately 20 days. A grade III injury requires anywhere from 3 to 6 weeks.

Strengthening should be performed unilaterally, continuing the exercises from phase II. Most phase III activities are performed in the weight room and include unilateral leg press to 90 degrees, step-downs from a 2- to 4-inch step height, unilateral leg extensions, squats to 90 degrees performed in a squat rack, lunges, and stair machine.

Easy agility drills are initiated at this time and should be completed with a hinged knee brace. Activities should include jump rope, backward running, lateral slides, cariocas, cutting movements, and a jogging to sprinting progression.

Successful completion of a functional progression constitutes the end of this phase. At this time, the patient can return to full activity. A functional knee brace is used depending on the demands of the individual's activity or sport and degree of injury. The patient needs to continue a regular strengthening program even after full return to activity.

Lateral Collateral Ligament Sprain

Pathomechanics

Fortunately, the lateral aspect of the knee is well supported by secondary stabilizers, and isolated injury to the LCL is rare. When it does occur, the clinician must rule out other ligamentous injuries. Isolated sprain of the LCL is the least common of all knee ligament sprains.[112] LCL sprains result in disruption at the fibular head either with or without an avulsion in approximately 75% of the cases, with 20% occurring at the femur, and only 5% as midsubstance tears.[156] It is not uncommon to see associated injuries of the peroneal nerve because the nerve courses around the head of the fibula. A complete disruption of the LCL often involves injury to the posterolateral joint capsule, as well as the PCL, and occasionally the ACL.

The amount of laxity evident on a varus stress test determines the severity of injury to the LCL. Grading the extent of LCL laxity follows the same I to III grading scale as the MCL.

Mechanism of Injury

An isolated LCL injury is almost always the result of a varus stress applied to the medial aspect of the knee. Occasionally, a varus stress may occur during weight bearing when weight is shifted away from the side of injury, creating stress on the lateral structures. Patients report hearing or feeling a pop and immediate lateral pain. Swelling is immediate and extraarticular, with no intraarticular joint effusion unless there is an associated meniscus or capsular injury.

Rehabilitation Concerns

Grade I injuries may be progressed as tolerated with or without the use of a hinged knee brace. Grade II injuries can be progressed as tolerated, depending on the patient's signs and symptoms. These injuries display increased varus laxity but retain a firm end point. A hinged knee brace can be used early in the rehabilitation, although an immobilizer may be used for patient comfort. Grade III injuries may be managed nonoperatively with bracing for 4 to 6 weeks, limited to 0 to 90 degrees of motion; however, grade III LCL tears with associated ligamentous injuries that result in rotational instabilities are usually managed by surgical repair or reconstruction. This is certainly the case if the patient has chronic varus laxity and intends to continue participation in athletics, or if there is a displaced avulsion.

Rehabilitation Progression

The rehabilitation progression following LCL sprains should follow the same course as was previously described for MCL sprains. In the case of a grade III LCL sprain that involves multiple ligamentous injury with associated instability that is surgically repaired or reconstructed, the patient should be placed in a postoperative brace, with partial weight bearing for 4 to 6 weeks. At 6 weeks, a rehabilitation program involving a carefully monitored gradual sport-specific functional progression should begin. In general, the patient may return to full activity at about 6 months.

Anterior Cruciate Ligament Sprain

Pathomechanics

The healing potential of a torn ACL is very poor.[47] Healing potential for a partially torn ACL can be favorable when certain conditions exist, but only 15% of all ACL injuries are partial tears.[39] Because of the poor healing conditions, the torn ACL often leads to anterior laxity, rotary instability, and meniscal tears when left untreated. Furthermore, untreated ACL injuries lead to functional deficits,[54,66,105] and an increased risk of second ACL injury.[123] Very few athletes can participate at a high level with a nonfunctional ACL.[64] Giving-way episodes are often the result, damaging the meniscus and articular cartilage within the joint.

Convincing evidence suggests that an active individual with a torn ACL is susceptible to meniscal injury.[22] Results of ACL reconstruction 9 years after surgery strongly correlated with the status of the meniscus and articular cartilage.[140] Patients who undergo ACL reconstruction without meniscal tears requiring or removal of articular cartilage damage had significantly better long-term results compared to patients who had surgery with meniscus removal or severe articular cartilage damage. Patients with normal meniscus and articular cartilage at the time of surgery had subjective scores equal to a normal control group without knee injuries.

The temporary stability of a nonoperated ACL tear is often referred to as the "honeymoon period." When treated nonoperatively, an active individual will likely become symptomatic. The present laxity will lead to instability, causing giving-way episodes with ensuing swelling and pain. Damage to the meniscus and articular cartilage is highly probable following such episodes. Meniscal damage is associated with half of acute cases and 90% of chronic ACL deficiencies of greater than 10 years' duration.[39] Thirty percent of acute ACL injuries and 70% of ACL-deficient knees at 10 years postinjury display articular cartilage lesions.[39] The relationship of long-term joint arthrosis to ACL deficiency is not fully understood. However, the alteration of knee biomechanics can lead to areas of overload, causing articular cartilage breakdown. Depending on the length of follow-up, detectable osteoarthritis in ACL injuries ranges from 15 to 65%.[31,44]

As with MCL and LCL sprains, the severity of the injury is indicated by the degree of laxity or instability. Rotational instability is present if indicated by a positive pivot shift. Patients most often report feeling and hearing a pop and a feeling that the knee "gave out." There is also significant pain, and hemarthrosis occurs within 1 to 2 hours.

Mechanism of Injury

The most common injury mechanism to the ACL involves a noncontact valgus and external rotation stress to the knee as the foot is planted on the ground. The classic example of this mechanism happens in football when a running back plants the foot to make a cut and avoid being tackled. Occasionally, the mechanism of injury involves deceleration, valgus stress, and internal rotation. Knee hyperextension combined with internal rotation can also produce a tear of the ACL.

External contact forces to the tibiofemoral joint can result in a combined knee injury of which an ACL rupture is a component. Typically, this injury is a result of lateral or hyperextension force to the knee, which frequently results in complete rupture of both the ACL and MCL, plus a longitudinal tear of the lateral meniscus, all of which require surgical reconstruction. Another common mechanism occurs when an athlete is unexpectedly bumped right before landing from a jump, causing a premature contraction of the quadriceps and landing upon an anteriorly translated tibia. Chapter 31 discusses ACL injuries in athletic females.

Rehabilitation Concerns

Although successful treatment options exist following ACL injury, an appropriate evidence-based plan of care is still under debate. For the sedentary individual, a more conservative approach may be considered in which the acute phase of the injury is allowed to pass followed by a vigorous rehabilitation program. If normal function does not return and the knee remains unstable, then reconstructive surgery is considered.

Most active and athletic patients prefer a more aggressive approach. The ideal patient is a young, motivated, and skilled athlete who is willing to make the personal sacrifices necessary to successfully complete the rehabilitation process. Thus, successful outcomes following surgical repair and reconstruction are dependent to a large extent upon patient selection.

In the case of a partially torn ligament, the medical community is split on treatment approach. Some feel that a partially damaged ACL is incompetent and should be viewed as if the ligament were completely gone. Others prefer a prolonged initial period of immobilization and limited motion, hoping that the ligament will heal and remain functional. Decisions for nonoperative treatment should be based on the individual's preinjury status and a willingness of the patient to engage only in activities such as jogging, swimming, or cycling that will not place the knee at high risk. This is clearly a case where the patient may seek several opinions before choosing the treatment course.

Surgical technique is crucial to a successful outcome. The improper placement of the tendon graft can prevent the return of normal motion. The type of graft chosen also affects postoperative rehabilitation in terms of tensile strength, harvest site comorbidity, and revascularization.

Traditional rehabilitation following ACL reconstruction is based on the work of Paulos et al[124] in which phases of rehabilitation correspond to healing time frames of animal models. The traditional model emphasized limited ROM and weight bearing, as well as delayed strengthening and return to activity. Return to sports typically occurred within 6 to 12 months. In 1990, Shelbourne and Nitz[141] reported positive outcomes with an accelerated rehabilitation program that emphasized immediate ROM and full extension, immediate weight bearing as tolerated, early CKC strengthening, and return to sporting activities by 2 months and to full competition within 4 to 6 months.

The following rehabilitation progression is based on the accelerated program.

Rehabilitation Progression

(Table 24-1 outlines the following discussion)

Phase I: Preoperative The preoperative phase objectives focus on physically preparing the knee for surgery and mentally preparing the patient to deal with the surgery and postoperative rehabilitation. Restoration of full ROM and normal strength prior to reconstruction are key components of this phase, with emphasis on obtaining full ROM before strengthening. To achieve full ROM, swelling must also be reduced. The clinician can educate the patient on the basic principles of rehabilitation, including maintenance of full hyperextension and full flexion, early weight bearing, and OKC and CKC strengthening.[101,104]

Preoperative testing provides a baseline for objective comparison in later phases. Bilateral ROM, including full terminal knee extension, a KT-1000 ligament arthrometer and an isokinetic strength evaluation, isometric leg press, and single-leg hop test on the noninvolved leg are all performed prior to surgery.

Gaining full ROM is the first goal during this period. Extension exercises include heel props, towel stretches, and prone hangs. An extension board or other extension device can be used if gaining full extension is difficult. Exercises aimed at gaining flexion include heel slides, wall slides, and supine flexion hangs. In conjunction with ROM exercises, activities to develop quadriceps control are initiated. Active heel lifts and standing knee lockouts produce quadriceps strength and develop early extension habits. Once full ROM with minimal

Table 24-1 **Postoperative Rehabilitation After ACL Reconstruction**

Phase	Days – Weeks	Goals	Restrictions	Treatment	Clinical Milestones
Phase I: Preoperative	PO	Restore ROM both active and passive Quadriceps activation Decreased effusion Pain reduction	WBAT with bilateral axillary crutches Brace locked at 0 degrees	RICE Electrical stimulation Extension ROM Passive flexion ROM Glute/Quad/Ham sets Hip abduction/adduction Leg presses Minisquats Step-downs	Surgical reconstruction Full knee extension Restoration of strength Minimal effusion No increased pain
Phase II: Immediate PO Phase	PO Wks 0 to 2	WBAT bilateral axillary crutches locked in extension Full knee extension Quadriceps control Pain reduction Normal patellar mobility	Full WBAT brace locked in full extension × 1 week After week 1 PROM flexion can be started Brace still locked in extension for weight bearing until SLR with no extensor lag	Patellar mobilization Scar tissue mobilization PROM flexion and extension PROM flexion progressed to 110 degrees week 1 130 degrees week 2 Quadriceps sets Straight leg raises × 4 Ankle pumps CPM Weight shifts Cryotherapy	Previous milestones Clean incisions Good quadriceps recruitment SLR with minimal lag Normalized patellar mobility Weight bearing progressed without symptoms Minimal pain and effusion
Phase III: Intermediate PO Phase	PO Wks 2 to 4	Normalized quadriceps recruitment Normal patellar mobility No pain or effusion Restoration of motion Maintain full weight bearing Improve balance	Braced unlocked for weight bearing as tolerated Crutches discontinued at approximately 2 weeks	Progression of previous Isometric quad sets at 0, 60, and 90 degrees Squats and leg press 0 to 60 degrees Stationary bike Step-downs Calf raises Minisquats Balance drills Band exercises	Previous milestones Satisfactory clinical exam ROM 0 to 130 degrees Improved stability with unilateral stance No pain Normal gait
Phase IV: Strengthening Phase	PO Wks 4 to 12	Full bilateral ROM Increase strength and endurance No pain No swelling Preparation for activities	None	Previous strengthening Progress bilateral loading to single limb loading exercises Lunges 0 to 60 degrees Advanced balance activities Hip extension progressing to isolated hamstring exercises in 12 weeks	Previous milestones Full motion: 0 to 130 degrees Single leg stance × 30 sec Squat 60 degrees with equal weight bearing No pain or effusion

(continued)

Table 24-1 Postoperative Rehabilitation After ACL Reconstruction *(Continued)*

Phase	Days – Weeks	Goals	Restrictions	Treatment	Clinical Milestones
Phase V: Return to Activity Phase	PO Wks 12+	Restoration of full motion No swelling No pain Return of full activities	None	Previous strengthening Unilateral calf raises Progress CKC exercises Advance hamstring exercises Agility drills Advanced balance drills Sports specific drills	Previous milestones Full motion Full confidence in knee Functional testing >90% of uninvolved Isokinetic testing >90% of uninvolved

CKC, closed kinetic chain; CPM, continuous passive motion; PO, postoperative; RICE, rest, ice, compression, elevation; ROM, range of motion; SLR, straight-leg raise; WBAT, weight bearing as tolerated; Wks, weeks.

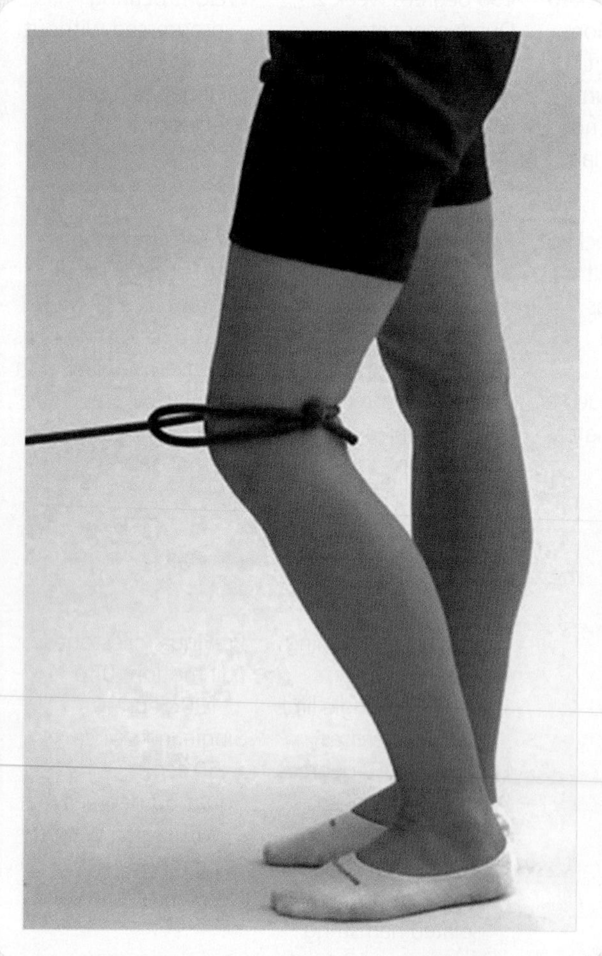

Figure 24-21 Standing knee lockout facilitates extension in weight bearing

swelling is obtained, CKC strengthening can begin. The patient can perform leg press, minisquat, step-down, stationary bike, and stair machine activities.

Phase II: Days 1 to 14 Phase II begins immediately after surgery to 2 weeks postoperatively. For those who may be likely to have motion problems, a CPM machine is utilized the day of surgery and is set from 0 to 30 degrees flexion (see Figure 24-11). A Cryo Cuff is donned immediately after surgery to control pain and swelling. During these first few weeks the patient is encouraged to fully weight bear as tolerated, with crutches if needed.

The patient generally begins formal therapy near the third postoperative day. Initially, extension exercises are performed 6 times daily. The knee is allowed to fully extend into terminal extension for 10 minutes during each bout with a heel prop. Towel stretches are also used to help gain extension. Knee flexion exercises are performed through a ROM of 110 degrees, completed 6 times daily. The patient can further increase flexion by pulling the leg toward the buttocks and holding for 3 minutes. Leg control is initiated with exercises that emphasize active quadriceps contractions such as quad sets, straight-leg raises, and active heel height.

Exercise progression for knee extension ROM becomes a critical factor during this time. The patient continues to push toward full hyperextension equal to the opposite leg by means of towel stretches, heel props, and prone hangs. A standing knee lock-out is performed by standing with the weight shifted to the reconstructed leg while fully locking the knee into extension by contracting the quadriceps (Figure 24-21). Obtaining full extension and normal gait early in the rehabilitation process enables the patient to regain quadriceps tone and leg control, setting the pace for the entire rehabilitation program. Once full knee extension and normal ambulation are obtained, more challenging leg control exercises such as minisquats and knee extensions are implemented. Knee flexion continues to progress through heel slides, wall slides, and supine flexion hangs.

Criteria for progression to phase III consist of full terminal extension, flexion to 130 degrees, minimal pain and swelling, soft-tissue healing, normalized gait, and the ability to lock the operated knee into full extension compared bilaterally.

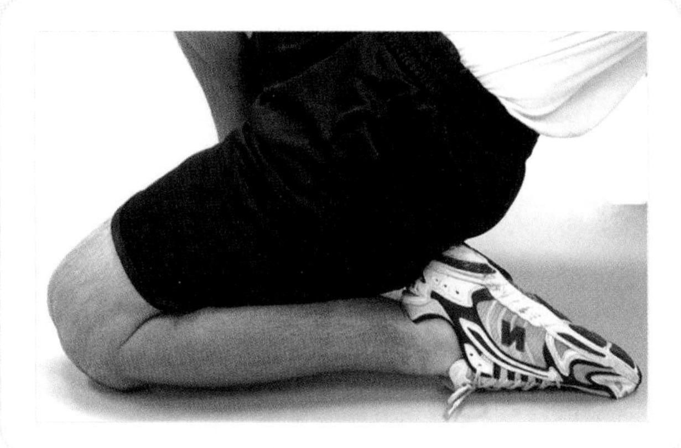

Figure 24-22 Sitting back on one's heels to achieve terminal knee flexion and assess flexion ROM

Phase III: Weeks 2 to 4 Clinical goals for phase III are full ROM, including terminal knee extension, and continued strengthening. The patient should work toward being able to sit back onto the heels. Again, ROM should be measured and documented at the end of this phase.

If full passive terminal extension or full flexion is not yet attained, other therapeutic methods should be taken to meet these goals. Because of the importance of attaining full ROM, especially extension, additional clinic visits may need to be scheduled. An extension board or other extension device can be used at home and during clinic visits to restore full extension. Supine flexion hangs are the most common method of regaining terminal flexion. The patient can gauge proximity to full terminal flexion by sitting back onto the heels (Figure 24-22).

Leg control through quadriceps strength is targeted with the addition of a progression of double leg squats to step-down exercises. Squats can begin bilaterally on a level surface progressing to a labile surface (Figure 24-23). High frequency and high repetitions are used to stimulate the patellar tendon graft harvest site. Progression to unilateral step-downs is determined by maintaining full ROM and minimal swelling.

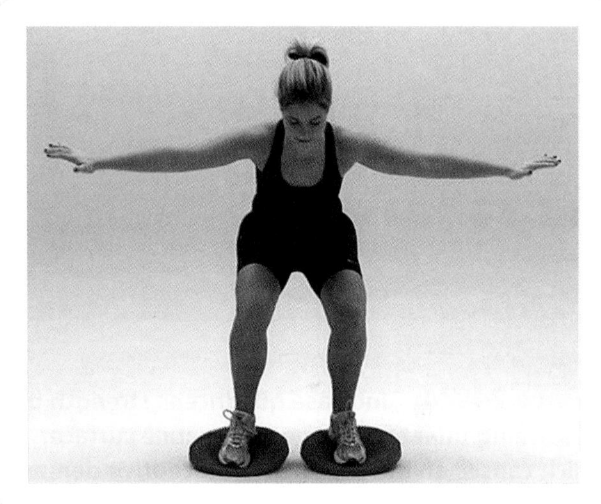

Figure 24-23 Increase quadriceps strength by performing bilateral squats on a labile surface, which causes an increase in proprioceptive demand

Progression to phase IV is achieved through equal motion bilaterally, a normal gait without assistive device, ability to stand on the surgical leg without assistance, and minimal pain and swelling. If these goals are not yet achieved, the athlete remains at phase III until the goals are met.

Phase IV: Weeks 4 to 12 Phase IV is characterized by improved strength and the initiation of functional activities. Full ROM including terminal extension should be maintained throughout this phase. Quadriceps tone should continue to improve with visible quadriceps definition returning. Once 70% quadriceps strength has been demonstrated, a proprioceptive and agility program can begin. A sport-specific functional progression can be set up toward the end of this phase.

Postoperative testing at 4 weeks includes a subjective knee questionnaire, bilateral ROM, and KT-1000 arthrometry. An isometric leg press test can also performed at this time. Near the 12-week postoperative date an isokinetic evaluation is performed at speeds of 60 degrees, 180 degrees, and 300 degrees per second.

During this period, strengthening exercises progress from bilateral to unilateral in an effort to emphasize strength of the quadriceps and patellar tendon graft site. The exercise

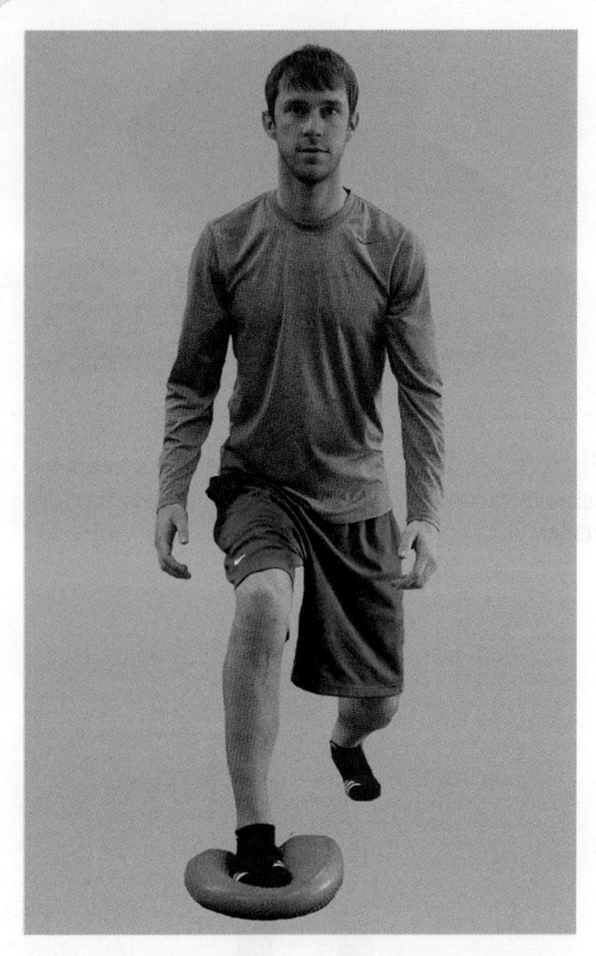

Figure 24-24 Increase quadriceps strength by performing unilateral lunges on a labile surface, which causes an increase in proprioceptive demand

regimen consists of unilateral leg presses, unilateral knee extensions, unilateral step-downs, and lunges on stable and unstable surfaces (Figure 24-24). Stair machines, stationary bicycles, and elliptical trainers can be used for aerobic conditioning and moderate speed strengthening.

Controlled agility training activities are initiated based upon the patient's subjective knee rating and strength-testing scores. Agility training and limited sports participation not only help the patient to regain quickness and functional movement patterns but also restore confidence in returning to previous functional status. Agility drills may include form running in shortened distances, backward running, lateral slides, crossovers, and single-leg hopping. Individual athletic drills should be sport specific, such as shooting a basketball or dribbling a soccer ball. For specifics on current jump training programs advocated for female athletes, refer to Chapter 31. This component of rehabilitation is not only for athletes, but should also be tailored to meet the demands each patient will face upon return to prior activity level.

Phase V: Week 12 and On Return to full activity is the focus of the final phase. The goals for the patient are to maintain full ROM, continue quadriceps strengthening, and increase activities as appropriate. Testing at this time includes a subjective knee questionnaire, bilateral ROM, KT-1000 arthrometry, isokinetic strength test, and isometric leg press. The single-leg hop test should be initiated now for a functional comparison of the legs. The single-leg hop is performed for distance with takeoff and landing from the same leg.

Exercises to maintain full ROM and continuous strength and conditioning are adjusted according to the patient's needs. A functional progression is integrated to meet the unique needs of each patient. The patient, family, coach, and athletic trainer need to be educated when and how to modify activity based upon subjective and objective knee findings. Return to full, nonrestricted activities is the ultimate goal of the patient and clinician in pursuit of a successful outcome. The patient will periodically follow up in the clinic for reassessment, strength testing, and research purposes.

Posterior Cruciate Ligament Sprain

Pathomechanics

Knowledge of anatomy and biomechanics of the PCL have been greatly expanded over the past 15 years. This increased understanding has led to a greater scientific basis for the design of rehabilitation approaches to this complicated ligament. Isolated injuries or tears of the PCL are uncommon and usually the result of a combined ligament injury. Most PCL tears occur on the tibia (70%), whereas 15% occur on the femur and 15% are midsubstance tears.[109] In the PCL-deficient knee, there is an increased likelihood of medial side meniscus lesions and chondral defects.[53]

As with other ligament sprains the severity of the injury is indicated by the degree of laxity. In a grade I injury, there will be 0 to 5 mm of posterior tibial translation but the tibial plateau will maintain its position anterior to the medial femoral condyle. A grade II sprain will have 5 to 10 mm of posterior translation of the tibial while the medial tibial plateau rests flush with the medial femoral condyle. A grade III sprain will demonstrate greater than 10 mm of posterior translation and the medial tibial plateau will fall posterior to the medial femoral condyle. Additionally with grades II and III sprains there will be increased laxity with the posterior drawer, posterior sag, and reverse pivot shift tests when compared to the opposite knee. Increased laxity is typically associated with combined ligament injuries and meniscus tears.

Mechanism of Injury

In athletics, the most common mechanism of injury to the PCL is with the knee in a position of forced hyperflexion with the foot plantar flexed. The PCL may also be injured when the tibia is forced posteriorly on the fixed femur or the femur is forced anteriorly on the fixed tibia. It is also possible to injure the PCL when the knee is hyperflexed and a downward force is applied to the thigh. Forced hyperextension and combined rotational forces will usually result in injury to both the PCL and ACL. If an anteromedial force is applied to a hyperextended knee, the posterolateral joint capsule may also be injured. If enough valgus or varus force is applied to the fully extended knee to rupture either collateral ligament, it is possible that the PCL may also be torn. When torn the ligament normally fails at its midsubstance, however, avulsions of the tibial or femoral attachments can occur. An isolated tear will occur during athletics, while combined injuries are more likely after traumatic high-energy trauma such as dislocations.

After PCL injury, the patients will likely indicate that they heard a pop. Unlike ACL injuries, patients sustaining injury to the PCL will often feel that the injury was minor and that they can return to activity immediately. There will be mild-to-moderate swelling occurring within 2 to 6 hours.

Rehabilitation Concerns

Perhaps the greatest concern in rehabilitating a patient with an injured PCL is altered joint arthrokinematics, which may eventually lead to degeneration of both the medial compartment and the patellofemoral joint. Van de Velde et al found that in patients with PCL-deficient knees there is a shift of tibiofemoral contact location and increased medial compartment cartilage deformation beyond 75 degrees of knee flexion.[157] Logan et al found that a ruptured PCL leads to an increase in passive sagittal laxity in the medial compartment, resulting in a persistent posterior subluxation of the medial tibia so that the femoral condyle rides up the anterior upslope of the medial tibial plateau.[94] Interestingly the kinematics of the lateral compartment are not altered by PCL rupture.

The treatment of PCL injuries remains unclear because of the uncertainty about the natural history and because of the lack of consistent and reproducible surgical results. Patients sustaining grade I or II PCL injuries should initially undergo nonoperative treatment as most athletes return to functional activity independent of degree of laxity. In addition, nonoperative treatment results are often similar to those for operative treatment. Many patients with an isolated PCL tear do not seem to exhibit any functional performance limitations and can continue to compete athletically, whereas others occasionally are limited in performing normal daily activities.[53] Parolie and Bergfield[122] reported a success rate of greater than 80% with nonoperative treatment and that knee stability was not related to return to sport or patient satisfaction.

Nonoperative treatment of PCL should follow a course of rehabilitation similar to that of the general progression presented earlier. For grades I and II injuries a more rapid progression with minimal immobilization can be undertaken. Rehabilitation following a grade III injury may be more reserved with a slower progression. In the early phase of grades I and II injuries, hamstring exercises should be avoided and knee extension should be performed in an arc of 0 to 60 degrees to prevent increased tibiofemoral shear forces. Bracing may be useful to prevent subtle subluxation in patients who report pain during rehabilitation, but is generally not recommended. For patients with a significant sag sign, it may be necessary to splint the knee in extension in order to promote healing in a shortened position. Often, there is minimal functional limitation and the patient may progress rapidly through the rehabilitative process with minimal pain and swelling. Because outcomes following nonoperative treatment of grade III injuries are less predictable, a more conservative approach is recommended. With these injuries a short course of immobilization with passive rather than active motion early may be required.

Operative treatment of acute or chronic grade II or III isolated PCL tears remains controversial. Furthermore, there are typically associated ligamentous injuries with increased posterior laxity. Therefore, PCL reconstructions are most often performed secondary to combined ligamentous instability, making the rate of performing isolated PCL reconstruction minimal. The decision to undergo operative treatment should be based on the functional participation status of the individual and associated risk factors that may produce arthritic changes.

Posterior Cruciate Ligament Rehabilitation Progression

Table 24-2 outlines the following discussion.

Phase I: Preoperative Phase I includes preoperative rehabilitation and objective testing. The goals of this phase include restoring full ROM and quadriceps strength, minimizing swelling and pain, and educating the patient in the basic principles of PCL

Table 24-2 Postoperative Rehabilitation After PCL Reconstruction

Phase	Days – Weeks	Goals	Restrictions	Treatment	Clinical Milestones
Phase I: Preoperative	PO	Restore ROM both active and passive Quadriceps activation Decreased effusion Pain reduction	WBAT with bilateral axillary crutches Brace locked at 0 degrees No isolated hamstring exercises	RICE Electrical stimulation Extension ROM Passive flexion ROM to 60 degrees Glute sets Quad sets Hip abduction/adduction	Surgical reconstruction Full knee extension Restoration of strength Minimal effusion No increased pain
Phase II: Immediate PO Phase	PO Wks 0 to 2	WBAT bilateral axillary crutches locked in extension Full knee extension Quadriceps control Pain reduction Normal patellar mobility	Full WBAT brace locked in full extension × 1 week After week 1 PROM flexion can be started Brace still locked in extension for weight bearing × 4 weeks No isolated hamstring exercises	Patellar mobilization Scar tissue mobilization PROM flexion and extension PROM flexion progressed to 60 degrees Quadriceps sets Straight leg raises × 4 Ankle pumps	Previous milestones Clean incisions Good quadriceps recruitment SLR with minimal lag Normalized patellar mobility Weight bearing progressed without symptoms Minimal pain and effusion

(continued)

Table 24-2 Postoperative Rehabilitation After PCL Reconstruction *(Continued)*

Phase	Days – Weeks	Goals	Restrictions	Treatment	Clinical Milestones
Phase III: Intermediate PO Phase	PO Wks 2 to 6	Normalized quadriceps recruitment Normal patellar mobility No pain or effusion Restoration of motion Maintain full weight bearing Improve balance	Braced unlocked for weight bearing at 4 weeks Brace allowed open to 100 degrees Crutches discontinued at 6 weeks No isolated hamstring exercises	Progression of previous PROM flexion progressed to 100 degrees Isometric quad sets at 0, 60, and 90 degrees Squats and leg press 0 to 60 degrees Stationary bike Step-downs Calf raises Balance drills	Previous milestones Satisfactory clinical exam ROM 0 to 120 degrees Improved stability with unilateral stance No pain Normal gait
Phase IV: Strengthening Phase	PO Wks 6 to 12	Increase strength and endurance No pain Preparation for activities	No isolated hamstring exercises	Previous strengthening Progress bilateral loading to single limb loading exercises Lunges 0 to 60 degrees Advanced balance activities Hip extension progressing to isolated hamstring exercises in 12 weeks	Previous milestones Full motion: 0 to 135 degrees Single-leg stance × 30 sec Squat 60 degrees with equal weight bearing No pain or effusion
Phase V: Return to Activity Phase	PO Wks 12+	Restoration of full motion No swelling No pain Return of full activities	Isolated hamstring exercises can begin at 12 weeks	Previous strengthening Unilateral calf raises Progress CKC exercises Advance hamstring exercises Agility drills Advanced balance drills Sports specific drills	Previous milestones Full motion Full confidence in knee Functional testing >90% of uninvolved Isokinetic testing >90% of uninvolved

CKC, closed kinetic chain; PO, postoperative; PROM, passive range of motion; RICE, rest, ice, compression, elevation; ROM, range of motion; SLR, single-leg raise; WBAT, weight bearing as tolerated; wks, weeks.

rehabilitation. Unlike patients with ACL injury, most patients with an isolated PCL injury do not have preoperative ROM limitations, quadriceps atrophy and weakness, or significant effusion. A functional PCL brace may be worn to assist in preventing posterior tibiofemoral shear forces. Strengthening exercises can progress as in the general progression with caution against hamstring dominated exercises and active knee flexion beyond

60 degrees. Preoperative testing consists of bilateral ROM, ligament arthrometry, and isokinetic strength evaluation.

Phase II: Days 1 to 14 The goals of phase II include controlling swelling and pain through the use of cryotherapy, improving gait quality, improving quadriceps control, and gradually returning flexion ROM.

The patient wears a Cryo Cuff and compression garment immediately postoperative through the first week. Cryotherapy can be weaned to 6 to 8 times per day after the first week of surgery. The patient will ambulate with crutches and a brace locked into extension, progressing from weight bearing as tolerated to full-weightbearing throughout the first 2 weeks. The brace should be unlocked several times per day for ROM but should remain locked in extension for 4 weeks. Extension ROM is maintained by laying the leg flat for 10 minutes, 3 to 4 times per day. The patient can work on passive flexion from 0 to 60 degrees, 3 to 4 times per day. Strengthening exercises to facilitate the early return of quadriceps control include quad sets, straight-leg raises, and knee extensions from 0 to 60 degrees of knee flexion. The patient is seen in the clinic 1 week postoperation to evaluate and modify the rehabilitation program as needed.

Phase III: Weeks 2 to 6 The goals of phase III include attaining symmetrical hyperextension, increasing flexion to 90 degrees, improving quadriceps strength, restoring patellar mobility, and restoring normal gait.

Cryotherapy is continued 4 to 6 times per day and a compression garment is worn in order to minimize residual swelling and pain. To avoid stretching the graft, the patient gradually begins to increase knee flexion passively up to 90 degrees, which can be done in a sitting position by placing a small bolster in the popliteal crease and gently pulling the distal tibia back. This technique ensures anterior placement of the tibia during flexion. Heel props or prone hangs can begin approximately 3 times per day in order to obtain symmetrical hyperextension. At the 4-week time frame, the brace can be opened up to 100 degrees for ambulation and ROM exercises. Patellar mobilization is also initiated in order to restore normal patellar glide and prevent contracture. Restoration of normal hyperextension and superior patellar glide is essential for proper patellofemoral biomechanics.

The patient may begin CKC strengthening that includes minisquats, calf raises, step-ups/-downs, and leg presses in addition to the strengthening exercises of phase II. The goals of strength training in this phase include muscle reeducation and protection of healing tissue. Active knee flexion and hamstring strengthening or activation must be avoided in this phase. Gait quality is assessed and progressed from full-weightbearing with a functional PCL brace locked at 100 degrees of flexion after 4 weeks.

Neuromuscular control drills at this time can be started to improve balance and coordination. Early exercises, such as weight-shifting to the involved leg progressing to unilateral stand on a stable surface, can be initiated in phase III.

Phase IV: Weeks 6 to 12 Goals of phase IV include gradual return of full flexion and aggressive strengthening. Cryotherapy is continued as needed. The flexion block on the PCL brace may be removed at this time. Full symmetrical ROM should be obtained by the end of weeks 10 to 12. Extension ROM is maintained by performing heel props, while full flexion is obtained by using the popliteal bolster and performing heel slides. The bolster may be removed once 120 degrees of flexion is achieved. The intensity of the current OKC and CKC strengthening exercises may be increased, and isolated hamstring strengthening can be initiated at the end of this phase if needed. Start hamstring strengthening by OKC hip extension progressing to isolated hamstring maneuvers (Figure 24-25). Step machine may be initiated using the PCL brace, and swimming may also begin following adequate healing of the incision. Exercises include squats, unilateral step-ups, and leg presses. ROM is measured during each clinical visit, and knee ligament arthrometry is conducted at the sixth postoperative week.

Neuromuscular control drills can progress in this phase to include unilateral balance activities on an unstable surface such as foam or balance board. Between weeks 6 and 12 perturbations can be added to the balance board, as well as sport-specific activities, such as catching a ball or swinging a racket, while balancing.

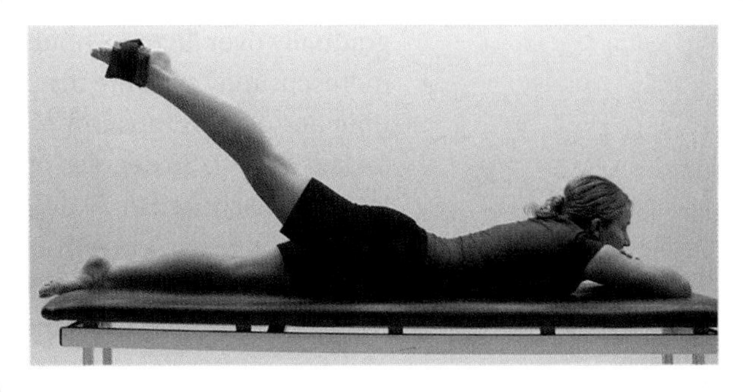

Figure 24-25 Initiation of hamstring exercises by combining with gluteus maximus during OKC hip extension

Phase V: Week 12 and On Phase V consists of weeks 12 through the first postoperative year. The goals of phase V include restoration of normal flexibility and a gradual return to sports, emphasizing return of power and endurance. Typically, the patient will experience a gradual return to full activity between 6 and 12 months postoperation.

Once full ROM is obtained, a comprehensive flexibility program is begun on a daily basis. The functional PCL brace may be removed and the aforementioned CKC strengthening exercises are performed with increased intensity, three times per week. Isotonic hamstring strengthening may be begun if rendered appropriated by the clinician. The principle of specificity is very important for preparing the athlete for the high-speed movements, jumping, and rapid changes in direction required by individual sports. Proprioceptive training needs to be addressed to improve static and dynamic balance deficiencies. Training for proprioception should be progressed from slow to fast speeds, low to high stress, and controlled to uncontrolled activities. Because real-life sport situations require response to rapid unknown or anticipated destabilizing loads to the knee, exercises that incorporate protective responses rapidly are helpful. This may require that quick, unanticipated, random destabilization loads be imparted to the patient's knee during rehabilitation drills.

Jogging and running are initiated once the patient has a strength of at least 75% compared to the uninvolved side. This usually does not occur until approximately 6 months after surgery. Running can begin in a pool, with progression to a treadmill and then to regular, level surface, dry land running.

Functional strength deficits need to be addressed if they are encountered in this phase, once the patient has achieved 80% of quadriceps strength compared to the uninvolved side. Agility drills are introduced in the 6- to 9-month postoperative time frame. These drills include change of direction, forward and backward running, lateral slides, shuttle drills, cutting, spinning, and carioca drills. The patient must safely pass a functional progression before a return to sports is allowed.

During periodic therapy visits at 6 months and 1 year, a subjective knee questionnaire, ROM, ligament arthrometry, isometric strength evaluation, and once strength is appropriate single-leg hop tests are performed at each of these visits. These tests are useful to make an informed decision regarding the safe return of the athlete to physical activity.

Meniscal Injury

Pathomechanics

The medial meniscus has a much higher incidence of injury than the lateral meniscus, which may be attributed to the coronary ligaments that attach the meniscus peripherally to the tibia and also to the capsular ligament. The lateral meniscus does not attach to the capsular ligament and is more mobile during knee movement. Because of the attachment to the medial structures, the medial meniscus is prone to disruption from valgus and torsional forces.

A meniscus tear often results in immediate joint-line pain with an effusion developing gradually over 48 to 72 hours. Initially, pain is described as a "giving-way" feeling. The torn meniscus may become displaced and wedge itself between the articulating surfaces of the tibia and femur, thus imposing a chronic locking or "catching" of the joint. A knee that is locked at 10 to 30 degrees of flexion may indicate a tear of the medial meniscus, whereas a knee that is locked at 70 degrees or more may indicate a tear of the posterior portion of the lateral meniscus. A positive McMurray test usually indicates a tear in the posterior horn of the meniscus.

Chronic meniscal lesions may also display recurrent swelling and obvious muscle atrophy around the knee. The patient may complain of an inability to perform a full squat or to change direction quickly without pain when running, a sense of the knee collapsing, or a "popping" sensation. Displaced meniscal tears can eventually lead to serious articular degeneration with major impairment and disability. Such symptoms and signs usually warrant surgical intervention.

Mechanism of Injury

Acute meniscus injuries are most often caused by coupled compression and rotation. As a result of these forces, the meniscus becomes pinched within the tibiofemoral joint and tears. Noncontact mechanisms include a plant and cut maneuver or jumping, common in sporting activities. A contact mechanism is usually the result of a direct blow or force to the knee that causes a valgus, varus, or hyperextension force combined with rotation while the knee is in a weightbearing position. Additional mechanisms during routine activities of daily living include squatting and pivoting in and out of a car.

Meniscal lesions can be longitudinal, oblique, or transverse. Stretching of the anterior and posterior horns of the meniscus can produce a vertical–longitudinal or "bucket-handle" tear. A longitudinal tear may also occur by forcefully extending the knee from a flexed position, while the femur is internally rotated. During extension, the medial meniscus is suddenly pulled back, causing the tear. In contrast, the lateral meniscus can sustain an oblique tear by a forceful knee extension with the femur externally rotated.

Rehabilitation Concerns

Three surgical treatment choices are possible for the patient with a damaged meniscus: partial meniscectomy, meniscal repair, or meniscal transplantation. Historically, it was an accepted surgical treatment for a torn meniscus to involve total removal of the damaged meniscus. However, total meniscectomy has been shown to cause premature degenerative arthritis. With the advent of arthroscopic surgery, the need for total meniscectomy has been virtually eliminated. Surgical management of meniscal tears should include every effort to minimize loss of any portion of the meniscus.

The location of the meniscal tear often dictates whether surgical treatment will involve a partial meniscectomy or a meniscal repair. Tears that occur within the avascular inner one-third of the meniscus will have to be resected because they are unlikely to heal, even with surgical repair. Because of adequate vascular supply, tears in the middle one-third of the meniscus, and particularly in the outer one-third, may heal well following surgical repair. Partial meniscectomy is much more common than meniscal repair.

Meniscus Repair Rehabilitation Progression

Table 24-3 outlines the following discussion.

As a result of soft-tissue healing restraint time frames, rehabilitation following meniscus repair techniques are usually different than that of meniscectomy. Stresses, such as loaded unrestricted weight bearing and knee flexion, that may be tolerable in a patient with meniscectomy, may be intolerable in a meniscus repair patient.

Table 24-3 Postoperative Rehabilitation After Meniscus Repair

Phase	Days – Weeks	Goals	Restrictions	Treatment	Clinical Milestones
Phase I: Immediate PO Phase	PO Wks 0 to 4	Quadriceps activation Decreased effusion Wound healing Pain reduction Begin proximal strengthening	WBAT with bilateral axillary crutches Brace locked at 0 degrees ROM 0 to 60 degrees flexion × 4 wks	RICE Electrical stimulation Glute sets Quad sets AAROM flexion to 60 degrees Hip abduction/adduction	Full knee extension ROM 0 to 60 degrees knee flexion Minimal effusion No increased pain Single limb stance
Phase II: Intermediate PO Phase	PO Wks 4 to 6	WBAT bilateral axillary crutches Quadriceps control Pain reduction Normal patellar mobility Progress to CKC exercises	Full WBAT brace opened to 0 to 90 degrees Discontinue crutches as tolerated	Exercises as previous Patellar mobilization Scar tissue mobilization AROM progressed to 90 degrees Heel raises Minisquats Step-ups Flexibility exercises Balance and proprioception	Previous milestones Good quadriceps recruitment Normalized patellar mobility Full weight bearing without symptoms Normal gait
Phase III: Advanced Strengthening Phase	PO Wks 6 to 10	Increase strength, power and endurance Normalized quadriceps recruitment Normal patellar mobility No pain or effusion Preparation for advanced activities	Knee flexion motion not greater than 130 degrees No pivoting	Progression of previous Advanced balance training Leg presses Endurance exercises Swimming and cycling	Previous milestones Satisfactory clinical exam Full ROM Improved stability with unilateral stance No pain Equal hip strength bilaterally
Phase IV: Return to Activity Phase	PO Wks 11 to 16+	Increase power and endurance Return to sports and ADLs Return to unrestricted activities	Avoidance of loaded full hyperflexion	Previous strengthening Endurance drills Agility drills Plyometrics Initiation of running progression Sports specific drills	Previous milestones Full confidence in knee Functional testing >90% of uninvolved Isokinetic testing >90% of uninvolved

ADLs, activities of daily living; AAROM, active assistive range of motion; CKC, closed kinetic chain; PO, postoperative; RICE, rest, ice, compression, elevation; ROM, Range of motion; WBAT, weight bearing as tolerated; Wks, weeks.

Phase I: Weeks 0 to 4 The goals of phase I include increasing quadriceps activation, decreasing effusion and pain and to begin proximal strengthening for full lower-extremity control. During the initial 4 weeks, weight bearing is allowed as tolerated as long as the brace is locked in full extension. Weightbearing forces may be beneficial to the repaired meniscus as it applies "hoop stress" to the meniscus, which actually pushes the meniscus peripherally, approximating the injured healing tissue. ROM during this time is limited to 0 to 60 degrees of flexion. It is thought that this is the safe range that does not allow undue shear stress to the healing tissue. Although flexion ROM is limited initially, extension is allowed to be full and expected to be equal to the uninvolved side.

Exercises that are tolerated at this time include quadriceps setting, gluteal sets, active assistive range of motion from 0 to 60 degrees flexion, ankle pumps, and straight-leg raises in all planes as tolerated. Modalities can be used judiciously for decreasing postoperative pain and swelling.

Criteria to progress to phase II include obtaining full knee extension equal to uninvolved side, ROM 0 to 60 degrees of flexion, minimal joint effusion and pain, and ability to stand on single leg without compensation or pain.

Phase II: Weeks 4 to 6 The goals of phase II are to gain better quadriceps control, restore normal patellar mobility, and progress closed kinetic exercises as tolerated. At 4 weeks, the brace can be opened to 0 to 90 degrees for activities and crutches can be discontinued if they are still used. Patellar mobility should be assessed and use of mobilizations is allowed to ensure full patellar motion is regained. Additionally at this time, incisions or portal sites should receive scar mobilization as needed to return full soft-tissue excursion.

In addition to previous exercises, CKC exercises can be initiated, including heel raises, minisquats, and step-ups. If CKC exercises cannot be performed in full weight bearing with proper form, they can be initially done on a total gym or leg press machine to offload some of the weight. Balance and proprioception exercises can also be started, including use of tilt boards. Balance exercises should always be started easy, with bilateral weight shifts progressing to harder exercises in a gradual, safe progression.

Criteria to move to phase III include previous milestones and good quadriceps recruitment, normal patellar mobility, ability to fully bear weight without pain or increased symptoms, and a normalized gait pattern without limp or antalgia.

Phase III: Weeks 6 to 10 Phase III goals are to begin working on strength, power and endurance. If Fq is not normalized by this time, it should be symmetrical to the uninvolved before this phase is over. This phase is to allow the patient to prepare for advanced activities of their sport or vocation.

At 6 weeks postoperation, if above criteria are met, the brace is allowed to be opened to 130 degrees. However, complete unrestricted hyperflexion and pivoting are not yet allowed. Advanced balance training drills are allowed. These include single-leg perturbation-type exercises with eyes open followed by eyes closed, if tolerated. Loaded leg presses, lunges, and squats are also allowed now. Swimming and cycling are started as tolerated, with gradual progressions of intensity and distance.

Criteria for phase IV include full motion and improved stability with unilateral stance. There should be no knee pain or swelling and proximal strength should also be equal bilaterally to allow forces that will be applied in the return to activity phase.

Phase IV: Weeks 11 to 16+ Phase IV goals are to continue to work on strength, power, and endurance, and to return the patient to sports or unrestricted activities of daily living. The limitation of no pivoting is lifted at this time, but full loaded hyperflexion is limited until 6 months.

Exercises include advancement of endurance drills and initiation of sport-specific or work-specific drills. Agility drills are advanced per patient needs. Plyometric activities can commence, as can a gradual running progression.

Before returning to sports or work, the patient should have full self-confidence in knee, have strength tests demonstrating 90% of uninvolved, and functional tests demonstrating 90% of uninvolved or age-matched normal.

Rehabilitation following meniscal repair commands restricted joint motion through 6 weeks to allow for soft-tissue healing. An upper body ergometer can be used to maintain cardiorespiratory endurance during this period. During this period, weight bearing is either limited, or allowed as tolerated with the knee locked in full extension, as per physician recommendations. Early strengthening can include quad sets and OKC hip exercises. Early, restricted, weightbearing exercise can be accomplished in an aquatic environment, when incisional healing allows. Chapter 16 has more details on aquatic rehabilitation. ROM exercises should focus on attaining flexion and extension within the restrictions. Partial weight bearing on crutches should progress to full weight bearing after 6 weeks. Once the brace can be removed, rehabilitation progresses similar to the general progression to regain full ROM and normal muscle strength. Generally, the patient can return to full activity around 3 months.

Not all meniscus tears require surgery. Some meniscus tears may heal or become asymptomatic without surgical intervention. When a tear remains symptomatic, surgery is recommended. Rehabilitation varies depending on the course of treatment and type of meniscal injury. Nonoperative rehabilitation aims to reduce swelling, restore full ROM, and normalize gait before returning to normal activities. The specific rehabilitation exercises for nonoperative rehabilitation are similar to those prescribed here for partial meniscectomy.

Partial Meniscectomy Rehabilitation Progression

Table 24-4 outlines the following discussion.

Phase I: Days 1 to 7 Clinical goals of phase I are to control swelling and inflammation, increase ROM, normalize gait, and improve quadriceps control. The clinician will test bilateral ROM during this phase.

A Cryo Cuff or other form of cryotherapy is applied 6 to 8 times per day to control pain and swelling. Cold application is particularly important following exercise. Use of a compression garment during the first postoperative week will help control swelling. However, with a partial meniscectomy a postoperative splint or motion control brace is not needed. The patient should keep the leg elevated as much as possible the first few days following surgery.

Regaining full extension is a critical factor in this phase. The patient is encouraged to push extension and regain full flexion through towel extensions, prone hangs, and heel slides. Extension can be assisted through a standing knee lockout with weight shifted to the operated leg.

The patient should begin partial to full weight bearing with bilateral axillary crutches. Use of crutches can be discontinued once gait is normalized. In most instances, the patient will be full weight bearing by 2 weeks. The patient may be non-weightbearing for a period of time if an osteochondral lesion is present on a weightbearing surface.

Quadriceps strengthening exercises are initiated to facilitate early return to normal strength. Strengthening should include straight-leg raises, knee extensions, and calf raises.

Phase II: Weeks 1 to 3 Phase II goals include attaining full ROM, normal gait, no swelling, and an early return to agility and sport-specific activities as tolerated. The clinician again measures ROM.

Cryotherapy should be continued 3 to 4 times per day and always after exercise. If the patient does not have full extension or flexion, ROM exercises are continued. Exercises should include unilateral one-quarter squats, unilateral step-downs, unilateral calf raises, and lunges. These exercises should not be performed if pain or crepitus exists.

Bicycle and stair machine workouts can begin in this phase. Initial workouts should be 10 to 15 minutes in length and progress to 30 minutes with moderate to high resistance. Toward the end of this phase, the patient can perform short sprints in 5-minute intervals.

Table 24-4 Postoperative Rehabilitation After Partial Meniscectomy

Phase	Days – Weeks	Goals	Restrictions	Treatment	Clinical Milestones
Phase I: Immediate PO Phase	PO Week 1	Independent ambulation Quadriceps activation Decreased effusion Wound healing Pain reduction	WBAT with bilateral axillary crutches as needed	RICE Glute sets Quad sets AAROM flexion to 60 degrees	Full extension No limp No increased effusion No increased pain
Phase II: Intermediate PO Phase	PO Weeks 1 to 3	Quadriceps control Pain reduction Normal patellar mobility Increased ROM Begin proximal strengthening	Full WBAT Discontinue crutches as tolerated	Exercises as previous Patellar mobilization Scar tissue mobilization Minisquats Step-ups Flexibility exercises Balance and proprioception	Previous milestones Full ROM Good quadriceps recruitment Normalized patellar mobility Full passive knee extension Full weight bearing without symptoms
Phase III: Advanced Strengthening Phase	PO Weeks 3 to 6	Normalized quadriceps recruitment Normal patellar mobility Full active ROM No pain No effusion	None at this time	Progression of previous Advanced balance training Leg presses Endurance exercises	Previous milestones Satisfactory clinical exam Improved stability with unilateral stance No pain Equal hip strength bilaterally
Phase IV: Return to Activity Phase	PO Weeks 6 to 8+	Return to sports and ADLs	None at this time	Previous strengthening Endurance drills Agility drills Plyometrics Initiation of running progression Sport-specific drills	Previous milestones Functional testing >90% of uninvolved Isokinetic testing >90% of uninvolved

ADLs, activities of daily living; AAROM, active assistive range of motion; PO, postoperative; RICE, rest, ice, compression, elevation; ROM, range of motion; WBAT, weight bearing as tolerated.

Freestyle and flutter kick swimming can be performed as well, but breaststroke is not encouraged. A jogging-to-sprinting progression can be performed in chest-deep water.

Proprioceptive and balance exercises to help improve neuromuscular control can begin in phase II and usually is advanced rapidly. Balance exercises can begin bilateral on a balance board progressing to unilateral as the patient is able to tolerate following the general principles of simple before complex exercises.

Once full ROM is regained and the patient has sufficient leg control, weight-room activities can be initiated. Exercises include unilateral leg presses, unilateral knee extensions, calf raises, and hamstring curls. Once tolerable, agility and sport-specific activities can commence toward the end of this phase.

Phase III: Weeks 3 to 6+ The focus of phase III is on a functional return to prior activity level. The patient is to maintain full ROM and no swelling. If weakness is noted, strengthening should continue to address the specific deficit. The clinician tests bilateral ROM and isokinetic strength if a specific athletic goal is desired. Implementation of a sport-specific functional progression is appropriate at this time.

Articular Cartilage

Articular cartilage covers the ends of bones of synovial joints. Water is the primary component (65% to 80%) of articular cartilage and provides for load deformation properties and gives cartilage its ability to absorb stress and compressive forces.[76] The reminder of articular cartilage components includes proteoglycans and noncollagenous proteins (10% to 15%) and collagen (10% to 15%). Articular cartilage provides a wear-resistant, accommodative surface that can withstand high compressive and shear loads during physical activities and movement. Because of synovial fluid and the properties of articular cartilage, a low coefficient of friction allows ease of movement between joint surfaces.

Pathomechanics

Hunter, in 1743, described articular cartilage as "a troublesome thing and once destroyed, it is not repaired."[70] Because of the prevalence of articular cartilage in the human body, injuries incurred to articular cartilage resulted in an estimated 385,000 procedures to repair articular cartilage defect in the United States in the year 1995 with numbers continuing to increase. A retrospective review assessing more than 25,000 knee arthroscopies found that 63% involved articular chondral lesions, with the most common location being the patellar articular surface (36%), with the medial femoral condyle a very close second (34%).[166]

Mechanism of Injury

Articular cartilage can be injured in multiple ways. Injury can be incurred during trauma or sports activities through direct blunt trauma to the knee such as landing on the ground or other hard surface or from a contusion between knee and helmet during a tackle in football. An indirect injury to the bone and overlying articular cartilage can occur during a twisting or torsional maneuver, such as occurs when making a plant-and-cut pattern to fake an opponent in soccer or basketball, that ultimately injures the ACL. Lastly, prolonged immobilization of a joint creates a loss of joint movement and synovial fluid production, and the fluid becomes stagnant and the nutrients in the synovial fluid depleted. Without this movement and constant flow of fresh synovial fluid necrosis of the articular cartilage occurs.[98-100] The significance of articular cartilage atrophy and degeneration is related to the magnitude and duration of joint immobilization. Joint contact surfaces suffer greater degenerative changes than noncontact areas of articular cartilage.[98-100]

Rehabilitation Concerns

A primary problem with articular cartilage injuries to the knee is that the injuries most commonly occur in the area of the patella or femoral condyle that makes contact between 30 and 70 degrees of knee flexion.[134] This commonly affected ROM is used for almost all activities of daily living, including normal gait, ascending and descending stairs, and sitting and rising from chairs.

An injury to vascularized tissue incites a cascade of events characterized by hemorrhage, inflammation, and fibrin clot formation. This reaction is almost nonexistent as articular cartilage is a nonhomogeneous and avascular tissue that lacks the ability to stimulate, regulate, or organize intrinsic repair.[3] Furthermore, mechanisms that hamper cartilage repair include both cell apoptosis and the presence of catabolic enzymes. These mechanisms impede the ability of differentiated chondrocytes to multiply sufficiently in tissue or to reach the site of injury by migration in extracellular matrix.[97,146] Without a vascular response, articular cartilage cannot form a fibrin scaffold or mobilize cells to repair the defect. Chondrocytes are trapped within the dense extracellular matrix and are incapable of mobilizing the damage site via vascular access channels.[100]

Surgical Procedures

In general, there are 2 broad forms of surgical treatment for articular cartilage injury. The first are marrow-stimulating techniques involving utilizing one's own body's pluripotent marrow stem cells to create reparative tissue consisting of fibrocartilage, which consists of primarily type 1 collagen.[113] These techniques include procedures such as microfracture, abrasion chondroplasty, and subchondral drilling to allow marrow stem cells to repopulate the area devoid of articular cartilage. These procedures are still commonly used because they can be done arthroscopically, cost very little, and are thought to relieve symptoms. The drawback seems to be that the cartilage that returns is usually fibrocartilage, the repair tissue that does not have the robust wear characteristics of the original hyaline type tissue.

The second group of procedures aims to restore the injured area with normal or near-normal articular cartilage. These procedures are called *cartilage replacement techniques* and include those such as osteochondral autografts and autologous chondrocyte implantation procedures. The main goals of these techniques are to restore normal articular cartilage contour of the joint and provide a superior wear surface more like the original articular cartilage that is being replaced. These procedures are, however, more demanding and incur not only increased cost, but longer rehabilitation and potentially more complications.

Rehabilitation following articular cartilage procedures is still in its infancy. Little is known regarding optimal treatment. Although like other knee postoperative rehabilitation early motion and progression to closed chain activity is needed, the optimal time frame for progression is not yet standardized due to varied procedures and surgeon own rehabilitation philosophy. Until specific guidelines are determined to be optimal, it is crucial that the surgeon and therapist have excellent communication regarding extent of damage, durability of the surgical procedure, size of defect, location of lesion, and specific restrictions placed upon the patient.[106]

Articular Cartilage Rehabilitation Progression

Table 24-5 outlines the following discussion.

Phase I: Weeks 1 to 6 The first phase of rehabilitation following articular cartilage procedures is the *Proliferation Phase* in which healing constraints are placed upon the patient to protect the repair.[16,17,169] Although advances allow some early weight bearing in isolated cases, usually there is some form of controlled partial weight bearing initially. Therefore, it is important to gradually increase passive motion, increase weight bearing, and decrease swelling and enhance motor control of the quadriceps muscles.

Because of the movement of synovial fluid in the knee joint, passive ROM is performed to create diffusion of the synovial fluid and provide stimulation for reparative cells to be produced.[19,20,161] Passive ROM exercises can be done via CPM device or with a physical therapist. This passive movement of the knee is started immediately after surgery to help nourish healing articular cartilage and prevent intraarticular scar adhesions from forming. Some have recommended the use of CPM for 8 hours per day for up to 6 to 8 weeks.[132] If a CPM device is not available, the judicious use of active assisted or passive ROM is recommended for the reasons listed above. In addition to knee joint, passive ROM emphases should be

Table 24-5 **Postoperative Rehabilitation after Microfracture and ACI**

Phase	Weeks	Goals	Restrictions	Treatment	Clinical Milestones
Phase I: Early PO Phase	PO 0 to 6	Independent ambulation Quadriceps activation Decreased effusion Wound healing Pain reduction	NWB or TTWB with bilateral axillary crutches	RICE Glute sets Quad sets in ROM that does not engage lesion PROM and AAROM in range restriction that does not engage lesion site per surgeon orders Full extension × 1 week Full flexion × 6 weeks OKC exercises light resistance in ROM that does not engage lesion × 4 weeks Patellar mobilization Scar tissue mobilization No CKC exercises	Full extension Independent use of ambulatory device No increased effusion No increased pain
Phase II: Intermediate PO Phase	PO 6 to 12	Quadriceps control Pain reduction Normal patellar mobility Increased ROM Begin CKC exercises Begin proximal strengthening Increased balance	DC crutches gradually as tolerated at 8 weeks May use pool or unweighting devices to transition to full weight bearing	Exercises as previous Begin CKC exercises Restrict range that does not engage lesion Minisquats Step-ups Flexibility exercises Balance and proprioception	Previous milestones Full ROM extension and flexion Good quadriceps recruitment Normalized patellar mobility Full passive knee extension Full weight bearing without symptoms
Phase III: Return to Activity Phase	PO 12+	Normalized quadriceps recruitment Normal patellar mobility Full active ROM No pain No effusion	Continue to increase tolerance to OKC, CKC exercises as tolerated limiting to ranges that do not engage lesion or cause symptoms	Progression of previous Advanced balance training Leg presses Endurance exercises Agility and sports specific exercises should begin at 50% effort progressing to full as tolerated Running delayed until 6 months	Previous milestones Satisfactory clinical exam Improved stability with unilateral stance No pain Equal hip strength bilaterally Quadriceps and hamstring strength to within 90% bilaterally

ADLs, activities of daily living; AAROM, active assistive range of motion; CKC, closed kinetic chain; NWB, non-weightbearing; OKC, open kinetic chain; PO, postoperative; PROM, passive range of motion; RICE, rest, ice, compression, elevation; ROM, range of motion; TTWB, touch-toe weightbearing.

placed on performance of patellar mobilization and passive movement, as a loss of motion across the extensor mechanism could be deleterious to normal knee function.

Because weight bearing is limited initially in the proliferative phase, early strengthening exercises are directed toward quadriceps volitional neuromuscular motor control rather than strict muscle strengthening. Because of weightbearing limitations, exercises are limited to those of an open-chain nature, including quadriceps setting and straight-leg raises in all planes. Any quadriceps exercise can be supplemented with electrical stimulation if there is a lack of neuromuscular control during active contraction. In some limited instances, depending on the location of the lesion, partial weight bearing may be allowed with the use of a rehabilitation brace locked in full extension.[43] The surgeon should include on the physical therapy referral form the type of surgical procedure, the location of the lesion, and any restrictions in ROM and weight bearing. A diagram of the lesion site is also helpful, as it enables the therapist to adhere to the ROM limitations and ensure that the lesion is not engaged during exercise.[43]

Phase II: Weeks 6 to 12 Weeks 6 to 12 are known as the *Transition Phase*.[16,17,169] Usually by 6 weeks the lesion has begun to fill in with immature cartilage tissue and is able to tolerate an increased progression of weight bearing and therapeutic exercises. It is at this time that the patient progresses from partial weight bearing to full weight bearing. Progression of weight bearing has been called into question lately as it is felt by some that although an "excessive" approach to weight bearing may risk graft delamination, whereas a too "conservative" approach may not provide adequate biomechanical graft stimulus.[35,36] The physical therapist should watch for signs of regression if the therapist sees an increase in patient pain or knee joint effusion with weightbearing increases. If this occurs, it may be an indication that the articular lesion is being harmed and both ROM and progression of weight bearing may need to be decreased until symptoms have subsided. It is usually during the 6- to 12-week time frame that patients believe they can begin to return to normal activities of daily living without the substantial restrictions that were imposed by weightbearing limitations and motion restriction in the previous phase.

Two ways in which exercise progression can be graded during this phase of increased weight bearing and stress are to begin using cardinal planes of movement before multiple planes and using bilateral exercise prior to unilateral loading exercises. Weightbearing exercises, such as squats, lunges, and weight shifting, should begin in cardinal planes, moving either in anterior-posterior or medial-lateral directions before using multiple plane-type movements, such as diagonals and rotation movements. Additionally, these exercises should always be done with 2 legs prior to progressing to a single leg. Utilization of this simple-to-complex progression of exercises ensures a gradual progression of applied loads and stress so as not to overload or damage healing cartilage tissue.

Phase III: Months 3 to 6 Postoperative months 3 to 6 are called the *Remodeling Phase*.[16,17,169] It is thought that during this phase there is an ongoing remodeling of the cartilage tissue that allows it to gain strength and durability. In this phase, activities can be increased to allow light functional activities. Patients without symptoms in this phase should continue all previous exercises from the prior stage but can begin more functional loading activities also. Low-to-moderate impact activities, including recreational walking on level ground, bicycle riding, and golfing, may begin as tolerated. High-impact activities are still not advisable at this point; however, with select patients and surgeon approval, adapted high-impact activities, such as jogging in a pool or use of an Alter G Antigravity Treadmill (Fremont, CA), may be permitted.

Phase IV: Months 6 to 18 The final phase, called the *Maturation Phase*, runs from 6 months to approximately 18 months postsurgery.[16,17,169] Full maturation of the articular cartilage defect depends on multiple factors, including health of patient, age of patient, size of defect, location of defect, and surgical procedure performed. Just like previous phases, impact loading should be done slowly and gradually, in a progressively gradient manner. These activities should be always patient specific based on their presentation and varied needs or requirements.

General Rehabilitation Progression for Patellofemoral Pathology

Table 24-6 outlines the following discussion.

A patient with patellofemoral pain should initially be treated with a tailored conservative rehabilitation program. An effective rehabilitation program takes into consideration the anatomy of the joints, the stage of healing, and the patient's response to treatment. Chapter 31 presents additional discussion of patellofemoral considerations in athletic

Table 24-6 General Rehabilitation for Patellofemoral Pathology

Phase	Weeks	Goals	Precautions	Treatment	Clinical Milestones
Phase I: Acute Phase	1	Independent ambulation Decreased effusion Pain and inflammation reduction	Avoid kneeling, deep squatting, prolonged positioning, and other aggravating activities	Relative rest Cryotherapy, antiinflammatory modalities LE stretching Grade I and II mobilizations	Full ROM Normalized gait Minimal effusion Minimal pain
Phase II: Intermediate Phase	2 to 6	Pain reduction Normal patellar mobility Normal LE flexibility LE strengthening, including thigh, hip, and calf musculature Maintenance of cardiovascular conditioning	Avoid kneeling, deep squatting, flexed-posture cycling, running (especially hills), and other aggravating activities	Continued cryotherapy and modalities as indicated Patellar glides and tilts LE stretching IT band, quadriceps, hamstrings, calf LE and core progressive strengthening Quadriceps, hip abduction, hip ER, and hip extension strengthening OKC exercises 60 to 90 degrees CKC exercises 0 to 45 degrees Orthotic needs evaluation Proprioceptive and cardiovascular training	>80% LE strength, balance, and proprioception Normalized patellar mobility and LE flexibility
Phase III: Advanced Phase	6+	Return to pain-free ADL Full LE strength, balance, and proprioception Tolerance for return-to-sport progression initiation	Avoid hill running and aggravating activities	Advanced strength and balance training Continued flexibility exercises Endurance exercises Bracing or taping as indicated	No pain during ADL Equal LE strength, balance, and proprioception bilaterally Return to sport

ADL, activities of daily living; CKC, closed kinetic chain; ER, external rotation; IT, iliotibial; LE, lower extremity; OKC, open kinetic chain; ROM, range of motion.

females. A general 3-phase rehabilitation program for patellofemoral injury is presented, with specific techniques for defined patellofemoral conditions to follow. The time frames of each phase varies, depending on pathology severity and patient activities, such as vocational necessities.

Phase I: Days 0 to 7

Phase I goals are to control pain and inflammation of the involved soft-tissue structures, restore normal ROM and gait, and educate the patient about the rehabilitation progression and safety considerations. Controlling pain and inflammation allows the patient to progress comfortably through the rehabilitation process. Full knee ROM and normal gait mechanics are essential to return to typical daily activities and initiate functional rehabilitation exercises.

Cryotherapy in the form of ice bags or ice massage, 3 to 4 times per day, is effective in reducing pain and controlling inflammation. Other physical modalities including ultrasound, iontophoresis, and electrical stimulation may also help control patellofemoral symptoms. Physician-prescribed nonsteroidal antiinflammatory medication can be useful as well. Active and active-assistive ROM exercise, a partial to full weightbearing progression, and the use of assistive devices as needed will aid restoration of knee ROM and normal ambulation. The patient should be educated to modify or avoid activities that exacerbate patellofemoral pain (such as kneeling, deep squatting, or prolonged positioning), and encouraged to manage symptoms with modalities or rest as they occur.

Phase II: Weeks 2 to 6

The emphasis of phase II is flexibility, advanced strengthening, proprioception, and cardiovascular conditioning. Exercise intensity and stress on the patellofemoral joint should be kept low in an effort to progress through rehabilitation without increasing symptoms. The clinician should conduct a dynamic biomechanical evaluation once ROM and gait are normal to determine the underlying cause of dysfunction. By the end of phase II, the patient should have improved flexibility of tightened structures, improved lower-extremity strength and proprioception, and maintained level of cardiovascular conditioning. In addition, the patient's biomechanical abnormalities should be addressed.

Flexibility

Flexibility exercises addressing deficits in the quadriceps, hamstrings, ITB, and gastrocnemius–soleus complex must be initiated. Evidence demonstrates abnormal joint stress if these tissues lack flexibility.[110,164] The frequency and duration of such stretching is controversial. Studies of individuals with limited hamstring flexibility (a 30-degree loss of knee extension at 90 degrees of hip flexion) have examined the differences of 30- and 60-second duration stretches.[10,11] The studies were in agreement that no increase in flexibility occurred when the duration of stretching was increased from 30 to 60 seconds; however, the average age of these subjects was 26 years. Research on stretching duration in elderly people has revealed that optimal stretching protocols may be age dependent. A study by Feland et al indicated that 60-second stretches were more effective than 15- or 30-second stretches for groups of elderly subjects with tight hamstrings during a 6-week stretching routine.[40] Nonetheless, lower-extremity tissue flexibility must be optimized to reduce abnormal loading of the patellofemoral joint.

In addition to muscular flexibility, patellar mobility should be incorporated to address imbalances in the passive soft tissue stabilizers. The patient can be instructed in self-mobilization techniques to correct an abnormal patellar glide or tilt (Figure 24-26).

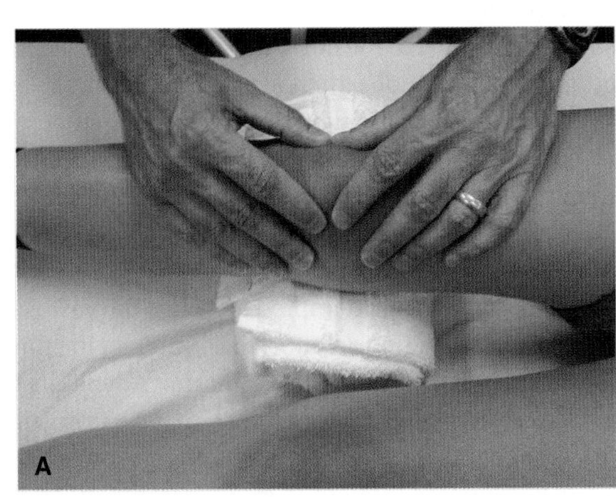

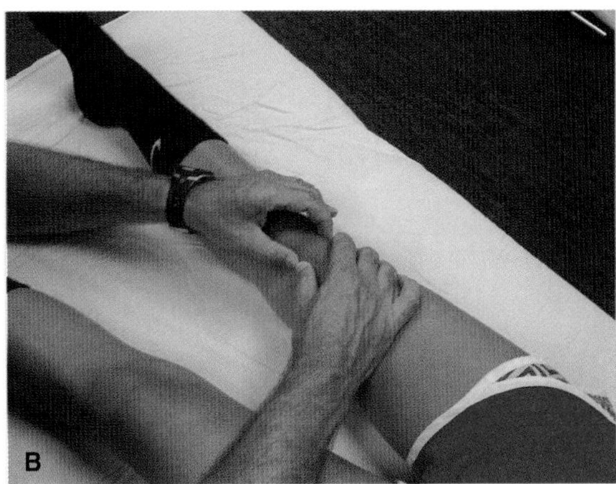

Figure 24-26 **Mobilization for the patella**

A. To mobilize the patella for a restricted medial glide, instruct the patient to long sit with knees straight and quadriceps relaxed. **B.** To mobilize the patella for a restricted lateral tilt (tight deep medial retinacular fibers), push laterally and anteriorly on the undersurface of the medial edge of the patella with the thumbs and push posteriorly on the lateral edge of the patella with the fingertips, titling laterally.

OKC and CKC Strengthening

Strengthening exercises for patients with patellofemoral dysfunction have shifted from non-weightbearing OKC exercises to more functional CKC exercises. This change is a result of reports that CKC exercise causes less patellofemoral joint stress and may, therefore, be more tolerable for patients with patellofemoral dysfunction.

A study by Steinkamp et al[126] demonstrated that patellofemoral joint stresses for leg press and leg extension exercises intersect at 48 degrees of knee flexion. Patellofemoral stress at 0 and 30 degrees of knee flexion was significantly less during the CKC leg press exercise than OKC leg extension exercise. Conversely, at 60 and 90 degrees of knee flexion, patellofemoral stress was significantly greater during the leg press exercise than during the leg extension exercise.

Similarly, Escamilla et al[38] showed that patellofemoral stress during the leg press exercise progressively increases as the knee flexion angle increases. During OKC knee extension, the results revealed progressively increasing patellofemoral stress until approximately 60 degrees of knee flexion, at which point patellofemoral stress was inversely related to knee flexion angles as the knee continued to flex. Escamilla et al recommended CKC exercise in between 0 and 50 degrees of knee flexion, and OKC exercise at lower (0 to 30 degrees) or higher (75 to 90 degrees) knee flexion angles.

In 2000, Witvrouw et al[172] performed the first prospective, randomized study comparing the efficacy of OKC versus CKC exercises in the management of patellofemoral pain. The group using a CKC protocol had significant improvements in pain and function compared to the OKC group. However, both protocols showed increased quadriceps strength and function, and decreased pain. As a result, Witvrouw et al suggest using both OKC and CKC strengthening in the treatment of patellofemoral pain.

An evidence-based approach to OKC and CKC exercises for the patient with patellofemoral pain will include both interventions. OKC exercises, such as leg extensions, appear produce less stress between 60 and 90 degrees of knee flexion, and CKC exercises appear to produce less joint stress between 0 and 45 degrees of knee flexion (Figure 24-27). The safest ROM will undoubtedly be different for each patient. The patient and clinician should

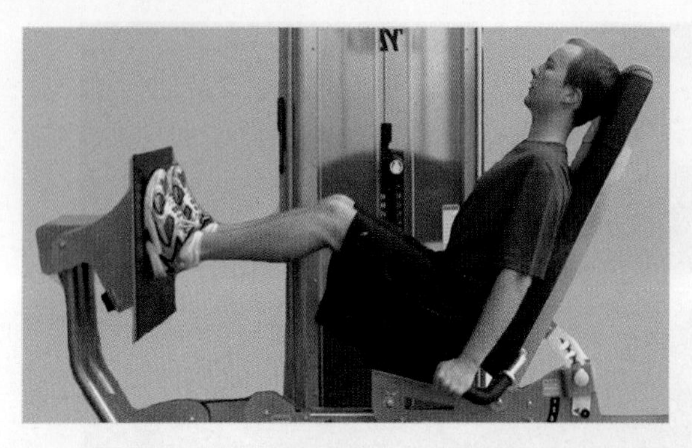

Figure 24-27 CKC exercises, such as the leg press, produce less patellofemoral joint stress between 0 and 45 degrees of knee flexion than greater degrees of flexion

be conscious of pain, crepitus, and the location of patellar articular surface lesions during exercise. An optimal progression includes increases in repetitions, external loads, and ROM per patient's tolerance. Activities may also be advanced by transitioning from bilateral to unilateral stance, with or without perturbation or labile surfaces.

Role of the Vastus Medialis Obliquus

Clinicians have long attempted to isolate the vastus medialis obliquus (VMO) in an effort to counteract the pull of the vastus lateralis and subsequently improve dynamic patellar tracking. Mirzabeigi et al[111] studied the electromyographic (EMG) activity of the separate quadriceps muscles during 9 sets of exercises thought to target VMO recruitment. The results showed that EMG activity of the VMO was not significantly greater than the other muscles tested, suggesting that the VMO cannot be significantly isolated during these exercises. Some studies have, however, shown that high levels of VMO EMG activity relative to vastus lateralis can be produced during leg press, lateral step-up, terminal knee extension, quad set, and hip adduction exercises.[28,75,145,168]

A review of the evidence shows that altering lower-limb joint orientation or adding a cocontraction does not preferentially enhance VMO activity over the vastus lateralis, but more well-designed studies are required.[147] Regardless, recruitment and strengthening of the VMO occurs in conjunction with general strengthening of the entire quadriceps, and is essential for rehabilitation of the patient with patellofemoral pathology.[111] The benefit of quadriceps strengthening has been emphasized in several studies of patients with patellofemoral pain.[15,78,127] Cowen et al[27] reported delayed onset of VMO EMG activity during stair climbing in patients with patellofemoral pain compared to controls. Chiu et al[25] reported that lower-limb strength training 3 times per week for 8 weeks, including knee extension exercises, significantly increased patellofemoral joint contact area in patients with patellofemoral pain syndrome, effectively reducing mechanical stress to the joint. Additionally, Natri et al[115] performed a 7-year prospective follow-up study of patients with chronic patellofemoral pain that found extension strength to be a significant predictor of successful outcomes.

Distal Factors

The role of foot mechanics in patellofemoral joint dysfunction has been theorized for quite some time. Buchbinder et al[18] proposed that prolonged pronation would internally rotate the lower extremity, producing a medially displaced patella. Tiberio[155] similarly contended that excessive subtalar joint pronation produces excessive internal rotation of the femur, causing increased lateral patellofemoral joint contact forces.

As a result, clinicians have attempted to limit the amount of tibial internal rotation and coupled femoral internal rotation in an effort to decrease the Q angle and resultant lateral patellofemoral joint contact forces. Klingman et al[82] reported that a medial wedge orthosis was capable of producing a mean medial displacement of the patella relative to the femoral trochlear groove of 1.08 mm. Sutlive et al[152] found that the best predictors of improvement in patients with patellofemoral pain using an off-the-shelf foot orthosis and modified activity were forefoot valgus alignment of 2 degrees or more, passive great toe extension of 78 degrees or less, or navicular drop of 3 mm or less. A more recent study suggests that age older than 25 years, height less than 65 inches, and maximum pain level on a visual analog scale of less than 53.25 mm are also strongly predictive of benefit from foot orthoses.[159]

A complete lower-extremity biomechanical examination in weightbearing and nonweightbearing positions is important. Literature supports an association between excessive pronation, lower-extremity internal rotation, and altered patellofemoral mechanics. Patients demonstrating excessive foot pronation or excessive lower-extremity internal rotation may benefit from a foot orthosis as part of a comprehensive rehabilitation program. Chapter 26 discusses examination and prescription of foot orthotics.

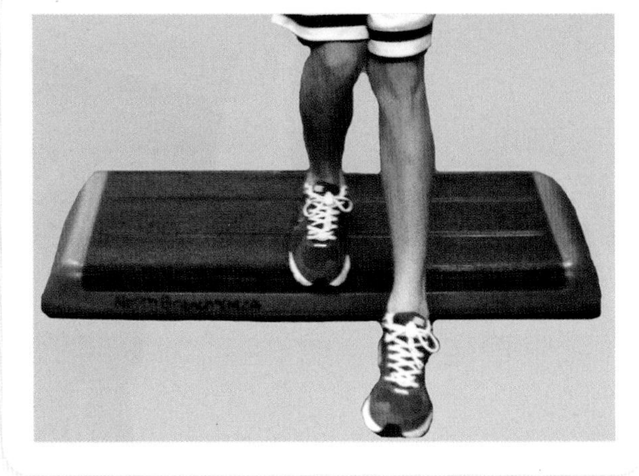

Figure 24-28 Femoral adduction and internal rotation collapse during weightbearing activities

Proximal Factors

Patients with patellofemoral pain who demonstrate a lack of adduction and internal rotation control during weight-bearing activities are candidates for hip strengthening (Figure 24-28). Internal rotation of the femur causes the trochlear groove to rotate underneath the patella, generating increased lateral patellofemoral joint stress as a result of the relative lateral position of the patella.[87]

Several studies demonstrate that patients with patellofemoral pain have hip strength deficits including abduction, external rotation, and extension.[108] Ireland et al[74] reported that subjects with patellofemoral pain were 26% weaker in hip abduction and 36% weaker in hip external rotation compared to a control group. Moreover, several studies have shown significant decreases in pain and increases in function following hip abductor and external rotator strengthening in patients with patellofemoral pain.[49,81,114]

Assessment of the hip and pelvis must be a priority in patients with suspected proximal weakness or lack of dynamic pelvic control, but the flexibility of proximal tissues must also be examined. Iliotibial band tightness is especially correlated with patellofemoral pathology; therefore, stretches to optimize the tissue's flexibility should be implemented.[65,67,171]

Proprioception and Cardiovascular Conditioning

The pain and abnormal tissue stresses present in patellofemoral dysfunction may lead to proprioception deficits. Baker et al[8] found that joint position sense was significantly decreased in knees with patellofemoral pain compared to the control group, decreased between the symptomatic and asymptomatic knees in the test group, and decreased between the asymptomatic knees in the test group compared to the control group. Whether or not proprioception deficits precede or result from patellofemoral pain, proprioception must be addressed during rehabilitation.

Maintaining cardiovascular conditioning is another important objective when treating a patient with patellofemoral pain. The clinician should strive to provide the patient with alternative training methods that allow pain-free knee ROM and minimize patellofemoral stress for return to prior activity level. Depending on the cause of patellofemoral pain and involved tissues, options for cardiovascular conditioning include jogging, swimming, bicycling on raised seats, and upper body ergometry or other forms of endurance exercise equipment. A recent study by Roos et al demonstrates that backward running produces 25% less patellofemoral joint compression forces compared to forward running; therefore, it may be preferred as a unique way to maintain cardiovascular conditioning.[133]

Phase III: Week 7 and On

The goal of phase III is to return the patient to the prior level of activity. A maintenance program of cryotherapy, lower-extremity flexibility, and lower-extremity strengthening should be continued 3 times per week to maintain the gains of phase II. Prior to full return

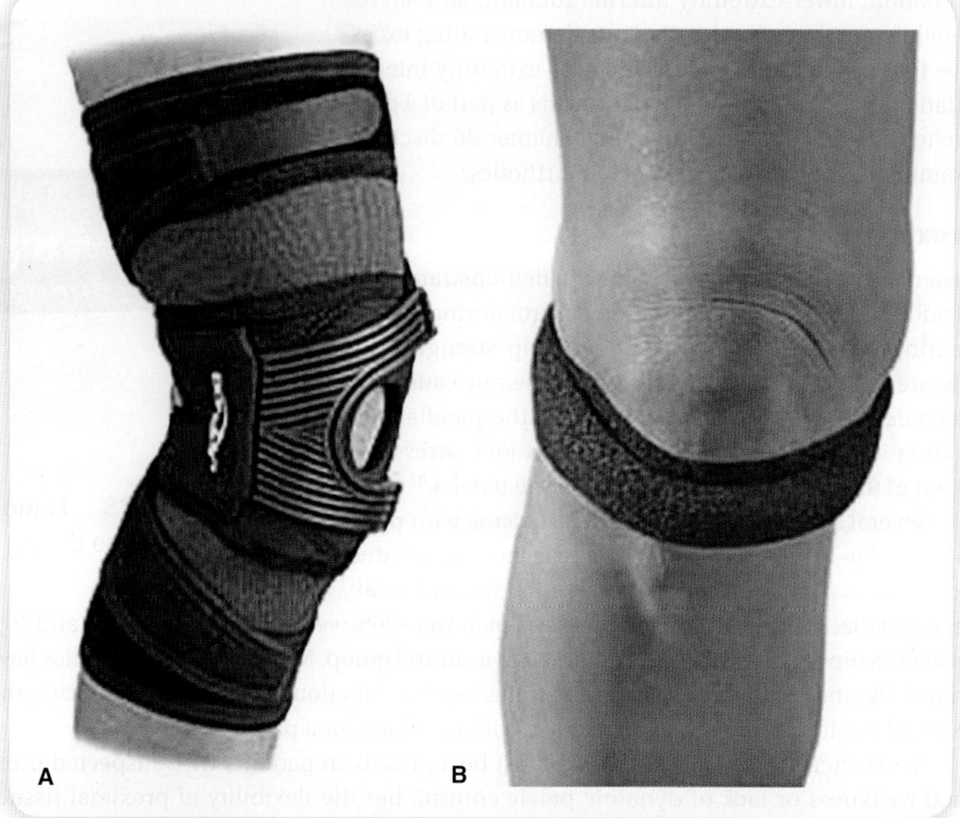

Figure 24-29 **External supports**

A. Patellar sleeve with lateral J buttress and straps for patellar subluxation or lateral patellar alignment. **B.** Infrapatellar band for patellar tendinitis and traction apophysitis.

to activity, an activity-specific functional progression should be performed with the use of external support as needed. The importance of abdominal stability is also applicable during this phase, especially for athletes and active individuals. Suboptimal core muscle function has been correlated with knee pathomechanics in multiple studies.[1,175]

Bracing and Taping

Many external supports (Figure 24-29) have been designed to augment the return to pain-free activity through helping to maintain patellar alignment or decrease soft-tissue stresses. Patellar braces are typically made of an elastic wrap or neoprene sleeve with various cutouts and pads to help control patellar positioning and tracking. An infrapatellar strap placed around the patellar tendon has been advocated for patellar tendinitis or traction apophysitis, and an ITB strap placed around the distal ITB for ITB friction syndrome. These straps apply compression near the site of irritation and act as a "counterforce" to decrease stress at the tendinous insertion. Although research on patellar straps is scant, similar braces have been shown to increase pain threshold and affect proprioception in patients with lateral epicondylitis.[116]

Although wearing a brace appears to be effective in reducing pain, radiographic studies show that decreases in pain are not the result of improvement in patellar alignment.[128] Powers et al[125] found a significant reduction in pain immediately upon application of patellar bracing and a significant increase in total patellofemoral joint contact area, as well as small but significant changes in lateral patellar displacement. Their results suggest that increases in patellofemoral joint contact area may decrease patellofemoral pain by decreasing joint stress. Powers et al[130] again supported this theory with a study that showed bracing significantly decreased patellofemoral stress during free and fast walking when compared to the nonbraced condition.

Bracing appears to provide some patients with a decrease in pain, improved patellofemoral joint contact, and the allowance of an adequate quadriceps strengthening and exercise progression.[129] The pain reduction secondary to wearing a brace may be the edge a patient needs to continue with rehabilitation exercises and return to sport activity. However, a brace should not be a substitution for a comprehensive rehabilitation program. A recent review reports moderate evidence for no additive effectiveness of knee braces to exercise therapy on pain and conflicting evidence on function.[153] A popular adjunct to treating patellofemoral pain is taping (Figure 24-30). In 1986, McConnell[107] published the taping methods for the treatment of patellar chondromalacia. The theory behind the McConnell taping technique is a passive correction of the abnormal glide, tilt, and rotational components of patellar maltracking to allow pain-free rehabilitation and facilitate VMO recruitment.

Much like bracing, numerous studies support that taping provides pain relief. However, alteration in patellar alignment or facilitation of the VMO has also been disputed. Pfeiffer et al[126] showed that McConnell medial glide taping resulted in significant medial glide of the patellofemoral joint before, but not after, a running and agility task. Ng and Cheng[117] reported a significant decrease in pain with patellar taping, but also reported a decrease in the relative activity of the VMO. A randomized controlled trial by Wittingham et al[165] found that the combination of taping and exercise was superior to placebo taping and exercise and exercise alone in treating patients with patellofemoral pain. A multicenter study by Wilson et al[170] found that patellar taping provided an immediate decrease in pain regardless of how the taping was applied, supporting that it is unlikely that taping works by altering patellar position. Cowan et al[29] found that individuals receiving therapeutic patellar taping improved in both EMG onset of vasti muscle contraction and pain in a stair-stepping task when compared with placebo taping and no tape. In conclusion, a review of therapeutic taping on patellofemoral pain syndrome suggests that, although patellar taping appears to decrease pain and improve function during activities of daily living and rehabilitation exercise, strong evidence to identify the underlying mechanisms remains unavailable.[5]

Clinically, taping and bracing offer significant pain relief in treating patients with patellofemoral pain despite the unknown mechanism by which either works. Whether or not changes occur in vasti muscle recruitment is debatable, but less muscle inhibition is expected with reduced pain. Evidence shows that the benefits from external patellar

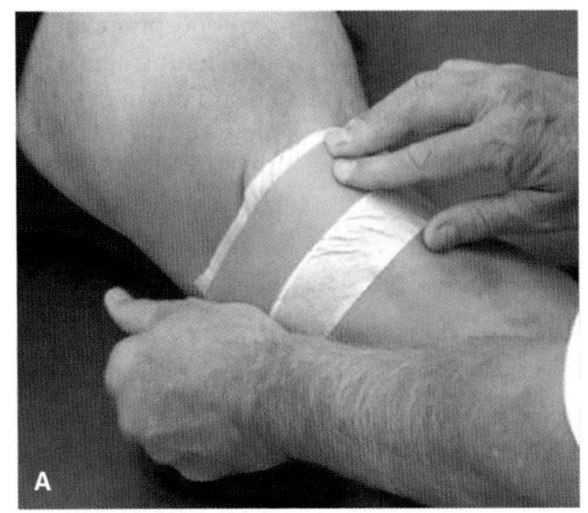

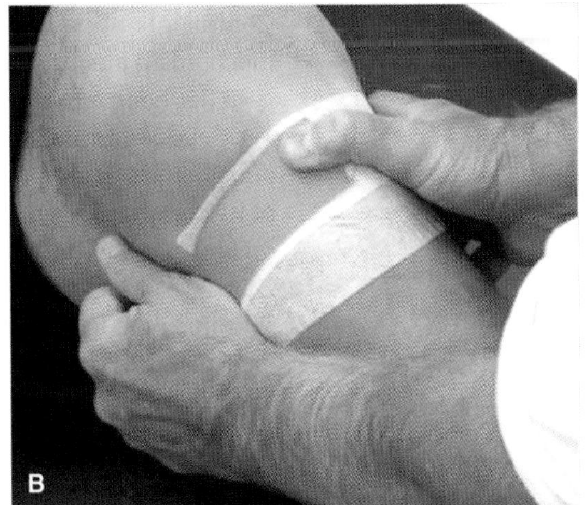

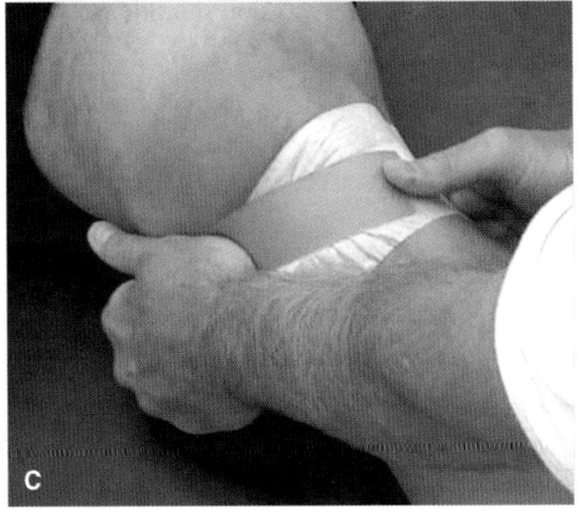

Figure 24-30 Patellofemoral taping

A. McConnell technique gliding the patella medially for an abnormal lateral glide. **B.** McConnell technique tilting the patella medially for an abnormal lateral tilt. **C.** McConnell technique internally rotating the patella for an abnormal external rotation.

supports probably do not occur from changes in patellar tracking or alignment. Changes in proprioception, increases in patellofemoral joint compression that decrease peak stresses, and shifting contact from sensitive to less irritated areas are more plausible explanations. Regardless of the mechanism by which patients experience relief through these applications, the use of external patellar supports can be a useful adjunct to quadriceps strengthening and exercise progression.

Specific Rehabilitation Techniques for Patellofemoral Injuries

Classification of Patellofemoral and Extensor Mechanism Injuries

Complaints of pain and disability associated with the patellofemoral joint and extensor mechanism are exceedingly common. The terminology used to describe this anterior knee pain has been a source of some confusion and requires clarification.

Several authors have proposed classification systems for patellofemoral disorders.[41,50,58,72,85,109,167] We choose to use the classification proposed by Wilk et al[167] because of its comprehensive and clearly defined diagnostic categories. The classification system divides patellofemoral disorders into the following: (a) patellar compression syndrome (PCS), (b) patellar instability, (c) biomechanical dysfunction, (d) direct patellar trauma, (e) soft-tissue lesions, (f) overuse syndromes, (g) osteochondritis diseases, and (h) neurologic disorders. However, the scope of this chapter does not feature management for direct patellar trauma, osteochondritis diseases, or neurologic disorders.

In general, the majority of patellofemoral injuries can follow the general patellofemoral rehabilitation progression. However, rehabilitation techniques and concerns unique to each disorder exist and are presented with the corresponding phases. The general progression should be referenced if a particular phase is not described.

Patellar Compression Syndromes

Pathomechanics

PCS is characterized by a patella overconstrained by the surrounding soft tissue, causing grossly restricting patellar mobility.[167] Typically, PCS occurs on the lateral side, but it can also occur globally, in which case patellar mobility is restricted both medially and laterally. PCS signs and symptoms often include peripatellar pain and crepitus with squatting or stair climbing, synovial irritation, decreased patellar mobility (laterally or globally), patellar malalignment or maltracking, and strength deficits or imbalance.[154] If left untreated, the abnormal pressure will have a deleterious effect on patellofemoral articular cartilage.

Rehabilitation Progression

Phase I Pain modulation and inflammatory control must begin immediately. Cryotherapy and activity modification should be used to manage these symptoms. Grades I and II patellar mobilizations can be used for pain control via large fiber input, and may be preceded by the use of a moist hot pack for patient comfort. In the case of severe lateral compression, patellar taping can be applied to unload the lateral patellofemoral articulation by providing a low-load, long-duration stretch. Patient education is critical to modify and avoid painful activities and manage symptoms.

Phase II The primary focus of phase II is the stretching of tightened lateral structures. This can be accomplished through patellar mobilization, prolonged tape application, and ITB stretching. Inflexibility of the hamstrings, quadriceps, and gastrocnemius should also be addressed. With global PCS, usually secondary to trauma or immobilization, normal patellar mobility and full knee ROM must be restored before initiating further therapy. Grades III and IV patellar mobilizations should be used to address specific limitations. Moreover, both patellar tilts and glides should be implemented to ensure adequate flexibility of both deep and superficial retinacular fibers, respectively. The most restricted motion should be addressed first, and retinacular stretching may be performed between 1 and 10 minutes at a time.[173] An emphasis on medial patellar tilts and deep retinacular fibers should be given to the patient with lateral compressive symptoms.

Quadriceps strengthening should be pain-free and may be augmented by patellar taping. The clinician must determine appropriate resistance and ROM with which to perform exercises to maintain pain-free strengthening. The focus of strengthening should not be on eliciting activation of the VMO, but rather the quadriceps as a whole. Once normal patellar mobility is restored, the patient can advance to an increased activity progression. Again, care should be taken to restore normal mobility before any aggressive exercises to prevent advancement of articular cartilage degeneration.

Patellar Instability

Pathomechanics

Patellar instability is the partial or complete lateral displacement of the patella, and is often associated with injury to medial soft-tissue structures. Patellofemoral joint stability depends on the architecture of the trochlea and patella, limb alignment, surrounding muscle function, and the integrity of soft-tissue constraints. In full extension, the patella has minimal contact with the femur. Upon knee flexion, the patella finds increasing stability within the trochlear groove. Trochlear dysplasia (abnormal shape and depth of the trochlear groove) and patella alta (an abnormally high-riding patella) encourage patellar instability. Higher Q angles create larger lateral vectors and increased the risk of lateral dislocation as well. Persistent lateral patellar deviation, also caused by VMO weakness, causes lateral structures such as the ITB to contract, resulting in further deviation and greater lateral subluxation. It was recently noted that the primary pathoanatomy associated with lateral patellar dislocation is injury to the medial patellofemoral ligament (MPFL).[37,137]

The MPFL is the primary static soft-tissue restraint to lateral patellar displacement.[26] The ligament originates near the medial epicondyle and adductor tubercle, coursing medially to attach to the upper one-half or two-thirds of the medial patella, as well as the deep fascia of the VMO tendon.[9] The MPFL resists lateral patellar displacement greatest in full knee extension, losing tension upon knee flexion as the trochlea and VMO take over stabilization of the patella within the trochlear groove.[6] It has been shown to provide 50% to 60% of restraint to lateral patellar translation during 0 to 20 degrees of knee flexion.[33] In a recent study of nearly 200 patients with lateral patellar dislocation, rupture of the MPFL at the patella attachment site occurred in 47% of knees, at the femoral attachment in 26%, and at both sites in 13%.[61] Attenuation of the MPFL without rupture occurred in 13% of knees.

Mechanism of Injury

In the absence of extensive medial-sided injury, nonoperative treatment is often recommended for primary patellar dislocations. However, a high percentage of associated pathology, other than injury to the MPFL, accompanies lateral patellar dislocation, including loose bodies (13%), meniscus tears (21%), patella fractures (7%), MCL sprains/tears (21%), and osteochondral lesions (49%).[61]

The classic noncontact mechanism involves a plant and cut maneuver during which the thigh internally rotates, promoting knee valgus. A simultaneous contraction of the quadriceps pulls the patella superiorly and creating a force to displace the patella. As a rule, displacement occurs laterally with the patella shifting over the lateral femoral condyle. Pain, swelling, and subsequent restriction of ROM are likely to occur in addition to palpable tenderness at the attachment site of medial retinaculum near the adductor tubercle.

The patella can also dislocate with contact, forcing the patella laterally. The patient reports a painful giving-way episode. The patient experiences a complete loss of knee function, pain, and swelling, with the patella remaining in an abnormal lateral position. If voluntary relocation does not occur, a physician should immediately reduce the dislocation by applying mild pressure on the patella with the knee extended as much as possible The rate of recurrent dislocation after primary dislocation and nonoperative treatment is 15% to 44%.[63] The rate of recurrent dislocation increases after a second dislocation to 50%.[42] Chronically subluxing patellae will place abnormal stress on the patellofemoral joint and medial restraints.

Rehabilitation Progression

Table 24-7 outlines the following discussion.

Phase I The goals of phase I are to control pain and inflammation and to restore full ROM and normal gait. Acutely following patellar dislocation, the knee may be braced or immobilized in extension for 3 to 6 weeks. The patient will require use of crutches for ambulation until full ROM and normal gait are attained. Treatment of chronic instability or subluxation requires less drastic efforts to manage pain, inflammation, and effusion

Table 24-7 **Postoperative Rehabilitation After MPFL Reconstruction**

Phase	Days – Weeks	Goals	Restrictions	Treatment	Clinical Milestones
Phase I: Protective Phase	Day 1 to Wk 6	Protect the surgical repair Decrease pain and inflammation Prevent the negative effects of immobilization Restore normal knee arthrokinematics Prevent primary/secondary hypomobility Promote dynamic stability Prevent reflex inhibition and secondary muscle atrophy	Brace locked in full extension weeks 0 to 2; weight bearing as tolerated in locked brace Discontinue brace at night at week 4 Discontinue brace at 6 weeks (per physician approval) if straight-leg raise can be performed without extensor lag	Total leg strengthening, including hip strengthening (in all planes), foot and ankle, trunk and core strengthening Patellofemoral joint mobilization in all planes Cryotherapy and modalities as needed for pain control Obtain full knee extension immediately Progress knee motion 0 to 90 degrees by week 4 (full ROM by week 10) Advance to mini squats, mini lunges, hamstring curls, step downs, and supine core/hip exercises in weeks 5 to 6	Full knee extension No pain No effusion 4/5 quadriceps, hamstring, and hip strength

(continued)

Table 24-7 Postoperative Rehabilitation After MPFL Reconstruction *(Continued)*

Phase	Days – Weeks	Goals	Restrictions	Treatment	Clinical Milestones
Phase II: Moderate Protection Phase	PO Wks 7 to 12	Progressively restore ROM (full by week 10) Maintain repair Progressively restore motion, strength, and balance	Discontinue brace at 6 weeks (per physician approval) if straight-leg raise can be performed without extensor lag Avoid activities that provoke pain	Continue to progress AROM/PROM (full by week 10) Progress previous LE strengthening exercises by altering intensity, speed, and/or proprioception Bosu/dynadisc lunges Bosu/box stepovers	Full knee flexion and extension (by week 10) No pain No swelling 5/5 quadriceps, hamstring and hip strength
Phase III: Minimum Protection Phase/ Advanced Strengthening Phase	PO Wks 13 to 16	Full non painful AROM/PROM Restoration of muscle strength, power and endurance No pain or tenderness Full balance and proprioception Gradual initiation of functional activities	Avoid activities that provoke pain	Maintain full ROM Increase intensity and decrease repetitions of standard exercises Double-leg jumping in place Double-leg jumping multiple planes Single-leg hopping in place Initiation of light functional/ plyometric activities: double-legs progressing to single (ie, ladder drills)	Full symmetrical AROM/PROM No pain No swelling Full balance and proprioception 5/5 isometric knee manual muscle test 5/5 isometric hip manual muscle test
Phase IV: Return to Full Activity Phase	PO Wks 17 to 20+	Maintain muscle strength, power and endurance Maintain knee motion Maintain balance and proprioception Progress functional activities Return to unrestricted sports activity	None	Continue previous exercises Initiate more advanced single-leg plyometric training Advanced sport-specific training Progress interval sports programs	Return to activity and/or sport

AROM, active range of motion; LE, lower extremity; PO, postoperative; PROM, passive range of motion; ROM, range of motion; Wks, weeks.

compared to acute instability. Nonetheless, irritation can be controlled by icing and avoidance of aggravating activities.

Phase II The emphasis of phase II is dynamic patellar stabilization through lower-extremity strengthening and stretching. If lateral tracking of the patella is involved in the instability, correction of lower-extremity alignment or tightened lateral structures such as the ITB must be addressed. Also, if lateral tracking is the result of abnormal adduction and internal rotation of the thigh, gluteus maximus and medius strengthening must be addressed. Maintaining cardiorespiratory endurance of the lower-extremity musculature is also important. As the condition of the knee improves, activities can be gradually advanced. Care should still be taken to minimize swelling during this stage, as it has a detrimental effect on quadriceps activity.

Phase III With advanced exercise and a functional progression, the use of a patellar stabilization brace may be used to encourage patellar stability and patient confidence. Quadriceps and gluteal strengthening should be advanced. Agility and sport-specific drills can also be introduced as appropriate. Athletes should practice cutting and jumping with biomechanical cues before returning to sport, including a focus on flexed knees upon landing or planting without femoral internal rotation or knee valgus.

If conservative treatments fail to return patients to their desired level of activity without continued symptoms of giving way, surgical treatment is an option. MPFL reconstruction rehabilitation should follow a structured guideline to ensure that excessive stress is not placed on graft tissue.[103]

Biomechanical Dysfunction

Pathomechanics

Biomechanical dysfunction is an alteration in the normal biomechanics of the lower extremity. The alteration is often subtle but can have a profound effect via repetition or intense activity. Individuals who develop patellofemoral pathology have been shown to be significantly weaker on measures of hip abduction, knee flexion, and knee extension strength, and commonly display greater navicular drop.[13] Leg length discrepancies, lower-extremity flexibility deficits, and weakness of the hip, core, ankle, and foot are also common causes of biomechanical dysfunction. Proximal and distal factors affecting patellofemoral biomechanics were previously discussed.

Rehabilitation Progression

Phase I Treatment of biomechanical dysfunction of the lower extremity rarely involves a focus on the source of pain. Excessive subtalar joint pronation or other intrinsic imbalances of the foot that result in altered patellofemoral articulation should be addressed with strengthening, footwear, or orthotics. A true or functional limb length discrepancy can cause pronation and other gait deviations; therefore, a shoe lift or manual correction may be indicated. Flexibility deficiencies can also lead to pronation, increased stress on the extensor mechanism, changes in gait, and lateral displacement of the patella. The clinician should restore any loss of flexibility in the gastrocnemius–soleus complex, quadriceps, hamstrings, ITB, and hip rotators. In addition, weakened gluteal muscles that result in an unstable pelvis and uncontrolled hip adduction and internal rotation during dynamic activities must be functionally strengthened. One study of hip and core muscle EMG activity during exercise suggests side-bridging and unilateral supine bridging are largely effective for activation of the gluteus medius and maximus, respectively, in addition to core musculature (Figures 24-31 and 24-32).[34]

Soft-Tissue Lesions

Pathomechanics

A soft-tissue lesion involves pain and inflammation of the numerous soft-tissue structures that surround the knee. Commonly involved tissues include bursa, plica, infrapatellar fat pad, distal ITB, and MPFL. Soft-tissue lesions may be the result of direct trauma, repeated activity, or biomechanical abnormality.

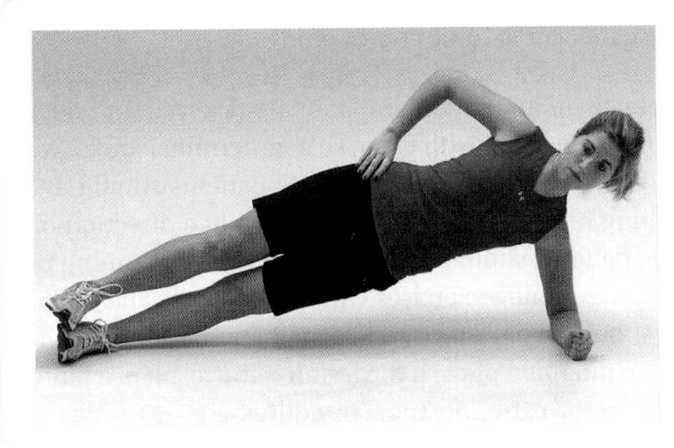

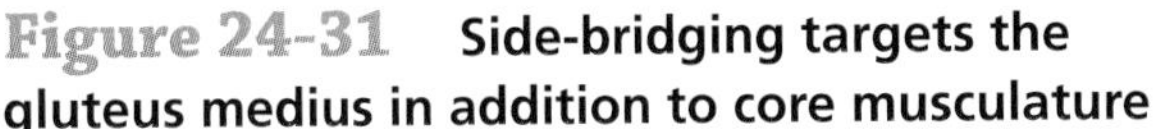

Figure 24-31 Side-bridging targets the gluteus medius in addition to core musculature

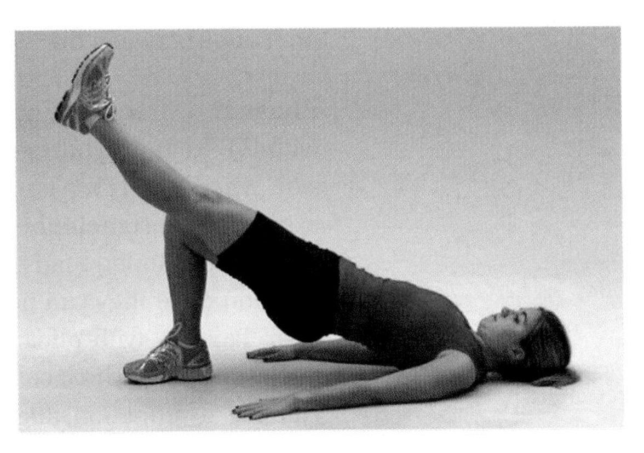

Figure 24-32 Unilateral supine bridging targets the gluteus maximus in addition to core musculature

Bursitis in the knee can be acute, chronic, or recurrent, and is usually the result of a direct trauma. Although any of the knee bursae can become inflamed, the prepatellar, deep infrapatellar, and suprapatellar bursae have the highest incidence of irritation in sports and among blue collar workers with heavy workloads and frequent kneeling.[88] Swelling is localized to the location of injury.

The medial patellar plica is also subject to injury. This bandlike tissue can bowstring across the anterior aspect of the medial femoral condyle, impinging between the articular cartilage and the medial patellar facet during knee flexion. Consequently, it has been seen to play a mechanical role in the development of medial femoral chondropathy, which confirms that excision of a plica is an appropriate prophylactic procedure during knee arthroscopy.[23] The patient may feel or hear a snap and report painful pseudolocking, although an intermittent dull pain is the most common symptom.[4] Inflammation of the plica, at times induced by acute trauma, leads to fibrosis and thickening with a loss of extensibility. When present, the majority of plicae are pliable and asymptomatic.

The distal ITB is injured while repetitively crossing the lateral femoral condyle during flexion and extension of the knee. Several studies suggest this pathology is especially prevalent among athletes.[45,151,171] Pain will radiate laterally toward the proximal tibia, becoming increasingly severe with continued activity. Increased tension of the ITB may be the result of hip weakness; leg length discrepancy; tightness in the tensor fasciae latae, hamstrings, and quadriceps; genu varum; excessive pronation; internal tibial torsion; or restricted dorsiflexion.

Rehabilitation Progression

Phase I During phase I of the rehabilitation process, iontophoresis, phonophoresis, and ice massage can be used to control pain and inflammation for numerous soft-tissue lesions. None of these modalities will be effective, however, unless the patient is educated and complies with appropriate activity modification. Also emphasized are a nonantalgic gait and full ROM. In the case of chronic bursitis, a compression wrap should be worn continuously. Medial plica syndrome requires ample stretching of the quadriceps, hamstrings, and gastrocnemius.[4] With chronic ITB syndrome, transverse friction massage administered by a therapist of via the use of a foam roller can be useful to create localized inflammation and promote collagen realignment. Isolated stretches, including contract-relax techniques, should precede muscle strengthening and reeducation. For athletes with ITB syndrome, both running and cycling should be avoided during the acute phase.[46] Swimming with a pool buoy between the legs is an alternative for aerobic conditioning.

Phase II Strengthening can begin once inflammation and pain are resolved. In patients with ITB friction syndrome, caution must be taken with exercise near terminal knee extension where the ITB passes over the lateral femoral condyle. These patients should avoid exercising on stairclimbers and running hills (especially downhill), in one direction on a track, or on sloped roads.[46] Moreover, patients should only begin a return-to-running progression once they can perform all strengthening exercises with proper form and without pain. Patients with plica syndrome should avoid exercise with full knee flexion, such as deep squatting, which can compress an inflamed plica. If the lesion is the result of a biomechanical dysfunction, alignment of the lower-extremity must be addressed.

Overuse Syndromes

Pathomechanics

Overuse syndromes are the result of excessive activity or stress to the extensor mechanism and include patellar tendinitis and traction apophysitis. Tendinitis of the extensor mechanism can occur at the superior patellar pole (quadriceps tendinitis), the tibial tubercle, or, most commonly, at the distal pole of the patella. Patellar tendinitis usually develops in patients involved in activities that require repetitive jumping and is frequently given the name "jumper's knee." Point tenderness on the posterior aspect of the inferior pole of the patella is the hallmark symptom. This condition is typically related to the eccentric shock-absorbing function that the quadriceps provides upon landing from a jump.

Traction apophysitis is a common adolescent condition that results from repeated stress of the patellar tendon at the apophysis of either the tibial tubercle or inferior patellar pole. The condition is characterized by pain and swelling that increases with activity and decreases with rest. Osgood-Schlatter disease occurs over the tibial tuberosity while Larsen-Johansson disease, although much less common, occurs at the inferior pole of the patella.

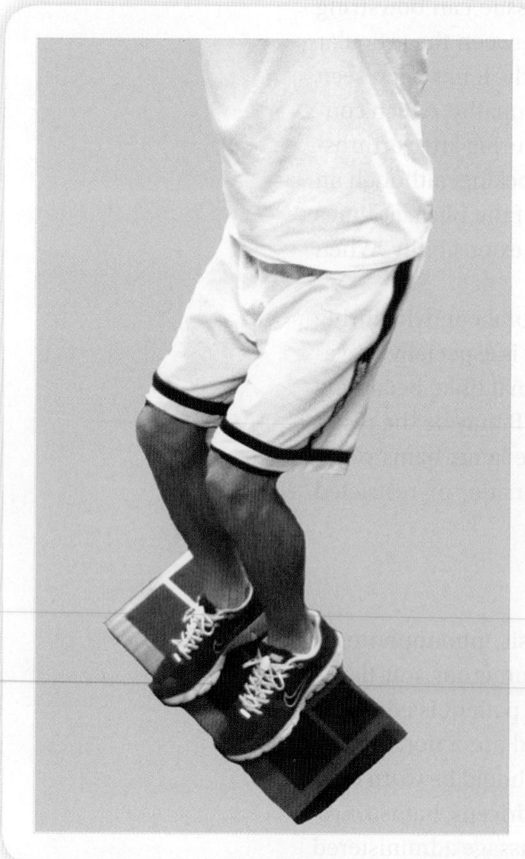

Figure 24-33 Eccentric quadriceps training on a 25-degree decline board

Rehabilitation Progression

Phase I Ice massage and iontophoresis can be used to control pain and inflammation during this stage of rehabilitation. Avoidance of jumping, kicking, running, and sudden deceleration that can cause undue stress on the extensor mechanism is warranted. Transverse friction massage can be used to facilitate the healing process of patellar tendinitis, but should not be performed in conjunction with antiinflammatory modalities. Ultrasound can reasonably be excluded as treatment for patellar tendinopathy.[86]

Phase II Therapeutic exercise, especially eccentric strengthening, is strongly supported by evidence as effective treatment for patellar tendinopathy.[86] Exercises can be progressed from low velocity to high velocity, and bilaterally to unilaterally. Several studies suggest standing on a 25-degree decline board while performing eccentric training of the quadriceps (Figure 24-33).[160] Evidence suggest patellar tendon strain is significantly greater, stop angles of the ankle and hip joints are significantly smaller, and EMG amplitudes of the knee extensor muscles are significantly greater during exercise on the decline board compared with standard squats.[83] Moderate evidence exists for more conservative, heavy, slow resistance training of the quadriceps.[86] Reducing body weight, increasing upper-leg flexibility, and the use of orthotics may also be beneficial treatment options for the intermediate phase of rehabilitation.[158]

Phase III Using a patellar strap can be beneficial in controlling pain when returning to intense activity. Controlled sports-specific exercise usually begins in this advanced stage of rehabilitation, although several studies report benefit from eccentric exercise rehabilitation programs targeting tendinopathy while continuing sports participation.[138] Activities for patients with traction apophysitis, an often self-limiting condition, can be progressed if the patient remains pain-free.

REFERENCES

1. Abt JP, Smoliga JM, Brick MJ, Jolly JT, Lephart SM, Fu FH. Relationship between cycling mechanics and core stability. *J Strength Cond Res.* 2007;21(4):1300-1304.
2. Aglietti P, Insall JN, Cerulli G. Patellar pain in incongruence I: measurements of incongruence. *Clin Orthop Relat Res.* 1983;176:217-224.
3. Alford JW, Cole BJ. Cartilage restoration, part 1: basic science, historical perspective, patient evaluation, and treatment options. *Am J Sports Med.* 2005;33(2)295-306.
4. Al-Hadithy N, Gikas P, Mahapatra AM, Dowd G. Review article: plica syndrome of the knee. *J Orthop Surg (Hong Kong).* 2011;19(3):354-358.
5. Aminaka N, Gribble PA. A systematic review of the effects of therapeutic taping on patellofemoral pain syndrome. *J Athl Train.* 2005;40(4):341-351.
6. Amis AA, Firer P, Mountney J, Senavongse W, Thomas NP. Anatomy and biomechanics of the medial patellofemoral ligament. *Knee.* 2003;10(3):215-220.
7. Arnoczky SP, Warren RF. Microvasculature of the human meniscus. *Am J Sports Med.* 1982;10:90-95.
8. Baker V, Bennell K, Stillman B, et al. Abnormal knee joint position sense in individuals with patellofemoral pain syndrome. *J Orthop Res.* 2002;20:208-214.
9. Baldwin JL. The anatomy of the medial patellofemoral ligament. *Am J Sports Med.* 2009;37(12):2355-2361.
10. Bandy WD, Irion JM. The effect of time on static stretch on the flexibility of the hamstring muscles. *Phys Ther.* 1994;79:845-850.
11. Bandy WD, Irion JM, Briggler M. The effect of time and frequency of static stretching on flexibility of the hamstring muscles. *Phys Ther.* 1997;77:1090-1096.
12. Beynnon BD, Fleming BC, Johnson RJ, et al. Anterior cruciate ligament strain behavior during rehabilitation exercise in vivo. *Am J Sports Med.* 1995;23:24-34.
13. Boling MC, Padua DA, Marshall SW, Guskiewicz K, Pyne S, Beutler A. A prospective investigation of biomechanical risk factors for patellofemoral pain syndrome: the Joint Undertaking to Monitor and Prevent ACL Injury (JUMP-ACL) cohort. *Am J Sports Med.* 2009;37(11):2108-2116.
14. Boucher JP, King MA, Lefebvre R, et al. Quadriceps femoris muscle activity in patellofemoral pain syndrome. *Am J Sports Med.* 1992;20:527-732.
15. Bizzini M, Childs JD, Piva SR, et al. Systematic review of the quality of randomized controlled trials for patellofemoral pain syndrome. *J Orthop Sports Phys Ther.* 2003;33:4-20.
16. Brittberg M, Lindahl A, Nilsson A, Ohlsson C, Isaksson O, Peterson L. Treatment of deep cartilage defects in the knee with autologous chondrocyte transplantation. *N Engl J Med.* 1994;331(14):889-895.
17. Brittberg M, Nilsson A, Lindahl A, Ohlsson C, Peterson L. Rabbit articular cartilage defects treated with autologous cultured chondrocytes. *Clin Orthop Relat Res.* 1996;326:270-283.
18. Buchbinder MR, Napora NJ, Biggs EW. The relationship of abnormal pronation to chondromalacia of the patella in distance runners. *J Am Podiatry Assoc.* 1979;69:159-162.
19. Buckwalter JA. Articular cartilage: injuries and potential for healing. *J Orthop Sports Phys Ther.* 1998;28(4): 192-202.
20. Buckwalter JA, Mankin HJ. Articular cartilage: tissue design and chondrocyte-matrix interactions. *Instr Course Lect.* 1998;47:487-504.
21. Butler DL, Noyes FR, Grood ES. Ligamentous restraints to anterior-posterior drawer in the human knee: a biomechanical study. *J Bone Joint Surg Am.* 1980;62:259-270.
22. Caborn DN, Johnson BM. The natural history of the anterior cruciate ligament-deficient knee: a review. *Clin Sports Med.* 1993;12:625-636.
23. Calpur OU, Tan L, Gürbüz H, Moralar U, Copuroğlu C, Ozcan M. Arthroscopic mediopatellar plicaectomy and lateral retinacular release in mechanical patellofemoral

disorders. *Knee Surg Sports Traumatol Arthrosc.* 2002;10(3):177-183.

24. Cavagna GA, Saibene FP, Margaria R. Mechanical work in running. *J Appl Physiol.* 1964;19:249-256.
25. Chiu JK, Wong YM, Yung PS, Ng GY. The effects of quadriceps strengthening on pain, function, and patellofemoral joint contact area in persons with patellofemoral pain. *Am J Phys Med Rehabil.* 2012;91(2): 98-106.
26. Colvin AC, West RV. Patellar instability. *J Bone Joint Surg Am.* 2008;90:2751-2762.
27. Cowan SM, Bennell KL, Crossley KM, et al. Delayed onset of electromyographic activity of vastus medialis obliquus relative to vastus lateralis in patients with patellofemoral pain syndrome. *Arch Phys Med Rehabil.* 2001;82:183-189.
28. Cowan SM, Bennell KL, Crossley KM, et al. Physical therapy alters recruitment of the vasti in patellofemoral pain syndrome. *Med Sci Sports Exerc.* 2002;34:1879-1885.
29. Cowan SM, Bennell KL, Hodges PW. Therapeutic patellar taping changes the timing of vasti muscle activation in people with patellofemoral pain syndrome. *Clin J Sport Med.* 2002;12:339-347.
30. Cox JS. Patellofemoral problems in runners. *Clin Sports Med.* 1985;4:699-715.
31. Daniel DM, Stone ML, Dobson BE, et al. Fate of the ACL-injured patient: a prospective outcome study. *Am J Sports Med.* 1994;22:632-644.
32. De Carlo MS, Sell KE. Normative data for range of motion and single-leg hop in high school athletes. *J Sport Rehabil.* 1997;6:246-255.
33. Desio SM, Burks RT, Bachus KN. Soft tissue restraints to lateral patellar translation in the human knee. *Am J Sports Med.* 1998;26(1):59-65.
34. Donatelli RA, Carp KC, Ekstrom RA. Electromyographic analysis of core trunk, hip, and thigh muscles during nine rehabilitation exercises. *J Orthop Sports Phys Ther.* 2007;37(12):754-762.
35. Ebert JR, Robertson WB, Lloyd D, Zheng MH, Wood DJ, Ackland T. A prospective, randomized comparison of traditional and accelerated approaches to postoperative rehabilitation following autologous chondrocyte implantation: 2-year clinical outcomes. *Cartilage.* 2010;1(3):180-187.
36. Ebert JR, Fallon M, Robertson WB, et al. Radiological assessment of accelerated versus traditional approaches to postoperative rehabilitation following matrix-induced autologous chondrocyte implantation. *Cartilage.* 2011;2(1):2011.
37. Elias DA, White LM, Fithian DC. Acute lateral patellar dislocation at MR imaging: injury patterns of medial patellar soft-tissue restraints and osteochondral injuries of the inferomedial patella. *Radiology.* 2002;225:736-743.
38. Escamilla RF, Fleisig GS, Zheng N, et al. Biomechanics of the knee during closed kinetic chain and open kinetic chain exercises. *Med Sci Sports Exerc.* 1998;30:556-569.
39. Evans NA, Chew HF, Stanish WD. The natural history and tailored treatment of ACL injury. *Phys Sportsmed.* 2001;29:19-34.
40. Feland JB, Myrer JW, Schulthies SS, Fellingham GW, Measom GW. The effect of duration of stretching of the hamstring muscle group for increasing range of motion in people aged 65 years or older. *Phys Ther.* 2001;81(5):1110-1117.
41. Ficat RP, Philippe J, Hungerford DS. Chondromalacia patellae: a system of classification. *Clin Orthop Relat Res.* 1979;144:55-62.
42. Fithian DC, Paxton EW, Stone ML, et al. Epidemiology and natural history of acute patellar dislocation. *Am J Sports Med.* 2004;32:1114-1121.
43. Fitzgerald GK, Irrgang JJ. Articular cartilage procedures of the knee. In: Brotzman SB, Manske RC, eds. *Clinical Orthopaedic Rehabilitation: An Evidence-Based Approach.* 3rd ed. St. Louis, MO: Mosby.
44. Frank CB, Jackson DW. The science of reconstruction of the anterior cruciate ligament. *J Bone Joint Surg Am.* 1997;79:1556-1576.
45. Fredericson M, Cookingham CL, Chaudhari AM, Dowdell BC, Oestreicher N, Sahrmann SA. Hip abductor weakness in distance runners with iliotibial band syndrome. *Clin J Sport Med.* 2000;10(3):169-175.
46. Fredericson M, Wolf C. Iliotibial band syndrome in runners: innovations in treatment. *Sports Med.* 2005;35(5):451-459.
47. Fu FH, Bennett CH, Lattermann C, et al. Current trends in anterior cruciate ligament reconstruction. Part 1: biology and biomechanics of reconstruction. *Am J Sports Med.* 1999;27:821-830.
48. Fukubayashi T, Kurosawa H. The contact area and pressure distribution pattern of the knee: a study of normal and osteoarthrotic knee joints. *Acta Orthop Scand.* 1980;51:871-879.
49. Fukuda TY, Rossetto FM, Magalhães E, Bryk FF, Lucareli PR, de Almeida Aparecida Carvalho N. Short-term effects of hip abductors and lateral rotators strengthening in females with patellofemoral pain syndrome: a randomized controlled clinical trial. *J Orthop Sports Phys Ther.* 2010;40(11):736-742.
50. Fulkerson JP, Kalenak A, Rosenberg TD, et al. Patellofemoral pain. *Instr Course Lect.* 1992;41:57-71.
51. Fullerton LR, Andrews JR. Mechanical block to extension following augmentation of the anterior cruciate ligament: a case report. *Am J Sports Med.* 1984;12:166-169.
52. Gardiner JC, Weiss JA, Rosenberg TD. Strain in the human medial collateral ligament during valgus loading of the knee. *Clin Orthop Relat Res.* 2001;391:266-274.
53. Geissler W, Whipple T. Intraarticular abnormalities in association with PCL injuries. *Am J Sports Med.* 1993;21:846-849.
54. Girgis FG, Marshall JL, Monajem A. The cruciate ligaments of the knee joint. Anatomical, functional and experimental analysis. *Clin Orthop Relat Res.* 1975;106:216-231.

55. Gollehon DL, Torzilli PA, Warren RF. The role of the posterolateral and cruciate ligaments in the human knee stability: a biomechanical study. *Trans Orthop Res Soc.* 1985;10:270.
56. Goodfellow J, Hungerford DS, Zindel M. Patello-femoral joint mechanics and pathology. I: functional anatomy of the patellofemoral joint. *J Bone Joint Surg Br.* 1976;58:287-290.
57. Grana WA, Kriegshauser LA. Scientific basis of extensor mechanism disorders. *Clin Sports Med.* 1985;4:247-257.
58. Grelsamer RP. Classification of patellofemoral disorders. *Am J Knee Surg.* 1997;10:96-100.
59. Grelsamer RP, Klein JR. The biomechanics of the patellofemoral joint. *J Orthop Sports Phys Ther.* 1998;28:286-298.
60. Grood ES, Noyes FR, Butler DL, et al. Ligamentous and capsular restraints preventing straight medial and lateral laxity in intact human cadaver knees. *J Bone Joint Surg Am.* 1981;63:1257-1269.
61. Guerrero P, Li X, Patel K, Brown M, Busconi B. Medial patellofemoral ligament injury patterns and associated pathology in lateral patella dislocation: an MRI study. *Sports Med Arthrosc Rehabil Ther Technol.* 2009;1(1):17.
62. Hardy MA. The biology of scar formation. *Phys Ther.* 1989;69:1014-1024.
63. Hawkins RJ, Bell RH, Anisette G. Acute patellar dislocations. The natural history. *Am J Sports Med.* 1986;14:117-120.
64. Hawkins RJ, Misamore GW, Merritt TR. Followup of the acute nonoperated isolated anterior cruciate ligament tear. *Am J Sports Med.* 1986;14:205-210.
65. Herrington L, Rivett N, Munro S. The relationship between patella position and length of the iliotibial band as assessed using Ober's test. *Man Ther.* 2006;11(3):182-186.
66. Hopper DM, Strauss GR, Boyle JJ, Bell J. Functional recovery after anterior cruciate ligament reconstruction: a longitudinal perspective. *Arch Phys Med Rehabil.* 2008;89:1535-1541.
67. Hudson Z, Darthuy E. Iliotibial band tightness and patellofemoral pain syndrome: a case-control study. *Man Ther.* 2009;14(2):147-151.
68. Hughston JC, Eilers AF. The role of the posterior oblique ligament in repairs of acute medial ligament tears of the knee. *J Bone Joint Surg Am.* 1973;55:923-940.
69. Hungerford DS, Barry M. Biomechanics of the patellofemoral joint. *Clin Orthop Relat Res.* 1979;144:9-15.
70. Hunter W. On the structure and diseases of articulating cartilage. *Philos Trans R Soc Lond B Biol Sci.* 1743;9:267.
71. Indelicato PA, Non-operative treatment of complete tears of the medial collateral ligament of the knee. *J Bone Joint Surg.* 1983;65A:323-329.
72. Insall J. "Chondromalacia patellae": patellar malalignment syndrome. *Orthop Clin North Am.* 1979;10:117-127.
73. Insall JN, Falvo KA, Wise DW. Chondromalacia patellae: a prospective study. *J Bone Joint Surg Am.* 1976;58:1-8.
74. Ireland ML, Willson JD, Ballantyne BT, et al. Hip strength in females with and without patellofemoral pain. *J Orthop Sports Phys Ther.* 2003;11:671-676.
75. Irish SE, Millward AJ, Wride J, Haas BM, Shum GL. The effect of closed-kinetic chain exercises and open-kinetic chain exercise on the muscle activity of vastus medialis oblique and vastus lateralis. *J Strength Cond Res.* 2010;24(5):1256-1262.
76. Jaffe FF, Mankin HJ, Weiss H, et al. Water binding in the articular cartilage of rabbits. *J Bone Joint Surg Am.* 1974;56:1031-1039.
77. Johnson RJ, Kettelkamp DB, Clark W, et al. Factors effecting late results after meniscectomy. *J Bone Joint Surg Am.* 1974;56:719-729.
78. Kannus P, Natri A, Paakkala T, et al. An outcome study of chronic patellofemoral pain syndrome: Seven-year follow-up of patient in a randomized, controlled trial. *J Bone Joint Surg Am.* 1999;81:355-363.
79. Kaufer H. Mechanical function of the patella. *J Bone Joint Surg Am.* 1971;53:1551-1560.
80. Kendall FP, McCreary EK, Provance PG. *Muscles: Testing and Function.* 4th ed. Baltimore, MD: Williams & Wilkins; 1993.
81. Khayambashi K, Mohammadkhani Z, Ghaznavi K, Lyle MA, Powers CM. The effects of isolated hip abductor and external rotator muscle strengthening on pain, health status, and hip strength in females with patellofemoral pain: a randomized controlled trial. *J Orthop Sports Phys Ther.* 2012;42(1):22-29.
82. Klingman RE, Liaos SM, Hardin KM. The effect of subtalar joint posting on patellar glide position in subjects with excessive rearfoot pronation. *J Orthop Sports Phys Ther.* 1997;25:185-191.
83. Kongsgaard M, Aagaard P, Roikjaer S, et al. Decline eccentric squats increases patellar tendon loading compared to standard eccentric squats. *Clin Biomech (Bristol, Avon).* 2006;21(7):748-754.
84. Kovachevick R, Shah JP, Arens AM, Stuart MH, Dahm DL, Levy BA. Operative management of the medial collateral ligament in the multi-ligament injured knee: an evidence-based systematic review. *Knee Surg Sports Traumatol Arthrosc.* 2009;17:823-829.
85. Larson RL, Cabaud HE, Slocum DB, et al. The patellar compression syndrome: surgical treatment by lateral retinacular release. *Clin Orthop Relat Res.* 1978;134:158-167.
86. Larsson ME, Käll I, Nilsson-Helander K. Treatment of patellar tendinopathy—a systematic review of randomized controlled trials. *Knee Surg Sports Traumatol Arthrosc.* 2012;20(8):1632-1646.
87. Lee TQ, Morris G, Csintalan RP. The influence of tibial and femoral rotation on patellofemoral contact and pressure. *J Orthop Sports Phys Ther.* 2003;11:686-693.
88. Le Manac'h AP, Ha C, Descatha A, Imbernon E, Roquelaure Y. Prevalence of knee bursitis in the workforce. *Occup Med (Lond).* 2012;62(8):658-660.

89. Levine J. Chondromalacia patellae. *Phys Sportsmed.* 1979;7:41-49.
90. Levy IM, Torzilli PA, Gould JD, et al. The effect of lateral meniscectomy on motion of the knee. *J Bone Joint Surg Am.* 1989;71:401-406.
91. Levy IM, Torzilli PA, Warren RF. The effect of medial meniscectomy on anterior-posterior motion of the knee. *J Bone Joint Surg Am.* 1982;64:883-888.
92. Lieb FJ, Perry J. Quadriceps function: an anatomical and mechanical study using amputated limbs. *J Bone Joint Surg Am.* 1968;50:1535-1548.
93. Lipke JM, Janecki CJ, Nelson CL, et al. The role of incompetence of the anterior cruciate and lateral ligaments in anterolateral and anteromedial instability: a biomechanical study of cadaver knees. *J Bone Joint Surg Am.* 1981;63:954-960.
94. Logan M, Williams A, Lavelle J, Gedroyc W, Freeman M. The effect of posterior cruciate ligament deficiency on knee kinematics. *Am J Sports Med.* 2004;32(8):1915-1922.
95. Lutz GE, Stuart MH, Sim FH. Rehabilitation techniques for athletes after reconstruction of the anterior cruciate ligament. *Mayo Clin Proc.* 1990;65:1322-1329.
96. MacIntyre DL, Robertsone DG. Quadriceps muscle activity in women runners with and without patellofemoral pain syndrome. *Arch Phys Med Rehabil.* 1992;73:10-14.
97. Mankin H. The response of articular cartilage to mechanical injury. *J Bone Joint Surg Am.* 1982;64:460-466.
98. Mankin HJ. The water of articular cartilage. In: Simon WH, ed. *The Human Joint in Health and Disease.* Philadelphia, PA: University of Pennsylvania Press; 1973; Miller MD. *Review of Orthopaedics.* Philadelphia, PA: Saunders; 1992.
99. Mankin JH, Mow VC, Buckwalter JA, et al. Articular cartilage repair and osteoarthritis. In: Buckwalter JA, Einhorn TA, Simon SR, eds. *Orthopaedic Basic Science, Biology, and Biomechanics.* 2nd ed. Rosemount, IL: American Academy of Orthopaedic Surgeons; 2000.
100. Mankin HJ, Mow VC, Buckwalter JA, et al. Articular cartilage structure composition and function. In: Buckwalter JA, Einhorn TA, Simon SR, Eds. *Orthopaedic Basic Science, Biology, and Biomechanics.* 2nd ed. Rosemount, IL: American Academy of Orthopaedic Surgeons; 2000.
101. Manske RC, Davies GJ, DeCarlo M, Paterno M. Rehabilitation concepts: historical to present following ACL repair. *Orthopaedic Knowledge Update: Sports Medicine 4.* Rosemount, IL: American Academy of Orthopaedic Surgeons; 2008.
102. Manske RC, Ellenbecker TS, Rohrberg J, Reiman M, Rogers M, Lehecka BJ. *Functional Therapeutic Progressions and Return to Function Following Surgery.* Orthopedic Section of the American Physical Therapy Association. La Crosse, WI: 2011.
103. Manske RC, Lehecka BJ, Prohaska D. *Medial Patellofemoral Ligament Reconstruction Rehabilitation. The Knee Monograph Series 2011.* Sports Section of the American Physical Therapy Association Series. Indianapolis, IN: 2011.
104. Manske RC, Prohaska D, Lucas B. Evidence-based rehabilitation following anterior cruciate ligament reconstruction: rehabilitation perspectives: critical reviews in rehabilitation medicine. *Curr Rev Musculoskelet Med.* 2012;5(1):59-71.
105. Mattacola CG, Perrin DH, Gansneder BM, Gieck JH, Saliba EN, McCue FC III. Strength, functional outcome, and postural stability after anterior cruciate ligament reconstruction. *J Athl Train.* 2002;37:262-268.
106. McAdams TR, Mithoefer K, Scopp JM, Mandelbaum BR. Articular cartilage injury in athletes. *Cartilage.* 2010;1(3):165-179.
107. McConnell J. The management of chondromalacia patellae: a long term solution. *Aust J Physiother.* 1986;32:215-223.
108. Meira EP, Brumitt J. Influence of the hip on patients with patellofemoral pain syndrome: a systematic review. *Sports Health.* 2011;3(5):455-465.
109. Merchant AC. Classification of patellofemoral disorders. *Arthroscopy.* 1988;4:235-240.
110. Merican AM, Amis AA. Iliotibial band tension affects patellofemoral and tibiofemoral kinematics. *J Biomech.* 22;2009;42(10):1539-1546.
111. Mirzabeigi E, Jordan C, Gronley JK, et al. Isolation of the vastus medialis oblique muscle during exercise. *Am J Sports Med.* 1999;27:50-53.
112. Miyasaka KC, Daniel D, Stone M. The incidence of knee ligament injuries in general population. *Am J Knee Surg.* 1991;4:3-8.
113. Moyad TF. Cartilage injuries in the adult knee: evaluation and management. *Cartilage.* 2011;2(3):226-236.
114. Nakagawa TH, Muniz TB, Baldon Rde M, Dias Maciel C, de Menezes Reiff RB, Serrão FV. The effect of additional strengthening of hip abductor and lateral rotator muscles in patellofemoral pain syndrome: a randomized controlled pilot study. *Clin Rehabil.* 2008;22(12):1051-1060.
115. Natri A, Kannus P, Jarvinen M. Which factors predict the long-term outcome in chronic patellofemoral pain syndrome? A 7-yr prospective follow-up study. *Med Sci Sports Exerc.* 1998;30:1572-1577.
116. Ng GY, Chan HL. The immediate effects of tension of counterforce forearm brace on neuromuscular performance of wrist extensor muscles in subjects with lateral humeral epicondylosis. *J Orthop Sports Phys Ther.* 2004;34:72-78.
117. Ng GY, Cheng JM. The effect of patellar taping on pain and neuromuscular performance in subjects with patellofemoral pain syndrome. *Clin Rehabil.* 2002;16:821-827.
118. O'Donoghue DH. Surgical treatment of fresh injuries to the major ligaments of the knee. *J Bone Joint Surg Am.* 1950;32:721-737.
119. O'Donoghue DH. An analysis of end results of surgical treatment of major ligaments of the knee. *J Bone Joint Surg Am.* 1955;37:1-12.

120. Oster A, Okholm K, Hulgaard J. Operative treatment of rupture in the medial collateral ligament. *Acta Orthop Scand.* 1971;42(5):439.

121. Palmer I. On the injuries to the ligaments of the knee joint: a clinical study. *Acta Chir Scand Suppl.* 53:?, 1938.

122. Parolie J, Bergfeld J. Long-term results of non-operative treatment of PCL injuries in the patient. *Am J Sports Med.* 1986;14:35-38.

123. Paterno MV, Schmitt LC, ford KR, et al. Biomechanical measures during landing and postural stability predict second anterior cruciate ligament injury after anterior cruciate ligament reconstruction and return to sport. *Am J Sports Med.* 2010;38:1968-1978.

124. Paulos LE, Wnorowski DC, Greenwald AE. Infrapatellar contracture syndrome: Diagnosis, treatment and long-term follow up. *Am J Sports Med.* 1994;22(4):440-449.

125. Paulos LE, Rusche K, Johnson C, et al. Patellar malalignment: a treatment rationale. *Phys Ther.* 1980;60:1624-1632.

126. Pfeiffer RP, DeBeliso M, Shea KG, et al. Kinematic MRI assessment of McConnell taping before and after exercise. *Am J Sports Med.* 2004;32:621-628.

127. Powers CM, Perry J, Hsu A, et al. Are patellofemoral pain and quadriceps femoris muscle torque associated with locomotor function? *Phys Ther.* 1997;77:1063-1078.

128. Powers CM, Shellock FG, Beering TV, et al. Effect of bracing on patellar kinematics in patients with patellofemoral joint pain. *Med Sci Sports Exerc.* 1999;31:1714-1720.

129. Powers CM, Ward SR, Chan L, et al. The effect of bracing on patella alignment and patellofemoral joint contact area. *Med Sci Sports Exerc.* 2004;36:1226-1232.

130. Powers CM, Ward SR, Chen Y, et al. The effect of bracing on patellofemoral joint stress during free and fast walking. *Am J Sports Med.* 2004;32:224-231.

131. Rivera JE. Open versus closed kinetic chain rehabilitation of the lower extremity: a functional and biomechanical analysis. *J Sport Rehabil.* 1994;3:154-167.

132. Rodrigo JJ, Steadman JR, Sillman JF. Improvement of full-thickness chondral defect healing in the human knee after debridement and microfracture using continuous passive motion. *Am J Knee Surg.* 1994;7:109-116.

133. Roos PE, Barton N, van Deursen RW. Patellofemoral joint compression forces in backward and forward running. *J Biomech.* 2012;45(9):1656-1660.

134. Rosenberg TD, et al. The forty-five-degree postero-anterior flexion weight-bearing radiograph of the knee. *J Bone Joint Surg Am.* 1988;70:1479-1483.

135. Rubinstein RA, Shelbourne KD, Van Meter CD, et al. Effect on knee stability if full hyperextension is restored immediately after autogenous bone-patellar tendon-bone anterior cruciate ligament reconstruction. *Am J Sports Med.* 1993;23:365.

136. Sachs RA, Daniel DM, Stone ML. Patellofemoral problems after ACL reconstruction. *Am J Sports Med.* 1990;19:957-964.

137. Sallay PI, Poggi J, Speer KP, Garett WE. Acute dislocation of the patella: a correlative pathoanatomic study. *Am J Sports Med.* 1996;24:52-60.

138. Saithna A, Gogna R, Baraza N, Modi C, Spencer S. Eccentric exercise protocols for patella tendinopathy: should we really be withdrawing athletes from sport? A systematic review. *Open Orthop J.* 2012;6:553-557.

139. Seering WP, Piziali RL, Nagel DA, et al. The function of the primary ligaments of the knee in varus-valgus and axial rotation. *J Biomech.* 1980;13:785-794.

140. Shelbourne KD, Gray T. Results of anterior cruciate ligament reconstruction based on the meniscus and articular cartilage status at the time of surgery: five- to fifteen-year evaluations. *Am J Sports Med.* 2000;28:446-452.

141. Shelbourne KD, Nitz P. Accelerated rehabilitation after anterior cruciate ligament reconstruction. *Am J Sports Med.* 1990;18(3):292-299.

142. Shelbourne KD, Patel DV. Management of combined injuries of the anterior cruciate and medial collateral ligaments. *J Bone Joint Surg Am.* 1995;77:800-806.

143. Shelbourne KD, Patel DV, Martini DJ. Classification and management of arthrofibrosis of the knee following anterior cruciate ligament reconstruction. *Am J Sports Med.* 1996;24:857.

144. Shelbourne KD, Wilckens JH, Mollabashy A, et al. Arthrofibrosis in acute anterior cruciate ligament reconstruction: The effect of timing of reconstruction and rehabilitation. *Am J Sports Med.* 1991;19:332-336.

145. Simoneau GG, Wilk KE. Electromyographic activity of vastus medialis and lateralis during four exercises [abstract]. *Phys Ther.* 1993;73:580.

146. Smith AV. Survival of frozen chondrocytes isolated from cartilage of adult mammals. *Nature.* 1965;205:782-784.

147. Smith TO, Bowyer D, Dixon J, Stephenson R, Chester R, Donell ST. Can vastus medialis oblique be preferentially activated? A systematic review of electromyographic studies. *Physiother Theory Pract.* 2009;25(2):69-98.

148. Souza DR, Gross MT. Comparison of vastus medialis obliquus: vastus lateralis muscle integrated electromyographic ratios between healthy subjects and patients with patellofemoral pain. *Phys Ther.* 1991;71:310-320.

149. Steinkamp LA, Dillingham MF, Markel MD, et al. Biomechanical considerations in patellofemoral joint rehabilitation. *Am J Sports Med.* 1993;21:438-444.

150. Sullivan D, Levy IM, Heskler S. Medial restraints to anterior-posterior motion of the knee. *J Bone Joint Surg Am.* 1984;66:930-936.

151. Sutker AN, Barber FA, Jackson DW, Pagliano JW. Iliotibial band syndrome in distance runners. *Sports Med.* 1985;2(6):447-451.

152. Sutlive TG, Mitchell SD, Maxfield SN, et al. Identification of individuals with patellofemoral pain whose symptoms improved after a combined program of foot orthosis use and modified activity: A preliminary investigation. *Phys Ther.* 2004;84:49-61.

153. Swart NM, van Linschoten R, Bierma-Zeinstra SM, van Middelkoop M. The additional effect of orthotic devices on exercise therapy for patients with patellofemoral pain syndrome: a systematic review. *Br J Sports Med.* 2012;46(8):570-577.

154. Terry GC. The anatomy of the extensor mechanism. *Clin Sports Med.* 1989;8:163-177.

155. Tiberio D. The effect of excessive subtalar joint pronation on patellofemoral mechanics: a theoretical model. *J Orthop Sports Phys Ther.* 1999;9:160-165.

156. Tria A, Klein K. *An Illustrated Guide to the Knee*. New York, NY: Churchill Livingstone; 1991.

157. Van de Velde SK, Bingham JT, Gill TJ, Li G. Analysis of tibiofemoral cartilage deformation in the posterior cruciate ligament-deficient knee. *J Bone Joint Surg Am.* 2009;91(1):167-175.

158. van der Worp H, van Ark M, Roerink S, Pepping GJ, van den Akker-Scheek I, Zwerver J. Risk factors for patellar tendinopathy: a systematic review of the literature. *Br J Sports Med.* 2011;45(5):446-452.

159. Vicenzino B, Collins N, Cleland J, McPoil T. A clinical prediction rule for identifying patients with patellofemoral pain who are likely to benefit from foot orthoses: a preliminary determination. *Br J Sports Med.* 2010;44(12):862-866.

160. Visnes H, Bahr R. The evolution of eccentric training as treatment for patellar tendinopathy (jumper's knee): a critical review of exercise programmes. *Br J Sports Med.* 2007;41(4):217-223.

161. Waldman SD, Spiteri CG, Grynpas MD, Pilliar RM, Hong J, Kandel RA. Effect of biomechanical conditioning on cartilaginous tissue formation in vitro. *J Bone Joint Surg Am.* 2003;85 (Suppl 2):101-105.

162. Warren RF, Marshall JL. The supporting structures and layers on the medial side of the knee. *J Bone Joint Surg Am.* 1979;61:56-72.

163. Weber MD, Woodall WR. Knee rehabilitation. In: Andrews JR, Harrelsn GL, Wilk KE, eds. *Physical Rehabilitation of the Injured Athlete.* 4th ed. St. Louis, MO: Elsevier; 2012:377-425.

164. Whyte EF, Moran K, Shortt CP, Marshall B. The influence of reduced hamstring length on patellofemoral joint stress during squatting in healthy male adults. *Gait Posture.* 2010;31(1):47-51.

165. Whittingham M, Palmer S, Macmillan F. Effects of taping on pain and function in patellofemoral pain syndrome: a randomized controlled trial. *J Orthop Sports Phys Ther.* 2004;34:504-510.

166. Widuchowski W, Widuchowski J, Trzaska T. Articular cartilage defects: study of 25,124 knee arthroscopies. *Knee.* 2007;14:177-182.

167. Wilk KE, Davies GJ, Mangine RE, et al. Patellofemoral disorders: a classification system and clinical guidelines for nonoperative rehabilitation. *J Orthop Sports Phys Ther.* 1998;28:307-322.

168. Wilk KE, Escamilla RF, Fleisig GS, et al. A comparison of tibiofemoral joint forces and electromyographic activity during open and closed kinetic chain exercises. *Am J Sports Med.* 1996;24:518-527.

169. Wilk KE, Macrina LC, Reinold MM. Rehabilitation following microfracture of the knee. *Cartilage.* 2010;1:96-97.

170. Wilson T, Carter N, Thomas G. A multicenter, single-masked study of medial, neutral, and lateral patellar taping in individuals with patellofemoral pain syndrome. *J Orthop Sports Phys Ther.* 2003;33:437-443.

171. Winslow J, Yoder E. Patellofemoral pain in female ballet dancers: correlation with iliotibial band tightness and tibial external rotation. *J Orthop Sports Phys Ther.* 1995;22(1):18-21.

172. Witvrouw E, Lysens R, Bellemans J, et al. Open versus closed kinetic chain exercises for patellofemoral pain: a prospective, randomized study. *Am J Sports Med.* 2000;28:687-694.

173. Woo SL-Y, Buckwalter JA. *Injury and Repair of the Musculoskeletal Soft Tissues*. Park Ridge, IL: American Academy of Orthopedic Surgeons; 1988.

174. Woo SL, Inoue M, McGurk-Burleson E, et al. Treatment of the medial collateral ligament injury. II: structure and function of canine knees in response to differing treatment regimens. *Am J Sports Med.* 1987;15:22-29.

175. Zazulak BT, Hewett TE, Reeves NP, Goldberg B, Cholewicki J. The effects of core proprioception on knee injury: a prospective biomechanical-epidemiological study. *Am J Sports Med.* 2007;35(3):368-373.

25

Rehabilitation of Lower-Leg Injuries

Christopher J. Hirth

OBJECTIVES

After completion of this chapter, the physical therapist should be able to do the following:

- Discuss the functional anatomy and biomechanics of the lower leg during open-chain and weightbearing activities such as walking and running.
- Identify the various techniques for regaining range of motion, including stretching exercises and joint mobilizations.
- Discuss the various rehabilitative strengthening techniques, including open- and closed-chain isotonic exercise, balance/proprioceptive exercises, and isokinetic exercise for dysfunction of the lower leg.
- Identify common causes of various lower-leg injuries and provide a rationale for treatment of these injuries.
- Discuss criteria for progression of the rehabilitation program for various lower-leg injuries.
- Describe and explain the rationale for various treatment techniques in the management of lower-leg injuries.

Functional Anatomy and Biomechanics

The lower leg consists of the tibia and fibula and 4 muscular compartments that either originate on or traverse various points along these bones. Distally the tibia and fibula articulate with the talus to form the talocrural joint. Because of the close approximation of the talus within the mortise, movement of the leg will be dictated by the foot, especially upon ground contact. This becomes important when examining the effects of repetitive stresses placed upon the leg with excessive compensatory pronation secondary to various structural lower-extremity malalignments.[78,79] Proximally the tibia articulates with the femur to form the tibiofemoral joint, as well as serving as an attachment site for the patellar tendon, the distal soft-tissue component of the extensor mechanism. The lower leg serves to transmit ground reaction forces to the knee as well as rotatory forces proximally along the lower extremity that may be a source of pain, especially with athletic activities.[56]

Compartments of the Lower Leg

All muscles work in a functionally integrated fashion in which they eccentrically decelerate, isometrically stabilize, and concentrically accelerate during movement.[50] The muscular components of the lower leg are divided anatomically into 4 compartments. In an open-kinetic-chain position, these muscle groups are responsible for movements of the foot, primarily in a single plane. When the foot is in contact with the ground, these muscle–tendon units work both concentrically and eccentrically to absorb ground reaction forces, control excessive movements of the foot and ankle to adapt to the terrain, and, ideally, provide a stable base to propel the limb forward during walking and running.

The anterior compartment is primarily responsible for dorsiflexion of the foot in an open-kinetic-chain position. Functionally these muscles are active in early and midstance phase of gait, with increased eccentric muscle activity directly after heel strike to control plantarflexion of the foot and pronation of the forefoot.[21] Electromyographic studies have noted that the tibialis anterior is active in more than 85% of the gait cycle during running.[54]

The deep posterior compartment is made up of the tibialis posterior and the long toe flexors and is responsible for inversion of the foot and ankle in an open kinetic chain. These muscles help control pronation at the subtalar joint and internal rotation of the lower leg.[21,54] Along with the soleus, the tibialis posterior will help decelerate the forward momentum of the tibia during midstance phase of gait.

The lateral compartment is made up of the peroneus longus and brevis, which are responsible for eversion of the foot in an open kinetic chain. Functionally, the peroneus longus plantarflexes the first ray at heel off, while the peroneus brevis counteracts the supinating forces of the tibialis posterior to provide osseous stability of the subtalar and midtarsal joints during the propulsive phase of gait. This is a prime example of muscles working synergistically to isometrically stabilize during movement. Electromyographic studies of running report an increase in peroneus brevis activity when the pace of running is increased.[54]

The superficial posterior compartment is made up of the gastrocnemius and soleus muscles, which in open-kinetic-chain position are responsible primarily for plantarflexion of the foot. Functionally these muscles are responsible for acting eccentrically, controlling pronation of the subtalar joint and internal rotation of the leg in the midstance phase of gait and acting concentrically during the push-off phase of gait.[21,54]

Rehabilitation Techniques for the Lower Leg

Strengthening Techniques

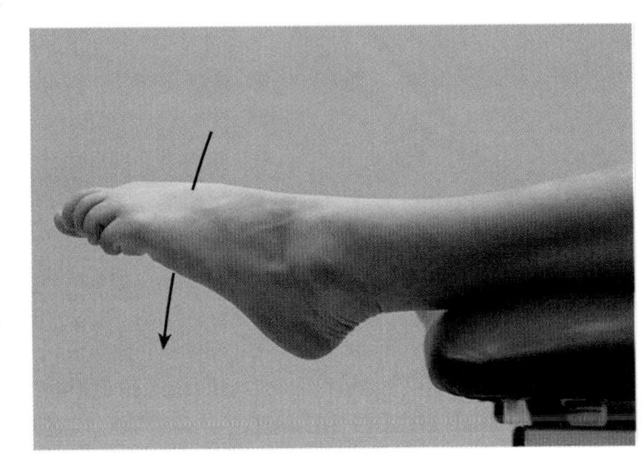

Figure 25-1 **Active range of motion ankle plantarflexion**

Used to activate the primary and secondary ankle plantarflexor muscle-tendon units after a period of immobilization or disuse. This exercise can be performed in a supportive medium such as a whirlpool.

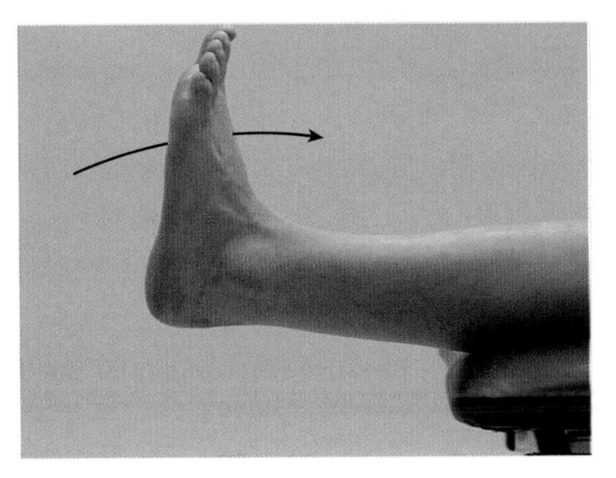

Figure 25-2 **Active range of motion ankle dorsiflexion**

Used to activate the tibialis anterior, extensor hallucis longus, and extensor digitorum longus muscle-tendon units after a period of immobilization or disuse.

Isotonic Open-Kinetic-Chain Exercises

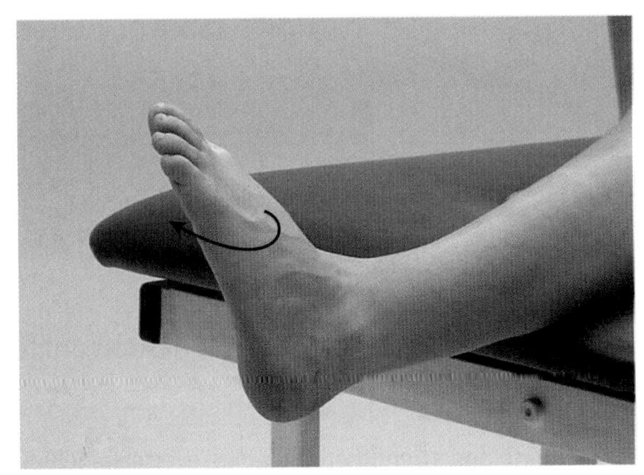

Figure 25-3 **Active range of motion ankle inversion**

Used to activate the tibialis posterior, flexor hallucis longus, and flexor digitorum longus muscle-tendon units after a period of immobilization or disuse.

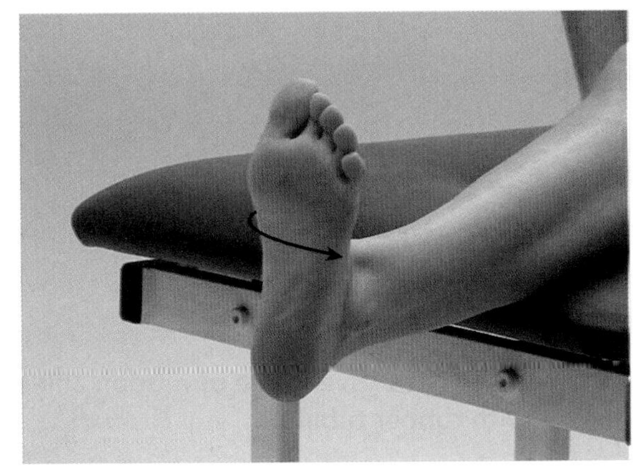

Figure 25-4 **Active range of motion ankle eversion**

Used to activate the peroneus longus and brevis muscle–tendon units after a period of immobilization or disuse.

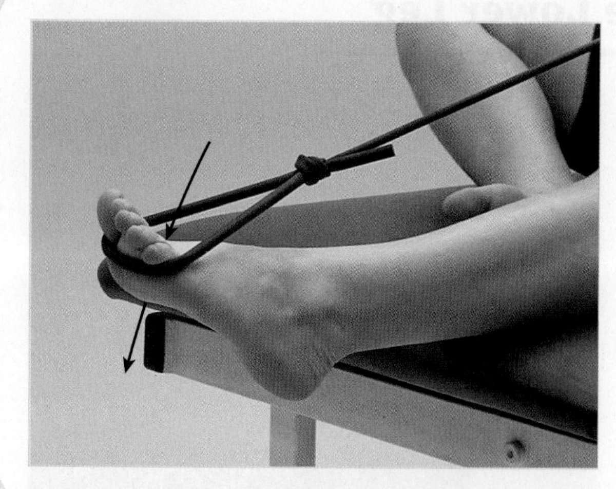

Figure 25-5 Resistive range of motion ankle plantarflexion with rubber tubing

Used to strengthen the gastrocnemius, soleus, and secondary ankle plantarflexors, including the peroneals, flexor hallucis longus, flexor digitorum longus, and tibialis posterior, in an open chain. This exercise will also place a controlled concentric and eccentric load on the Achilles tendon.

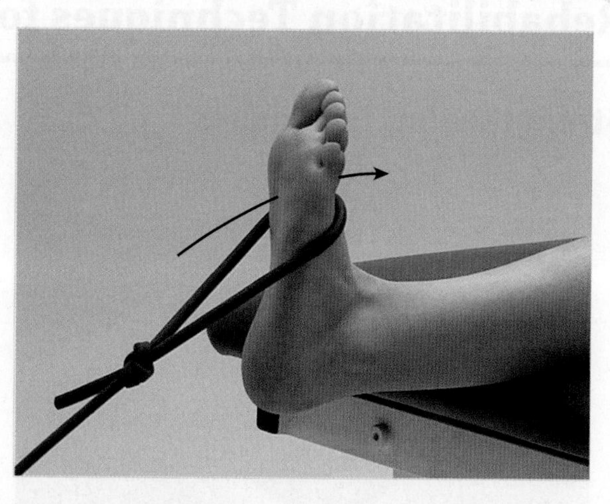

Figure 25-6 Resistive range of motion ankle dorsiflexion with rubber tubing

Used to isolate and strengthen the ankle dorsiflexors, including the tibialis anterior, extensor hallucis longus, and extensor digitorum longus, in an open chain.

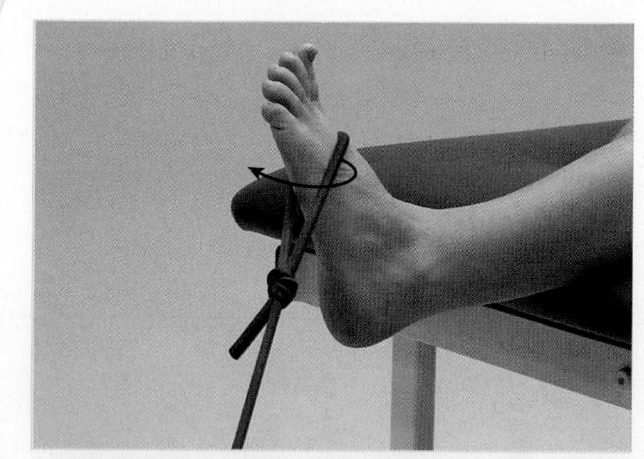

Figure 25-7 Resistive range of motion ankle inversion with rubber tubing

Used to isolate and strengthen the ankle inverters, including the tibialis posterior, flexor hallucis longus, and flexor digitorum longus, in an open chain.

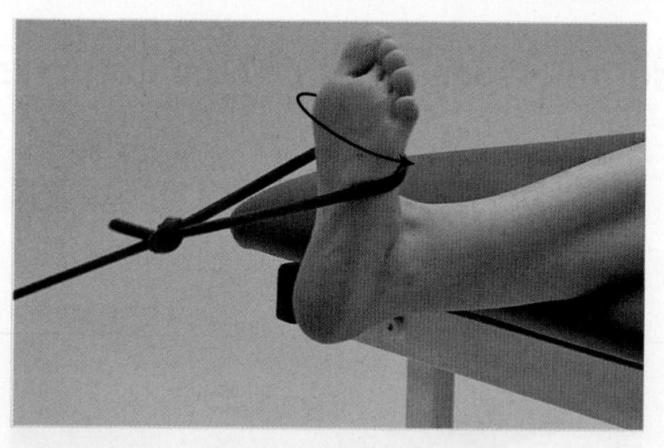

Figure 25-8 Resistive range of motion ankle eversion with rubber tubing

Used to isolate and strengthen the ankle everters, including the peroneus longus and peroneus brevis, in an open chain.

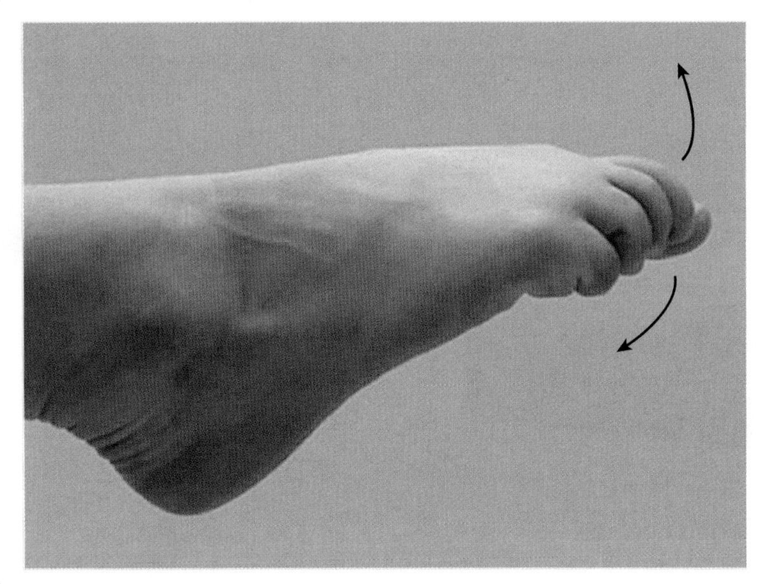

Figure 25-9 **Active range of motion toe flexion/extension**

Used to activate the long toe flexors, extensors, and foot intrinsic musculature. This exercise will also help to improve the tendon-gliding ability of the extensor hallucis longus, extensor digitorum longus, flexor hallucis longus, and flexor digitorum longus tendons after a period of immobilization.

Closed-Kinetic-Chain Strengthening Exercises

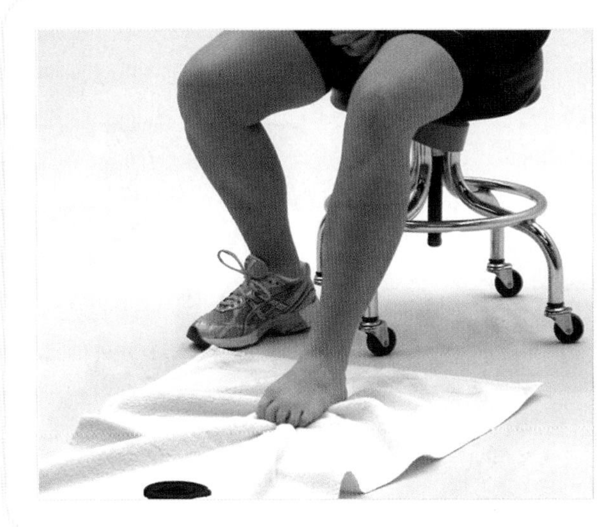

Figure 25-10 **Towel-gathering exercise**

Used to strengthen the foot intrinsics and long toe flexor and extensor muscle-tendon units. A weight can be placed on the end of the towel to require more force production by the muscle-tendon unit as range of motion and strength improve.

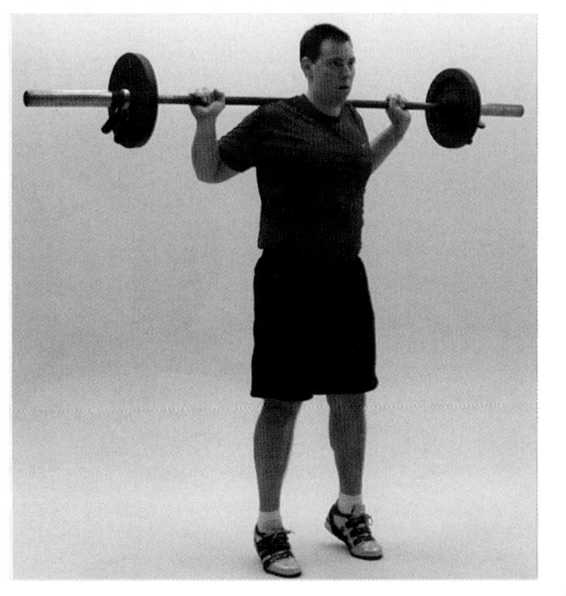

Figure 25-11 **Heel raises**

Used to strengthen the gastrocnemius musculature and will directly load the Achilles tendon.

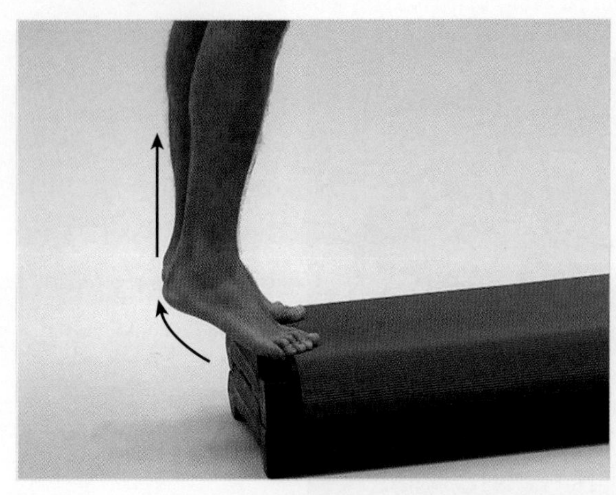

Figure 25-12 **Two-legged heel raise**

Used to strengthen the gastrocnemius when the knee is extended and the soleus when the knees are flexed. The flexor hallucis longus, flexor digitorum longus, tibialis posterior, and peroneals will also be activated during this activity. The patient can modify concentric and eccentric activity depending on the type and severity of the condition. For example, if an eccentric load is not desired on the involved side, the patient can raise up on both feet and lower down on the uninvolved side until eccentric loading is tolerated on the involved side.

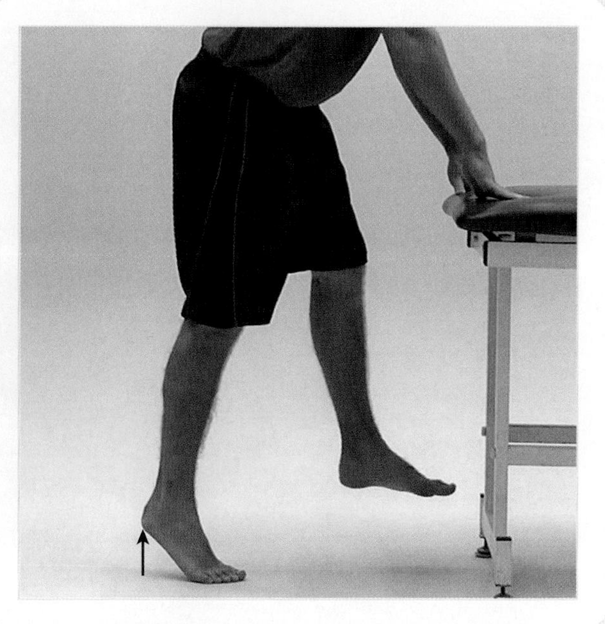

Figure 25-13 **One-legged heel raise**

Used to strengthen the gastrocnemius and soleus muscles when the knee is extended and flexed, respectively. This can be used as a progression from the two-legged heel raise.

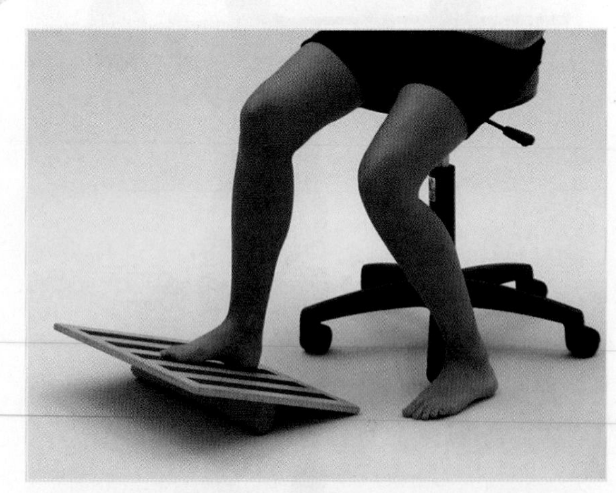

Figure 25-14 **Seated closed-chain ankle dorsiflexion/plantarflexion active ROM**

Used to activate the ankle dorsiflexor/plantarflexor musculature in a closed-chain position.

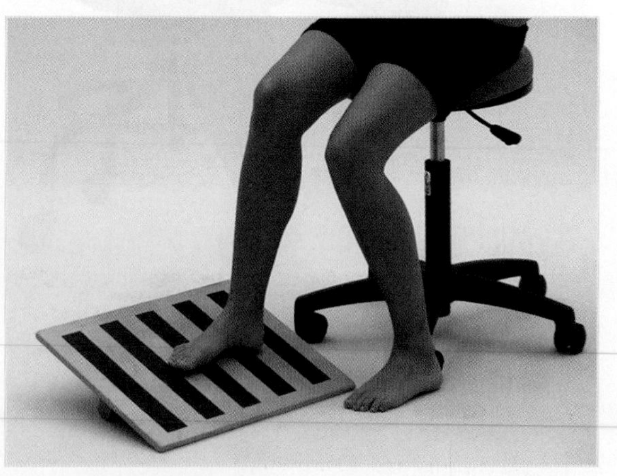

Figure 25-15 **Seated closed-chain ankle inversion/eversion active ROM**

Used to activate the ankle inverter/everter musculature in a closed-chain position.

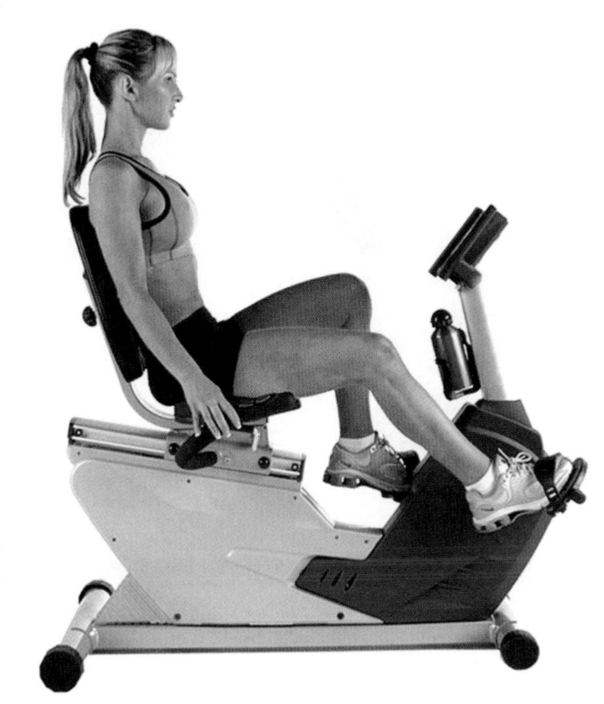

Figure 25-16 **Stationary cycle**

Used to reduce impact of weightbearing forces on the lower extremity while also maintaining cardiovascular fitness levels.

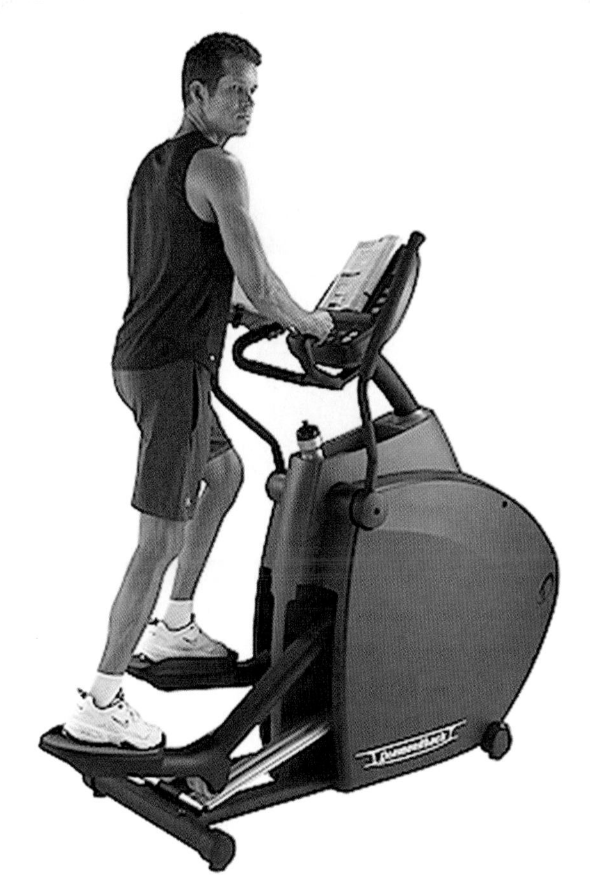

Figure 25-17 **Stair-stepping machine**

Used to progressively load the lower extremity in a closed-chain as well as maintain and improve cardiovascular fitness.

Stretching Exercises

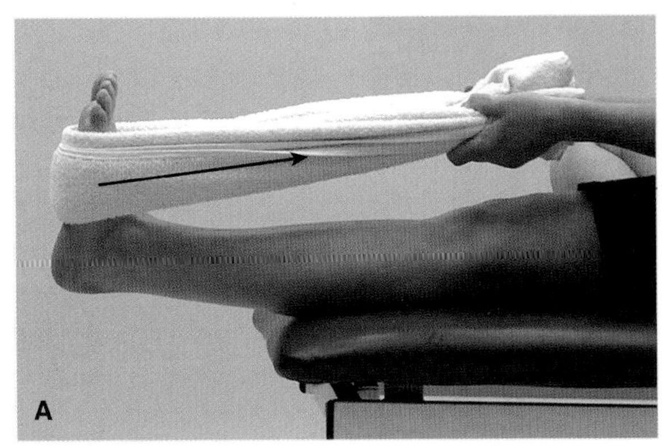

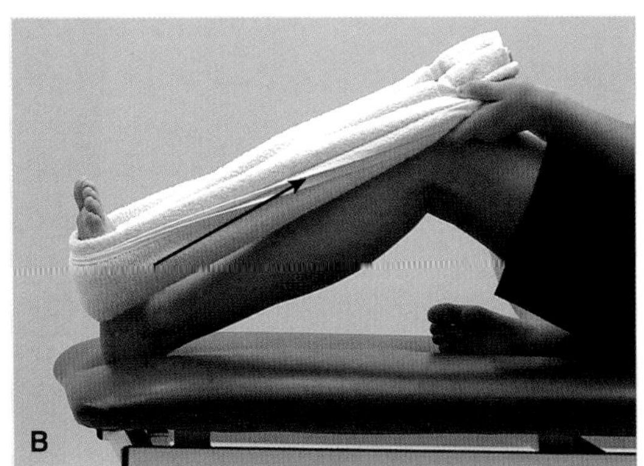

Figure 25-18 **Ankle plantarflexors towel stretch**

A. Used to stretch the gastrocnemius when the knee is extended and (**B**) the soleus when the knee is flexed. The Achilles tendon will be stretched with both positions. The patient can hold the stretch for 20 to 30 seconds.

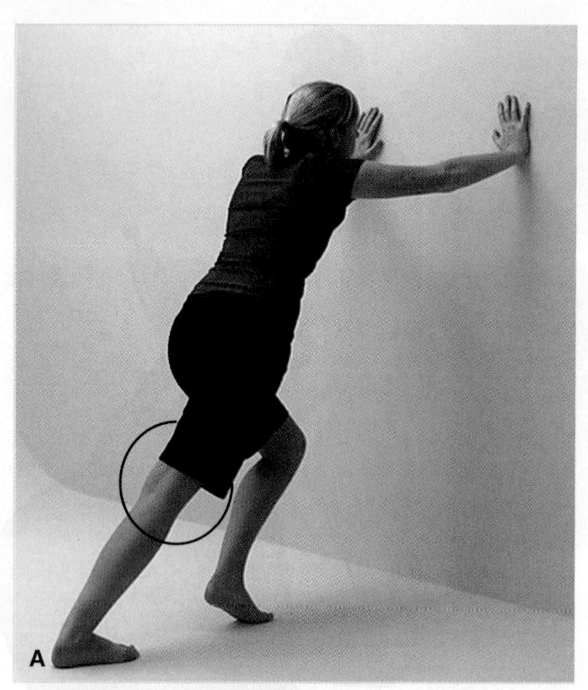

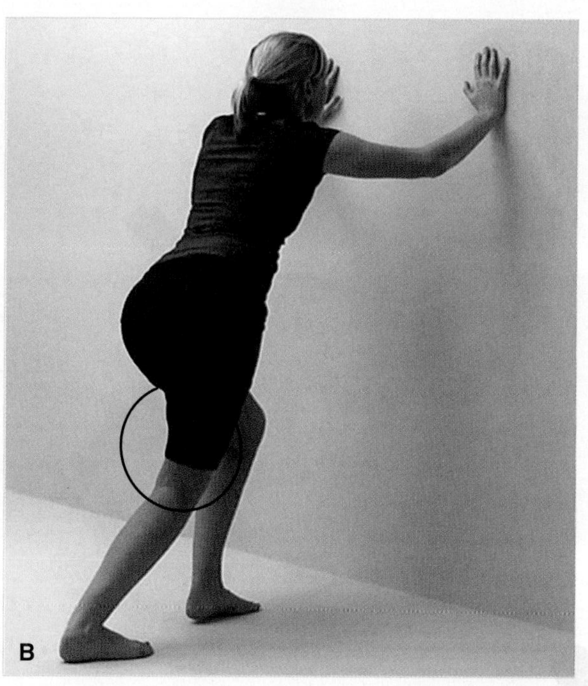

Figure 25-19

A. Standing gastrocnemius stretch. Used to stretch the gastrocnemius muscle. The Achilles tendon will also be stretched. **B.** Standing soleus stretch. Used to stretch the soleus muscle. The Achilles tendon will also be stretched.

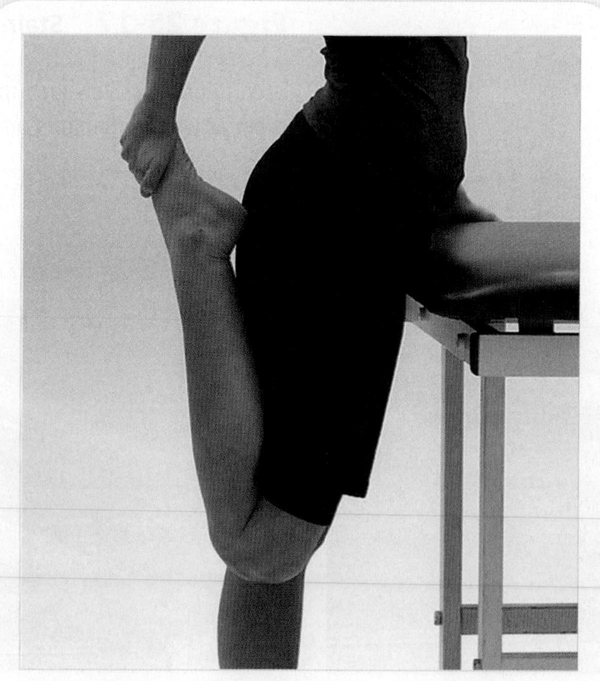

Figure 25-20 **Standing ankle dorsiflexor stretch**

Used to stretch the extensor hallucis longus, extensor digitorum longus, tibialis anterior, and anterior ankle capsule.

Exercises to Reestablish Neuromuscular Control

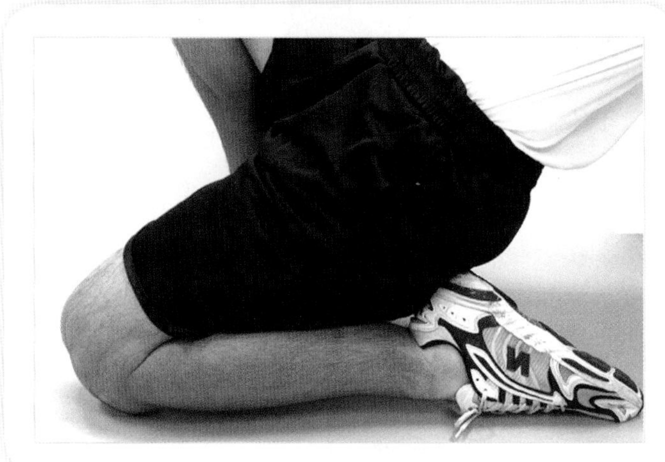

Figure 25-21 **Kneeling ankle dorsiflexor stretch**

Used to stretch the extensor hallucis longus, extensor digitorum longus, tibialis anterior, and anterior ankle capsule. This is an aggressive stretch that can be used in the later stages of rehabilitation to gain endrange-of-motion ankle dorsiflexion.

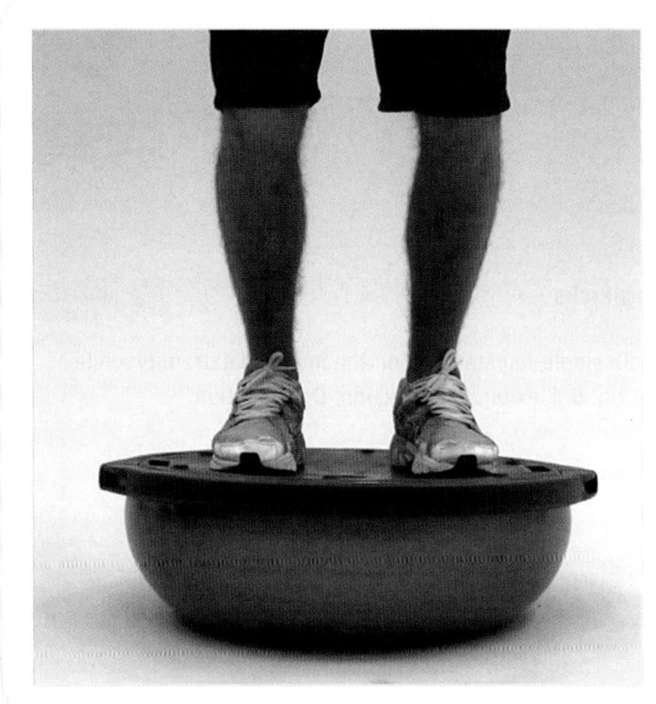

Figure 25-22 **Standing double-leg balance on BOSU Balance Trainer**

Used to activate the lower-leg musculature and improve balance and proprioception in the lower extremity.

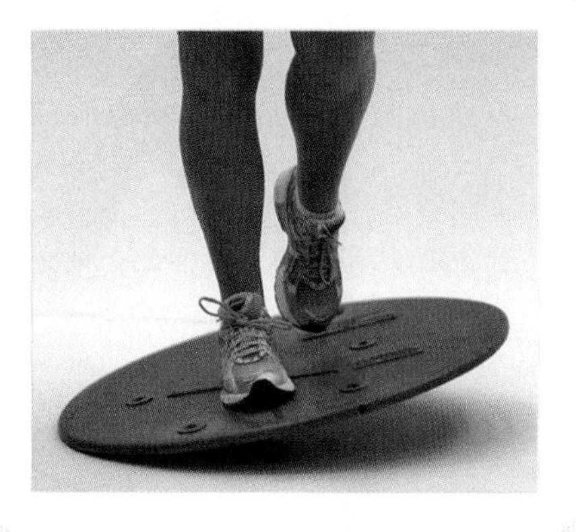

Figure 25-23 **Standing single-leg balance board activity**

Used to activate the lower-leg musculature and improve balance and proprioception in the involved extremity.

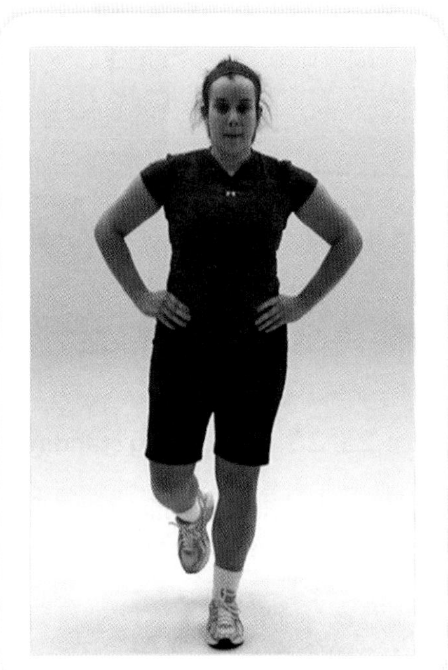

Figure 25-24 **Static single-leg standing balance progression**

Used to improve balance and proprioception of the lower extremity. This activity can be made more difficult with the following progression: (a) single-leg stand, eyes open; (b) single-leg stand, eyes closed; (c) single-leg stand, eyes open, toes extended so only the heel and metatarsal heads are in contact with the ground; (d) single-leg stand, eyes closed, toes extended.

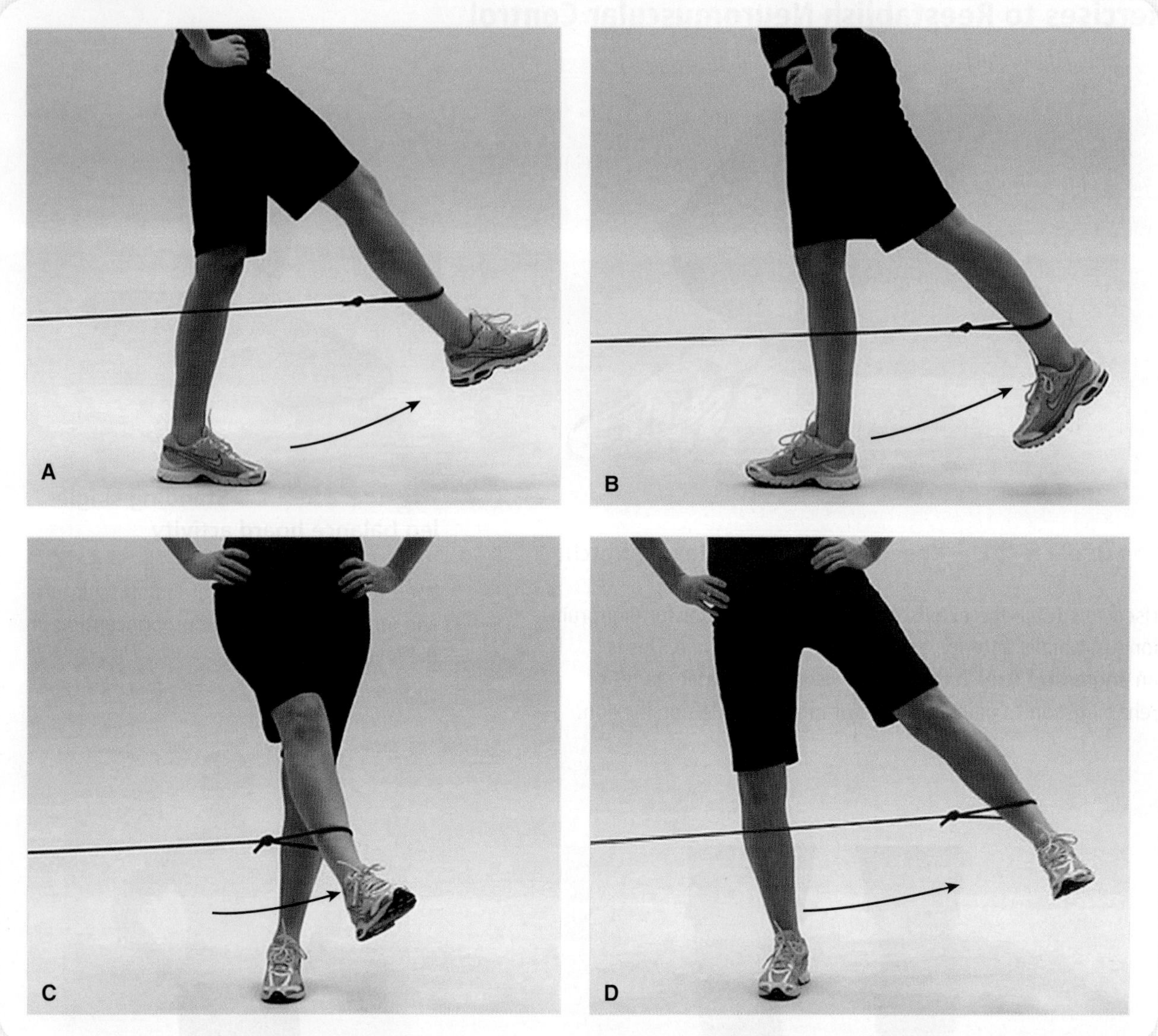

Figure 25-25 **Single-leg standing rubber-tubing kicks**

Used to improve muscle activation of the lower leg to maintain single-leg standing on the involved extremity while kicking against the resistance of the rubber tubing. **A.** Extension. **B.** Flexion. **C.** Adduction. **D.** Abduction.

Exercises to Improve Cardiorespiratory Endurance

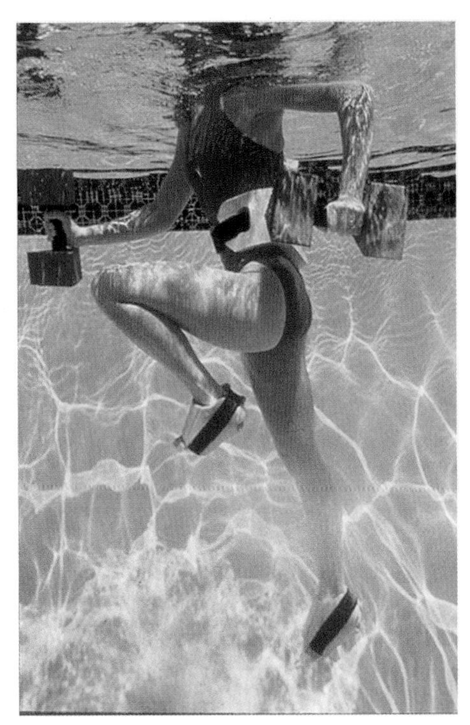

Figure 25-26 **Pool running with flotation device**

Used to reduce impact weightbearing forces on the lower extremity while maintaining cardiovascular fitness level and running form.

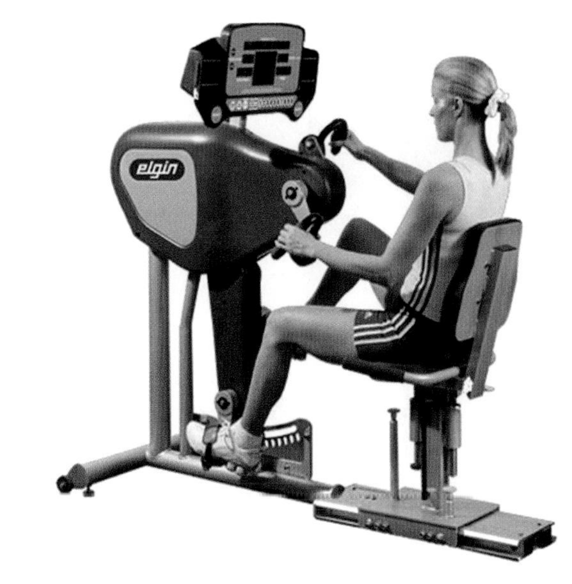

Figure 25-27 **Upper-body ergometer**

Used to maintain cardiovascular fitness when lower-extremity ergometer is contraindicated or too difficult for the patient to use.

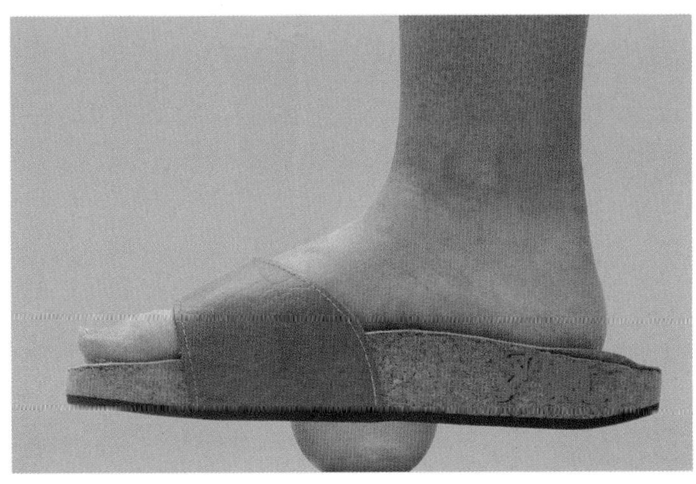

Figure 25-28 **Exercise sandals (OPTP, Minneapolis, MN)**

Wooden sandals with a rubber hemisphere located centrally on the plantar surface.

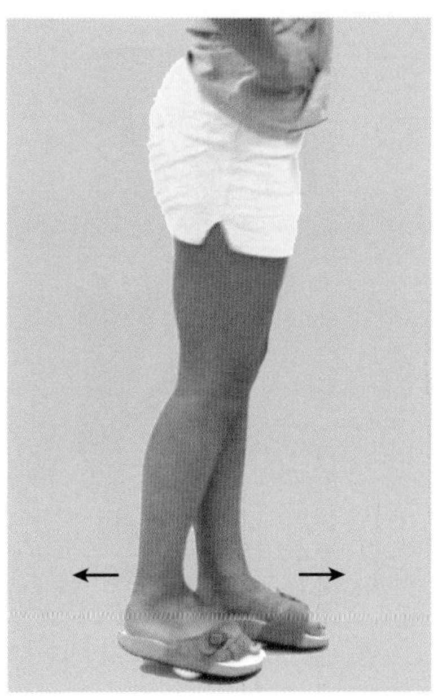

Figure 25-29 **Exercise sandal forward and backwards walking**

Used to enhance balance and proprioception and increase muscle activity in the foot intrinsics, lower-leg musculature, and gluteals. The patient takes small steps forward and backwards.

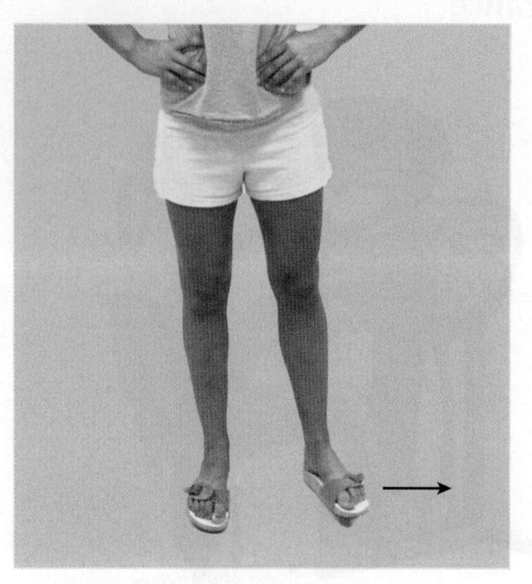

Figure 25-30 Exercise sandals sidestepping

Used to enhance balance and proprioception in the frontal plane. Increases muscle activity of the lower-leg musculature and foot intrinsics. The patient moves directly to the left or right along a straight line with the toes pointed forward.

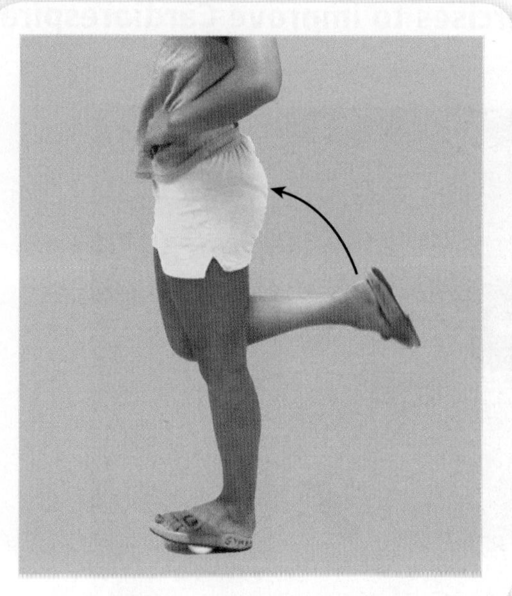

Figure 25-31 Exercise sandals butt kicks

Used to promote balance and proprioception along with increased muscle activity of the foot intrinsics, lower-leg musculature, and gluteals. This exercise enhances single-leg stance in the exercise sandals.

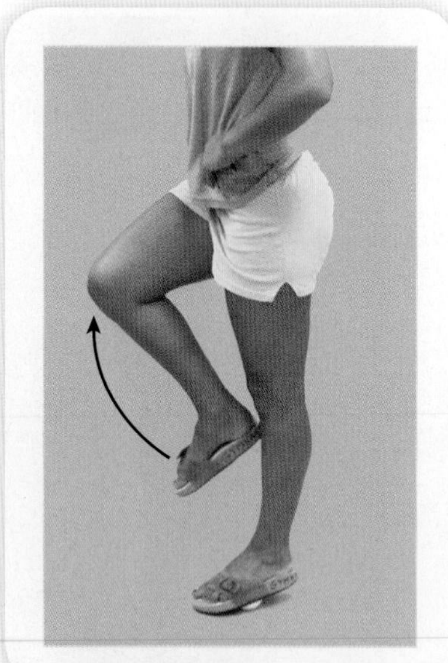

Figure 25-32 Exercise sandals high knees

Used to enhance balance and proprioception and muscle activity of the foot intrinsics, lower-leg musculature, and especially the gluteals. The patient should maintain an upright posture and avoid trunk flexion with hip flexion. This exercise promotes single-leg stance progression for a short period of time.

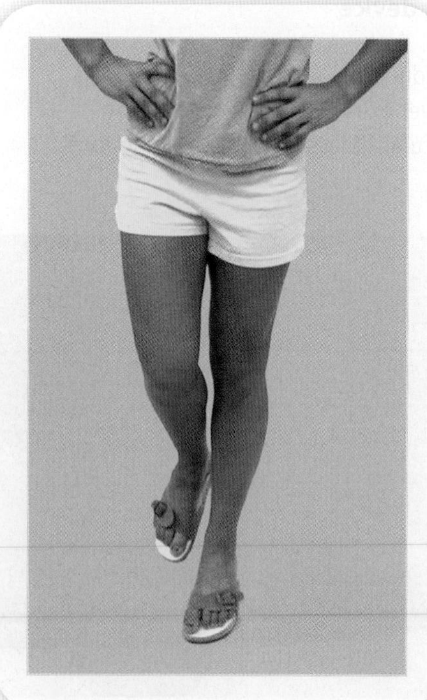

Figure 25-33 Exercise sandals single-leg stance

Used to enhance balance, proprioception, and muscle activity in the entire lower extremity. This exercise is the most demanding in the exercise sandal progression.

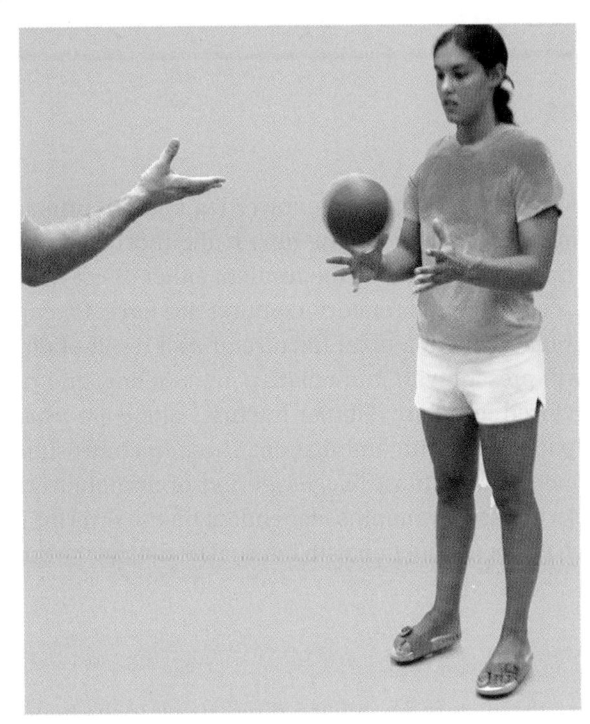

Figure 25-34 Exercise sandal ball catch

Used to enhance balance, proprioception, and lower-leg muscle activity. The patient focuses on catching and throwing the ball to the therapist while moving laterally to the left or right.

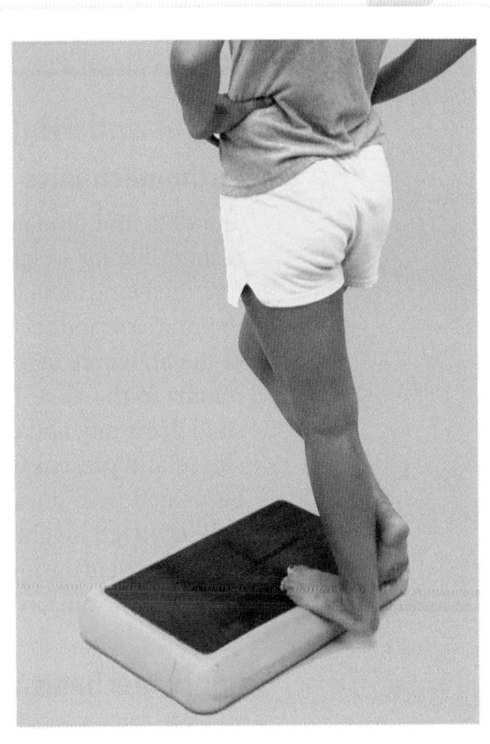

Figure 25-35 Achilles tendon eccentric muscle loading

Used to enhance gastrocnemius (knee straight) and soleus (knee bent) strength and Achilles tendon tensile strength. The patient uses the uninvolved side to elevate onto the patient's toes and then places all weight on toes of the involved side to eccentrically lower. Initially, the patient lowers to the step and then progresses below the level of the step. Extra weight can be added via a backpack.

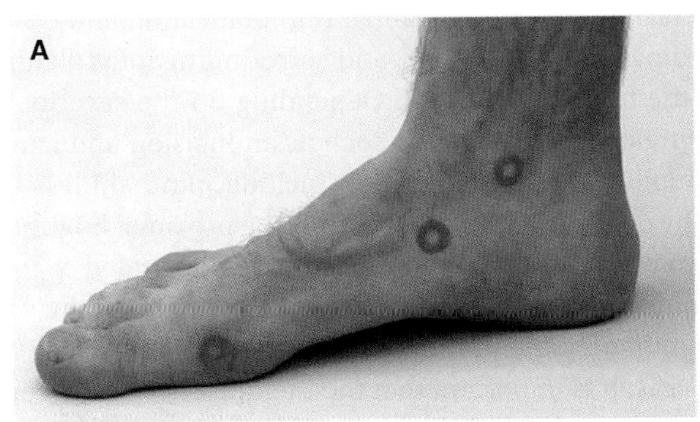

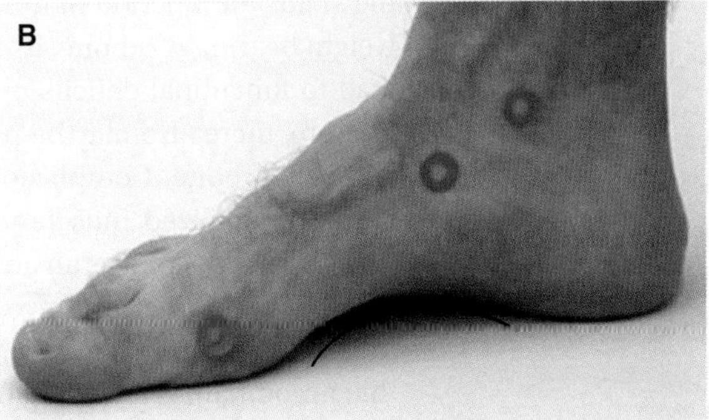

Figure 25-36 Short foot concept

Used to enhance and strengthen the foot intrinsic muscles. The patient is instructed to shorten the foot from front to back while keeping the toes straight. The metatarsal heads should stay in contact with the ground. The therapist can palpate the foot intrinsics and will notice a raised longitudinal arch with a flexible foot type. The shortened foot should be maintained at all times while in the exercise sandals.

Rehabilitation Techniques for Specific Injuries

Tibial and Fibular Fractures

Pathomechanics

The tibia and fibula constitute the bony components of the lower leg and are primarily responsible for weight bearing and muscle attachment. The tibia is the most commonly fractured long bone in the body, and fractures are usually the result of either direct trauma to the area or indirect trauma such as a combination rotatory/compressive force. Fractures of the fibula are usually seen in combination with a tibial fracture or as a result of direct trauma to the area. Tibial fractures will present with immediate pain, swelling, and possible deformity and can be open or closed in nature. Fibular fractures alone are usually closed and present with pain on palpation and with ambulation. These fractures should be treated with immediate medical referral and most likely a period of immobilization and restricted weight bearing for weeks to possibly months, depending on the severity and involvement of the injury. Surgery such as open reduction with internal fixation of the bone, usually of the tibia, is common.

Injury Mechanism

The 2 mechanisms of a traumatic lower-leg fracture are either a direct insult to the bone or indirectly through a combined rotatory/compressive force. Direct impact to the long bone, such as from a projectile object or the top of a ski boot, can produce enough damaging force to fracture a bone. Indirect trauma from a combination of rotatory and compressive forces can be manifested in sports when an athlete's foot is planted and the proximal segments are rotated with a large compressive force. An example of this could be a football running back attempting to gain more yardage while an opposing player is trying to tackle him from above the waist and applying a superincumbent compressive load. If the patient's foot is planted and immovable and the lower extremity is rotated, the superincumbent weight of the defender may be enough to cause a fracture in the tibia. A fibular fracture may accompany the tibial fracture.

Rehabilitation Concerns

Tibial and fibular fractures are usually immobilized and placed on a restricted weightbearing status for a period of time to facilitate fracture healing. Immobilization and restricted weight bearing of a bone, its proximal and distal joints, and surrounding musculature will lead to functional deficits once the fracture is healed. Depending on the severity of the fracture, there also may be postsurgical considerations such as an incision and hardware within the bone. Complications following immobilization include joint stiffness of any joints immobilized, muscle atrophy of the lower leg and possibly the proximal thigh and hip musculature, as well as an abnormal gait pattern. Bullock-Saxton demonstrated changes in gluteus maximus electromyographic muscle activation after a severe ankle sprain.[13] Proximal hip muscle weakness is magnified by the immobility and non-weightbearing action that accompanies lower-leg fractures. It is important that the therapist perform a comprehensive evaluation of the patient to determine all potential rehabilitation problems, including range of motion, joint mobility, muscle flexibility, strength and endurance of the entire involved lower extremity, balance, proprioception, and gait. The therapist must also determine the functional demands that will be placed on the patient upon return to competition and set up short- and long-term goals accordingly. Upon cast removal it is important to address range-of-motion (ROM) deficits. This can be managed with passive, then active, ROM exercises in a supportive medium such as a warm whirlpool (Figures 25-1 to 25-4, 25-9, 25-14, 25-15, 25-16, and 25-17). Joint stiffness can be addressed via joint mobilization to any joint that was immobilized (see Figures 13-61 to 13-68). It is possible to have post-traumatic edema in the foot and ankle after cast removal that can be reduced with massage. Strengthening exercises can help facilitate muscle firing, strength, and endurance (Figures 25-5 to 25-8 and 25-10 to 25-17). Balance and proprioception can be improved with single-leg standing activities and balance board activities (Figures 25-22 to 25-25). Cardiovascular endurance can be addressed with pool activities including swimming and pool running with a flotation device, stationary cycling, and the use of an upper-body ergometer (see Figures 25-16, 25-26 and 25-27). A stair stepper is also an excellent way to address cardiovascular needs as well as lower-extremity strength, endurance, and weight bearing (Figure 25-17).

Once the patient demonstrates proficiency in static balance activities on various balance modalities, more dynamic neuromuscular control activities can be introduced. Exercise sandals (OPTP, Minneapolis, MN) can be incorporated into rehabilitation as a closed-kinetic-chain functional exercise that places increased proprioceptive demands on the patient. The exercise sandals are wooden sandals with a rubber hemisphere located centrally on the plantar surface (Figure 25-28). The patient can be progressed into the exercise sandals once they demonstrate proficiency in barefoot single-leg stance. Prior to using the exercise sandals the patient is instructed in the short-foot concept—a shortening of the foot in an anteroposterior direction while the long toe flexors are relaxed, thus activating the short toe flexors and foot the intrinsics (see Figure 25-36).[37] Clinically, the short foot appears to enhance the longitudinal and transverse arches of the foot. Once the patient can perform the short-foot concept in the sandals, the patient is progressed to walking in place and forward walking with short steps (Figure 25-29). The patient is instructed to assume a good upright posture while training in the sandals. Initially, the patient may be limited to 30 to 60 seconds while acclimating to the proprioceptive demands. Once the patient appears safe with walking in place and small-step forward walking, the patient can follow a rehabilitation progression (Table 25-1 and Figures 25-30 to 25-34).

The exercise sandals offer an excellent means of facilitating lower-extremity musculature that can be affected by tibial and fibular fractures. Bullock-Saxton et al noted increased gluteal muscle activity with exercise sandal training after 1 week.[14] Myers et al also demonstrated increased gluteal activity, especially with high-knees marching in the exercise sandals.[48] Blackburn et al have shown increased activity in the lower-leg musculature, specifically the tibialis anterior and peroneus longus, while performing the exercise sandal progression activities.[11] The lower-leg musculature is usually weakened and atrophied, from being so close to the trauma. The exercise sandals offer an excellent means of increasing muscle activation of the lower-leg musculature in a functional weightbearing manner.

Table 25-1 Exercise Sandal Progression

1. Walking in place
2. Forward/backward walking—small steps
3. Sidestepping
4. Butt kicks
5. High knees
6. Single-leg stance—10 to 15 seconds
7. Ball catch—sidestepping
8. Sport-specific activity
   - Each activity can be performed for 30 to 60 seconds with rest between each activity.
   - All exercises should be performed with short-foot and good standing posture except where sport-specific activity dictates otherwise.

Rehabilitation Progression

Management of a postimmobilization fracture requires good communication with the physician to determine progression of weightbearing status, any assistive devices to be used during the rehabilitation process, such as a walker boot, and any other pertinent information that can influence the rehabilitation process. It is important to address ROM deficits immediately with active range of motion (AROM), passive stretching, and skilled joint mobilization. Isometric strengthening can be initiated and progressed to isotonic exercises once ROM has been normalized. After weightbearing status is determined, gait training to normalize walking should be initiated. Assistive devices should be utilized as needed. Strengthening of the involved lower extremity can be incorporated into the rehabilitation process, especially for the hip and thigh musculature. It is important for the therapist to identify and address this hip muscular weakness early on in rehabilitation through open- and closed-chain strengthening. Balance and proprioceptive exercises can begin once there is full pain-free weightbearing on the involved lower extremity.

As ROM, strength, and walking gait are normalized, the patient can be progressed to a walking/jogging progression and a sport-related functional progression. It must be realized that the rate of rehabilitation progression will depend on the severity of the fracture, any surgical involvement, and length of immobilization. The average healing time for uncomplicated nondisplaced tibial fractures is 10 to 13 weeks; for displaced, open, or comminuted tibial fracture, it is 16 to 26 weeks.[67]

Fibular fractures may be immobilized for 4 to 6 weeks. Again, an open line of communication with the physician is required to facilitate a safe rehabilitation progression for the patient.

Criteria for Full Return

The following criteria should be met prior to the return to full activity: (a) full ROM and strength, compared to the uninvolved side; (b) normalized walking, jogging, and running gait; (c) ability to hop for endurance and 90% hop for distance as compared to the uninvolved side, without complaints of pain or observable compensation; and (d) successful completion of a sport-specific functional test.

Tibial and Fibular Stress Fractures

Pathomechanics

Stress fractures of the tibia and fibula are common in sports. Studies indicate that stress fractures of the tibia occur at a higher rate than those of the fibula.[7,8,45] Stress fractures in the lower leg are usually the result of the bone's inability to adapt to the repetitive loading response during training and conditioning of the athlete. The bone attempts to adapt to the applied loads initially through osteoclastic activity, which breaks down the bone. Osteoblastic activity, or the laying down of new bone, will soon follow.[53,77] If the applied loads are not reduced during this process, structural irregularities will develop within the bone, which will further reduce the bone's ability to absorb stress and will eventually lead to a stress fracture.[8,27]

Repetitive loading of the lower leg with a weightbearing activity such as running is usually the cause of tibial and fibular stress fractures. Romani reports that repetitive mechanical loading seen with the initiation of a stressful activity may cause an ischemia to the affected bone.[58] He reports that repetitive loading may lead to temporary oxygen debt of the bone, which signals the remodeling process to begin.[58] Also, microdamage to the capillaries further restricts blood flow, leading to more ischemia, which again triggers the remodeling process—leading to a weakened bone and a setup for a stress fracture.[58]

Stress fractures in the tibial shaft mainly occur in the mid anterior aspect and the posteromedial aspect.[7,45,55,77] Anterior tibial stress fractures usually present in patients involved in repetitive jumping activities with localized pain directly over the mid anterior tibia. The patient will complain of pain with activity that is relieved with rest. The pain can affect activities of daily living (ADL) if activity is not modified. Vibration testing using a tuning fork will reproduce the symptoms, as will hopping on the involved extremity. A triple-phase technetium-99 bone scan can confirm the diagnosis faster than an X-ray, as it can take a minimum of 3 weeks to demonstrate radiographic changes.[53,55,77] Posteromedial tibial pain usually occurs over the distal one-third of the bone with a gradual onset of symptoms.

Focal point tenderness on the bone will help differentiate a stress fracture from medial tibial stress syndrome (MTSS), which is located in the same area but is more diffuse upon palpation. The procedures listed above will be positive and will implicate the stress fracture as the source of pain. Fibular stress fractures usually occur in the distal one-third of the bone with the same symptomatology as for tibial stress fractures. Although less common, stress fractures of the proximal fibula are noted in the literature.[45,73,88]

Injury Mechanism

Anterior tibial stress fractures are prevalent in patients involved with jumping. Several authors have noted that the tibia will bow anteriorly with the convexity on the anterior aspect.[18,53,56,77] This places the anterior aspect of the tibia under tension that is less than ideal for bone healing, which prefers compressive forces. Repetitive jumping will place greater tension on this area, which has minimal musculotendinous support and blood supply. Other biomechanical factors may be involved, including excessive compensatory pronation at the subtalar joint to accommodate lower-extremity structural alignments such as forefoot varus, tibial varum, and femoral anteversion. This excessive pronation might not affect the leg during ADL or with moderate activity, but might become a factor with increases in training intensity, duration, and frequency, even with sufficient recovery time.[30,77] Increased training may affect the surrounding muscle–tendon unit's ability to absorb the impact of each applied load, which places more stress on the bone. Stress fractures of the distal posteromedial tibia will also arise from the same problems as listed above, with the exception of repetitive jumping. Excessive compensatory pronation may play a greater role with this type of injury. This hyperpronation can be accentuated when running on a crowned road; such is the case of the uphill leg.[60] Also, running on a track with a small radius and tight curves will tend to increase pronatory stresses on the leg that is closer to the inside of the track.[60] Excessive pronation may also play a role with fibular stress fractures. The repeated activity of the ankle everters and calf musculature pulling on the bone may be a source of this type of stress fracture.[53] Training errors of increased duration and intensity along with wornout shoes will only accentuate these problems.[60] Other factors, including menstrual irregularities, diet, bone density, increased hip external rotation, tibial width, and calf girth, also have been identified as contributing to stress fractures.[8,29]

Rehabilitation Concerns

Immediate elimination of the offending activity is most important. The patient must be educated on the importance of this to prevent further damage to the bone. Many patients will express concerns about fitness level with loss of activity. Stationary cycling and running in the deep end of the pool with a flotation device can help maintain cardiovascular fitness (see Figures 25-16 and 25-26). Eyestone et al demonstrated a small, but statistically significant, decrease in maximal aerobic capacity when water running was substituted for regular running.[23] This was also true with using a stationary bike.[23] These authors recommend that intensity, duration, and frequency be equivalent to regular training. Wilder et al note that water provides a resistance that is proportional to the effort exerted.[84] These authors found that cadence, via a metronome, gave a quantitative external cue that with increased rate showed high correlation with heart rate.[84] Nonimpact activity in the pool or on the bike will help maintain fitness and allow proper bone healing. Proper footwear that matches the needs of the foot is also important. For example, a high arched or pes cavus foot type will require a shoe with good shock-absorbing qualities. A pes planus foot type or more pronated foot will require a shoe with good motion control characteristics. Recent evidence-based reviews indicate that shock-absorbing insoles can have a preventative effect with tibial stress fractures.[65] A detailed biomechanical exam of the lower extremity, both statically and dynamically, may reveal problems that require the use of a custom foot orthotic. Stretching and strengthening exercises can be incorporated in the rehabilitation process. The use of ice and electrical stimulation to control pain is also recommended. The utilization of an Aircast with patients who have diagnosed stress fractures has produced positive results.[20] Dickson and Kichline speculate that the Aircast unloads the tibia and fibula enough to allow healing of the stress fracture with continued participation.[20] Swenson et al reported that patients with tibial stress fractures who used an Aircast returned to full unrestricted activity in 21 ± 2 days; patients who used traditional regimen returned in 77 ± 7 days.[76] Fibular and posterior medial tibial stress fractures will usually heal without residual problems if the above-mentioned concerns are addressed. Stress fractures of the mid anterior tibia can take much longer, and residual problems might exist months to years after the initial diagnosis, with attempts at increased activity.[18,22,55,56] Initial treatment may include a short leg cast and non–weight bearing for 6 to 8 weeks. Batt et al noted that use of a pneumatic brace in those individuals allowed for return to unrestricted activity, an average of 12 months from presentation.[4] The proposed hypothesis for use of a pneumatic brace is that elevated osseous hydrostatic and venous blood pressure produces a positive piezoelectric effect that stimulates osteoblastic activity and facilitates fracture healing.[87] Rettig et al used rest from the offending activity as well as electrical stimulation in the form of a pulsed electromagnetic field for a period of 10 to 12 hours per day. The authors noted an average of 12.7 months from the onset of symptoms to return to full activity with this regimen.[56] They recommended using this program for 3 to 6 months before considering surgical intervention.[56] Chang and Harris noted good to excellent results with a surgical procedure involving intramedullary nailing of the tibia with individuals with delayed union of this type of stress fracture.[18] Surgical procedures involving bone grafting have also been recommended to improve healing of this type of stress fracture.

Rehabilitation Progression

After diagnosis of the stress fracture, the patient may be placed on crutches, depending on the amount of discomfort with ambulation. Ice and electrical stimulation can be used to reduce local inflammation and pain. The patient can immediately begin deep-water running with the same training parameters as their regular regimen if they are pain-free. Stretching exercises for the gastrocnemius–soleus musculature can be performed 2 to 3 times per day (Figure 25-19). Isotonic strengthening exercises with rubber tubing can begin as soon as tolerated on an every-other-day basis, with an increase in repetitions and sets as the therapist sees fit (see Figures 25-5 to 25-8). Strengthening of the gastrocnemius can be done initially in an open chain and eventually be progressed to a closed chain (see Figures 25-5, 25-12, and 25-13). The patient should wear supportive shoes during the day and avoid shoes with a heel, which can cause adaptive shortening of the gastrocnemius-soleus complex and increase strain on the healing bone. Custom foot orthotics can be fabricated for motion control in order to prevent excessive pronation for those patients who need it. Foot orthotics can also be fabricated for a high-arched foot to increase stress distribution throughout the plantar aspect of the whole foot versus the heel and the metatarsal heads. Shock-absorbing materials can augment these orthotics to help reduce ground reaction forces. The exercise sandal progression can also be introduced to help facilitate lower-leg muscle activity and strength (see Figures 25-29 to 25-34 and 25-36). As the symptoms subside over a period of 3 to 4 weeks and X-rays confirm that good callus formation is occurring, the patient may be progressed to a walking/jogging progression on a surface suitable to that patient's needs. The patient must demonstrate pain-free ambulation prior to initiating a walk/jog program. A quality track or grass surface may be the best choice to begin this progression. The patient may be instructed to jog for 1 minute, then walk for 30 seconds for 10 to 15 repetitions. This can be performed on an every-other-day basis with high-intensity/long-duration cardiovascular training occurring daily in the pool or on the bike. The patient should be reminded that the purpose of the walk/jog progression is to provide a gradual increase in stress to the healing bone in a controlled manner. If tolerated, the jogging time can be increased by 30 seconds every 2 to 3 training sessions until the patient is running 5 minutes without walking. The above progression is a guideline and can be modified based on individual needs.

Romani has developed a 3-phase plan for stress fracture management.[58] Phase 1 focuses on decreasing pain and stress to the injured bone while also preventing deconditioning. Phase 2 focuses on increasing strength, balance, and conditioning, and normalizing function, without an increase in pain. After 2 weeks of pain-free exercise in phase 2, running and functional activities of phase 3 are introduced. Phase 3 has functional phases and rest phases. During the functional phase, weeks 1 and 2, running is progressed; in the third week, or rest phase, running is decreased. This is done to mimic the cyclic fashion of bone growth. During the first 2 weeks, as bone is resorbed, running will promote the formation of trabecular channels; in the third week, while the osteocytes and periosteum are maturing, the impact loading of running is removed.[58] This cyclic progression is continued over several weeks as the patient becomes able to perform sport-specific activities without pain.[58]

Criteria for Full Return

The patient can return to full activity when: (a) there is no tenderness to palpation of the affected bone and no pain of the affected area with repeated hopping; (b) plain films demonstrate good bone healing; (c) there has been successful progression of a graded return to running with no increase in symptoms; (d) gastrocnemius–soleus flexibility is within normal limits; (e) hyperpronation has been corrected or shock-absorption problems have been decreased with proper shoes and foot orthotics if indicated; and (f) all muscle strength and muscle length issues of the involved lower extremity have been addressed.

Compartment Syndromes

Pathomechanics and Injury Mechanism

Compartment syndrome is a condition in which increased pressure within a fixed osseofascial compartment causes compression of muscular and neurovascular structures within the compartment. As compartment pressures increase, the venous outflow of fluid decreases and eventually stops, causing further fluid leakage from the capillaries into the compartment. Eventually arterial blood inflow also ceases secondary to rising intracompartmental pressures.[82] Compartment syndrome can be divided into 3 categories: acute compartment syndrome, acute exertional compartment syndrome, and chronic compartment syndrome. Acute compartment syndrome occurs secondary to direct trauma to the area and is a medical emergency.[38,74,82] The patient will complain of a deep-seated aching pain, tightness, and swelling of the involved compartment. Reproduction of the pain will occur with passive stretching of the involved muscles. Reduction in pedal pulses and sensory changes of the involved nerve can be present, but are not reliable signs.[82,86] Intracompartmental pressure measurements will confirm the diagnosis. Emergency fasciotomy is the definitive treatment.

Acute exertional compartment syndrome occurs without any precipitating trauma. Cases have been cited in the literature in which acute compartment syndrome has evolved with minimal to moderate activity. If not diagnosed and treated properly, it can lead to poor functional outcomes for the patient.[24,86] Again, intracompartmental pressures will confirm the diagnosis, with emergency fasciotomy being the treatment of choice. Chronic compartment syndrome (CCS) is activity-related in that the symptoms arise rather consistently at a certain point in the activity. The patient complains of a sensation of pain, tightness, and swelling of the affected compartment that resolves upon stopping the activity. Studies indicate that the anterior and deep posterior compartments are usually involved.[6,57,64,75,85] Upon presentation of these symptoms, intracompartmental pressure measurements will further define the severity of the condition. Pedowitz et al developed modified criteria using a slit-catheter measurement of the intracompartmental pressures. These authors consider 1 or more of the following intramuscular pressure criteria as diagnostic of CCS: (a) preexercise pressure greater than 15 mm Hg; (b) a 1-minute postexercise pressure of 30 mm Hg; (c) a 5-minute postexercise pressure greater than 20 mm Hg.[51]

Rehabilitation Concerns

Management of CCS is initially conservative with activity modification, icing, and stretching of the anterior compartment and gastrocnemius–soleus complex (see Figures 25-21 to 25-23). A lower-quarter structural exam along with gait analysis might reveal a structural variation that is causing excessive compensatory pronation and might benefit from the use of foot orthotics and proper footwear. However, these measures will not address the issue of increased compartment pressures with activity. Cycling has been shown to be an acceptable alternative in preventing increased anterior compartment pressures when compared to running and can be utilized to maintain cardiovascular fitness.[2] If conservative measures fail, fasciotomy of the affected compartments has produced favorable results in a return to higher level of activity.[57,61,82,85]

The patient should be counseled regarding the outcome expectations after fasciotomy for CCS. Howard reported a clinically significant improvement in 81% of the anterior/lateral releases and a 50% improvement in deep posterior compartment releases with CCS.[36] Slimmon et al noted that 58% of the subjects responding to a long-term follow-up study for CCS fasciotomy reported exercising at a lower level than before the injury.[68] Micheli et al noted that female patients may be more prone to this condition and that for reasons unclear, they did not respond to the fasciotomy as well as their male counterparts.[46]

Rehabilitation Progression

Following fasciotomy for CCS, the immediate goals are to decrease postsurgical pain, swelling with RICE (rest, ice, compression, elevation), and assisted ambulation with the use of crutches. After suture removal and soft-tissue healing of the incision has progressed, AROM and flexibility exercises should be initiated (see Figures 25-1 to 25-4, 25-18 to 25-21). Weight bearing will be progressed as ROM improves. Gait training should be incorporated to prevent abnormal movements in the gait pattern secondary to joint and soft-tissue stiffness or muscle guarding. AROM exercises should be progressed to open-chain exercises with rubber tubing (see Figures 25-5 to 25-8). Closed-kinetic-chain activities can also be initiated to incorporate strength, balance, and proprioception that may have been affected by the surgical procedure (see Figures 25-11 to 25-15 and 25-22 to 25-25). Lower-extremity structural variations that lead to excessive compensatory pronation during gait should be addressed with foot orthotics and proper footwear after walking gait has been normalized. These measures should help control excessive movements at the subtalar joint/lower leg and thus theoretically decrease muscular activity of the deep posterior compartment, which is highly active in controlling pronation during running.[54] Cardiovascular fitness can be maintained and improved with stationary cycling and running in the deep end of a pool with a flotation device (see Figures 25-16 and 25-26). When ROM, strength, and walking gait have normalized, a walking/jogging progression can be initiated.

Criteria for Returning to Full Activity

The patient may return to full activity when: (a) there is normalized ROM and strength of the involved lower leg; (b) there are no gait deviations with walking, jogging, and running; and (c) the patient has completed a progressive jogging/running program with no complaints of CCS symptoms. It should be noted that patients undergoing anterior compartment fasciotomy may not return to full activity for 8 to 12 weeks after surgery, and patients undergoing deep posterior compartment fasciotomy may not return until 3 to 4 months postsurgery.[40,61]

Muscle Strains

Pathomechanics

The majority of muscle strains in the lower leg occur in the medial head of the gastrocnemius at the musculotendinous junction.[28] The injury is more common in middle-aged patients and occurs in activities requiring ballistic movement, such as tennis and basketball. The patient may feel or hear a pop as if being kicked in the back of the leg. Depending on the severity of the strain, the athlete may be unable to walk secondary to decreased ankle dorsiflexion in a closed kinetic chain, which passively stretches the injured muscle and causes pain during the push-off phase of gait. Palpation will elicit tenderness at the site of the strain, and a palpable divot may be present, depending on the severity of the injury and how soon it is evaluated.

Injury Mechanism

Strains of the medial head of the gastrocnemius usually occur during sudden ballistic movements. A common scenario is the patient lunging with the knee extended and the ankle dorsiflexed. The ankle plantar flexes, in this case the medial head of the gastrocnemius, are activated to assist in push-off of the foot. The muscle is placed in an elongated position and activated in a very short period of time. This places the musculotendinous junction of the gastrocnemius under excessive tensile stress. The muscle–tendon junction, a transition area of one homogeneous tissue to another, is not able to endure the tensile loads nearly as well as the homogeneous tissue itself, and tearing of the tissue at the junction occurs.

Rehabilitation Concerns

The initial management of a gastrocnemius strain is ice, compression, and elevation. It is important for the patient to pay special attention to compression and elevation of the lower extremity to avoid edema in the foot and ankle that can further limit ROM and prolong the rehabilitation process. Gentle stretching of the muscle–tendon unit should be initiated early in the rehabilitation process (see Figure 25-18). Ankle plantar flexor strengthening with rubber tubing can also be initiated when tolerated (see Figure 25-5). Weight bearing may be limited to an as-tolerated status with crutches. The foot/ankle will prefer a plantar flexed position, and closed-kinetic-chain dorsiflexion of the foot and ankle, which is required during walking, will stress the muscle and cause pain. Pulsed ultrasound can be utilized early in the rehabilitation process and eventually progressed to continuous ultrasound for its thermal effects. A stationary cycle can be used for an active warm-up as well as cardiovascular fitness. A heel lift may be placed in each shoe to gradually increase dorsiflexion of the foot and ankle as the patient is progressed off crutches. Standing, stretching, and strengthening can be added as soft-tissue healing occurs and ROM and strength improve. Eventually the patient can be progressed to a walking/jogging program and sport-specific activity. It is important that the patient warm up and stretch properly before activity, to prevent reinjury.

Rehabilitation Progression

Early management of a medial head gastrocnemius strain focuses on reduction of pain and swelling with ice, compression, and elevationand modified weight bearing. The patient is encouraged to perform gentle towel stretching for the affected muscle group several times per day (see Figure 25-18). AROM of the foot and ankle in all planes will also facilitate movement and act to stretch the muscle (see Figures 25-1 to 25-4). With mild muscle strains, the patient may be off crutches and performing standing calf stretches and strengthening exercises by about 7 to 10 days with a normal gait pattern (see Figures 25-12, 25-13, and 25-19). Moderate to severe strains may take 2 to 4 weeks before normalization of ROM and gait occur. This is usually because of the excessive edema in the foot and ankle. Strengthening can be progressed from open- to closed-chain activity as soft-tissue healing occurs (see Figures 25-14, 25-15, and 25-22 to 25-25). As walking gait is normalized, the patient is encouraged to begin a graduated jogging program in which distance and speed are modulated throughout the progression. Most soft-tissue injuries demonstrate good healing by 14 to 21 days postinjury. In the case of mild muscle strain, as the patient becomes more comfortable with jogging and running, plyometric activities can be added to the rehabilitation process. Plyometric activities should be introduced in a controlled fashion with at least 1 to 2 days of rest between activities to allow for muscle soreness to diminish. As the patient adapts to the plyometric exercises, sport-specific training should be added. Care should be taken to save sudden, ballistic activities for when the patient is warmed up and the gastrocnemius is well stretched.

Criteria for Full Return

The patient may return to full activity when the following criteria have been met: (a) full ROM of the foot and ankle; (b) gastrocnemius strength and endurance are equal to the uninvolved side; (c) ability to walk, jog, run, and hop on the involved extremity without any compensation; and (d) successful completion of a sport-specific functional progression with no residual calf symptoms.

Medial Tibial Stress Syndrome

Pathomechanics

MTSS is a condition that involves increasing pain about the distal two-thirds of the posterior medial aspect of the tibia.[27,70] The soleus and tibialis posterior have been implicated as muscular forces that can stress the fascia and periosteum of the distal tibia during running activities.[2,26,64] In a cadaveric dissection study, Beck and Osternig implicated the soleus, and not the tibialis posterior, as the major contributor to MTSS.[5] Magnusson et al noted reduced bone mineral density at the site of MTSS, but could not ascertain whether this was the cause or the result.[42] Bhatt reported abnormal histologic appearance of bone and periosteum in longstanding MTSS.[10] Pain is usually diffuse about the distal medial tibia and the surrounding soft tissues and can arise secondary to a combination of training errors, excessive pronation, improper footwear, and poor conditioning level.[16,66] Initially, the area is diffusely tender and might hurt only after an intense workout. As the condition worsens, daily ambulation may be painful and morning pain and stiffness may be present. There is limited evidence in the literature that interventions used in rehabilitation are effective at preventing MTSS.[19,88] Rehabilitation of this condition must be comprehensive for each individual and address several factors, including musculoskeletal, training, and conditioning, as well as proper footwear and orthotics intervention.

Injury Mechanism

Many sources have linked excessive compensatory pronation as a primary cause of MTSS.[16,26,64,70,80] Bennett et al reported that a pronatory foot type was related to MTSS. The authors noted that the combination of a patient's gender and navicular drop test measures provided an accurate prediction for the development of MTSS in high school runners.[9] Subtalar joint pronation serves to dissipate ground reaction forces upon foot strike in order to reduce the impact to proximal structures. If pronation is excessive, or occurs too quickly, or at the wrong time in the stance phase of gait, greater tensile loads will be placed on the muscle–tendon units that assist in controlling this complex triplanar movement.[31,78] Lower-extremity structural variations, such as a rearfoot and forefoot varus, can cause the subtalar joint to pronate excessively in order to get the medial aspect of the forefoot in contact with the ground for push-off.[70] The magnitude of these forces will increase during running, especially with a rearfoot striker. Sprinters may present with similar symptoms but with a different cause, that being overuse of the plantarflexors secondary to being on their toes during their event. Training surfaces including embankments and crowned roads can place increased tensile loads on the distal medial tibia, and modifications should be made whenever possible.

Rehabilitation Concerns

Management of this condition should include physician referral to rule out the possibility of stress fracture via the use of bone scan and plain films. Activity modification along with measures to maintain cardiovascular fitness should be set in place immediately.

Correction of abnormal pronation during walking and running can be addressed with antipronation taping and temporary orthotics to determine their effectiveness. Vicenzino et al reported that these measures were helpful in controlling excessive pronation.[83] If the above measures are helpful, a custom foot orthotic can be fabricated. Masse' Genova and Gross noted that foot orthotics significantly reduced maximum calcaneal eversion and calcaneal eversion at heel rise with abnormal pronators during treadmill walking.[44] Proper footwear, especially running shoes with motion-control features, can also be very helpful in dealing with MTSS. Although the above-mentioned measures provide passive support to address abnormal pronation, exercise sandals may provide a dynamic approach to managing excessive pronation issues. Michell et al noted a trend in reduced rearfoot eversion angles in 2-dimensional rearfoot kinematics during barefoot treadmill walking with abnormal pronators in subjects who trained in the exercise sandals for 8 weeks.[47] The subjects also demonstrated improved balance in a single-leg stance and subjectively noted improved foot function.[47] These improvements might be a result of increased muscle activity of the foot intrinsics via the short-foot concept and increased activity of the lower-leg musculature that may assist in controlling pronation. Also, the exercise sandals appear to place the foot in a more supinated position, which may enhance the cuboid pulley mechanism and its effects on the function of the first ray during the push-off phase of gait.[35] Ice massage to the affected area may help reduce localized pain and inflammation. A flexibility program for the gastrocnemius–soleus musculature should be initiated.

Rehabilitation Progression

Running and jumping activities may need to be completely eliminated for the first 7 to 10 days after diagnosis. Pool workouts with a flotation device will help maintain cardiovascular fitness during the healing process. Gastrocnemius–soleus flexibility is improved with static stretching (see Figure 25-19). Ice and electrical stimulation can be used to reduce inflammation and modulate pain in the early stages. As the condition improves, general strengthening of the ankle musculature with rubber tubing can be performed along with calf muscle strengthening (see Figures 25-5 to 25-8, 25-12, and 25-13). These exercises may cause muscle fatigue but should not increase the patient's symptoms. The exercise sandal progression can be introduced to enhance dynamic pronation control at the foot and ankle (see Table 25-1; Figures 25-29 to 25-34, and 25-36). An isokinetic strengthening program of the ankle inverters and everters can be utilized to improve strength and has been shown to reduce pronation during treadmill running (see Figure 25-24).[25] As mentioned previously, it is imperative that all structural deviations that cause pronation be addressed with a foot orthotic or at least proper motion-control shoes. As pain to palpation of the distal tibia resolves, the patient should be progressed to a jogging/running program on grass with proper footwear. This may involve beginning with a 10- to 15-minute run and progressing by 10% every week. In the case of track athletes, a pool or bike workout can be implemented for 20 to 30 minutes after the run to produce a more demanding workout. The patient needs to be compliant with a gradual progression and should be educated to avoid doing too much, too soon, which could lead to a recurrence of the condition or possibly a stress fracture.

Criteria for Returning to Full Activity

The patient may return to full activity when: (a) there is minimal to no pain to palpation of the affected area; (b) all causes of excessive pronation have been addressed with an orthotic and proper footwear; (c) there is sufficient gastrocnemius–soleus musculature flexibility; and (d) the patient has successfully completed a gradual running progression and a sport-specific functional progression without an increase in symptoms.

Achilles Tendinitis

Pathomechanics

Achilles tendinitis is an inflammatory condition that involves the Achilles tendon and/or its tendon sheath, the paratenon. Often there is excessive tensile stress placed on the tendon repetitively, as with running or jumping activities, that overloads the tendon, especially on its medial aspect.[49,63] This condition can be divided into Achilles paratenonitis or peritendinitis, which is an inflammation of the paratenon or tissue that surrounds the tendon, and tendinosis, in which areas of the tendon consist of mucinoid or fatty degeneration with disorganized collagen.[63] The patient often complains of generalized pain and stiffness about the Achilles tendon region that when localized is usually 2- to 6-cm proximal to the calcaneal insertion. Uphill running or hill workouts and interval training will usually aggravate the condition. There may be reduced gastrocnemius and soleus muscle flexibility in general that may worsen as the condition progresses and adaptive shortening occurs. Muscle testing of the above muscles may be within normal limits, but painful, and a true deficit may be observed when performing toe raises to fatigue as compared to the uninvolved extremity.

Injury Mechanism

Achilles tendinitis will often present with a gradual onset over a period of time. Initially the patient might ignore the symptoms, which might present at the beginning of activity and resolve as the activity progresses. Symptoms may progress to morning stiffness and discomfort with walking after periods of prolonged sitting. Repetitive weightbearing activities, such as running, or early season conditioning in which the duration and intensity are increased too quickly with insufficient recovery time, will worsen the condition. Excessive compensatory pronation of the subtalar joint with concomitant internal rotation of the lower leg secondary to a forefoot varus, tibial varum, or femoral anteversion will increase the tensile load about the medial aspect of the Achilles tendon.[32,63] Decreased gastrocnemius–soleus complex flexibility can also increase subtalar joint pronation to compensate for the decreased closed-kinetic-chain dorsiflexion needed during early and midstance phase of running. If the patient continues to train, the tendon will become further inflamed and the gastrocnemius–soleus musculature will become less efficient secondary to pain inhibition. The tendon may be warm and painful to palpation, as well as thickened, which may indicate the chronicity of the condition. Crepitans may be palpated with AROM plantar and dorsiflexion and pain will be elicited with passive dorsiflexion.

Rehabilitation Concerns

Achilles tendinitis can be resistant to a quick resolution secondary to the slower healing response of tendinous tissue. It has also been noted that an area of hypovascularity exists within the tendon that may further impede the healing response. It is important to create a proper healing environment by reducing the offending activity and replacing it with an activity that will reduce strain on the tendon. Studies have shown that the Achilles tendon force during running approaches 6 to 8 times body weight.[63] Addressing structural faults that may lead to excessive pronation or supination should be done through proper footwear and foot orthotics, as well as flexibility exercises for the gastrocnemius–soleus complex. Soft-tissue manipulation of the gastrocnemius–soleus with a foam roller can be helpful prior to stretching. Modalities such as ice can help reduce pain and inflammation early on, and ultrasound can facilitate an increased blood flow to the tendon in the later stages of rehabilitation. Cross-friction massage may be used to break down adhesions that may have formed during the healing response and further improve the gliding ability of the paratenon. Strengthening of the gastrocnemius–soleus musculature must be progressed carefully so as not to cause a recurrence of the symptoms. Lastly a gradual progression must be made for a safe return to activity to avoid having the condition becoming chronic.

Rehabilitation Progression

Activity modification is necessary to allow the Achilles tendon to begin the healing process. Swimming, pool running with a flotation device, stationary cycling, and use of an upper-body ergometer are all possible alternative activities for cardiovascular maintenance (see Figures 25-16, 25-26, and 25-27). It is important to reduce stresses on the Achilles tendon that may occur with daily ambulation. Proper footwear with a slight heel lift, such as a good running shoe, can reduce stress on the tendon during gait. Structural biomechanical abnormalities that manifest with excessive pronation or supination should be addressed with a custom foot orthotic. Placing a heel lift in the shoe or building it into the orthotic can reduce stress on the Achilles tendon initially, but should be gradually reduced so as not to cause an adaptive shortening of the muscle-tendon unit. Gentle pain-free stretching can be performed several times per day and can be done after an active or passive warm-up with exercise or modalities such as superficial heat or ultrasound (see Figures 25-18 and 25-19). Open-kinetic-chain strengthening with rubber tubing can begin early in the rehabilitation process and should be progressed to closed-kinetic-chain strengthening in a concentric and eccentric fashion utilizing the patient's body weight with modification of sets, repetitions, and speed of exercise to intensify the rehabilitation session (see Figures 25-5, 25-12, and 25-13). Recent studies report excellent results with the use of eccentric training of the gastrocnemius–soleus musculature with chronic Achilles tendinosis over a 12-week period.[1,52,59] The patient should be progressed to a regimen of isolated eccentric loading of the Achilles tendon using body weight (Figure 25-35). A walking–jogging progression on a firm but forgiving surface can be initiated when the symptoms have resolved and ROM, strength, endurance, and flexibility have been normalized to the uninvolved extremity. The patient must be reminded that this progression is designed to improve the affected tendon's ability to tolerate stress in a controlled fashion and not to improve fitness level. Studies show that cardiovascular fitness can be maintained with biking and swimming.[23] Finally, it is important to educate the patient on the nature of the condition in order to set realistic expectations for a safe return without recurrence of the condition.

REHABILITATION PLAN

ACHILLES TENDINITIS

INJURY SITUATION A 17-year-old male lacrosse player presents with pain in his right Achilles. He notes that the pain has been present for the past week, secondary to an increase in preseason conditioning that has included long runs on asphalt, hill running, and interval training on the track. He currently has morning stiffness and pain with walking, especially up hills and going down stairs. The patient is concerned that the pain will affect his conditioning for the lacrosse season, which will start in 3 weeks.

SIGNS AND SYMPTOMS The patient stands in moderate subtalar joint pronation with mild tibial varum. His single-leg stance balance is poor, with an increase in subtalar joint pronation and internal rotation of the entire lower extremity. Observation of the tendon reveals slight thickening. Palpation reveals mild crepitus with pain 4 cm proximal to the calcaneal insertion on the medial side of the tendon. ROM testing reveals tightness in both the gastrocnemius and soleus musculature versus the uninvolved side. A 6-inch lateral step-down demonstrates restricted closed-kinetic-chain ankle dorsiflexion that is painful, with compensation at the hip to get the opposite heel to touch the ground. The patient is able to perform 10 heel raises on the right with pain and 20 on the left without pain. Walking gait reveals increased pronation during the entire stance phase of gait. A 12-degree forefoot varus is noted on the right with the athlete in a prone subtalar joint neutral position.

MANAGEMENT PLAN The goal is to decrease pain, address the issues of abnormal pronation, and provide a protected environment for the tendon to heal. Eventually address ROM and strength deficits that are preventing the athlete from functioning at his expected level.

PHASE ONE Acute Inflammatory Stage

GOALS: Modulate pain, address abnormal pronation, and begin appropriate therapeutic exercise.

Estimated Length of Time (ELT): Day 1 to Day 4

Use ice and electrical stimulation to decrease pain. Nonsteroidal antiinflammatory drugs could help reduce inflammation. A foot orthotic could be fabricated to address the excessive pronation, which may be placing increased tensile stress on the medial aspect of the Achilles tendon. A heel lift could be built into the foot orthotic. It might be recommended that the patient wear a motion-control running shoe to address pronation and provide a heel lift. The patient could begin gentle, pain-free towel stretching for the gastrocnemius and soleus musculature several times per day. Conditioning could be done in a pool or on a bike.

PHASE TWO Fibroblastic Repair Stage

GOALS: Increase gastrocnemius–soleus flexibility, gain strength, and improve single-leg stance (SLS) balance and single-leg stance closed-kinetic-chain functional activity.

Criteria for Full Return

The patient may return to full activity when: (a) there has been full resolution of symptoms with ADL and minimal or no symptoms with sport-related activity; (b) ROM, strength, flexibility, and endurance are equal to the opposite uninvolved extremity; and (c) all contributing biomechanical faults have been corrected during walking and running gait analysis with proper footwear and/or custom foot orthotics.

Achilles Tendon Rupture

Pathomechanics

The Achilles tendon is the largest tendon in the human body. It serves to transmit force from the gastrocnemius and soleus musculature to the calcaneus. Tension through the Achilles tendon at the end of stance phase is estimated at 250% of body weight.[63] Rupture of the Achilles tendon usually occurs in an area 2 to 6 cm proximal to the calcaneal insertion, which has been implicated as an avascular site prone to degenerative changes.[17,34,39] The injury presents after a sudden plantarflexion of the ankle, as in jumping or accelerating with a sprint. The patient will often feel or hear a pop and note a sensation of being kicked in the back of the leg. Plantarflexion of the ankle will be painful and limited but still possible with the

Estimated Length of Time (ELT): Days 5 to 14

As signs of inflammation decrease, the use of ultrasound could be introduced, first at a pulsed level and then at a continuous level. Stretching could be progressed to standing on a flat surface. Strengthening could be started with isometrics and progressed to open-kinetic-chain isotonics with rubber tubing. As the patient improves, standing double-leg heel raises can be introduced. Single-leg stance activity could be added, focusing on control of the lower extremity, especially foot pronation and lower-leg internal rotation. Conditioning at the end of this stage could be upgraded to weightbearing activity, such as the elliptical trainer with the foot flat on the pedal, avoiding ankle plantarflexion.

PHASE THREE Maturation Remodeling Stage

GOALS: Complete elimination of pain and full return to activity.

Estimated Length of Time (ELT): Week 3 to Full Return

As ROM and strength improve, the athlete could be progressed to gastrocnemius–soleus stretching on a slant board and single-leg heel raises, with an increased focus on eccentric loading of the involved side. Dynamic muscle loading via double-leg hopping on a yielding surface such as jumping rope for short periods of time could be added. A running program on a flat, yielding surface such as grass or track could be initiated with good running shoes and the foot orthotic in place. The program should be sport-specific and initially should be done every other day to allow the tendon to recover. A sport-specific functional program could also begin when straight running and sprinting are tolerated by the patient. Other forms of conditioning could also be continued to maintain fitness levels. Achilles taping may be of benefit when the athlete returns to training on a daily basis to reduce excess load to the tendon over the next several weeks.

Criteria for Returning to Competitive Lacrosse

1. No pain with walking, ADL, and running.
2. Gastrocnemius–soleus flexibility and strength are equal to the uninvolved extremity.
3. Improved single-leg stance balance, closed-kinetic-chain function (step-down, squat, lunge).

DISCUSSION QUESTIONS

1. Why would an orthotic be helpful in this case?
2. Why would closed-kinetic-chain activities such as a single-leg stance and reach and a step-down be painful and limited with this condition?
3. Explain what training errors may have caused this condition to arise with this patient.
4. Explain what intrinsic factors may have contributed to this condition occurring with this patient.
5. Explain why an Achilles tendon taping would benefit this patient during his sporting activity.

assistance of the tibialis posterior and the peroneals. A palpable defect will be noted along the length of the tendon, and the Thompson test will be positive. The patient will require the use of crutches to continue ambulation without an obvious limp.

Injury Mechanism

Achilles tendon rupture is usually caused by a sudden forceful plantarflexion of the ankle. It has been theorized that the area of rupture has undergone degenerative changes and is more prone to rupture when placed under higher levels of tensile loading.[34,49,62,63] The degenerative changes may be a result of excessive compensatory pronation at the subtalar joint to accommodate for structural deviations of the forefoot, rearfoot, and lower leg during walking and running. This pronation can place an increased tensile stress on the medial aspect of the Achilles tendon. Also, a chronically inflexible gastrocnemius–soleus complex will reduce the available amount of dorsiflexion at the ankle joint, and excessive subtalar joint pronation will assist in accommodating this loss. The above mechanisms may result in tendinitis symptoms that precede the tendon rupture, but this is not always the case. Fatigue of the deconditioned patient or weekend warrior may also contribute to tendon rupture, as well as improper warm-up prior to ballistic activities such as basketball or racquet sports.[33]

Rehabilitation Concerns

After an Achilles tendon rupture, the question of surgical repair versus cast immobilization will arise. Cetti et al report that surgical repair of the tendon is recommended to allow the patient to return to previous levels of activity.[17] Surgical repair of the Achilles tendon may require a period of immobilization for 6 to 8 weeks to allow for proper tendon healing.[15,34,43] The deleterious effects of this lengthy immobilization include muscle atrophy, joint stiffness including intra-articular adhesions and capsular stiffness of the involved joints, disorganization of the ligament substance, and possible disuse osteoporosis of the bone.[15] Isokinetic strength deficits for the ankle plantarflexors, especially at lower speeds, have been documented with periods of cast immobilization for 6 weeks.[41] Steele et al noted significant deficits isokinetically of ankle plantarflexor strength after 8 weeks of immobilization.[68] Some feel that the primary limiting factor that influences functional outcome might be the duration of postsurgical immobilization.[72] Several studies have been done using early controlled ankle motion and progressive weight bearing without immobilization.[3,15,34,43,63,69,71,81] It is important not only to regain full ROM without harming the repair, but also to regain normal muscle function through controlled progressive strengthening. This can be performed through a variety of exercises, including isometrics, isotonics, and isokinetics (see Figures 25-1 to 25-13). Open- and closed-kinetic-chain activities can be incorporated into the progression to gradually increase weightbearing stress on the tendon repair, as well as to improve proprioception (see Figures 25-11, 25-14, 25-15, and 25-22 to 25-25). Cardiovascular endurance can be maintained with stationary biking and pool running with a flotation device. Gait normalization for walking and running can be performed using a treadmill.

Rehabilitation Progression

It is important for the therapist to have an open line of communication with the physician in charge of the surgical repair. Decisions about length and type of immobilization, weightbearing progression, allowable ROM, and progressive strengthening should be thoroughly discussed with the physician. Excellent results have been reported with early and controlled mobilization with the use of a splint that allows early plantarflexion ROM and that slowly increases ankle dorsiflexion to neutral and full dorsiflexion over a 6- to 8-week period of time.[15,34] More recent studies have noted excellent functional results with early weight bearing and ROM. Aoki et al reported a full return to sports activity in 13.1 weeks.[3] Controlled progressive weight bearing based on percentages of the patient's body weight can be done over 6 to 8 weeks postoperatively, with full weight bearing by the end of this time frame. During the early stages of rehabilitation, ice, compression, and elevation are used to decrease swelling. A variety of ROM exercises are done to increase ankle ROM in all planes as well as initiate activation of the surrounding muscles (see Figures 25-1 to 25-4, 25-9, 25-10, 25-14, 25-15, 25-18, and 25-20). By 4 to 6 weeks postoperatively, strengthening exercises with rubber tubing can be progressed to closed-chain exercises utilizing a percentage of the patient's body weight with heel raises on a Total Gym apparatus (see Figures 25-5, 25-8, and 25-11). It is important to do more concentric than eccentric loading initially, so as not to place excessive stress on the repair. Gradual increases in eccentric loading can occur from 10 to 12 weeks postoperatively. Also at this time, isokinetic exercise can be introduced with submaximal high-speed exercise and be progressed to lower concentric speeds gradually over time (see Figures 24-24 and 24-25). By 3 months, full-weightbearing heel raises can be performed (see Figures 25-12 and 25-13). At the same time a walking/jogging program can be initiated. Isokinetic strength testing can be done between 3 and 4 months to determine if any deficits in ankle plantarflexor strength exist. The number of single-leg heel raises performed in a specified amount of time as compared to the uninvolved extremity can also be utilized to determine functional plantar flexor strength and endurance. Sport-related functional activities can be initiated at 3 months along with a progressive jogging program. A full return to unrestricted athletic activity can begin after 6 months, once the patient successfully meets all predetermined goals.

Criteria for Full Return

The patient can return to full activity after the following criteria have been met: (a) full AROM of the involved ankle as compared to the uninvolved side; (b) isokinetic strength of the ankle plantarflexors at 90% to 95% of the uninvolved side; (3) 90% to 95% of the number of heel raises throughout the full ROM in a 30-second period as compared to the uninvolved side; and (4) the ability to walk, jog, and run without an observable limp and successful completion of a sport-related functional progression without any Achilles tendon irritation.

Retrocalcaneal Bursitis

Pathomechanics

The retrocalcaneal bursae is a disc-shaped object that lies between the Achilles tendon and the superior tuberosity of the calcaneus.[12,63] The patient will report a gradual onset of pain that may be associated with Achilles tendinitis. Careful palpation anterior to the Achilles tendon will rule out involvement of the tendon. Pain is increased with AROM/passive ROM ankle dorsiflexion and relieved with plantarflexion. Depending on the severity and swelling associated, it may be painful to walk, especially when attempting to attain full closed-kinetic-chain ankle dorsiflexion during the midstance phase of gait.

Injury Mechanism

Loading the foot and ankle in repeated dorsiflexion, as in uphill running, can be a cause of this condition. When the foot is dorsiflexed, the distance between the posterior/superior calcaneus and the Achilles tendon will be reduced, resulting in a repeated mechanical compression of the retrocalcaneal bursae. Also, structural abnormalities of the foot may lead to excessive compensatory movements at the subtalar joint, which may cause friction of the Achilles tendon on the bursae with running.

Rehabilitation Concerns

Because of the close proximity of other structures, it is important to rule out involvement of the calcaneus and Achilles tendon with careful palpation of the area. Rest and activity modification in order to reduce swelling and inflammation is necessary. If walking is painful, crutches with weight bearing as tolerated is recommended for a brief period. Gentle but progressive stretching and strengthening should be added as tolerated, with care being taken not to increase pain with gastrocnemius–soleus stretching (see Figures 25-5, 25-12, 25-13, 25-18, and 25-19). If excessive compensatory pronation is noted during gait analysis, recommendations on proper footwear should be made, especially in regard to the heel counter, and foot orthotics should be considered.

Rehabilitation Progression

The early management of this condition requires all measures to reduce pain and inflammation, including ice, rest from offending activity, proper footwear, and modified weight bearing with crutches if necessary. Cardiovascular fitness can be maintained with pool running with a flotation device. Gentle stretching of the gastrocnemius–soleus needs to be introduced slowly because this will tend to increase compression of the retrocalcaneal bursae. As pain resolves and ROM and walking gait are normalized, the patient may begin a progressive walking/jogging program. The patient can progress back to activity as the condition allows. Heel lifts in both shoes may be necessary in the early return to activity, with gradual weaning away from them as AROM/passive ROM dorsiflexion improves. The condition may allow full return in 10 days to 2 weeks if treated early enough. If the condition persists, 6 to 8 weeks of rest, activity modification, and treatment may be needed before a successful result is attained with conservative care.

Criteria for Return to Full Activity

The following criteria need to met before return to full activity: (a) no observable swelling and minimal to no pain with palpation of the area at rest or after daily activity; (b) full ankle dorsiflexion AROM and normal pain-free strength of the gastrocnemius and soleus musculature; and (c) normal and pain-free walking and running gait.

SUMMARY

1. Although some injuries in the region of the lower leg are acute, most injuries seen in an athletic population result from overuse, most often from running.
2. Tibial fractures can create long-term problems for the patient if inappropriately managed. Fibular fractures generally require much shorter periods for immobilization. Treatment of these fractures involves immediate medical referral and most likely a period of immobilization and restricted weight bearing.
3. Stress fractures in the lower leg are usually the result of the bone's inability to adapt to the repetitive loading response during training and conditioning of the patient and are more likely to occur in the tibia.
4. CSSs can occur from acute trauma or repetitive trauma of overuse. They can occur in any of the 4 compartments, but are most likely in the anterior compartment or deep posterior compartment.
5. Rehabilitation of MTSS must be comprehensive and address several factors, including musculoskeletal, training, and conditioning, as well as proper footwear and orthotics intervention.
6. Achilles tendinitis often presents with a gradual onset over a period of time and may be resistant to a quick resolution secondary to the slower healing response of tendinous tissue.
7. Perhaps the greatest question after an Achilles tendon rupture is whether surgical repair or cast immobilization is the best method of treatment. Regardless of treatment method, the time required for rehabilitation is significant.
8. With retrocalcaneal bursitis the athlete will report a gradual onset of pain that may be associated with Achilles tendinitis. Treatment should include rest and activity modification in order to reduce swelling and inflammation.

REFERENCES

1. Alfredson H, Pietila T, Jonsson P, et al. Heavy-load eccentric calf muscle training of the treatment of Achilles tendinosis. *Am J Sports Med.* 1998;26(3): 360-366.
2. Andrish J, Work J. How I manage shin splints. *Phys Sportsmed.* 1990;18(12):113-114.
3. Aoki M, Ogiwara N, Ohta T, et al. Early active motion and weightbearing after cross stitch Achilles tendon repair. *Am J Sports Med.* 1998;26(6):794-800.
4. Batt M, Kemp S, Kerslake K. Delayed union stress fracture of the tibia: conservative management. *Br J Sports Med.* 2001;35:74-77.

5. Beck B, Osternig L. Medial tibial stress syndrome. *J Bone Joint Surg Am.* 1994;76(7):1057-1061.
6. Beckham S, Grana W, Buckley P, et al. A comparison of anterior compartment pressures in competitive runners and cyclists. *Am J Sports Med.* 1993;21(1):36-40.
7. Bennell K, Malcolm S, Thomas S, et al. The incidence and distribution of stress fractures in competitive track and field athletes: a twelve-month prospective study. *Am J Sports Med.* 1996;24(2):211-217.
8. Bennell K, Malcolm S, Thomas S, et al. Risk factors for stress fractures in track and field athletes: a twelve-month prospective study. *Am J Sports Med.* 1996;24(6):810-817.
9. Bennett J, Reinking M, Pleumer B, et al. Factors contributing to the development of medial tibial stress syndrome in high school runners. *J Orthop Sports Phys Ther.* 2001;31(9):504-511.
10. Bhatt R, Lauder I, Allen M, et al. Correlation of bone scintigraphy and histological findings in medial tibial stress syndrome. *Br J Sports Med.* 2000;34:49-53.
11. Blackburn T, Hirth C, Guskiewicz K. EMG comparison of lower leg musculature during functional activities with and without balance shoes. *J Athl Train.* 2002;38(3):198-203.
12. Bordelon R. The heel. In: DeLee J, Drez D, eds. *Orthopaedic and Sports Medicine: Principles and Practice.* Philadelphia, PA: WB Saunders; 1994.
13. Bullock-Saxton J. Local sensation changes and altered hip muscle function following severe ankle sprain. *Phys Ther.* 1994;74(1):17-31.
14. Bullock-Saxton J, Janda V, Bullock M. Reflex activation of gluteal muscles in walking. *Spine (Phila Pa 1976).* 1993;21(6):704-708.
15. Carter T, Fowler P, Blokker C. Functional postoperative treatment of Achilles tendon repair. *Am J Sports Med.* 1992;20(4):459-462.
16. Case W. Relieving the pain of shin splints. *Phys Sportsmed.* 1994;22(4):31-32.
17. Cetti R, Christensen S, Ejsted R, et al. Operative versus nonoperative treatment of Achilles tendon rupture: a prospective randomized study and review of the literature. *Am J Sports Med.* 1993;21(6):791-799.
18. Chang P, Harris R. Intramedullary nailing for chronic tibial stress fractures: a review of five cases. *Am J Sports Med.* 1996;24(5):688-692.
19. Craig D. Medial tibial stress syndrome: evidence-based prevention. *J Athl Train.* 2008;43(3):316-318.
20. Dickson T, Kichline P. Functional management of stress fractures in female athletes using a pneumatic leg brace. *Am J Sports Med.* 1987;15(1):86-89.
21. Donatelli R. Normal anatomy and biomechanics. In: Donatelli R, Wolf S, eds. *The Biomechanics of the Foot and Ankle.* Philadelphia, PA: FA Davis; 1990.
22. Ekenman I, Tsai-Fellander L, Westblad P, et al. A study of intrinsic factors in patients with stress fractures of the tibia. *Foot Ankle.* 1996;17(8):477-482.
23. Eyestone E, Fellingham G, George J, Fisher G. Effect of water running and cycling on maximum oxygen consumption and 2-mile run performance. *Am J Sports Med.* 1993;21(1):41-44.
24. Fehlandt A, Micheli L. Acute exertional anterior compartment syndrome in an adolescent female. *Med Sci Sports Exerc.* 1995;27(1):3-7.
25. Feltner M, Macrae H, Macrae P, et al. Strength training effects on rearfoot motion in running. *Med Sci Sports Exerc.* 1994;26(8):102-107.
26. Fick D, Albright J, Murray B. Relieving painful shin splints. *Phys Sportsmed.* 1992;20(12):105-113.
27. Fredericson M, Bergman A, Hoffman K, Dillingham M. Tibial stress reaction in runners: A correlation of clinical symptoms and scintigraphy with a new magnetic resonance imaging grading system. *Am J Sports Med.* 1995;23(4):472-481.
28. Garrick J, Couzens G. Tennis leg: how I manage gastrocnemius strains. *Phys Sportsmed.* 1992;20(5):203-207.
29. Giladi M, Milgrom C, Simkin A, et al. Stress fractures: identifiable risk factors. *Am J Sports Med.* 1991;19(6):647-652.
30. Goldberg B, Pecora C. Stress fractures: a risk of increased training in freshmen. *Phys Sportsmed.* 1994;22(3):68-78.
31. Gross M. Lower quarter screening for skeletal malalignment: suggestions for orthotics and shoeware. *J Orthop Sports Phys Ther.* 1995;21(6):389-405.
32. Gross M. Chronic tendinitis: pathomechanics of injury factors affecting the healing response and treatment. *J Orthop Sports Phys Ther.* 1992;16(6):248-261.
33. Hamel R. Achilles tendon ruptures: making the diagnosis. *Phys Sportsmed.* 1992;20(9):189-200.
34. Heinrichs K, Haney C. Rehabilitation of the surgically repaired Achilles tendon using a dorsal functional orthosis: a preliminary report. *J Sport Rehabil.* 1994;3:292-303.
35. Hirth C. *Rehabilitation Strategies in the Management of Foot and Ankle Dysfunction: Research and Practical Applications.* Paper presented at the National Athletic Trainers Association 52nd Annual Meeting and Clinical Symposium, Los Angeles, CA, 19-23 June 2001.
36. Howard J, Mohtadi N, Wiley J. Evaluation of outcomes in patients following surgical treatment of chronic exertional compartment syndrome in the leg. *Clin J Sport Med.* 2000;10(3):176-184.
37. Janda V, VaVrova M. Sensory motor stimulation [video]. Brisbane, Australia: Body Control Systems; 1990.
38. Kaper B, Carr C, Shirreffs T. Compartment syndrome after arthroscopic surgery of knee: a report of two cases managed nonoperatively. *Am J Sports Med.* 1997;25(1):123-125.
39. Karjalainen P, Aronen H, Pihlajamaki H, et al. Magnetic resonance imaging during healing of surgically repaired Achilles tendon ruptures. *Am J Sports Med.* 1997;25(2):164-171.
40. Kohn H. Shin pain and compartment syndromes in running. In: Guten G, ed. *Running Injuries.* Philadelphia, PA: WB Saunders; 1997.

41. Leppilahti J, Siira P, Vanharanta H, et al. Isokinetic evaluation of calf muscle performance after Achilles rupture repair. *Int J Sports Med.* 1996;17(8):619-623.
42. Magnusson H, Westlin N, Nyqvist F, et al. Abnormally decreased regional bone density in athletes with medial tibial stress syndrome. *Am J Sports Med.* 2001;29(6):712-715.
43. Mandelbaum B, Myerson M, Forster R. Achilles tendon ruptures: a new method of repair, early range of motion, and functional rehabilitation. *Am J Sports Med.* 1995;23(4):392-395.
44. Masse' Genova J, Gross M. Effect of foot orthotics in calcaneal eversion during standing and treadmill walking for subjects with abnormal pronation. *J Orthop Sports Phys Ther.* 2000;30(11):664-675.
45. Matheson G, Clement B, McKenzie C, et al. Stress fractures in athletes: a study of 320 cases. *Am J Sports Med.* 1987;15(1):46-58.
46. Micheli L, Solomon K, Solomon R, et al. Surgical treatment for chronic lower leg compartment syndrome in young female athletes. *Am J Sports Med.* 1999;27:197-201.
47. Michell T, Guskiewicz K, Hirth C, et al. *Effects of Training in Exercise Sandals on 2-D Rearfoot Motion and Postural Sway in Abnormal Pronators* [undergraduate honors thesis]. Chapel Hill: University of North Carolina; 2000.
48. Myers R, Padua D, Prentice W, et al. *Electromyographic Analysis of the Gluteal Musculature During Closed Kinetic Chain Exercises* [masters thesis]. Chapel Hill: University of North Carolina; 2002.
49. Myerson M, McGarvey W. Instructional course lectures, The American Academy of Orthopaedic Surgeons: disorders of the insertion of the Achilles tendon and Achilles tendinitis. *J Bone Joint Surg.* 1998;80:1814-1824.
50. National Academy of Sports Medicine. *Performance Enhancement Specialist Online Manual.* Callabassus, CA: Author; 2002.
51. Pedowitz R, Hargens A, Mubarek S, et al. Modified criteria for the objective diagnosis of chronic compartment syndrome of the leg. *Am J Sports Med.* 1990;18(1):35-40.
52. Petersen W, Welp R, Rosenbaum D. Chronic Achilles tendinopathy: a prospective randomized study comparing the therapeutic effect of eccentric training, the Air Heel Brace and a combination of both. *Am J Sports Med.* 2007;35:1659-1667.
53. Puddu G, Cerullo G, Selvanetti A, DePaulis F. Stress fractures. In: Harries M, Williams C, Stanish W, Micheli L, eds. *Oxford Textbook of Sports Medicine.* New York, NY: Oxford University Press; 1994.
54. Reber L, Perry J, Pink M. Muscular control of the ankle in running. *Am J Sports Med.* 1993;21(6):805-810.
55. Reeder M, Dick B, Atkins J, et al. Stress fractures: current concepts of diagnosis and treatment. *Sports Med.* 1996;22(3):198-212.
56. Rettig A, Shelbourne K, McCarrol J, et al. The natural history and treatment of delayed union stress fractures of the anterior cortex of the tibia. *Am J Sports Med.* 1988;16(3):250-255.
57. Rettig A, McCarroll J, Hahn R. Chronic compartment syndrome: surgical intervention in 12 cases. *Phys Sportsmed.* 1991;19(4):63-70.
58. Romani W. Mechanisms and management of stress fractures in physically active persons. *J Athl Train.* 2002;37(3):306-314.
59. Roos E, Engstrom M, Lagerquist A, et al. Clinical improvement after 6 weeks of eccentric exercise in patients with mid-portion Achilles tendinopathy: a randomized trial with 1 year follow-up. *Scand J Med Sci Sports.* 2004;14:286-295.
60. Sallade J, Koch S. Training errors in long distance runners. *J Athl Train.* 1992;27(1):50-53.
61. Schepsis A, Martini D, Corbett M. Surgical management of exertional compartment syndrome of the lower leg: long-term followup. *Am J Sports Med.* 1993;21(6):811-817.
62. Schepsis A, Wagner C, Leach R. Surgical management of Achilles tendon overuse injuries: a long-term follow-up study. *Am J Sports Med.* 1994;22(5):611-619.
63. Schepsis A, Jones H, Haas H. Achilles tendon disorders in athletes. *Am J Sports Med.* 2002;30(2):287-305.
64. Schon L, Baxter D, Clanton T. Chronic exercise-induced leg pain in active people: more than just shin splints. *Phys Sportsmed.* 1992;20(1):100-114.
65. Shaffer S, Uhl T. Preventing and treating lower extremity stress reactions and fractures in adults. *J Athl Train.* 2006;41(4):466-469.
66. Shwayhat A, Linenger J, Hofher L, et al. Profiles of exercise history and overuse injuries among United States Navy Sea, Air, and Land (SEAL) recruits. *Am J Sports Med.* 1994;22(6):835-840.
67. Simon R. The tibial and fibular shaft. In: Simon R, Koenigshnecht S, eds. *Emergency Orthopedics: The Extremities.* 3rd ed. Norwalk, CT: Appleton-Lange; 1995.
68. Slimmon D, Bennell K, Bruker P, et al. Long-term outcome of fasciotomy with partial fasciectomy for chronic exertional compartment syndrome of the lower leg. *Am J Sports Med.* 2002;30:581-588.
69. Solveborn S, Moberg A. Immediate free ankle motion after surgical repair of acute Achilles tendon ruptures. *Am J Sports Med.* 1994;22(5):607-610.
70. Sommer H, Vallentyne S. Effect of foot posture on the incidence of medial tibial stress syndrome. *Med Sci Sports Exerc.* 1995;27(6):800-804.
71. Speck M, Klaue K. Early full weightbearing and functional treatment after surgical repair of acute Achilles tendon rupture. *Am J Sports Med.* 1998;26:789-793.
72. Steele G, Harter R, Ting A. Comparison of functional ability following percutaneous and open surgical repairs of acutely ruptured tendons. *J Sport Rehabil.* 1993;2:115-127.
73. Strudwick W, Stuart G. Proximal fibular stress fracture in an aerobic dancer: a case report. *Am J Sports Med.* 1992;20(4):481-482.

74. Stuart M, Karaharju T. Acute compartment syndrome: recognizing the progressive signs and symptoms. *Phys Sportsmed.* 1994;22(3):91-95.
75. Styf J, Nakhostine M, Gershuni D. Functional knee braces increase intramuscular pressures in the anterior compartment of the leg. *Am J Sports Med.* 1992;20(1):46-49.
76. Swenson E, DeHaven K, Sebastianelli J, et al. The effect of a pneumatic leg brace on return to play in athletes with tibial stress fractures. *Am J Sports Med.* 1997;25(3):322-338.
77. Taube R, Wadsworth L. Managing tibial stress fractures. *Phys Sportsmed.* 1993;21(4):123-130.
78. Tiberio D. Pathomechanics of structural foot deformities. *Phys Ther.* 1988;68(12):1840-1849.
79. Tiberio D. The effect of excessive subtalar joint pronation on patellofemoral mechanics: a theoretical model. *J Orthop Sports Phys Ther.* 1987;9(4):160-165.
80. Thacker S, Gilchrist J, Stroup D, et al. The prevention of shin splints in sports: a systematic review of literature. *Med Sci Sports Exerc.* 2002;34(1):32-40.
81. Twaddle B, Poon P. Early motion for Achilles tendon ruptures: is surgery important. *Am J Sports Med.* 2007;35:2033-2038.
82. Vincent N. Compartment syndromes. In: Harries M, Williams C, Stanish W, Micheli L, eds. *Oxford Textbook of Sports Medicine.* New York, NY: Oxford University Press; 1994.
83. Vincenzino B, Griffiths S, Griffiths L, et al. Effect of antipronation tape and temporary orthotics on vertical navicular height before and after exercise. *J Orthop Sports Phys Ther.* 2000;30(6):333-339.
84. Wilder R, Brennan D, Schotte D. A standard measure for exercise prescription for aqua running. *Am J Sports Med.* 1993;21(1):45-48.
85. Wiley J, Clement D, Doyle D, et al. A primary care perspective of chronic compartment syndrome of the leg. *Phys Sportsmed.* 1987;15(3):111-120.
86. Willy C, Becker B, Evers H. Unusual development of acute exertional compartment syndrome due to delayed diagnosis: a case report. *Int J Sports Med.* 1996;17(6):458-461.
87. Whitelaw G, Wetzler M, Levy A, et al. A pneumatic leg brace for the treatment of tibial stress fractures. *Clin Orthop.* 1991;270:301-305.
88. Yasuda T, Miyazaki K, Tada K, et al. Stress fracture of the right distal femur following bilateral fractures of the proximal fibulas: a case report. *Am J Sports Med.* 1992;20(6):771-774.

26

Rehabilitation of the Ankle and Foot

Scott Miller, Stuart L. (Skip) Hunter, and William E. Prentice

OBJECTIVES **After completion of this chapter, the physical therapist should be able to do the following:**

- Discuss the biomechanics and functional anatomy of the foot and ankle.
- Discuss the various injuries that occur at the ankle and foot.
- Discuss the various treatment options for rehabilitating the ankle and foot.
- Discuss the various functional exercises and appropriate progressions.
- Discuss the effect of first ray position, forefoot varus, forefoot valgus, and calcaneal varus on the foot and lower extremity.
- Describe a biomechanical examination of the foot.
- Describe techniques for orthosis fabrication.
- Discuss appropriate running footwear options.
- Identify specific pathomechanics and/or pathology associated with the foot and ankle and the appropriate treatment options.

Functional Anatomy and Biomechanics

Talocrural Joint

The ankle or talocrural joint is a hinge joint formed by articular facets on the distal tibia, the medial malleolus, and the lateral malleolus, which articulate with the talus. The talus is the second largest tarsal bone and main weightbearing bone of the articulation linking the lower leg to the foot. The relatively square shape of the talus allows the ankle only 2 movements about the transverse axis: plantarflexion and dorsiflexion. Because the talus is wider on the anterior aspect than posteriorly, the most stable position of the ankle is dorsiflexion as the talus fits tighter between the malleoli. In contrast, as the ankle moves into plantarflexion, the wider portion of the tibia is brought into contact with the narrower posterior aspect of the talus, creating a less-stable position than dorsiflexion.[5]

The lateral malleolus of the fibula extends further distally so that the bony stability of the lateral aspect of the ankle is more stable than the medial. Motion at the talocrural joint ranges from 20 degrees of dorsiflexion to 50 degrees of plantarflexion, depending on the patient. An individual requires 20 degrees of plantarflexion and 10 degrees of dorsiflexion for walking, and up to 25 degrees of plantarflexion for running for normal gait.[2,3]

Talocrural Joint Ligaments

The ligamentous support of the ankle consists of the articular capsule, 3 lateral ligaments, 2 ligaments that connect the tibia and fibula, and the medial or deltoid ligament (Figure 26-1). The 3 lateral ligaments include the anterior talofibular, posterior talofibular, and calcaneofibular ligaments. The anterior and posterior tibiofibular ligaments bridge the tibia and fibula and form the distal portion of the interosseous membrane. The thick deltoid ligament provides primary resistance to foot eversion. A thin articular capsule encases the ankle joint.

Talocrural Joint Muscles

The muscles passing posterior to the lateral malleolus will produce ankle plantarflexion along with toe flexion. Anterior muscles serve to dorsiflex the ankle and to produce toe extension. The anterior muscles include the extensor hallucis longus, the extensor digitorum longus, the peroneus tertius, and the tibialis anterior. The posterior muscle group falls

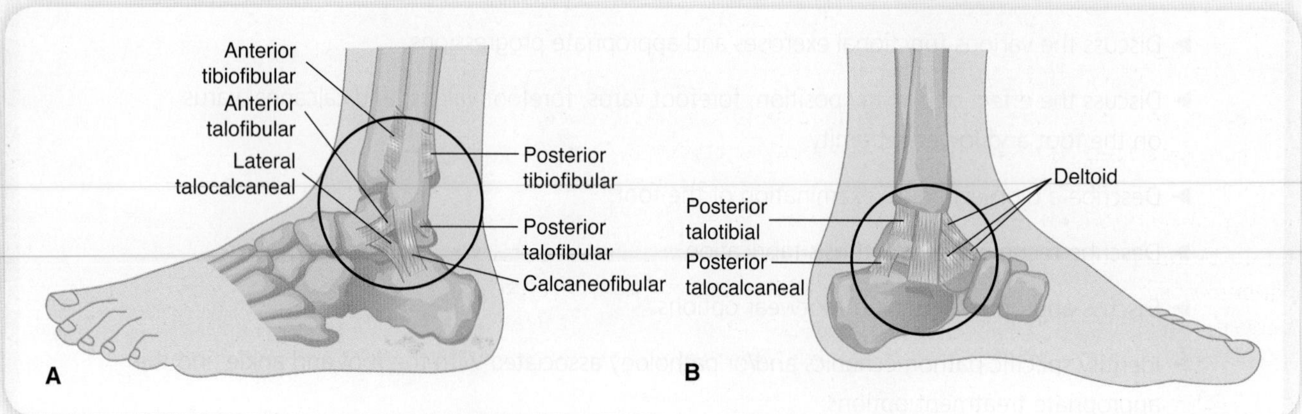

Figure 26-1 Ligaments of the talocrural joint

A. Lateral aspect. **B.** Medial aspect.

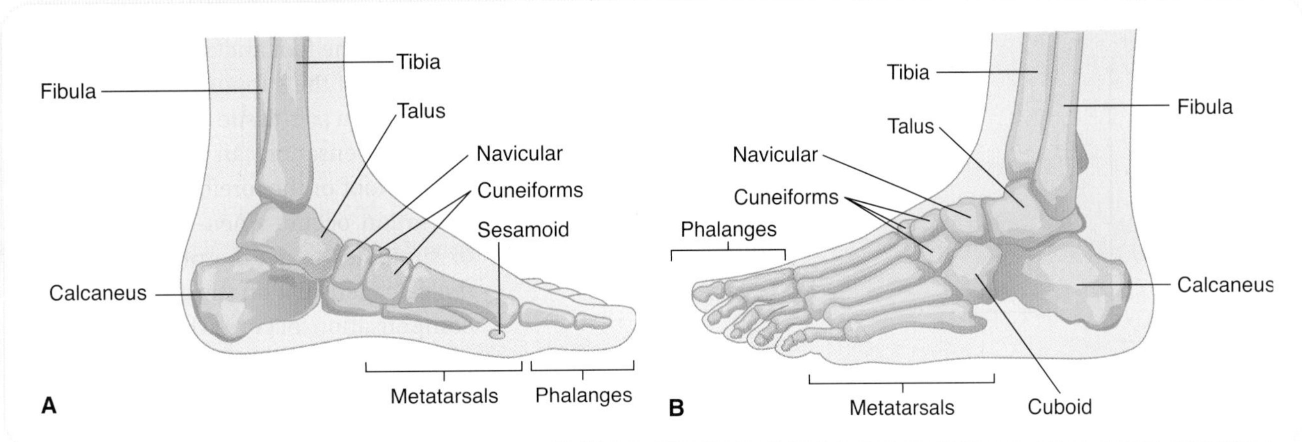

Figure 26-2 **Bones of the foot**

A. Medial aspect. B. Lateral aspect.

into 3 layers: at the superficial layer is the gastrocnemius; the middle layer includes the soleus and the plantaris; and the deep layer contains the tibialis posterior, flexor digitorum longus, and flexor hallucis longus.[5]

Subtalar Joint

The subtalar joint (STJ) consists of the articulation between the talus and the calcaneus (Figure 26-2).[97] Supination and pronation are normal movements that occur at the STJ. These movements are triplanar movements, that is, movements that occur in all 3 planes simultaneously.[28,73,84] In non-weight bearing, pronation is the composite motion of abduction, dorsiflexion, and calcaneal eversion. Supination is the composite motion of adduction, plantarflexion, and calcaneal inversion.[2,28,73,110,118]

In weight bearing, the STJ also acts as a torque convertor to translate the pronation or supination into leg rotation.[2,110,118] STJ pronation creates tibial internal rotation when the knee flexes (unlocks), whereas supination facilitates tibial external rotation when the knee extends. The movements of the talus during pronation and supination have profound effects on the lower extremity, both proximally and distally.

Effects of Rearfoot and Forefoot Alignment and Mobility on STJ Position

The evaluation of rearfoot and forefoot alignment and mobility to determine if there are primary abnormalities of the foot is essential in the treatment of any lower-extremity overuse injury. This assessment is performed in a subtalar joint neutral (STJN) position, most commonly with the patient in a prone position. Once STJN is attained, the evaluator looks for deviations from intrinsic normalcy, which can be described as the bisection of the calcaneus (posteriorly) being parallel with the bisection of the lower third of the lower leg between the tibia and fibula. Next, the posterior bisection of the calcaneus is perpendicular to the line bisecting the second through fifth metatarsal heads. Finally, metatarsal's 2 through 5 should be in the same plane as the first metatarsal.[2,3]

When alignment abnormalities are present in the forefoot or rearfoot, compensation for these alignment faults occur. Compensation can be defined as the movement of one body part in order to neutralize the effects of a movement or alignment of another body part. Normal compensation allows for normal function of the foot and ankle. However,

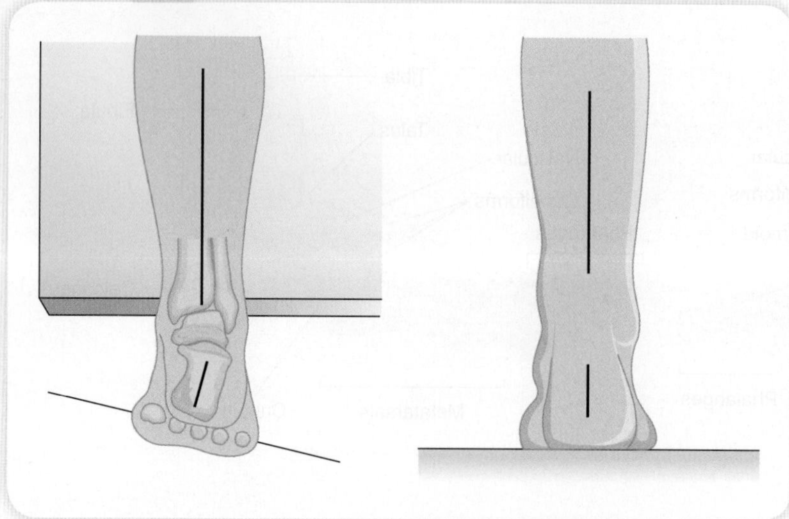

Figure 26-3 Compensated subtalar or calcaneal varus

Comparing non–weightbearing neutral to weightbearing resting position.
(Figure used with permission of Brian Hoke, American Physical Rehabilitation Network.)

excessive compensation occurs when the motion of the foot and ankle surpasses the tolerance of the supportive tissues, which can result in soft-tissue damage.

Compensation can take place at either the rearfoot or the forefoot. Rearfoot compensation occurs when the STJ pronates or supinates to get the plantar surface of the calcaneus flat on the ground. Forefoot compensation occurs when the STJ and midtarsal joint (MTJ) pronate or supinate to get the metatarsal heads flat on the ground. A foot is described as uncompensated when the rearfoot or forefoot does not reach flat contact to the ground, usually because of lack of STJ motion or extreme abnormal alignment in the lower extremity.[2,3]

Compensated subtalar (calcaneal) varus is present when the calcaneus is inverted and the forefoot is in neutral in a non-weightbearing position. In weight bearing, compensation is then noted with increased STJ pronation bringing the plantar surface of the calcaneus flat to the ground (Figure 26-3). Uncompensated subtalar (calcaneal) varus is evident when there is insufficient motion of the STJ to compensate for the deformity and the calcaneus remains inverted (Figure 26-4).[2,3]

Compensated forefoot varus is present when the calcaneus is neutral and the forefoot is in a varus position (first metatarsal more cephalad as compared to the fifth) in a non-weightbearing position. In weight bearing, compensation occurs secondary to increased STJ pronation bringing the forefoot into contact with the ground (Figure 26-5). Typically, this compensation involves excessive forefoot mobility and the STJ remains pronated throughout stance phase. Uncompensated forefoot varus is evident when there is insufficient motion at the STJ, MTJ, or first ray to bring the forefoot into contact with the ground (Figure 26-6).[2,3]

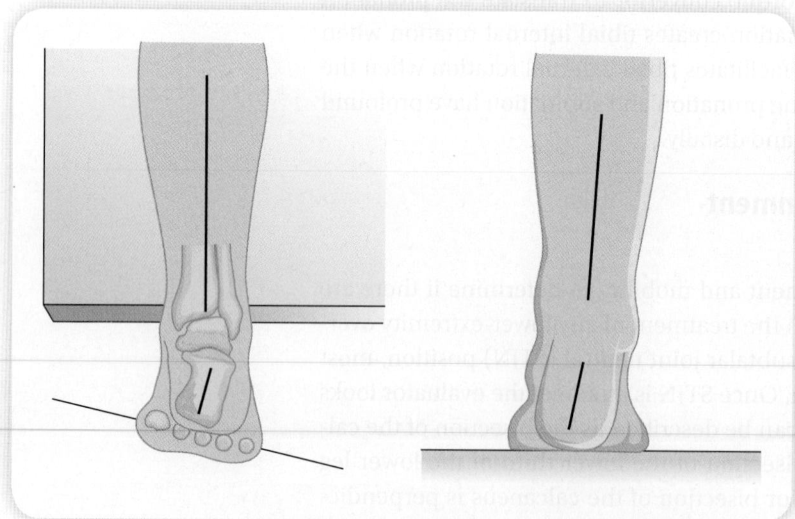

Figure 26-4 Uncompensated subtalar or calcaneal varus

Comparing non–weightbearing neutral to weightbearing resting position.
(Figure used with permission of Brian Hoke, American Physical Rehabilitation Network.)

Compensated forefoot valgus is present when the calcaneus is neutral and the forefoot is in a valgus position (first metatarsal more caudal as compared to the fifth) in a non-weightbearing position. In weight bearing, compensation occurs when the calcaneus moves into an inverted position (Figure 26-7). In this condition, there is often decreased mobility of the first ray and the STJ resupinates before the foot flat phase of stance due to the premature loading of the medial forefoot.[2,3]

It is less typical, but not uncommon to have combinations of subtalar varus with either a forefoot varus or valgus. Mobility of the rearfoot, forefoot, and first ray play a key role in whether compensation is noted or not.

Midtarsal Joint

The MTJ consists of 2 distinct joints with 2 different axes that function simultaneously: the calcaneocuboid joint laterally and the talocalcaneonavicular joint medially.[2,3] The MTJ depends primarily on ligamentous and muscular tension to maintain position and integrity. The midtarsal region comprises 2 joint axes: an oblique and a longitudinal. The axes can undergo independent motion in a non–weightbearing position; however, the movements of the axes in a weightbearing position are controlled by the STJ. This is considered a constrained system and the stability of the MTJ is directly related to the position of the STJ. Furthermore, as the MTJ becomes more or less mobile, it has an overall direct effect on the distal portion of the foot as a result of the articulations at the tarsometatarsal joint.[78]

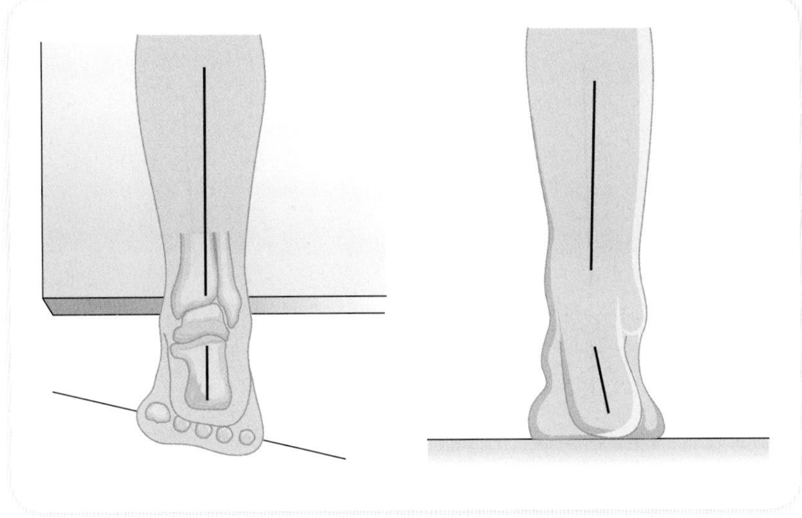

Figure 26-5 Compensated forefoot varus

Comparing non–weightbearing neutral to weightbearing resting position.
(Figure used with permission of Brian Hoke, American Physical Rehabilitation Network.)

Effects of Midtarsal Joint Position During Pronation

During pronation, the talus adducts and plantar flexes and makes the joint articulations of the MTJ more congruous. The planes of the oblique and longitudinal axes of the talocalcaneonavicular and calcaneocuboid joints become more parallel, thus allowing increased mobility so the foot becomes more supple. The resulting foot is in a loose pack position and often referred to as a "loose bag of bones."[28,97] This normal function of the MTJ allows the foot to accommodate both even and uneven surfaces.

As more motion occurs at the MTJ, the lesser tarsal bones, particularly the first metatarsal and first cuneiform, become more mobile. These bones comprise a functional unit known as the first ray. With pronation of the MTJ, the first ray is more mobile because of its articulations with that joint. One of the original descriptions was Morton's paper describing the now classic Morton toe.[79] The first ray is also stabilized by the attachment of the long peroneal tendon, which attaches to the base of the first metatarsal. The long peroneal

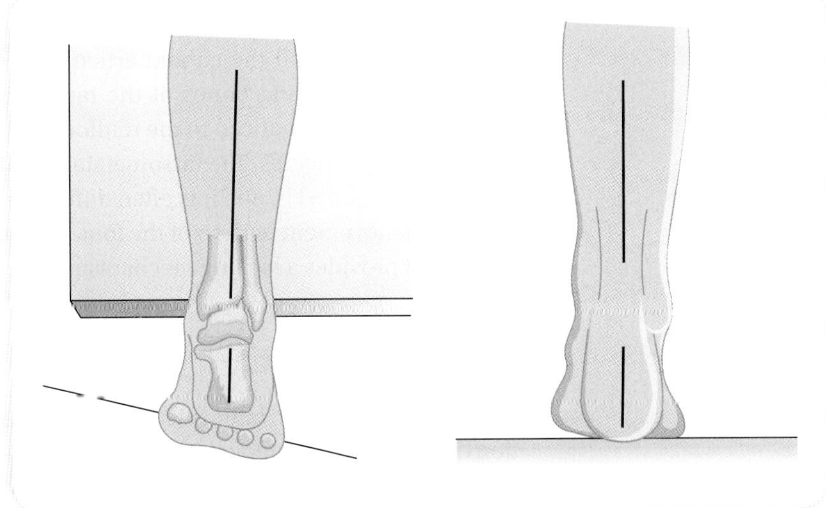

Figure 26-6 Uncompensated forefoot varus

Comparing non–weightbearing neutral to weightbearing resting position.
(Figure used with permission of Brian Hoke, American Physical Rehabilitation Network.)

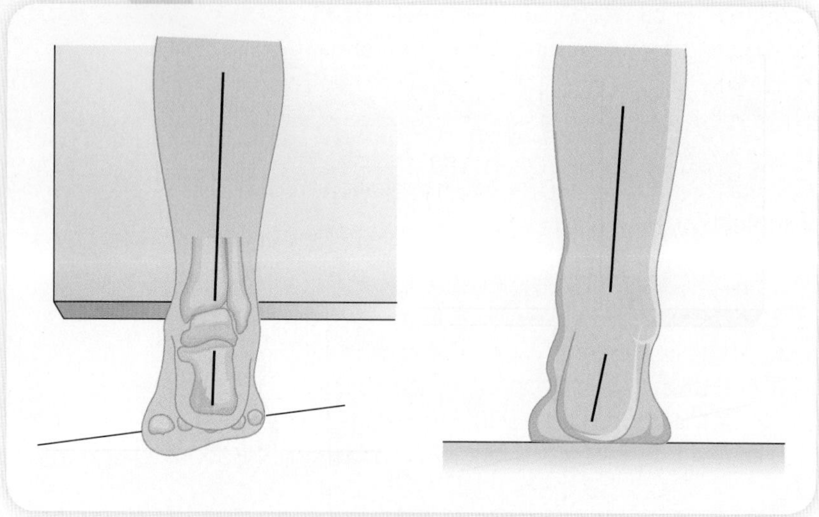

Figure 26-7 Compensated forefoot valgus

Comparing non–weightbearing neutral to weightbearing resting position.
(Figure used with permission of Brian Hoke, American Physical Rehabilitation Network.)

tendon passes posteriorly around the base of the lateral malleolus and then through a notch in the cuboid to cross the foot to the first metatarsal. The cuboid functions as a pulley to increase the mechanical advantage of the peroneal tendon. Stability of the cuboid is essential in this process. In the pronated position, the cuboid loses much of its mechanical advantage as a pulley; therefore the peroneal tendon no longer stabilizes the first ray effectively. This condition creates hypermobility of the first ray and increases pressure on the other metatarsals.

Effects of Midtarsal Joint Position During Supination

During supination, the talus abducts and dorsi flexes, which raises the level of the talonavicular joint superior to that of the calcaneocuboid joint and allows less congruency of both joint articulations.[95] The planes of the oblique and longitudinal axes of the joints become more oblique or nonparallel. This position of the axes causes increased stability of the foot, making the foot more rigid and stable. Because less movement occurs at the calcaneocuboid joint, the cuboid becomes hypomobile. The long peroneal tendon has a greater amount of tension because the cuboid has less mobility and thus will not allow hypermobility of the first ray. In this case the majority of the weight is borne by the first and fifth metatarsals. This normal effect of the MTJ allows the foot to become a more rigid lever for more efficient push off during late stance phase.

Tarsometatarsal Joint

The tarsometatarsal joint comprises the 4 proximal tarsal bones of the first, second, and third cuneiforms, and the cuboid articulating distally with the bases of the 5 metatarsal bones. The articulating bones of the tarsometatarsal joint allow for accommodation of rotational forces introduced to the midfoot and forefoot region when the foot is engaged in weightbearing activities. The tarsometatarsal joints move as a unit and work in unison with the midtarsal and STJs, and it is often difficult to distinguish the individual contributions to the overall movement pattern of the foot.[72] Also known as the Lisfranc joint, the tarsometatarsal joint provides a locking mechanism that also aids in foot stability.

Metatarsal Joints

Together with subtalar, talonavicular, and tarsometatarsal interrelationships, foot stabilization depends on the interaction between the metatarsal joints. The first ray moves independently from the other metatarsal bones. As a main functional weightbearing unit, the first ray is necessary for body propulsion. Stabilization depends on the peroneus longus muscle, which attaches on the medial aspect of the first ray. As with the other segments of the foot, stability of the first metatarsal bone depends on the relative position of the subtalar and talonavicular joints. Control of the first ray with orthotic therapy has shown to be effective in the management of lower-extremity overuse injuries.[2]

The fifth metatarsal bone, like the first metatarsal bone, moves independently. With plantarflexion, the first metatarsal moves into abduction and eversion while the fifth moves into adduction and inversion. Conversely, with dorsiflexion, the first metatarsal moves into adduction and inversion while the fifth moves into abduction and eversion.[2,49]

The second ray is the most stable of the 5 rays because of the secure connection with the tarsals. The second ray functions as the pivot point, as the other rays undergo a torsional twist during the motions of foot pronation and supination.[72]

Biomechanics of Normal Gait

The functions of the foot during the gait cycle are adaptation, shock absorption, rigid support for leverage, and torque conversion. The action of the lower extremity during walking gait can be divided into 2 basic phases (Figure 26-8*A*). The first is the stance, or support phase, which starts with the initial contact at heel strike and ends at toe-off. Stance phase can be subdivided into 3 defined events: contact, midstance, and propulsion. The second is the swing or recovery phase, which can also be subdivided into 3 defined events: early swing, mid swing, and late swing. This represents the time immediately after toe-off in which the leg is moved from behind the body to a position in front of the body in preparation for heel strike.[2,3]

The action of the lower extremity during running gait can also be divided into 2 basic phases (see Figure 26-8*B*). The first is the support phase, which starts with the initial contact and ends at takeoff. Support phase can be subdivided into 3 different events: foot contact, mid support, and toe-off. The second is swing phase, which can be subdivided into 3 defined events: follow through, forward swing, and foot descent.

There are distinct differences in the gait cycle of an individual who is walking, jogging, or running. These differences include speed, vertical ground reaction force (GRF), stance time and foot contact. Speed of gait can be defined for various forms of gait, including

Stance			Swing		
Contact	Mid stance	Propulsion	Early swing	Mid swing	Late swing

A

Support			Swing		
Foot contact	Mid support	Toe off	Follow through	Forward swing	Foot descent

B

Figure 26-8 Gait cycle

A. Walking. B. Running. (Adapted from American Physical Rehabilitation Network, 2000.)

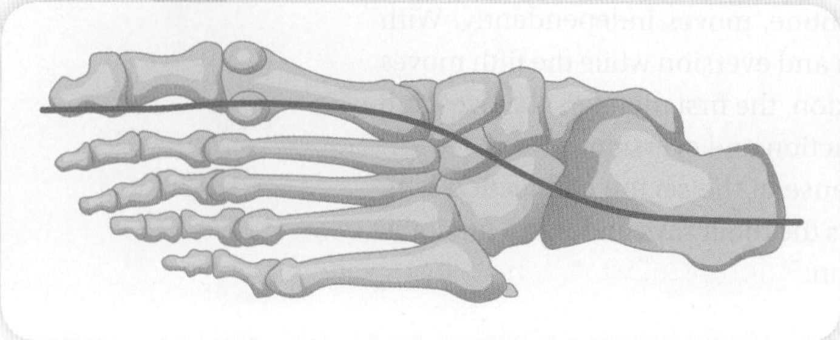

Figure 26-9 **Center of weightbearing forces**

(Adapted from American Physical Rehabilitation Network, 2000.)

walking at a pace of 15 to 30 minutes per mile (2 to 4 mph), jogging at a pace of 7 to 14 minutes per mile (5 to 9 mph), and running at a pace of 6 minutes per mile or faster (10+ mph).[3]

There is variability in GRF data between the left and right foot of an individual, as well as between individuals. Generally speaking, with walking, peak GRF at initial contact is less than body weight (BW) and exceeds BW near the end of contact. Peak GRF then diminishes at midstance but exceeds BW to the highest peak value during propulsion. During jogging, peak GRF at initial contact is 1.5 to 2 times BW, which increases to approximately 2 to 3 times BW during propulsion. With running, there is no peak GRF at initial contact, but a single peak of 2 to 3 times BW occurs during propulsion, which is actually less than jogging (Figure 26-9).[3]

The time an individual spends in each phase depends on whether the individual is walking, jogging, or running. One complete gait cycle is defined as initial contact of left foot through the initial contact of the left foot again. The duration of the gait cycle is approximately 1.0 second for walking, 0.7 seconds for jogging, and 0.6 seconds for running. The start of the gait cycle is described by heel strike during walking, and either heel, midfoot, or forefoot strike with jogging or running. The part of the foot that strikes during jogging or running depends on the speed and cadence of the activity. With walking, there is a period of time, called the *double-limb support phase,* in which there is an overlap between stance phase of one limb and stance phase of the opposite limb. This phase constitutes the first 12% and the last 12% of each stance phase. During jogging and running, there is no double-limb support phase. There is actually a *nonsupportive* or *float phase* with running and jogging. The duration of stance is also reduced as an individual progresses from walking to running, with walking stance duration approximately 0.6 seconds, jogging 0.23 seconds, and running 0.17 seconds. When comparing walking to running, the ratio of stance to swing changes with the percentage of stance phase diminishing and the percentage of swing phase increasing.[3]

Cadence is defined as the number times (step frequency) both feet hit the ground in a 60-second period of time. More specific to running, the "ideal" cadence is 180 steps per minute. This number is based on elite runners and is used more as a guide than an absolute. Cadence manipulation is one technique to facilitate the transition to a forefoot strike pattern with running from a heel strike pattern.[46,47] Several studies have looked at the higher incidence of running injuries with the presence of an impact peak in the vertical GRF.[12,25,27,64,76,105] An impact peak is more prevalent with a heel strike pattern as compared to a forefoot strike pattern. Heiderscheit et al concluded that runners who increased their step frequency by 5% demonstrated a decreased in vertical excursion of the center of mass (COM) and decrease in braking impulse. A 10% increased increase in step frequency demonstrated a decrease in GRF at the hip and knees.[46,47] Even though this particular study did not address the effect of GRF specifically to the ankle and foot, assumptions can be made to the benefit of cadence manipulation on the entire kinetic chain.

The foot's function during the support phase of running is twofold. At initial contact, the foot acts as a shock absorber to the impact forces and then adapts to the uneven surfaces. At push-off, the foot functions as a rigid lever to transmit the explosive force from the lower extremity to the running surface.

Despite the noted differences observed in walking versus running, there are a number of similarities in the gait cycle. In a heel-strike pattern with walking or running gait, initial contact of the foot is on the lateral aspect of the calcaneus with the STJ in supination.[8]

Associated with this supination of the STJ is an obligatory external rotation of the tibia. As the foot is loaded, the STJ moves into a pronated position until the forefoot is in contact with the ground. The change in subtalar motion occurs between initial heel strike and 20% into the support or stance phase. As pronation occurs at the STJ, there is obligatory internal rotation of the tibia. Transverse plane rotation occurs at the knee joint because of this tibial rotation.[8] Pronation of the foot unlocks the MTJ and allows the foot to assist in shock absorption and to adapt to uneven surfaces. It is important during initial impact to reduce the GRFs and to distribute the load evenly on many different anatomic structures throughout the foot and leg. Pronation is normal and allows for this distribution of forces to as many structures as possible to avoid excessive loading on just a few structures. The STJ remains in a pronated position until 55% to 85% of the support phase with maximum pronation is concurrent with the body's center of gravity passing over the base of support.[5] Maximal pronation is approximately 6 to 8 degrees for walking and 9 to 12 degrees for running.[3]

The foot begins to resupinate and will approach the neutral subtalar position at 70% to 90% of the support phase. In supination, the MTJs are locked and the foot becomes stable and rigid to prepare for push-off. This rigid position allows the foot to exert a great amount of force from the lower extremity to the walking or running surface.[55]

Pathomechanics of Gait Associated with Running Form

Although barefoot running isn't a new concept, there has been a great deal of publicity since the book *Born to Run* was released in 2008, and the push toward a more "natural or minimalistic" running style. In conjunction with the rise in interest within the running community, there is an increase in evidence to support the potential benefits to transitioning to a midfoot style running approach as compared to the more traditional heel strike pattern.[12,25,27,64,76,96,105] Moving away from shod (or traditional shoe) running toward barefoot and/or the use of minimalistic footwear is one "tool" to promote this type of running approach. As a note for clarification, this shift toward a midfoot strike pattern pertains more directly to the distance running athlete, as compared to a sprinting athlete whose running is performed predominately by striking on the forefoot.

To briefly summarize the research, the following have been described as potential benefits to barefoot running[12,25,27,64,76,96,105]:

- Less contact time (foot moves off of the ground faster)
- Lower flight time (correlates with higher cadence)
- Lower passive vertical peak impact forces
- Increased preactivation of triceps surae (stored elastic energy)
- Increased vertical stiffness (results in less COM displacement)
- Barefoot runners exhibit more forefoot and midfoot striking patterns
- Shod running is associated with significantly increased peak torque forces at the hip, knee, and ankle joints

Another concept that also needs to be taken into consideration when discussing midfoot versus heel-strike patterns is the foot position relative to the runners COM. Dicharry showed that runners who performed a midfoot landing pattern, but out in front of their COM, had significantly higher vertical loading rate and impact peaks as compared to those who performed a heel-strike pattern with the foot position near their COM.[26]

Despite the proposed benefits to barefoot/forefoot running, care needs to be taken in the implementation, utilization, and progression of barefoot running, use of minimalistic footwear, or cadence manipulation. It should be noted that despite the studied differences in barefoot/minimalistic footwear/midfoot landing style, calcaneal and tibial movement patterns do not substantially differ when compared to shod/heel-strike landing style.[106] However, excessive or dysfunctional movement patterns at the calcaneus or tibia are common biomechanical factors in overuse injuries in all runners.

Anecdotally, one author has seen a significant rise in lower-extremity injures in runners who present to the clinic since 2008. Specific to the foot and ankle, Achilles tendinopathy, plantar fasciitis, and lateral metatarsal stress fractures seem to be the most common injuries associated with runners who have changed their running form or undergone modification/removal of traditional footwear.[42,75] It is theorized that the increased demand on the soft tissue and preactivation levels of the triceps surae may be one reason for the rise in injuries. Another reason for the increase in overuse injuries is related to the rapid increase in either the rate or volume of running training.

It should be noted that some runners may not be candidates for barefoot/minimalistic techniques or use of the midfoot landing pattern. Numerous anatomical factors should be considered, including the presence of a cavus (high-arch) foot, leg-length discrepancies, and muscle weakness, which may preclude someone from successful barefoot running or the use of minimalistic footwear.[15,60,81,96,111] Furthermore, if a runner is experiencing any of the previously noted injuries commonly seen with barefoot or midfoot landing style, allowing the runner to continue with a heel-strike pattern may be advantageous during the runner's rehabilitation process.

A review of the running literature published (of papers in English from 1980 to 2011) by Lorenz and Pontillo[65] indicated that while minimal data exist that definitively support barefoot running, there are data to support the argument that runners should use a forefoot (midfoot) strike versus heel-strike pattern. Whether there is a positive or negative effect on injury rate is yet to be determined. Unquestionably, more research is definitely needed to assist in the development of an evidence-based approach to reduce the frequency of running-related injuries. However, there is agreement in the literature that a few common factors exist in reducing the risk for injury, including: slow progression using minimalistic footwear or barefoot training techniques; consideration of foot intrinsic strength; adequate proximal stability of hip abductors and flexors; and a thorough lower extremity assessment with a gait biomechanical evaluation.[31,81,94,96]

Pathomechanics of Gait Associated with Primary Abnormalities of the Foot

STJ motion can be analyzed throughout all phases of gait with significant differences noted between the previously described abnormalities of the forefoot and rearfoot, most effectively through slow motion video analysis. Having an understanding of these differences will assist in proper treatment and management of lower-extremity overuse injuries. STJ is evaluated during the contact, midstance, and propulsion stages of stance phase.

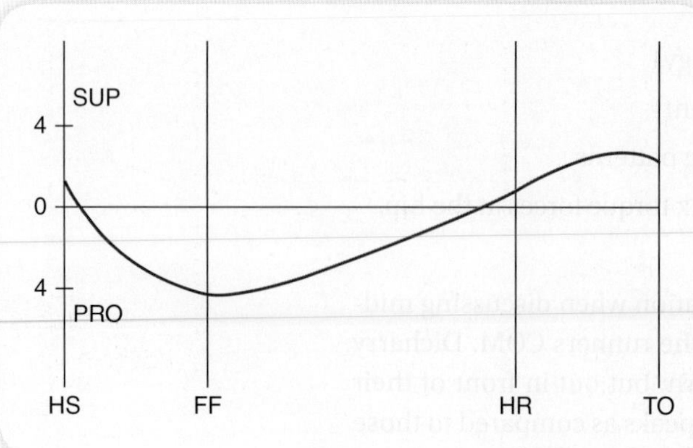

Figure 26-10 Subtalar joint motion analysis

Intrinsic normalcy. (Figure used with permission from Brian Hoke, American Physical Rehabilitation Network.)

With intrinsic normalcy (Figure 26-10), during contact the STJ is slightly supinated at heel strike (HS) and pronates to 3 to 5 degrees of pronation by foot flat (FF). During midstance, the STJ resupinates to neutral or slight supination by heel rise (HR). During propulsion, the STJ continues to supinate to toe-off (TO).[2,3]

With compensated subtalar varus (Figure 26-11), during contact the calcaneus is inverted more than normal at initial HS, thus the STJ must excessively pronate to

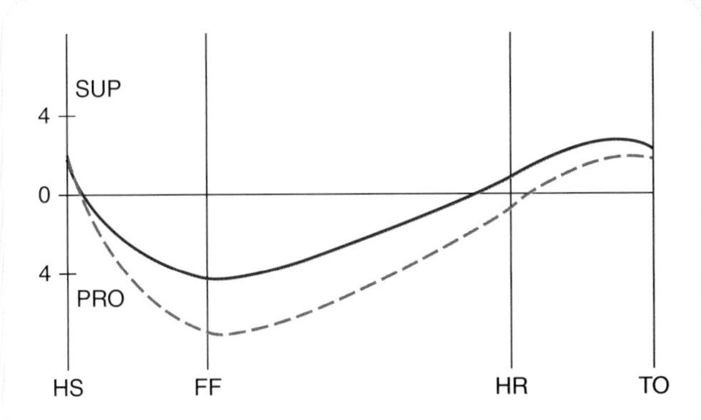

Figure 26-11 **Subtalar joint motion analysis**

Compensated subtalar or calcaneal varus. (Figure used with permission from Brian Hoke, American Physical Rehabilitation Network.)

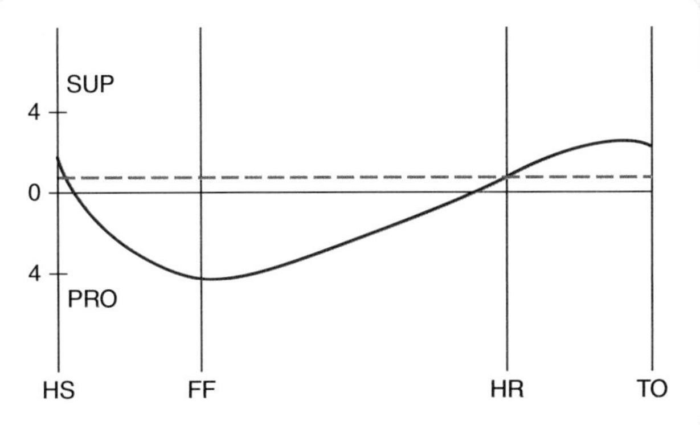

Figure 26-12 **Subtalar joint motion analysis**

Uncompensated subtalar or calcaneal varus. (Figure used with permission from Brian Hoke, American Physical Rehabilitation Network.)

compensate for this abnormality. During midstance, the STJ will resupinate as the weight shifts from the heel; however, there is a lag as compared to normal as HR approaches. Because of this lag, there is associated delayed tibial external rotation. During propulsion, the STJ continues to TO.[2,3]

With uncompensated subtalar varus (Figure 26-12), during contact the calcaneus is again inverted more than normal at heel strike; however, in this situation the STJ motion is insufficient to compensate for the deformity. The calcaneus remains inverted throughout midstance and propulsion toward TO. Weight bearing is more lateral than normal during midstance, but will shift medially as the heel rises.[2,3]

With compensated forefoot varus (Figure 26-13), during contact the STJ reacts the same as in intrinsic normalcy. However, during midstance, the STJ continues to pronate to compensate for the forefoot alignment. Because of the continued pronation, this mechanism unlocks the MTJ creating excessive forefoot mobility at HR. During propulsion, the STJ remains pronated throughout the remainder of stance. This is described as either late pronation or delayed resupination, and typically there is associated excessive tibial internal rotation.[2,3]

With uncompensated forefoot varus (Figure 26-14), during contact the STJ is slightly supinated at heel strike; however, it usually pronates less than the normal 3 to 5 degrees. During midstance, the STJ motion is insufficient to compensate for the forefoot alignment and weight bearing stays on the lateral forefoot. During propulsion, there is a small amount of continued pronation at the STJ and no resupination as the foot approaches TO. These individuals are classified as neither an overpronator nor supinator, just lacking sufficient motion at the STJ.[2,3]

Finally, with compensated forefoot valgus (Figure 26-15), during contact the STJ pronates, but this motion may be limited to premature loading of the first ray. As a result, during midstance, the STJ rapidly resupinates as a result of the influence of the normal or rigid first ray. During propulsion, when the heel begins to rise, potential STJ pronation occurs to achieve the necessary

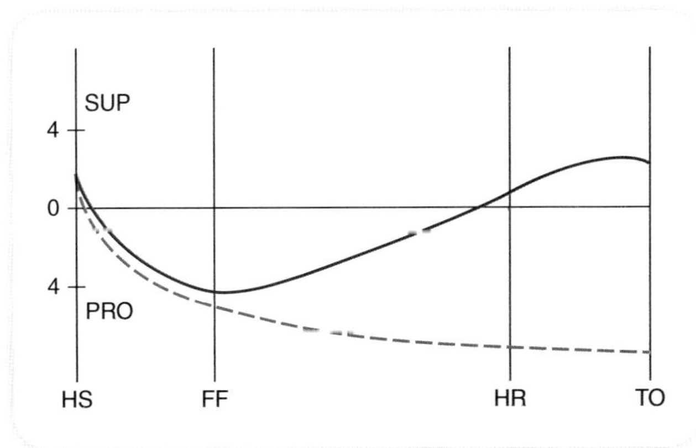

Figure 26-13 **Subtalar joint motion analysis**

Compensated forefoot varus. (Figure used with permission from Brian Hoke, American Physical Rehabilitation Network.)

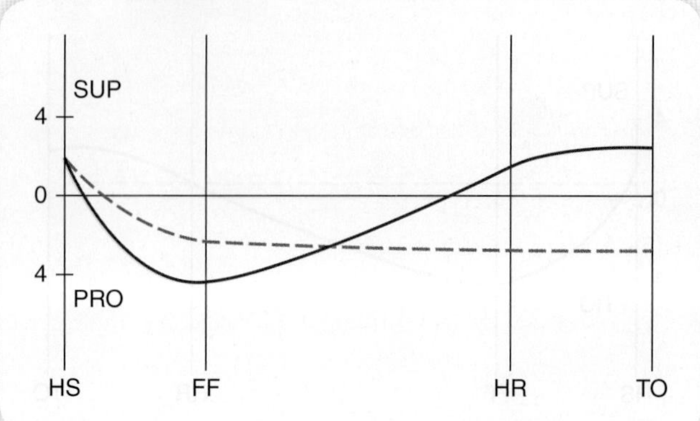

Figure 26-14 Subtalar joint motion analysis

Uncompensated forefoot varus. (Figure used with permission from Brian Hoke, American Physical Rehabilitation Network.)

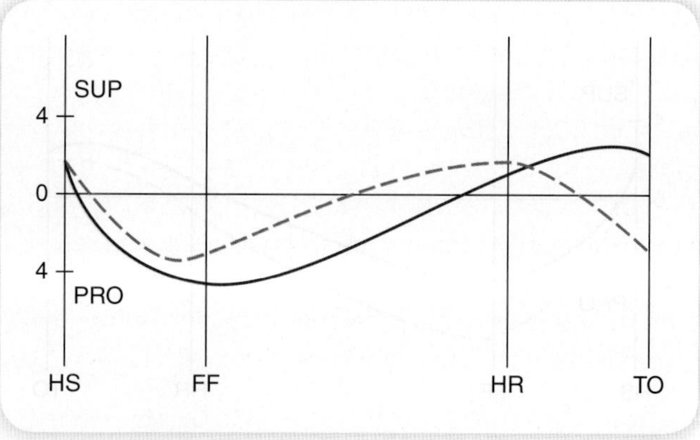

Figure 26-15 Subtalar joint motion analysis

Compensated forefoot valgus. (Figure used with permission from Brian Hoke, American Physical Rehabilitation Network.)

weight shift from the lateral aspect of the stance foot to the contralateral limb. This is typically observed when the foot snaps back into pronation late in the stance phase.[2,3]

Rehabilitation Techniques for Specific Injuries

Ankle Sprains

Pathomechanics and Injury Mechanism

Ankle sprains are among the more common musculoskeletal injuries.[10,21,23,120] Injuries to the ligaments of the ankle may be classified either according to their location or by the mechanism of injury.

Inversion Sprains An inversion ankle sprain is the most common and often results in injury to the lateral ligaments. The anterior talofibular ligament is the weakest of the 3 lateral ligaments. Its major function is to stop forward subluxation of the talus. It is injured in an inverted, plantar flexed, and internally rotated position.[57,113] The calcaneofibular and posterior talofibular ligaments are also likely to be injured in inversion sprains as the force of inversion is increased. Increased inversion force is needed to tear the calcaneofibular ligament. Because the posterior talofibular ligament prevents posterior subluxation of the talus, injuries to it only occur with severe trauma, such as complete dislocations.[11] The deltoid ligament may also be contused in inversion sprains due to impingement between the fibular malleolus and the calcaneus.

Eversion Sprains The eversion ankle sprain is less common than the inversion ankle sprain, largely because of the bony and ligamentous anatomy. As mentioned previously, the fibular malleolus extends further inferiorly than does the tibial malleolus. This, combined with the strength of the thick deltoid ligament, prevents excessive eversion. More often, eversion injuries may involve an avulsion fracture of the tibia before the deltoid ligament tears.[18] Despite the fact that eversion sprains are less common, the severity is such that these sprains may take longer to heal than inversion sprains.[86]

Syndesmotic Sprains Isolated injuries to the distal tibiofemoral joint are referred to as syndesmotic sprains. The anterior and posterior tibiofibular ligaments are found between the distal tibia and fibula and extend up the lower leg as the interosseous ligament or syndesmotic ligament. Sprains of the ligaments are more common than has been realized in the past. These ligaments are torn with increased external rotational or forced dorsiflexion and are often injured in conjunction with a severe sprain of the medial and lateral ligament complexes.[112] Initial rupture of the ligaments occurs distally at the tibiofibular ligament above the ankle mortise. As the force of disruption is increased, the interosseous ligament is torn more proximally. Sprains of the syndesmotic ligaments are extremely hard to treat and often take months to heal. Treatments for this problem are essentially the same as for medial or lateral sprains, with the difference being an extended period of immobilization. Rehabilitation will likely require a longer period of time than for the inversion or eversion sprains.

Severity of the Sprain There are several factors involved with the severity of an ankle sprain, including previous history, intrinsic and extrinsic abnormalities, velocity, and mechanism of injury. In a grade I sprain, there is some stretching or perhaps minimal tearing of some of the ligamentous fibers, with little or no joint instability. Mild pain, little swelling, and joint stiffness may be apparent. With a grade II sprain, there is some tearing and separation of the ligamentous fibers and moderate instability of the joint. Moderate-to-severe pain, swelling, and joint stiffness should be expected.

Grade III sprains involve total rupture of the ligament, manifested primarily by gross instability of the joint. Severe pain may be present initially, followed by little or no pain caused by total disruption of nerve fibers. Swelling may be profuse, and thus the joint tends to become very stiff some hours after the injury. A grade III sprain with marked instability usually requires some form of immobilization lasting several weeks. Frequently, the force producing the ligament injury is so great that other ligaments or structures surrounding the joint may also be injured. With cases in which there is injury to multiple ligaments, surgical repair or reconstruction may be necessary to correct instability.

Rehabilitation Concerns

During the initial phase of ankle rehabilitation, the major goals are reduction of postinjury swelling, bleeding, and pain, and protection of the already healing ligament. As is the case in all acute musculoskeletal injuries, initial treatment efforts should be directed toward limiting the amount of swelling.[89] This is perhaps more true in the case of ankle sprains than with any other injury. Controlling initial swelling is the single most important treatment measure that can be taken during the entire rehabilitation process. Limiting the amount of acute swelling can significantly reduce the time required for rehabilitation. Initial management includes compression, ice, elevation, rest, and protection.

Compression Immediately following injury and evaluation, a compression wrap should be applied to the sprained ankle. An elastic bandage should be firmly and evenly applied, wrapping distal to proximal. It is also recommended that the elastic bandage be wet in order to facilitate the passage of cold. To add more compression, a horseshoe-shaped felt pad may be inserted under the wrap over the area of maximum swelling.

Following initial treatment, open Gibney taping may be applied under an elastic wrap to provide additional compression and support. Care should be taken not to compartmentalize this treatment by placing tape across the top and bottom of the open area of the open Gibney (Figure 26-16). Uneven pressure or uncovered areas over any part of the extremity may allow the swelling to accumulate.

Other devices are available that apply external compression to the ankle to control or reduce swelling. External compression should be used both initially and throughout the rehabilitative process. Most of these devices use either air or cold water within an enclosed bag to provide pressure to reduce swelling. One commonly used device is the intermittent compression unit, such as a Jobst, or other pneumatic pump, or the Cryo Cuff (Figure 26-17).

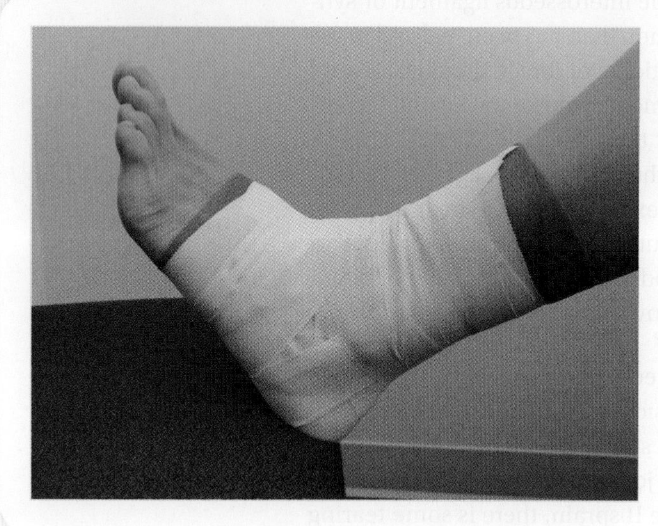

Figure 26-16 Closed basket weave taping

Ice The use of ice on acute injuries has been well documented in the literature. Initially, ice and compression should be used together, because this treatment regimen is more effective than ice alone.[104] The initial use of ice is indicated for constricting superficial blood flow to prevent hemorrhage as well as in reducing the hypoxic response to injury by decreasing cellular metabolism. Long-term benefits may be from reduction of pain and guarding.[5] Garrick suggests the use of ice for a minimum of 20 minutes once every 4 waking hours.[36] Ice should not be used longer than 30 minutes, especially over superficial nerves such as the peroneal and ulnar nerves. Prolonged use of ice in such areas may produce transient nerve palsy.[30]

Current literature suggests that ice can be used during all phases of rehabilitation,[61] but is most effective if used immediately after injury.[89] Ice can certainly do no harm if used properly, but heat, if applied too soon after injury, may lead to increased swelling. Often the switch from ice to heat cannot be made for days or weeks, if necessary at all.

Elevation Elevation is an essential part of edema control. Pressure in any vessel below the level of the heart is increased, which may lead to increased edema accumulation.[19] Elevation allows gravity to work with the lymphatic system rather than against it. Elevation decreases hydrostatic pressure to decrease fluid loss and also assists venous and lymphatic return through gravity.[89] Patients should be encouraged to maintain an elevated position as often as possible, particularly during the first 24 to 48 hours following injury. An attempt should be made to treat in the elevated position rather than the gravity-dependent position. Any treatment performed in the dependent position will allow edema to increase.[89,102]

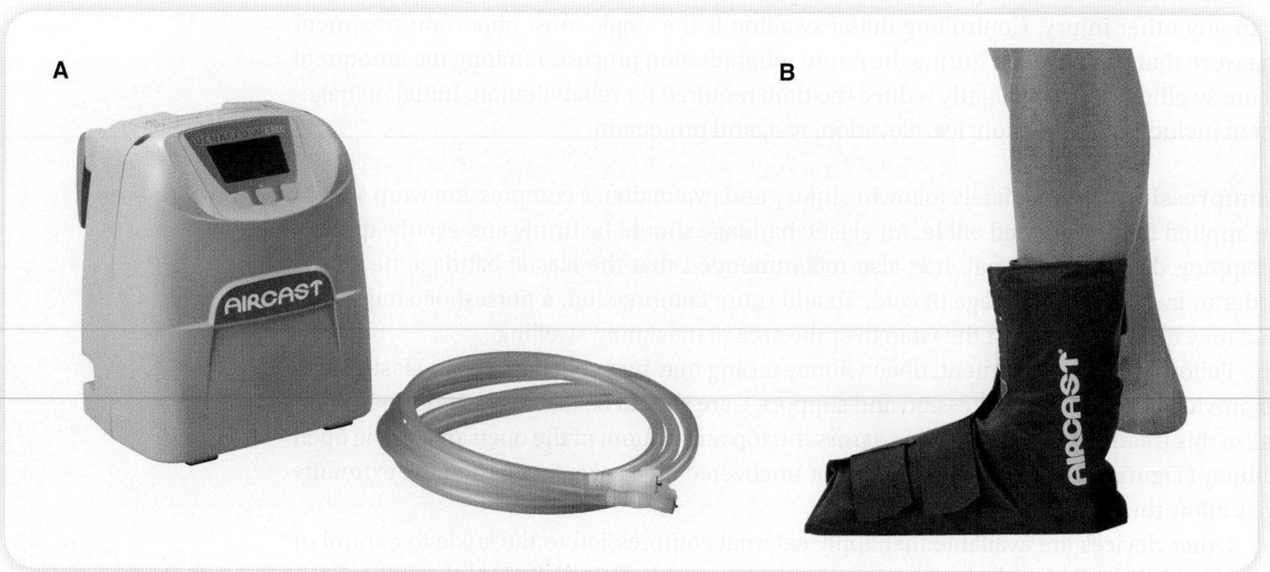

Figure 26-17

A. Jobst intermittent air compression device. B. Cryo Cuff.

Rest It is important to allow the inflammatory process to run its course during the first 24 to 48 hours before incorporating aggressive exercise techniques. However, rest does not mean that the injured patient does nothing. Contralateral exercises may be performed to obtain cross-transfer effects on the muscles of the injured side.[59] Isometric exercises may be performed very early in dorsiflexion, plantarflexion, inversion, and eversion (see Exercises 26-1 to 26-4). These types of exercises may be performed to prevent atrophy without fear of further injury to the ligament. Active plantarflexion and dorsiflexion may be initiated early because they also do not endanger the healing ligament as long as they are done in a pain-free range. Active plantarflexion and dorsiflexion can be done while the patient is iced and elevated. Inversion and eversion are to be avoided, because they might initiate bleeding and further traumatize ligaments.

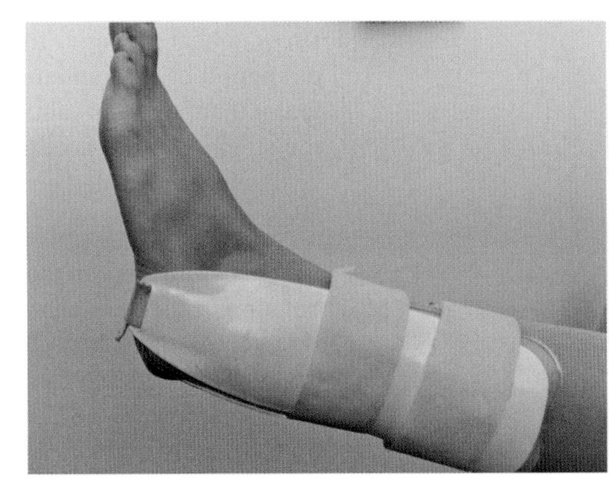

Figure 26-18 Commercially available Aircast ankle stirrup

Protection Several appliances are available to accomplish this early protected motion. Quillen[90] recommends the ankle stirrup, which allows motion in the sagittal plane while limiting movement of the frontal plane and thus avoids stressing the injured ligaments through inversion and eversion (Figure 26-18). Several commercially available braces accomplish this goal and also apply cushioned pressure to help with edema.[107] When a commercially available product is not feasible, a similar protective device may be fashioned from thermoplastic materials such as Hexalite or Orthoplast (Figure 26-19).

The open Gibney taping technique also provides early medial and lateral protection while allowing plantarflexion and dorsiflexion, in addition to being an excellent mechanism of edema control (see Figure 26-16).

Gross et al compared the effectiveness of a number of commercial ankle orthoses and taping in restricting eversion and inversion. All of these support methods significantly reduced inversion and eversion immediately after initial application and following an exercise bout when compared to preapplication measures. Of the support systems tested, taping provided the least amount of support after exercise.[45] Early application of these devices allows for early ambulation.

Rehabilitation Progression

In the early phase of rehabilitation, vigorous exercise is discouraged. The injured ligament must be maintained in a stable position so that healing can occur.[82] Thus, during the period of maximum protection following injury, the patient should be either non–weight bearing or perhaps partial weight bearing on crutches.

Partial weight bearing with crutches helps control several complications to healing. Muscle atrophy, proprioceptive loss, and circulatory stasis are all reduced when even limited weight bearing is allowed. Weight bearing also inhibits contracture of the tendons, which may lead to tendinitis. For these reasons, early ambulation, even if only touchdown weight bearing, is essential.[68]

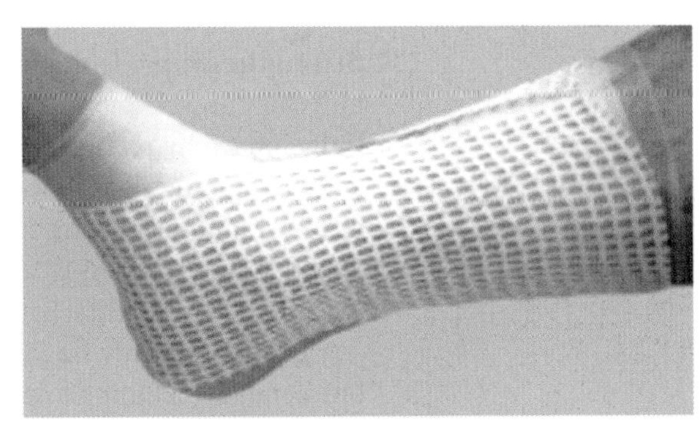

Figure 26-19 Molded Hexalite ankle stirrup

It has been clearly demonstrated that a healing ligament needs a certain amount of stress to heal properly. The literature suggests that early limited stress following the initial period of inflammation may promote faster and stronger healing.[11,82] These studies found that protected motion facilitated proper collagen reorientation and thus increased the strength of the healing ligament. Once swelling and pain decrease, indicating that ligaments have healed enough to tolerate limited stress, rehabilitation can become more aggressive.

Range of Motion In the early stages of the rehabilitation, inversion and eversion should be minimized. Light joint mobilization concentrating on dorsiflexion and plantarflexion should be initiated first.[67] Range of motion (ROM) can be improved by manual joint mobilization techniques. It can also be improved through exercises such as towel stretching for the plantarflexors (see Exercise 26-27) and standing or kneeling stretches for the dorsiflexors (see Exercise 26-29). Patients are encouraged to do these exercises slowly, without pain, and to use high repetitions (2 to 3 sets of 30 to 40 repetitions).

As tenderness over the ligament decreases, inversion-eversion exercises may be initiated in conjunction with plantarflexion and dorsiflexion exercises. Early exercises include pulling a towel from one side to the other by alternatively inverting and everting the foot and alphabet drawing in an ice bath, which should be done in capital letters to ensure that full range is used.

Exercises performed on a BAPS (biomechanical ankle platform system) (Board Spectrum Therapy Products, Inc.) board, Fitter Rocker board, Fitter Wobble board, or the BOB may be beneficial for ROM as well as a beginning exercise for regaining neuromuscular control.[114] These exercises typically should first be performed in a seated position, progressing to partial and then full weight bearing.

Initially, the patient should start in the seated position with Fitter Rocker board in the plantarflexion-dorsiflexion direction. As pain decreases and ligament healing progresses, the board may be turned in the inversion-eversion direction (see Exercises 26-25*A* and *B*). As the patient performs these movements easily, the patient could start weight bearing active-assisted ROM in the plantarflexion-dorsiflexion direction with the BOB (see Exercise 26-11). A seated BAPS board or Fitter Wobble board may be used for full ROM exercises, including clockwise and counter clockwise directions (see Exercise 26-33*A*). When seated exercises are performed with ease, progression to partial weightbearing exercises should be initiated, utilizing a leg-press machine or Total Gym. Finally, progression to full weightbearing exercises is initiated, focusing on ROM and balance retraining (see Exercises 26-33*B* and *C*).

Vigorous pain-free heel cord stretching for the gastrocnemius and soleus should be initiated as soon as possible, utilizing either static or dynamic multiplanar techniques (see Exercises 26-26, 26-28, and 26-11). McCluskey et al[70] found that the heel cord acts as a bowstring when tight and may increase the chance of ankle sprains.

Strengthening Isometrics may be done in the 4 major ankle motion planes, frontal and sagittal (see Exercises 26-1 to 26-4). They may be accompanied early in the rehabilitative phase by plantarflexion and dorsiflexion isotonic exercises, which do not endanger the healing ligaments (see Exercises 26-7, 26-8, and 26-10). As the ligaments heal and ROM increases, strengthening exercises may be initiated in all planes of motion (see Exercises 26-5 and 26-6). Care must be taken when exercising the ankle in inversion and eversion to avoid tibial rotation as a substitute movement.

During the early stages of rehabilitation, foot intrinsic strengthening exercises are recommended, including towel curls (see Exercise 26-12) and arch raises (see Exercise 26-13).

Pain should be the basic guideline for deciding when to start inversion-eversion isotonic exercises. Light resistance with high repetitions has fewer detrimental effects on the ligaments (2 to 4 sets of 15 to 25 repetitions). Resistive tubing exercises, ankle weights around the foot, and a multidirectional Elgin ankle exerciser (see Exercise 26-9) are excellent methods of strengthening inversion and eversion. Tubing has advantages in that it may be used both eccentrically and concentrically.

Isokinetics have advantages in that more functional speeds may be obtained (see Exercises 26-19 and 26-20). Proprioceptive neuromuscular facilitation strengthening exercises, which isolate the desired motions at the talocrural joint, can also be used (see Exercises 26-21 to 26-24).

Proprioception and Neuromuscular Control The role of proprioception in repeated ankle trauma has been questioned.[17,32,35,80] The literature suggests that proprioception is certainly a factor in recurrent ankle sprains. Rebman[92] reported that 83% of patients experienced a reduction in chronic ankle sprains after a program of proprioceptive exercises. Glencross and Thornton[43] found that the greater the ligamentous disruption, the greater the proprioceptive loss.

Early weightbearing has previously been mentioned as a method of reducing proprioceptive loss. During the early rehabilitation phase, standing on both feet with side-to-side and heel-to-toes weight shifting is recommended, as well as double-limb stance with eyes closed. Next progression would be single-leg stance on a stable surface starting with eyes open working toward eyes closed including performing this with additional weight shifting toward the heel (see Exercises 26-31). This exercise series can be progressed to single-limb stance on unstable surfaces, which should be done initially with support from the hands, using such commercial devices as foam rollers, Fitter Wobble board, Fitter Rocker board, DynaDisc (Exertools), BOSU (DW Fitness, LLC) Balance Trainer, or KAT system. Once the patient demonstrates good control on a specific device, the patient can progress to free standing and controlling the board through all ranges (see Exercise 26-32). To further challenge the patient's neuromuscular control and incorporate more functional activities, perturbations can be introduced via the upper extremities using tubing, medicine balls, or the Body Blade while in a single-limb stance position (see Exercise 26-34).

Other closed kinetic chain exercises may be functionally beneficial. The leg press (see Exercise 26-36), miniform squats (see Exercise 26-38*A*), or minilunges (see Exercise 26-39) are each examples of closed kinetic chain exercises. Initially, start any of the closed kinetic chain exercises in double-limb stance and progress to single limb (see Exercise 26-37) or to unstable surfaces (see Exercise 26-38*B*). Single-leg standing kicks using abduction, adduction, extension, and flexion of the uninvolved side, while weight bearing on the affected side, will increase both strength and proprioception. This may be accomplished either by free standing (see Exercise 26-35) or while having the patient stand on an unstable surface.

Additional information on impaired neuromuscular control and reactive neuromuscular training can be referenced in Chapter 9.

Proximal Stability This chapter focuses on the foot and ankle. However, it is essential that when managing a patient with foot and ankle pathology or pathomechanics, that proximal stability is addressed, specifically that of the knee, hip, and trunk musculature. As already discussed, ROM, strength, flexibility, and neuromuscular control are all key components. More detailed information is available in several previous chapters, including those on the core, hip, and knee.

To further expand on strengthening exercises, when a patient has weightbearing restrictions, initiating mat table exercises for proximal trunk and hip stability early in the rehabilitation process are recommended. For example, exercises for gluteus medius, hip lateral rotators, trunk extensors, and gluteus maximus can be initiated against gravity, against resistance or using an exercise ball. Once weight bearing is progressed to full and pain-free, then a more functional program can be implemented.

Finally, it is important when managing a patient with a proximal movement-related dysfunction or diagnosis, to examine the foot and ankle. It is well accepted that when the foot comes into contact with the ground, there is a biomechanical influence up the kinetic chain.[2,3] Thus, the assumption can be made that overuse injuries involving knees, hips, or back could be related to foot or ankle pathomechanics.

Cardiorespiratory Endurance Cardiorespiratory conditioning should be maintained during the entire rehabilitation process. A stationary bike, NuStep (NuStep Inc.), or elliptical trainer are all appropriate forms of no impact, partial to full-weightbearing activities as long as pain-free motion is achieved (see Exercises 26-42 to 26-44). An upper-extremity ergometer or Air-Dyne (Schwinn Fitness) bike with the hands (see Exercise 26-41) provides excellent cardiovascular exercise without placing stress on the lower extremities. Pool activities such as running using a float vest or swimming are also good cardiovascular exercises (see Exercise 26-40). Further information on aquatic therapy in rehabilitation is available in Chapter 16.

Functional Progressions Functional progressions may be as complex or simple as needed. The more severe the injury, the greater the need for a detailed functional progression. The typical progression begins early in the rehabilitation process as the patient becomes partial weight bearing. Full weightbearing activities should be started when ambulation can be performed without a limp. Running may be initiated as soon as ambulation is pain-free. Pain-free hopping on the affected side may also be a guideline to determine when running is appropriate.

Exercising in a pool allows for early running. The patient is placed in the pool in a swim vest that supports the body in water. The patient then runs in place without touching the bottom of the pool. Proper running form should be stressed. Eventually the patient is moved into shallow water so that more weight is placed on the ankle. More detail on varied aquatic exercises is found in Chapter 16.

Progression is then to running on a smooth, flat surface, ideally a track. Initially, the patient should jog straight and walk the curves, and then progress to jogging the entire track. Initially, a time-based progression is easier for the patient to follow as the patient may start as low as 5 minutes of running for the first time. For the first 4 weeks, the patient may increase the running time after two successful runs at the allowed time. It is also important during the first 4 weeks to run every other day with a rest day in between. Rest does not necessarily mean doing nothing. It is recommended that cross-training take place on the off days as previously described in the "Cardiorespiratory Endurance" section above. After 4 weeks of pain-free running, the patient is then allowed to start running 2 days in a row with a day off in between. General guidelines for return to running include 10% to 15% increase in total mileage or time per week. Once a pain-free running base has been reestablished, speed may be increased to a sprint in a straight line.

Movement in directions other than straight planes is necessary for return to sport. The cutting sequence should begin with circles of diminishing diameter. Cones may be set up for the patient to run figure-8s as the next cutting progression. The crossover or side step is next.[4] The patient sprints to a predesignated spot and cuts or sidesteps abruptly. When this progression is accomplished, the cut should be done without warning on the command of another person. Jumping and hopping exercises should be started on both legs simultaneously, and gradually reduced to only the injured side.

The patient may perform at different levels for each of these functional sequences. One functional sequence may be done at half speed while another is done at full speed. An example of this is the patient who is running full speed on straights of the track while doing figure-8s at only half speed. Once the upper levels of all the sequences are reached, the patient may return to limited practice, which may include early teaching and fundamental drills.

It has been estimated that 30% to 40% of all inversion injuries result in reinjury.[32,52,53,69,99] In the past, patients were simply allowed to return to their normal activities once the pain was low enough to tolerate the activity. The contemporary rehabilitative process should include a gradual progression of functional activities that slowly increase the stress on the ligaments.[58]

It is common practice that some type of ankle support be worn initially. It appears that ankle taping does have a stabilizing effect on unstable ankles[37,115] without interfering with motor performance.[33,70] McCluskey et al[69] suggest taping the ankle and also taping the shoe onto the foot to make the shoe and ankle function as a single functional unit. High-topped footwear may further stabilize the ankle.[48] An Aircast or some other supportive ankle brace can also be worn for support as a substitute for taping (see Figure 26-18).

Subluxation and Dislocation of the Peroneal Tendons

Pathomechanics

The peroneus brevis and longus tendons pass posterior to the fibula in the peroneal groove under the superior peroneal retinaculum. Peroneal tendon dislocation may occur because of rupture of the superior retinaculum or because the retinaculum strips the periosteum away from the lateral malleolus, creating laxity in the retinaculum. It appears that there is no anatomic correlation between peroneal groove size or shape and instability of the peroneal tendons.[56] An avulsion fracture of the lateral ridge of the distal fibula may also occur with a subluxation or dislocation of the peroneal tendons.

Injury Mechanism

Subluxation of peroneal tendons can occur from any mechanism causing sudden and forceful contraction of the peroneal muscles that involves dorsiflexion and eversion of the foot.[56] This forces the tendons anteriorly, rupturing the retinaculum and potentially causing an avulsion fracture of the lateral malleolus. The patient will often hear or feel a "pop." In differentiating peroneal subluxation from a lateral ligament sprain or tear, there will be tenderness over the peroneal tendons and swelling and ecchymosis in the retromalleolar area. During active eversion, the subluxation of the peroneal tendons may be observed and palpated. This is easier to observe when acute symptoms have subsided. The patient will typically complain of chronic "giving way" or "popping." If the tendon is dislocated on initial evaluation, it should be reduced using gentle inversion and plantarflexion with pressure on the peroneal tendon.[56]

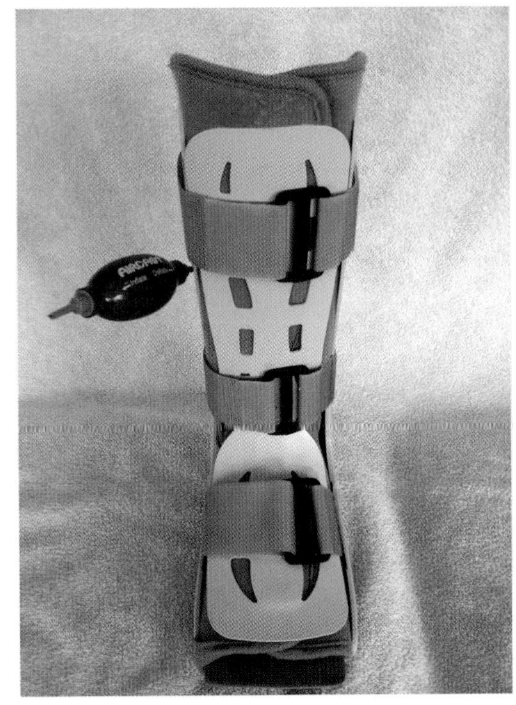

Figure 26-20 Short-leg walking cast

Rehabilitation Concerns and Progression

Following reduction, the patient should be initially placed in a compression dressing with a felt pad cut in the shape of a keyhole strapped over the lateral malleolus, placing gentle pressure on the peroneal tendons. Once the acute symptoms abate, the patient should be placed in a short leg cast in slight plantarflexion and non–weight bearing for 5 to 6 weeks (Figure 26-20). Aggressive ankle rehabilitation, as previously described, is initiated after cast removal.

In the case of an avulsion injury, or when this becomes a chronic problem, conservative treatment is unlikely to be successful and surgery is needed to prevent the problem from recurring. A number of surgical procedures have been recommended, including repair or reconstruction of the superior peroneal retinaculum, deepening of the peroneal groove, or rerouting the tendon. Following surgery, the patient should be placed in a non-weightbearing short-leg cast for approximately 4 weeks. The course of rehabilitation is similar to that described for ankle fractures with increased emphasis on strengthening of the peroneal tendons in eversion.[56] The patient may require approximately 10–12 weeks for rehabilitation.

Tendinopathy

Pathomechanics and Injury Mechanism

Inflammation of the tendons surrounding the ankle joint is common. The tendons most commonly involved are the posterior tibialis tendon behind the medial malleolus, the anterior tibialis under the extensor retinaculum on the dorsal surface of the ankle, and the peroneal tendons both behind the lateral malleolus and at the base of the fifth metatarsal.[112]

Tendinitis or tendinopathy of these tendons may result from one specific cause or from a variety of mechanisms, including faulty foot mechanics (discussed later in the section entitled Excessive Pronation and Supination); inappropriate or poor footwear that can create faulty foot mechanics; acute trauma to the tendon; tightness in the plantarflexor complex; or training errors in the athletic population. Training errors include training at too great of an intensity, training too frequently, changing training surfaces, and changes in activities within the training program.[112] Patients who develop a tendinopathy are likely to complain of pain both with active movement and passive stretching; swelling around the area of the tendon because of inflammation of the tendon and the tendon sheath; crepitus on movement; and stiffness and pain following periods of inactivity, but particularly in the morning.

Rehabilitation Concerns and Progression

In the early stages of rehabilitation, exercises are used to produce increased circulation and thus increased lymphatic flow. This will not only facilitate removal of fluid and the by-products of the inflammatory process, but will also increase nutrition to the healing tendon. In addition, exercise should also be used to limit atrophy, which may occur with disuse, and to minimize loss of strength, proprioception, and neuromuscular control.

Techniques should be incorporated into rehabilitation that act to reduce or eliminate inflammation, including rest, using therapeutic modalities (ice or iontophoresis), and use of antiinflammatory medications as prescribed by a physician.

If faulty foot mechanics are a cause of tendinitis, it may be helpful to construct an appropriate orthotic device to correct the foot and ankle biomechanics. Taping of the foot may also be helpful in temporarily reducing stress on the tendons.

In many instances, if the mechanism causing the irritation and inflammation of the tendon is removed, and the inflammatory process runs its normal course, the tendinopathy will often resolve within 10 days to 2 weeks. This is particularly true if rest and treatment are begun as soon as the symptoms begin. Unfortunately, as is most often the case, if treatment does not begin until the symptoms have been present for several weeks or even months, the tendinopathy will take much longer to resolve. This is because of longstanding inflammation, during which the tendon thickens, making the period of time required for that tendon to remodel significantly greater.

In our experience, it is better to allow the patient to rest for a sufficient period of time so that tendon healing can take place. With tendinopathy, an aggressive approach that does not allow the tendon to first eliminate the inflammatory response and then begin tissue realignment and remodeling will not allow the tendon to heal. This may potentially exacerbate the existing inflammation and lead to chronic inflammation. Thus, the rehabilitation progression must be slow and controlled, with full return when the patient is free of tendon pain.

Ankle Fractures and Dislocation

Pathomechanics and Injury Mechanism

When dealing with fractures of the ankle or tibial and fibular malleoli, the therapist must always be cautious about suspecting an ankle sprain when a fracture actually exists. A fracture of the malleoli will generally result in immediate swelling. Ankle fractures can occur from several mechanisms that are similar to those seen for ankle sprains. In an inversion injury, medial malleolar fractures are often accompanied by a sprain of the lateral ligaments of the ankle. A fracture of the lateral malleolus is often more likely to occur than a sprain if an eversion force is applied to the ankle. This is because the lateral malleolus extends as far as the distal aspect of the talus. With a fracture of the lateral malleolus, however, there may also be a sprain of the deltoid ligament. Fractures result from either avulsion or compression forces. With avulsion injuries, it is often the injured ligaments that prolong the rehabilitation period.[44]

Osteochondral fractures are sometimes seen in the talus. These fractures may also be referred to as dome fractures of the talus. Generally, they will be either nondisplaced or compression fractures.[44]

Although sprains and fractures are very common, dislocations in the ankle and foot are rare. They most often occur in conjunction with fractures and require open reduction and internal fixation.[98]

Rehabilitation Concerns

Generally, nondisplaced ankle fractures should be managed with rest and protection until the fracture has healed, whereas displaced fractures are treated with open reduction and internal fixation. Nondisplaced fractures are treated by casting the limb in a short-leg walking cast for 6 weeks with early weight bearing. The course of rehabilitation following this period of immobilization is generally the same as for ankle sprains. Following surgery for displaced or unstable fractures, the patient may be placed in a removable walking cast; however, it is essential to closely monitor the rehabilitation process to make certain that the patient is compliant.[44]

If an osteochondral fracture is displaced and there is a fragment, surgery is required to remove the fragment. In other cases, if the fragment has not healed within a year, surgery may be considered to remove the fragment.[44]

Rehabilitation Progression

Following open reduction and internal fixation, a posterior splint with the ankle in neutral should be applied, and the patient should be non-weight bearing for approximately 2 weeks. During this period efforts should be directed at controlling swelling and wound management.

At 2 to 3 weeks, the patient may be placed in a short-leg walking brace (see Figure 26-20), which allows for partial weight bearing, for 6 weeks. Active ROM plantarflexion and dorsiflexion exercises can begin and should be done 2 or 3 times a day, along with general strengthening exercises for the rest of the lower extremity.

At 6 weeks, the patient can be weight bearing in the walking brace and this should continue for 2 to 4 weeks more. Isometric exercises (see Exercises 26-1 to 26-4) can be performed initially without the brace, progressing to isotonic strengthening exercises (see Exercises 26-5 to 26-8 and 26-10), which concentrate on eccentrics. Stretching exercises

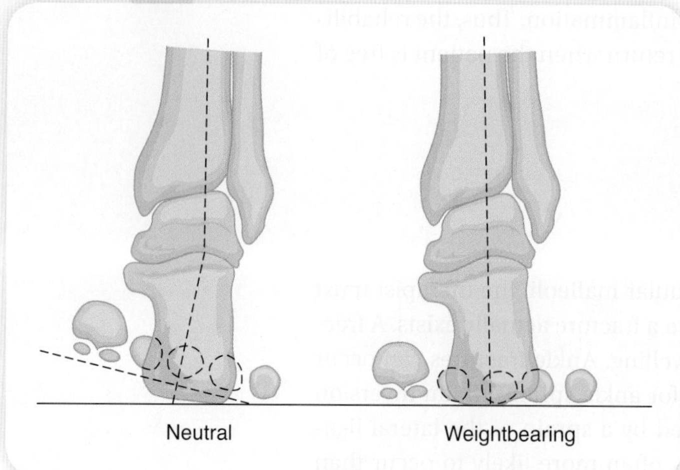

Figure 26-21 **Subtalar or calcaneal varus**

Comparing weightbearing neutral and resting positions.

can also be incorporated (see Exercises 26-11 and 26-25 to 26-29). If there are specific joint restrictions at the ankle and foot, mobilization techniques by a therapist may be used to reduce capsular tightness.

Exercises to regain proprioception and neuromuscular control, as previously described in the "Ankle Sprains" section, can be progress from sitting to standing and from stable to unstable surfaces as tolerated (see Exercises 26-25 and 26-31 to 26-35). As strength and neuromuscular control continue to increase, more functional, closed kinetic chain-strengthening activities can begin (see Exercises 26-14 to 26-18 and 26-36 to 26-39).

Excessive Pronation and Supination

Pathomechanics and Injury Mechanism

Often when we hear the terms *pronation* or *supination*, we automatically think of some pathological condition related to gait. It must be reemphasized that pronation and supination of the foot and STJ are normal movements that occur during the support phase of gait. However, if pronation or supination is excessive, delayed, or prolonged, overuse injuries may develop. Excessive or prolonged supination or pronation at the STJ is likely to result from some structural or functional deformity in the foot or leg. The structural deformity forces the STJ to compensate in a manner that will allow the weightbearing surfaces of the foot to make stable contact with the ground and get into a weightbearing position. Thus, excessive pronation or supination is a compensation for an existing structural deformity. Three of the most common structural deformities of the foot as previously described are subtalar or calcaneal varus (Figure 26-21), forefoot varus (Figure 26-22), and forefoot valgus (Figure 26-23).

Structural calcaneal varus and forefoot varus deformities are usually associated with excessive pronation. A structural forefoot valgus usually causes excessive supination. The deformities usually exist in 1 plane, but the triplane STJ will interfere with the normal functions of the foot and make it more difficult to act as a shock absorber, adapt to uneven surfaces, and act as a rigid lever for push off. The compensation rather than the deformity itself usually causes overuse injuries.

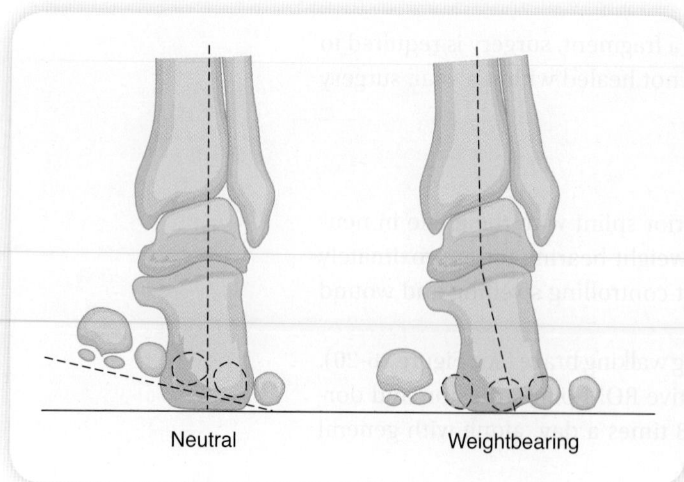

Figure 26-22 **Forefoot varus**

Comparing weightbearing neutral and resting positions.

Excessive, delayed, or prolonged pronation of the STJ during the support phase of running is a major cause of stress injuries. Overload of specific structures results when excessive pronation is produced in the support phase or when pronation is prolonged into the propulsive phase of running.

Excessive pronation during the support phase will cause compensatory STJ motion such that the MTJ remains unlocked, resulting in an excessively loose foot. There is also an increase in tibial rotation, which forces the knee joint to absorb more transverse rotation motion. Delayed or late pronation of the STJ is when the motion initially is not excessive, but because of the continued pronation during stance phase, a similar result exists as with excessive pronation. Prolonged pronation of the STJ will not allow the foot to resupinate in time to provide a rigid lever for push off, resulting in a less powerful and efficient force. Thus, various foot and leg problems will occur with excessive, delayed, or prolonged pronation during the support phase, including callus formation under the second metatarsal, stress fractures of the second metatarsal, bunions because of hypermobility of the first ray, plantar fasciitis, posterior tibial tendinitis, Achilles tendinitis, tibial stress syndrome, iliotibial band friction syndrome, or medial knee pain.

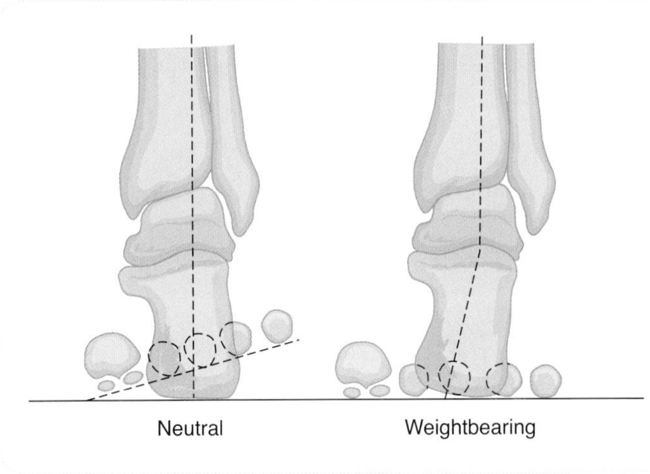

Figure 26-23 Forefoot valgus

Comparing weightbearing neutral and resting positions.

Several extrinsic keys may be observed that indicate disproportionate pronation,[97] including excessive eversion of the calcaneus during the stance phase (Figure 26-24) and excessive or prolonged internal rotation of the tibia. This internal rotation may cause increased symptoms in the shin or knee.[24] A lowering of the medial arch accompanies pronation. It may be measured as the navicular differential[71]—the difference between the height of the navicular tuberosity from the floor in a non-weightbearing position versus a weightbearing position (Figure 26-25). As previously discussed, the talus plantar flexes and adducts with pronation. This may present as a visually discernible medial bulging of the talar head (Figure 26-26). This same talar adduction causes increased concavity below the lateral malleolus in a posterior view while the calcaneus everts (Figure 26-27).[73]

Prolonged or excessive supination at heel strike and the resultant compensatory movement at the STJ will not allow the MTJ to unlock, causing the foot to remain excessively rigid. Thus, the foot cannot absorb the GRFs efficiently. Excessive supination limits tibial internal rotation. Injuries typically associated with excessive supination include fifth metatarsal stress fractures, Achilles tendinopathy, inversion ankle sprains, tibial stress syndrome, peroneal tendinitis, iliotibial band friction syndrome, or trochanteric bursitis.

Structural deformities originating outside the foot also require compensation by the foot for a proper weightbearing position to be attained. Tibial varum is the common bowleg deformity.[73] The distal tibia is medial to the proximal tibia (Figure 26-28).[28] This measurement is taken weight bearing with the foot in neutral position.[50] The angle of deviation

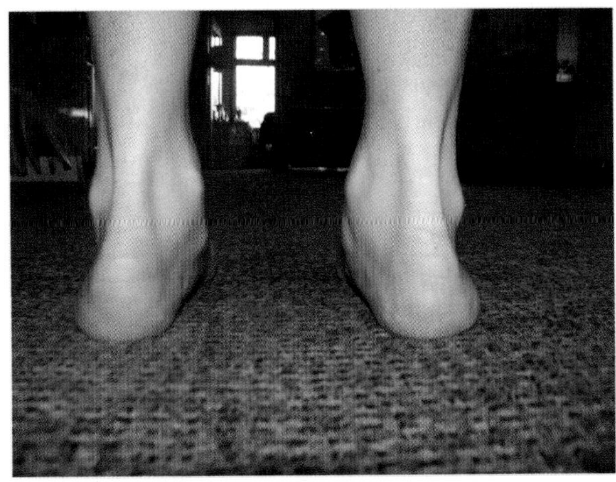

Figure 26-24 Eversion of the calcaneus, indicating pronation

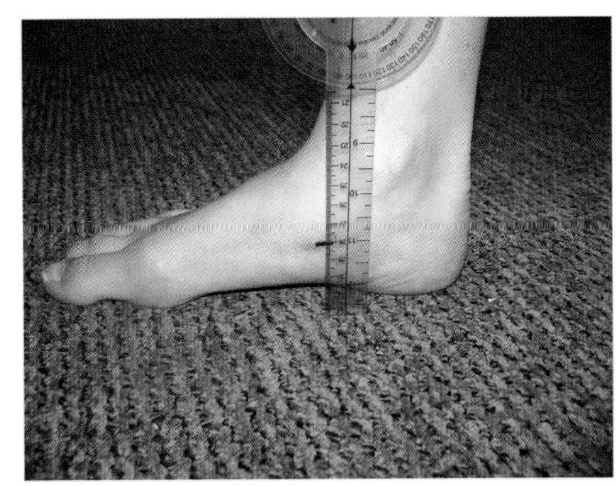

Figure 26-25 Measurement of the navicular differential

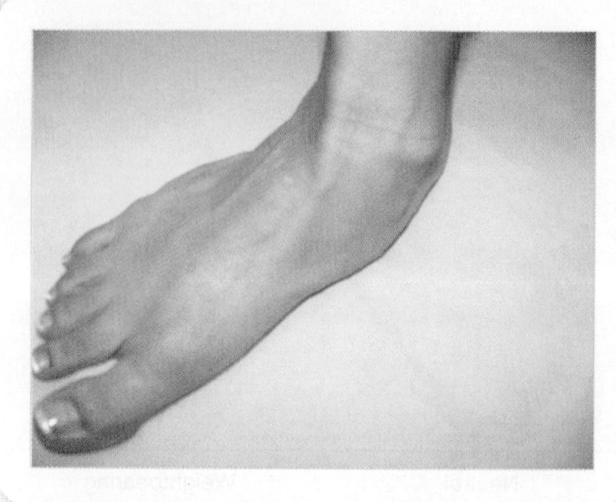

Figure 26-26 Medial bulge of the talar head of the left foot, indicating pronation

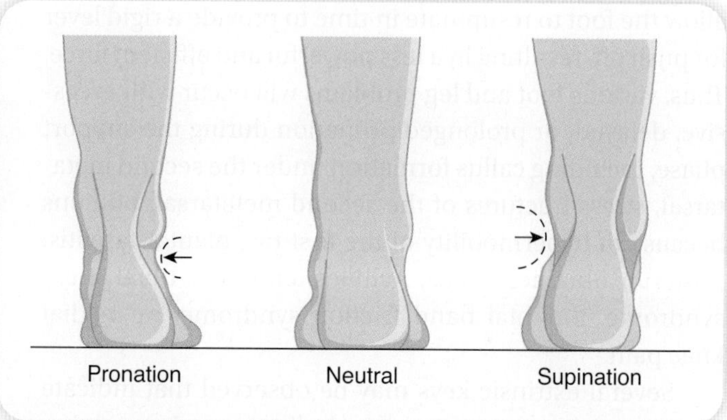

Figure 26-27 Concavity below the lateral malleolus, indicating pronation. Concavity below the medial malleolus, indicating supination

of the distal tibia from a perpendicular line from the calcaneal midline is considered tibial varum.[39] Tibial varum increases pronation to allow proper foot function.[13] At heel strike, the calcaneus must evert to attain a perpendicular position.[110]

Ankle joint equinus is another extrinsic deformity that may require abnormal compensation. It may be considered an extrinsic or intrinsic problem, but is typically a result of loss of talocrural joint ROM into dorsiflexion. The key compensator is the oblique MTJ. If the MTJ is hypermobile or unstable, there will be increased dorsiflexion and forefoot abduction at the MTJ. If the MTJ is hypomobile or stable, there will be early heel rise during propulsion with continued forced pronation.

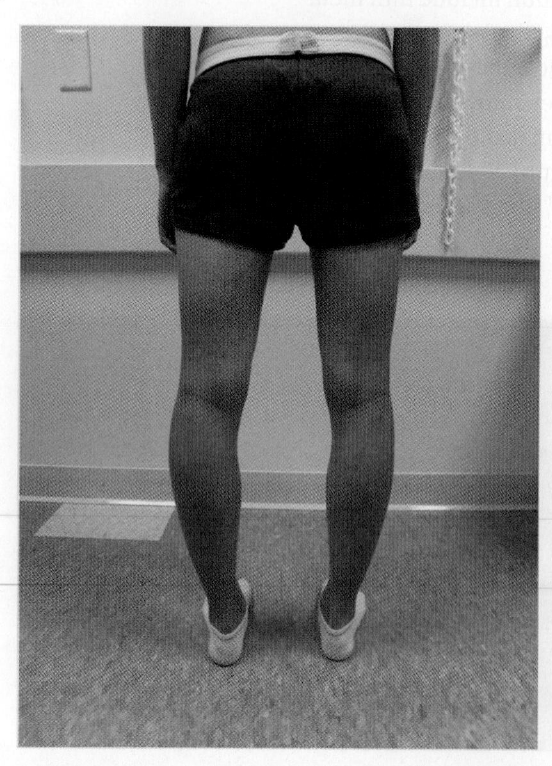

Figure 26-28 Tibial varum or bow-leg deformity

During normal gait, the tibia must move anterior to the talar dome. Approximately 10 degrees of dorsiflexion for walking and 15 to 20 degrees for running are required (Figure 26-29).[73] Lack of dorsiflexion may cause compensatory pronation of the foot with resultant foot and lower-extremity pain. Often, this lack of dorsiflexion results from tightness of the posterior leg muscles. Forefoot equinus, in which the plane of the forefoot is below the plane of the rearfoot, is another cause.[73] It occurs in many high-arched feet. This deformity requires more ankle dorsiflexion. When enough dorsiflexion is not available at the ankle, the additional movement is required at other sites, such as dorsiflexion of the MTJ and rotation of the leg.

Rehabilitation Concerns

In individuals who excessively pronate or supinate, the goal of treatment is quite simply to correct the faulty biomechanics that occur as a result of the existing structural deformity. An accurate biomechanical analysis of the foot and lower extremity should identify those deformities that require abnormal compensatory movements. In the majority of cases, faulty biomechanics can be corrected by constructing an appropriate orthotic device.

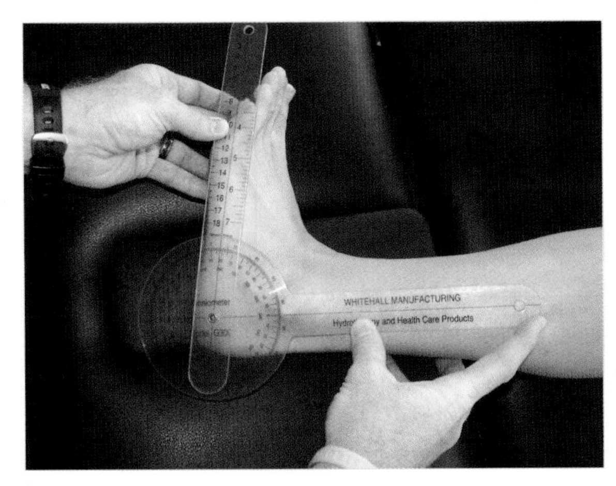

Figure 26-29 **Dorsiflexion of 10 degrees is necessary for normal walking gait**

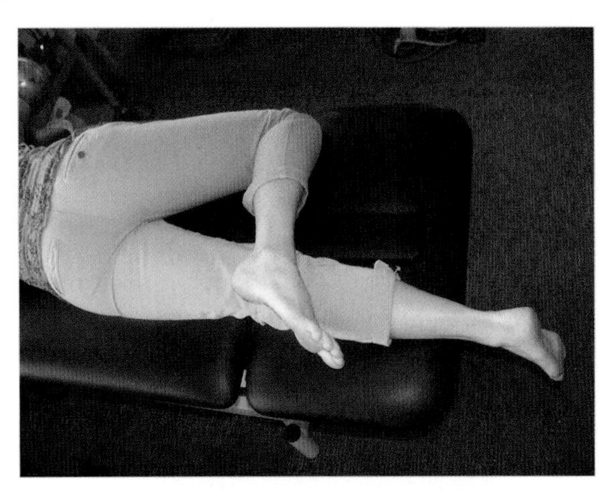

Figure 26-30 **Examination position for STJN position**

Despite arguments in the literature, the authors have found orthotic therapy to be of tremendous value in the treatment of many lower-extremity problems. This view is supported in the literature by several clinical studies. Donatelli[28] found that 96% of patients reported pain relief from orthotics and 52% would not leave home without the devices in their shoes. McPoil et al found that orthotics were an important treatment for valgus forefoot deformities only.[72] Riegler reported that 80% of patients experienced at least a 50% improvement with orthotics.[93] This same study reported improvements in sports performance with orthotics. Hunt reported decreased muscular activity with orthotics.[50]

The process for evaluating the foot biomechanically, constructing an orthotic device, and selecting the appropriate footwear is given in detail in next section.

Examination The first step in the evaluation process is to establish a position of STJN. The patient should be prone with the distal third of the leg hanging off the end of the table (Figure 26-30). A line should be drawn bisecting the posterior lower leg and posterior calcaneus (Figure 26-31).[112] With the patient still prone and the left foot as the example, the therapist palpates the talus with the right hand while the forefoot is inverted or everted using the left hand. One finger should palpate the talus near the anterior aspect of the fibula and the thumb near the anterior portion of the medial malleolus (Figure 26-32). The position at which the talus is equally prominent on both sides is considered neutral subtalar position.[54] Root et al[97] describe this as the position of the STJ where it is neither pronated or supinated. It is the standard position in which the foot should be placed to examine deformities.[84] In this position, the lines on the lower leg and calcaneus should form a straight line. Any variance is considered to be a rearfoot valgus or varus deformity. The most common deformity of the foot is a rearfoot varus deformity.[77] A varus deviation of 2 to 3 degrees is normal.[117]

Another method of determining STJN position involves using the lines that were drawn on the leg and back of the heel in a different manner. With the patient prone, the calcaneus is moved into full eversion and inversion, with angle measurements taken at the end range of each position. Neutral position is then considered to be two-thirds of the total STJ ROM away from maximum inversion or one-third of the total STJ motion away from maximum eversion. For example, from a neutral position, if the foot inverts 27 degrees and everts 3 degrees, the total STJ ROM equals 30 degrees. Thus, the position at which this foot is neither pronated nor supinated is that point at which the calcaneus is inverted 7 degrees,

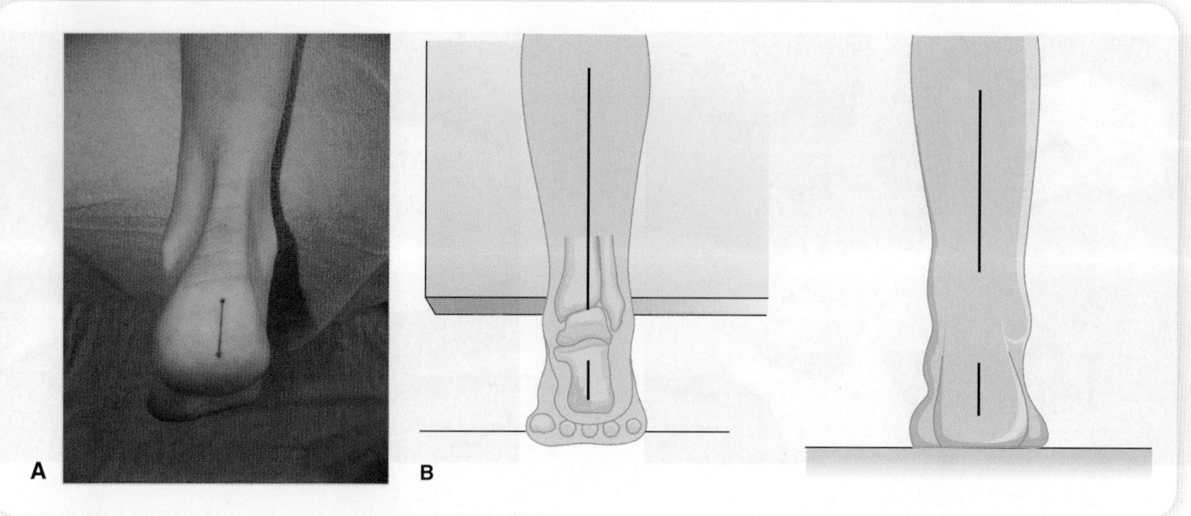

Figure 26-31

A. Line bisecting the posterior leg and calcaneus. **B.** Comparing non–weightbearing neutral to weightbearing resting position. (Figure used with permission from Brian Hoke, American Physical Rehabilitation Network.)

which is calculated by subtracting 20 degrees (two-thirds of 30 degrees) from maximal inversion (27 degrees). The normal foot pronates 6 to 8 degrees from neutral.[97]

Once the STJ is placed in a neutral position, mild dorsiflexion should be applied to the forefoot at the fifth metatarsophalangeal joint while observing the metatarsal heads (specifically second to fifth) in relation to the plantar surface of the calcaneus. First metatarsal position is evaluated independently of the other metatarsals. Forefoot varus is an osseous deformity in which the medial metatarsal heads are inverted in relation to the plane of the calcaneus (see Figure 26-22). Forefoot varus is the most common cause of excessive pronation, according to Subotnick.[108] Forefoot valgus is a position in which the lateral metatarsals are everted in relation to the rearfoot (see Figure 26-23). These forefoot deformities benign in a non-weightbearing position, but in stance the foot or metatarsal heads must somehow get to the floor to bear weight. This compensated movement is accomplished by the talus rolling down and in and the calcaneus everting for a forefoot varus. For the forefoot valgus, the calcaneus inverts and the talus abducts and dorsiflexes. McPoil et al[73] report that forefoot valgus is the most common forefoot deformity in their sample group.

In a calcaneal varus deformity, when the foot is in STJN position non-weight bearing, the calcaneus is in an inverted position; however, the metatarsals are still in a relative perpendicular position to the calcaneus. To get to foot flat in weight bearing, the STJ must pronate (see Figure 26-21). Minimal osseous deformities of the forefoot have little effect on the function of the foot. When either forefoot varus or valgus is too large, the foot compensates through abnormal movements to bear weight.

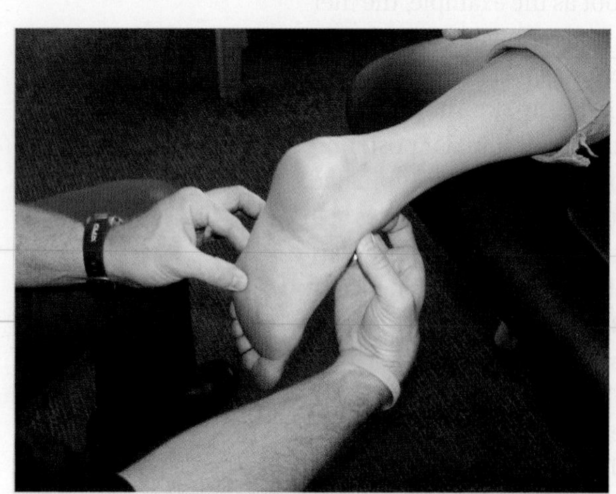

Figure 26-32 Palpation of the talus to determine STJN position

Further consideration for the position and mobility of the first ray is necessary. The first ray in relationship to the remainder of the metatarsals can either be dorsiflexed, neutral, or plantarflexed. Clinically, a neutral or plantarflexed first ray is most commonly seen. Mobility of the first ray is an important predictor in pathomechanics and injury mechanism.[2,3] For example, a rigid plantarflexed first ray will respond differently in weight bearing than a mobile plantarflexed first ray. This distinction in mobility is important when making recommendations for orthosis fabrication in regard to forefoot correction. With a flexible first ray, a medial post may be used directly under the first ray only. With a more rigid first ray, medial posting material will extend more laterally to encompass additional metatarsals (Figure 26-33). There is further discussion on specific orthotic construction in the section entitled Orthosis Materials and Fabrication.

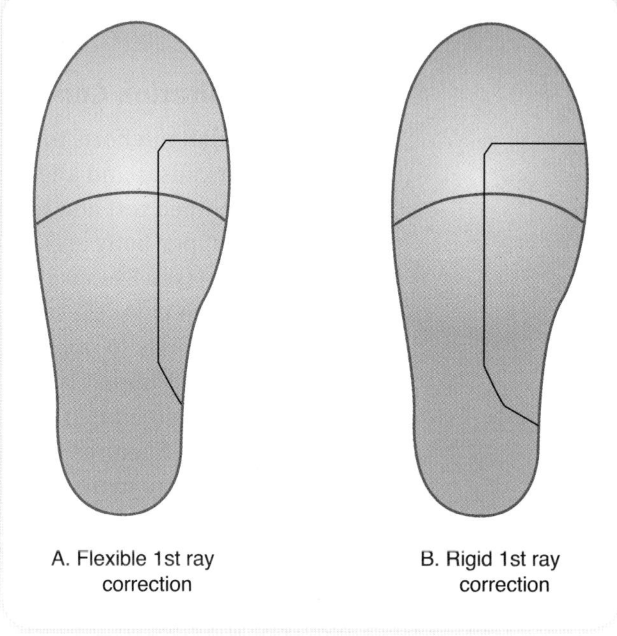

Figure 26-33 **First ray correction for a foot orthosis**

Stress Fractures in the Foot

Pathomechanics and Injury Mechanism

The most common stress fractures in the foot involve the navicular, second metatarsal (March fracture), and diaphysis of the fifth metatarsal (Jones fracture). Navicular and second metatarsal stress fractures are likely to occur with excessive foot pronation, whereas fifth metatarsal stress fractures tend to occur in a more rigid pes cavus foot.

Navicular Stress Fractures Individuals who excessively pronate during running gait are likely to develop a stress fracture of the navicular. This is attributed most commonly to individuals with either a compensated calcaneal and/or forefoot varus. Because of the compensatory movement and increased stress at the talonavicular joint of the tarsal bones, it is most likely to have a stress fracture.

Second Metatarsal Stress Fractures Second metatarsal stress fractures occur most often in running and jumping sports. As is the case with other injuries in the foot associated with overuse, the most common causes include calcaneal varus and/or forefoot varus structural deformities in the foot that result in excessive pronation, flexible first ray, training errors, changes in training surfaces, and wearing inappropriate shoes. The base of the second metatarsal extends proximally into the distal row of tarsal bones and is held rigid and stable by the bony architecture and ligament support. In addition, the second metatarsal is particularly subjected to increased stress with excessive pronation, which causes a hypermobile foot. In addition, if the second metatarsal is longer than the first, as seen with a Morton toe, it is theoretically subjected to greater bone stress during running. A bone scan, as opposed to a standard radiograph, is frequently necessary for diagnosis.

Fifth Metatarsal Stress Fractures Fifth metatarsal stress fractures can occur from overuse, acute inversion, or high-velocity rotational forces. A Jones fracture occurs at the diaphysis of the fifth metatarsal most often as a sequela of a stress fracture.[98] The patient will complain of a sharp pain on the lateral border of the foot and will usually report hearing a "pop." Because of documented poor blood supply and a history of delayed healing, a Jones fracture may result in nonunion, requiring an extended period of rehabilitation. A common foot type seen with this injury is more of a supinatory foot, or those patients with a forefoot valgus or a rigid plantarflexed first ray. The patient spends more time laterally, thus increasing stresses to the fifth metatarsal. As previously mentioned, this injury has been cited in the literature as a possible result of transitioning to barefoot or minimalistic footwear too quickly.[42,75]

Rehabilitation Concerns

Rehabilitation efforts for stress fractures should focus on determining the precipitating cause or causes and alleviating them. Second metatarsal stress fractures tend to do well with modified rest and non–weightbearing exercises, such as pool running (see Exercise 26-40), upper-body ergometer (see Exercise 26-41), stationary bike (see Exercise 26-42), or NuStep (see Exercise 26-43) to maintain the patient's cardiorespiratory fitness for 2 to 4 weeks. An elliptical trainer may be utilized to transition the patient from non-weightbearing activity to nonimpact weightbearing exercise. This is followed by a progressive return to full-impact activities of running and jumping functional activities over a 2- to 3-week period, potentially using appropriately constructed orthoses and modified footwear. Stress fractures of both the navicular of the proximal shaft of the fifth metatarsal usually require more aggressive treatment; requiring non–weightbearing short-leg casts for 6 to 8 weeks for nondisplaced fractures. With cases of delayed union, nonunion, or especially displaced fractures, both the Jones and navicular fractures require internal fixation, with or without bone grafting. In the highly active patient, immediate internal fixation should be recommended.

Plantar Fasciitis/Fasciosis

Pathomechanics

Heel pain is a very common problem that may be attributed to several etiologies, including heel spurs, plantar fascia irritation (acute or chronic), and bursitis. Plantar fasciitis is a "catch-all term" that is commonly used to describe pain in the proximal arch and heel. However, when truly defining whether someone has plantar fasciitis, it is important to consider the absence or presence of inflammation. If histologic findings indicate the presence of inflammation, the diagnosis of plantar fasciitis is appropriate and subsequent treatment appropriate for acute inflammation should be considered.[21] However, if findings include myxoid degeneration with fragmentation and degeneration of the plantar fascia, as well as bone marrow vascular ectasia, the diagnosis can be made of degenerative fasciosis without inflammation, not fasciitis.[63] Thus, treatment intervention should be varied when treating chronic versus acute conditions.

The plantar fascia (plantar aponeurosis) runs the length of the sole of the foot. It is a broad band of dense connective tissue that is attached proximally to the medial surface of the calcaneus. It fans out distally, with fibers and their various small branches attaching to the metatarsophalangeal articulations and merging into the capsular ligaments. Other fibers, arising from well within the aponeurosis, pass between the intrinsic muscles of the foot and the long flexor tendons of the sole and attach themselves to the deep fascia below the bones. The function of the plantar aponeurosis is to assist in maintaining the stability of the foot and in securing or bracing the longitudinal arch.[112]

Tension develops in the plantar fascia both during extension of the toes and depression of the longitudinal arch as the result of weight bearing. When the weight is principally on the heel, as in ordinary standing, the tension exerted on the fascia is negligible. However, when the weight is shifted to the ball of the foot (on the heads of the metatarsals), fascial tension is increased. In running, because the push-off phase involves both a forceful extension of the toes and a powerful push-off thrust off the metatarsal heads, fascial tension is increased to approximately twice the BW.

Patients who have a mild pes cavus foot type are particularly prone to fascial strain. Modern street shoes, by nature of their design, take on the characteristics of splints and tend to restrict foot action to such an extent that the arch may become somewhat rigid. This occurs because of shortening of the ligaments and other mild abnormalities. The patient, when changing from dress shoes to softer, more flexible athletic shoes, often develops irritation of the plantar fascia. Trauma may also result from poor running technique or improper running footwear. Excessive lumbar lordosis—a condition in which an increased forward tilt of the pelvis produces an unfavorable angle of foot strike when there is considerable force exerted on the ball of the foot—can also contribute to this problem.

Injury Mechanism

A number of anatomic and biomechanical conditions have been studied as possible causes of plantar fasciitis. They include leg-length discrepancy, excessive pronation of the STJ, inflexibility of the longitudinal arch, and tightness of the gastrocnemius–soleus unit. Wearing shoes without sufficient arch support, an overlengthened stride during running, transition to midfoot or forefoot landing pattern too quickly, and running on soft surfaces are also potential causes of plantar fasciitis.

The patient complains of pain in the anteromedial aspect of the heel, usually at the attachment of the plantar fascia to the calcaneus, which eventually moves more centrally into the central portion of the plantar fascia. This pain is particularly troublesome upon arising in the morning or upon bearing weight after sitting for a prolonged period of time. However, the pain typically decreases after a few steps. Pain also will be intensified when the toes and forefoot are forcibly dorsiflexed, particularly with terminal stance phase in weight bearing.

Rehabilitation Concerns

With respect to the treatment of heel pain or plantar fasciitis/fasciosis, research has not indicated any consensus on a specific treatment regimen that has proven to resolve heel pain with any statistical significance. However, Gill[41] states that there is agreement that nonsurgical treatment is ultimately effective in approximately 90% of patients. Despite the uncertainty in the literature regarding a specific treatment, there are several different interventions that have proven to be beneficial in the acute and chronic management of heel pain.

Orthotic therapy is very useful in the treatment of this problem. The authors have found that semiflexible orthoses addressing the patient's specific biomechanical and structural concerns, in combination with exercises, can significantly reduce the pain level of these patients (Figure 26-34).

A semiflexible orthosis tends to be more effective than a rigid orthotic device, particularly in a more active patient or athlete, because it allows for forefoot and rearfoot correction for decreasing pathomechanical compensation with appropriate shock absorption. An extra-deep heel cup could also be built into the orthosis to provide improved calcaneal and subsequent STJ control. The orthosis should be worn at all times, especially upon arising from bed in the morning. The patient should be encouraged to wear a supportive shoe with the prescribed orthosis, rather than ambulating barefooted.[14] When soft orthoses are not feasible, longitudinal arch taping may reduce the symptoms. A simple arch taping or alternative taping technique often allows pain-free ambulation.[120] For those patients who have a distended calcaneal fat pad, the use of a heel cup will help to reapproximate the lateral margins of the fat pad under the calcaneus, reestablishing the natural cushion under the area of irritation.

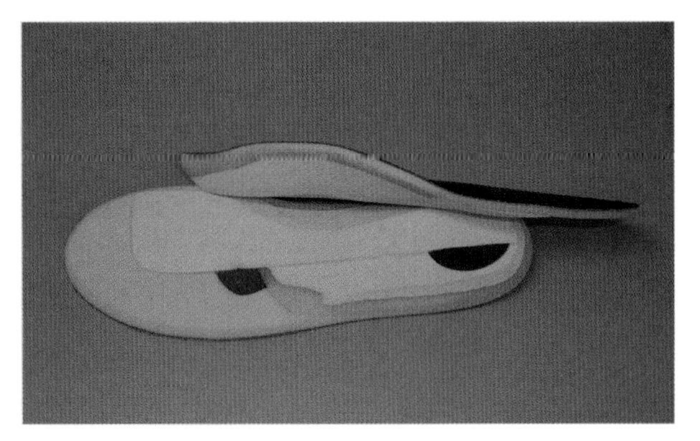

Figure 26-34 Semiflexible full-length custom orthosis

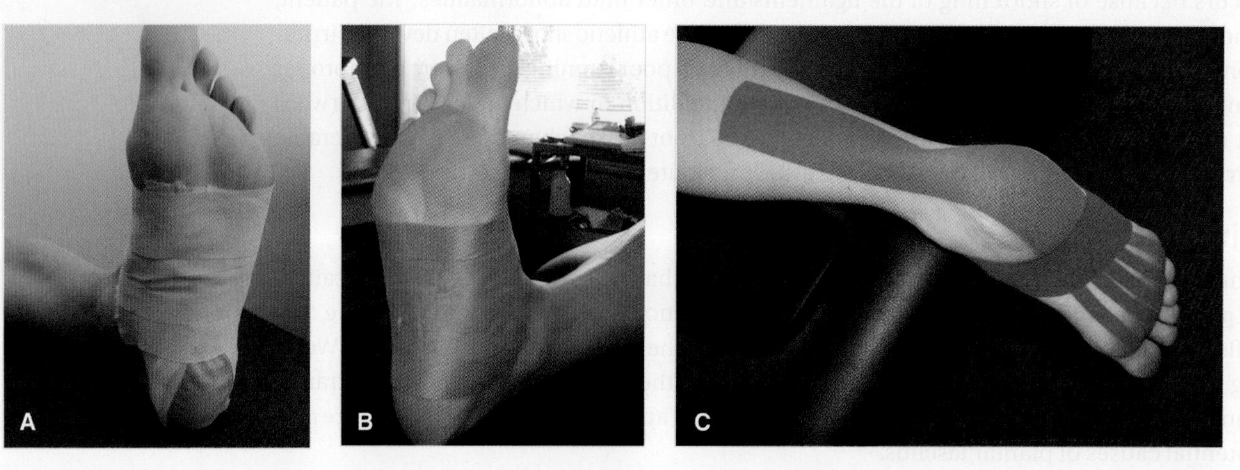

Figure 26-35

A. Low-dye arch taping. **B.** Leukotape P taping technique. **C.** Kinesiotape technique.

The use of low-dye longitudinal arch taping[121] (Figure 26-35*A*) or Leukotape P technique (Figure 26-35*B*) has been shown to unload the plantar aponeurosis in weightbearing situations. Kinesio TEX can be utilized for pain management (Figure 26-35*C*) as described by the Kinesio Taping Method. In more chronic or severe cases, it may be necessary to use a night splint to maintain a position of static stretch while sleeping or a short-leg walking cast during the day for 4 to 6 weeks.

Pain-free heel cord stretching should be used, along with an exercise to stretch the plantar fascia in the arch (see Exercises 26-30*B* and *C*) if these tissues are tight. During the acute phase, or if there is pain with passive stretching of heel cords or plantar fascia, dynamic stretching can be done (see Exercises 26-28). Exercises or manual therapy techniques that help to increase dorsiflexion of the great toe also may be of benefit to this problem (see Exercises 26-26 and 26-30*A*). Passive stretching should be performed using the principle of a low load, prolonged stretch and performed at least 3 times a day.[100] Effective stretching is most effective with "consistency versus intensity."

As for the use of antiinflammatory intervention, it is important to consider the stage of healing (acute versus chronic). In the acute phase, nonsteroidal antiinflammatory medications may be beneficial. Steroidal injection may be warranted at some point if symptoms fail to resolve, although review of the literature is inconclusive as to the efficacy of injections for long-term benefits.[1,34,38,62,63,74,85,86,88,101] Concerns regarding the use of steroid injection for management of heel pain or plantar fasciitis or fasciosis include the potential for calcaneal fat pad deterioration, plantar fascia rupture, decreased plantar fascia tension, reduced arch height, ineffectiveness of subsequent extracorporeal shock wave therapy, and the potential development of several other foot problems.[1,62,85,86] Lemont[63] suggests that treatment regimens, such as corticosteroid injections into the plantar fascia, should be reevaluated in the absence of inflammation.

Other possible interventions include ultrasound, iontophoresis with acetic acid or dexamethasone, extracorporeal shock wave therapy, or surgery. Preliminary research in the literature has shown that extracorporeal shock wave therapy has been successful in managing plantar fasciosis.[74,86,91]

Management of plantar fasciitis generally requires an extended period of treatment. It is not uncommon for symptoms to persist for as long as 8 to 12 weeks. Persistence on the part of the patient in doing the recommended stretching and foot intrinsic strengthening exercises is critical, along with addressing any biomechanical or structural concerns. As with many of the foot and ankle injuries cited in this chapter, orthotic therapy, activity modification, appropriate footwear, and addressing any proximal neuromusculoskeletal concerns are also keys to successfully managing plantar fasciitis or fasciosis.

Cuboid Subluxation

Pathomechanics and Injury Mechanism

A condition that often mimics plantar fasciitis is cuboid subluxation. Pronation and trauma have been reported to be prominent causes of this syndrome.[119] Displacement of the cuboid causes pain along the fourth and fifth metatarsals, as well as directly over the cuboid. The primary reason for pain is the stress placed on the long peroneal muscle when the foot is in pronation. In this position, the long peroneal muscle allows the cuboid bone to move downward and medially. This problem often refers pain to the heel area as well. Many times this pain is increased upon arising after a prolonged non-weightbearing period.

Rehabilitation Considerations

Dramatic treatment results may be obtained by manipulation technique to restore the cuboid to its natural position. The manipulation is done with the patient prone (Figure 26-36*A*). The plantar aspect of the forefoot is grasped by the thumbs with the fingers supporting the dorsum of the foot. The thumbs should be over the cuboid. The manipulation should be a thrust downward to move the cuboid into its more dorsal position. Often a pop is felt as the cuboid moves back into place. Once the cuboid is manipulated, an orthosis or taping technique is required to support it in its proper position (Figure 26-36*B*).

If manipulation is successful, quite often the patient can return to normal function immediately with little or no pain. It should be recommended that the patient wears an appropriately constructed orthosis to reduce the chances of recurrence, along with specific foot intrinsic strengthening exercises (see Exercise 26-13).

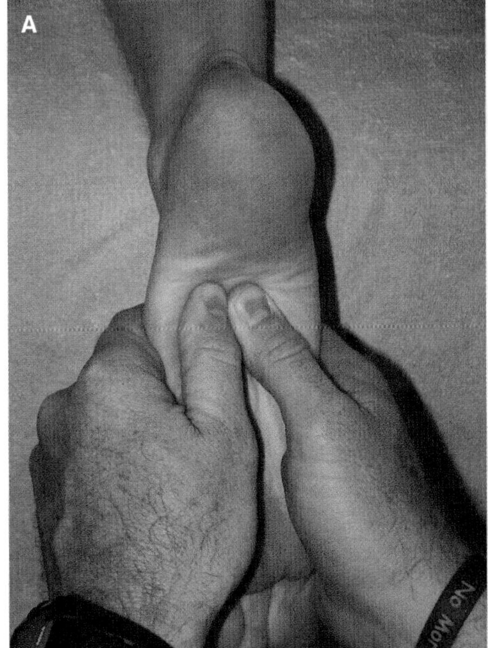

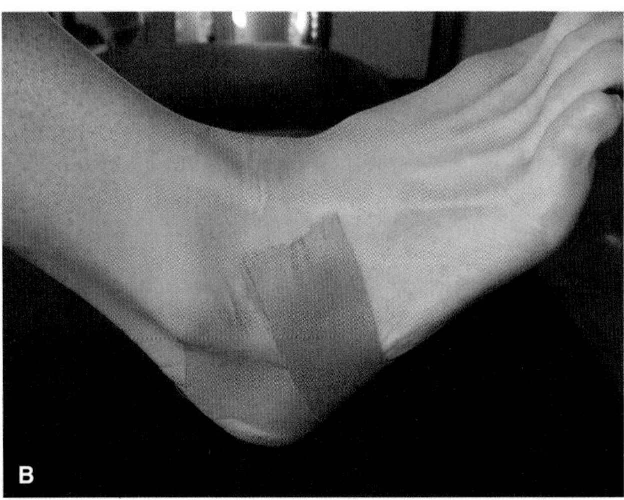

Figure 26-36

A. Prone position for cuboid manipulation.
B. Corrective cuboid taping technique.

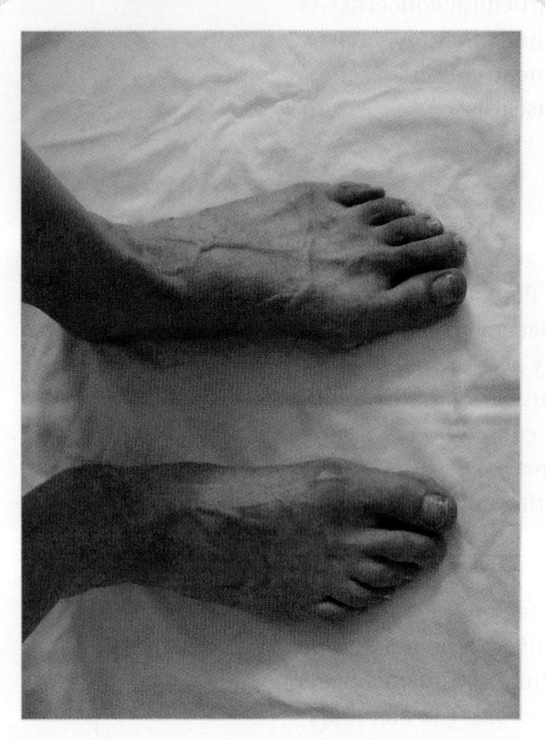

Figure 26-37 Hallux valgus deformity with a bunion

Peelen describes an alternate way of manipulating a subluxated cuboid using a specific sequence for mobilizing the other bones of the foot first in order to effectively remobilize the cuboid. He states that it is rare that only 1 or 2 bones of the foot are dysfunctional in isolation. By first mobilizing the talus, calcaneus, navicular, cuneiforms, and metatarsals, the necessary space to reduce the cuboid under the distal lip of the calcaneus is achieved.[87]

Hallux Valgus Deformity (Bunions)

Pathomechanics and Injury Mechanism

A bunion is a deformity of the head of the first metatarsal in which the large toe assumes a valgus position (Figure 26-37). A bunion is commonly associated with a structural forefoot varus or flexible first ray. The result of the outward splaying of the first ray is an increased pressure on the first metatarsal head. The bursa over the first metatarsophalangeal joint becomes inflamed and eventually thickens. The joint becomes enlarged and the great toe becomes malaligned, moving laterally toward the second toe, sometimes to such an extent that it eventually overlaps the second toe. This type of bunion may also be associated with a depressed or flattened transverse arch. Often the bunion occurs from wearing shoes that are pointed, too narrow, too short, or have high heels.

A bunion is one of the most frequent painful deformities of the great toe. As the bunion is developing, there is typically associated tenderness, swelling, and enlargement with calcification of the head of the first metatarsal. Shoes that fit poorly can increase the irritation and pain of the bunion.

Rehabilitation Concerns

Prevention is the key; however if the condition progresses, a custom orthosis is recommended to help normalize foot mechanics. Often an orthotic designed to correct a structural fore-foot varus or flexible first ray can help increase stability and significantly reduce the symptoms and progression of a bunion. Shoe selection may also play an important role in the treatment of bunions. Shoes of the proper width cause less mechanical irritation to the bunion. Local therapy, including moist heat, soaks, iontophoresis, or ultrasound, may alleviate some of the acute symptoms of a bunion. Protective devices, such as wedges, pads, and tape, can also be used. Surgery to correct the hallux valgus deformity is very common during the later stages of this condition, but the potential of postoperative stiffness or loss of motion is a concern.

Morton Neuroma

Pathomechanics and Injury Mechanism

A neuroma is a mass occurring about the nerve sheath of the common plantar nerve while it divides into the 2 digital branches to adjacent toes. It occurs most commonly between the metatarsal heads and is the most common nerve problem of the lower extremity. A Morton neuroma is located between the third and fourth metatarsal heads where the nerve is the thickest, receiving both branches from the medial and lateral plantar nerves. The patient complains of severe intermittent pain radiating from the distal metatarsal heads to the tips of the toes and is often relieved when non-weight bearing. Irritation increases with the collapse of the transverse arch of the foot, putting the transverse metatarsal ligaments under stretch and thus compressing the common digital nerve and vessels. Excessive foot pronation can also be a predisposing factor, with more metatarsal shearing forces occurring with the prolonged forefoot abduction.

The patient complains of a burning paresthesia in the forefoot that is often localized to the third web space and radiating to the toes.[110] Hyperextension of the toes on weightbearing—as in squatting, stair climbing, or running—can increase the symptoms. Wearing shoes with a narrow toe box or high heels can increase the symptoms. If there is prolonged nerve irritation, the pain can become constant. A bone scan is often necessary to rule out a metatarsal stress fracture.

Rehabilitation Concerns

Orthotic therapy is essential to reduce the shearing movements of the metatarsal heads. To reduce this shearing effect, often either a metatarsal bar is placed just proximal to the metatarsal heads or a teardrop-shaped pad is placed between the heads of the third and fourth metatarsals in an attempt to have these splay apart with weightbearing (Figure 26-38). The goal of the orthosis with placement of additional pads such as these is to decrease pressure on the affected area.

Therapeutic modalities such as ultrasound or iontophoresis can be used to help reduce inflammation. Shoe selection also plays an important role in treatment of neuromas. Narrow shoes, particularly women's shoes that are pointed in the toe area and certain men's boots, may squeeze the metatarsal heads together and exacerbate the problem. A shoe that is wide in the toe-box area should be selected. A straight-laced shoe often provides increased space in the toe box.[103] Firm-soled, inflexible shoes (such as clogs) can assist in managing this problem by inhibiting hyperextension of the toes during gait. Often, appropriate soft orthotic padding or a gel pad will markedly reduce pain. On a rare occasion surgical excision may be required.

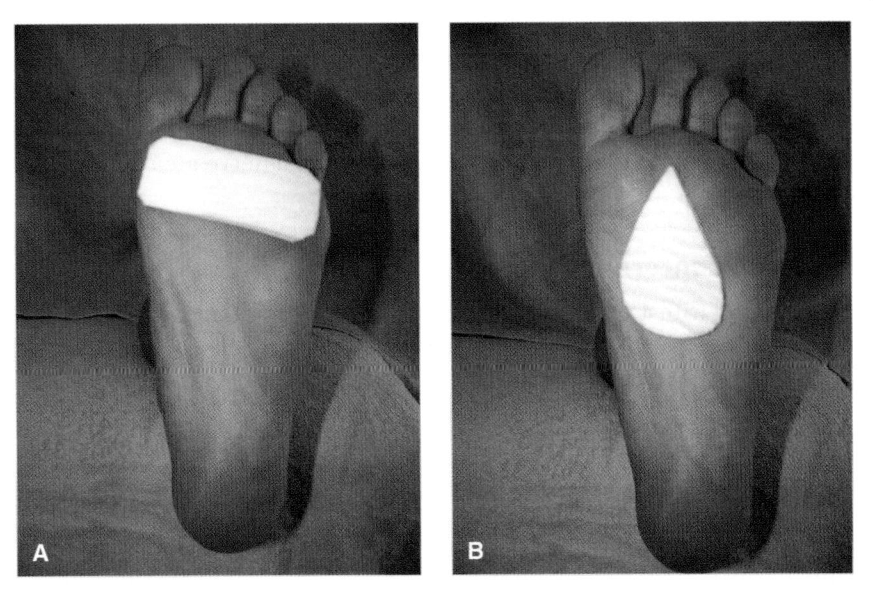

Figure 26-38

A. Metatarsal bar. **B.** Teardrop pad.

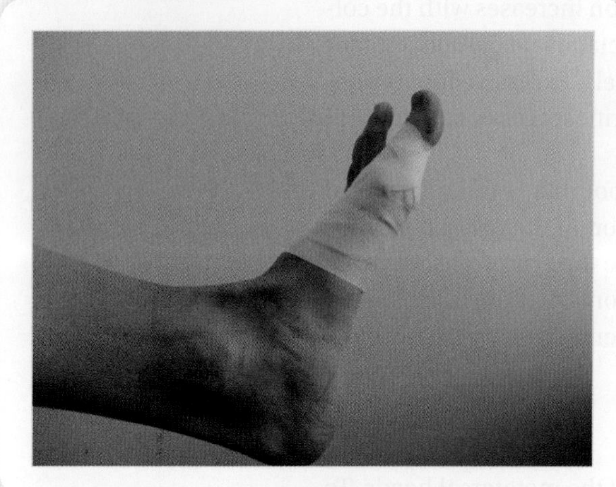

Figure 26-39 Turf toe taping

Turf Toe

Pathomechanics and Injury Mechanism

Turf toe is a hyperextension injury that usually occurs in the athletic population and results in a sprain of the metatarsophalangeal joint of the great toe, either from repetitive overuse or trauma.[116] Typically, this injury occurs on unyielding synthetic turf, although it can occur on grass or hard court surfaces as well. Many of these injuries occur because artificial turf shoes often are more flexible and allow more dorsiflexion of the great toe.

Rehabilitation Concerns

Some shoe companies have addressed this problem by adding steel or other materials to the forefoot of their turf shoes to stiffen them. Flat insoles that have thin sheets of steel under the forefoot are also available. When commercially made products are not available, a thin, flat piece of Orthoplast may be placed under the shoe insole or may be molded to the foot.[116] Taping the toe to prevent dorsiflexion may be done separately or with one of the shoe-stiffening suggestions (Figure 26-39).

Modalities of choice include ice, iontophoresis, and ultrasound. One key component for the acute management for turf toe is rest and protection.

In less-severe cases, patient can continue normal activities with the addition of a rigid insole. With more severe sprains, 3 to 4 weeks may be required for pain to reduce to the point where the patient can push off on the great toe.

Tarsal Tunnel Syndrome

Pathomechanics and Injury Mechanism

The tarsal tunnel is a loosely defined area about the medial malleolus that is bordered by the retinaculum, which binds the tibial nerve.[40] Overpronation, overuse conditions, and trauma may cause neurovascular problems in the ankle and foot. Symptoms may vary with pain, numbness, and paresthesia reported along the medial ankle and into the sole of the foot.[9] Tenderness may be present over the tibial nerve area behind the medial malleolus.

Rehabilitation Concerns

Neutral foot control with a custom orthosis may alleviate symptoms in less involved cases. Surgery is often performed if symptoms do not respond to conservative treatment or if weakness occurs in the flexors of the toes.[9]

Rehabilitation Techniques Summary

The ankle and foot can be a complicated and confusing region to manage with success. Thus, with any ankle or foot injury, it is important to "treat what you find," and evaluate "above and below" the joint. Furthermore, address any imbalances in strength, flexibility, mobility, or neuromuscular control both proximally and distally, as well as biomechanical and gait considerations. Finally, help the patient to help themselves with the skills and knowledge available to reach their functional goals.

Orthosis and Footwear Recommendations

Philosophy of Orthotic Therapy

Almost all problems of the lower extremity have been treated using orthotic therapy. The use of an orthosis (commonly referred to as "orthotic") for control of foot deformities has been recommended by various health care professionals for many years.[7,20,22,29,40,54,95,108,110,118] The normal foot functions most efficiently when no deformities are present that predispose it to injury or exacerbation of existing injuries. Orthoses are used to control abnormal compensatory movements of the foot by "bringing the floor to the foot."[51]

The foot functions most efficiently in an STJN position. By providing support so that the foot does not have to move abnormally, an orthosis should help prevent compensatory problems.

For problems that have already occurred, the orthosis provides a platform of support so that soft tissues can heal properly without undue stress. In summary, the goal is to create a biomechanically balanced kinetic chain by using a device capable of controlling motion pathology in the foot and leg by maintaining the foot in or close to STJN position. Basically, there are 2 types of orthoses:

- Biomechanical orthosis—a hard device (Figure 26-40) or semiflexible device (see Figures 26-34 and 26-41) capable of controlling movement-related pathology by attempting to guide the foot into functioning at or near STJN. This device consists of a shell (or module) that is either rigid or flexible with noncompressible posting (wedges) angled in degrees that will address both forefoot and rearfoot deformities (Figure 26-42). The rigid style shell is fabricated from carbon graphite, acrylic Rohadur, or (polyethylene) hard plastic. The control acquired is high, while shock absorption is sacrificed somewhat. The flexible shell is fabricated from thermoplastic, rubber, or leather and is the preferred device for the more active or sports-specific patient. The semirigid device takes advantage of various types of materials that provide both shock absorption and motion control under increased loading while retaining their original shape. The rigid devices take the opposite approach and are designed to firmly restrain foot motion and alter its position with nonyielding materials. Both the rigid and flexible shells are molded from a neutral cast and allow control for most overuse symptoms.[2,3,51,66,110]
- Accommodative orthosis—a device that does not attempt to establish foot function around the STJN but instead allows the foot to compensate. These devices are designed for patients who are deemed to be poor candidates for biomechanical control because of congenital malformations, restricted motions at foot or leg, neuromuscular dysfunctions, insensitive feet, illness, or physiologic old age. The materials used to fabricate the shell are softer that will yield to foot forces rather than resist them. Compressible wedges are used to bias the foot.[2,3]

Although not considered a true orthosis, oftentimes pads and soft, flexible felt or gel supports (Figure 26-43) can be readily fabricated for situations when shoe space is compromised (eg, running spikes) or when shoes are not worn (eg, ballet dancing). This type of foot correction is advocated for mild overuse syndromes.

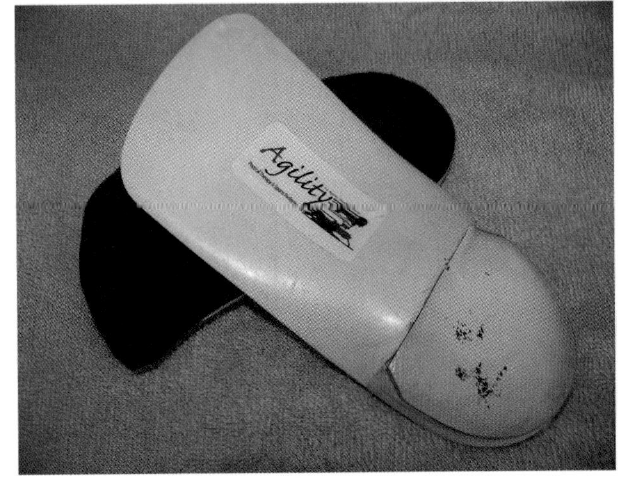

Figure 26-40 Hard orthosis

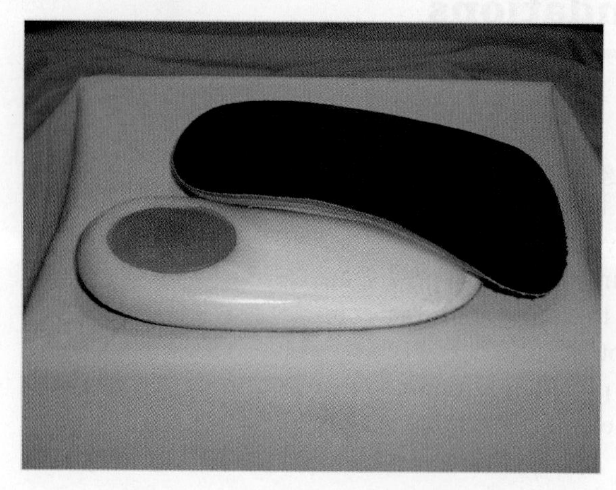

Figure 26-41 Semiflexible three-quarter–length custom orthosis

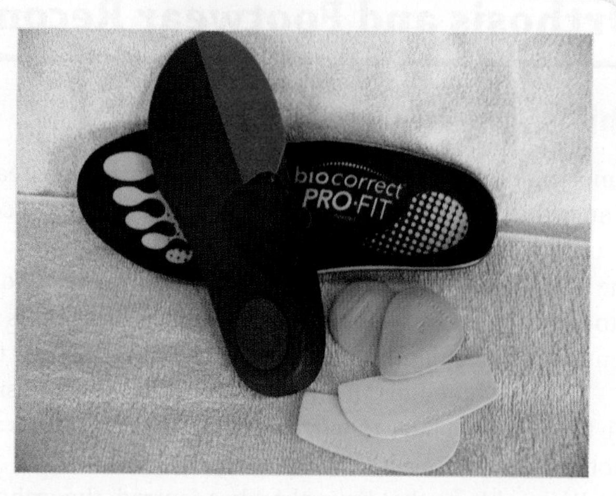

Figure 26-42 Foot orthosis semiflexible shell with noncompressible posting attached underneath

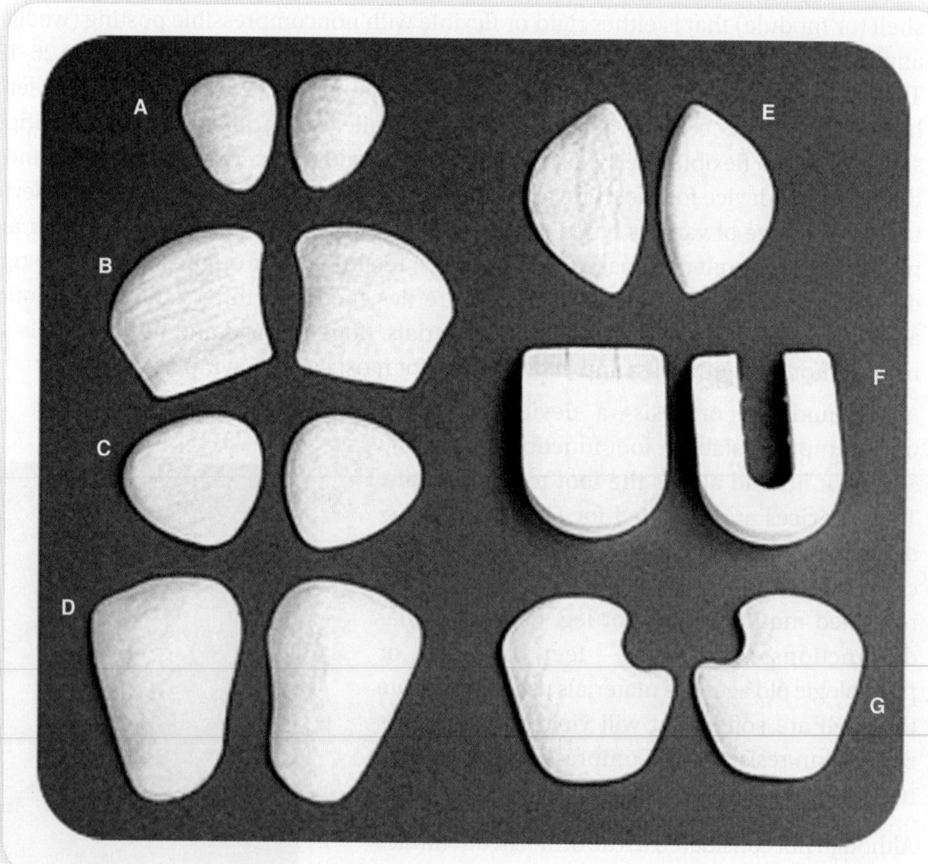

Figure 26-43 Felt pads

A. Metatarsal pads. **B.** Metatarsal bars. **C.** Metatarsal cookies. **D.** Longitudinal metatarsal pads. **E.** Scaphoid pads. **F.** Horseshoe heel cushions. **G.** Dancer pads.

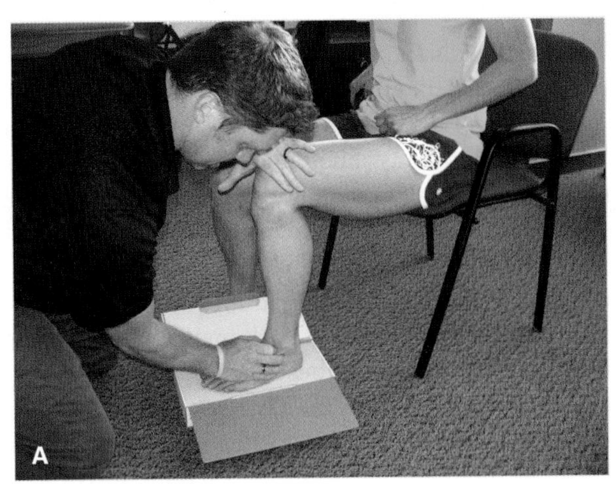

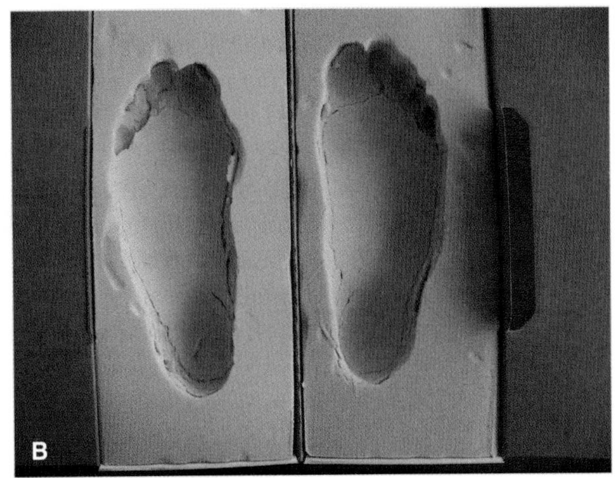

Figure 26-44 **Foam-box impression**

A. Impression taken in the seated position. **B.** Foam impressions used for construction of the orthosis.

Negative Foot Impression

Some therapists will make a negative impression of the patient's foot using a foam box or slipper casting using plaster strips or a commercial casting product. This negative impression is mailed to an orthotic laboratory, where it is fabricated utilizing therapist recommendations or laboratory discretion. Others like to complete the entire orthosis from start to finish, which requires a much more skilled evaluator and technician, as well as the necessary equipment and supplies. There are obvious cost advantages and disadvantages to in-office fabrication.

No matter which method is chosen, the first step is the fabrication of the negative impression, which is done with the patient in a STJN. If using the foam-box impression method, the patient is placed in a seated position with the knee directly over the foot. The patient's foot is gently placed on the foam box. The therapist will then place the foot in an STJN position. While maintaining this semi-weightbearing alignment, the therapist will apply a downward force through the knee and the forefoot toward the floor until the heel is seated in the foam. Finally, the toes are seated into the foam avoiding overcompression of the foam. The foot is carefully removed from the foam box by lifting the heel first. This is then repeated on the contralateral side (Figure 26-44).

The other method of developing the negative mold is using the slipper cast technique. Once STJN is found in a non-weightbearing position, 3 layers of plaster splints are applied to the plantar surface and sides of the foot. STJN position is maintained as pressure is applied on the fifth metatarsal area in a dorsiflexion direction until the MTJ is locked. This position is held until the plaster dries. At this point the plaster cast may be sent out to have the orthosis fabricated by the lab or ready for the next step by the therapist. If it is mailed out, the appropriate measurements of forefoot and rearfoot positions should be sent, along with any extrinsic measurements.

The next step is making the positive mold by pouring plaster of Paris into the cast or foam-box impression. When working with the cast molds, the inside of the plaster should be liberally lined with talc or powder.

No special preparation is required when using the foam-box impressions.

Orthosis Materials and Fabrication

Many different materials may be used in the fabrication of a custom orthosis, including the shell (or module), top covers, posting materials, or any type of additional padding or inserts (eg, gel heel insert). The specific type of materials used by a therapist or orthotist depends on the preference of that individual. Considerations should include long-term goal of the device, what material has proven to be successful, availability of the material, and ease of working with the material. Other considerations include color, stiffness (durometer), durability, and shock absorption.

One author uses one-eigth-inch Aliplast covering (Alimed Inc., Boston) with a one-quarter-inch Plastazote underneath. A rectangular piece of each material large enough to completely encompass the lower third of the mold is cut. These 2 pieces are placed in a convection oven at approximately 275°F. At this temperature, the 2 materials bond together and become moldable in approximately 5 to 7 minutes. At this time, the materials are removed from the oven and placed on the positive mold. Ideally, a form or vacuum press should be used to form the orthosis to the mold.[51]

If the patient is present and once cooled, the uncut orthosis is placed under the foot while the patient sits in a chair. Excess material is then trimmed from the sides of the orthosis with scissors. Any material that can be seen protruding from either side of the foot should be trimmed to provide the proper width of the orthosis. The length should be trimmed so that the end of the orthosis bisects the metatarsal heads. This style is slightly longer than traditional sulcus length orthosis, but one author has found that this length provides better comfort.[51]

Next, a third layer of medial Plastazote may be glued to the arch to fill that area to the floor. Grinding begins with the sides of the orthosis, which should be ground so that the sides are slightly beveled inward to allow better shoe fit. The bottom of the orthosis is leveled so that the surface is perpendicular to the bisection of the calcaneus. Grinding is continued until very little Plastazote remains under the Aliplast at the heel. The forefoot is posted by selectively attaching and/or grinding Plastazote just proximal to the metatarsal heads. Forefoot varus is posted by grinding more laterally than medially. Forefoot valgus requires grinding more medially than laterally. With the metatarsal length orthosis, the final step is to grind the distal portion of the orthosis so that only a very thin piece of Aliplast is under the area where the orthosis ends. This prevents discomfort under the forefoot where the orthosis stops. If the patient feels that this area is a problem and the metatarsal length device has already been fabricated, a full insole of Spenco or other material may be used to cover the orthosis to the end of the shoe to eliminate the dropoff sometimes felt as the orthosis ends.

Another author has developed a measurement system in conjunction with an orthotic laboratory (Biocorrect Custom Foot Orthotics Laboratory, Kentwood, MI) to determine the amount of forefoot and rearfoot posting required for the needed biomechanical corrections. Having already performed the lower leg and calcaneal bisection and the non–weightbearing assessment, weightbearing measurements are taken using an inclinometer in an STJN position, resting position, and end-range dorsiflexed position of 25 degrees (Figure 26-45*A* and *B*). The end-range measurements are then used to prescribe the recommended rearfoot posting (0 to 3 degrees maximum) and forefoot posting (0 to 6 degrees maximum). When making recommendations to an orthotics laboratory, other considerations need to be made including materials used for shells, posting, top covers, length of orthosis, cutouts, deep heel cups, gel heel inserts, metatarsal pads or bars, or external flanges. The length of an orthosis can be described as a full, sulcus, or metatarsal device. A full-length device starts at the calcaneus and extends past the distal phalanges. A metatarsal length device extends distal to the metatarsal phalangeal joints, whereas the sulcus length device stops just proximal to the metatarsal phalangeal joints. An external flange, not routinely used, is an extension of the shell and rearfoot posting to provide additional motion or position control. Finally, the thickness of the orthosis needs to be considered depending on its use and the footwear into which the device is going to be placed.

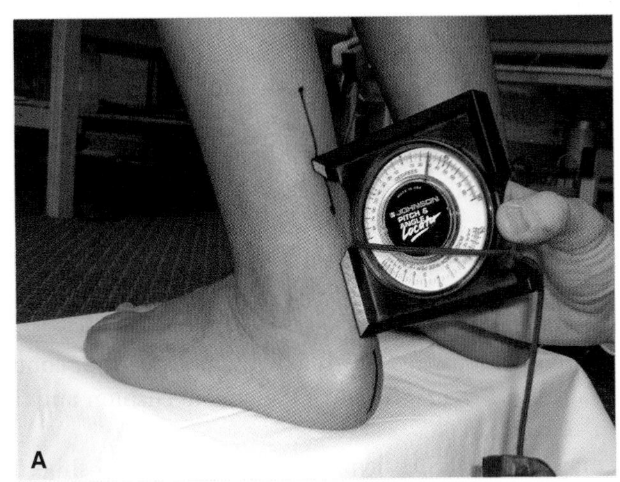

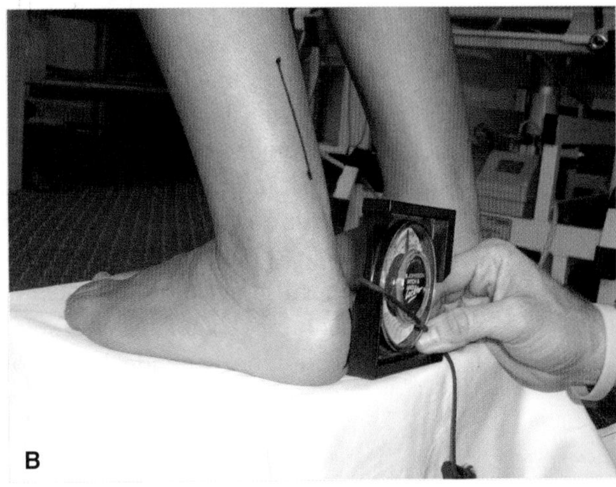

Figure 26-45

A. End-range dorsiflexion (25 degrees). **B.** Rear foot measurement with inclinometer.

In the majority of cases, a full-length orthosis that allows for forefoot and first ray correction along with the standard rearfoot correction is suggested. Exact corrections will be determined depending on the patient's biomechanical issues.

Biocorrect Custom Foot Orthotics Laboratory recommends a high-density (1 to 3 mm) polyethylene shell, which is lightweight and high-impact resilient (JMS Plastics Supply Inc., Neptune, NJ). Various top covers (ACOR Inc., Cleveland, OH) are available using one-eighth-inch Vinair, leather, or Neosponge in combination with one-sixteenth-inch to three-sixteenths-inch P-Cell or Micro-cell Puff ethylene vinyl acetate (EVA) material for additional shock absorption (Figure 26-46). A firmer EVA (45 to 50 durometers) material (JMS Plastics Supply Inc.) is used for the extrinsic forefoot/rearfoot posting and arch support.

The process is essentially the same as previously described, except the patient does not need to be present to determine the necessary forefoot, rearfoot, or first ray corrections. These prescribed corrections have already been established during the evaluation process. Once all of the specific materials have been attached or glued to the shell, the necessary grinding will take place to complete the finished orthosis.

Time must be allowed for proper break-in. The patient should wear the orthosis for 3 to 4 hours the first day, 6 to 8 hours the next day, and then all day on the third day. Physical activities should be started with the orthosis only after it has been worn all day for several days.[49]

Sometimes corrections or adjustments are necessary to the orthosis. Orthotic therapy is "an art and a science," so it is important to be able to make corrections or adjustments quickly and easily. This may influence a clinician as to whether they choose an out-of-state versus a local laboratory, or make the investment of having a full or partial in-house laboratory.

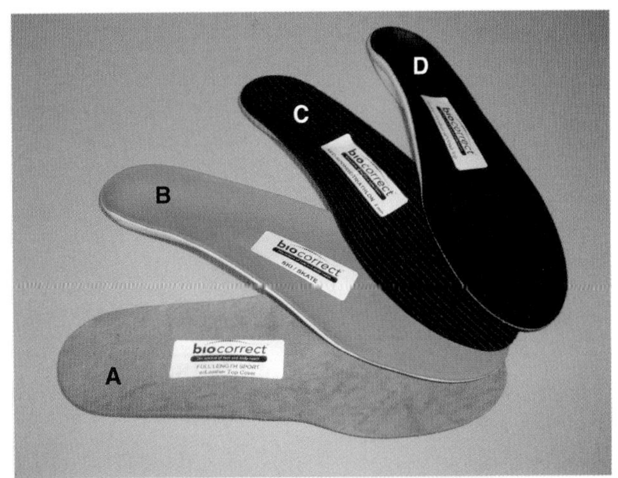

Figure 26-46 **Various top cover materials**

A. Leather top cover. **B.** Microcell Puff top cover. **C.** Neosponge top cover. **D.** Vinair top cover.

Shoe Selection

Shoes are one of the biggest considerations in treating a foot problem successfully.[109] Even a properly made orthosis is less effective if placed in a poorly constructed or an inappropriate shoe for the patient. It is critical that the shoe–orthosis interface matches the anatomical alignment and biomechanics of each individual. In many cases related to walking or running, improper shoe and/or orthotic can be a primary cause of lower extremity overuse injuries, ranging from the hip to the foot.

As noted, pronation is usually a problem of hypermobility. Thus, pronatory foot types need stability and firmness to reduce excess movement. Research indicates that forefoot compression of the outer sole of the shoe may actually increase pronation versus a barefoot condition.[6] The ideal shoe for a pronated foot is less flexible with good rearfoot control. Conversely, supinated feet are usually more rigid. Shoes with adequate cushion and flexibility benefit this type of foot.

Several construction factors may influence the firmness and stability of a shoe. The basic form upon which a shoe is built is called the *last* (Figure 26-47).[3,6] The upper is fitted onto a last in several ways. Each method has its own flexibility and control characteristics. A central slip-lasted shoe is sewn together like a moccasin and is very flexible. A peripheral (Strobel or California) lasted shoe has similar characteristics as the central slip, except the stitching is along the outside of the shoe. Board-lasting provides a piece of fiberboard upon which the upper is attached, which provides a very firm, inflexible base for the shoe. A combination-lasted shoe is boarded in the back half of the shoe and slip-lasted in the front, which provides rear-foot stability with forefoot mobility. The shape of the last may also be used to assist with shoe selection. The 3 different types of shapes are straight lasted, curved lasted, and semicurved lasted and are usually consistent with the construction of a shoe. The shape and the construction of the last are typically consistent

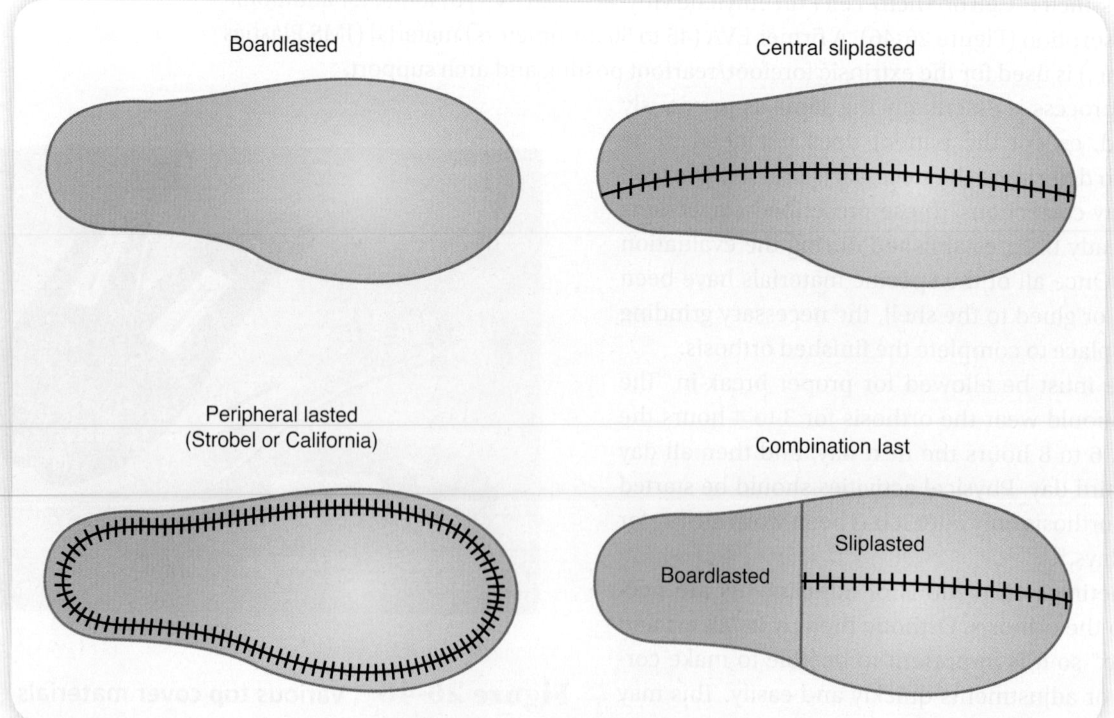

Figure 26-47 Shoe last construction

with one another. Most patients with excessive pronation perform better in a straight-lasted shoe,[3,6] that is, a shoe in which the forefoot does not curve inward in relation to the rear-foot.

In comparing all of the dress and athletic shoes available to the consumer, running shoes have the greatest investment in money and resources by the manufactures for research and development with respect to controlling the motion of the foot. Thus, when it comes to providing a patient with specific footwear recommendations for running or walking, running shoes have the largest selection of options to choose from. There are several different categories of running shoes available with a specific purpose in mind. Some are designed more for training, while others geared for performance. Since 2008, there has been a resurgence of shoes developed to promote the minimalistic or barefoot trend in running. Within each category, there are several different brands with their own unique cushioning and control systems. The general categories can be defined as: Motion Control, Stability, Guidance, Straight-lasted Cushion, Neutral Cushion, Minimalistic/Performance, Minimalistic/Specialty (Figures 26-48 and 26-49), Spikes, and Trail Runner.

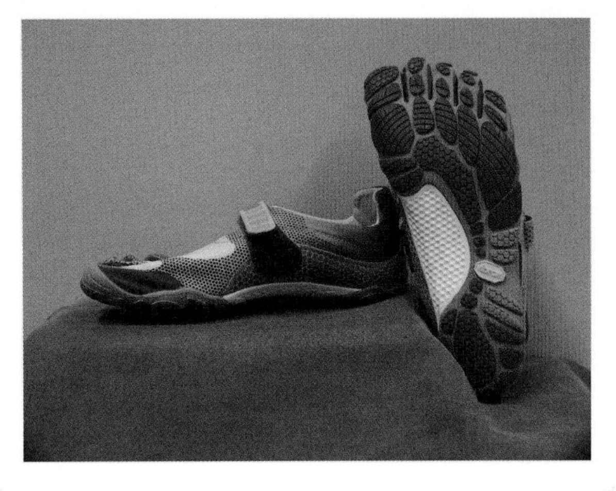

Figure 26-48 Minimalistic/Specialty shoe (Vibram Five Finger)

Midsole design plays the biggest role in the amount of cushion or stability inherently built into the shoe. There are several features of the midsole that define each shoe, including EVA density, stability systems, last shape and drop. The midsole is what separates the upper portion of the shoe from the outsole (bottom of the shoe).[3,16] EVA is one of the most commonly used materials in the midsole.[3,86] The higher the density of the EVA is (measured by Durometer scale), the more stiff the midsole of a shoe will be. In the Guidance, Stability, and Motion Control categories, a dual-density EVA is often times utilized. A higher density EVA, often times colored differently to show that it is denser, is placed under within the less dense EVA material along the medial aspect of the midsole to assist with pronation control. Also, in an effort to control rearfoot movement, many shoe manufacturers have reinforced the heel counter both internally and externally, often in the form of extra plastic along the outside of the heel counter.[3,71] Each manufacturer has a unique, patented stability system to promote more pronation control (eg, Brooks Progressive Diagonal Rollbar found in their Adrenaline 12). A straighter-lasted shoe will be inherently more stable than a semi- or curve lasted shoe just be the geometry of the midsole. Finally, the drop of the shoe (measured in millimeters from the heel to the toe) plays a role in performance of the shoe. It is theorized that a smaller drop from heel to toe will encourage a more mid-foot strike pattern as compared to a heel-strike pattern. The newer line of Minimalistic category range from a zero, 4- or 8-mm drop shoe, whereas the more traditional footwear (Neutral Cushion through Motion Control) range from 8- to 12-mm drop shoes.

Other factors that may affect the performance of a shoe are the outsole contour and composition, lacing systems, and forefoot wedges (for specific details, refer to Table 26-1).

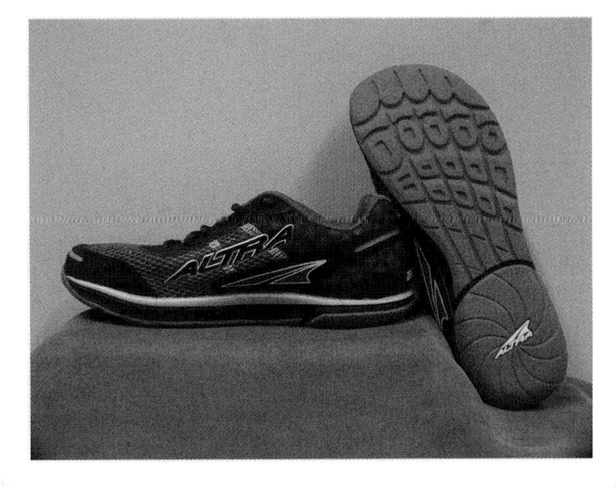

Figure 26-49 Minimalistic/Specialty shoe (Ultra Zero Drop)

Table 26-1 General Classification and Characteristics of Running Shoe Types

Motion Control Shoe
- Indications: Severe overpronator
- Straighter last shape
- Board or combination last construction[a]
- Midsole materials (EVA or Polyeurethane (PU)) depend on BW
- Firmer dual-density medial midsole or stabilization device and typically runs from heel counter up into forefoot
- Reinforced and/or extended heel counter
- Will sometimes use higher medial side versus lateral side (wedge) for increased early motion control

Stability Shoe
- Indications: Moderate over-pronator
- Semicurved last shape
- Combination or peripheral last construction
- Midsole materials (EVA or PU) dependent on BW
- Firmness of dual-density medial midsole or stabilization device dependent of range of stability shoe and typically runs from the heel counter up past the arch
- Firm heel counter

Guidance Shoe
- Indications: mild overpronator
- Semicurved last shape
- Combination or peripheral last construction
- Midsole materials usually a lighter weight EVA
- Firmness of dual-density medial midsole or stabilization device dependent of range of stability shoe that typically runs under the arch
- Firm heel counter

Straight-Lasted Cushion Shoe
- Indication: Neutral to supinatory foot that is unstable
- Newer *transition* shoe that bridges the gap between cushion and stability mostly with the geometry of the shoe
- Straighter last shoe
- Midsole materials (EVA or PU) dependent on BW, but usually lean to lighter-weight EVA
- Single density midsole
- May utilize stability pillars (eg, Brooks Dyad series)
- Firmer heel counter

Neutral Cushion Shoe
- Indication: Neutral to supinatory foot
- Typically more curve last shape
- Central or peripheral slip last construction
- Midsole materials (EVA or PU) dependent on BW, but usually lean to lighter-weight EVA
- Single density midsole
- Midsole cushioning units (rearfoot and forefoot)

Minimalistic/Performance Shoe
- Indication: neutral to supinatory foot
- Recommended use: short distance training or racing
- Typically more curve last shape
- Central or peripheral slip last construction
- Midsole materials (EVA or PU) dependent on BW, but usually lean to lighter-weight EVA
- Single density midsole with minimal to zero drop from heel to toe
- Midsole cushioning units (rearfoot and forefoot)

[a]Board last combination primarily used with older running shoes and basketball shoes. Combination last primarily used with newer running shoes.

Source: Rob Lillie, General Manager at Gazelle Sports, Kalamazoo, Michigan.

Shoe Wear Evaluation

Shoe wear patterns can sometimes give the therapist helpful information about the patient's biomechanical considerations and potential movement dysfunctions. Patients with excessive pronation often wear out the front of the running shoe under the second metatarsal (Figure 26-50). Shoe wear patterns are commonly misinterpreted by patients who think they must be pronators because they wear out the back outside edges of their heels. Actually, most people who wear out the back outside edges of their shoes are consistent with lateral heel strike at initial contact. Just before heel strike, the anterior tibial muscle fires to prevent the foot from slapping forward. The anterior tibialis muscle not only dorsiflexes the foot but also slightly inverts it, hence the wear pattern on the back edge of the shoe. For those runners who are midfoot to forefoot strikers, typically less lateral heel wear is evident. The key to inspection of wear patterns on shoes is observation of the heel counter and the forefoot.

There are 3 simple tests that can be utilized to determine the structural integrity of a running shoe. The first test is used to determine if the individual is placing an exceptional amount of torsional torque on the shoe, specifically through the midfoot region. By simply placing the shoe on a flat surface, and pushing down on the front of the toe box in the center, observe the natural movement pattern of the shoe. If the shoe veers medially or laterally, this is indicative of increased torsion on the shoe. This may indicate that a more stable shoe is required to counteract the force, or an orthosis is necessary to create improved balance throughout stance phase. The second test is to determine excessive wear of the shoe. If it is possible to bend the toe of the shoe in half to touch the heel collar of the shoe, the shoe no longer has the necessary structural integrity to function properly. In most cases, the shoe's cushioning properties have been broken down to a point where the shoe would be more likely to cause injury than to prevent injury. The third test is also utilized to determine if the shoe's structural stability is solid enough to support the runner. Simply, bend the shoe in a "figure 8" pattern. In this test, if you can twist the shoe around the central axis, the structural integrity is broken down enough to increase the possibility of injury.

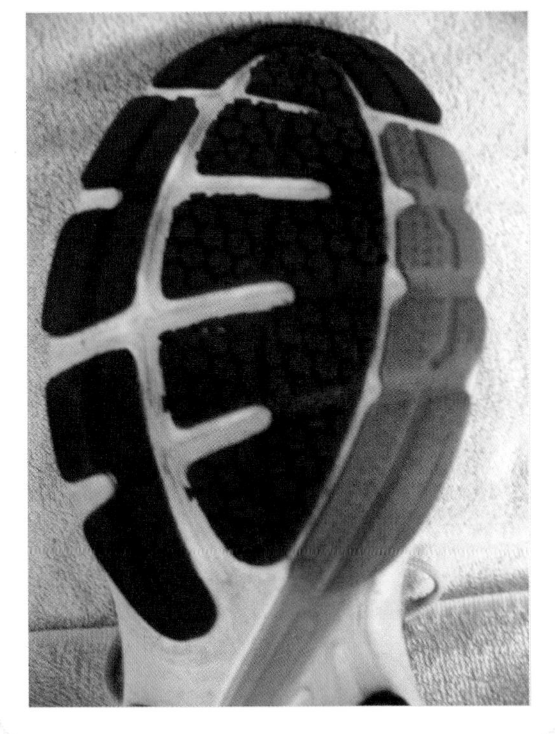

Figure 26-50 **Front forefoot of a running shoe showing the typical wear pattern of a pronator**

Finally, running shoes are currently being designed with the primary goal of having the lightest weight shoe possible. Newer materials are being used to decrease weight while attempting to maintain some stability and cushioning properties. The result of this trend is that the life expectancy of shoes drastically decreases. Runners, for the most part, should be looking at changing their running shoes after 300 total miles of running, rather than the old adage of 450 to 500 miles.

Another evaluation technique for footwear is to determine if the patient is placing an exceptional amount of torsional torque on the shoe, specifically through the midfoot region. By simply placing the shoe on a flat surface, and pushing down on the front of the toe box in the center, observe the natural movement pattern of the shoe. If the shoe veers medially or laterally, this is indicative of increased torsion on the shoe. This may indicate that a more stable shoe is required to counteract the force, or an orthosis is necessary to create improved balance throughout stance phase.

Exercises

Rehabilitation Techniques

Strengthening Exercises

Isometric Strengthening Exercises

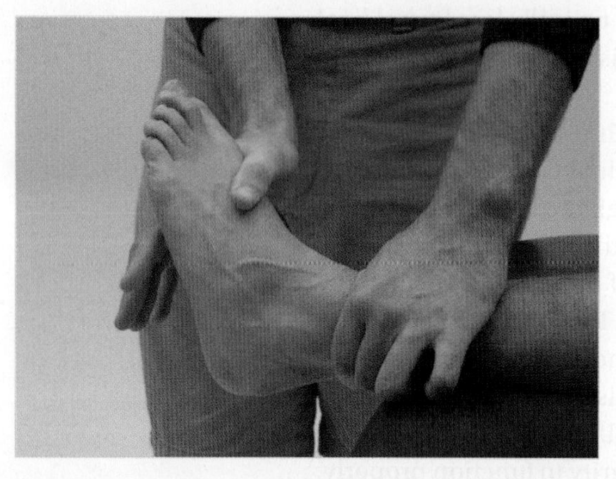

Exercise 26-1

Isometric inversion against a stable object. Used to strengthen the posterior tibialis, flexor digitorum longus, and flexor hallucis longus.

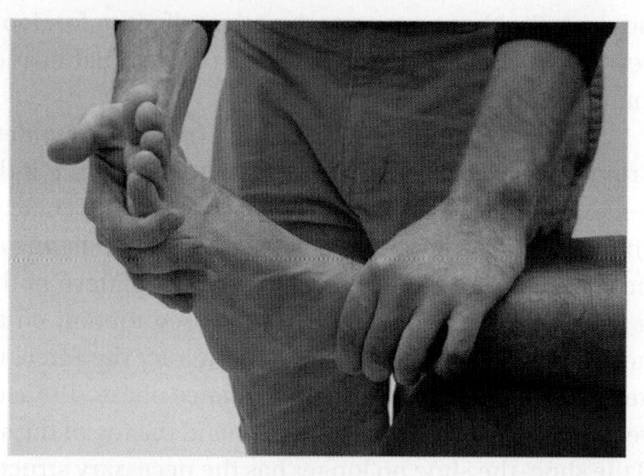

Exercise 26-2

Isometric eversion against a stable object. Used to strengthen the peroneus longus, brevis, tertius, and extensor digitorum longus.

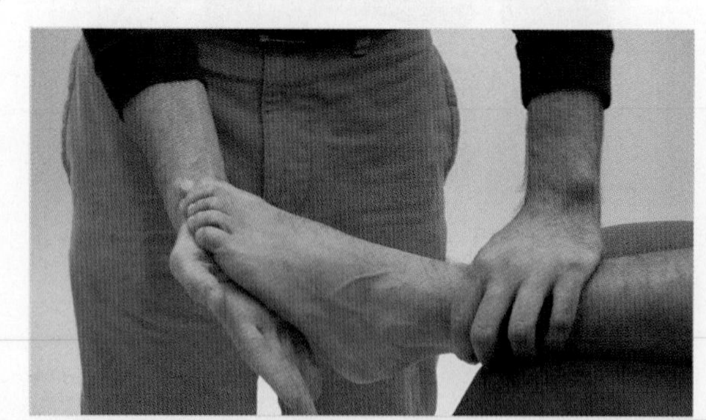

Exercise 26-3

Isometric plantarflexion against a stable object. Used to strengthen the gastrocnemius, soleus, posterior tibialis, flexor digitorum longus, flexor hallucis longus, and plantaris.

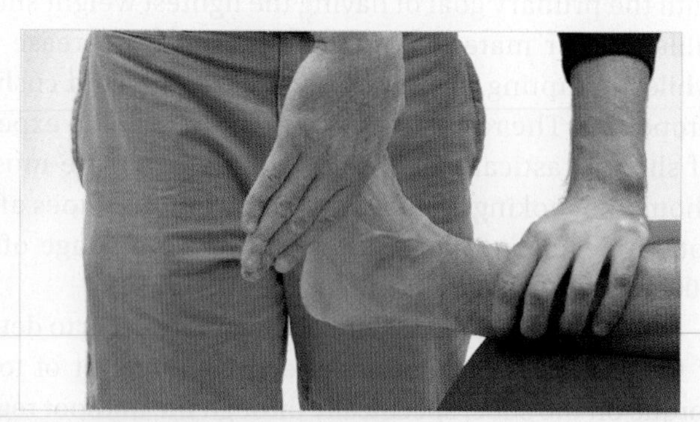

Exercise 26-4

Isometric dorsiflexion against a stable object. Used to strengthen the anterior tibialis and peroneus tertius.

Isotonic Open-Chain Strengthening Exercises

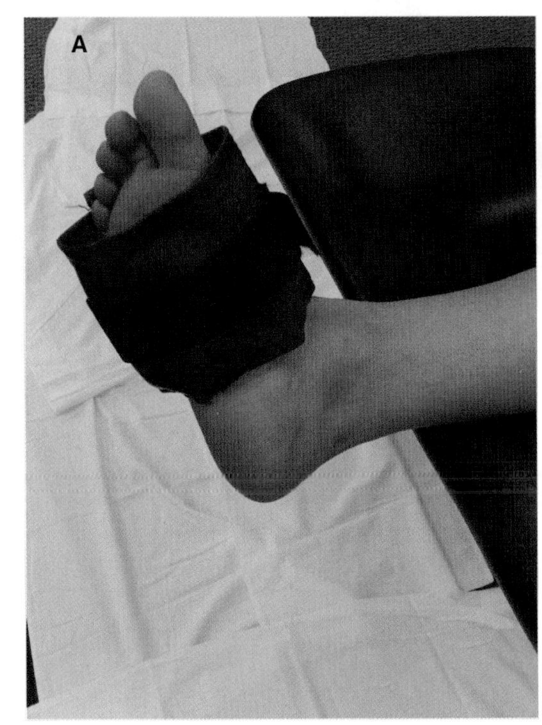

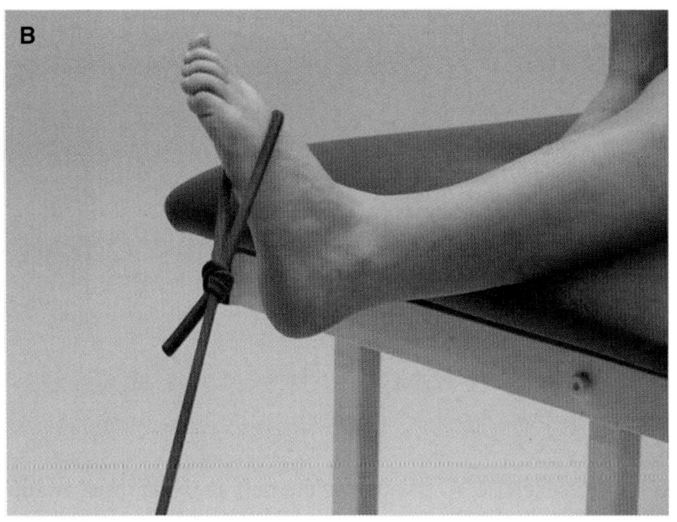

Exercise 26-5

Inversion exercise. **A.** Using a weight cuff. **B.** Using resistive tubing. Used to strengthen the posterior tibialis, flexor digitorum longus, and flexor hallucis longus.

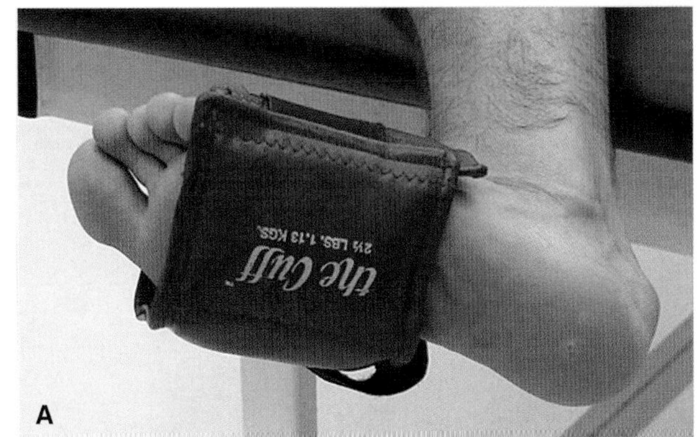

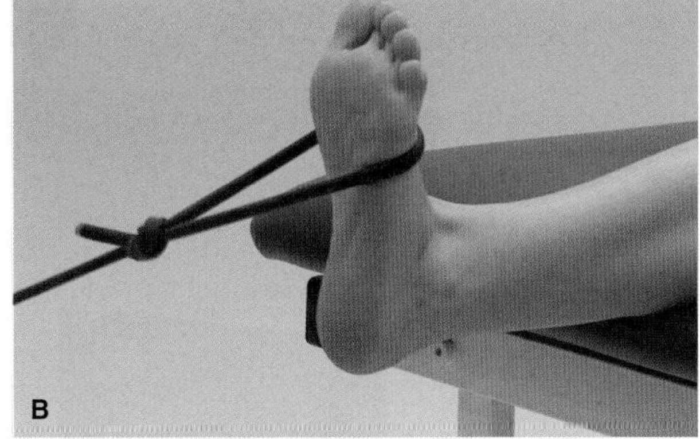

Exercise 26-6

Eversion exercise. **A.** Using a weight cuff. **B.** Using resistive tubing. Used to strengthen the peroneus longus, brevis, tertius, and extensor digitorum longus.

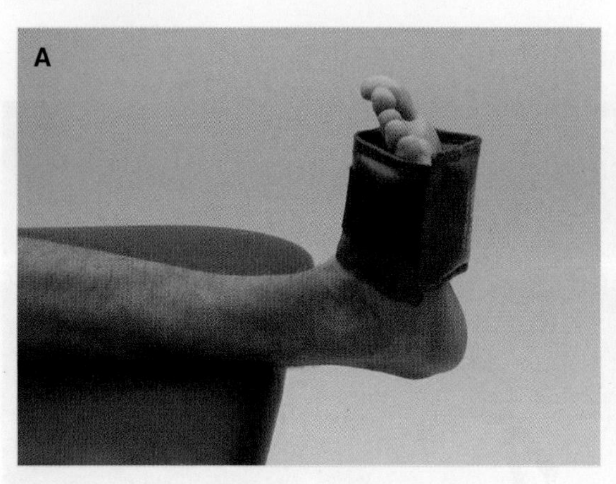

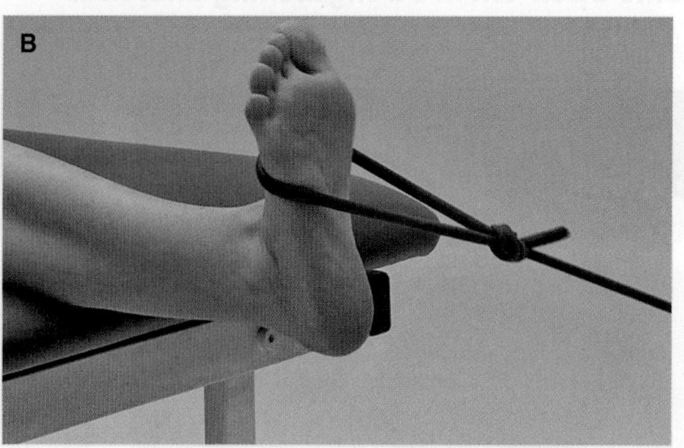

Exercise 26-7

Dorsiflexion exercise. **A.** Using a weight cuff. **B.** Using resistive tubing. Used to strengthen the anterior tibialis and peroneus tertius.

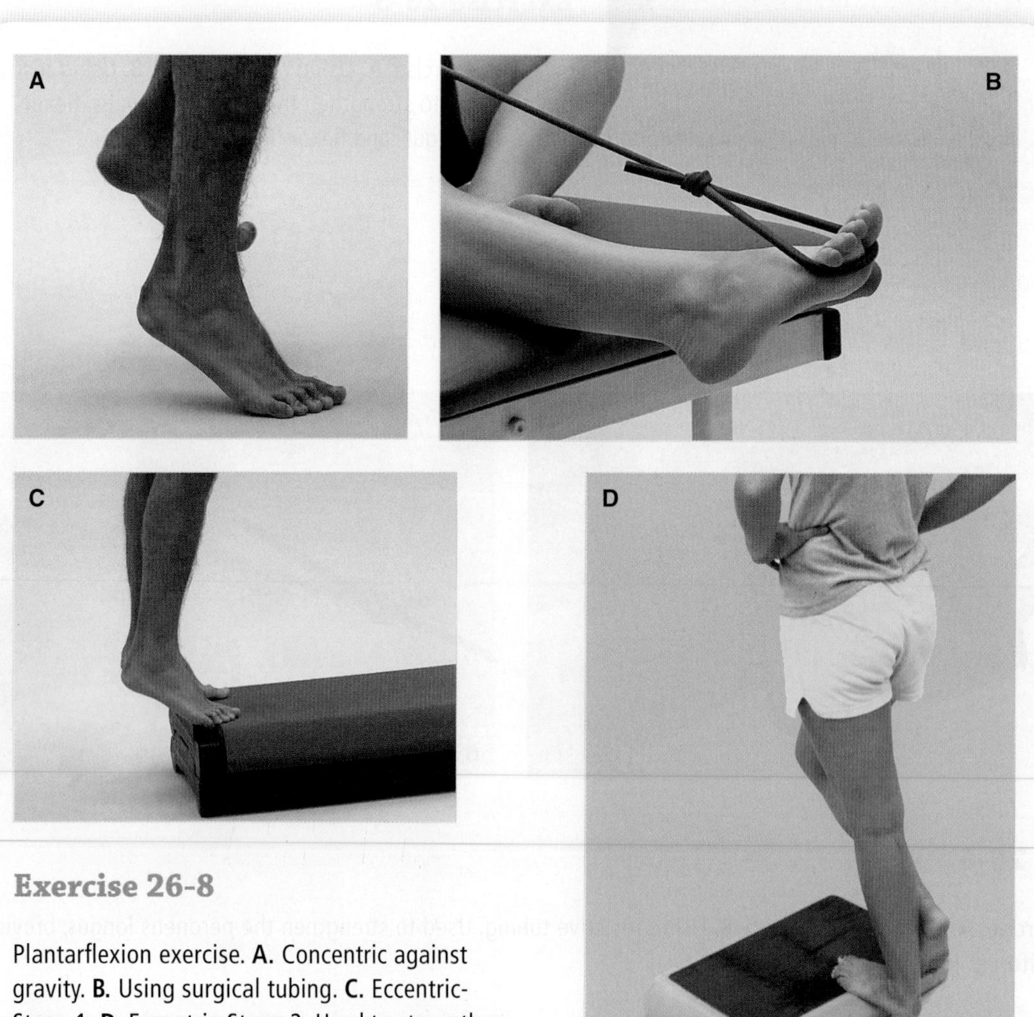

Exercise 26-8

Plantarflexion exercise. **A.** Concentric against gravity. **B.** Using surgical tubing. **C.** Eccentric-Stage 1. **D.** Eccentric-Stage 2. Used to strengthen the gastrocnemius, soleus, posterior tibialis, flexor digitorum longus, flexor hallucis longus, and plantaris.

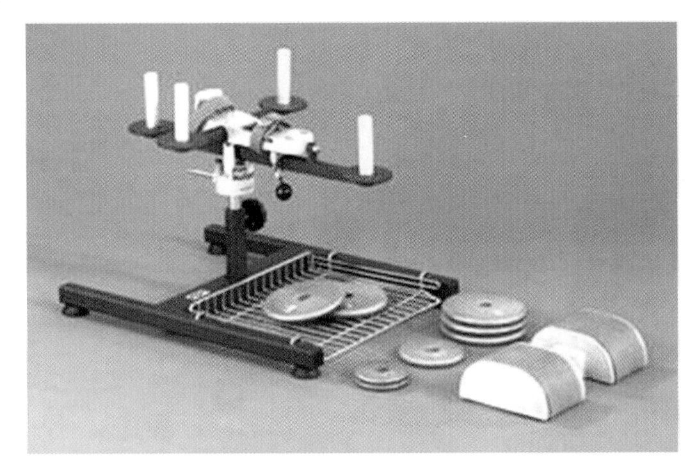

Exercise 26-9

Multidirectional Elgin ankle exerciser.

Closed-Chain Strengthening Exercises

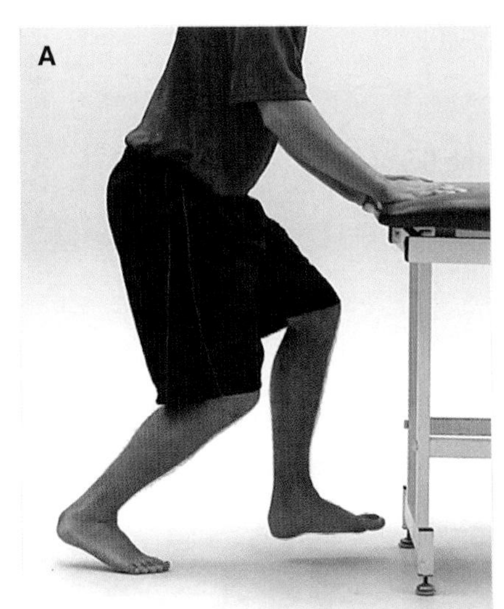

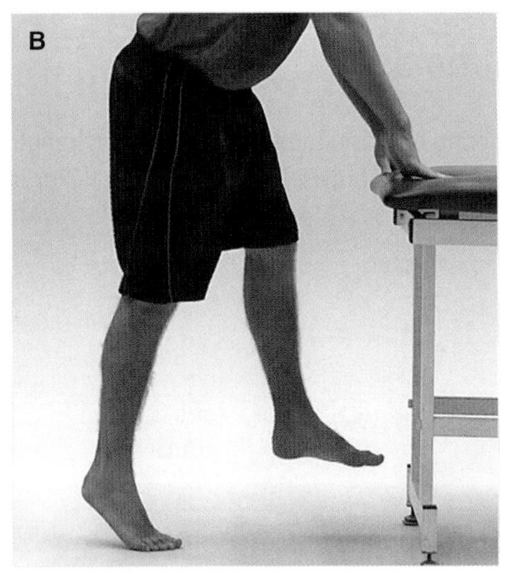

Exercise 26-10

Isolated toe raises. **A.** Toe raises with extended knee strengthens the gastrocnemius. **B.** Toe raises with flexed knee strengthens the soleus.

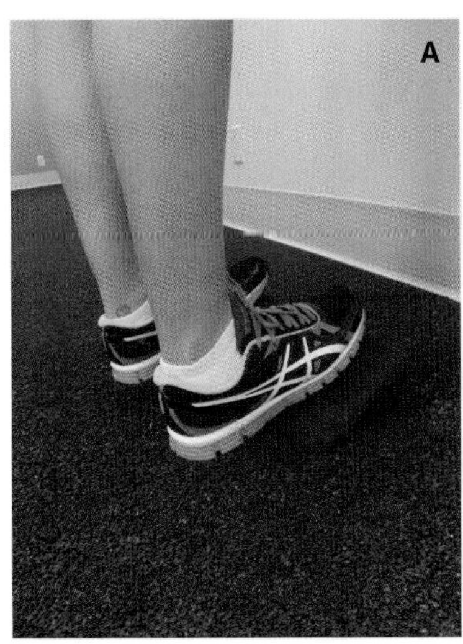

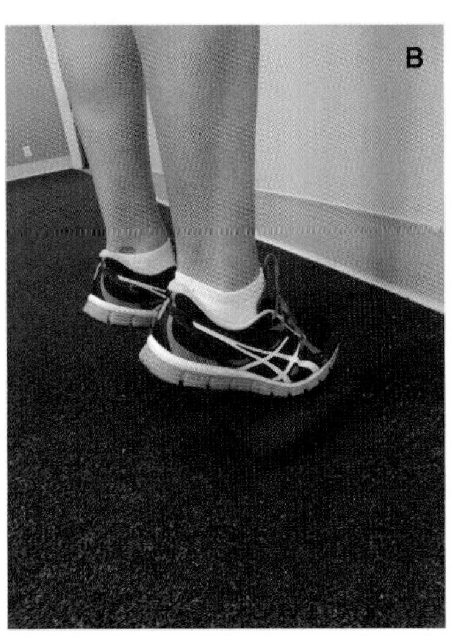

Exercise 26-11

Active-assisted plantarflexion using the BOB (Caledonia, MI). **A.** Starting position. **B.** Finishing position. Can also use as a static stretch by holding end range positions.

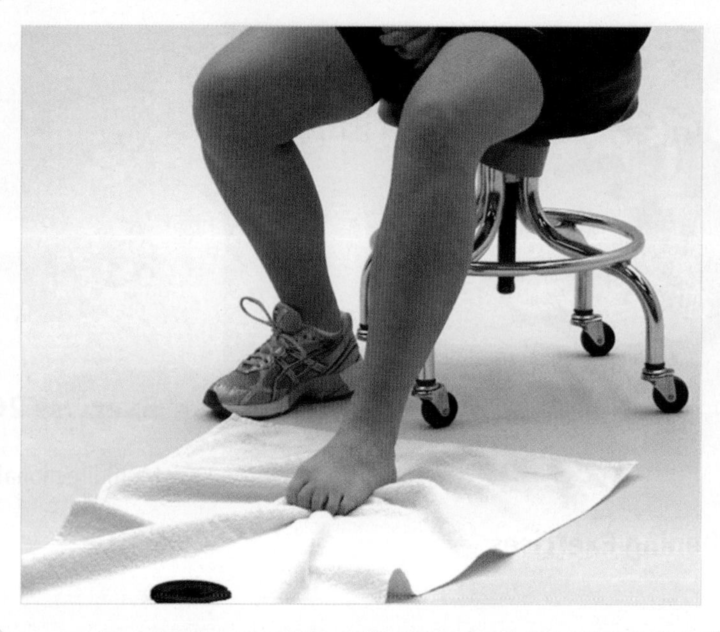

Exercise 26-12

Towel gathering exercise. Toe flexion. Used to strengthen the flexor digitorum longus and brevis, lumbricales, and flexor hallucis longus.

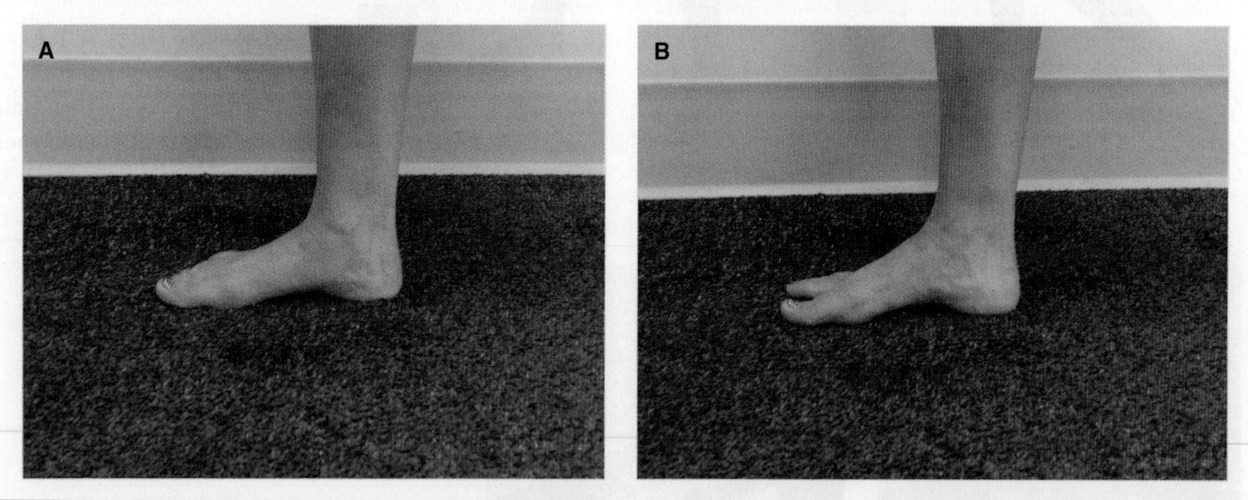

Exercise 26-13

Foot intrinsic strengthening. **A.** Starting position, relaxed foot. **B.** End position, with actively drawn up arch.

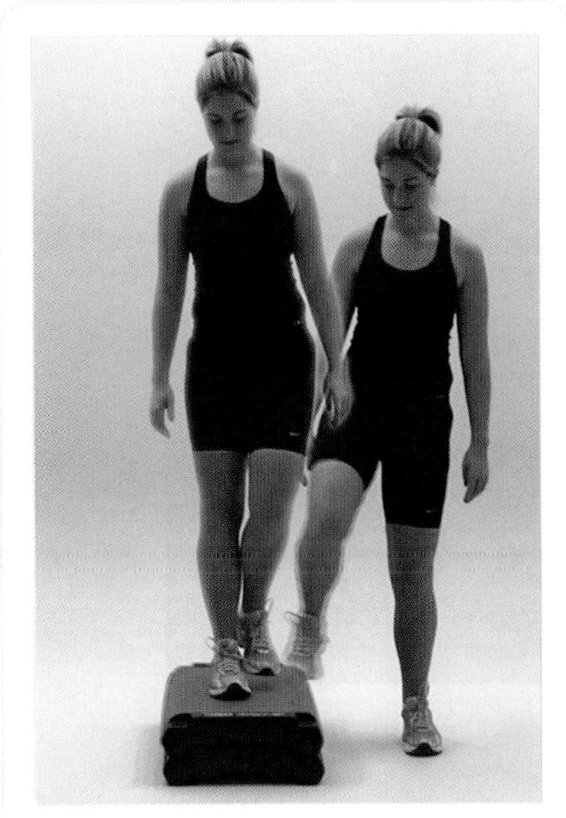

Exercise 26-14

Lateral step-ups.

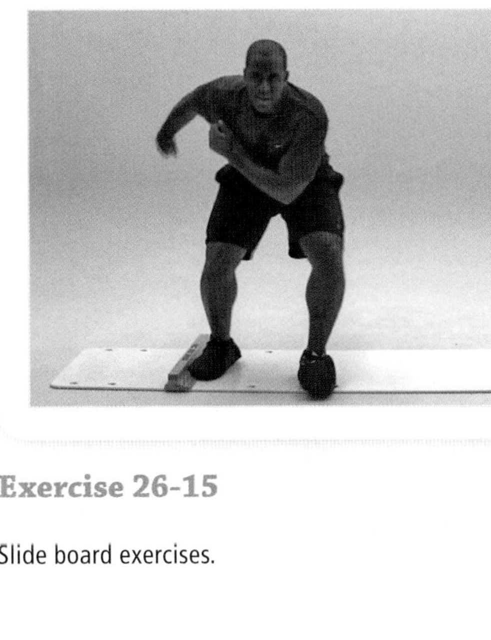

Exercise 26-15

Slide board exercises.

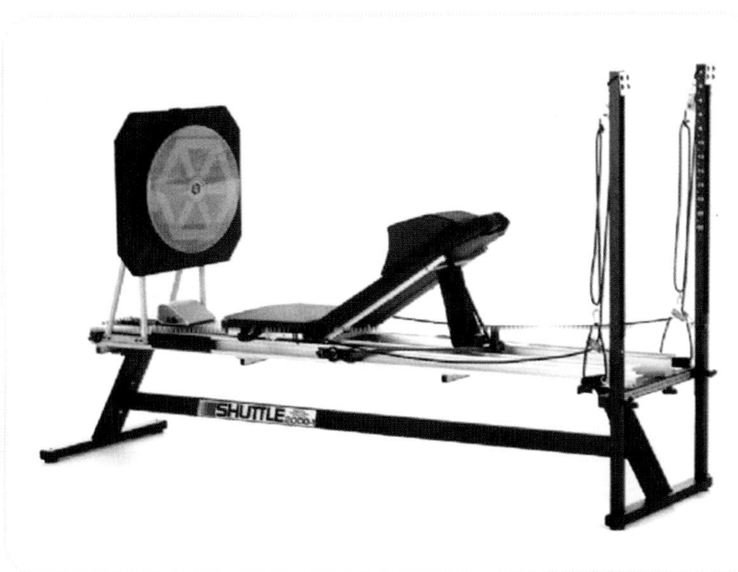

Exercise 26-16

Shuttle exercise machine.

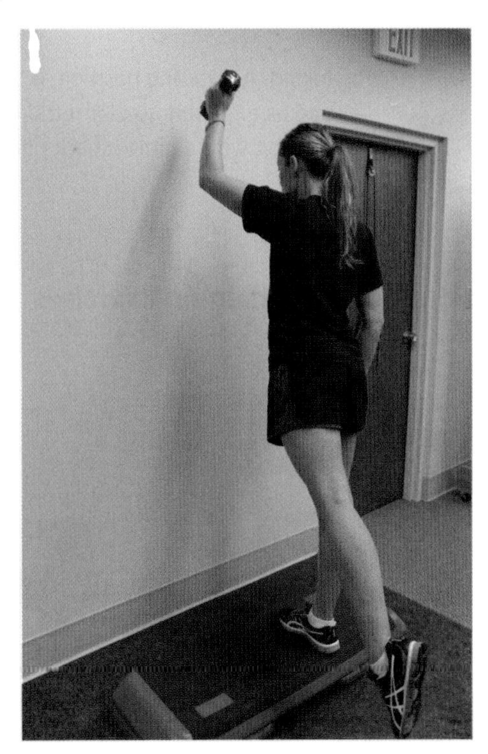

Exercise 26-17

Forward step-up with alternate arm raise using a dumbbell. Used for cross-over strengthening of gluteus maximus and balance/neuromuscular control as well as contralateral dorsal musculature associated with thoracolumbar fascia.

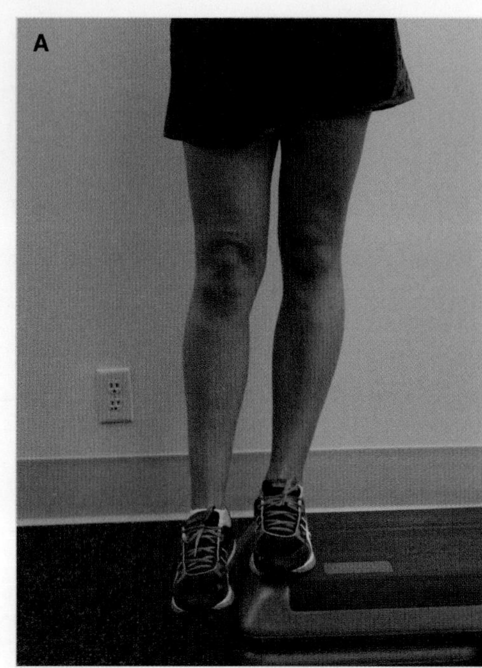

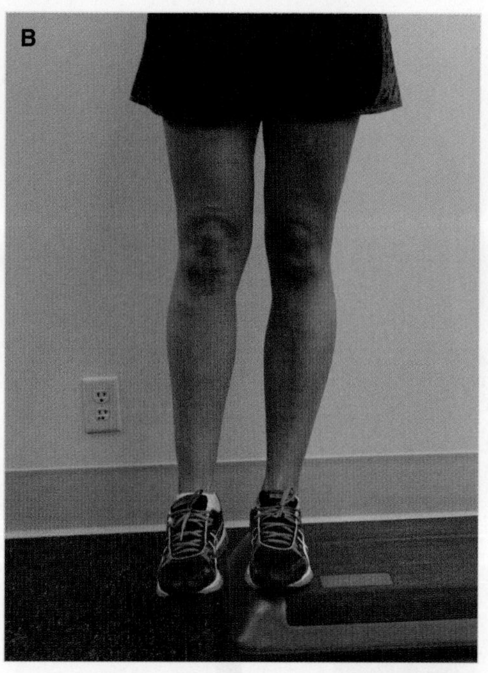

Exercise 26-18

Hip hiking. **A.** Starting position. **B.** Finishing position. Used to strengthen gluteus medius. Can also be used as a neuromuscular retraining exercise having the patient stop when pelvis is level or in conjunction with a biofeedback unit over gluteus medius for proper recruitment.

Isokinetic Strengthening Exercises

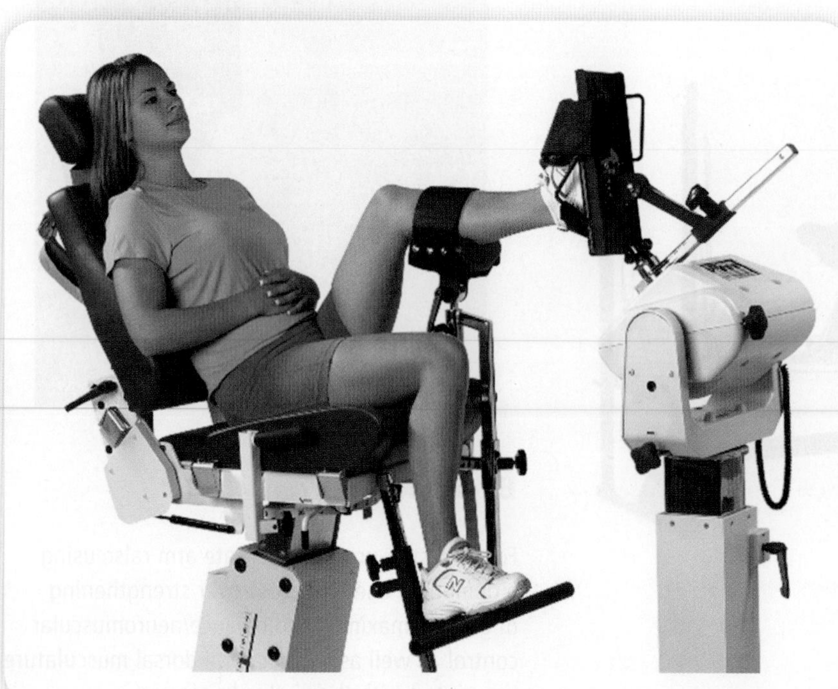

Exercise 26-19

Isokinetic inversion/eversion exercise. Used to improve the strength and endurance of the ankle inverters and everters in an open chain. Also can provide an objective measurement of muscular torque production.

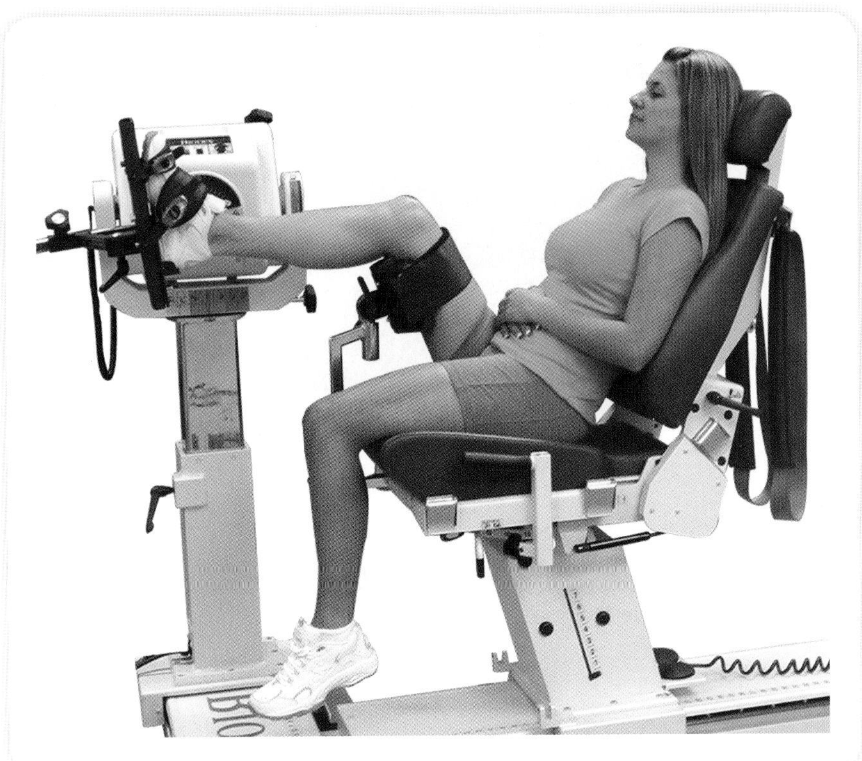

Exercise 26-20

Isokinetic plantarflexion/dorsiflexion exercise. Used to improve the strength and endurance of the ankle dorsiflexors and plantarflexors in an open chain. Also can provide an objective measurement of torque production.

Proprioceptive Neuromuscular Facilitation Strengthening Exercises

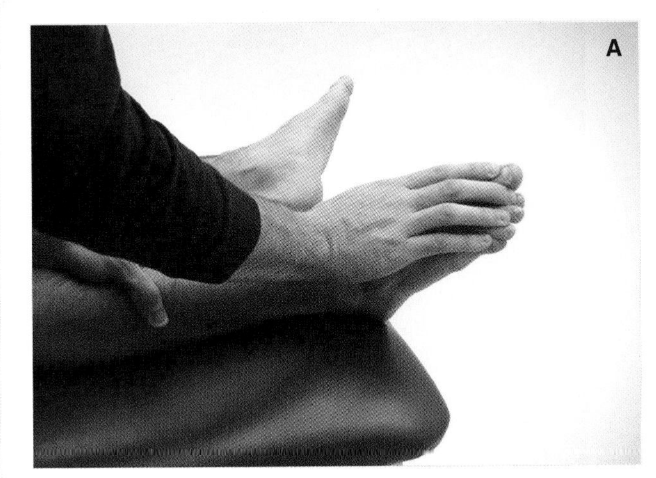

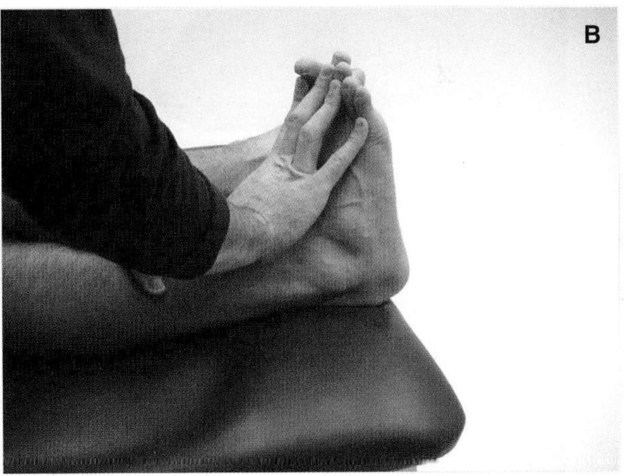

Exercise 26-21

Diagonal 1 (D1) pattern moving into flexion. **A.** Starting position: ankle plantar flexed, foot everted, toes flexed. **B.** Terminal position: ankle dorsiflexed, foot inverted, toes extended.

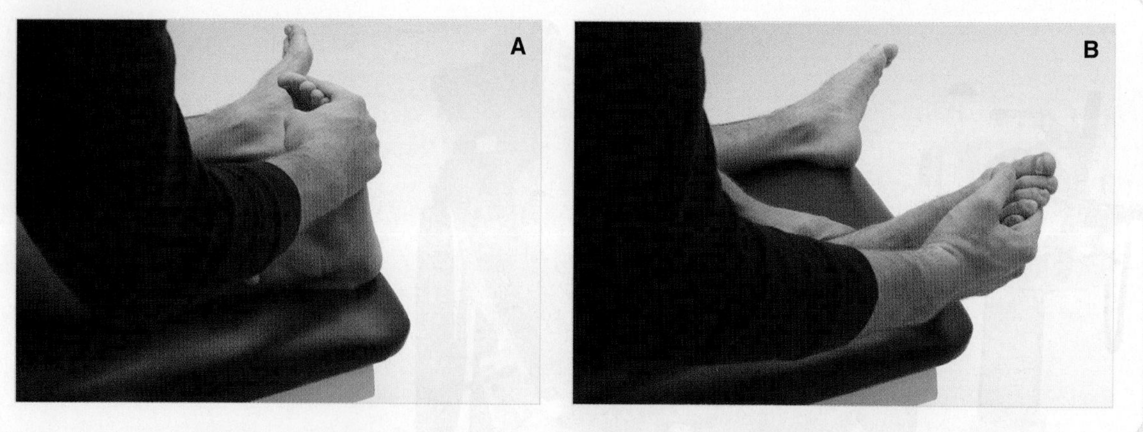

Exercise 26-22

Diagonal 1 (D1) pattern moving into extension. **A.** Starting position: ankle dorsiflexed, foot inverted, toes extended. **B.** Terminal position: ankle plantar flexed, foot everted, toes flexed.

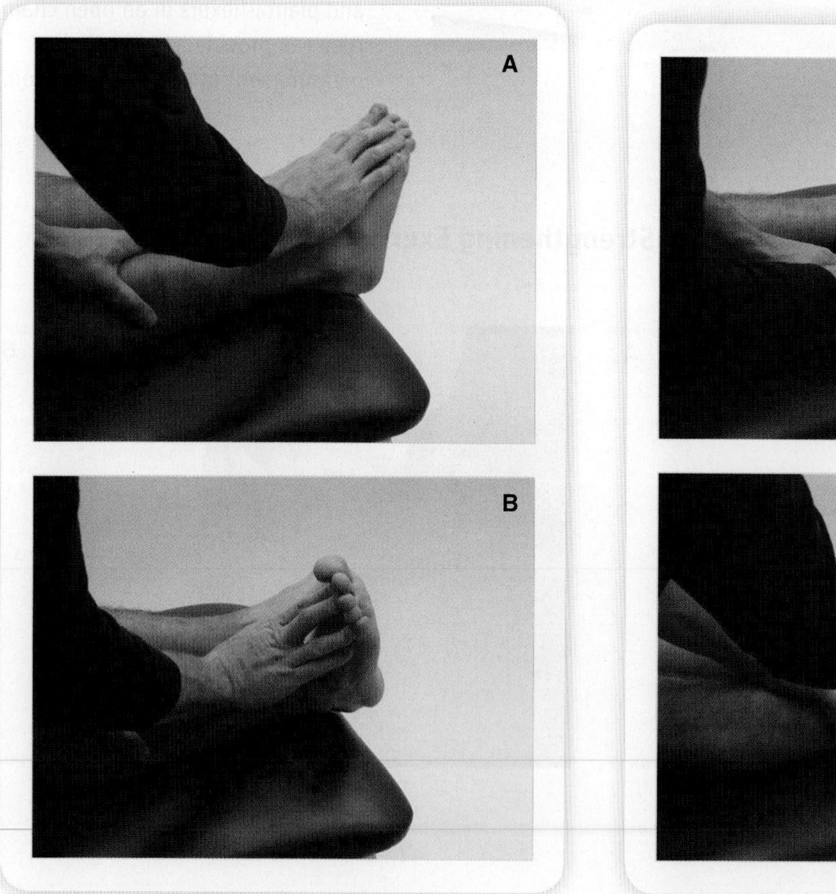

Exercise 26-23

Diagonal 2 (D2) pattern moving into flexion. **A.** Starting position: ankle plantar flexed, foot inverted, toes flexed. **B.** Terminal position: ankle dorsiflexed, foot everted, toes extended.

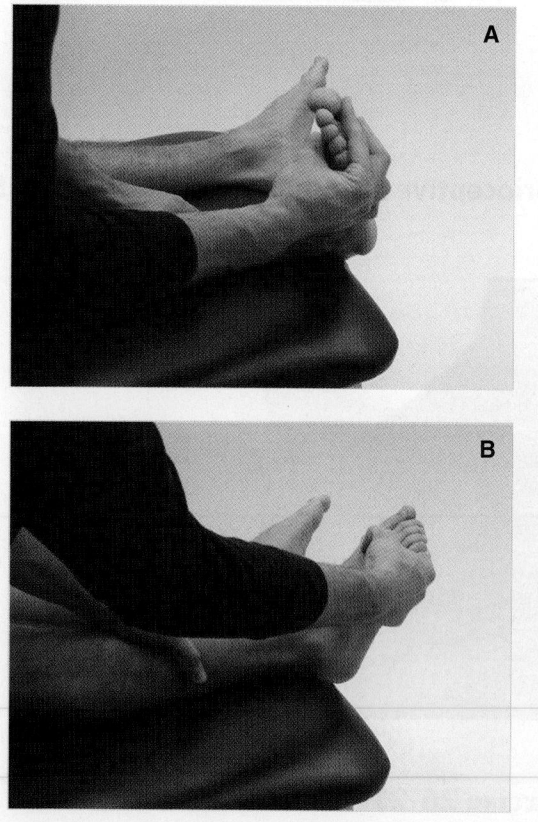

Exercise 26-24

Diagonal 2 (D2) pattern moving into extension. **A.** Starting position: ankle dorsiflexed, foot everted, toes extended. **B.** Terminal position: ankle plantar flexed, foot inverted, toes flexed.

Stretching Exercises

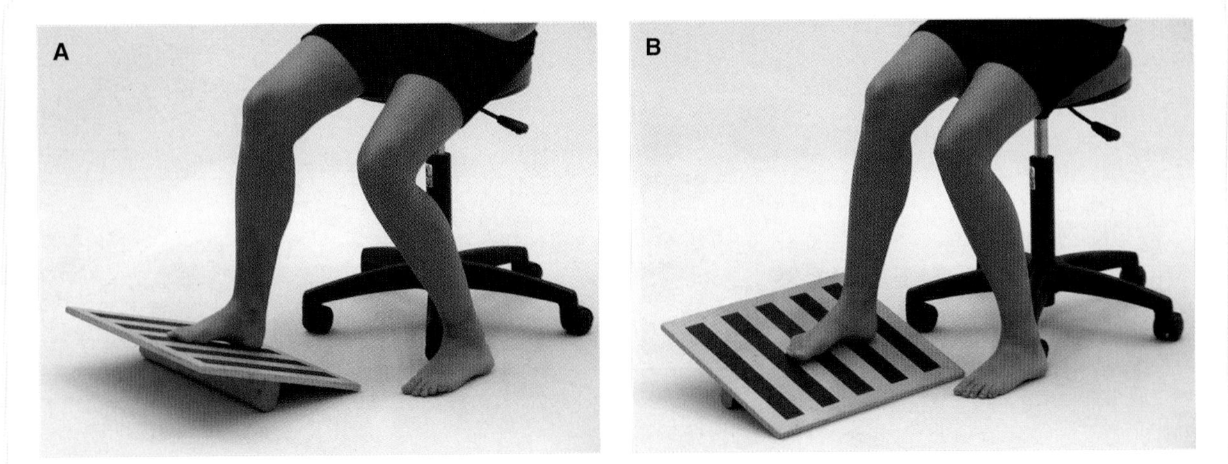

Exercise 26-25

Fitter Rocker board exercises are an active range of motion exercise, useful in regaining normal ankle motion and early neuromuscular retraining. **A.** Seated plantarflexion—dorsiflexion. **B.** Seated inversion—eversion. Both can be progressed to standing, in partial or full weight bearing conditions.

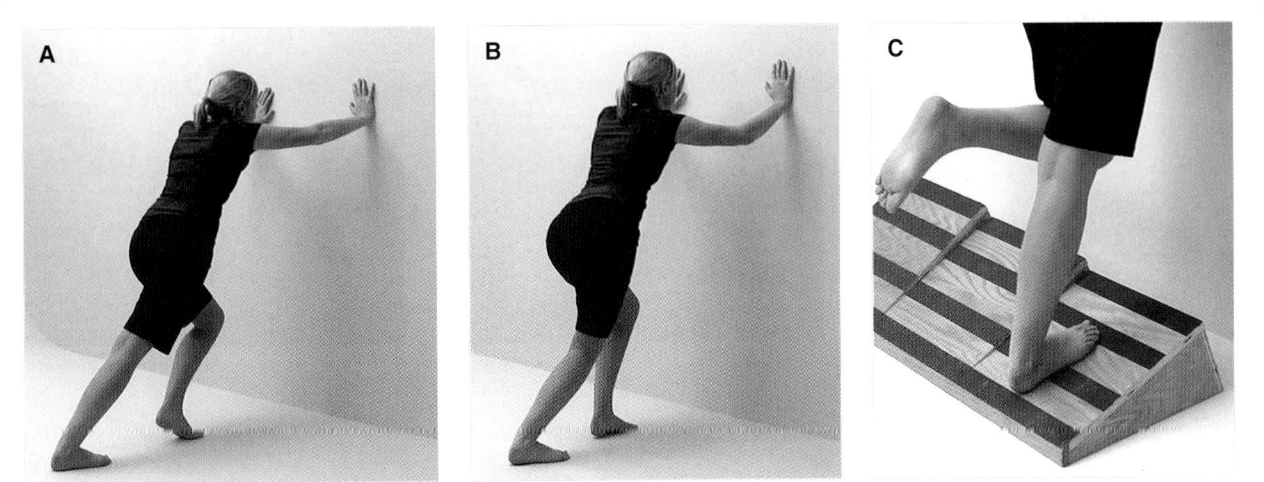

Exercise 26-26

Standing heel cord stretch. **A.** Gastrocnemius. **B.** Soleus. **C.** Gastrocnemius stretch using a slant board.

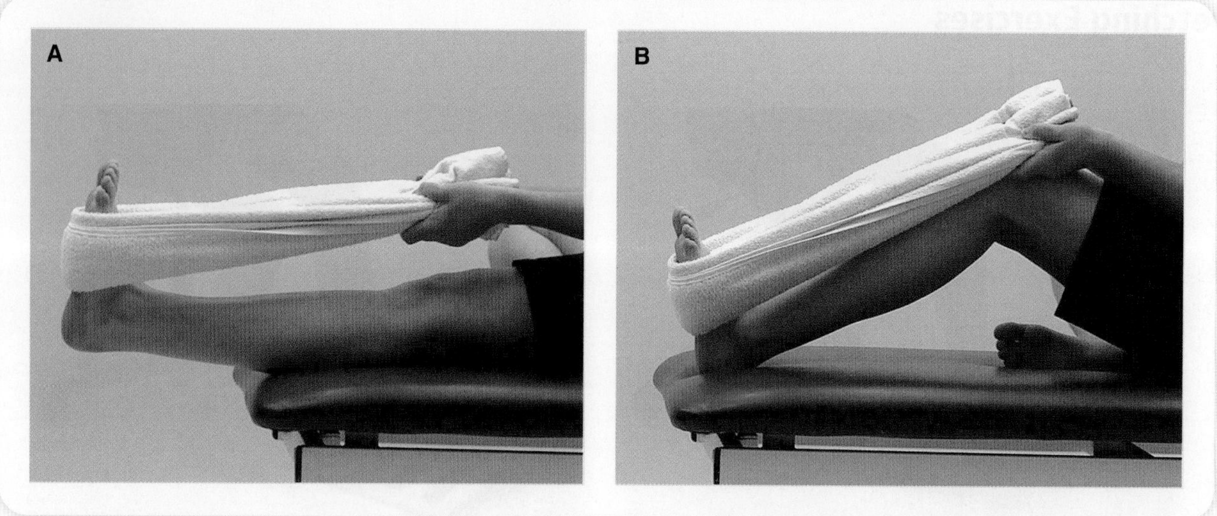

Exercise 26-27

Seated heel cord stretch using a towel. **A.** Gastrocnemius. **B.** Soleus.

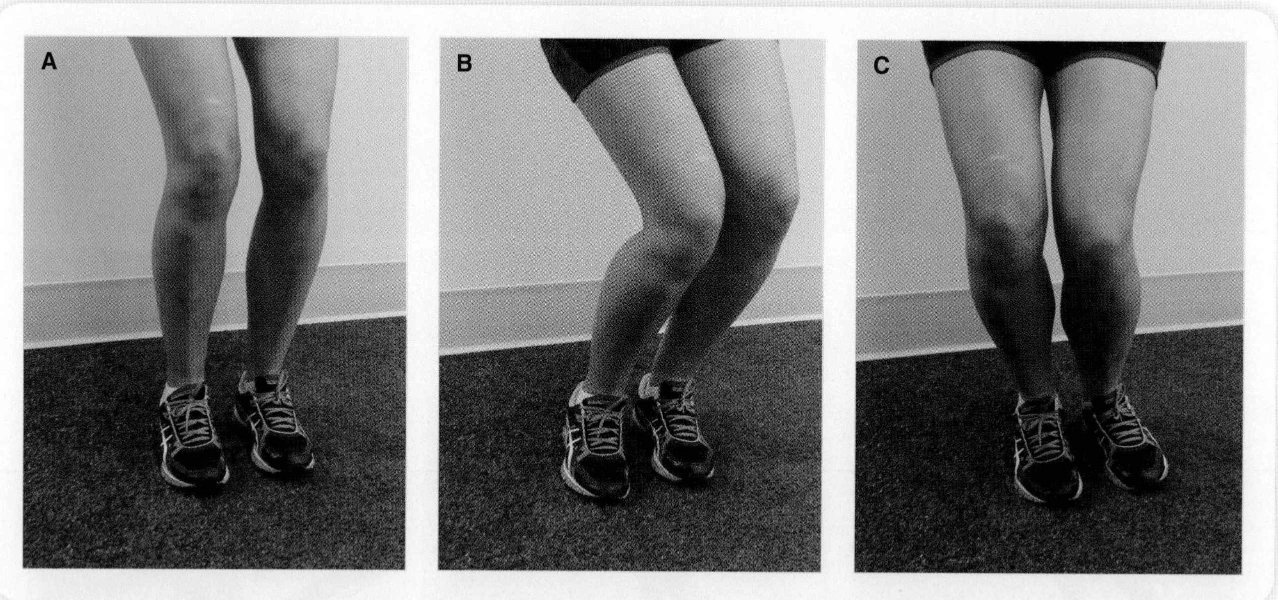

Exercise 26-28

Dynamic heel cord stretch. **A.** Position 1. **B.** Position 2. **C.** Position 3. Varied positions offer different dynamic challenges to the ankle and foot musculature, in addition to stretching the heel cord.

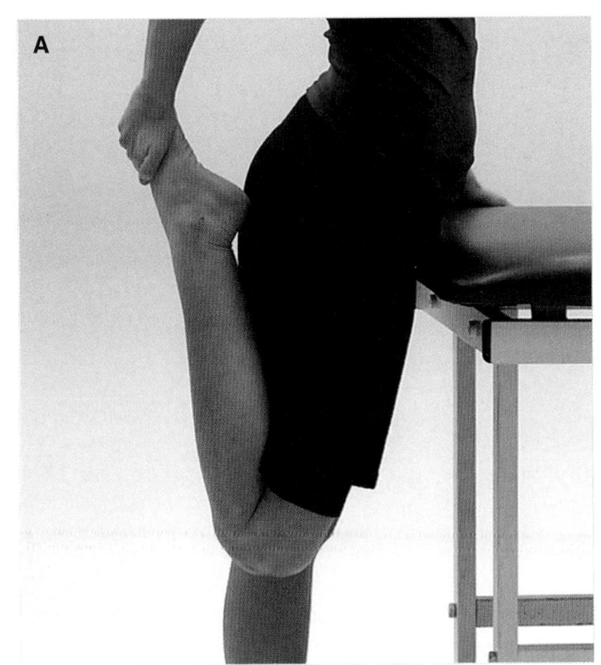

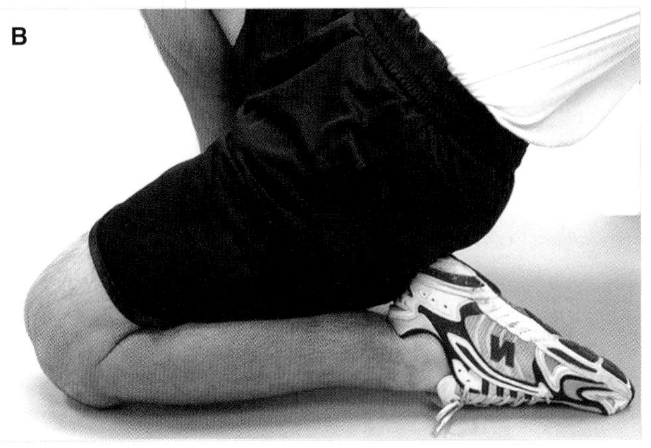

Exercise 26-29

Ankle plantarflexion stretch for the anterior tibialis. **A.** Standing. **B.** Kneeling.

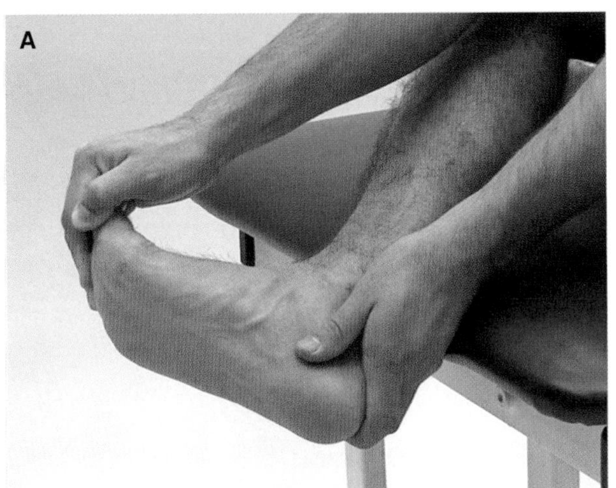

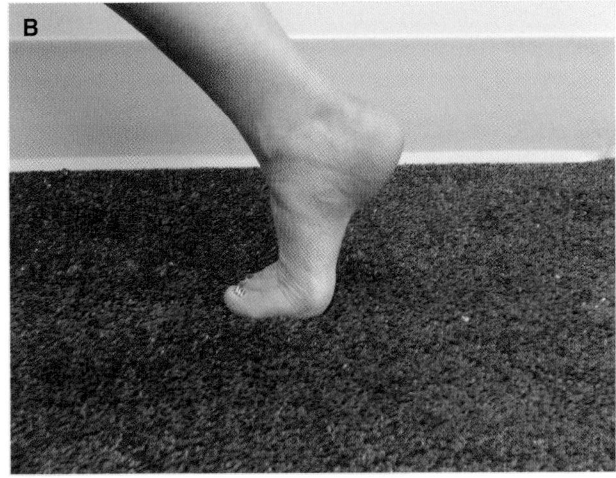

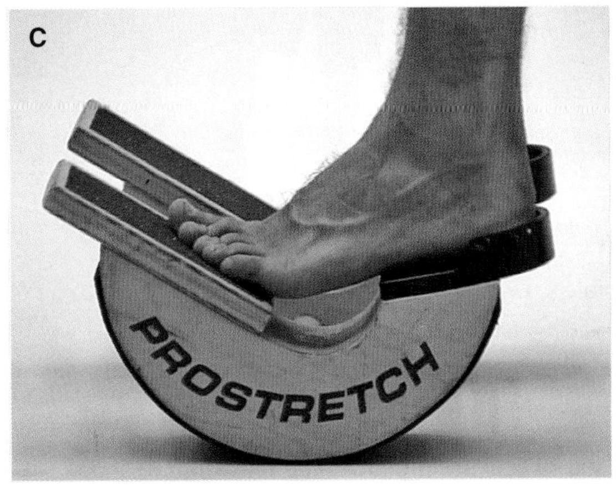

Exercise 26-30

Plantar fascia stretches. **A.** Manual. **B.** Floor stretch. **C.** Prostretch.

Exercises to Reestablish Neuromuscular Control

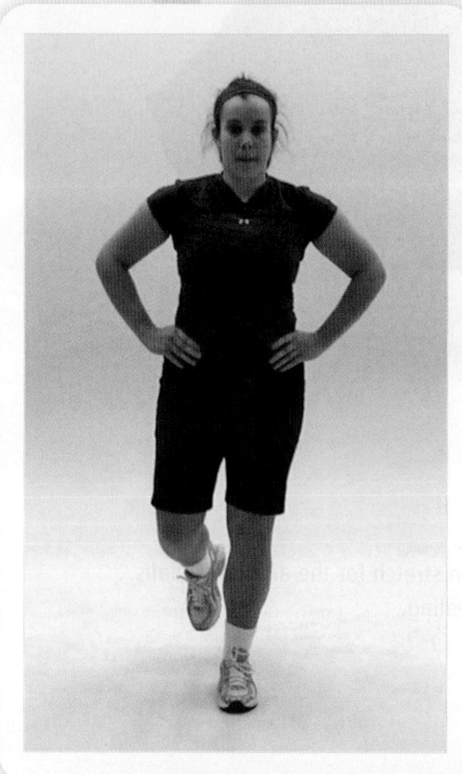

Exercise 26-31

Static single-leg standing balance progression. Used to improve balance and proprioception of the lower extremity. This activity can be made more difficult with the following progression: (a) single-leg standing with eyes open; (b) single-leg standing with eyes closed; (c) single-leg standing with eyes open and toes extended so only the heel and metatarsal heads are in contact with the ground; and (d) single-leg standing with eyes closed and toes extended.

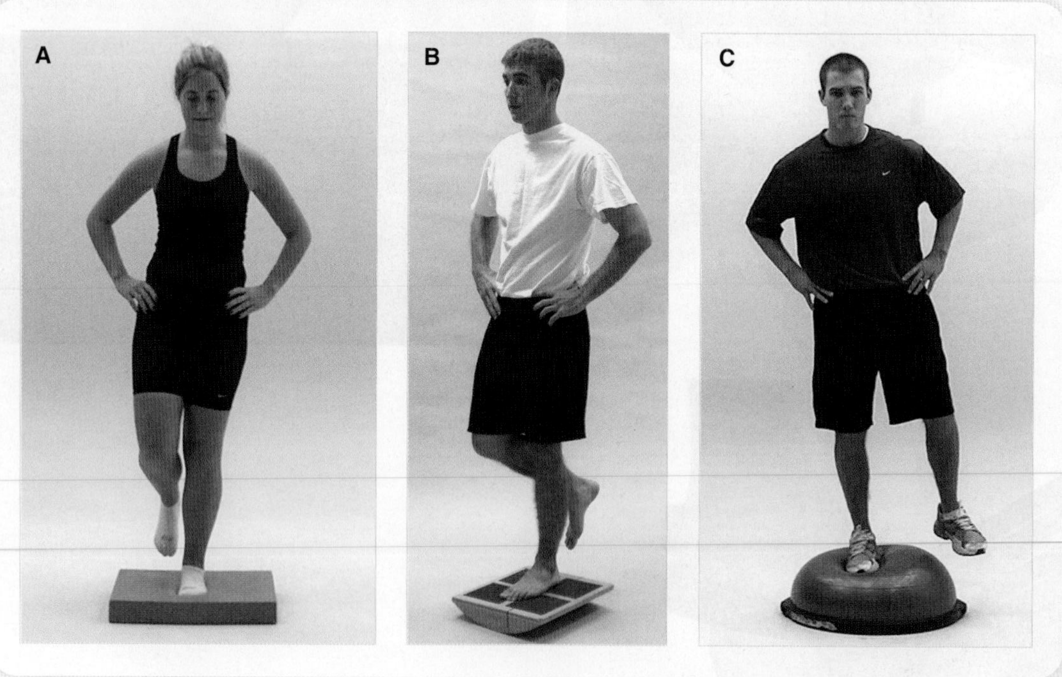

Exercise 26-32

Standing single-leg balance activities of increasing difficulty. Used to activate the lower-leg musculature and improve balance and proprioception of the involved extremity. **A.** Wedge board. **B.** BAPS board. **C.** BOSU ball.

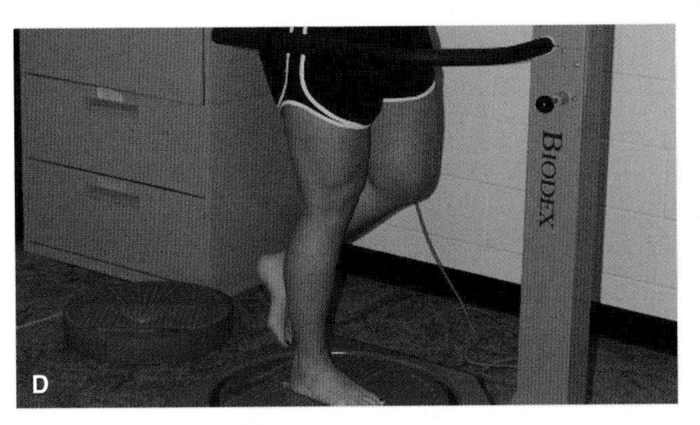

Exercise 26-32 (*Continued*)

D. Biodex Stability System™.

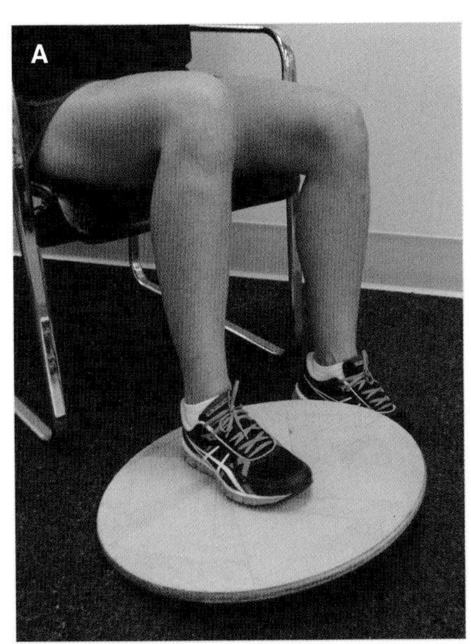

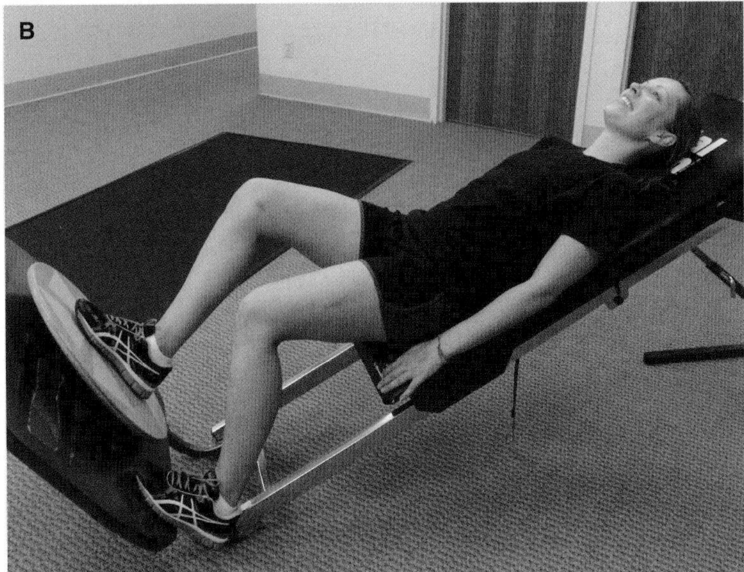

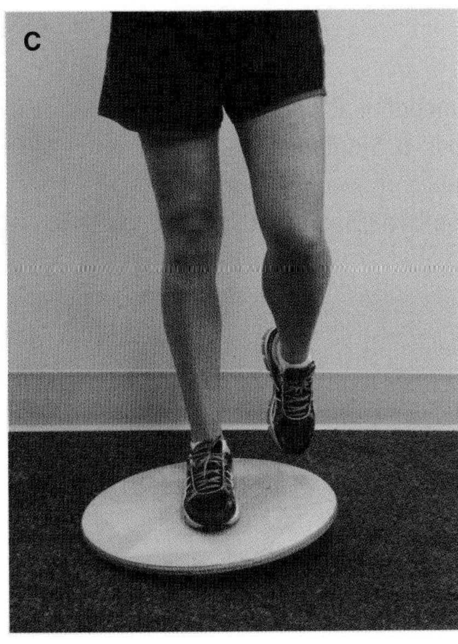

Exercise 26-33

Fine motor-control activity in multiple planes using the Fitter wobble board for weightbearing progressions. **A.** Seated. **B.** Total Gym. **C.** Standing.

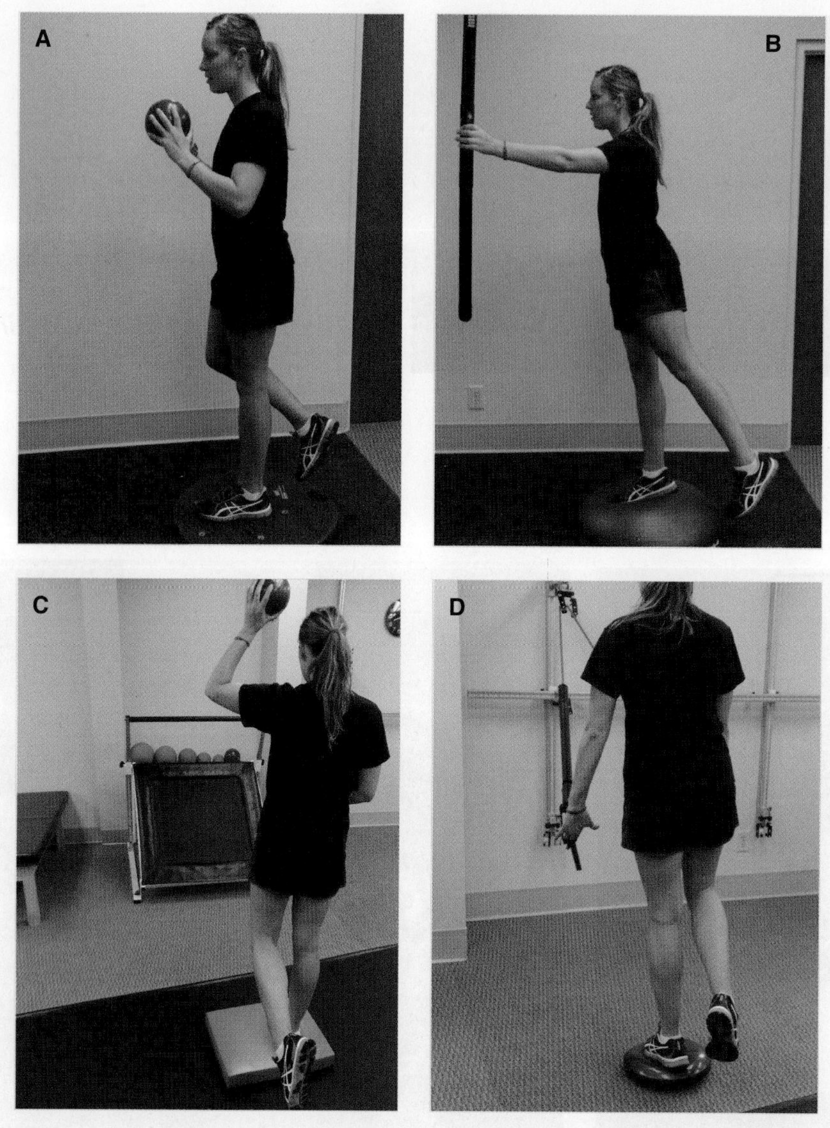

Exercise 26-34

Single-leg stance on an unstable surface while performing functional activities. **A.** Single-limb stance on BAPS™ board with medicine ball toss. **B.** Single-limb stance on BOSU™ ball with Body Blade™. **C.** Single-limb stance on Airex™ foam pad with Plyoback medicine ball toss. **D.** Single-limb stance on DynaDisc™ with tubing self-perturbations (forward).

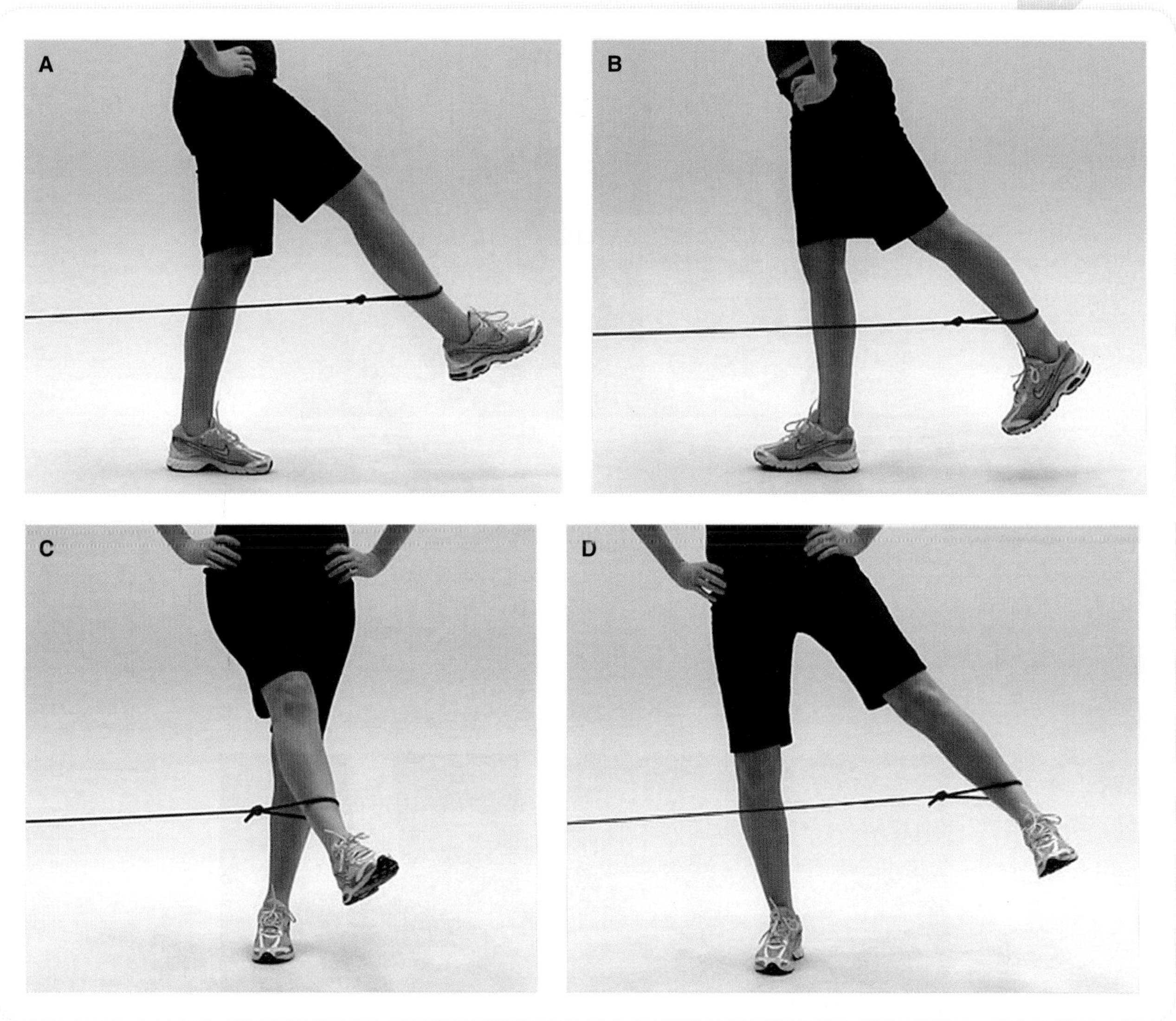

Exercise 26-35

Single-limb stance tubing kicks. Resisted kicks with the tubing around the uninvolved side while weight bearing on the involved side will challenge neuromuscular control. Four directions: **A.** Flexion. **B.** Extension. **C.** Adduction. **D.** Abduction.

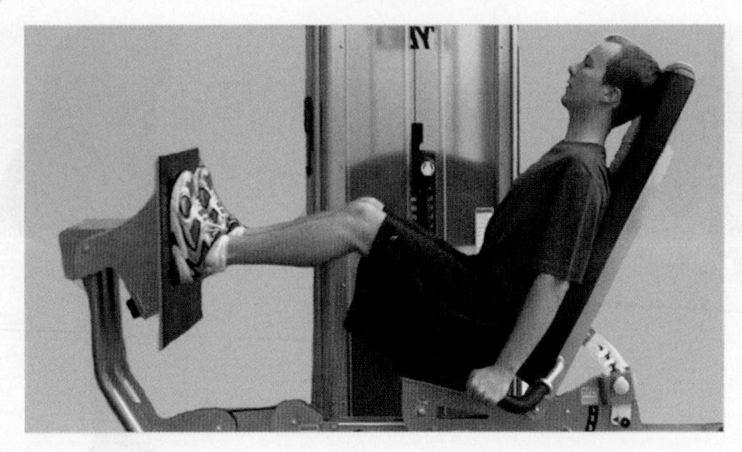

Exercise 26-36

Double-leg press.

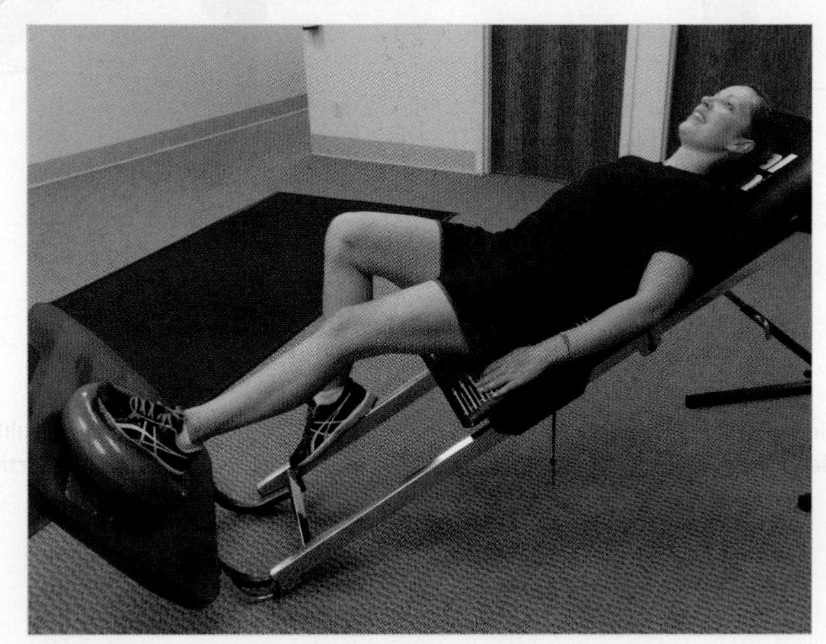

Exercise 26-37

Single-leg press on Total Gym using a DynaDisc.

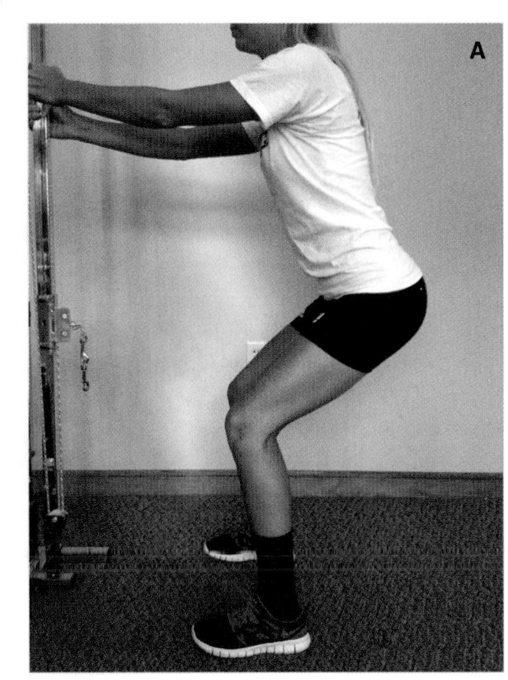

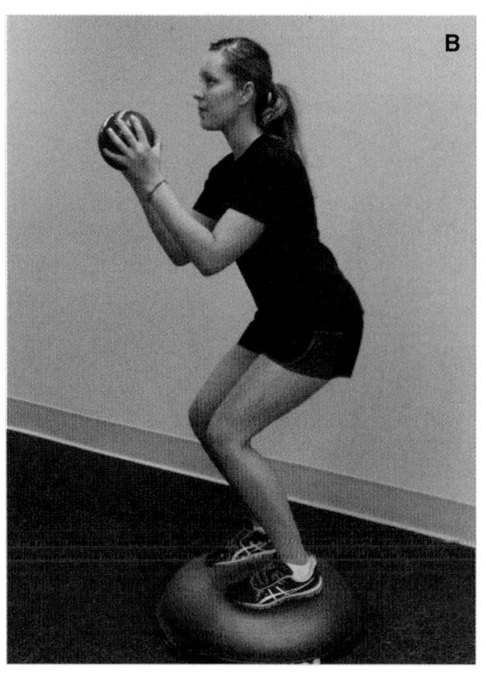

Exercise 26-38

A. Mini form squats. **B.** Mini form squats on BOSU™ ball with medicine ball lift to increase difficulty as a result of perturbation offered by the upper-extremity movement and weighted medicine ball.

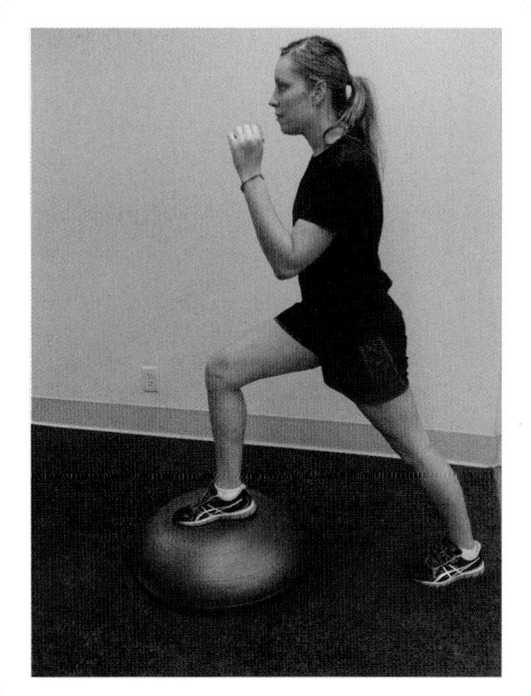

Exercise 26-39

Mini-lunge to unstable surface (BOSU™ ball).

Exercises to Improve Cardiorespiratory Endurance

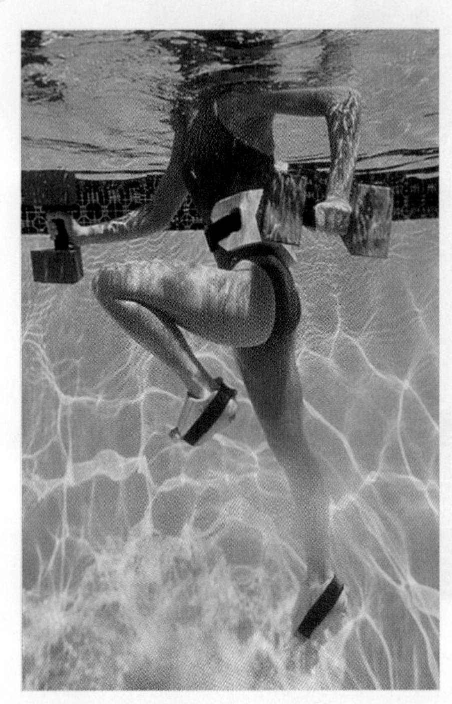

Exercise 26-40

Pool running with flotation device. Used to reduce the impact of weightbearing forces on the lower extremity while maintaining cardiovascular fitness level and running form.

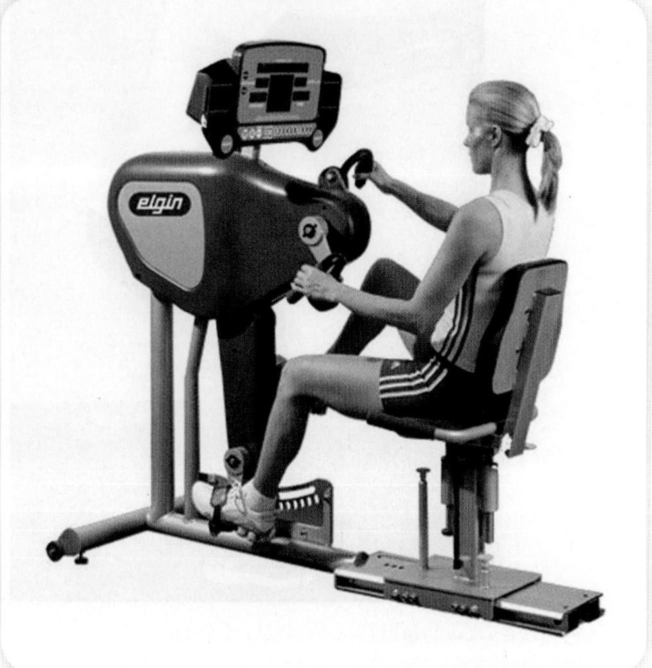

Exercise 26-41

Upper body ergometer used to maintain cardiovascular fitness when LE exercise is too painful or too difficult. Note: This brand of upper extremity ergometer also has LE pedals for alternate use.

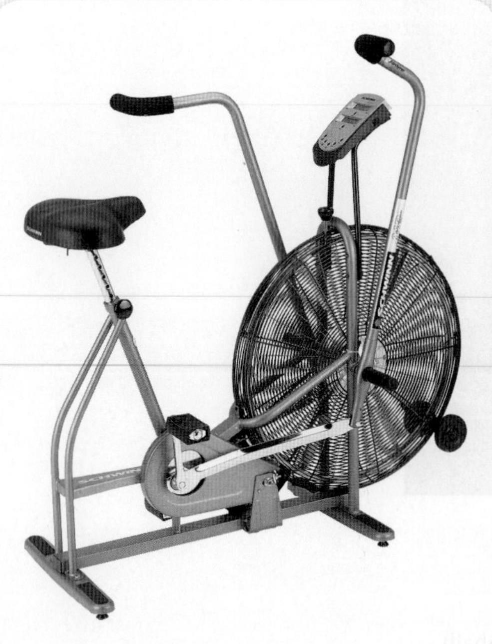

Exercise 26-42

AirDyne stationary exercise bicycle. Used to maintain cardiovascular fitness when lower-extremity weight bearing is difficult.

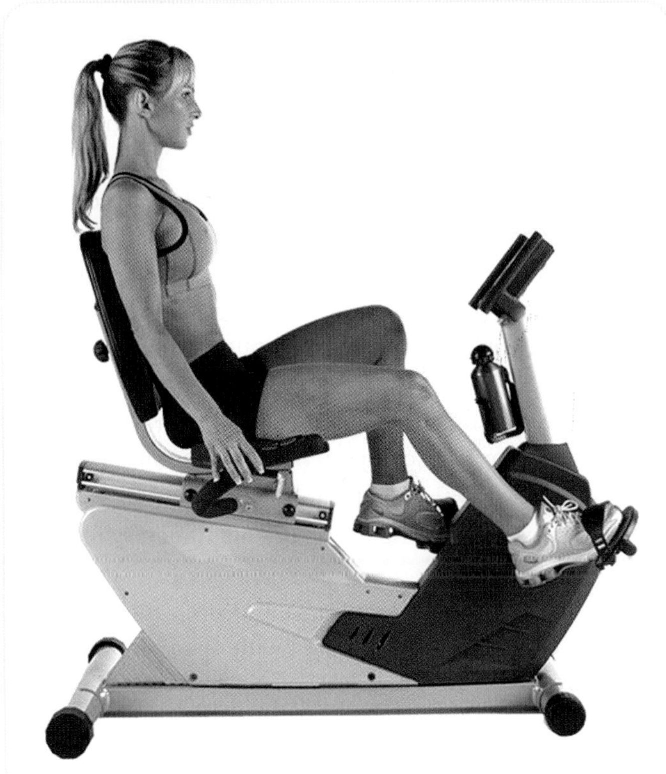

Exercise 26-43

Recumbant bicycle.

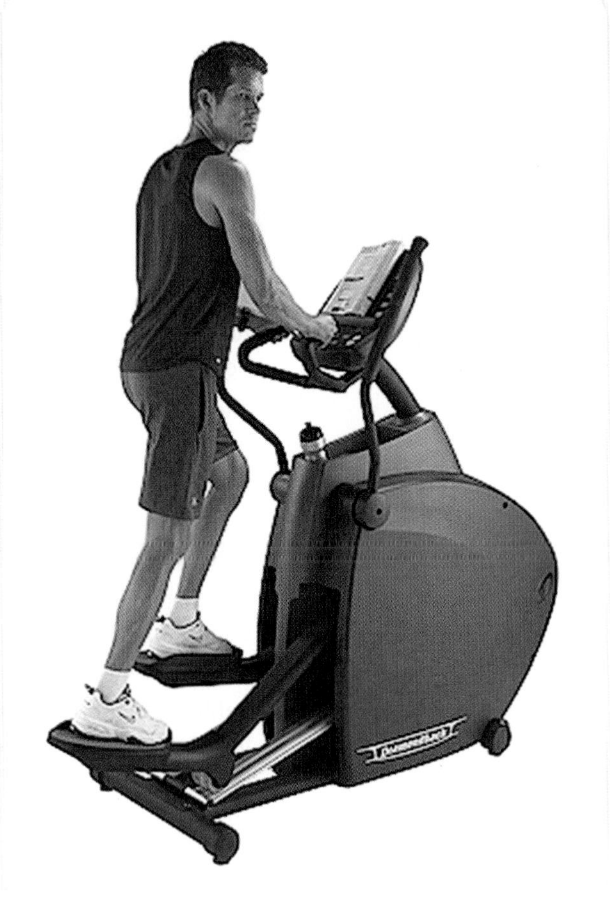

Exercise 26-44

Elliptical trainer. Used to maintain cardiovascular fitness when weight bearing, no impact activity is recommended.

SUMMARY

1. The movements that take place at the talocrural joint are ankle plantarflexion and dorsiflexion. Inversion and eversion occur at the STJ.
2. The position of the STJ determines whether the MTJs will be hypermobile or hypomobile. Dysfunction at either joint may have a profound effect on the foot and lower extremity.
3. Ankle sprains are very common. Inversion sprains usually involve the lateral ligaments of the ankle, and eversion sprains frequently involve the medial ligaments of the ankle. Rotational injuries often involve the tibiofibular and syndesmotic ligaments and may be very severe.
4. The early phase of treatment of ankle sprains includes use of ice, compression, elevation, rest, and protection, all of which are critical components in preventing swelling.
5. Early weight bearing following ankle sprain is beneficial to the healing process. Rehabilitation may become more aggressive following the acute inflammatory response phase of healing.
6. Nondisplaced ankle fractures should be managed with rest and protection until the fracture has healed, whereas displaced fractures are treated with open reduction and internal fixation.
7. Subluxation of peroneal tendons can occur from any mechanism causing sudden and forceful contraction of the peroneal muscles that involves dorsiflexion and eversion of the foot. In the case of an avulsion injury or when this becomes a chronic problem, conservative treatment is unlikely to be successful and surgery is needed to prevent the problem from recurring.
8. Tendinitis in the posterior tibialis, anterior tibialis, and the peroneal tendons may result from one specific cause or from a collection of mechanisms. Techniques should be incorporated into rehabilitation that acts to reduce or eliminate inflammation, including rest, using therapeutic modalities (ice, ultrasound, iontophoresis), and using antiinflammatory medications as prescribed by a physician.
9. Excessive or prolonged supination or pronation at the STJ is likely to result from some structural or functional deformity, including forefoot varus, a forefoot valgus, or a rearfoot varus, which forces the STJ to compensate in a manner that will allow the weightbearing surfaces of the foot to make stable contact with the ground and get into a weightbearing position.
10. Orthotics are used to control abnormal compensatory movements of the foot by "bringing the floor to the foot." By providing support so that the foot does not have to move abnormally, an orthotic should help prevent compensatory problems.
11. Shoe selection is an important parameter in the treatment of foot problems. The type of foot will dictate specific shoe features.
12. The most common stress fractures in the foot involve the navicular, second metatarsal (March fracture), and diaphysis of the fifth metatarsal (Jones fracture). Navicular and second metatarsal stress fractures are likely to occur with excessive foot pronation, whereas fifth metatarsal stress fractures tend to occur in a more rigid pes cavus foot.
13. A number of anatomic and biomechanical conditions have been studied as possible causes of plantar fasciitis. There is pain in the anterior medial heel, usually at the attachment of the plantar fascia to the calcaneus. Orthotics in combination with stretching exercises can significantly reduce pain.
14. Subluxation of the cuboid will create symptoms similar to plantar fasciitis and can be corrected with manipulation.

15. A bunion is a deformity of the head of the first metatarsal in which the large toe assumes a valgus position that is commonly associated with a structural forefoot varus in which the first ray tends to splay outward, putting pressure on the first metatarsal head.
16. In treating a Morton neuroma, a metatarsal bar is placed just proximal to the metatarsal heads or a teardrop-shaped pad is placed between the heads of the third and fourth metatarsals in an attempt to have these splay apart with weight bearing.
17. Turf toe is a hyperextension injury resulting in a sprain of the metatarsophalangeal joint of the great toe.

REFERENCES

1. Acevedo JI, Beskin JL. Complications of plantar fascia rupture associated with corticosteroid injection. *Foot Ankle Int.* 1998;2:91-97.
2. American Physical Rehabilitation Network. *When the Feet Hit the Ground...Everything Changes. Program Outline and Prepared Notes—A Basic Manual.* Sylvania, OH; 2000.
3. American Physical Rehabilitation Network. *When the Feet Hit the Ground...Take the Next Step. Program Outline and Prepared Notes—An Advanced Manual.* Sylvania, OH; 1994.
4. Andrews JR, McClod W, Ward T, et al. The cutting mechanism. *Am J Sports Med.* 1977;5:111-121.
5. Arnheim D, Prentice W. *Principles of Athletic Training.* New York, NY: McGraw-Hill; 2000.
6. Baer T. Designing for the long run. *Mech Eng.* 1984;6:67-75.
7. Bates BT, Osternig L, Mason B, et al. Foot orthotic devices to modify selected aspects of lower extremity mechanics. *Am J Sports Med.* 1979;7:338.
8. Baxter D. *The Foot and Ankle in Sport.* St. Louis, MO: Mosby; 1995.
9. Birnham JS. *The Musculoskeletal Manual.* New York, NY: Academic Press; 1982.
10. Bosien WR, Staples OS, Russell SW. Residual disability following acute ankle sprains. *J Bone Joint Surg Am.* 1955;37:1237.
11. Bostrum L. Treatment and prognosis in recent ligament ruptures. *Acta Chir Scand.* 1966;132:537-550.
12. Braunstein B, Arampatzis A, Eysel P, Brüggemann GP. Footwear affects the gearing of the ankle and knee joints during running. *J Biomech.* 2010;43:2120-2125.
13. Brody DM. Techniques in the evaluation and treatment of the injured runner. *Orthop Clin North Am.* 1982;13:541.
14. Brotzman B, Brasel J. Foot and ankle rehabilitation. In: Brotzman B, ed. *Clinical Orthopaedic Rehabilitation.* St. Louis, MO: Mosby; 1996.
15. Brunet ME, Cook SD, Brinker MR, Dickinson JA. A survey of running injuries in 1505 competitive and recreational runners. *J Sports Med Phys Fitness.* 1990;30:307-315.
16. Brunwich T, Wischnia B. Battle of the midsoles. *Runner's World,* April 1987:47.
17. Burgess PR, Wei J. Signalling of kinesthetic information by peripheral sensory receptors. *Annu Rev Neurosci.* 1982;5:171-187.
18. Calliet R. *Foot and Ankle Pain.* Philadelphia, PA: Davis; 1968.
19. Canoy WF. *Review of Medical Physiology,* 7th ed. Los Altos, CA: Lange; 1975.
20. Cavanaugh PR. *An Evaluation of the Effects of Orthotics Force Distribution and Rearfoot Movement During Running.* Paper presented at meeting of American Orthopedic Society for Sports Medicine, Lake Placid, 1978.
21. Choi J. Acute conditions: Incidence and associated disability. *Vital Health Stat 10.* 1978;120:10.
22. Collona P. Fabrication of a custom molded orthotic using an intrinsic posting technique for a forefoot varus deformity. *Phys Ther Forum.* 1989;8:3.
23. Cutler JM. Lateral ligamentous injuries of the ankle. In: Hamilton WC, ed. *Lateral Ligamentous Injuries of the Ankle.* New York, NY: Springer-Verlag; 1984.
24. Delacerda FG. A study of anatomical factors involved in shinsplints. *J Orthop Sports Phys Ther.* 1980;2:55-59.
25. De Wit B, De Clercq D, Aerts P. Biomechanical analysis of the stance phase during barefoot and shod running. *J Biomech.* 2000;33:269-278.
26. Dicharry J. Kinematics and kinetics of gait: from lab to clinic. *Clin Sports Med.* 2010;29:347-364.
27. Divert C, Mornieux G, Baur H, Mayer F, Belli A. Mechanical comparison of barefoot and shod running. *Int J Sports Med.* 2005;26:593-598.
28. Donatelli R. Normal biomechanics of the foot and ankle. *J Orthop Sports Phys Ther.* 1985;7:91-95.
29. Donatelli R, Hurlbert C, Conaway D, et al. Biomechanical foot orthotics: a retrospective study. *J Orthop Sports Phys Ther.* 1988;10:205-212.
30. Drez D, Faust D, Evans P. Cryotherapy and nerve palsy. *Am J Sports Med.* 1981;9:256-257.

31. Fredericson M, Cookingham CL, Chaudhari AM, Dowdell BC, Oestreicher N, Sahrmann SA. Hip abductor weakness in distance runners with iliotibial band syndrome. *Clin J Sport Med.* 2000;10:169-175.
32. Freeman M, Dean M, Hanhan I. The etiology and prevention of functional instability at the foot. *J Bone Joint Surg Br.* 1965;47:678-685.
33. Fumich RM, Ellison A, Guerin G, et al. The measured effect of taping on combined foot and ankle motion before and after exercise. *Am J Sports Med.* 1981;9:165-169.
34. Fury JG. Plantar fasciitis. The painful heel syndrome. *J Bone Joint Surg Am.* 1975;5:672-673.
35. Garn SN, Newton RA. Kinesthetic awareness in subjects with multiple ankle sprains. *Phys Ther.* 1988;68:1667-1671.
36. Garrick JG. When can I...? A practical approach to rehabilitation illustrated by treatment of an ankle injury. *Am J Sports Med.* 1981;9:67-68.
37. Garrick JG, Requa RK. Role of external supports in the prevention of ankle sprains. *Med Sci Sports Exerc.* 1977;5:200.
38. Gene H, Saracoglu M, Nacir B, et al. Long-term ultrasonographic follow-up of plantar fasciitis patients treated with steroid injection. *Joint Bone Spine.* 2005;72(1):61.
39. Giallonardo LM. Clinical evaluation of foot and ankle dysfunction. *Phys Ther.* 1988;68:1850-1856.
40. Gill E. Orthotics. *Runner's World.* February 1985:55-57.
41. Gill LH. Plantar fasciitis: diagnosis and conservative management. *J Am Acad Orthop Surg.* 1997;2:109-117.
42. Giuliani J, Masini B, Alitz C, Owens BD. Barefoot-simulating footwear associated with metatarsal stress injury in 2 runners. *Orthopedics.* 2011;34:320-323.
43. Glencross D, Thornton E. Position sense following joint injury. *J Sport Med Phys Fitness.* 1981;21:23-27.
44. Glick J, Sampson T. Ankle and foot fractures in athletics. In: Nicholas J, Hershman E, eds. *The Lower Extremity and Spine in Sports Medicine.* St. Louis, MO: Mosby; 1996.
45. Gross M, Lapp A, Davis M. Comparison of Swed-O-Universal ankle support and Aircast Sport Stirrup orthoses and ankle tape in restricting eversion—inversion before and after exercise. *J Orthop Sports Phys Ther.* 1991;13:11-19.
46. Heiderscheit BC, Chumanov ES, Michalski MP, Wille CM, Ryan MB. Effects of step manipulation on joint mechanics during running. *Med Sci Sports Exerc.* 2011;43:296-302.
47. Heiderscheit BC. Gait retraining for runners: in search of the ideal. *J Orthop Sports Phys Ther.* 2011;41: 909-910.
48. Hirata I. Proper playing conditions. *J Sports Med.* 1974;4: 228-234.
49. Hoppenfield S. *Physical Examination of the Spine and Extremities.* New York, NY: Appleton-Century-Crofts; 1976.
50. Hunt G. Examination of lower extremity dysfunction. In: Gould J, Davies G, eds. *Orthopedic and Sports Physical Therapy,* Vol. 2. St. Louis, MO: Mosby; 1985.
51. Hunter S, Dolan M, Davis M. *Foot Orthotics in Therapy and Sports.* Champaign, IL: Human Kinetics; 1996.
52. Isakov E, Mizrahi J, Solzi P, et al. Response of the peroneal muscles to sudden inversion of the ankle during standing. *Int J Sports Biomech.* 1986;2:100-109.
53. Itay S. Clinical and functional status following lateral ankle sprains: follow-up of 90 young adults treated conservatively. *Orthop Rev.* 1982;11:73-76.
54. James SL. Chondromalacia of the patella in the adolescent. In: Kennedy SC, ed. *The Injured Adolescent.* Baltimore, MD: Lippincott Williams & Wilkins; 1979.
55. James SL, Bates BT, Osternig LR. Injuries to runners. *Am J Sports Med.* 1978;6:43.
56. Jones D, Singer K. Soft-tissue conditions of the foot and ankle. In: Nicholas J, Hershman E, eds. *The Lower Extremity and Spine in Sports Medicine.* St. Louis, MO: Mosby; 1996.
57. Kelikian H, Kelikian AS. *Disorders of the Ankle.* Philadelphia, PA: Saunders; 1985.
58. Kergerris S. The construction and implementation of functional progressions as a component of athletic rehabilitation. *J Orthop Sports Phys Ther.* 1983;5:14-19.
59. Klein KK. A study of cross transfer of muscular strength and endurance resulting from progressive resistive exercises following surgery. *J Assoc Phys Ment Rehabil.* 1955;9:5.
60. Korpelainen R, Orava S, Karpakka J, Siira P, Hulkko A. Risk factors for recurrent stress fractures in athletes. *Am J Sports Med.* 2001;29:304-310.
61. Kowal MA. Review of physiologic effects of cryotherapy. *J Orthop Sports Phys Ther.* 1983;5:66-73.
62. Leach R, Jones R, Silva T. Rupture of the plantar fascia in athletes. *J Bone Joint Surg Am.* 1978;4:44-46.
63. Lemont H, Ammirati KM, Usen N. Plantar fasciitis: a degenerative process (fasciosis) without inflammation. *J Am Podiatr Med Assoc.* 2003;3:234-237.
64. Lieberman DE, Venkadesan M, Werbel WA, et al. Foot strike patterns and collision forces in habitually barefoot versus shod runners. *Nature.* 2010;463: 531-535.
65. Lorenz DS, Pontillo M. Is there evidence to support a forefoot strike pattern in barefoot runners? A Rreview. *Sports Health: A Multidisciplinary Approach.* 2012;4(6):480-484.
66. Loudin J, Bell S. The foot and ankle: an overview of arthrokinematics and selected joint techniques. *J Athl Train.* 1996;31:173-178.
67. Mandelbaum BR, Finerman G, Grant T, et al. Collegiate football players with recurrent ankle sprains. *Phys Sportsmed.* 1987;15:57-61.
68. Mayhew JL, Riner WF. Effects of ankle wrapping on motor performance. *Athl Train.* 1974;3:128-130.
69. McCluskey GM, Blackburn TA, Lewis T. Prevention of ankle sprains. *Am J Sports Med.* 1976;4:151-157.
70. McPoil TG. Footwear. *Phys Ther.* 1988;68:1857-1865.
71. McPoil TG, Adrian M, Pidcoe P. Effects of foot orthoses on center of pressure patterns in women. *Phys Ther.* 1989;69:149-154.

72. McPoil TG, Brocato RS. The foot and ankle: Biomechanical evaluation and treatment. In: Gould J, Davies G, eds. *Orthopedic and Sports Physical Therapy*. St. Louis, MO: Mosby; 1985.
73. McPoil TG, Knecht HG, Schmit D. A survey of foot types in normal females between the ages of 18 and 30 years. *J Orthop Sports Phys Ther.* 1988;9:406-409.
74. Melegati G, Tornese D, Bandi M, et al. The influence of local steroid injections, body weight and the length of symptoms in the treatment of painful subcalcaneal spurs with extracorporeal shock wave therapy. *Clin Rehabil.* 2002;7:789-794.
75. Milgrom C, Finestone A, Sharkey N, et al. Metatarsal strains are sufficient to cause fatigue during cyclic overloading. *Foot Ankle Int.* 2002;23:230-235.
76. Morley JB, Decker LM, Dierks T, Blanke D, French JA, Stergiou N. Effects of varying amounts of pronation on the mediolateral ground reaction forces during barefoot versus shod running. *J Appl Biomech.* 2010;26:205-214.
77. Morris JM. Biomechanics of the foot and ankle. *Clin Orthop.* 1977;122:10-17.
78. Morton DJ. Foot disorders in general practice. *JAMA.* 1937;109:1112-1119.
79. Nawoczenski DA, Owen M, Ecker M, et al. Objective evaluation of peroneal response to sudden inversion stress. *J Orthop Sports Phys Ther.* 1985;7:107-119.
80. Nicholas JA, Hershman EB. *The Lower Extremity and Spine in Sports Medicine*. St. Louis, MO: Mosby; 1990.
81. Niemuth PE, Johnson RJ, Myers MJ, Thieman TJ. Hip muscle weakness and overuse injuries in recreational runners. *Clin J Sport Med.* 200515:14-21.
82. Noyes FR. Functional properties of knee ligaments and alterations induced by immobilization: a correlative biomechanical and histological study in primates. *Clin Orthop.* 1977;123:210-243.
83. Oatis CA. Biomechanics of the foot and ankle under static conditions. *Phys Ther.* 1988;68:1815-1821.
84. Ogden J, Alvarez RG, Cross GL, et al. Plantar fasciopathy and orthotripsy: the effect of prior contisone injection. *Foot Ankle Int.* 2005;3:231-233.
85. Ogden J, Alvarez RG, Levitt, RL, et al. Electrohydraulic high-energy shock-wave treatment for chronic plantar fasciitis. *J Bone Joint Surg Am.* 2004;10:2216-2228.
86. Pagliano JN. Athletic footwear. *Sports Med Digest.* 1988;10:1-2.
87. Peeland A. The relationship of pedal osseous malalignment to pain in other body segments. *Current Podiatric Medicine.* May, 1998.
88. Porter MD, Shadbolt B. Intralesional corticosteroid injection versus extracorporeal shock wave therapy for plantar fasciopathy. *Clin J Sport Med.* 2005;3:119-124.
89. Prentice W. *Therapeutic Modalities in Sports Medicine.* Dubuque, IA: WCB/McGraw-Hill; 1999.
90. Quillen S. Alternative management protocol for lateral ankle sprains. *J Orthop Sports Phys Ther.* 1980;12:187-190.
91. Rajkumar P, Schmitgen GF. Shock waves do more than just crush stones: extracorporeal shockwave therapy in plantar fasciitis. *Int J Clin Pract.* 2002;10:735-737.
92. Rebman LW. Ankle injuries: clinical observations. *J Orthop Sports Phys Ther.* 1986;8:153-156.
93. Riegler HF. Orthotic devices for the foot. *Orthop Rev.* 1987;16:293-303.
94. Robbins SE, Hanna AM. Running-related injury prevention through barefoot adaptations. *Med Sci Sports Exerc.* 1987;19:148-156.
95. Rogers MM, LeVeau BF. Effectiveness of foot orthotic devices used to modify pronation in runners. *J Orthop Sports Phys Ther.* 1982;4:86-90.
96. Rothschild C. Running barefoot or in minimalist shoes: evidence or conjecture? *Strength Cond J.* 2012;34:8-17.
97. Root ML, Orien WP, Weed JH. *Normal and Abnormal Functions of the Foot.* Los Angeles, CA: Clinical Biomechanics; 1977.
98. Sammarco JG. *Rehabilitation of the Foot and Ankle.* St. Louis, MO: Mosby; 1995.
99. Sammarco JG. Biomechanics of foot and ankle injuries. *Athl Train.* 1975;10:96.
100. Sapega AA, Quedenfeld TC, Moyer RA, et al. Biophysical factors in range-of-motion exercise. *Phys Sportsmed.* 1981;12:57-64.
101. Sellman JR. Plantar fascia ruptures associated with corticosteroid injection. *Foot Ankle Int.* 1994;7:376-381.
102. Sims D. Effects of positioning on ankle edema. *J Orthop Sports Phys Ther.* 1986;8:30-33.
103. Sims DS, Cavanaugh PR, Ulbrecht JS. Risk factors in the diabetic foot. *Phys Ther.* 1988;68:1887-1901.
104. Sloan JP, Guddings P, Hain R. Effects of cold and compression on edema. *Phys Sportsmed.* 1988;16:116-120.
105. Squadrone R, Gallozzi C. Biomechanical and physiological comparison of barefoot and two shod conditions in experience barefoot runners. *J Sports Med Phys Fitness.* 2009;49:6-13.
106. Stacoff A, Nigg BM, Reinschmidt C, van den Bogert AJ, Lundberg A. Tibiocalcaneal kinematics of barefoot versus shod running. *J Biomech.* 2000;33:1387-1395.
107. Stover CN, York JM. Air stirrup management of ankle injuries in the patient. *Am J Sports Med.* 1980;8:360-365.
108. Subotnick SI. The flat foot. *Phys Sportsmed.* 1981;9:85-91.
109. Subotnick SI. *The Running Foot Doctor*. Mt. Vias, CA: World; 1977.
110. Subotnick SI, Newell SG. *Podiatric Sports Medicine.* Mt. Kisco, NY: Futura; 1975.
111. Thijs Y, Van Tiggelen D, Roosen P, De Clercq D, Witvrouw E. A prospective study on gait-related intrinsic risk factors of patellofemoral pain. *Clin J Sport Med.* 2007;17:437-445.
112. Tiberio D. Pathomechanics of structural foot deformities. *Phys Ther.* 1988;68:1840-1849.
113. Tippett SR. A case study: the need for evaluation and reevaluation of acute ankle sprains. *J Orthop Sports Phys Ther.* 1982;4:44.
114. Tropp H, Askling C, Gillquist J. Prevention of ankle sprains. *Am J Sports Med.* 1985;13:259-266.

115. Vaes P, DeBoeck H, Handleberg F, et al. Comparative radiologic study of the influence of ankle joint bandages on ankle stability. *Am J Sports Med.* 1985;13:46-49.
116. Visnich AL. A playing orthoses for "turf toe." *Athl Train.* 1987;22:215.
117. Vogelbach WD, Combs LC. A biomechanical approach to the management of chronic lower extremity pathologies as they relate to excessive pronation. *Athl Train.* 1987;22:6-16.
118. Williams JGP. The foot and chondromalacia—a case of biomechanical uncertainty. *J Orthop Sports Phys Ther.* 1980;2:50-51.
119. Woods A, Smith W. Cuboid syndrome and the techniques used for treatment. *Athl Train.* 1983;18:64-65.
120. Yablon IG, Segal D, Leach RE. *Ankle Injuries.* New York, NY: Churchill Livingstone; 1983.
121. Zylks DR. Alternative taping for plantar fasciitis. *Athl Train.* 1987;22:317.

Rehabilitation Protocols

Achilles Tendon Repair Program*

- Surgical indications: Rupture of the Achilles tendon from the insertion on the calcaneus.
- Surgical interventions: Surgical fixation of the Achilles tendon to the anatomical insertion on the calcaneus.

Acute Phase

Beginning of Week 3 Postoperatively

1. Weightbearing status: Non–weight bearing
2. Patient education in protection of surgical site
3. ROM exercises:
   a. Out-of-splint active ROM (AROM)
   b. Plantarflexion and/or dorsiflexion (2 sets of 5 repetitions 3 times per day)
4. Strengthening:
   a. Initiate non–weightbearing proximal strengthening activities for lower extremities and core stabilizers (3 sets of 15 repetitions)
5. Proprioceptive/neuromuscular reeducation exercises:
   a. Seated rocker board for plantarflexion and dorsiflexion (Exercise 26-25A)

Week 4 Postoperatively

1. Weightbearing status: Non–weight bearing
2. ROM exercises:
   a. Out-of-splint AROM
   b. Plantarflexion and/or dorsiflexion (2 sets of 20 repetitions)
   c. Inversion and/or eversion (2 sets of 20 repetitions)
   d. Circumduction in both directions (2 sets of 20 repetitions)
3. Strengthening exercises:
   a. Isometric inversion and/or eversion in neutral (2 sets of 20 repetitions) (Exercises 26-1 and 26-2)
   b. Toe curls with towel and weight (Exercise 26-12)

*The Achilles Tendon Repair Program modified and used with permission from Orthopaedic Associates of Grand Rapids, PC, Grand Rapids, MI.

   c. Continue with non-weightbearing proximal strengthening for lower extremities and core stabilizers (3 sets of 15 repetitions)

4. Proprioceptive/neuromuscular re-education exercises:
   a. Seated rocker board for plantarflexion-dorsiflexion and inversion-eversion (Exercises 26-25*A* and *B*)
   b. Seated wobble board for clockwise and counterclockwise circumduction (Exercise 26-33*A*)
5. Physical therapy adjuncts:
   a. Gentle manual mobilization of scar tissue
   b. Cryotherapy with caution of any open areas

Week 5 Postoperatively

1. Weightbearing status: Progressive partial-weight bearing in walker splint
2. ROM exercises:
   a. Previous AROM exercises continued
   b. Begin gentle passive stretching into dorsiflexion with towel (Exercise 26-27*A*)
3. Strengthening exercises:
   a. Isometric inversion and/or eversion (2 sets of 20 repetitions) (Exercises 26-1 and 26-2)
   b. Isometric plantarflexion (initially 2 sets of 10 repetitions, progressing to 2 sets of 20 repetitions over the course of the week) (Exercise 26-3)
   c. Thera-Band inversion and/or eversion (2 sets of 10 repetitions) (Exercises 26-5*B* and 26-6*B*)
   d. Thera-Band plantarflexion and/or dorsiflexion (2 sets of 10 repetitions) (Exercises 26-7*B* and 26-8*B*)
   e. Continue with proximal strengthening for lower extremity and core stabilizers in non- or partial-weight bearing in walker splint (3 sets of 15 repetitions)
4. Proprioceptive/neuromuscular re-education exercises:
   a. Standing rocker board for plantarflexion-dorsiflexion and inversion-eversion maintaining weightbearing restrictions (Exercises 25*A* and *B*, progressed to PWB in standing)
   b. Standing wobble board for clockwise and counterclockwise circumduction maintaining weightbearing restrictions (Exercise 26-33*C*)
5. Conditioning activities:
   a. Stationary bicycling begins, 7 to 12 minutes, minimal resistance (Exercise 26-42)
   b. Water therapy can begin under total buoyant conditions with use of a floatation device (Aqua-jogger vest) (Exercise 26-40)
   c. In the water, ankle ROM and running/walking activities can be initiated
6. Physical therapy adjuncts:
   a. Manual mobilization of scar and cryotherapy continues
   b. Manual mobilization of ankle and foot joints (if necessary)
   c. Gentle passive manual stretching (unless patient already has 10 degrees of dorsiflexion)

Intermediate Phase

Weeks 6 to 8 Postoperatively

1. **Weightbearing status:** Progressive partial- to full-weight bearing by week 7 or 8
2. **ROM exercises:**
   - **a.** Previous ROM exercises decreased to one set of 10 repetitions each direction
   - **b.** Passive stretching continues into dorsiflexion with progressively greater efforts (knee in full extension and flexed to 35 to 40 degrees) (Exercises 26-27*A* and *B*)
   - **c.** Begin standing calf stretch with full extension and flexed at week 7 (Exercises 26-26*A* and *B*)
3. **Strengthening exercises:**
   - **a.** Decrease isometrics to 1 set of 10 repetitions for inversion and/or eversion and plantarflexion
   - **b.** Progress Thera-Band resistance for inversion, eversion, plantarflexion, and dorsiflexion (3 sets of 20 repetitions)
   - **c.** Continue with proximal lower-extremity and core-stability exercises progressing to full-weight bearing after week 7 (Exercises 26-18*A* and *B*)
4. **Conditioning exercises:**
   - **a.** Stationary bicycling to 20 minutes with minimal resistance (Exercise 26-42)
   - **b.** Water therapy exercises continue in totally buoyant state
5. **Proprioceptive/neuromuscular reeducation exercises:**
   - **a.** Continue with previous wobble board and rocker board exercises
   - **b.** *Once full-weight bearing achieved*, can initiate single-leg balance activities on stable surfaces
6. **Physical therapy adjuncts:**
   - **a.** Gentle cross-fiber massage to Achilles tendon to release adhesions between tendon and peritendon soft-tissue structures
   - **b.** Continue with previous manual therapy techniques if needed
   - **c.** Cryotherapy continues; ultrasound and electrical stimulation may be added for chronic swelling or excessive scar formation

Advanced Phase

Weeks 8 to 14 Postoperatively

1. **Weightbearing status:** Full-weight bearing with heel lift (high top shoes)
2. **ROM exercises:**
   - **a.** Further progressed with standing calf stretch
   - **b.** Add dynamic heel cord stretching in multiple planes (Exercises 26-28*A* to *C*)
3. **Strengthening exercises:**
   - **a.** Discontinue isometric exercises
   - **b.** Continue with progressive resistance Thera-Band ankle strengthening in all directions
   - **c.** Begin double-leg heel raises (plantarflexion) with BW as tolerated (Exercises 26-8*C* and 26-11*A* and *B*)

   d. Continue with proximal lower-extremity and core-stability exercises in full-weight bearing (Exercises 26-35*A* to *D*)
4. Proprioceptive/neuromuscular re-education exercises:
   a. Initiate single-leg balance activities on unstable surfaces, including rocker board, wobble board, foam rollers, DynaDisc, BOSU Balance Trainer, or KAT system as tolerated (Exercises 26-32*A* to *D*)
   b. Progress single-leg balance activities on unstable surfaces with perturbations by therapist or using medicine balls, dumb bell weights, Theratubing, or Body Blade (Exercises 26-34*A* to *D*)
5. Conditioning activities:
   a. Stationary cycling
   b. Treadmill walking
   c. StairMaster
   d. Elliptical trainer (Exercise 26-44)
   e. NuStep (Exercise 26-43)
   f. Water therapy exercises in chest-deep water
6. Therapy adjunct:
   a. Previously described if needed

Return to Function Phase

Weeks 14 and Beyond Postoperatively

1. Strengthening exercises:
   a. Heel raises should progress to use additional weight at least as great as BW, and in the case of athletes, up to 1.5 times BW
   b. Initiate single-leg heel raises as tolerated, possibly eccentric first, the progressing to concentric (Exercises 26-8*A* and *D*)
   c. Progress functional strengthening exercises specific to athletic activity as patient tolerates (Exercises 26-15 and 26-39)
2. Conditioning activities:
   a. Progress to jogging on trampoline and then to treadmill running via a walk-run program
   b. Eventually perform steady-state outdoor running up to 20 minutes before adding figure-8 or cutting drills
   c. Water therapy exercises performed in shallow (waist deep) water
   d. In the water, begin to include hopping, bounding, and jumping drills
3. Goals:
   a. The completely rehabilitated Achilles tendon repair allows 15 to 20 degrees of dorsiflexion and the ankle. This must be maintained with regular stretching of the gastrocnemius-soleus group. Caution must be considered not to *overstretch* the Achilles tendon. Do not want to continue manual or passive stretching once 20 degrees of dorsiflexion is achieved
   b. Strength and endurance are developed to preinjury levels, and continued strength and flexibility work is advised
   c. Once return to sporting activities allowed, patient can complete functional sports-specific drills without pain or compensation

Modified Brostrom Ankle Rehabilitation Program†

- Surgical indications: Chronic lateral ankle instability.
- Surgical interventions: A lateral incision is made to the ankle region, at which time the capsule and lateral ligament structures, including the anterior talofibular and calcaneofibular ligaments are tightened. Surgery may also include os calcis osteotomy.

Acute Phase

Weeks 0 to 6 Postoperatively

Prior to Start of Physical Therapy

1. Weightbearing status: Non-weight bearing progressing to full-weight bearing (depends on the physician orders)
2. Patient education in protection of surgical site

Intermediate Phase

Weeks 6 to 8 Postoperatively

1. Weightbearing status: Full-weight bearing
2. ROM exercises: *Protect inversion. Do not stretch out repair*
   a. Out-of-splint AROM
   b. Plantarflexion and/or dorsiflexion (2 sets of 20 repetitions)
   c. Eversion and limited inversion (2 sets of 20 repetitions)
   d. Circumduction in both directions (2 sets of 20 repetitions)
3. Strengthening exercises:
   a. Ankle isometrics in all directions or light manual resistance (2 sets of 20 repetitions) (Exercises 26-1 to 26-4)
   b. Initiate proximal lower-extremity strengthening activities for lower extremity and core stabilizers (3 sets of 15 repetitions) (Exercises 26-35*A* to *D*)
4. Stretching exercises:
   a. Pain-free gastrocnemius-soleus stretching (30 second hold × 3 sets) (Exercise 26-27)
5. Proprioceptive/neuromuscular reeducation exercises:
   a. Seated rocker board for plantarflexion and dorsiflexion (Exercise 26-25*A*)
   b. Seated rocker board for eversion and limited inversion (Exercise 26-25*B*)
   c. Seated wobble board for clockwise and counterclockwise circumduction (Exercise 26-33*A*)

   Single-leg balance activities on stable surface progressing to perturbations by therapist or using medicine balls, dumb bell weights, Theratubing, or Body Blade (Exercises 26-32*A* to *D* and 26-34*A* to *D*)
6. Physical therapy adjuncts:
   a. Gentle manual mobilization of scar tissue
   b. Manual therapy for joint mobility protecting surgical site (if needed)
   c. Modalities for pain and swelling control
   d. Gait training

†The Modified Brostrom Ankle Rehabilitation Program modified and used with permission from Orthopaedic Associates of Grand Rapids, PC, Grand Rapids, MI.

7. Conditioning exercises:
   a. Stationary bicycling to 20 minutes, minimal resistance
   b. Water therapy can begin under total buoyant conditions with use of a floatation device (Aqua-jogger vest) (Exercise 26-40)
   c. In the water, ankle ROM and running/walking activities can be initiated

Advanced Phase

Weeks 8 to 14 Postoperatively

1. Weightbearing status: Full-weight bearing
2. ROM exercises:
   a. As needed. *Do not stretch out repair*
3. Strengthening exercises:
   a. Concentric/eccentric strengthening in both open and closed kinetic chain positions
   b. Discontinue isometric exercises
   c. Initiate isokinetic strengthening (50% maximum effort) (Exercises 26-19 and 26-20)
   d. Continue with proximal lower-extremity and core-stability exercises in full-weight bearing
4. Proprioceptive/neuromuscular re-education exercises:
   a. Initiate single-leg balance activities on unstable surfaces, including rocker board, wobble board, foam rollers, DynaDisc, BOSU Balance Trainer, or KAT system as tolerated (Exercises 26-32*A* to *D*)
   b. Progress single-leg balance activities on unstable surfaces with perturbations by therapist or using medicine balls, dumb bell weights, Theratubing, or Body Blade (Exercises 26-34*A* to *D*)
5. Conditioning activities:
   a. Stationary cycling
   b. Treadmill walking
   c. Straight-line running progression program
   d. StairMaster
   e. Elliptical trainer
   f. NuStep
   g. Water therapy exercises in chest-deep water
6. Therapy adjunct:
   a. Previously described if needed

Return to Function Phase

Weeks 14 and Beyond Postoperatively

1. Strengthening exercises:
   a. Progress functional strengthening exercises specific to athletic activity as patient tolerates
2. Conditioning activities:
   a. Progress straight line running program to 20 minutes before adding figure 8 or cutting drills

b. Water therapy exercises performed in shallow (waist deep) water

c. In the water, begin to include hopping, bounding, and jumping drills

3. Goals:

a. The completely rehabilitated Modified Brostrom procedure allows for full ankle ROM maintaining protection into inversion not to *overstretch* the repair.

b. Strength and endurance are developed to preinjury levels, and continued strength and flexibility work is advised

c. Return to sporting activities allowed once patient cancomplete functional sports specific drills without pain or compensation

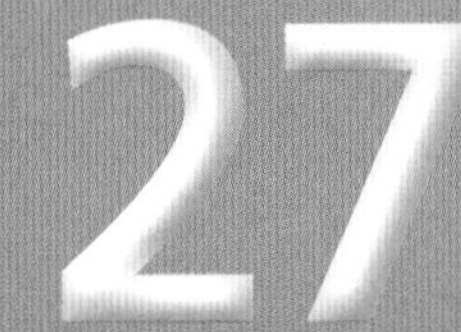

Cervical and Thoracic Spine

Terry L. Grindstaff and Eric M. Magrum

OBJECTIVES

After completion of this chapter, the physical therapist should be able to do the following:

- Discuss the functional anatomy and biomechanics of the cervical and thoracic spine.
- Compare and contrast the regional differences between the cervical and thoracic spine.
- Discuss the rehabilitation approach to conditions of the cervical spine.
- Discuss the rehabilitation approach to conditions of the thoracic spine.
- Explain the rationale for why therapeutic exercise programs for the cervical and thoracic spine would include neuromuscular control of the scapulothoracic joint or the lumbopelvic region.
- Describe why a comprehensive history and examination are necessary to develop a rehabilitation program for cervical and thoracic spine pathology.
- Compare and contrast common clinical presentations for cervical or thoracic spine pathologies.
- Explain the components of a comprehensive rehabilitation approach for the management of cervical or thoracic spine pathology.
- Incorporate the rehabilitation approach to specific conditions affecting the cervical or thoracic spine.

Functional Anatomy and Biomechanics

The cervical and thoracic spine are comprised of 19 vertebrae (7 cervical and 12 thoracic). Typically, components of the vertebrae include the body, pedicle, lamina, transverse processes and spinous process (Figures 27-1 and 27-2). The posterior aspect of the vertebral body, lamina, transverse processes and spinous process form the vertebral foramen. The spinal cord passes through the vertebral foramen with nerve roots that pass through the intervertebral foramen. The size of the vertebral foramen progressively decreases in a caudal direction as the spinal cord tapers in size. The intervertebral foramen are larger at the cervical and lumbar levels to accommodate the larger nerve roots at each level which are responsible for innervation of the limbs. The cervical nerve roots (C1-7) exit through the intervertebral foramen above the associated vertebral segment, while the other nerve roots exit below their associated vertebral segment (eg, C8 nerve root exits below C7, T1 nerve root exits below T1).

There are 2 major joints for each vertebral segment: the intervertebral and zygapophyseal (facet) joints. The intervertebral joint is a symphysis joint consisting of 2 vertebral bodies connected by an intervertebral disc. The zygapophyseal joint (right and left side) is a diarthrodial synovial joint with articulations between the inferior facet of a vertebral segment and the superior facet of the caudal segment.

The intervertebral disc transmits loads between segments and provides spacing between segments allowing motion to occur. There is a progressive increase in disc size from the cervical to the lumbar region. The anterior portion of the disc is wider and relatively stronger than the thinner posterior aspect of the disc. Each vertebral segment is separated by an intervertebral disc, with the exception of the atlantooccipital and atlantoaxial joints. The disc is comprised of 3 major structural components: nucleus pulposus, annulus fibrosus, and the vertebral end plate. The primary composition of these structures are water, collagen, and proteoglycans. The nucleus pulposus is the innermost aspect of the disc and has a higher water and proteoglycan content and lower collagen content relative to the annulus fibrosus and the vertebral end plate, which provides the ability to resist compressive loads between the segments. The supportive structure of the disc is provided by the annulus fibrosus and the vertebral end plate which have a higher collagen content than nucleus pulposus. The vertebral end plate serves as a cartilaginous attachment for the disc to the vertebral body and provides structure to the superior and inferior aspects of the nucleus pulposus. The annulus fibrosus also contains elastin, surrounding the periphery of the nucleus pulposus and attaching to the vertebral end plates. The anterior portion of the annulus fibrosus is stronger as a result of higher collagen content than the weaker posterior aspect of the annulus fibrosus. The higher collagen content and the presence of elastin provide circumferential support to the nucleus pulposus and is able to resist tensile forces. Nutrition and hydration of the intervertebral disc is primarily dependent on diffusion, which results from movement and compression of the vertebral segments. The outer third of the annulus fibrosus has a neurovascular supply and is innervated by the sinuvertebral nerve.[1] This indicates that the area can be a pain generator, as well as having the capability for tissue healing. Because the posterior aspect of the disc is in close proximity to the spinal cord and nerve roots, there is the potential for the disc to encroach on these tissues.

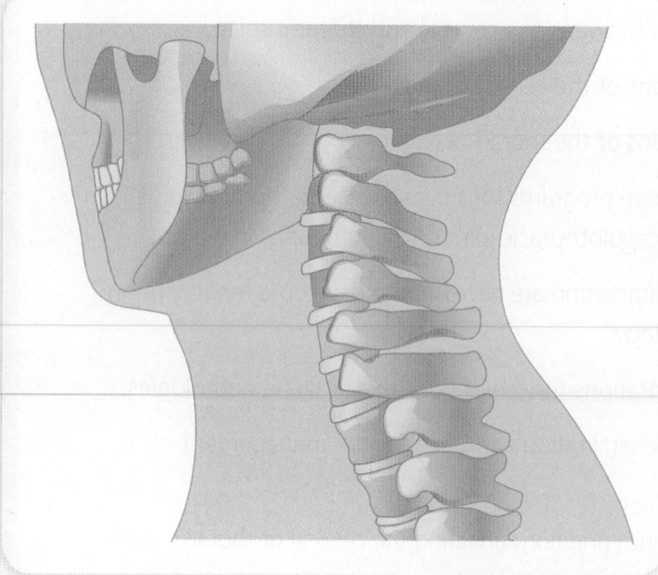

Figure 27-1 Cervical and thoracic vertebrae anatomy

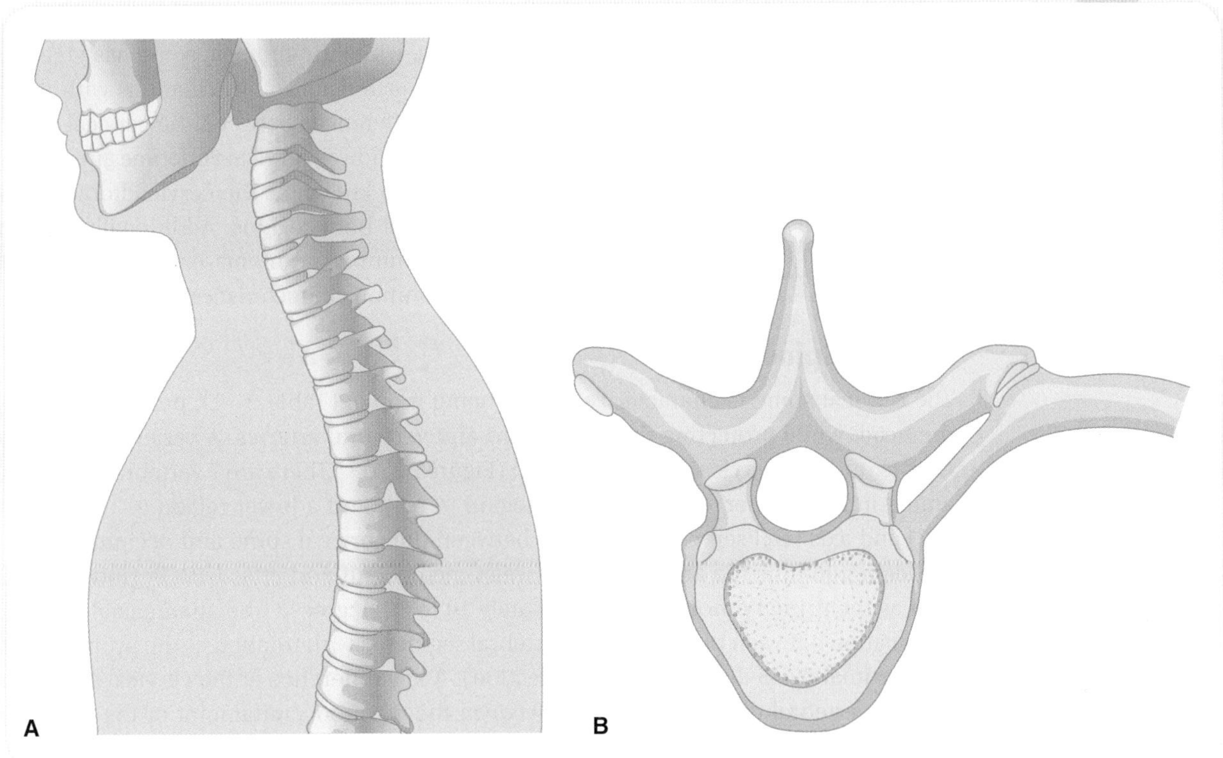

Figure 27-2 Cervical and thoracic vertebrae anatomy

Clinical Pearl

Discogenic referral pattern from the mid cervical region is to the medial border of the scapula.

Active motion is produced by coordinated interaction contractile tissues while accessory motion is influenced by contractile and noncontractile tissues. Available physiologic motion at the spine occurs in the 3 cardinal planes and includes flexion and extension, lateral flexion (side bending), and rotation. Three additional arthrokinematic motions occur at the spine and include lateral translation, compression/distraction, and anterior/posterior translation. These motions do not occur in isolation, but are a result of coupled segmental motion and contributions of adjacent vertebral segments.

Consistent with available motions at the spine, the cervical and thoracic spine are subject to forces including compression/tension, bending, torsion, and shear. Compression and tension produce an axial force through the vertebral body, intervertebral disc, and zygapophyseal joints. Bending forces cause compression and tension depending on if the tissues are approximated or separated. Torsion is caused during rotation with the intervertebral disc distributing the load. Shearing is caused by anterior/posterior translation of the vertebral segment with the load distributed by the intervertebral disc with minimal contribution from the surrounding musculature.

Regional Considerations

Although there are common structural and functional characteristics of the spinal regions, as described previously, there are also key structural and functional differences between the cervical and thoracic spine. There is a cephalocaudal increase in vertebral body size as each segment is responsible for greater weightbearing loads than the caudal segment. The cervical

Table 27-1 Cervical Spine Range of Motion

- Flexion 45 degrees
- Extension 45 degrees
- Rotation 80 to 90 degrees
- Side bending 45 degrees

spine bears less weight than the thoracic spinal segments and has greater mobility, while the thoracic spine has greater stability (less mobility) as a result of articulations with the ribs. Although there are differences between the cervical and thoracic spinal regions, the lower cervical vertebrae and the upper thoracic vertebrae, also known as the cervicothoracic region, share characteristics of both regions. Additionally, the lower thoracic and upper lumbar segments or the thoracolumbar region also share common characteristics.

Cervical Spine

The cervical spine is characterized by as being mobile (Table 27-1), providing control of the head, while protecting the spinal cord and vertebral arteries. A variety of techniques exist to quantify cervical range of motion (Figure 27-3).[2,3] There are 7 vertebrae (C1-7), separated into an upper, craniovertebral region (C1-2), and a lower region (C3-7). The atlas (C1) and axis (C2) serve as a junction between the cervical spine and occiput. The atlantooccipital joint is the articulation between the occiput and atlas with flexion and extension as the primary motion (approximately 10 to 30 degrees). The atlantoaxial joint is the articulation between the C1 and C2 vertebral segments with rotation as the primary motion (approximately 45 degrees in each direction). A key difference at the cervical spine is that an intervertebral disc is not present between the atlantooccipital joint or the atlantoaxial joint. The ratio of intervertebral disc height to vertebral body height is greater in the cervical spine relative to the thoracic spine. The greater proportional disc height in the cervical spine allows for greater motion, as well as the ability to accommodate the larger cervical nerve roots.

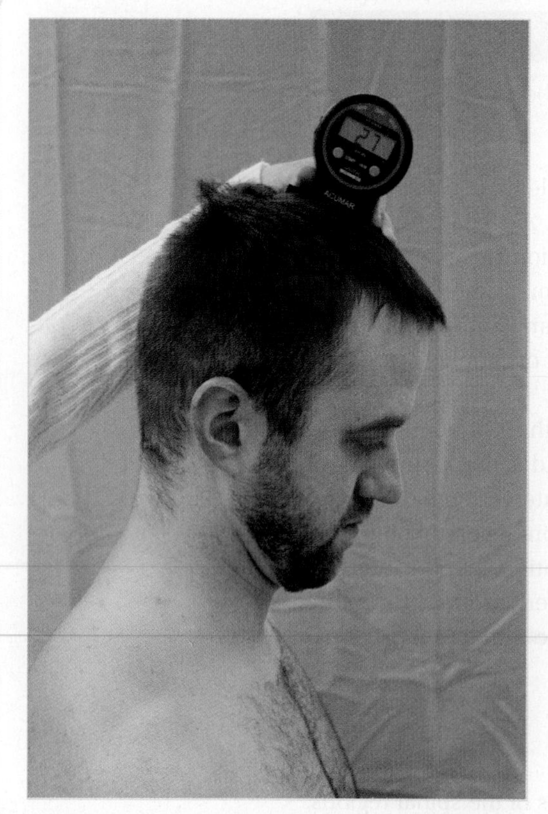

Figure 27-3 Cervical spine range of motion assessment with inclinometer

The zygapophyseal joints are oriented in the frontal plane (promotes flexion/extension) and have a larger joint capsule, which provides a greater availability of motion. Greater amounts of flexion and extension occur at the lower segments relative to the upper segments with maximum flexion and extension motion occurring at the C5-6 segment.[4] Lateral flexion (side bending) and rotation are coupled motions that occur in an ipsilateral manner (eg, left lateral flexion occurs in conjunction with left rotation). Forces across the cervical spine are dependent on position of the head and neck. The line of gravity falls anterior to the cervical spine, creating an external flexion moment and anterior shear. The vertebral body and intervertebral disc bear approximately two-thirds of the compressive load with the other one-third distributed across the zygapophyseal joints. Loads are highest at end ranges of motion.

The primary functions of muscles in the cervical spine region are to control the head and scapula, as well as to provide stability to the cervical spine. Because of the higher mobility of the cervical spine (as compared to other regions in the spine) and the relatively low contribution of noncontractile supportive structures (ligament, bony structures comprise approximately 20% of the mechanical stability), the surrounding musculature provides a considerable amount of stability.[5] Flexion of the cervical spine is produced primarily by the bilateral contraction of the sternocleidomastoid muscles and the scalene muscle group (anterior, middle, and posterior) on the anterior aspect of the neck (Figure 27-4). Smaller muscles, such as the longus

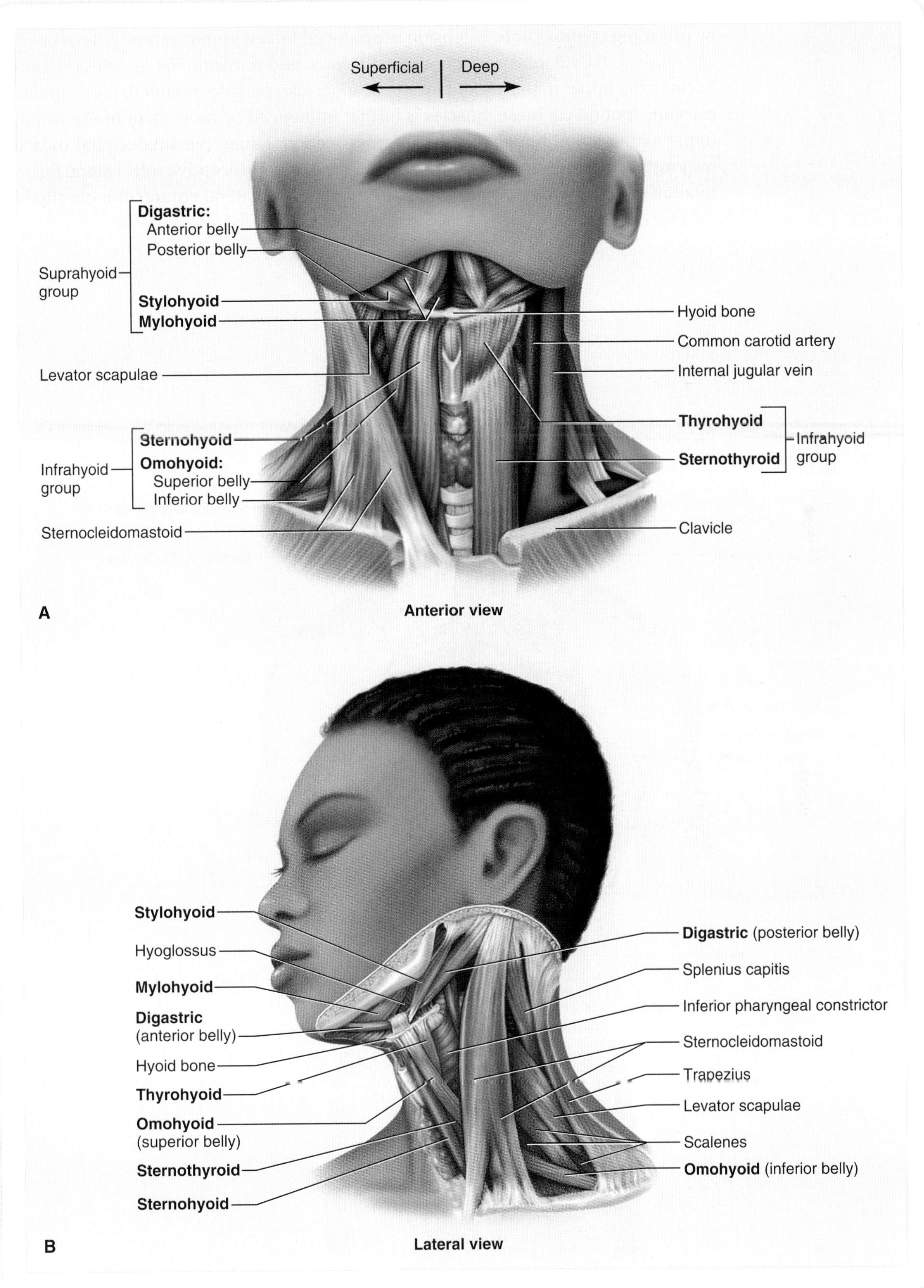

Figure 27-4 Anterior cervical spine musculature

capitis and longus colli, also contribute to spinal flexion, but have more of a stabilizing role by providing compression. Extension is produced by the upper trapezius, levator scapula, splenius capitis, splenius cervicis, erector spinae, and semispinalis muscles (Figure 27-5). Because the upper trapezius and levator scapula also provide motion to the scapula, cervical spine motion via these muscles is further influenced by movement of the scapula and upper extremity. Although smaller in cross-sectional area, the suboccipital muscles are responsible for extension of the occiput and have a proprioceptive role. Lateral flexion and rotation occur when a muscle contracts unilaterally. Bilateral contraction of muscle pairs

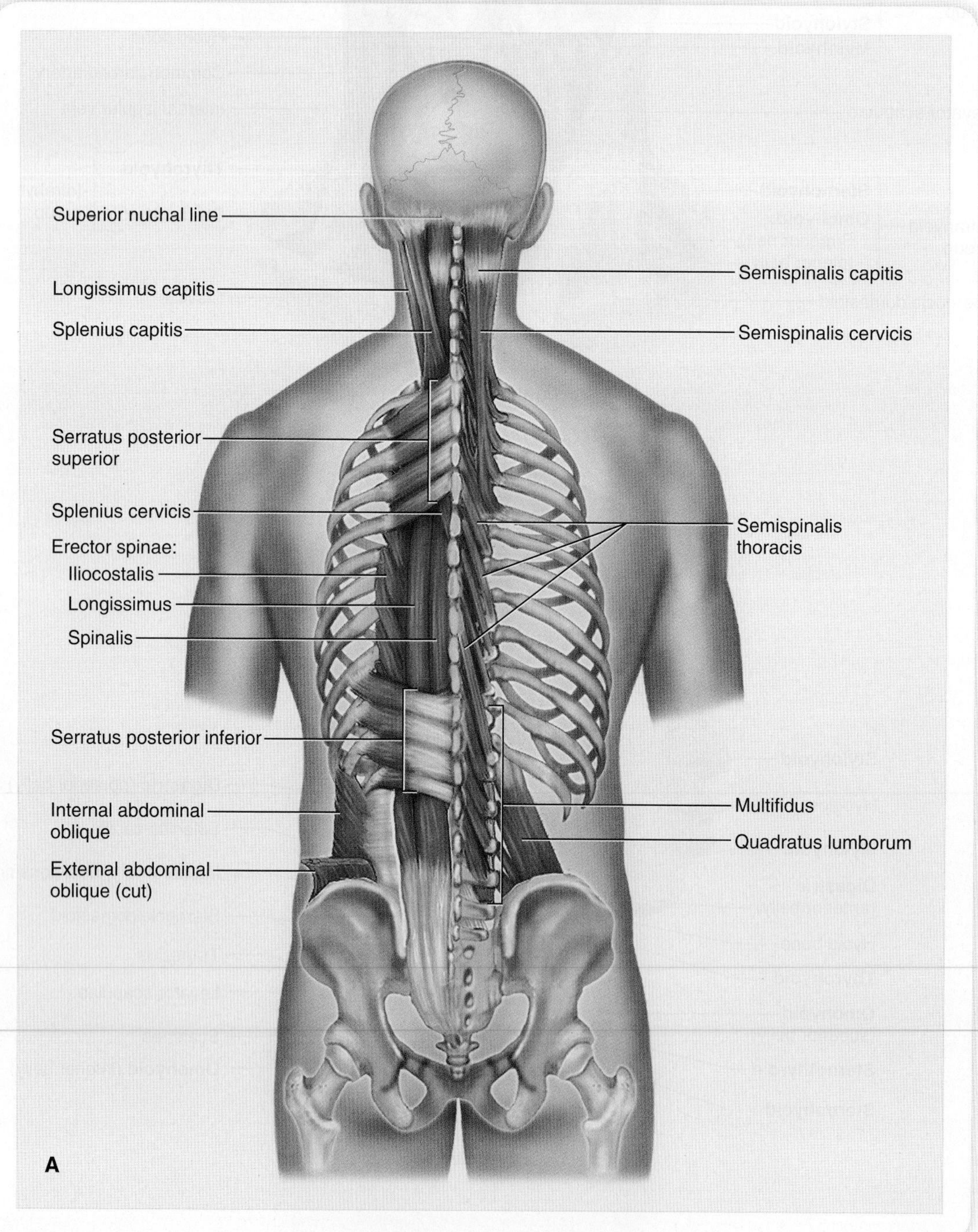

Figure 27-5 **A. Posterior cervical spine musculature**

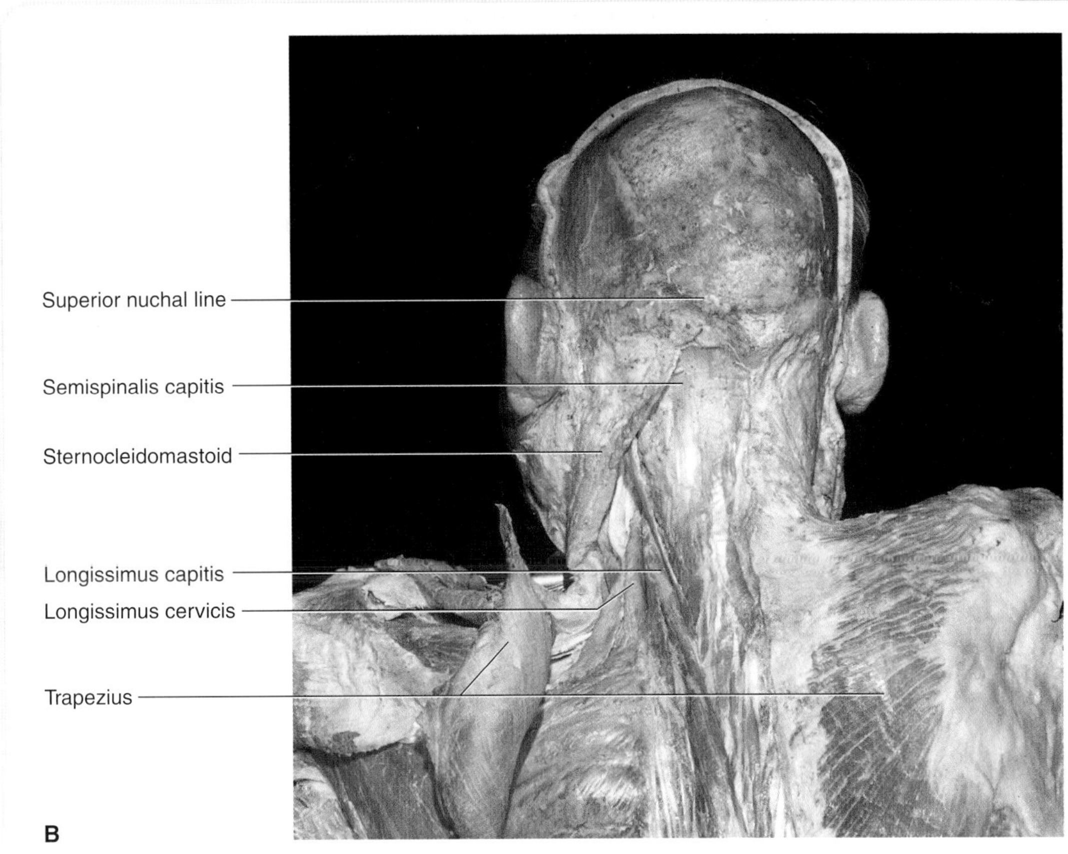

Figure 27-5 B. Posterior cervical musculature in anatomic dissection (*Continued*)

produces either flexion (ie, sternocleidomastoid) or extension (ie, upper trapezius). Ipsilateral lateral flexion (side bending) is produced by the scalenes, sternocleidomastoid, upper trapezius, levator scapula, and suboccipital muscles. Ipsilateral rotation is produced by the levator scapula, splenius capitis, splenius cervicis, erector spinae, semispinalis, and suboccipital muscles. Contralateral rotation is produced by the scalenes, sternocleidomastoid, and upper trapezius muscles.

Clinical Pearl

The upper trapezius and levator scapulae tend to get tight because they are countering the anterior shear forces of the head, created by the line of gravity. Tightness of these muscles is accentuated by a forward head posture.

Thoracic Spine

The degree of available motion (Table 27-2) at the thoracic spine is less than the cervical spine and primarily as a result of articulations with the ribs. A variety of techniques exist to quantify thoracic spine range of motion (Figures 27-6 and 27-7).[6,7] The vertebral bodies are more wedge shaped, with a larger posterior height relative to the anterior portion.

Table 27-2 Thoracic Spine Range of Motion

- Flexion 20 to 45 degrees
- Extension 20 to 45 degrees
- Rotation 35 to 50 degrees
- Side bending 20 to 40 degrees

This wedge shape contributes to the kyphotic curve of the thoracic spine. The thoracic intervertebral disc height to vertebral body height is less than the cervical spine and provides greater stability (less mobility). There are 2 ribs associated with each thoracic spine vertebrae. The thoracic vertebral body has demifacets that serve as an articulation with the head of the ribs known as the *costovertebral joint*. The transverse process also articulates with the ribs at the costotransverse joint. Structure and function of the thoracic spine are coupled with the ribs. Ribs 1 to 7 have a direct attachment to the sternum (true ribs), whereas ribs 8 to 10 have an indirect attachment with the sternum via costochondral cartilage, and ribs 11 and 12 are considered *floating* ribs and have no attachment to the sternum (see Figures 27-5 and 27-6). The upper thoracic segments are similar to lower cervical segments, and the lower thoracic segments are similar to the lumbar region. This overlap indicates that pathology of the cervical or lumbar spine can influence the thoracic region.

Clinical Pearl

Less mobility is available in the upper thoracic region as a result of direct attachment of the ribs to the sternum.

The joint capsule of the zygapophyseal joints is smaller and more taut than the cervical spine. The slightly lateral orientation of the upper thoracic (T1-6) facet joints from the frontal plane provides more lateral flexion and rotation relative to flexion and extension. Flexion of the thoracic spine is limited by tension of the posterior longitudinal ligament while extension is limited because of the wedge shape of the vertebral body and the larger spinous processes. This limitation is most pronounced in the upper thoracic segments (T1-6). Thoracic spine rotation and lateral bending are limited by articulations with the ribs. The line of gravity falls anterior to the thoracic spine, creating an external flexion moment, which is counteracted by posterior ligaments and musculature. The thoracic spine is also subject to increased compressive loads caused by the support of the head, neck, and upper extremities.

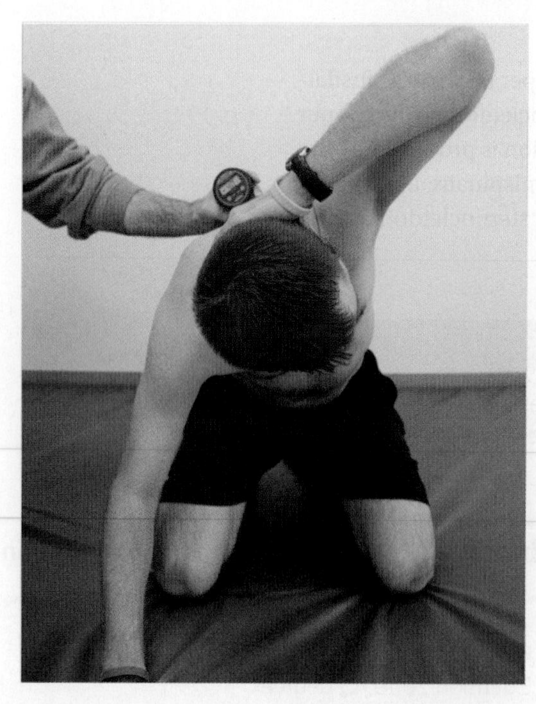

Figure 27-6 **Thoracic spine range of motion assessment with inclinometer**

Muscles within the thoracic spine region have a number of functions including respiration, movement of the thorax, movement of the upper extremity, and coupling with the cervical and lumbar spine. It is important to note that motion in the thoracic spine does not occur independently from other regions. Flexion of the thoracic spine is produced by gravity, the anterior abdominal musculature (rectus abdominis, obliques) and the psoas (Figure 27-8). Extension is produced by the erector spinae, semispinalis thoracis, multifidus, and quadratus lumborum (Figure 27-9). Similar to the cervical spine rotation, lateral flexion and rotation occur as a result of the unilateral action of the flexor and extensor musculature. Lateral flexion is produced by the external and internal obliques, quadratus lumborum, erector spinae, rhomboids, and serratus anterior. Rotation is produced by ipsilateral contraction of erector spinae, multifidus, splenius thoracis and external oblique and contralateral contraction of the internal oblique muscle. The intercostal muscles (external and internal) play a substantial role with breathing. The external intercostal muscles are responsible for rib elevation, while the internal intercostals are responsible for rib depression. Additionally, the scalene muscles have an attachment on the first (anterior and middle) and second (posterior) ribs. The scalenes assist with elevation of the sternum and ribs during breathing. During episodes of increased ventilatory demand the sternocleidomastoid, pectoralis major, subclavius, can all influence rib motion.

Motion of the ribs is coupled with motion of the thoracic spine segment. Flexion of the thoracic spine is coupled with posterior rib elevation and internal torsion while extension of the thoracic spine is coupled with posterior rib depression and external torsion.[8] Thoracic rotation causes the ipsilateral rib to rotate posteriorly (external torsion) and the contralateral rib to rotate anteriorly (internal torsion).[8] Lateral flexion (side bending) causes approximation of the ipsilateral ribs and separation of the contralateral ribs.[8]

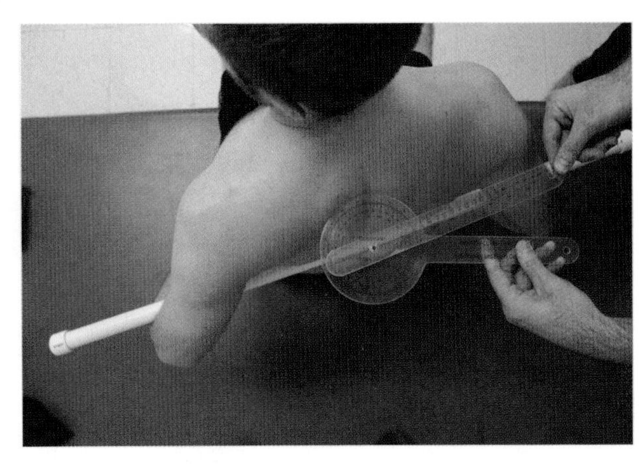

Figure 27-7 Thoracic spine range of motion assessment with goniometer

Importance and Purpose of Examination

In many instances, medical referral for rehabilitation does not include specific information regarding the underlying pathology (ie, neck pain). Although a specific diagnosis can provide the clinician with a better understanding of the underlying pathology, the clinician must still obtain a thorough history and perform a comprehensive examination. A systematic history and examination should be able to determine aggravating and easing factors, identify impairments which contribute to functional limitations and pain, establish baseline objective and subjective measures to monitor progress, and establish patient rapport, decrease anxiety, and increase patient compliance with the rehabilitation program. The clinician should also look at sites adjacent to the cervical and thoracic spine (eg, shoulder, lumbar spine) for potential contributing factors. Because of the proximity of vital organs (heart, lungs) and overlap with common areas of referred pain, it is important for the clinician to determine the source of pain (musculoskeletal vs. nonmusculoskeletal). Nonmusculoskeletal pain, such as cardiac, pulmonary, or visceral pain, should be referred to the appropriate health care provider.

Clinical Pearl

Visceral referral is common in the thoracic region. Poorly localized pain occurs secondary to projection to various parts of the central nervous system from this region.

Although examination techniques are not within the context of this chapter, interventions that are specific to addressing the underlying pathology are critical components of the rehabilitation plan and should be selected based on examination findings. Therapeutic exercise, manual therapy (joint mobilization, massage) and physical agents/modalities may be used to address patient impairments, functional limitations, and pain. The selection of interventions should have a specific purpose with appropriate

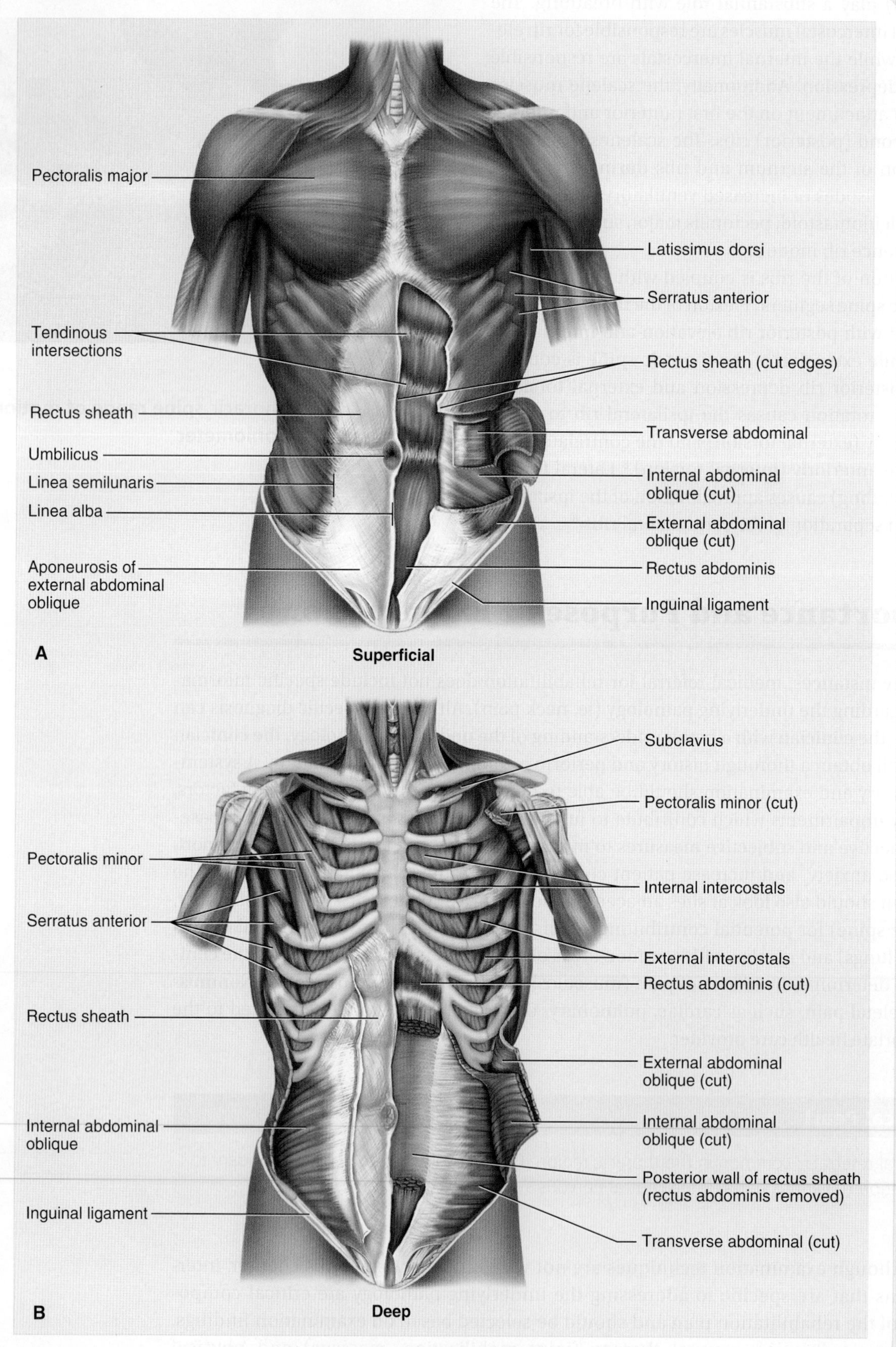

Figure 27-8 **Anterior thoracic spine musculature**

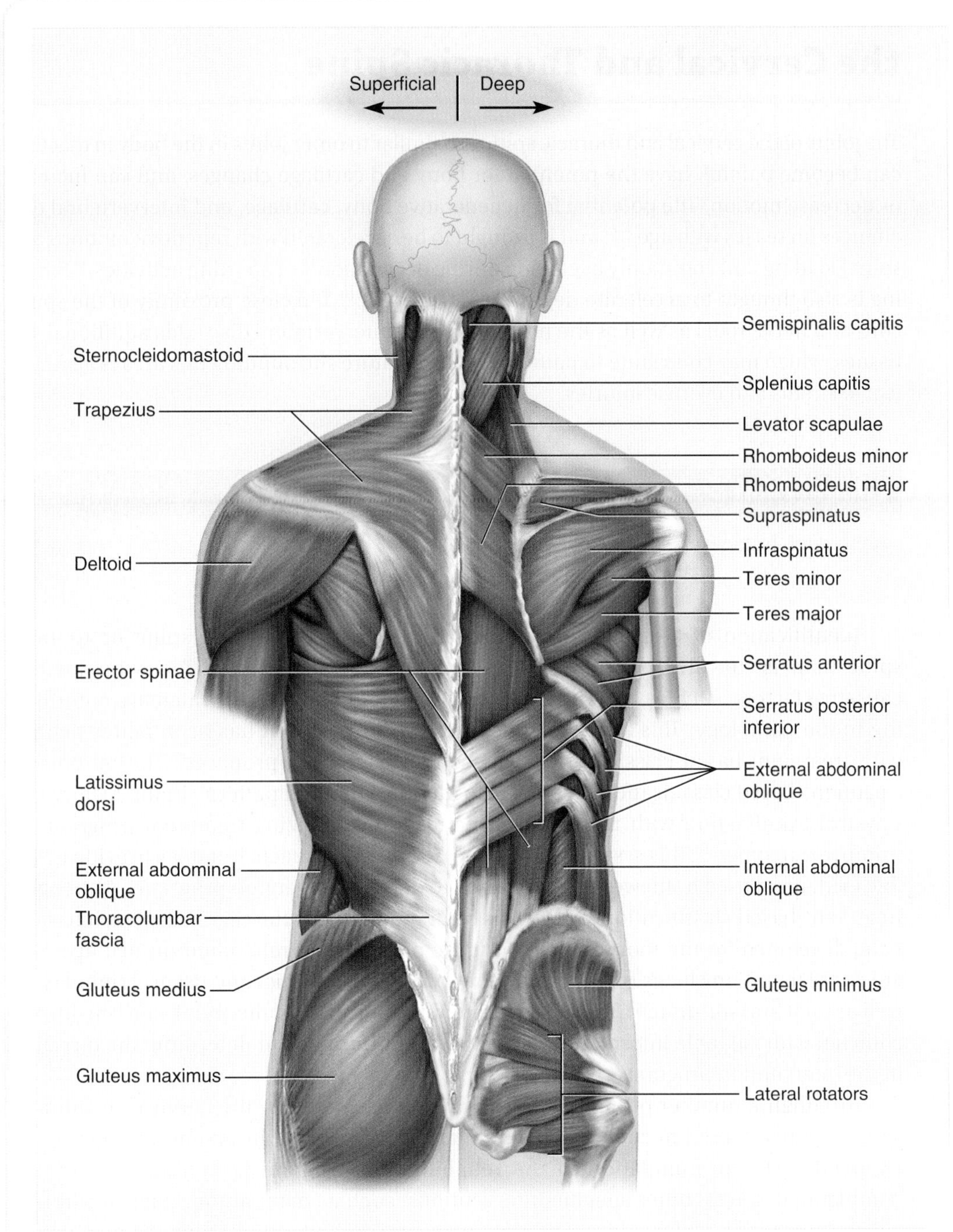

Figure 27-9 **Posterior thoracic spine musculature**

rationale and consideration of evidence-based practice. The clinician should consistently monitor patient progress and alter the program as needed. Although interventions listed within this chapter are specific to the cervical and thoracic spine, clinicians should appreciate that interventions focused on this region often have overlapped with therapeutic exercise programs for shoulder and lumbar spine pathology. Examples included interventions to improve neuromuscular control of the scapulothoracic joint or the lumbopelvic region.

Rehabilitation Considerations for the Cervical and Thoracic Spine

The joints of the cervical and thoracic spine are similar to other joints in the body in that they can become painful, have the potential for bony and cartilage changes, and can increase or decrease motion. The potential for degenerative bony, cartilage, and intervertebral disc changes increases with age,[9-12] and is thought to be accelerated with repetitive motions and spinal loading and commonly occurring during occupation[13] or sporting activities.[14] Smoking is also thought to accelerate degenerative changes.[10] The close proximity of the spinal cord and nerve roots as well as the presence of the intervertebral disc adds additional soft tissues, which may contribute to pathology. Musculature surrounding this area is also subject to strains and overuse injuries.

Clinical Pearl

A thorough history and comprehensive examination will help guide the intervention approach.

Identification of a specific pathoanatomical cause of cervical spine or thoracic spine pain is not always possible.[15-17] Thus, the clinician should focus on treating causative factors, such as impairments and functional limitations, which are contributing to the pathology. This approach is not new or unique, but has been better defined with treatment-based classification systems that have been proposed. The purpose of treatment-based classification systems is to identify common patterns in the history and physical examination with the intent of better individualizing treatment programs to improve outcomes.[18] This system is not a cookie cutter approach, but does provide a flexible evidence-based framework for clinicians to derive intervention programs. Although a treatment-based classification system has been proposed for the cervical spine, it has not been developed for the thoracic spine but the principles of rehabilitation management are consistent. Knowledge of symptom duration (acute, chronic) and tissue irritability, as well as joint and soft-tissue mobility (hypermobile, normal, hypomobile), can provide the clinician with valuable information, which is then prioritized to determine the direction of the intervention program.

Although a number of pathologies may be present within the cervical or thoracic spine regions, there are considerable similarities among the intervention approaches (Appendix 1). The foundation of the rehabilitation program is therapeutic exercise complemented with other specific interventions, such as manual therapies or physical agents/modalities, which address motion, pain, and radicular symptoms,[19,20] and patient education regarding contributing factors[19,20] and mechanisms of pain.[21] Acute conditions or conditions with highly irritable symptoms (pain) can be managed with relative rest, range of motion, physical agents/modalities, and lower intensity manual therapies. Conditions involving hypermobility or decreased neuromuscular control benefit from exercise interventions which improve stability and neuromuscular control. Hypomobility may be addressed with manual therapies such as joint mobilization and stretching. Radicular symptoms can be addressed with interventions that decrease mechanical or chemical stimuli that irritate nervous tissue and promote centralization of symptoms. Finally, headaches that have a musculoskeletal component may also be managed via impairment-based interventions directed at the cervical and thoracic region. Rehabilitation progression is based on resolution of symptoms and changes in impairments and function.

Clinical Pearl

Best available evidence for treatment of most musculoskeletal pathology: education, manual therapy, and exercise prescription.

Cervical Spine

Neck pain has an annual incidence rate of 15% with a recurrence rate of nearly 25%.[22,23] As previously stated, it is not always possible to identify a specific underlying pathoanatomical cause.[15-17] Females and individuals with high psychological stress are more at risk for neck pain.[15,24] Prolonged sitting, often associated with office or computer work, is also considered to be a risk factor, particularly when coupled with poor posture.[24] Participation in general fitness programs appear to decrease the risk of neck pain.[15]

The cervical spine is highly dependent on surrounding musculature for mechanical stability.[5] Following injury there is atrophy and decreased function of surrounding musculature, particularly the deeper stabilizing musculature.[25] These changes occur within a relatively short time period (<1 month) and also result in decreased joint position sense.[26] Individuals with neck pain tend to utilize the larger superficial muscles to a greater extent than the deeper cervical stabilizing muscles (longus capitis and longus colli),[27,28] which is evidenced by decreased performance of the craniocervical flexion test.[29] This muscle dysfunction is thought to persist despite symptom resolution[26] and is the rationale for inclusion of postural exercises, with low loads, targeting deep cervical neck flexors in therapeutic exercise programs.[20,30] Deficits of the deeper stabilizing musculature can be determined clinically using the craniocervical flexion test (Figure 27-10).[31]

Individuals with cervical spine pathology often present with characteristic history and physical examination findings that can help determine preferred treatment options (Table 27-3). These profiles are often part of a treatment-based classification system,[18] which identifies common patterns in the history and physical examination with the intent of better individualizing treatment programs to improve outcomes.[18] This provides a flexible evidence-based framework for clinicians to derive intervention programs.

The foundation of the rehabilitation program for cervical spine pathology is therapeutic exercise complemented with manual therapy or physical agents/modalities to address motion, pain, and radicular symptoms, and patient education to address potential causative factors (posture)[19,20] and mechanisms of pain.[21] Acute conditions or conditions with highly irritable symptoms (pain) can be managed with relative rest, range of motion, physical agents/modalities, and lower-intensity manual therapies. Conditions involving hypermobility or decreased neuromuscular control benefit from exercise interventions that improve stability and neuromuscular control. Manual therapies are indicated when there is a restriction in soft-tissue or joint mobility. Hypomobility may be addressed with manual therapies such as joint mobilization and stretching. Radicular symptoms can be addressed with interventions that

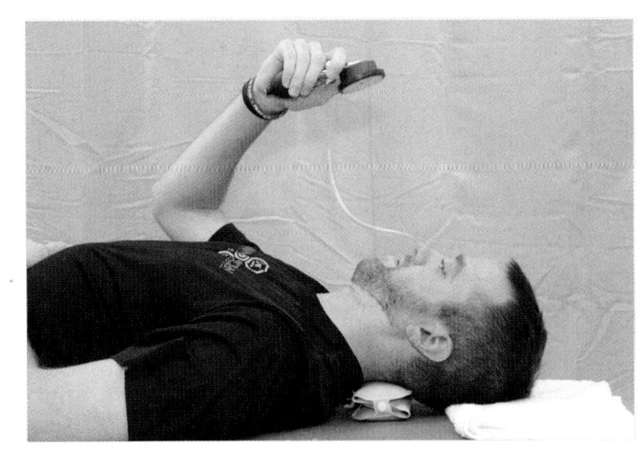

Figure 27-10 Craniocervical flexion test

Table 27-3 Treatment Based Classifications for Cervical Spine Pathology

Therapeutic exercise
Mobility and exercise
Centralization (nerve root compression)
Acute neck pain as a result of trauma (whiplash)
Cervicogenic headache

decrease mechanical or chemical stimuli that irritate nervous tissue and promote centralization of symptoms. Finally, headaches that have a musculoskeletal component may also be managed via impairment-based interventions directed at the cervical and thoracic region. Rehabilitation program progression is based on resolution of symptoms and changes in impairments and function. Clinicians are encouraged to reevaluate the patient and attempt to further identify the underlying cause of symptoms for cases that do not resolve with typical conservative management.

Degenerative Disc/Joint Disease, Spondylosis, and Stenosis

Pathomechanics and Injury Mechanism

Degenerative changes broadly include degenerative disc/joint disease, spondylosis, and stenosis. The typical patient with degenerative changes in cervical spine structures with or without radiculopathy is 30 to 50 years of age. Individuals older than 50 years of age are more likely to have stenosis (central or lateral). The progressive loss of intervertebral disc height is thought to place greater demands on articular surfaces, facilitating degenerative changes and contributing to ligamentous laxity. Degenerative changes and intervertebral disc pathology tend to occur more often between the C5 and C7 segments.[32]

Rehabilitation Concerns and Progression

Exercise intervention is a consistent component for the management of most cervical spine pathologies.[19,20] It is not clear whether a specific approach targeting cervical stabilizing muscles or a generalized approach to strengthen neck and upper extremity is more efficacious for symptom management.[20,33,34] It is suggested that exercises be selected to address specific impairments and functional limitations with regard to the stage of rehabilitation. Generally a specific approach targeting deeper cervical stabilizing muscles is used initially (Figures 27-11 to 27-15), then transitioned to a generalized approach as symptoms diminish and neuromuscular control improves (Figures 27-26 to 27-29). Lower-load exercises are also more likely to be tolerated during acute stages when structures are highly irritable (pain) than higher-load strengthening approaches.

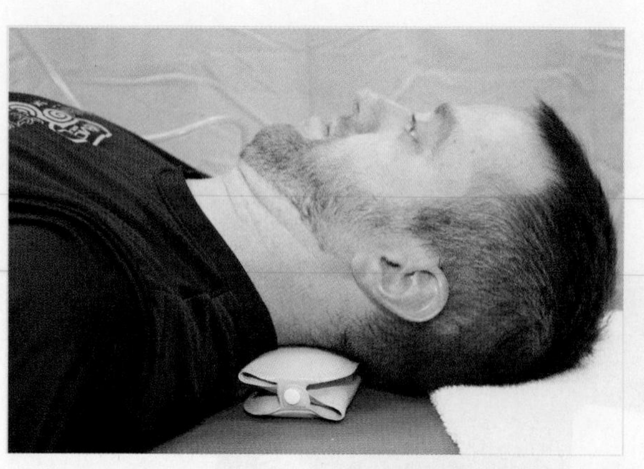

Figure 27-11 Chin tuck—supine with stabilizer

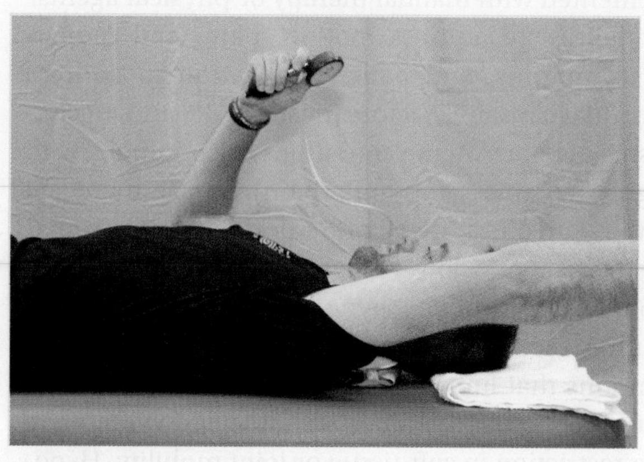

Figure 27-12 Chin tuck—supine with arm movement

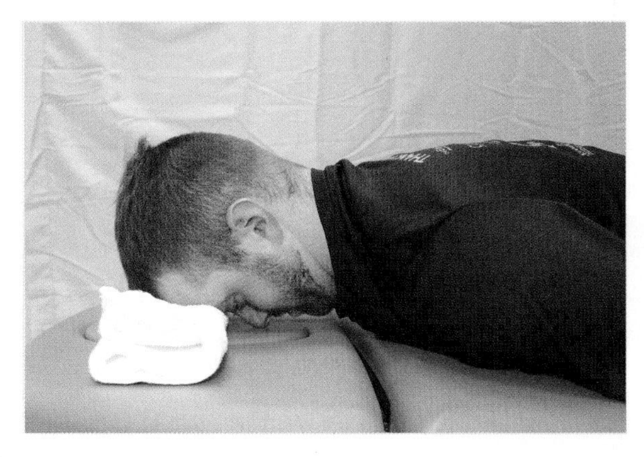

Figure 27-13 Chin tuck—prone

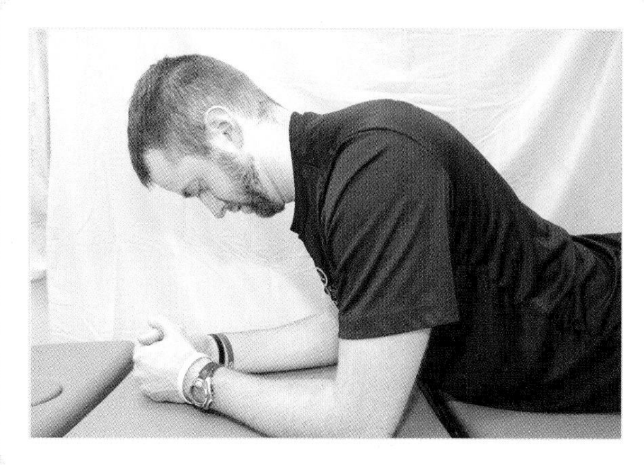

Figure 27-14 Chin tuck—prone on elbows

Lower-load exercises are also thought to better target deeper stabilizing musculature[35] and have been shown to decrease pain sensitivity.[36] Positional progression is usually from a supine (Figures 27-11 and 27-12), to a prone or 4-point kneeling position (Figures 27-13 and 27-14), to sitting or standing (Figures 27-16 to 27-18). Initial exercises focus on establishing neuromuscular control of the cervical spine in static positions (Figures 27-11, 27-13, and 27-16) and progress to incorporating surrounding musculature (eg, arm movement with cervical stabilization) (Figures 27-12, 27-18, and 27-23). Progression should also incorporate education of posture (Figure 27-33) and exercises that develop endurance (Figure 27-25) while incorporating tasks of daily living or mimicking recreational activities (Figures 27-28 and 27-30).

Centralization (Nerve Root Compression)

Pathomechanics and Injury Mechanism

Disc herniation and stenosis are the most common causes of cervical nerve root compression, with males affected more than females.[32] The incidence of radiculopathy is 83 per

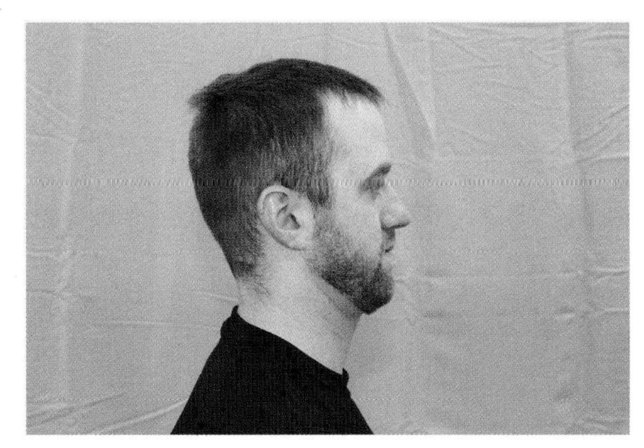

Figure 27-15 Chin tuck—seated

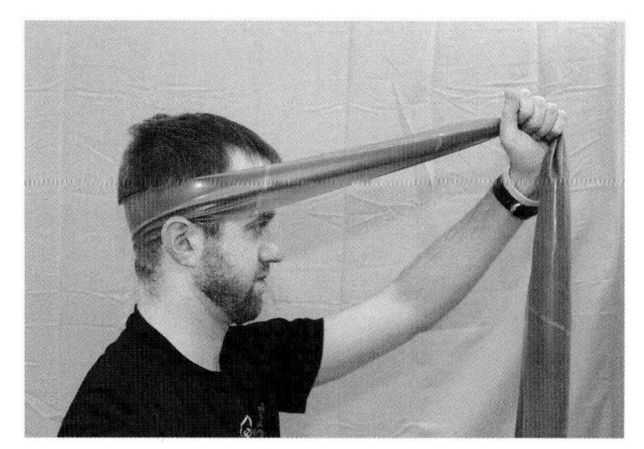

Figure 27-16 Isometric cervical spine extension with Thera-Band

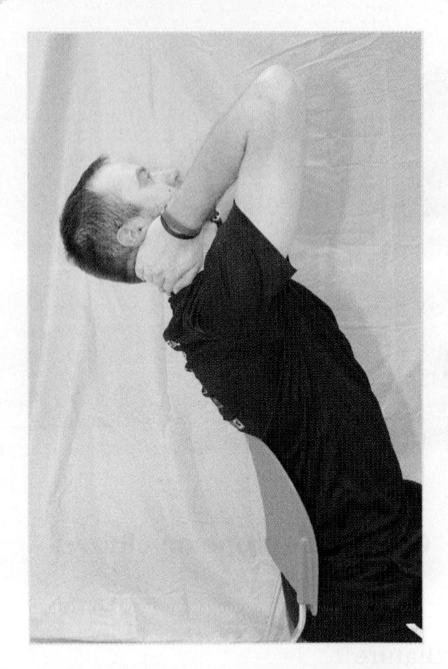

Figure 27-17 **Seated thoracic extension with chin tuck**

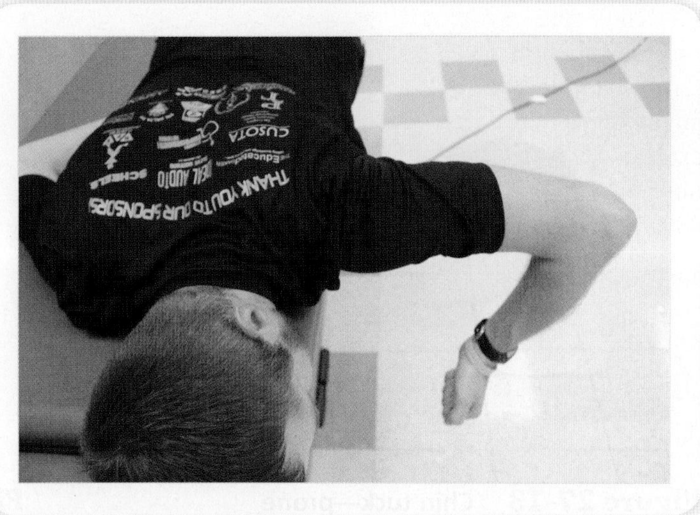

Figure 27-18 **Horizontal abduction—prone row**

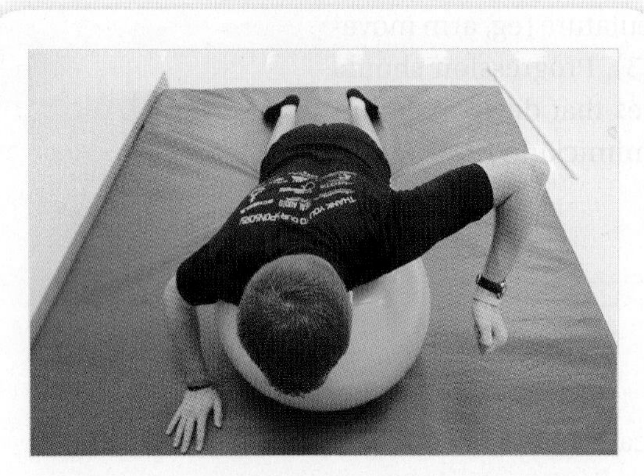

Figure 27-19 **Prone shoulder horizontal abduction on stability ball**

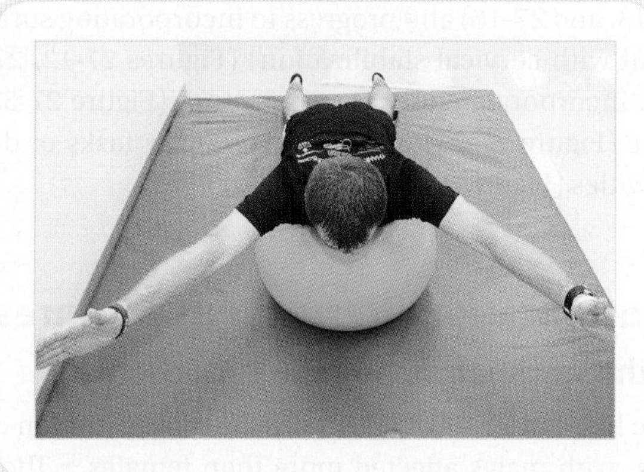

Figure 27-20 **Y on stability ball—shoulder flexion prone 135 degrees**

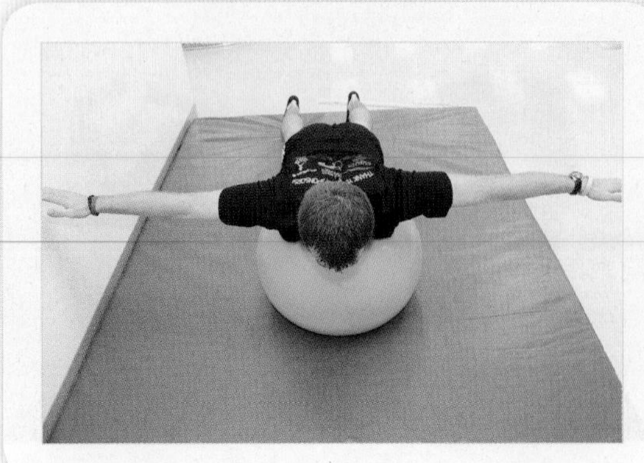

Figure 27-21 **T on stability ball—horizontal abduction**

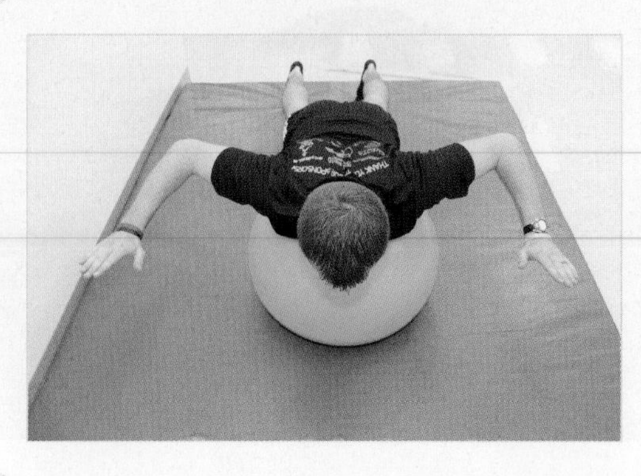

Figure 27-22 **W on stability ball**

100,000 people with individuals older than 50 years of age the most commonly affected.[32] Cervical nerve root compression causes radicular symptoms, specifically arm pain, and sensory and motor deficits. Individuals with nerve root compression and radiculopathy are more likely to demonstrate radicular symptoms with cervical spine motion, especially extension. Degenerative changes and intervertebral disc pathology tend to occur more often between the C5-7 segments.[32] Individuals with neurologic signs and symptoms indicative of cervical myelopathy (gait abnormality, positive Hoffmann or Babinski tests, abnormal reflexes) should be referred to a physician.[37]

Clinical Pearl

Clinical prediction rule for discogenic pathology: (+) Spurling test, (+) upper limb tension test, cervical rotation less than 60 degrees, (+) distraction test: positive likelihood ratio of 30.3.

Rehabilitation Concerns and Progression

Radicular symptoms can be addressed with interventions which decrease mechanical or chemical stimuli which are irritating nervous tissue and promote centralization of symptoms.[38] Centralization describes the migration distal symptoms toward the spine in response to movement or intervention. Peripheralization describes symptoms which become more distal with movement or provoking activities. The most common interventions are therapeutic exercise, traction (manual or mechanical), manual therapy, and patient education regarding posture.[20,39-42] Unfortunately, individuals with nerve root compression have a less-favorable prognosis compared to other cervical spine pathologies.[16] Individuals who meet at least 3 of the following 4 predictive criteria are thought to have the most favorable outcomes: participation in a comprehensive rehabilitation program, younger than 54 years of age, dominant arm not involved, and cervical flexion does not increase symptoms.[43] Cases that are not responsive to conservative management, involve a decline in quality of life, or have neurologic deficits (sensory/motor) may be considered for surgical intervention. It is estimated that approximately 25% of individuals with radiculopathy require surgical intervention.[32]

Initial management of nerve root compression should focus on centralization of symptoms. Interventions include traction (manual or mechanical) (Figures 27-34 and 27-35) and cervical retraction (Figures 27-36 and 27-37). Once pain decreases and symptoms begin to centralize, exercises that focus on neuromuscular control of the neck can be initiated in static positions (see Figures 27-11, 27-13, and 27-16) and progressed to incorporate surrounding musculature (eg, arm movement with cervical stabilization) (see Figures 27-12, 27-18, 27-23, and 27-38).[20,30] Deficits of the deeper stabilizing musculature can be determined clinically using the craniocervical flexion test (see Figure 27-10).[31] Because posture can contribute to neck pain, the patient should be educated on proper posture (see

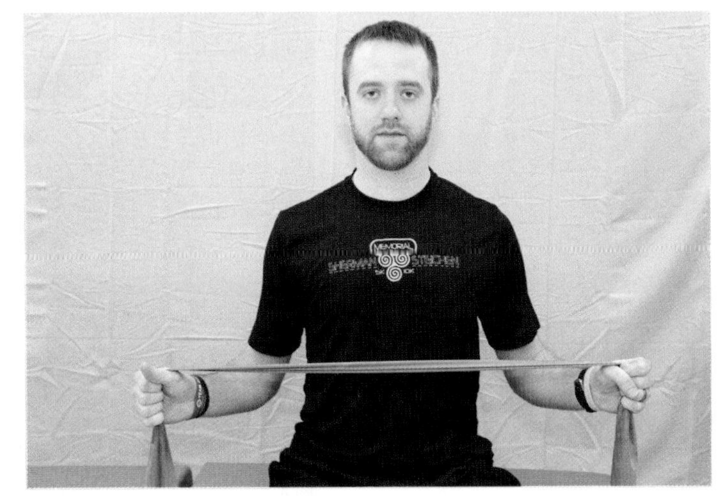

Figure 27-23 **Shoulder external rotation with tubing—bilateral**

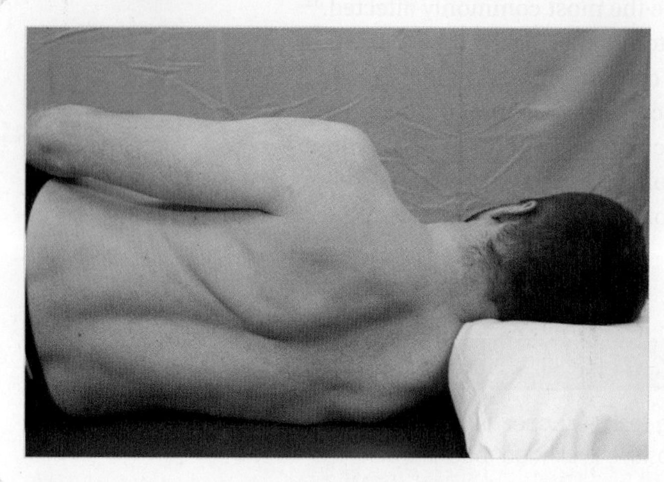

Figure 27-24 Scapular proprioceptive neuromuscular facilitation (PNF) pattern

Figure 27-33) and made aware of patterns that may contribute to dysfunction (eg, head forward, slumped, rounded shoulders). Exercises that involve the upper extremity can then be incorporated while maintaining a stable cervical spine (see Figures 27-12, 27-18, and 27-23). Examples include interventions to improve neuromuscular control of the scapulothoracic joint (see Figures 27-18 to 27-23, 27-28 to 27-32, and 27-55 to 27-66). Stretching exercises may also be incorporated to address muscular tightness identified during the examination (Figures 27-39 to 27-41). Progression should also incorporate education of posture (see Figure 27-33), and exercises that develop endurance (see Figure 27-25) while incorporating tasks of daily living or mimicking recreational activities (see Figures 27-28 and 27-30).

Acute Joint Pathology

Pathomechanics and Injury Mechanism

The person with acute cervical spine joint injury and intervertebral disc pathology tends to be a younger individual, 20 to 35 years of age. The Canadian C-Spine Rules can be used to determine if cervical spine imaging is necessary following neck injury.[44] Briefly, individuals who do not meet high- or low-risk criteria and can actively rotate the neck 45 degrees

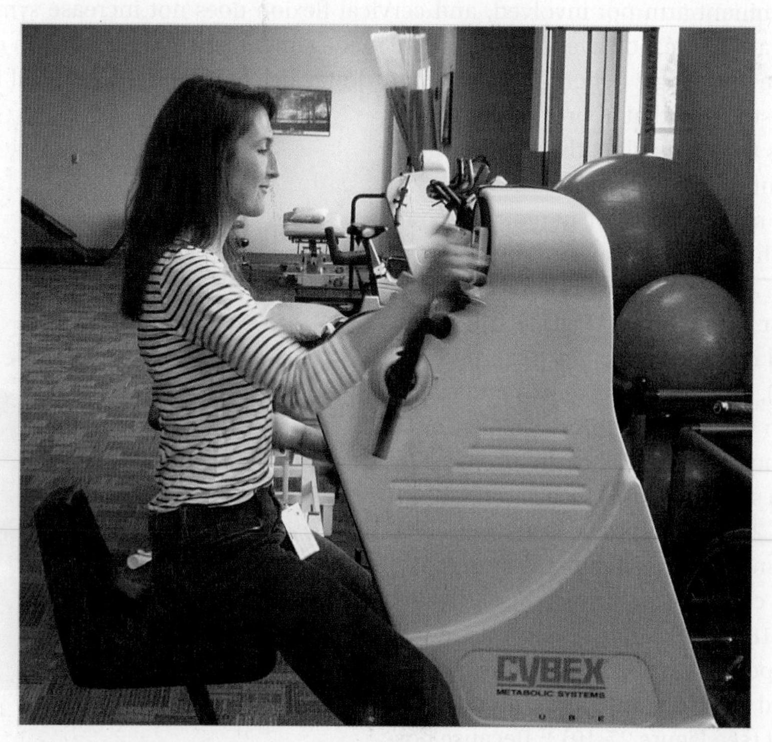

Figure 27-25 Upper body ergometer with proper posture

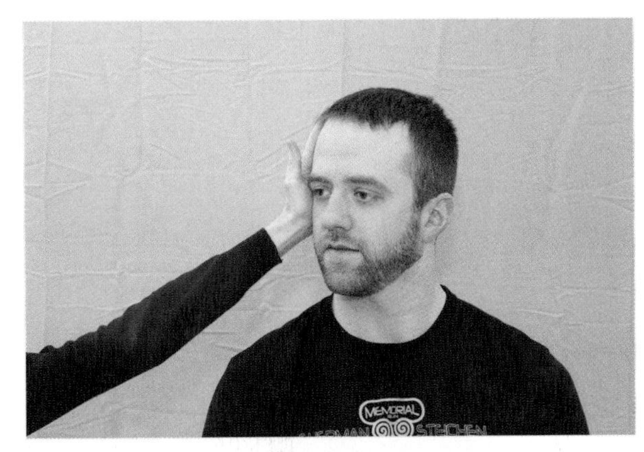

Figure 27-26 Neck rotation—resisted

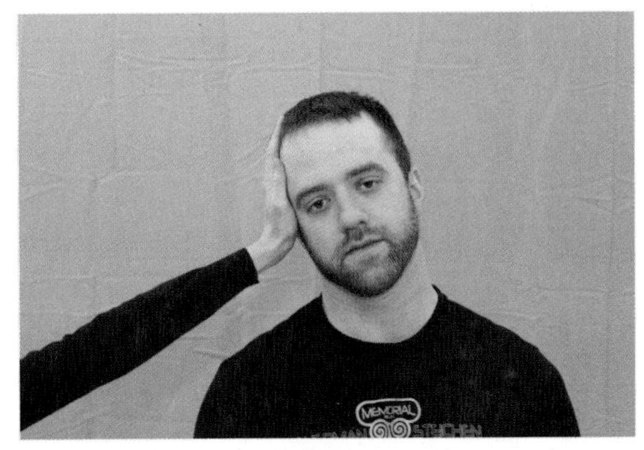

Figure 27-27 Neck sidebending—resisted

bilaterally are less likely to have a cervical spine fracture. As in any case, if there are suspicions of fracture, spinal cord involvement, or dislocation, the patient should be referred immediately to an emergency department. A cervical sprain usually results from a traumatic event (motor vehicle collision, collision sports). Muscles may also be strained with the traumatic event. There may be palpable tenderness over the transverse and spinous processes that serve as sites of attachment for the ligaments.[45]

Alternatively, acute joint pathology may have an insidious onset and is often first noticed after waking in the morning. This is typically isolated to a single vertebral segment and manifests as hypomobility and pain. Interventions may include physical agents/modalities to decrease pain and muscle spasm and be complemented with manual therapies to address joint hypomobility.

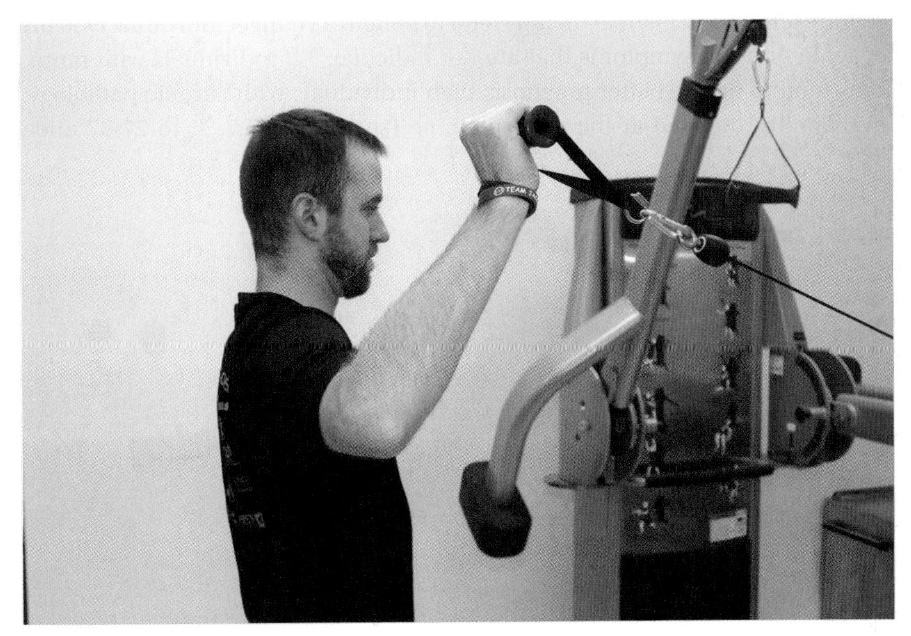

Figure 27-28 Shoulder external rotation with tubing—standing

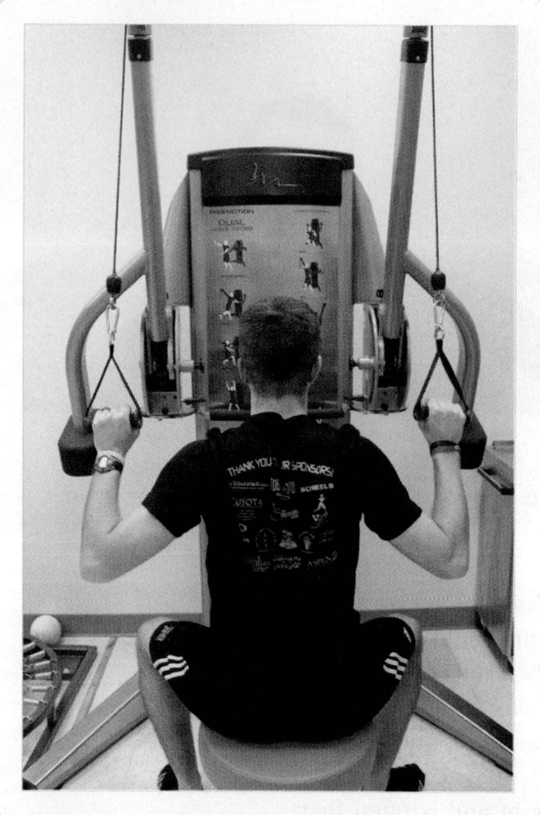

Figure 27-29 Lat pulldown

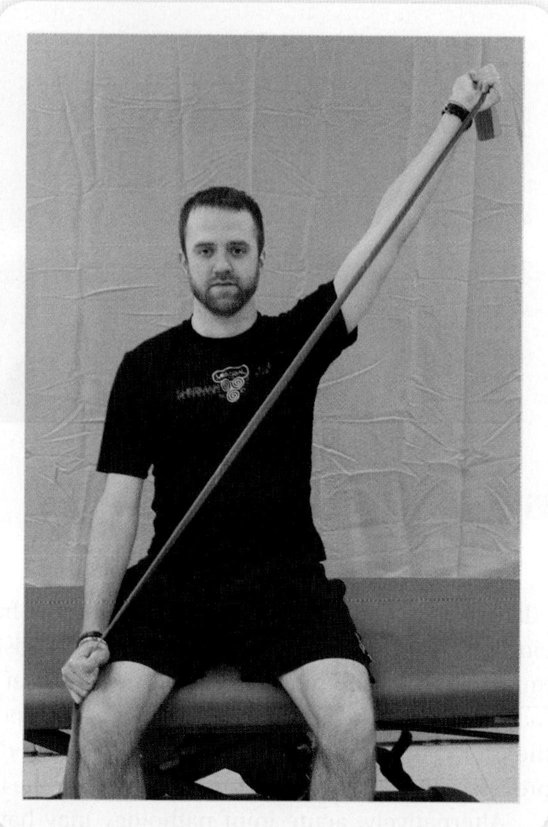

Figure 27-30 Proprioceptive neuromuscular facilitation (PNF) pattern with tubing

Rehabilitation Concerns and Progression

Therapeutic exercise and manual therapy tend to benefit a younger individual who presents with an acute onset of symptoms that are not radicular.[46-48] Individuals with more acute symptoms tend to have a better prognosis than individuals with chronic pathology.[16,22,49] Manual therapies directed at the cervical spine (see Figures 27-34 to 27-37 and 27-42

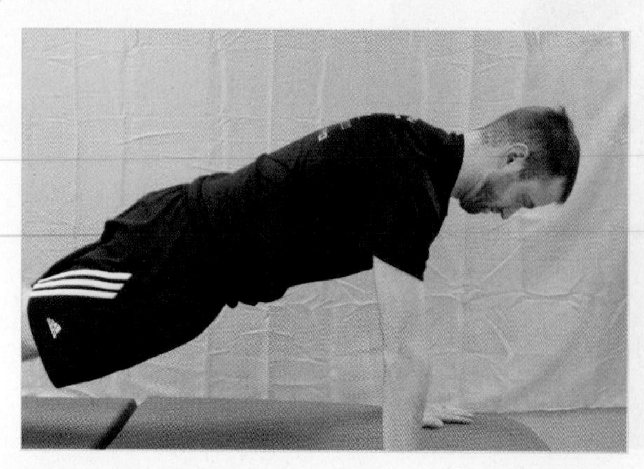

Figure 27-31 Pushup with cervical stabilization

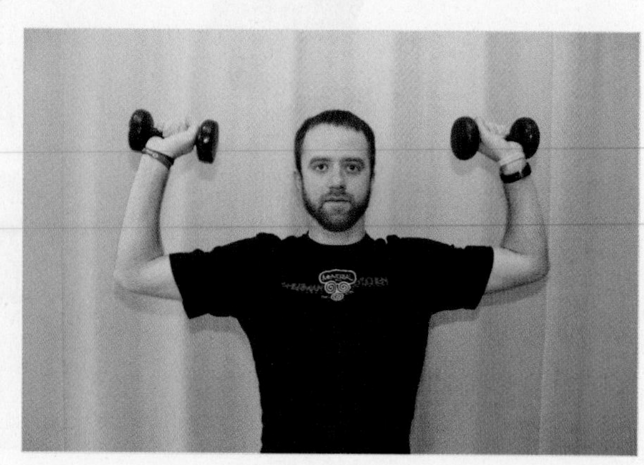

Figure 27-32 Shoulder press

to 27-47) have been shown to improve function[50] and range of motion,[51,52] and to decrease pain sensitivity.[53] These changes are thought to complement the hypoalgesia associated with therapeutic exercise.[36] Regarding the benefits of mobilization versus a manipulation approach, it does not appear that manipulation augments effects to a greater degree than mobilization.[54] Improvements in function, range of motion, and decreased pain can also be accomplished via manual therapy interventions directed at the thoracic spine (Figures 27-67 to 27-70) for individuals with cervical spine pathology.[55,56] Interventions directed at the thoracic spine may help to minimize some of the risks (craniocervical arterial dissection) associated with cervical spine manipulation,[57,58] but may not be as effective as interventions directed at the cervical spine.[59]

The use of therapeutic exercise in conjunction with manual therapy is thought to provide the greatest improvement in pain and function.[19,20,39,47,50] It is important to note that the comprehensive approach is thought to yield better outcomes than either therapeutic exercise or manual therapy performed in isolation.[20,50] Manual or mechanical traction (see Figures 27-34 and 27-35) may also be used to relieve pain and muscle guarding. If hypermobility is present, which is common following joint sprain, strengthening and stabilization exercises should be incorporated

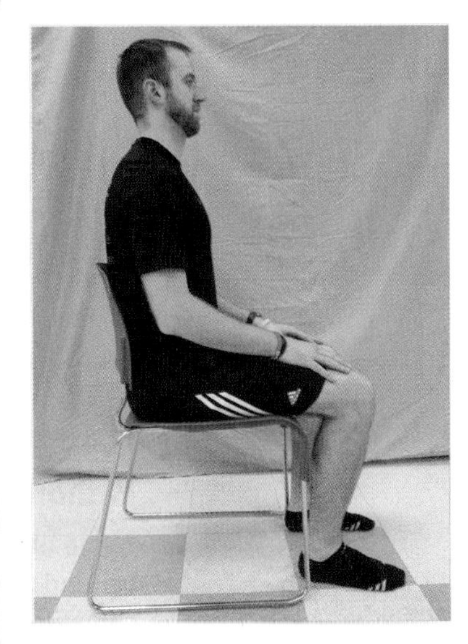

Figure 27-33 Proper sitting posture

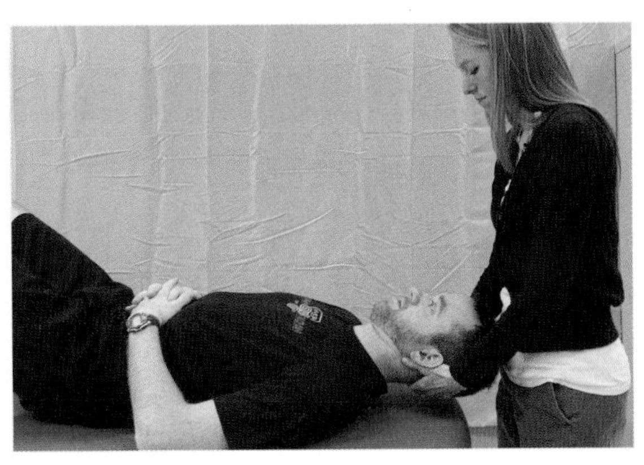

Figure 27-34 Manual traction

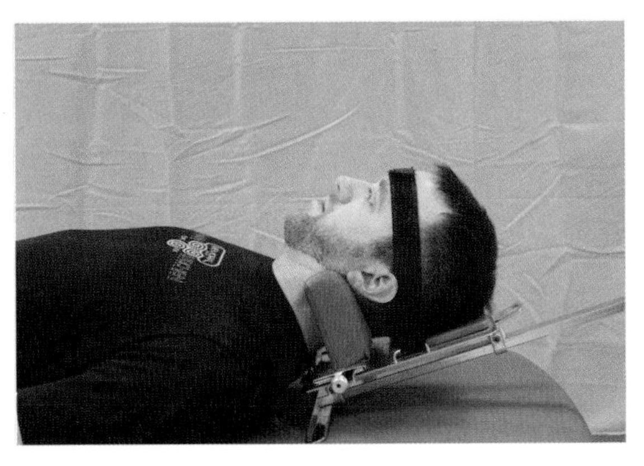

Figure 27-35 Mechanical traction

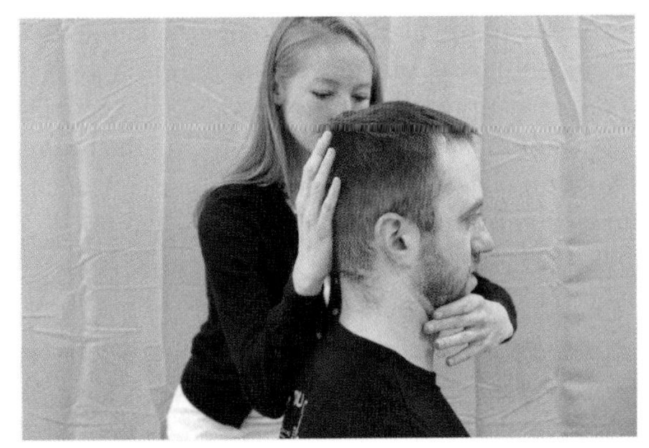

Figure 27-36 Cervical retraction mobilization

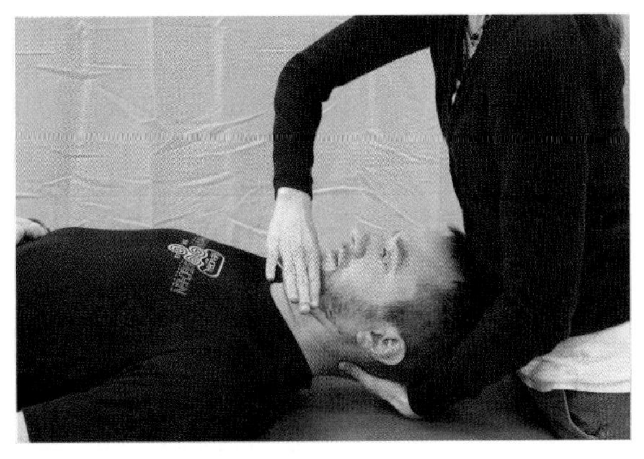

Figure 27-37 Supine cervical retraction

into the rehabilitation program.[45] Initial exercises should focus on neuromuscular control of the neck (see Figures 27-11 to 27-18). The deeper cervical stabilizing muscles (longus capitis and longus colli) are targeted using low loads and focusing on endurance.[20,30] Deficits of the deeper stabilizing musculature can be determined clinically using the craniocervical flexion test (see Figure 27-10).[31] The exercise progression includes exercises to improve neuromuscular control of the scapulothoracic joint (see Figures 27-18 to 27-23, 27-28 to 27-32, and 27-55 to 27-66) with emphasis placed on maintaining control of the cervical spine. Progression should also incorporate tasks of daily living or mimic recreational activities (see Figures 27-28 and 27-30).

Traumatic Neck Pain (Whiplash)

Pathomechanics and Injury Mechanism

Acute neck injuries are most commonly attributed to whiplash, which has both physical and emotional/psychological components. Whiplash is often the result of a motor vehicle collision[60] and has an incidence between 70 and 329 per 100,000 people.[49,50] Approximately 50% of individuals following acute whiplash injury develop chronic symptoms lasting at least 1 year.[61] Thus it is imperative to identify individuals at risk for prolonged symptoms and disability. The strongest predictors of prolonged pain (>6 months) include neck pain greater than 5.5/10 and a score on the Neck Disability Index greater than 14.5/50.[62]

Clinical Pearl

Impairments related to the aftereffects of whiplash can vary widely between individuals.

A variety of symptoms may be associated with whiplash, including neck pain, decreased range of motion, headache, dizziness, visual disturbances, radicular symptoms, and cognitive impairment.[63] A number of structures included the intervertebral disc, zygapophyseal joints, ligaments, and musculature may be damaged,[64] but specific pain-generating structures may not always be identified.[17] As a result of the number of potential structures involved, as well as the emotional/psychological components, it is evident that whiplash is not a homogeneous pathology. Careful consideration of examination findings and clinical presentation should be used to determine the structure of the rehabilitation program. Common impairments associated with whiplash are pain, a loss of cervical spine range of motion, and decreased proprioception.[65] Similar to general neck pain,[22,23] individuals with whiplash tend to utilize the larger superficial muscles to a greater extent than the deeper cervical stabilizing muscles.[66] The motor system dysfunction is thought to persist despite initial symptom resolution, potentially contributing to recurrent symptoms.[26] These persistent muscles imbalances provide the rationale for using low-load postural exercises targeting deep cervical neck flexors.[20,30] Deficits of the deeper stabilizing musculature can be determined clinically using the craniocervical flexion test.[31]

Clinical Pearl

Diminished or absent pain is not indicative of the resolution of motor impairments in patients who has sustained a whiplash injury. Additional interventions are required for a full return to function.

Rehabilitation Concerns and Progression

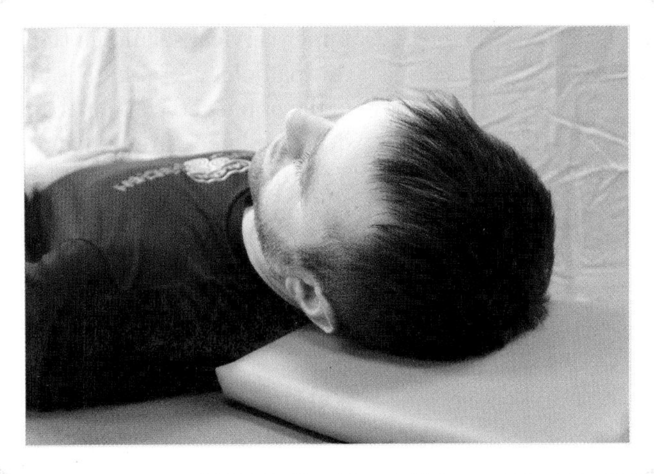

Figure 27-38 Cervical active range of motion with supine wedge

Following acute trauma, the recommendation is for the rehabilitation program to emphasize active range of motion through exercise and manual therapy[67] and improve neuromuscular control and proprioception with gaze stabilization and a cervical proprioceptive training progression.[68] The rehabilitation program should also minimize disability through patient education[67] and avoid immobilization via the use of a soft cervical collar.[67,69,70] The use of a soft collar (see Figure 27-47), although thought to facilitate healing, may actually prolong recovery. The use of physical agents/modalities may complement the exercise rehabilitation program to minimize pain and facilitate motion. Exercises that focus on neuromuscular control of the neck can be initiated in static positions (see Figures 27-11, 27-13, and 27-16) and progressed to incorporating surrounding musculature (eg, arm movement with cervical stabilization) (see Figures 27-12, 27-18, 27-23, and 27-38).[20,30] Deficits of the deeper stabilizing musculature can be determined clinically using the craniocervical flexion test (see Figure 27-10).[31] Sensorimotor training exercises to improve eye–neck coordination and gaze stability are also incorporated.[68] These exercises are initiated with the neck in a static position (stationary) and moving the eyes between 2 fixed targets. Progression involves eye movement to a fixed target followed by moving the head toward a fixed target.

Clinical Pearl

In patients with chronic whiplash-associated disorder, proprioceptive/sensorimotor training is commonly needed for a full return to function.

After acute symptoms begin to subside (usually 3 to 6 weeks), individuals should continue with a focused therapeutic exercise program.[71] Exercises that incorporate upper-extremity movement and require neuromuscular control of the neck and scapulothoracic joints (see Figures 27-18 to 27-23, 27-28 to 27-32, and 27-55 to 27-66) may be added as motor control improves. It is important to note that because patients may still experience symptoms, aggressive intervention programs may be counterproductive.[71] Exercises should continue to focus on neuromuscular control of the neck, as well as improving kinesthetic awareness of head position.[72] Advanced sensorimotor training exercises to improve neuromuscular control, eye–neck coordination, and gaze stability include performing coordinated eye and head movements during walking or while maintaining balance on an unstable surface.[68] Cases that progress to chronic symptoms may still derive short-term benefits from exercise and manual therapy, but the long-term efficacy is questionable.[73]

Cervicogenic Headache

Pathomechanics and Injury Mechanism

Cervicogenic headache has a prevalence of 1% to 4% and is thought to account for approximately 20% of all headaches.[74,75] Women have a greater prevalence than men.[76,77] Headache that originates from the cervical spine is known as *cervicogenic*.[78] The headache is characteristically unilateral, with a "ram horn" presentation, and is provoked by cervical spine motion.[79] Pain typically originates in the neck and then extends to the head. The upper cervical segments (C1-3), including facets and discs are thought to contribute to this pathology.[80,81] There is also tightness of the superficial neck musculature, tenderness of the upper cervical joints and surrounding musculature, decreased range of motion, and decreased neck strength and endurance.[80,82] Cervicogenic headache can be distinguished from other headaches with a comprehensive examination. The presence of restricted motion, hypomobility of the upper segments, and deficits of the deeper stabilizing musculature determined using the craniocervical flexion test were indicative of cervicogenic headache.[83] The signs and symptoms that indicate conservative management of cervicogenic headache include therapeutic exercise and manual therapy.[34]

Clinical Pearl

Convergence of the trigeminal nerve and the upper 3 cervical nerve roots in the trigeminocervical nucleus is likely to be a contributor to cervicogenic headaches.

Rehabilitation Concerns and Progression

Cervicogenic headaches are responsive to intervention programs that target cervical spine stabilizing muscles, improve strength of upper extremity musculature, and address hypomobility of the cervical or thoracic spine with manual therapy.[34,84,85] Cryotherapy is also thought to demonstrate benefit.[77] Initial management includes manual therapy interventions to decrease tenderness and facilitate motion in the upper cervical segments (see Figures 27-36, 27-37, and 27-42 to 27-44). Next, exercises that focus on neuromuscular control of the neck can be initiated. The deeper cervical stabilizing muscles (longus capitis and longus colli) are targeted using low loads and focusing on endurance (see Figures 27-11 to 27-15).[20,30] Deficits of the deeper stabilizing musculature can be determined clinically using the craniocervical flexion test (see Figure 27-10).[31] Exercises that involve the upper extremity can then be incorporated while maintaining a stable cervical spine (see Figures 27-12, 27-18, and 27-23). These exercises are then progressed to more challenging positions and are similar to exercises to improve neuromuscular control of the scapulothoracic joint (see Figures 27-18 to 27-23, 27-28 to 27-32, and 27-55 to 27-66). Progression should also incorporate tasks of daily living or mimic recreational activities (see Figures 27-28 and 27-30). Stretching exercises may also be incorporated to address muscular tightness identified during the examination (see Figures 27-39 to 27-41).

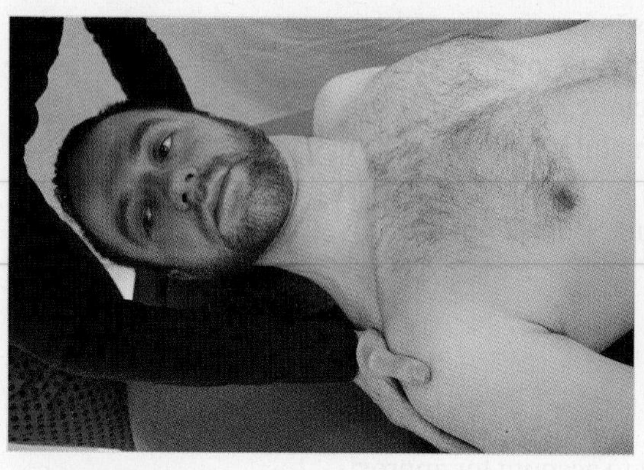

Figure 27-39 Synovial chondromatosis (SCM) stretch

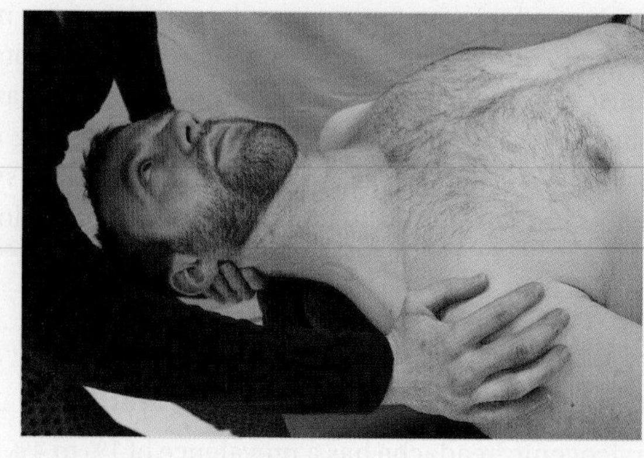

Figure 27-40 Scalene stretch

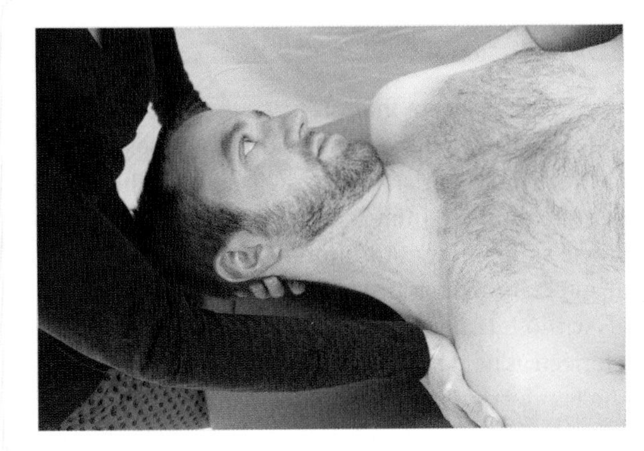

Figure 27-41 Levator scapulae stretch

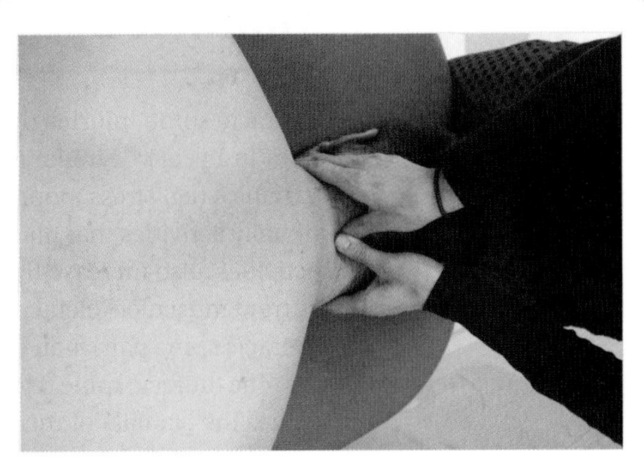

Figure 27-42 Mobilization prone cervical posteroanterior (PA)

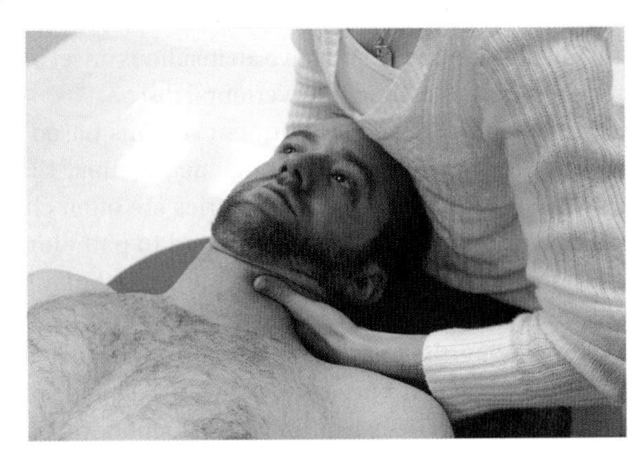

Figure 27-43 Mobilization cervical lateral glide

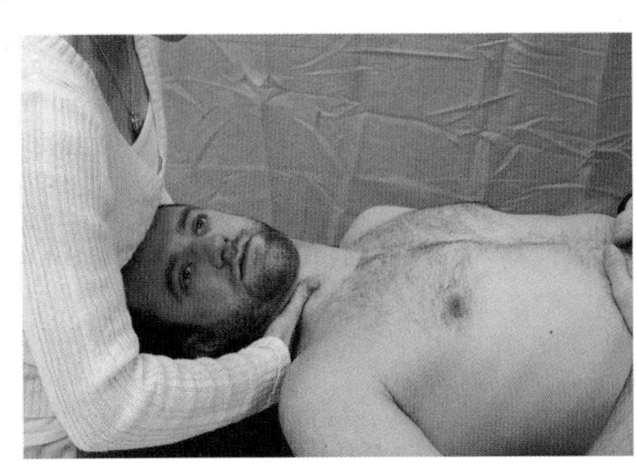

Figure 27-44 Mobilization cervical rotation

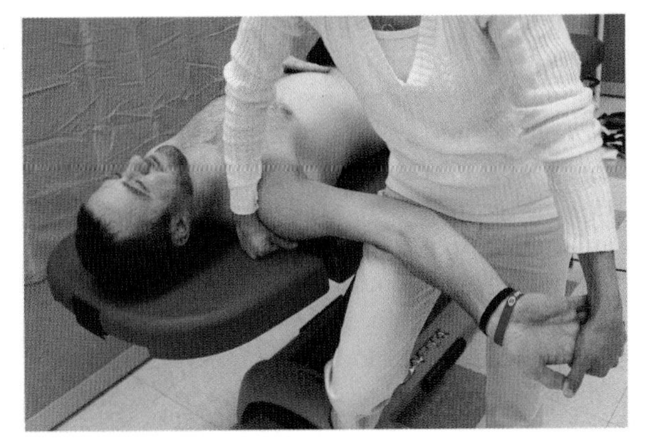

Figure 27-45 Neural mobilization or the upper limb tension test (ULTT).

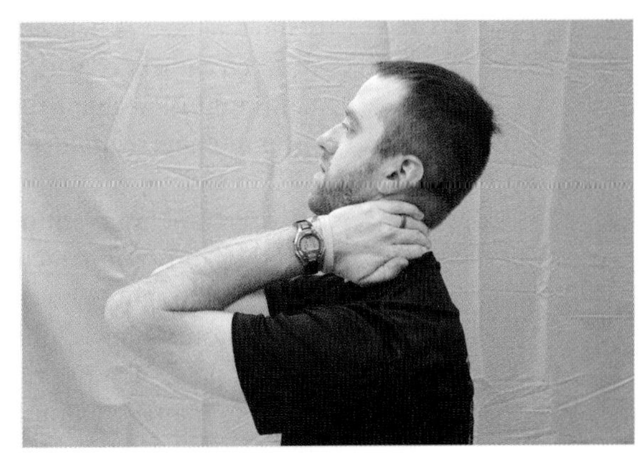

Figure 27-46 Cervical self-mobilization with fingers

Thoracic Spine

Thoracic spine injuries occur at a lower incidence rate than injuries to the cervical spine (10% in 1 year).[86] Similar to cervical spine injury, females and individuals with psychosocial variables (eg, stress, poor mental status) are more at risk for thoracic spine injury.[86] Additionally activities that place loads across the thoracic spine, such as sports or occupational activities, also increase the risk of thoracic spine injury. Additionally individuals with concurrent musculoskeletal pain (cervical spine, lumbar spine) also have a higher incidence of thoracic spine pain than do individuals without concurrent musculoskeletal pain.[86]

The thoracic spine region is characterized as being more stable than the adjacent cervical spine. The stability of the thoracic spine is provided by articulations with the ribs and sternum, lower thoracic intervertebral disc height to vertebral body height, and smaller, more taut zygapophyseal joints. Thoracic spine pathology can involve a number of structures and covers a much greater region than the cervical spine. Complexity is added as a result of the ribs and underlying structures of the thoracic cavity (heart, lungs). Pain in this region is often vague and may not include a specific mechanism of injury.[87] Thus it is important for the clinician to differentiate between musculoskeletal and nonmusculoskeletal (eg, cardiac, pulmonary) causes of thoracic spine pain. Acute (traumatic) injury often presents with a specific mechanism, such as contact with another individual or object resulting in fracture, contusion, or muscle strain. Most thoracic spine injures are nontraumatic and have an insidious onset from overuse affecting the surrounding bones, joints, muscles, and intervertebral disc.

Similar to the cervical spine, it is possible to determine treatment options based on injury mechanism, tissue involvement, and location of pain. Although acute injury (fracture, intercostal muscle strain) can occur at any segment, overuse injuries are often characterized by region. Additionally the thoracic spine may also be subjected to pathologies that are not the result of an injury, such as scoliosis or Scheuermann kyphosis, but may still have an impact on daily function and recreational activities. The first rib is often implicated in dysfunctional breathing and injuries involving the cervical spine and upper extremity, because it is an attachment site for muscles which have origins in the cervical spine (scalenes, subclavius). The midthoracic region (T2-8) is susceptible to costochondritis and rib stress fracture. Pain localized to the costochondral or costosternal joints may be associated with a costochondritis or Tietze syndrome. Both conditions are similar, except Tietze syndrome includes the presence of swelling, heat, or erythema.[88] Stress fractures of the ribs commonly occur in individuals who perform repetitive rotational activities that place loads across the ribs and thoracic spine.[88,89] These commonly occur in throwing sports (baseball, javelin), golf, and rowing. First rib stress fractures are thought to be caused by attachment of the scalenes, subclavius, and serratus anterior, whereas stress fractures of the other ribs are often associated with serratus anterior and external oblique involvement.[88-90] Additional contributing mechanisms include hypomobility of posterior spinal structures.[89,91,92] The lower thoracic segment (T8-12) is susceptible to intervertebral disc pathology.[93]

Management of most thoracic spine injuries involves relative rest from aggravating activities and interventions that facilitate the return to activity. Symptoms may persist for months[94] or become recurrent,[95] but are thought to resolve within a year.[96,97] Most conditions are thought to be self-limiting,[87,88] indicating that individuals may continue activity as symptoms allow. Conservative management is usually symptomatic[87-89] and includes reassurance.[88] The use of modalities,[87,98] analgesics,[88] or local injections[94,95] may be necessary to manage painful conditions. Initially loads and stress across the upper thoracic spine and ribs may be minimized with the use of an arm sling or cervical soft collar (see Figure 27-47), whereas loads across the lower segments can be minimized with the use of a rib/lumbar spine support belt (Figure 27-77). Relative rest is often 3 to 6 weeks in duration with a gradual progression back to activity.[87,88,90,99,100] Relative rest from aggravating factors can also minimize loads across the affected area. Exercise intervention is a consistent component for the management of thoracic spine pathology and often shares similarities between exercise programs that focus on scapula and lumbar stabilization. Many of the muscles with attachments in the thoracic spine have origins or insertions in the cervical, shoulder, or lumbar regions, thus similarities between programs are apparent. Manual therapies are indicated when there is a restriction in soft tissue or joint mobility. Program progression is based on resolution of symptoms and changes in impairments and function. Clinicians are encouraged to reevaluate the patient and attempt to further identify the underlying cause of symptoms for cases that do not resolve with typical conservative management.

Intercostal Muscle Strain

Pathomechanics and Injury Mechanism

Muscle strain is usually a result of heavy lifting or athletic events that involve the upper extremity (rowing, wrestling). Muscle strain may also be the result of recent illness that involves coughing or vomiting. Pain is usually isolated to the muscle belly, between the ribs, and is worse with movement. Muscle strains often have symptoms that overlap with rib injury. Intercostal muscle spasm can often accompany rib injury to immobilize the affect area.

Rehabilitation Concerns and Progression

Management typically involves relative rest, splinting if necessary, and avoidance of aggravating activities. Interventions to address discomfort such as cryotherapy or electrical stimulation can be used as needed. A cardiovascular conditioning program should be implemented to maintain physical fitness during the rehabilitative process. Because breathing can aggravate a costovertebral joint sprain, cardiovascular conditioning may need to be modified to avoid further injury aggravation. Acute management of intercostal muscle strain may include immobilization of the lower ribs with the use of a rib/lumbar spine support belt (see Figure 27-77) or with rib taping. Progression back to activity is often based on symptomatic criteria. As symptoms begin to subside range of motion exercises may be added to the rehabilitation program (Figures 27-73 to 27-75). If impairments in strength or neuromuscular control are present exercise interventions to address these impairments should be included as part of the rehabilitation program. The progression of exercises is similar shoulder and lumbar spine injuries. Exercises are first performed with trunk support and single plane movements (see Figures 27-18 to 27-23, 27-28 to 27-30, and 27-55). Exercise loads may be increased and further advanced using more challenging upper body exercises (see Figures 27-31, 27-32, 27-57, and 27-61) and incorporating kneeling and standing positions (see Figures 27-56, 27-58, and 27-60). Exercises, including upper extremity weight bearing using unstable surfaces, may require the greatest amount of scapulothoracic and lumbopelvic neuromuscular control (see Figures 27-59 to 27-66).

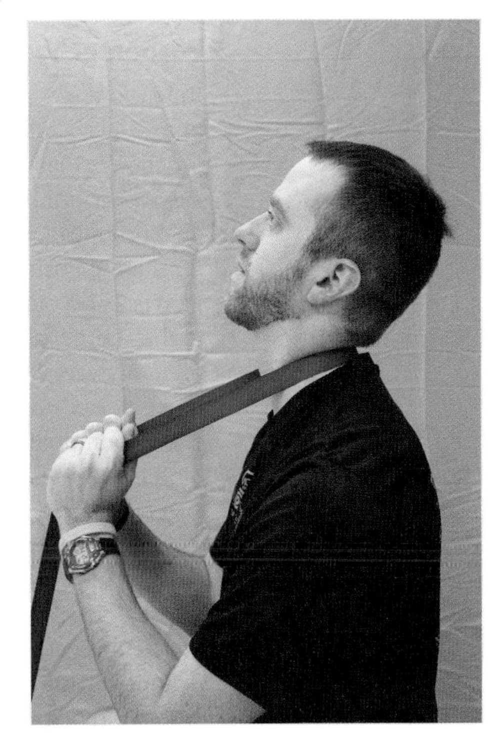

Figure 27-47 Cervical self-mobilization with strap

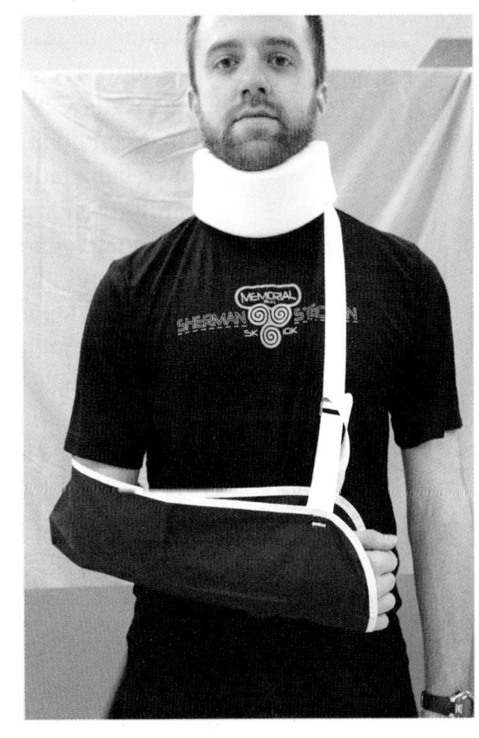

Figure 27-48 Arm sling and cervical collar

Costovertebral Arthralgia or Joint Sprain

Pathomechanics and Injury Mechanism

Injury to the costovertebral joints is often the result of repetitive stress placed through the joint. The costotransverse joint may also be involved as a result of the close proximity and function of these joints. Activities involving repetitive motion with upper-extremity loading, such as swimming and rowing, are thought to cause costovertebral joint sprain.[101] Pain may be reproduced with movement, breathing, coughing, or lying in a supine position. Pain in the supine position is further exacerbated with movement such as a sit up or bench press. Pain is usually localized to the costovertebral joint, but may radiate along the associated rib to the lateral or anterior chest wall. Costovertebral joint sprain typically involves a rib segment between T4-8, with ribs 6 to 7 the most commonly affected. Tenderness with palpation of the costovertebral joint or with a rib spring test is a hallmark sign.

Hypomobility of the affected segment may also be evident and determined with joint mobility testing. The associated hypomobility of the segment is likely why this injury may also be referred to as a costovertebral joint subluxation. Costovertebral joint sprain is often associated with decreased neuromuscular control of the lumbopelvic and scapulothoracic regions. It is possible that weakness or decreased neuromuscular control in these adjacent regions may place greater loads and demands on the costovertebral joint. Unfortunately, the definitive causes of costovertebral joint sprain and relationship with surrounding regions are not well understood. The signs and symptoms often mimic rib stress fracture and may precipitate rib stress fracture.

Rehabilitation Concerns and Progression

Rehabilitation should initially focus on symptom management and attempting to address underlying impairments which contributed to the injury. Relative rest from aggravating factors can also minimize loads across the affected area. Physical agents/modalities and oral analgesics may help diminish symptoms. The intervention program should include therapeutic exercise and manual therapies to address impairments. Hypomobile segments are addressed with manual therapy interventions such as joint mobilization/manipulation (see Figures 27-67 to 27-70), and self-mobilization (Figures 27-71 to 27-75). A cardiovascular conditioning program should be implemented to maintain physical fitness during the rehabilitative process. Because breathing can aggravate a costovertebral joint sprain, cardiovascular conditioning may need to be modified to avoid further injury aggravation. Interventions to improve strength and neuromuscular control of the scapulothoracic (see Figures 27-18 to 27-23, 27-28 to 27-32, and 27-55 to 27-66) and lumbopelvic regions (Figures 27-49 to 27-53) may begin as symptoms allow. This progression is similar to exercises for shoulder and lumbar spine injuries. Exercises are first performed with trunk support and single-plane movements (see Figures 27-18 to 27-23, 27-28 to 27-30, and 27-55). Exercise loads may be increased and further advanced using more challenging upper-body exercises (see Figures 27-31, 27-32, 27-57, and 27-61) and incorporating kneeling and standing positions (see Figures 27-56, 27-58, and 27-60). Exercises, including upper-extremity weight bearing using unstable surfaces, may require the greatest amount of scapulothoracic and lumbopelvic neuromuscular control (see Figures 27-59 to 27-66). Although relative rest and rehabilitation can diminish symptoms, the clinician should attempt to identify contributing factors to the initial injury in attempt to prevent further reoccurrence.

Costochondritis and Tietze's Syndrome

Pathomechanics and Injury Mechanism

Costochondritis and Tietze syndrome are localized to the costochondral or costosternal joints with a diagnosis based on clinical symptoms and examination findings.[88] These

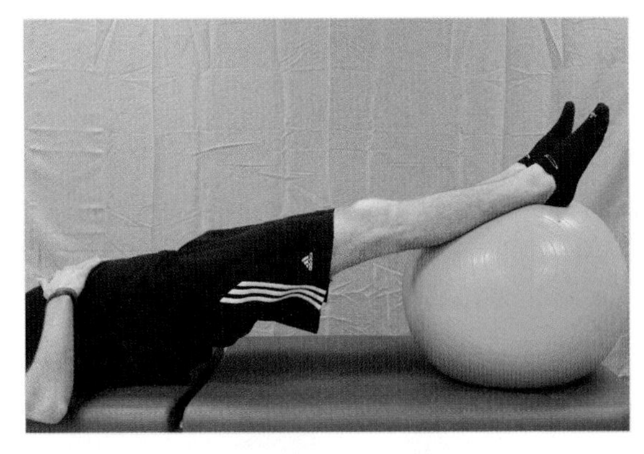

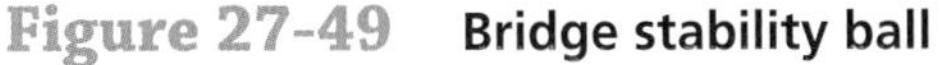

Figure 27-49 Bridge stability ball

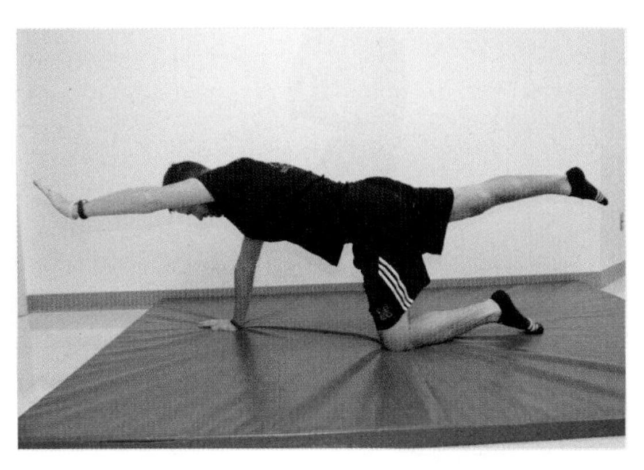

Figure 27-50 Alternating arm/leg extension

conditions tend to affect females more than males.[102] Symptoms tend to be localized to the anterior chest, lateral to the sternum (T2-5) at the costochondral joints. The conditions are relatively similar, except Tietze syndrome includes the presence of swelling, heat, or erythema.[88] Imaging studies offer little value in the diagnosis of costochondritis or Tietze syndrome.[103] Symptoms may be recurrent[95] and persist for months,[94] but are thought to typically resolve within 1 year.[96,97] The mechanism of injury may be a result of contraction of adjacent musculature,[89] repetitive arm adduction,[89] and hypomobility of posterior spinal structures and ribs.[89,91,92] Pain can be provoked palpation of the costochondral joint, rib springing, and with arm movement, especially shoulder horizontal adduction.[88] Identification of the underlying cause of costochondritis is necessary for appropriate management. Costochondritis and Tietze syndrome are thought to be self-limiting conditions,[88] allowing individuals to continue activity participation as symptoms allow.

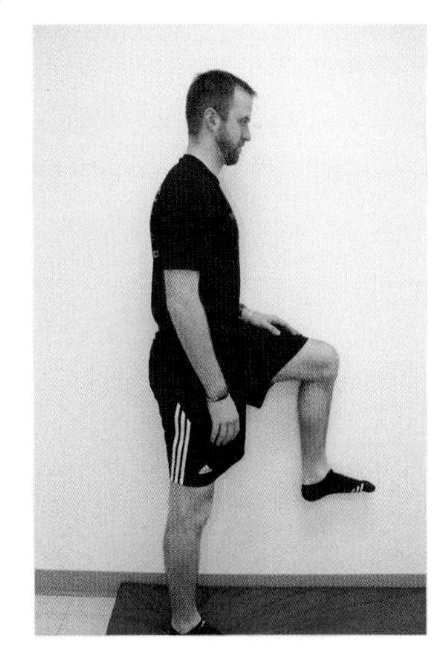

Figure 27-51 Hip abduction—standing

Rehabilitation Concerns and Progression

Rehabilitative management usually focuses on symptom resolution[87-89] and addressing contributing impairments. Because the condition is self-limiting, programs also typically include reassurance.[88] Interventions usually address

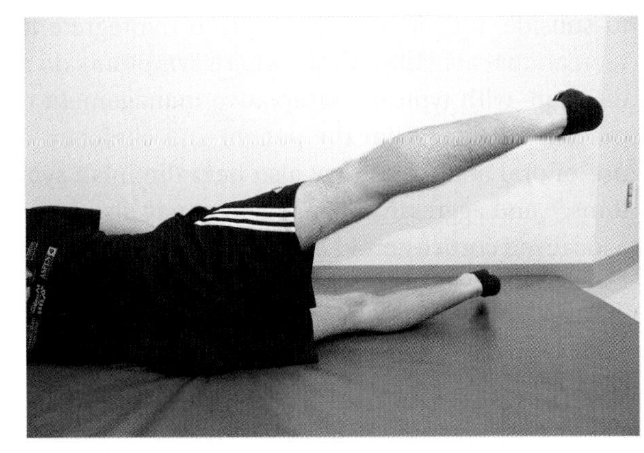

Figure 27-52 Hip abduction—sidelying

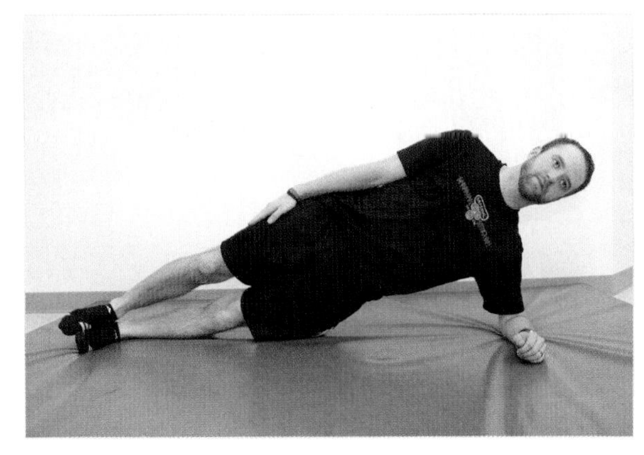

Figure 27-53 Side bridge

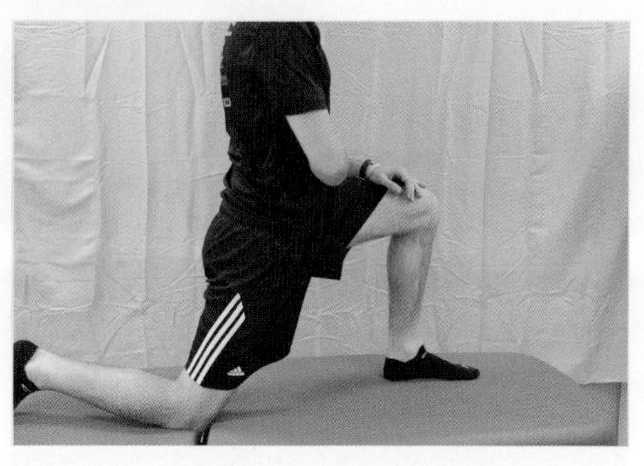

Figure 27-54 Hip flexor stretch

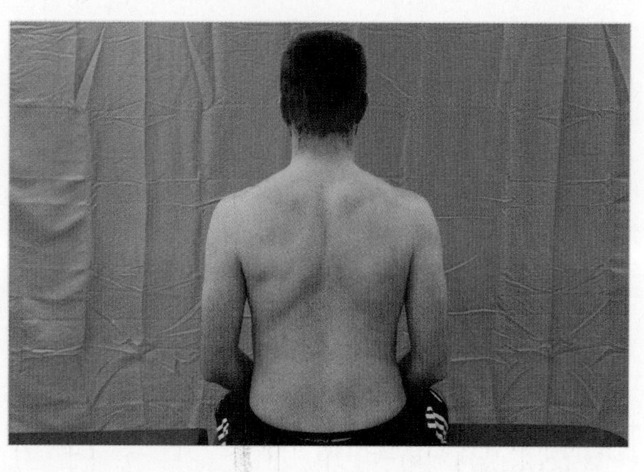

Figure 27-55 Bilateral scapular retraction (seated or standing)

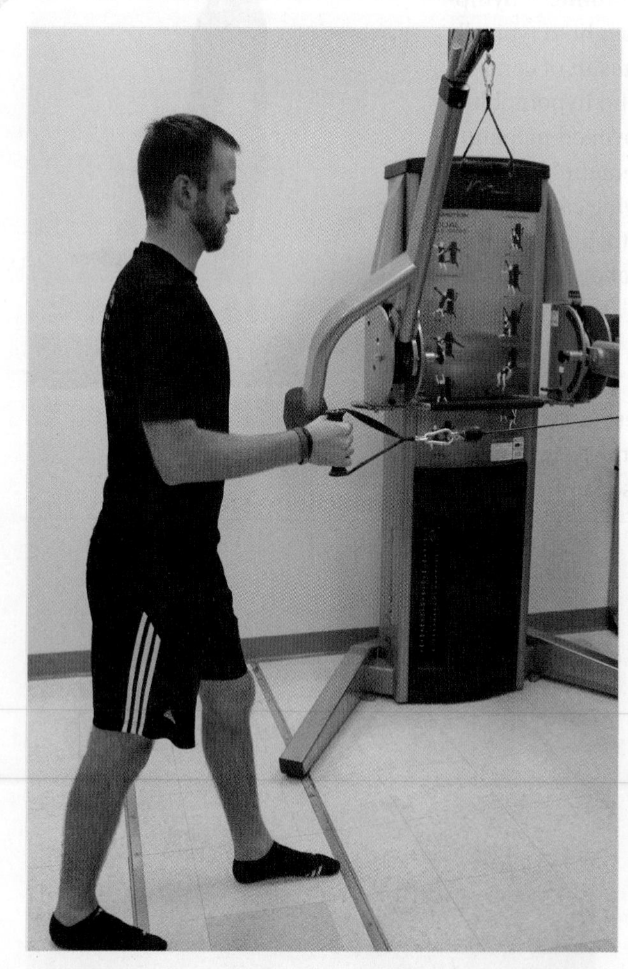

Figure 27-56 Standing row with cable/tubing—split stance

tightness of anterior chest musculature and promote extension of the thoracic spine and ribs (see Figures 27-67 to 27-73). Addressing anterior muscle tightness and thoracic spine hypomobility is thought to decrease loads placed on the joints of the anterior chest (costosternal joint).[98] Initial therapeutic exercises include postural correction (see Figure 27-33), cervical stabilization (see Figures 27-11 to 27-13), and scapular stabilization exercises (see Figures 27-18 to 27-23). Initial exercises can usually be advanced quickly as symptoms allow. Exercise loads may be increased and further advanced using more challenging upper-body exercises (see Figures 27-31, 27-32, 27-57, and 27-61) and incorporating kneeling and standing positions (see Figures 27-56, 27-58, and 27-60). Exercises, including upper-extremity weight bearing using unstable surfaces, may require the greatest amount of scapulothoracic and lumbopelvic neuromuscular control (see Figures 27-59 to 27-66). Once symptoms begin to subside, individuals can begin to reintegrate into recreational activities. Cases where symptoms do not dissipate with typical conservative management can present challenges for the patient and clinician. The use of oral analgesics may also help diminish symptoms,[88] and aggressive management may also include a localized corticosteroid injection.[94,95]

Rib Stress Fracture

Pathomechanics and Injury Mechanism

Stress fractures of the ribs commonly occur in individuals who perform repetitive overhead or rotational activities which place loads across the ribs and thoracic spine. These commonly occur in throwing sports (baseball, javelin), golf, and rowing. First rib stress fractures occur more often in overhead athletics (baseball, tennis)[99,100] are thought to be caused by attachment of the scalenes, subclavius, and serratus anterior. Stress fractures of the other ribs are often associated with serratus anterior and external oblique involvement,[88] and typically occur at ribs 4 to 8.[104] Females are thought to be at greater risk than males because of lower bone mineral density.[104] Stress fractures are usually precipitated by an increase in training volume and may also be a result of technique or changes in equipment. Pain may be specific to one area or may be vague, possibly radiating into the shoulder or upper back. Pain can be reproduced with palpation of the affected area and with breathing (worse with high rates or deep inspiration). Rib springing can reproduce pain and a bony callus may be palpable.

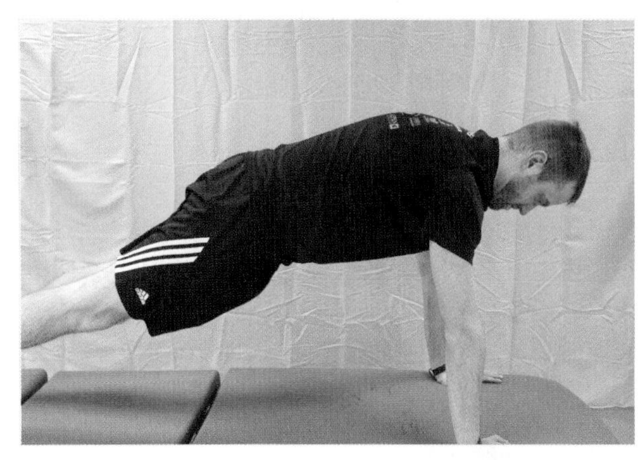

Figure 27-57 Pushup with plus

Decreased upper-extremity strength relative to lower-extremity strength and decreased neuromuscular control of the lumbopelvic region also may be risk factors for rib stress fracture.[105] It is possible that weakness or decreased neuromuscular control in these adjacent regions may place greater loads and demands on the thoracic spine and ribs. Unfortunately, the definitive causes of rib stress fracture and relationship with surrounding regions is not well understood. Similar to costovertebral joint sprain and costochondritis, there also may be hypomobility of posterior spinal structures and ribs.[89,91,92] It is hypothesized that this hypomobility results in a concurrent hypermobility of the rib, which usually occurs along the lateral rib margin.

Rehabilitation Concerns and Progression

Management of rib stress fracture is also guided by symptom resolution.[87-89] Initially, loads across the first rib may be minimized with the use of an arm sling or cervical soft collar (see Figure 27-48).[88] Lower ribs can be immobilized with the use of a rib/lumbar spine support

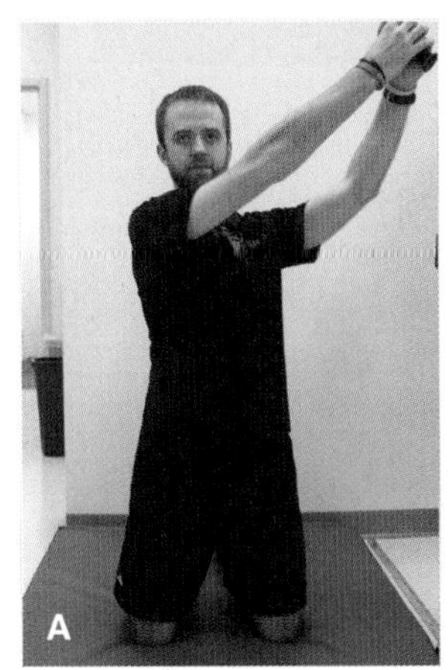

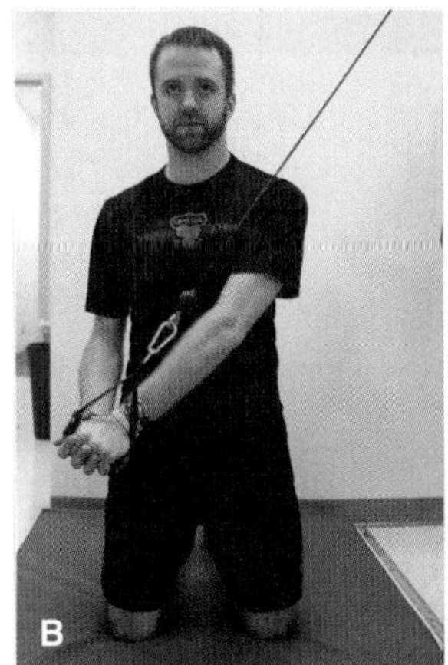

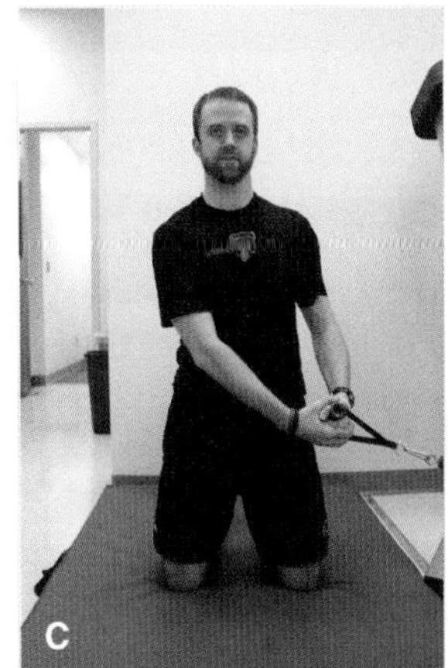

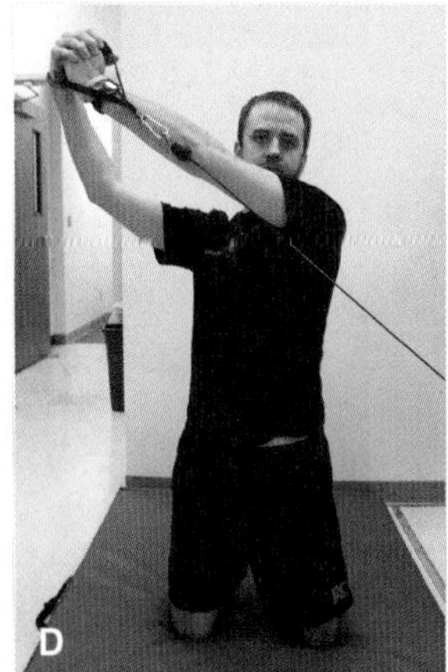

Figure 27-58 "Chop and lift with cable or Thera-Band (kneeling, tall kneeling, half kneeling)"

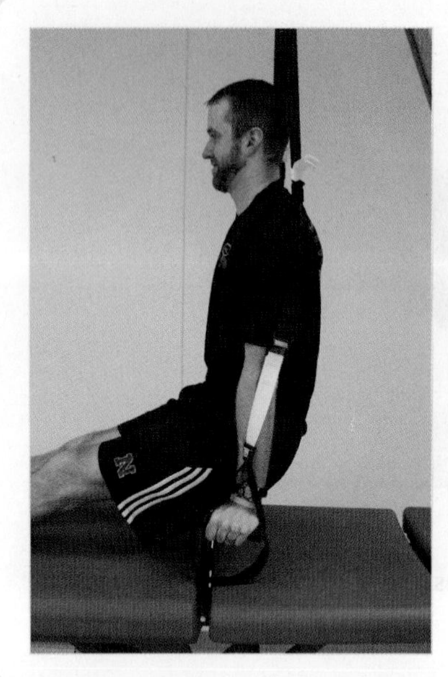

Figure 27-59 Press up TRX® Suspension Training, San Francisco, CA.

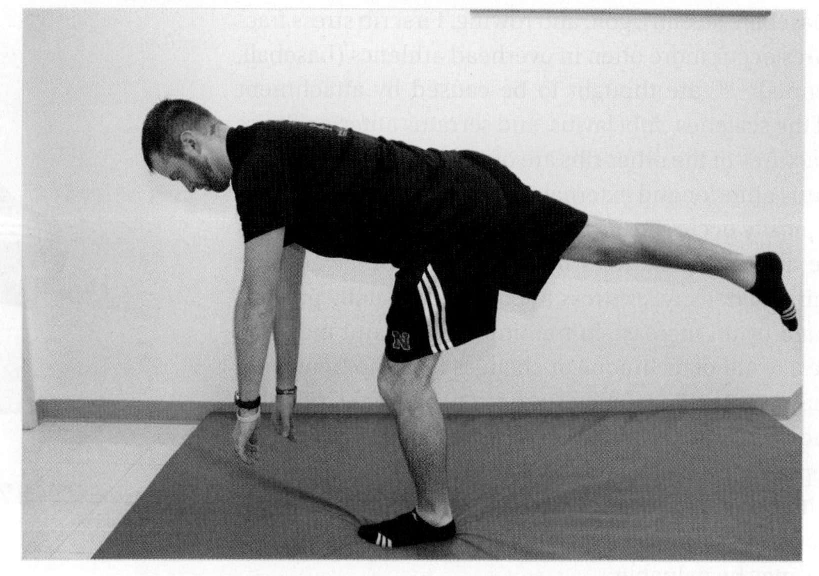

Figure 27-60 Single-leg Romanian deadlift

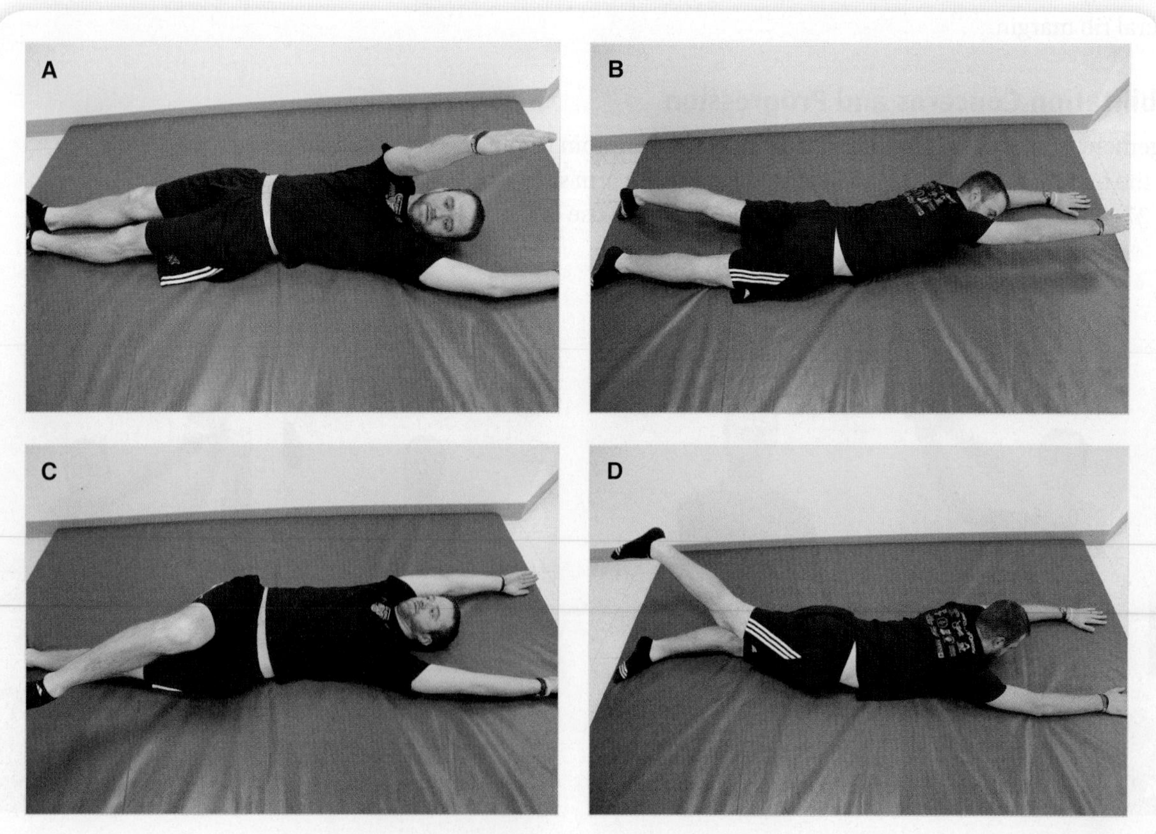

Figure 27-61 Rolling diagonals (upper extremity/lower extremity and flexion/extension)

belt (see Figure 27-77) or with rib taping.[106] Relative rest from aggravating factors can also minimize loads across the affected area. Relative rest is often 3 to 8 weeks in duration with a gradual progression back to activity.[87,88,99,100] Physical agents/modalities and oral analgesics may help diminish symptoms.[88] The intervention program should include therapeutic exercise and manual therapies to address impairments, as well as a cardiovascular conditioning program to maintain physical fitness during the rehabilitative process.[104] Hypomobile segments are address with manual therapy interventions such as joint mobilization/manipulation (see Figures 27-67 to 27-70) and self-mobilization (see Figures 27-71 to 27-75). Exercises are first performed with trunk support and single-plane movements (see Figures 27-18 to 27-23, 27-28 to 27-30, and 27-55). Exercise loads may be increased and further advanced using more challenging upper-body exercises (see Figures 27-31, 27-32, 27-57, and 27-61) and incorporating kneeling and standing positions (see Figures 27-56, 27-58, and 27-60). Exercises, including upper-extremity weight bearing using unstable surfaces, may require the greatest amount of scapulothoracic and lumbopelvic neuromuscular control (see Figures 27-59 to 27-66). It should be noted that because breathing can aggravate a rib stress fracture, cardiovascular conditioning may need to be modified to avoid further injury aggravation. After pain subsides, a gradual progression back to activity over the course of 1 to 2 weeks is advised.

Clinical Pearl

Stress fractures that are caused by technique (eg, golf, rowing) often reoccur if technical modifications are not part of the rehabilitation program.

Intervertebral Disc Pathology

Pathomechanics and Injury Mechanism

Although thoracic disc herniations are not as common as cervical or lumbar disc herniations, they can still have debilitating effects.[107] Most disc herniations are central or posterior lateral.[108] Posterolateral disc pathology manifests with pain localized to the paravertebral region, whereas anterior tears produce visceral pain. Pain may be reproduced or provoked with activities that increase intradiscal pressure (straining, sneezing) or place tension on neural structures (slump test, neck flexion). Disc pathology is determined using imaging such as MRI. Because of the kyphotic curvature of the thoracic spine, the spinal cord and nerve roots are in closer proximity to the intervertebral disc than the cervical and lumbar regions. Therefore, even small herniations may irritate or compress these neural structures highlighting the importance of a comprehensive neurological examination of the distal segments. Individuals with neurologic deficits such as bowel/bladder impairment or upper motor neuron signs, should be referred to a physician for further examination. Lower thoracic regions (T8-L1) are more likely to demonstrate disc pathology as this region has larger discs, bearing greater loads, with more mobile vertebral segments relative to the upper thoracic region.[109,110] **The segments T11-12 and T12-L1 are the most common for intervertebral disc pathology.**[110] Most individuals with thoracic spine intervertebral disc pathology will have favorable outcomes with conservative management.[108] It is also possible that the intervertebral disc herniation can be reabsorbed over time.[111]

Clinical Pearl

Thoracic intervertebral disc pathology is more common in lower thoracic segments than in the upper segments.

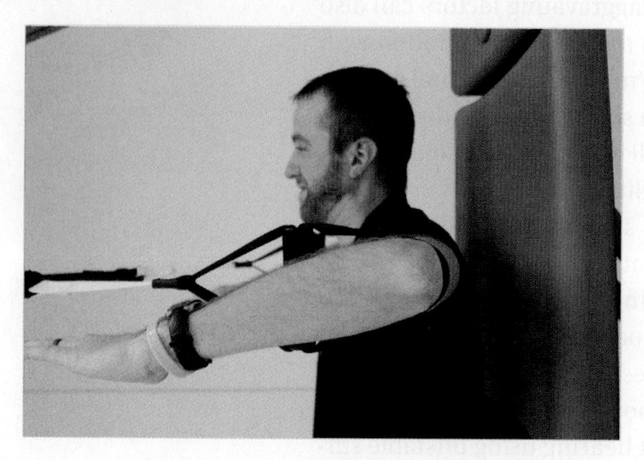

Figure 27-62 Scapular retraction TRX® Suspension Training, San Francisco, CA.

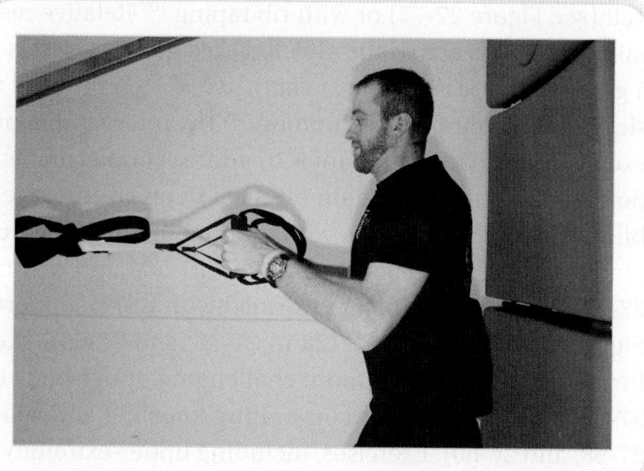

Figure 27-63 Supine row TRX® Suspension Training, San Francisco, CA.

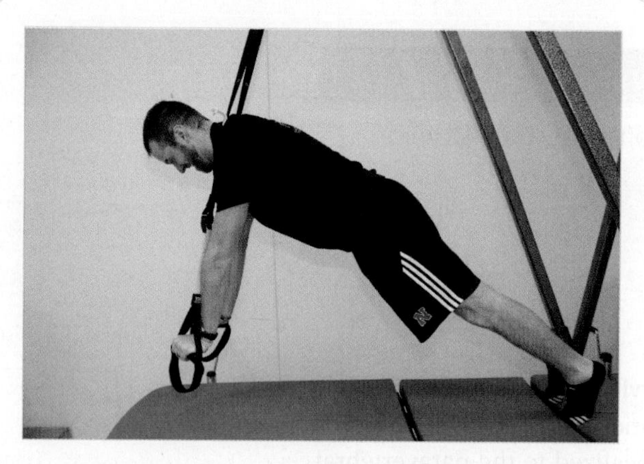

Figure 27-64 Pushup plus TRX® Suspension Training, San Francisco, CA.

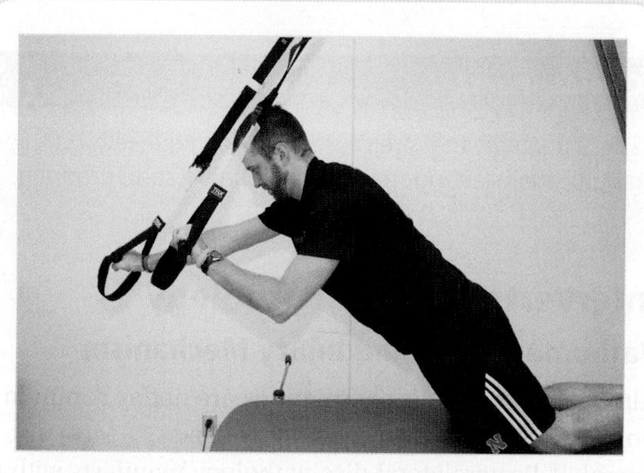

Figure 27-65 Shoulder protraction TRX® Suspension Training, San Francisco, CA.

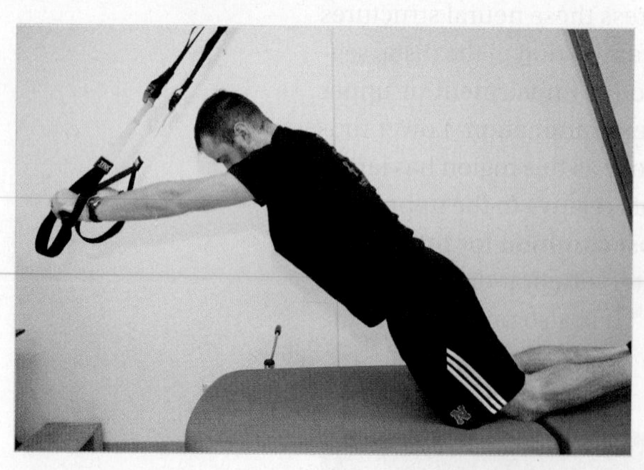

Figure 27-66 Shoulder extension TRX® Suspension Training, San Francisco, CA.

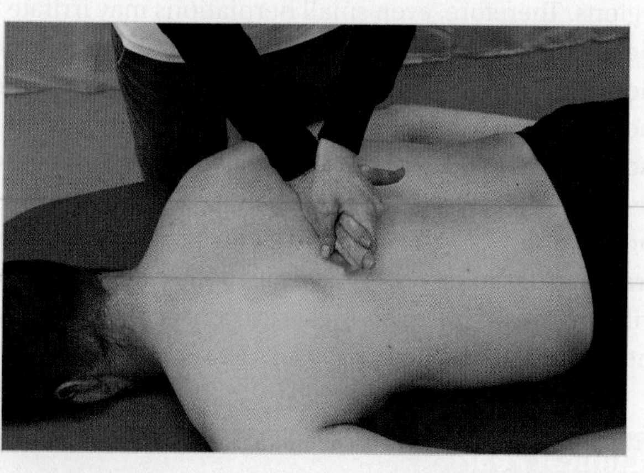

Figure 27-67 Mobilization prone thoracic posteroanterior (PA)

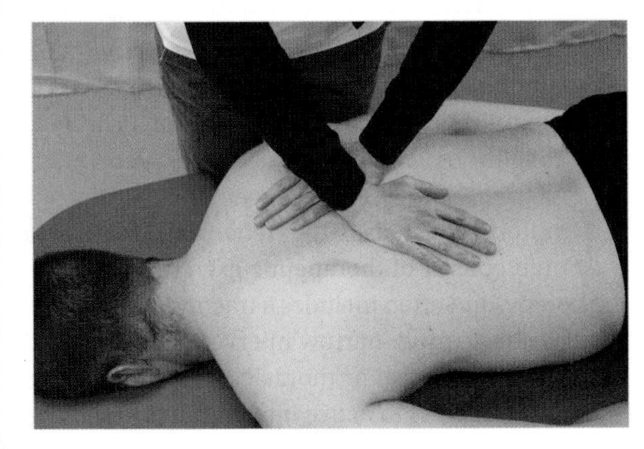

Figure 27-68 Mobilization prone midthoracic

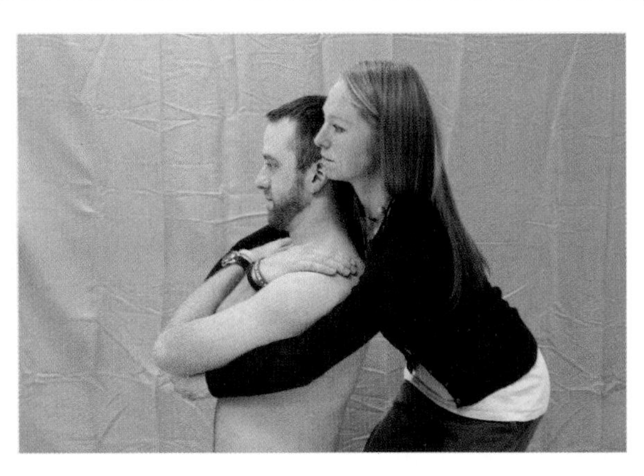

Figure 27-69 Mobilization seated midthoracic

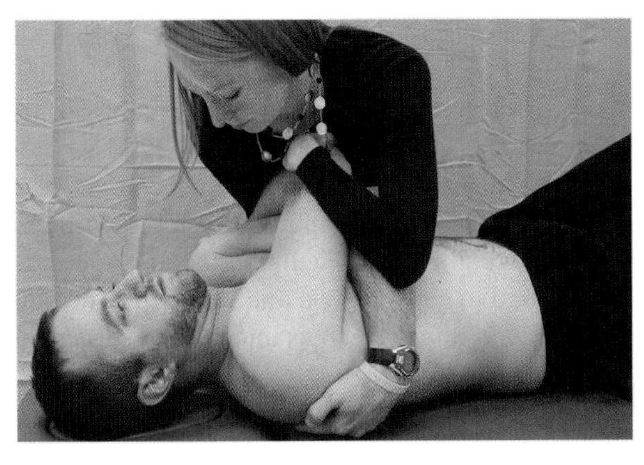

Figure 27-70 Mobilization supine upper or midthoracic

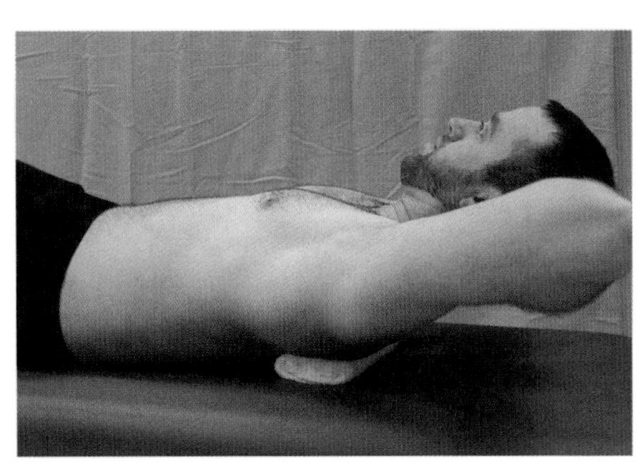

Figure 27-71 Thoracic self-mobilization with towel roll

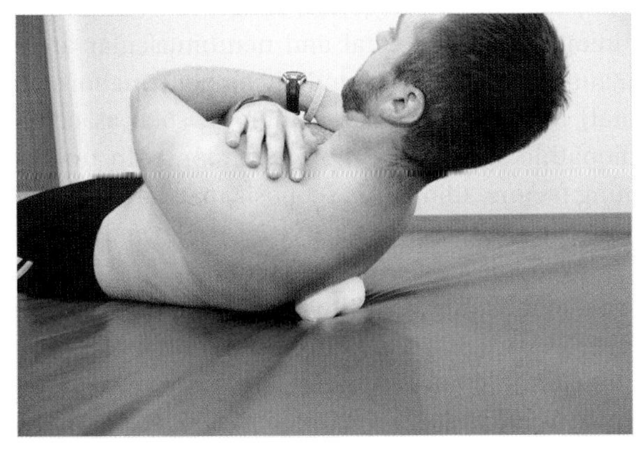

Figure 27-72 Thoracic self-mobilization with tennis balls

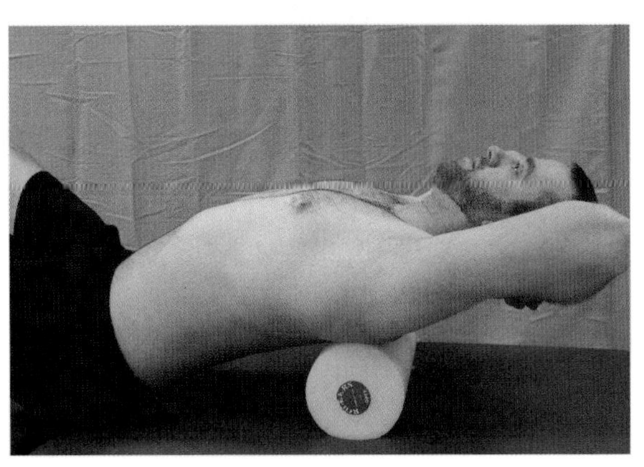

Figure 27-73 Thoracic self-mobilization with foam roller

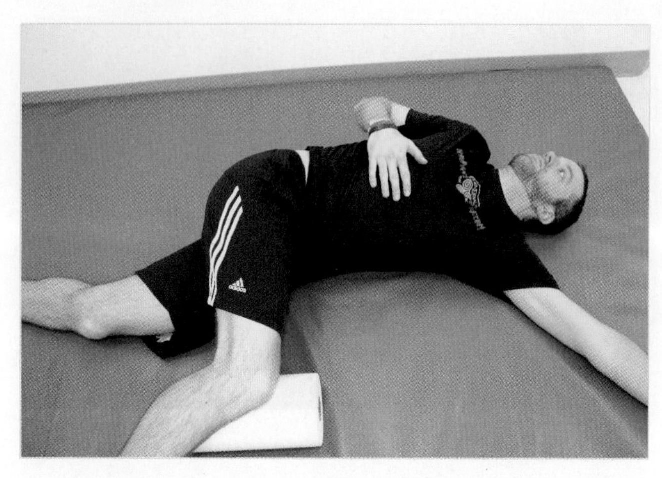

Figure 27-74 Thoracic side-lying rotation self-mobilization

Rehabilitation Concerns and Progression

Treatment is similar to disc pathology of the cervical or lumbar spine. Initial management of acute injury and pain should focus on activity modification and interventions which help decrease pain (analgesics, cryotherapy, physical agents). As initial acute symptoms decrease, the rehabilitation program should consist of therapeutic exercise and manual therapy, and often includes a traction component to address the more narrow intervertebral space relative to the cervical or thoracic spine. Interventions should progress to active interventions and include active range of motion (see Figures 27-71 to 27-75), stretching (Figure 27-76), and exercises to improve endurance and strength (see Figures 27-18 to 27-23, 27-28 to 27-30, and 27-55). Manual therapies should be utilized to promote thoracic extension (see Figures 27-67 to 27-75). Exercise loads may be increased and further advanced using more challenging upper-body exercises (see Figures 27-31, 27-32, 27-57, and 27-61) and incorporating kneeling and standing positions (see Figures 27-56, 27-58, and 27-60). Exercises, including upper-extremity weight bearing using unstable surfaces, may require the greatest amount of scapulothoracic and lumbopelvic neuromuscular control (see Figures 27-59 to 27-66). Cases that do not respond to conservative management may require more invasive interventions, such as injection or surgery, and warrant referral to a physician.

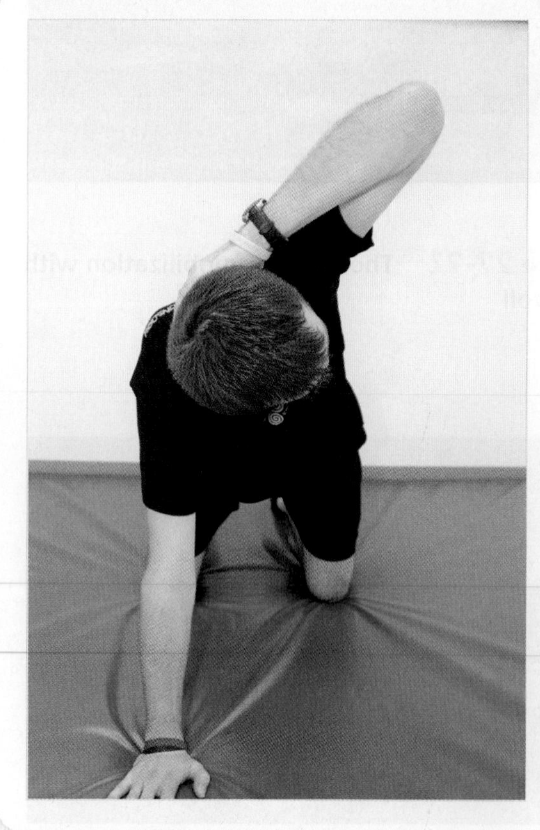

Figure 27-75 Thoracic kneeling rotation self-mobilization

Scoliosis

Pathomechanics and Injury Mechanism

A scoliosis is an abnormal curve (>10 degrees) that occurs in the coronal or frontal plane in the thoracic spine or in the lumbar spine, or in both regions simultaneously. Scoliosis may be classified into 3 categories: congenital, neuromuscular, and idiopathic. Congenital and neuromuscular are less common and are the result of underlying bony malformation (congenital) or neuromuscular pathology, such as cerebral palsy. Idiopathic scoliosis is more common with unknown contributing factors. Idiopathic scoliosis may be further subdivided into early onset (prior to 10 years of age) and late onset or adolescent. Adolescent scoliosis is thought to affect 1% to 3% of the general population, with females more affected than males.[112,113] Sports that involve unilateral rotation (ie, throwing) are thought to contribute to a higher risk of scoliosis.[114] The majority of individuals with scoliosis are asymptomatic, but seek care because of asymmetrical abnormalities. As the curvature progresses, back pain can develop, but is not thought to be at a greater rate than that of the general population.[115]

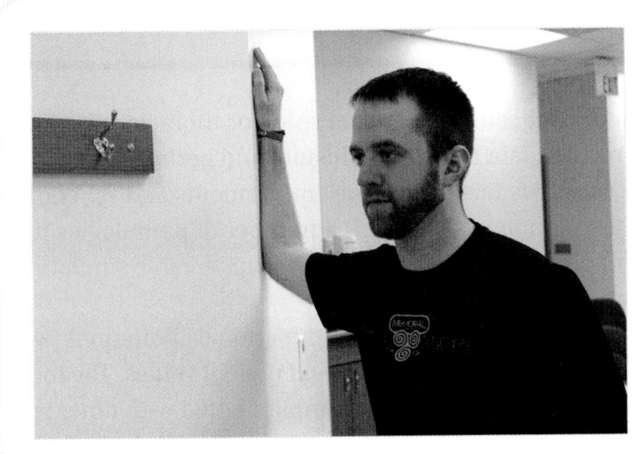

Figure 27-76 Pectoralis minor stretch

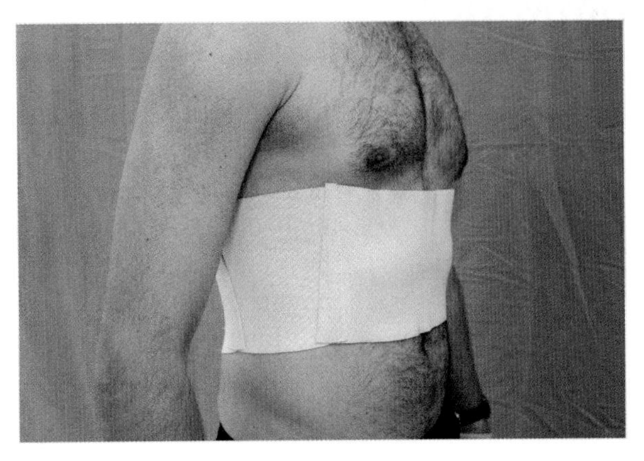

Figure 27-77 Rib/lumbar spine support belt

Cardiopulmonary function can be compromised if the chest is deformed as a consequence of the scoliosis (typically curves >50 degrees).[115]

Rehabilitation Concerns and Progression

Conservative management of scoliosis includes bracing, therapeutic exercise, and electrical stimulation to minimize curve progression. Bracing is usually considered with curves between 25 and 40 degrees, particularly if the patient is skeletally immature and the curve is likely to progress.[116] Bracing can minimize curve progression, but has limited high-quality evidence.[117] Therapeutic exercise and manual therapy can also reduce curvature progression, reduce brace wear, and improve strength and mobility,[118-120] but also has limited high quality evidence.[118,121,122] Aerobic training can improve cardiovascular function.[123] A common limitation of current studies is patient compliance.

Cases that are not responsive to conservative care are considered for surgical intervention. The most common reason for surgery is pain relief and to mitigate pulmonary complications. Surgery is typically recommended for curves greater than 50 degrees, especially in individuals who are skeletally immature. As surgical options are employed to minimize curvature progression, this usually involves multiple surgical procedures. Although surgical intervention has inherent risk, these risks are thought to be outweighed by the benefits gained in lung function and reduced deformity.[115]

A well-designed rehabilitation program can provide pain relief and improve function in many patients. Rehabilitation programs for scoliosis typically include therapeutic exercise, manual therapy, and postural education with visual and tactile biofeedback. Acute pain can be managed with activity modification and interventions that help decrease pain (analgesics, cryotherapy, physical agents). The rehabilitation program should also consist of therapeutic exercises (see Figures 27-50, 27-53 to 27-58, and 27-61) and manual therapies (see Figures 27-67 to 27-75) that target specific impairments identified in the examination and attempt to establish a normalized spinal curvature. Postural education and exercises should focus on sitting and standing postures (see Figure 27-33). Emphasis is placed on the posture of the shoulder and pelvic girdle and positions which unload the curve pattern. Therapeutic exercise is then performed in the corrected postural pattern to increase muscular endurance (see Figure 27-25) and to help reinforce the pattern. Cases that do not respond to conservative management may require more invasive interventions such as surgery.

SUMMARY

Identification of a specific pathoanatomical cause of cervical spine or thoracic spine pain is not always possible. The clinician must obtain a thorough history and perform a comprehensive examination to identify the causative factors such as impairments and functional limitations that are contributing to the pathology. Although a number of pathologies may be present within the cervical or thoracic spine regions, there are considerable similarities among the intervention approaches.

Interventions should address specific impairments and functional limitations with consideration of the available evidence, clinician experience, and patient values. The foundation of the rehabilitation program is therapeutic exercise complemented with other specific interventions that address motion, pain, and radicular symptoms. The clinician should consistently monitor patient progress and alter the program as needed. Rehabilitation progression is based on resolution of symptoms and changes in impairments and function.[19,20]

Sample Cases

Cervical Case 1: Cervical Radiculopathy

Background

The patient is a 35-year-old male attorney and recreational triathlete with a 2-week onset of right moderate (3/10), lateral, midcervical pain and severe (7/10), sharp, shooting pain in his lateral forearm with intermittent thumb/index finger paresthesia. Symptoms began following painting rooms, including ceilings, in his new house for 2 weeks after work and on weekends. Symptoms are aggravated in the AM/first rising; when sitting/driving for longer than 30 minutes; when looking up; and with right rotation. Symptoms are relieved with supine lying in flexion (2 pillows), arm resting on top of head, and nonsteroidal antiinflammatory drugs (NSAIDs). Neck Disability Index: 16/50. Objective findings: Limited cervical range of motion (ROM)—right rotation, right side bending, extension. (+) upper limb tension test (ULTT) 1 right; pain with Spurling test; reduction in symptoms with cervical distraction. His lateral cervical paraspinals are tender to palpation, with muscle spasm and guarding right > left. Normal myotomal strength, sensation to pin prick and light touch, muscle stretch reflexes.

Treatment[42,43,124]

Phase I: (acute—cervical + radicular pain mid ROM cervical sidebending (SB)/rotation/extension)

Manual Therapy: Cervical manual distraction in neutral, slight flexion (see Figures 27-34, and 27-36)

Thoracic extension mobilization/manipulation (see Figures 27-68 to 27-70)

Soft tissue mobilization—upper trapezius, scaleni, suboccipitals

Neural mobilization - ULLT1 (gentle, pain free) (see Figure 27-45)

Exercise: Deep neck flexor training (supine) (see Figures 27-11 and 27-12)

Mid ROM (pain free) cervical rotation (see Figure 27-38)

Postural correction—sitting (see Figures 27-17, 27-25, and 27-33)

Bilateral scapular retraction and external rotation (ER) (see Figure 27-55)

Education: Sitting posture—work station modifications/ergonomics (see Figure 27-33)

Phase II: (subacute—cervical rotation/SB/extension with radicular pain at end ROM)

Manual Therapy: Continue manual cervical distraction (see Figures 27-34 and 27-36)

Soft-tissue mobilization to cervical paraspinals

Cervical side glide mobilizations right C5-6 (see Figure 27-43)

Cervical rotational/opening mobilizations right C5-6 (see Figure 27-44)

Thoracic manipulation (see Figures 27-68 to 27-70)

Exercise: Prone cervical stabilization (deep neck flexors)—sagittal plane (see Figure 27-13)

Seated cervical stabilization—scapular stabilization (pulleys or tubing) (see Figure 27-23)

Prone scapular stabilization (see Figures 27-18 and 27-19)

Neural mobilizations—self (see Figure 27-45)

Phase III: (nonradicular signs and symptoms)

Manual Therapy: Cervical manual distraction (see Figures 27-34 and 27-36)

Cervical opening mobilizations/manipulation (see Figures 27-43 and 27-44)

Soft-tissue mobilization—cervical paraspinals

Exercise: Cervical stabilization (general cervical strengthening)—multiplanar/ multipositional (see Figures 27-26 and 27-27)

Scapular stabilization—prone stability ball (see Figures 27-19 to 27-22)

Phase IV: (symptom free, full active range of motion [AROM])

Exercise: Sport-specific cervical/scapular stabilization (see Figures 27-62 to 27-66)

Bike fit/postural assessment

Swimming stroke mechanic training

Return to gym exercises—review postural correction with progressive increase in resistance training (see Figures 27-29 and 27-32)

Cervical Case 2: Anterior Cervical Decompression/Fusion (ACDF) Postoperative Rehabilitation

Background

The patient is a 58-year-old female administrative assistant and recreational tennis player who presented with chronic neck pain and progressive myelopathy and who failed 12 weeks' of conservative management, including physical therapy, pharmacologic management, and epidural steroid injections × 3. She had a 2-level cervical decompression and anterior cervical instrumented fusion at C5-6.

Treatment/Postoperative Management[125-127]

Phase I (Postoperative weeks 4 to 8): following 4 weeks of cervical collar + progressive walking program (15 minutes 1×/day, progressing up to 30 minutes 2×/day)

Manual Therapy: Soft-tissue mobilization to cervical paraspinals, including anterior incision

Gentle cervical AROM exercises (supine) (see Figure 27-38)

Exercise: Upper body ergometry (postural correction) (see Figure 27-25)

Sensorimotor training: deep neck flexor activation (see Figures 27-11 and 27-12)

Scapular retraction exercise (prone—head supported) (see Figure 27-18)

Education: Posture (see Figure 27-33)

Relaxation/stress management/breathing

Pain physiology

Self-management/coping strategies

Self-efficacy

Phase II (Postoperative weeks 8 to 12):

Manual Therapy: Progression of cervical active ROM exercises to full

Passive range of motion (PROM)—progress cervical ROM to full

Grades II/III cervical side bend/side glide mobilizations (above/below C5/6) (see Figures 27-43 and 27-44)

Thoracic mobilizations (see Figures 27-67 to 27-70)

Exercise: Cervical stabilization exercises (seated) (see Figures 27-15 to 27-17)

Upper-extremity rowing, proprioceptive neuromuscular facilitation (PNF) diagonals (see Figures 27-24, 27-29, 27-30, 27-55, and 27-56)

Cervical motor control exercises through progressing ROM (supported to unsupported) (see Figures 27-13 to 27-17)

Education: Self-efficacy

Ergonomics—workstation design (see Figure 27-33)

Phase III (Postoperative weeks 12 to 16):

Exercise: Progress endurance of cervical stabilizers (deep neck flexors)

General strengthening—upper quarter with cervical stabilization/postural correction (see Figures 27-29 and 27-32)

Functional training: Scapular stabilization with standing sport-specific (tennis) movement patterns (see Figures 27-28 and 27-30)

Education: Postural correction with return to prior level of activity

Thoracic Case 1: Rib Stress Fracture

Background

Patient is an 18-year-old female collegiate-club-level rower (single sculler) with a 3-week history of anterior lateral lower rib cage pain that worsens with increased training/practice in the boat. Symptoms are aggravated by breathing, cough/sneeze; overhead upper-extremity use—flexion worse than abduction; trunk extension > flexion; transitional movements, especially sit-to-supine in bed; unable to row secondary to sharp pain. Symptoms are eased with rest, analgesics, ice. Bone scan (+) lateral seventh rib stress injury.

Treatment[104,105,128]

Phase I: Education: Rest × 3 weeks from all rowing

Analgesics (not NSAIDs)

Ice for pain management

Diet/caloric intake consultation/referral

Manual Therapy: Soft-tissue mobilization to regional myofascia-abdominals, obliques, intercostals, serratus

Grades II/III mobilizations to thoracic spine (see Figures 27-67 to 27-70)

Hip/lumbar flexion mobilization/stretching

Exercise: Lower-body cardiovascular training: cycling (upright posture)

Trunk/core stability (avoiding excessive abdominal loading/contraction) (see Figures 27-49, 27-50, and 27-53)

Lower quarter/hip strengthening (gluteals) (see Figures 27-51 and 27-52)

Stretching for lumbar/hip especially flexion (see Figure 27-54)

Phase II: Education: Gradual progressive return to rowing (on land/ergo meter)

Assess rowing mechanics—cuing to correct, especially simultaneous leg drive

Manual Therapy: Regional soft-tissue mobilization

Thoracic mobilization (grades II/III) to improve costovertebral, costotransverse, thoracic mobility (see Figures 27-67 to 27-75)

Exercise: Gradual progression of upper quarter cardiovascular training, including ergometry/rowing

Progress trunk/core stability using unstable surfaces and unilateral exercises (see Figures 27-49, 27-50, and 27-53)

Lower quarter strengthening, especially hip/knee extension, including squats and single-leg Romanian deadlift (see Figure 27-60)

Scapular stabilization—mid/lower trap strengthening, light resistance—serratus strengthening (see Figures 27-19 to 27-22, 27-55, and 27-56)

Phase III: Education: Continue progressive return to rowing—progress to boat

Rowing biomechanical assessment—cueing

Manual Therapy: Continue regional soft-tissue mobilization

Joint mobilizations: Thoracic, costotransverse, costovertebral joint mobilizations (grades III/IV) (see Figures 27-67 to 27-75)

Exercise: Progress scapular stabilization especially serratus anterior

Progress to eccentric serratus strengthening, including weightbearing exercises (see Figures 27-57 to 27-60)

Phase IV: Education: Continue to progress toward full practice load

Communicate with coaches to reinforce mechanics/technique recommendations

Manual Therapy: Soft-tissue mobilizations

Joint mobilizations as needed (see Figures 27-67 to 27-75)

Exercise: Continue to strengthen scapular stabilizers, especially eccentric serratus (see Figures 27-63 to 27-67)

Incorporate endurance training with emphasis on proper technique

Progress core/trunk stability incorporating more specific abdominal cocontraction into rowing specific strengthening and technique drills. Single-leg squats and single-leg Romanian deadlift (see Figure 27-60). Can incorporate unstable surfaces

REFERENCES

1. Rudert M, Tillmann B. Lymph and blood supply of the human intervertebral disc. Cadaver study of correlations to discitis. *Acta Orthop Scand.* 1993;64(1):37-40.
2. Audette I, Dumas JP, Cote JN, De Serres SJ. Validity and between-day reliability of the cervical range of motion (CROM) device. *J Orthop Sports Phys Ther.* 2010;40(5):318-323.
3. Cleland JA, Childs JD, Fritz JM, Whitman JM. Interrater reliability of the history and physical examination in patients with mechanical neck pain. *Arch Phys Med Rehabil.* 2006;87(10):1388-1395.
4. Dvorak J, Panjabi MM, Novotny JE, Antinnes JA. In vivo flexion/extension of the normal cervical spine. *J Orthop Res.* 1991;9(6):828-834.
5. Panjabi MM, Cholewicki J, Nibu K, Grauer J, Babat LB, Dvorak J. Critical load of the human cervical spine: An in vitro experimental study. *Clin Biomech (Bristol, Avon).* 1998;13(1):11-17.
6. Johnson KD, Grindstaff TL. Thoracic rotation measurement techniques: Clinical commentary. *N Am J Sport Phys Ther.* 2010;5:252-256.
7. Johnson KD, Kim KM, Yu BK, Saliba SA, Grindstaff TL. Reliability of thoracic spine rotation range-of-motion measurements in healthy adults. *J Athl Train.* 2012;47(1):52-60.
8. Lee D. Biomechanics of the thorax: a clinical model of in vivo function. *J Man Manip Ther.* 1993;1(1):13-21.
9. Gore DR, Sepic SB, Gardner GM. Roentgenographic findings of the cervical spine in asymptomatic people. *Spine (Phila Pa 1976).* 1986;11(6):521-524.
10. Matsumoto M, Okada E, Ichihara D, et al. Age-related changes of thoracic and cervical intervertebral discs in asymptomatic subjects. *Spine (Phila Pa 1976).* 2010;35(14):1359-1364.
11. Kato F, Yukawa Y, Suda K, Yamagata M, Ueta T. Normal morphology, age-related changes and abnormal findings of the cervical spine. Part II: magnetic resonance imaging of over 1,200 asymptomatic subjects. *Eur Spine J.* 2012;21(8):1499-1507.
12. Yukawa Y, Kato F, Suda K, Yamagata M, Ueta T. Age-related changes in osseous anatomy, alignment, and range of motion of the cervical spine. Part I: radiographic data from over 1,200 asymptomatic subjects. *Eur Spine J.* 2012;21(8):1492-1498.
13. Badve SA, Bhojraj S, Nene A, Raut A, Ramakanthan R. Occipito-atlanto-axial osteoarthritis: a cross sectional clinico-radiological prevalence study in high risk and general population. *Spine (Phila Pa 1976).* 2010;35(4):434-438.
14. Triantafillou KM, Lauerman W, Kalantar SB. Degenerative disease of the cervical spine and its relationship to athletes. *Clin Sports Med.* 2012;31(3):509-520.
15. Hush JM, Michaleff Z, Maher CG, Refshauge K. Individual, physical and psychological risk factors for neck pain in Australian office workers: a 1-year longitudinal study. *Eur Spine J.* 2009;18(10):1532-1540.
16. Borghouts JAJ, Koes BW, Bouter LM. The clinical course and prognostic factors of non-specific neck pain: a systematic review. *Pain.* 1998;77(1):1-13.
17. Matsumoto M, Okada E, Ichihara D, et al. Prospective ten-year follow-up study comparing patients with whiplash-associated disorders and asymptomatic subjects using magnetic resonance imaging. *Spine (Phila Pa 1976).* 2010;35(18):1684-1690.
18. Fritz JM, Brennan GP. Preliminary examination of a proposed treatment-based classification system for patients receiving physical therapy interventions for neck pain. *Phys Ther.* 2007;87(5):513-524.
19. Gross AR, Goldsmith C, Hoving JL, et al. Conservative management of mechanical neck disorders: A systematic review. *J Rheumatol.* 2007;34(5):1083-1102.
20. Kay Theresa M, Gross A, Goldsmith Charles H, et al. Exercises for mechanical neck disorders. *Cochrane Database Syst Rev.* 2012;(8):CD004250.
21. Louw A, Diener I, Butler DS, Puentedura EJ. The effect of neuroscience education on pain, disability, anxiety, and stress in chronic musculoskeletal pain. *Arch Phys Med Rehabil.* 2011;92(12):2041-2056.
22. Côté P, Cassidy JD, Carroll LJ, Kristman V. The annual incidence and course of neck pain in the general population: a population-based cohort study. *Pain.* 2004;112(3):267-273.
23. Hoy DG, Protani M, De R, Buchbinder R. The epidemiology of neck pain. *Best Pract Res Clin Rheumatol.* 2010;24(6):783-792.
24. Cagnie B, Danneels L, Van Tiggelen D, Loose V, Cambier D. Individual and work related risk factors for neck pain among office workers: a cross sectional study. *Eur Spine J.* 2007;16(5):679-686.
25. O'Leary S, Falla D, Elliott JM, Jull G. Muscle dysfunction in cervical spine pain: implications for assessment and management. *J Orthop Sports Phys Ther.* 2009;39(5):324-333.
26. Sterling M, Jull G, Vicenzino B, Kenardy J, Darnell R. Development of motor system dysfunction following whiplash injury. *Pain.* 2003;103(1-2):65-73.
27. Falla D, Farina D. Neural and muscular factors associated with motor impairment in neck pain. *Curr Rheumatol Rep.* 2007;9(6):497-502.
28. Falla D. Unravelling the complexity of muscle impairment in chronic neck pain. *Man Ther.* 2004;9(3):125-133.
29. Chiu TT, Law EY, Chiu TH. Performance of the craniocervical flexion test in subjects with and without chronic neck pain. *J Orthop Sports Phys Ther.* 2005;35(9):567-571.

30. Beer A, Treleaven J, Jull G. Can a functional postural exercise improve performance in the cranio-cervical flexion test?—A preliminary study. *Man Ther.* 2012;17(3):219-224.
31. Jull GA, O'Leary SP, Falla DL. Clinical assessment of the deep cervical flexor muscles: The craniocervical flexion test. *J Manipulative Physiol Ther.* 2008;31(7):525-533.
32. Radhakrishnan K, Litchy WJ, O'Fallon WM, Kurland LT. Epidemiology of cervical radiculopathy: a population-based study from Rochester, Minnesota, 1976 through 1990. *Brain.* 1994;117(2):325-335.
33. Ylinen J, Takala EP, Nykänen M, et al. Active neck muscle training in the treatment of chronic neck pain in women: a randomized controlled trial. *JAMA.* 2003;289(19):2509-2516.
34. Jull G, Trott P, Potter H, et al. A randomized controlled trial of exercise and manipulative therapy for cervicogenic headache. *Spine (Phila Pa 1976).* 2002;27(17):1835-1843.
35. O'Leary S, Falla D, Jull G, Vicenzino B. Muscle specificity in tests of cervical flexor muscle performance. *J Electromyogr Kinesiol.* 2007;17(1):35-40.
36. O'Leary S, Falla D, Hodges PW, Jull G, Vicenzino B. Specific therapeutic exercise of the neck induces immediate local hypoalgesia. *J Pain.* 2007;8(11):832-839.
37. Cook C, Brown C, Isaacs R, Roman M, Davis S, Richardson W. Clustered clinical findings for diagnosis of cervical spine myelopathy. *J Man Manip Ther.* 2010;18(4):175-180.
38. Werneke M, Hart DL, Cook D. A descriptive study of the centralization phenomenon: A prospective analysis. *Spine (Phila Pa 1976).* 1999;24(7):676-683.
39. Young IA, Michener LA, Cleland JA, Aguilera AJ, Snyder AR. Manual therapy, exercise, and traction for patients with cervical radiculopathy: a randomized clinical trial. *Phys Ther.* 2009;89(7):632-642.
40. Heintz MM, Hegedus EJ. Multimodal management of mechanical neck pain using a treatment based classification system. *J Man Manip Ther.* 2008;16(4):217-224.
41. Salt E, Wright C, Kelly S, Dean A. A systematic literature review on the effectiveness of non-invasive therapy for cervicobrachial pain. *Man Ther.* 2011;16(1):53-65.
42. Cleland JA, Whitman JM, Fritz JM, Palmer JA. Manual physical therapy, cervical traction, and strengthening exercises in patients with cervical radiculopathy: a case series. *J Orthop Sports Phys Ther.* 2005;35(12):802-811.
43. Cleland JA, Fritz JM, Whitman JM, Heath R. Predictors of short-term outcome in people with a clinical diagnosis of cervical radiculopathy. *Phys Ther.* 2007;87(12):1619-1632.
44. Stiell IG, Clement CM, McKnight RD, et al. The Canadian c-spine rule versus the nexus low-risk criteria in patients with trauma. *N Engl J Med.* 2003;349(26):2510-2518.
45. Zmurko MG, Tannoury TY, Tannoury CA, Anderson DG. Cervical sprains, disc herniations, minor fractures, and other cervical injuries in the athlete. *Clin Sports Med.* 2003;22(3):513-521.
46. Cleland JA, Childs JD, Fritz JM, Whitman JM, Eberhart SL. Development of a clinical prediction rule for guiding treatment of a subgroup of patients with neck pain: use of thoracic spine manipulation, exercise, and patient education. *Phys Ther.* 2007;87(1):9-23.
47. Hoving JL, Koes BW, de Vet HC, et al. Manual therapy, physical therapy, or continued care by a general practitioner for patients with neck pain. A randomized, controlled trial. *Ann Intern Med.* 2002;136(10):713-722.
48. Tseng Y-L, Wang WTJ, Chen W-Y, Hou T-J, Chen T-C, Lieu F-K. Predictors for the immediate responders to cervical manipulation in patients with neck pain. *Man Ther.* 2006;11(4):306-315.
49. Cleland JA, Mintken PE, Carpenter K, et al. Examination of a clinical prediction rule to identify patients with neck pain likely to benefit from thoracic spine thrust manipulation and a general cervical range of motion exercise: Multi-center randomized clinical trial. *Phys Ther.* 2010;90(9):1239-1250.
50. Gross AR, Hoving JL, Haines TA, et al. A Cochrane review of manipulation and mobilization for mechanical neck disorders. *Spine (Phila Pa 1976).* 2004;29(14):1541-1548.
51. Saavedra-Hernández M, Arroyo-Morales M, Cantarero-Villanueva I, et al. Short-term effects of spinal thrust joint manipulation in patients with chronic neck pain: a randomized clinical trial. *Clin Rehabil.* 2012;27(6):504-12.
52. Millan M, Leboeuf-Yde C, Budgell B, Descarreaux M, Amorim MA. The effect of spinal manipulative therapy on spinal range of motion: a systematic literature review. *Chiropr Man Therap.* 2012;20(1):23.
53. Vicenzino B, Collins D, Benson H, Wright A. An investigation of the interrelationship between manipulative therapy-induced hypoalgesia and sympathoexcitation. *J Manipulative Physiol Ther.* 1998;21(7):448-453.
54. Boyles RE, Walker MJ, Young BA, Strunce J, Wainner RS. The addition of cervical thrust manipulations to a manual physical therapy approach in patients treated for mechanical neck pain: a secondary analysis. *J Orthop Sports Phys Ther.* 2010;40(3):133-140.
55. Masaracchio M, Cleland JA, Hellman M, Hagins M. Short-term combined effects of thoracic spine thrust manipulation and cervical spine non-thrust manipulation in individuals with mechanical neck pain: a randomized clinical trial. *J Orthop Sports Phys Ther.* 2012.
56. Cross KM, Kuenze C, Grindstaff TL, Hertel J. Thoracic spine thrust manipulation improves pain, range of motion, and self-reported function in patients with mechanical neck pain: a systematic review. *J Orthop Sports Phys Ther.* 2011;41(9):633-642.
57. Thomas LC, Rivett DA, Attia JR, Parsons M, Levi C. Risk factors and clinical features of craniocervical arterial dissection. *Man Ther.* 2011;16(4):351-356.
58. Miley ML, Wellik KE, Wingerchuk DM, Demaerschalk BM. Does cervical manipulative therapy cause vertebral artery dissection and stroke? *Neurologist.* 2008;14(1):66-73.

59. Puentedura EJ, Landers MR, Cleland JA, Mintken PE, Huijbregts P, Fernández-de-Las-Peñas C. Thoracic spine thrust manipulation versus cervical spine thrust manipulation in patients with acute neck pain: A randomized clinical trial. *J Orthop Sports Phys Ther.* 2011;41(4):208-220.
60. Quinlan KP, Annest JL, Myers B, Ryan G, Hill H. Neck strains and sprains among motor vehicle occupants—United States, 2000. *Accid Anal Prev.* 2004;36(1):21-27.
61. Carroll LJ, Holm LW, Hogg-Johnson S, et al. Course and prognostic factors for neck pain in whiplash-associated disorders (WAD): results of the bone and joint decade 2000-2010 task force on neck pain and its associated disorders. *Spine (Phila Pa 1976).* 2008;33(4 Suppl):S83-S92.
62. Walton DM, Macdermid JC, Giorgianni AA, Mascarenhas JC, West SC, Zammit CA. Risk factors for persistent problems following acute whiplash injury: update of a systematic review and meta-analysis. *J Orthop Sports Phys Ther.* 2013;43(2):31-43.
63. Spitzer WO, Skovron ML, Salmi LR, et al. Scientific monograph of the quebec task force on whiplash-associated disorders: Redefining "whiplash" and its management. *Spine (Phila Pa 1976).* 1995; 20(8 Suppl):1S-73S.
64. Uhrenholt L, Grunnet-Nilsson N, Hartvigsen J. Cervical spine lesions after road traffic accidents: a systematic review. *Spine (Phila Pa 1976).* 2002;27(17):1934-1940.
65. Dall'Alba PT, Sterling MM, Treleaven JM, Edwards SL, Jull GA. Cervical range of motion discriminates between asymptomatic persons and those with whiplash. *Spine (Phila Pa 1976).* 2001;26(19):2090-2094.
66. Falla D, Bilenkij G, Jull G. Patients with chronic neck pain demonstrate altered patterns of muscle activation during performance of a functional upper limb task. *Spine (Phila Pa 1976).* 2004;29(13):1436-1440.
67. Teasell RW, McClure JA, Walton D, et al. A research synthesis of therapeutic interventions for whiplash-associated disorder (WAD): Part 2—interventions for acute wad. *Pain Res Manag.* 2010;15(5):295-304.
68. Kristjansson E, Treleaven J. Sensorimotor function and dizziness in neck pain: implications for assessment and management. *J Orthop Sports Phys Ther.* 2009;39(5):364-377.
69. Rosenfeld M, Gunnarsson R, Borenstein P. Early intervention in whiplash-associated disorders: a comparison of two treatment protocols. *Spine (Phila Pa 1976).* 2000;25(14):1782-1787.
70. McKinney LA. Early mobilisation and outcome in acute sprains of the neck. *BMJ.* 1989;299(6706):1006-1008.
71. Teasell RW, McClure JA, Walton D, et al. A research synthesis of therapeutic interventions for whiplash-associated disorder (WAD): Part 3—interventions for subacute wad. *Pain Res Manag.* 2010;15(5):305-312.
72. Jull GA. Considerations in the physical rehabilitation of patients with whiplash-associated disorders. *Spine (Phila Pa 1976).* 2011;36 Supplement(25S):S286-S291.
73. Teasell RW, McClure JA, Walton D, et al. A research synthesis of therapeutic interventions for whiplash-associated disorder (WAD): Part 4—noninvasive interventions for chronic wad. *Pain Res Manag.* 2010;15(5):313-322.
74. Evers S. Introduction: comparison of cervicogenic headache with migraine. *Cephalalgia.* 2008; 28(1 Suppl):16-17.
75. Sjaastad O. Cervicogenic headache: comparison with migraine without aura; Vågå study. *Cephalalgia.* 2008;28(Suppl 1):18-20.
76. Leone M, Cecchini A, Mea E, Tulio V, Bussone G. Epidemiology of fixed unilateral headaches. *Cephalalgia.* 2008;28(1 Suppl):8-11.
77. Knackstedt H, Bansevicius D, Aaseth K, Grande RB, Lundqvist C, Russell MB. Cervicogenic headache in the general population: the Akershus study of chronic headache. *Cephalalgia.* 2010;30(12):1468-1476.
78. Sjaastad O, Fredriksen TA, Pfaffenrath V. Cervicogenic headache: diagnostic criteria. The Cervicogenic Headache International Study Group. *Headache.* 1998;38(6):442-445.
79. Bogduk N, Govind J. Cervicogenic headache: an assessment of the evidence on clinical diagnosis, invasive tests, and treatment. *Lancet Neurol.* 2009;8(10):959-968.
80. Hall T, Robinson K. The flexion–rotation test and active cervical mobility—a comparative measurement study in cervicogenic headache. *Man Ther.* 2004;9(4):197-202.
81. Hall T, Briffa K, Hopper D, Robinson K. Reliability of manual examination and frequency of symptomatic cervical motion segment dysfunction in cervicogenic headache. *Man Ther.* 2010;15(6):542-546.
82. Dumas J-P, Arsenault A, Boudreau G, et al. Physical impairments in cervicogenic headache: traumatic vs. nontraumatic onset. *Cephalalgia.* 2001;21(9):884-893.
83. Jull G, Amiri M, Bullock-Saxton J, Darnell R, Lander C. Cervical musculoskeletal impairment in frequent intermittent headache. Part 1: subjects with single headaches. *Cephalalgia.* 2007;27(7):793-802.
84. Chaibi A, Russell M. Manual therapies for cervicogenic headache: a systematic review. *J Headache Pain.* 2012;13(5):351-359.
85. Ylinen J, Nikander R, Nykänen M, Kautiainen H, Häkkinen A. Effect of neck exercises on cervicogenic headache: a randomized controlled trial. *J Rehabil Med.* 2010;42(4):344-349.
86. Briggs AM, Smith AJ, Straker LM, Bragge P. Thoracic spine pain in the general population: prevalence, incidence and associated factors in children, adolescents and adults. A systematic review. *BMC Musculoskelet Disord.* 2009;10:77.
87. Karlson KA. Thoracic region pain in athletes. *Curr Sports Med Rep.* 2004;3(1):53-57.
88. Gregory PL, Biswas AC, Batt ME. Musculoskeletal problems of the chest wall in athletes. *Sports Med.* 2002;32(4):235-250.

89. Rumball JS, Lebrun CM, Di Ciacca SR, Orlando K. Rowing injuries. *Sports Med.* 2005;35(6):537-555.

90. Karlson KA. Rib stress fractures in elite rowers: A case series and proposed mechanism. *Am J Sports Med.* 1998;26(4):516-519.

91. Aspegren D, Hyde T, Miller M. Conservative treatment of a female collegiate volleyball player with costochondritis. *J Manipulative Physiol Ther.* 2007;30(4):321-325.

92. Ian Rabey M. Costochondritis: Are the symptoms and signs due to neurogenic inflammation. Two cases that responded to manual therapy directed towards posterior spinal structures. *Man Ther.* 2008;13(1):82-86.

93. Arce CA, Dohrmann GJ. Herniated thoracic disks. *Neurol Clin.* 1985;3(2):383-392.

94. Härkönen M. Tietze's syndrome. *Br Med J.* 1977;2(6094):1087-1088.

95. Freeston J, Karim Z, Lindsay K, Gough A. Can early diagnosis and management of costochondritis reduce acute chest pain admissions? *J Rheumatol.* 2004;31(11):2269-2271.

96. Brown RT, Jamil K. Costochondritis in adolescents: a follow-up study. *Clin Pediatr (Phila).* 1993;32(8):499-500.

97. Disla E, Rhim HR, Reddy A, Karten I, Taranta A. Costochondritis. A prospective analysis in an emergency department setting. *Arch Intern Med.* 1994;154(21):2466-2469.

98. Grindstaff TL, Beazell JR, Saliba EN, Ingersoll CD. Treatment of a female collegiate rower with costochondritis: a case report. *J Man Manip Ther.* 2010;18(2):64-68.

99. Coris EE, Higgins HW. First rib stress fractures in throwing athletes. *Am J Sports Med.* 2005;33(9):1400-1404.

100. Sakellaridis T, Stamatelopoulos A, Andrianopoulos E, Kormas P. Isolated first rib fracture in athletes. *Br J Sports Med.* 2004;38(3):e5-e5.

101. Thomas PL. Thoracic back pain in rowers and butterfly swimmers—costovertebral subluxation. *Br J Sports Med.* 1988:81a.

102. Disla E, Rhim HR, Reddy A, Karten I, Taranta A. Costochondritis. A prospective analysis in an emergency department setting. *Arch Intern Med.* 1994;154(21):2466-2469.

103. Mendelson G, Mendelson H, Horowitz SF, Goldfarb CR, Zumoff B. Can 99m technetium methylene diphosphonate bone scans objectively document costochondritis? *Chest.* 1997;111(6):1600-1602.

104. McDonnell L, Hume P, Nolte V. Rib stress fractures among rowers. *Sports Med.* 2011;41(11):883-901.

105. Vinther A, Kanstrup IL, Christiansen E, et al. Exercise-induced rib stress fractures: Potential risk factors related to thoracic muscle co-contraction and movement pattern. *Scand J Med Sci Sports.* 2006;16(3): 188-196.

106. Wajswelner H. Management of rowers with rib stress fractures. *Aust J Physiother.* 1996;42(2):157-161.

107. Mall NA, Buchowski J, Zebala L, Brophy RH, Wright RW, Matava MJ. Spine and axial skeleton injuries in the national football league. *Am J Sports Med.* 2012;40(8):1755-1761.

108. Vanichkachorn JS, Vaccaro AR. Thoracic disk disease: Diagnosis and treatment. *J Am Acad Orthop Surg.* 2000;8(3):159-169.

109. Sizer PS, Phelps V, Azevedo E. Disc related and non-disc related disorders of the thoracic spine. *Pain Practice.* 2001;1(2):136-149.

110. Rogers MA, Crockard HA. Surgical treatment of the symptomatic herniated thoracic disk. *Clin Orthop Relat Res.* 1994;(300):70-78.

111. Haro H, Domoto T, Maekawa S, Horiuchi T, Komori H, Hamada Y. Resorption of thoracic disc herniation. *Journal of Neurosurgery: Spine (Phila Pa 1976).* 2008;8(3):300-304.

112. Soucacos PN, Zacharis K, Soultanis K, Gelalis I, Xenakis T, Beris AE. Risk factors for idiopathic scoliosis: Review of a 6-year prospective study. *Orthopedics.* 2000;23(8):833-838.

113. Stirling AJ, Howel D, Millner PA, Sadiq SA, Sharples D, Dickson RA. Late-onset idiopathic scoliosis in children six to fourteen years old. A cross-sectional prevalence study. *The Journal of Bone & Joint Surgery.* 1996;78(9):1330-1336.

114. Swärd L. The thoracolumbar spine in young elite athletes. Current concepts on the effects of physical training. *Sports Med.* 1992;13(5):357-364.

115. Weinstein SI DLASKFPKKSMJPIV. Health and function of patients with untreated idiopathic scoliosis: A 50-year natural history study. *JAMA.* 2003;289(5):559-567.

116. Kim HJ, Blanco JS, Widmann RF. Update on the management of idiopathic scoliosis. *Curr Opin Pediatr.* 2009;21(1):55-64.

117. Negrini S, Minozzi S, Bettany-Saltikov J, et al. Braces for idiopathic scoliosis in adolescents. *Cochrane Database Syst Rev.* 2010(1). http://onlinelibrary.wiley.com/doi/10.1002/14651858.CD006850.pub2/abstract.

118. Fusco C, Zaina F, Atanasio S, Romano M, Negrini A, Negrini S. Physical exercises in the treatment of adolescent idiopathic scoliosis: An updated systematic review. *Physiother Theory Pract.* 2011;27(1):80-114.

119. Mooney V, Brigham A. The role of measured resistance exercises in adolescent scoliosis. *Orthopedics.* 2003;26(2):167-171.

120. Mooney V, Gulick J, Pozos R. A preliminary report on the effect of measured strength training in adolescent idiopathic scoliosis. *J Spinal Disord.* 2000;13(2):102-107.

121. Romano M, Minozzi S, Bettany-Saltikov J, et al. Exercises for adolescent idiopathic scoliosis. *Cochrane Database Syst Rev.* 2012(8). http://onlinelibrary.wiley.com/doi/10.1002/14651858.CD007837.pub2/abstract.

122. Mordecai S, Dabke H. Efficacy of exercise therapy for the treatment of adolescent idiopathic scoliosis: A review of the literature. *Eur Spine J.* 2012;21(3):382-389.

123. Bas P, Romagnoli M, Gomez-Cabrera M-C, et al. Beneficial effects of aerobic training in adolescent patients with moderate idiopathic scoliosis. *Eur Spine J.* 2011;20(3):415-419.
124. Wainner RS, Fritz JM, Irrgang JJ, Boninger ML, Delitto A, Allison S. Reliability and diagnostic accuracy of the clinical examination and patient self-report measures for cervical radiculopathy. *Spine (Phila Pa 1976).* 2003;28(1):52-62.
125. Peolsson A, Söderlund A, Engquist M, et al. Physical function outcome in cervical radiculopathy patients after physiotherapy alone compared with anterior surgery followed by physiotherapy: A prospective randomized study with a 2-year follow-up. *Spine (Phila Pa 1976).* 2013;38(4):300-307.
126. Forbush SW, Cox T, Wilson E. Treatment of patients with degenerative cervical radiculopathy using a multimodal conservative approach in a geriatric population: A case series. *J Orthop Sports Phys Ther.* 2011;41(10):723-733.
127. Waldrop M. Diagnosis and treatment of cervical radiculopathy using a clinical prediction rule and a multimodal intervention approach: A case series. *J Orthop Sports Phys Ther.* 2006;36(3):152-159.
128. Warden SJ, Gutschlag FR, Wajswelner H, Crossley KM. Aetiology of rib stress fractures in rowers. *Sports Med.* 2002;32(13):819-836.

Appendix 1

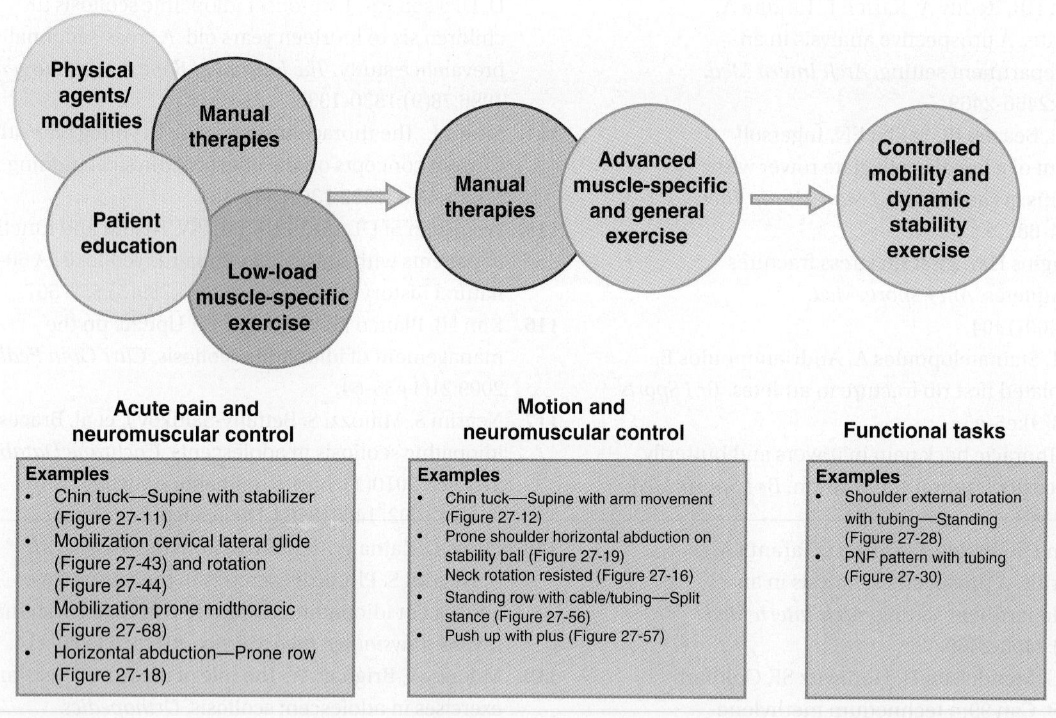

28

Rehabilitation of Injuries to the Lumbar and Sacral Spine

Daniel N. Hooker and William E. Prentice

OBJECTIVES

After completion of this chapter, the physical therapist should be able to do the following:

- Discuss the functional anatomy and biomechanics of the spine.
- Describe the difference between spinal segmental stabilization and core stabilization.
- Explain the rationale for using the different positioning exercises for treating pain in the spine.
- Conduct a thorough evaluation of the back before developing a rehabilitation plan.
- Compare and contrast the importance of using either joint mobilization or core stabilization exercises for treating spine patients.
- Differentiate between the acute versus reinjury versus chronic stage models for treating low back pain.
- Explain the eclectic approach for rehabilitation of back pain in the athletic population.
- Describe basic- and advanced-level training in the reinjury stage of treatment.
- Incorporate the rehabilitation approach to specific conditions affecting the low back.

Functional Anatomy and Biomechanics

From a biomechanical perspective, the spine is one of the most complex regions of the body, with numerous bones, joints, ligaments, and muscles, all of which are collectively involved in spinal movement. The proximity to and relationship of the spinal cord, the nerve roots, and the peripheral nerves to the vertebral column add to the complexity of this region. Injury to the cervical spine has potentially life-threatening implications, and low back pain is one of the most common ailments known to humans.

The 33 vertebrae of the spine are divided into 5 regions: cervical, thoracic, lumbar, sacral, and coccygeal. Between each of the cervical, thoracic, and lumbar vertebrae lie fibrocartilaginous intervertebral disks that act as important shock absorbers for the spine.

The design of the spine allows a high degree of flexibility forward and laterally, and limited mobility backward. The movements of the vertebral column are flexion and extension, right and left lateral flexion, and rotation to the left and right. The degree of movement differs in the various regions of the vertebral column. The cervical and lumbar regions allow extension, flexion, and rotation around a central axis. Although the thoracic vertebrae have minimal movement, their combined movement between the first and twelfth thoracic vertebrae can account for 20 to 30 degrees of flexion and extension.

As the spinal vertebrae progress downward from the cervical region, they grow increasingly larger to accommodate the upright posture of the body, as well as to contribute to weight bearing. The shape of the vertebrae is irregular, but the vertebrae possess certain characteristics that are common to all. Each vertebra consists of a neural arch through which the spinal cord passes, and several projecting processes that serve as attachments for muscles and ligaments. Each neural arch has 2 pedicles and 2 laminae. The pedicles are bony processes that project backward from the body of the vertebrae and connect with the laminae. The laminae are flat bony processes occurring on either side of the neural arch that project backward and inward from the pedicles. With the exception of the first and second cervical vertebrae, each vertebra has a spinous and transverse process for muscular and ligamentous attachments, and all vertebrae have multiple articular processes.

Intervertebral articulations are between vertebral bodies and vertebral arches. Articulation between the bodies is of the symphysial type. Besides motion at articulations between the bodies of the vertebrae, movement takes place at four articular processes that derive from the pedicles and laminae. The direction of movement of each vertebra is somewhat dependent on the direction in which the articular facets face. The sacrum articulates with the ilium to form the sacroiliac joint, which has a synovium and is lubricated by synovial fluid.

Ligaments

The major ligaments that join the various vertebral parts are the anterior longitudinal, the posterior longitudinal, and the supraspinous. The anterior longitudinal ligament is a wide, strong band that extends the full length of the anterior surface of the vertebral bodies. The posterior longitudinal ligament is contained within the vertebral canal and extends the full length of the posterior aspect of the bodies of the vertebrae. Ligaments connect one lamina to another. The interspinous, supraspinous, and intertransverse ligaments stabilize the transverse and spinous processes, extending between adjacent vertebrae. The sacroiliac joint is maintained by the extremely strong dorsal sacral ligaments. The sacrotuberous and the sacrospinous ligaments attach the sacrum to the ischium.

Muscle Actions

The muscles that extend the spine and rotate the vertebral column can be classified as either superficial or deep. The superficial muscles extend from the vertebrae to ribs. The erector spinae is a group of superficial paired muscles that is made up of 3 columns or bands, the longissimus group, the iliocostalis group, and the spinalis group. Each of these groups is further divided into regions, the cervicis region in the neck, the thoracis region in the middle back, and the lumborum region in the low back. Generally, the erector spinae muscles extend the spine. The deep muscles attach one vertebra to another and function to extend and rotate the spine. The deep muscles include the interspinales, multifidus, rotators, thoracis, and the semispinalis cervicis.

Flexion of the cervical region is produced primarily by the sternocleidomastoid muscles and the scalene muscle group on the anterior aspect of the neck. The scalenes flex the head and stabilize the cervical spine as the sternocleidomastoids flex the neck. The upper trapezius, semispinalis capitis, splenius capitis, and splenius cervicis muscles extend the neck. Lateral flexion of the neck is accomplished by all of the muscles on one side of the vertebral column contracting unilaterally. Rotation is produced when the sternocleidomastoid, the scalenes, the semispinalis cervicis, and the upper trapezius on the side opposite to the direction of rotation contract in addition to a contraction of the splenius capitis, splenius cervicis, and longissimus capitis on the same side of the direction of rotation.

Flexion of the trunk primarily involves lengthening of the deep and superficial back muscles and contraction of the abdominal muscles (rectus abdominis, internal oblique, external oblique) and hip flexors (rectus femoris, iliopsoas, tensor fasciae lata, sartorius). Seventy-five percent of flexion occurs at the lumbosacral junction (L5-S1), whereas 15% to 70% occurs between L4 and L5. The rest of the lumbar vertebrae execute 5% to 10% of flexion.[12] Extension involves lengthening of the abdominal muscles and contraction of the erector spinae and the gluteus maximus, which extends the hip. Trunk rotation is produced by the external obliques and the internal obliques. Lateral flexion is produced primarily by the quadratus lumborum muscle, along with the obliques, latissimus dorsi, iliopsoas, and the rectus abdominis on the side of the direction of movement.

Spinal segment stability is produced by the deep muscles of the spine (multifidi, medial quadratus lumborum, iliocostalis lumborum, interspinales, intertransversarii) working in concert with the transversus abdominis and internal abdominal oblique (Figure 28-1). Their location is close to the center of rotation of the spinal segment and their short muscle lengths are ideal for controlling each spinal segment. The transversus abdominis, because of its pull on the thoracolumbar fascia, and its ability to create increased intraabdominal pressure as it narrows the abdominal cavity, is a major partner in spinal segment stability (Figure 28-2). This combination creates a rigid cylinder and in concert with the deep spinal muscles provides significant segmental stability to the lumbar spine and pelvis.[20,33-35,58-60,62,67-69]

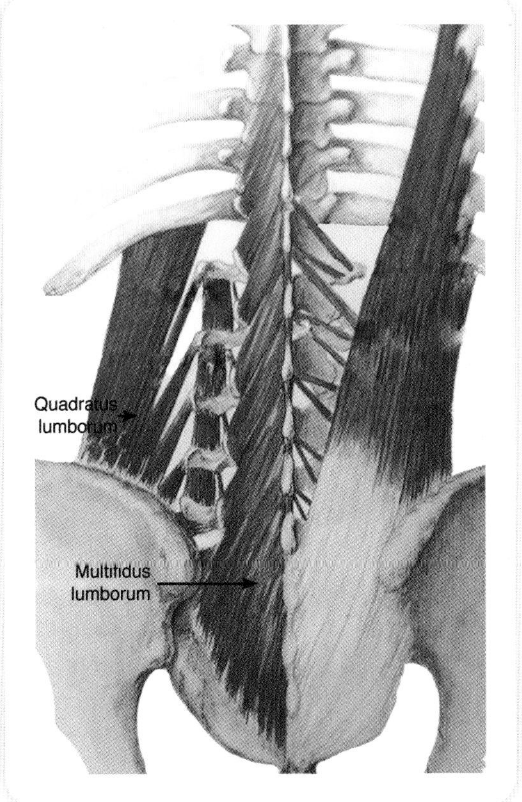

Figure 28-1 **Muscles of the low back**

The multifidus and the quadratus lumborum muscles.

Spinal Cord

The spinal cord is that portion of the central nervous system that is contained within the vertebral canal of the spinal column. Thirty-one pairs of spinal nerves extend from the sides of the spinal cord, coursing downward and outward through the intervertebral foramen passing near the articular facets of the vertebrae. Any abnormal movement of these facets, such as in a dislocation or a fracture, may expose the spinal nerves to injury. Injuries that occur below the third lumbar vertebra usually result in nerve root damage but do not cause spinal cord damage.

The spinal nerve roots combine to form a network of nerves, or a plexus. There are 5 nerve plexuses: cervical, brachial, lumbar, sacral, and coccygeal.

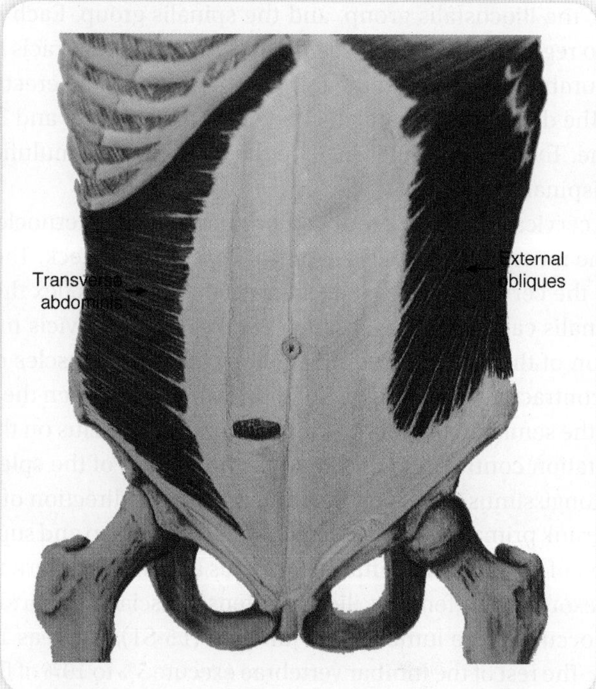

Figure 28-2 **The transverse abdominis and external oblique muscles**

The Importance of Evaluation in Treating Back Pain

In many instances after referral for medical evaluation, the patient returns to the therapist with a diagnosis of low back pain. Even though this is a correct diagnosis, it does not offer the specificity needed to help direct the treatment planning. The therapist planning the treatment would be better served with a more specific diagnosis, such as spondylolysis, disk herniation, quadratus lumborum strain, piriformis syndrome, or sacroiliac ligament sprain.

Regardless of the diagnosis or the specificity of the diagnosis, the importance of a thorough evaluation of the patient's back pain is critical to good care. The therapist should become an expert on this individual patient's back. Taking the time to perform a comprehensive evaluation will pay great rewards in the success of treatment and rehabilitation. The evaluation has 6 major purposes:

1. To clearly locate areas and tissues that might be part of the problem. The therapist should use this information to direct treatments and exercises.[31,34,50]
2. To establish the baseline measurements used to assess progress and guide the treatment progression and help the therapist make specific judgments on the progression of or changes in specific exercises. The improvement in these measurements also guides the return-to-activity decision and provides 1 measure of the success of the rehabilitation plan.[37,46,70]
3. To provide some provocative guidance to help the patients probe the limits of their condition, help them better understand their problem, present limitations, and understand the management of their injury problem.[37,46,70]
4. To establish confidence in the therapist. This increases the placebo effect of the therapist patient interaction.[86,87]

5. To decrease the anxiety of the patient. This increases the patient's comfort, which will increase the patient's compliance with the rehabilitation plan; a more positive environment is created, and the therapist and patient avoid the "no one knows what is wrong with me" trap.[17,53]
6. To provide information for making judgments on pads, braces, and corsets.

Table 28-1 provides a detailed scheme for evaluation of back pain.

Table 28-1 Lumbar and Sacroiliac Joint Objective Examination

1. Standing position
   a. Posture—alignment
   b. Gait
      i. Patient's trunk frequently bent laterally or hips shifted to one side
      ii. Walks with difficulty or limps
   c. Alignment and symmetry
      iii. Trochanteric levels
      iv. Posterior superior iliac spine (PSIS) and anterior superior iliac spine (ASIS) levels
      v. Levels of iliac crests
      Recent studies have raised the concern that these clinical assessments of alignment are not valid because of the small movements available at the sacroiliac joints. These tests should be used as a small part of the overall evaluation and not as standalone tests. In sacroiliac dysfunction, the ASIS, PSIS, and iliac crests may not appear to be in the same horizontal plane
   d. Lumbar spine active movements
      i. With sacroiliac dysfunction, the patient will experience exacerbation of pain with side bending toward the painful side
      ii. Often a lumbar lesion is present along with a sacroiliac dysfunction
   e. Single-leg standing with backwards bending is a provocation test and can provoke pain in cases of spondylolysis or spondylolisthesis
2. Sitting position
   a. Lumbar spine rotation range of motion
   b. Passive hip internal rotation and external rotation range of motion
      i. Piriformis muscle irritation would be provoked by internal rotation and could be present from sacroiliac joint dysfunctions or myofascial pain from overuse of this muscle
      ii. Limited range of motion of the hip can be a red flag for hip problems
   c. Sitting knee extension produces some stretch to the long neutral structures
   d. Slump sit is used to evaluate lumbar flexibility and neutral tension
3. Supine position
   a. Hip external rotation in a resting position may indicate piriformis muscle tightness
   b. Palpation of the transversus abdominis, as the patient is directed to contract, can help in the assessment of spinal segment control. Can the patient isolate this contraction from the other abdominal muscles?
   c. Palpation of the symphysis pubis for tenderness. Some sacroiliac problems create pain and tenderness in this area. Sometimes the presenting subjective symptoms mimic adductor or groin strain but the objective evaluation does not show pain or weakness on muscle contraction or muscle tenderness that would support this assessment
   d. Straight-leg raise (passive)
      i. Interpretation of straight-leg raise: pain provoked before
         - 30 degrees—hip problem or very inflamed nerve
         - 30 to 60 degrees—sciatic nerve involvement
         - 70 to 90 degrees—sacroiliac joint involvement
         - Neck flexion—exacerbates symptoms—disk or root irritation
         - Ankle dorsiflexion or Lasègue sign—exacerbated symptoms usually indicate sciatic nerve or root irritation

(continued)

Table 28-1 Lumbar and Sacroiliac Joint Objective Examination *(Continued)*

e. Sacroiliac loading test (compression, distraction, posterior shear or P4 Test, Gaenslen Scissor Stretch)—pain provoked by physical stress through the sacroiliac joints can be helpful in assessing for sacroiliac joint dysfunction
f. FABER (flexion, abduction, external rotation), also known as the Patrick test—at end range assesses irritability of the sacroiliac joint; hip muscle tightness can also be assessed using this test
g. FADIR (flexion, adduction, internal rotation) produces some stretch on the iliolumbar ligament
h. Bilateral knees to chest—will usually exacerbate lumbar spine symptoms as the sacroiliac joints move with the sacrum in this maneuver
i. Single knee to armpit can provoke pain from a variety of sources from sacroiliac joint to lumbar spine muscles and ligaments; make the patients be specific about their pain location and quality

4. Side-lying position
   a. Iliotibial band length—sacroiliac (SI) joint problems sometimes create tightness of the iliotibial band and stress to the iliotibial band will provoke pain in the SI joint area
   b. Quadratus lumborum stretch and palpation
   c. Hip abduction and piriformis muscle test

   Pain provocation in muscular locations with either of these tests indicates primary myofascial pain problems or secondary tightness, weakness, and pain from muscle guarding associated with different pathologies. Pain provocation in the SI joint area would help confirm an SI joint dysfunction

5. Prone position
   a. Palpation
      i. Well-localized tenderness medial to or around the PSIS indicates SI dysfunction
      ii. Tenderness lateral and superior to the PSIS indicates gluteus medius irritation or myofascial trigger point
      iii. Gluteus maximus area—sacrotuberous and sacrospinous ligaments are in this area, as well as piriformis muscle and sciatic nerve. Changes in tension and tenderness can help make the evaluation more specific
      iv. Tenderness around spinous processes or postural alignment faults from S-1 to T-10 could implicate some lumbar problems
   b. Anterior—posterior or rotational provocational stresses can be applied to the spinous processes
   c. Sacral provocation stress test—pain from anterior–posterior pressure at the center of the sacral base and/or on each side of the sacrum just medial to the PSIS may be indicative of SI joint dysfunction
   d. Hip extension—knee flexion stretch will provoke the L3 nerve root and create a nerve quality pain down the anterolateral thigh
   e. Anterior rotation stress to the sacroiliac joint can be delivered by using passive hip extension and PSIS pressure; pain in the SI joint area on either side would be indicative of SI dysfunction

6. Manual muscle test

   If the lumbar spine or posterior hip musculature is strained, active movement against gravity and/or resistance should provoke a pain complaint similar to patients' subjective description of their problem
   a. Hip extension
   b. Hip internal rotation
   c. Hip external rotation
   d. Hip flexion
   e. Hip adduction
   f. Trunk extension—arm and shoulder extension
   g. Trunk extension—arm, shoulder, and neck extension
   h. Trunk extension—resisted
   i. Multifidus activation and control
   j. Spinal segment coactivation of transversus abdominis and multifidi[29,44,52,69,70]

Rehabilitation Techniques for the Low Back

Positioning and Pain-Relieving Exercises

Most patients with back pain have some fluctuation of their symptoms in response to certain postures and activities. The therapist logically treats this patient by reinforcing pain-reducing postures and motions and by starting specific exercises aimed at specific muscle groups or specific ranges of motion. A general rule to follow in making these decisions is as follows: *Any movement that causes the back pain to radiate or spread over a larger area should not be included during this early phase of treatment.* Movements that centralize or diminish the pain are correct movements to include at this time.[50] Including some exercise during initial pain management generally has a positive effect on the patient. The exercise encourages them to be active in the rehabilitation plan and helps them to regain lumbar movement.[29,87]

When a patient relieves pain through exercise and attention to proper postural control, the patient is much more likely to adopt these procedures into a daily routine. A patient whose pain is relieved via some other passive procedure, and then is taught exercises, will not be able to readily see the connection between relief and exercise.[20,36,58,69]

The types of exercises that may be included in initial pain management include the following:

- Spinal segment control, transverse abdominis, and multifidus coactivation
- Lateral shift corrections
- Extension exercises—stretching and mobilization
- Flexion exercises—stretching and mobilization
- Postural traction positions
- Gentle rhythmic movements in flexion, extension, rotation, and sidebending
- Spinal manipulation

Spinal Segment Control Exercise

In devising exercise plans to address the different clinical problems of the lumbo-pelvic-hip complex, *the use of core-stabilizing exercises is a must for every problem for recovery, maintenance, and prevention of reinjury.* Clinically, the core stabilization rehabilitation exercise sequence begins with relearning the muscle activation patterns necessary for segmental spinal stabilization. This beginning exercise plan is based on the work of Richardson, Jull, Hodges, and Hides.[33-36,60,68,69]

The first step in segmental spinal stabilization is to reestablish separate control of the transversus abdominis and the lumbar multifidi (see Figures 28-1 and 28-2). The control and activation of these deep muscles should be separated from the control and activation of the global or superficial muscles of the core. Once the patients have mastered the behavior of coactivation of the transversus abdominis and multifidi to create and maintain a corset-like control and stabilization of the spinal segments, they may then progress to using the global muscles in the core stabilization sequence and more functional activities. Segmental spinal stabilization is the basic building block of core stabilization exercises and should be an automatic behavior to be used in every subsequent exercise and activity.[2,33,34,36,44,58,59]

The basic exercise that the patient must master is coactivation of the transversus abdominis and multifidi, isolating them from the global trunk muscles. This contraction should be of sufficient magnitude to create a small increase in the intraabdominal pressure.

This is a simple concept, but these muscle contractions are normally under subconscious automatic control; and in patients with low back pain, the subconscious control of timing and firing patterns become disturbed and the patient loses spinal segmental control.[34] To regain this vital skill and return the subconscious timing and firing patterns of these muscles, the patient will need individual instruction and testing to prove that the patient has mastered the conscious control of each muscle individually and in a coactivation pattern. The next step is to incorporate this coactivation pattern into functional exercise and other activities. The success of this exercise is dependent upon this muscular coactivation becoming a habitual postural control movement under both conscious and subconscious control.

A muscle contraction of 10% to 15% of the maximum voluntary contraction of the multifidus and the transversus abdominis is all that is necessary to create segmental spinal stability. Contraction levels greater than 20% of maximum voluntary contraction will cause overflow of activity to the more global muscles and negate the exercise's intent of isolating control of the transversus abdominis and multifidi.[36] Precision of contraction and control is the intent of these exercises; the ultimate goal is a change in the patient's behavior. As this behavior is incorporated into more daily activities and exercise, the strength and endurance of these muscle groups will also improve, and the core system will work more effectively and efficiently.[28,37,38,43,46,47]

Transversus Abdominis Behavior Exercise Plan

1. Test the patient's ability to consciously contract and control the transversus abdominis in isolation from the other abdominal muscles. The therapist can assess the contraction through observation and palpation. The patient is positioned in a comfortable relaxed posture: stomach-lying, back-lying, side-lying, or hand-knee position. The best palpation location is medial to the anterior superior iliac spine (ASIS) approximately 1.5 inches (Figure 28-3). The internal abdominal oblique has more vertical fibers and is closest to the ASIS, whereas the transversus fibers run horizontal from ilia to ilia. The therapist monitors the muscle with light palpation

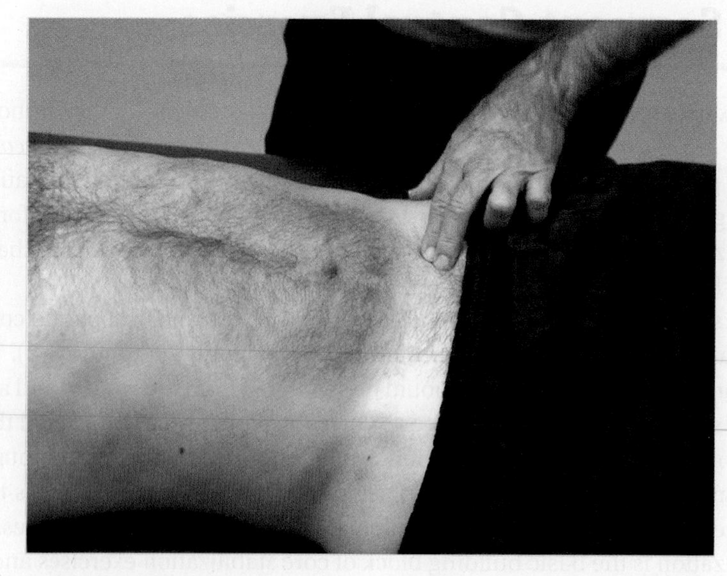

Figure 28-3

Palpation location to feel for isolated transversus abdominis contraction.

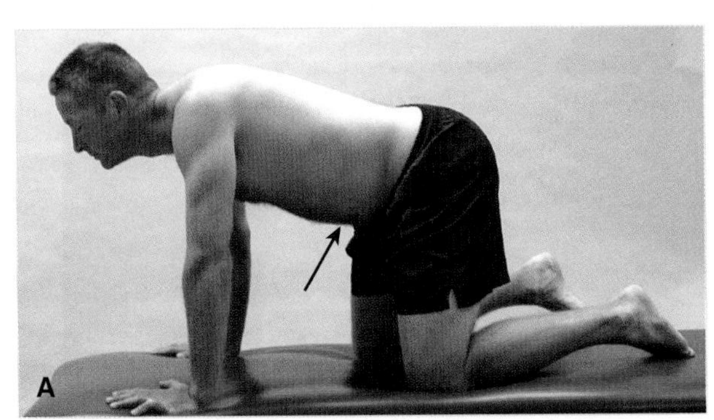

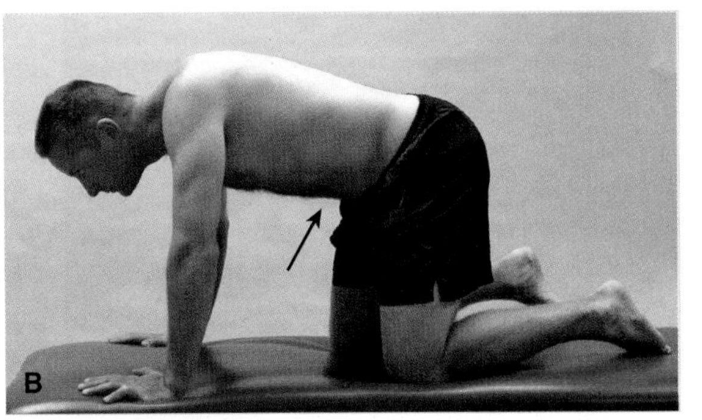

Figure 28-4

The quadrupeds position can be used to demonstrate and practice the isolated transversus abdominis contraction. The patient is instructed to (**A**) let the belly sag, and then (**B**) slowly and gently contract the pelvic floor muscles and practice holding this position for 10 seconds.

and instructs the patient to contract the muscle, feeling for the transversus drawing together across the abdomen. As the contraction increases, the internal oblique fibers and external oblique fibers will start to fire. If the patients cannot separate the firing of the transversus from the other groups and/or cannot maintain the separate contraction for 5 to 10 seconds, they will need individual instruction with various forms of feedback to regain control of this muscle behavior. In patients with low back pain, transversus contraction usually becomes more phasic and fires only in combination with the obliques or rectus.[36,69]

2. The patients are positioned in a comfortable pain-free position and instructed to breathe in and out gently, stop the breathing, and slowly, gently contract and hold the contraction of their transversus—and then resume normal light breathing while trying to maintain the contraction. Changes in body position (positions of choice are prone, side-lying, supine, or quadruped), verbal cues, and visual and tactile feedback will speed and enhance the learning process (Figure 28-4). The use of imaging ultrasound as visual biofeedback to visualize the contractions of these muscles provides visualization of the tendon movement and can help in isolating and bringing these muscle contractions under cognitive control.[36,69]
3. The lumbar multifidi contractions are taught with tactile pressure over the muscle bellies next to the spinous processes (Figure 28-5). The patient is asked to contract the muscle so that the muscle swells up directly under the finger pressure. The feeling should be a deep tension. A rapid superficial contraction or a contraction that brings in the global muscles is not acceptable, and continued trial and error with feedback is used until the desired contraction and control are achieved.[36,69]
4. As soon as cognitive control of the transversus and multifidi is achieved, more functional positions and exercises aimed at coactivation of both muscles are begun. The therapist should attempt to have the patient use the transversus and multifidi coactivation in a comfortable neutral lumbopelvic position with restoration of a normal lordotic curve so that the muscle coactivation strategies can start to be incorporated into the patient's daily life (Figure 28-6). Repetition improves the effectiveness of this contraction, and as it is used more, the cognitive control becomes less and the subconscious pattern of segmental spinal stabilization returns to normal.[36,69]

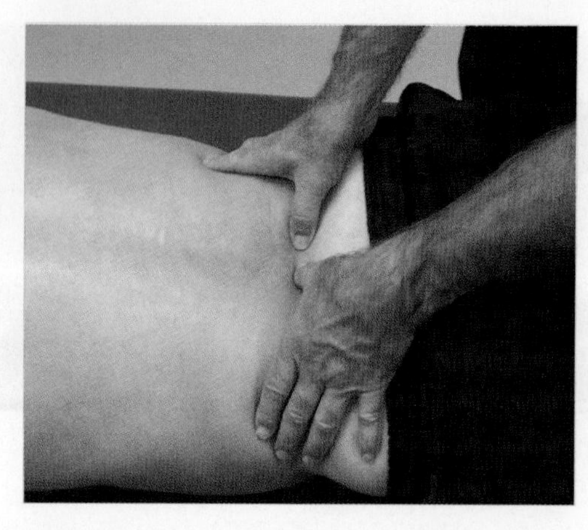

Figure 28-5

Palpation location to feel for isolated lumbar multifidi contractions.

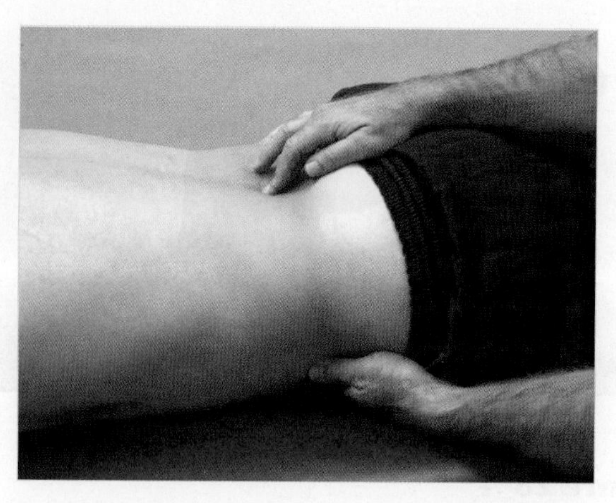

Figure 28-6

Palpation location to feel contractions, to give the patient feedback on the patient's ability to perform a coactivation segmental spinal stabilization contraction.

5. Incorporating the coactivation contraction back into activities is the next step and is accomplished by graduating the exercises to include increases in stress and control. Supine-lying with simple leg and arm movements is a good starting point. Using a pressure biofeedback unit for this phase will help the patients measure their ability to use the coactivation contraction effectively during increased exercise. The Stabilizer pressure biofeedback unit is inflated to a pressure of approximately 40 mm Hg. As the patient coactivates the transversus abdominis and multifidi, the pressure reading should stay the same or decrease slightly and remain at that level throughout the increased movement exercises (Figure 28-7). This is an indirect measure of the spinal

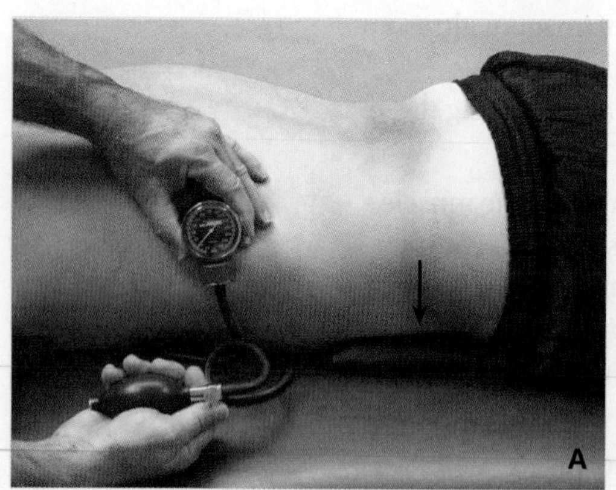

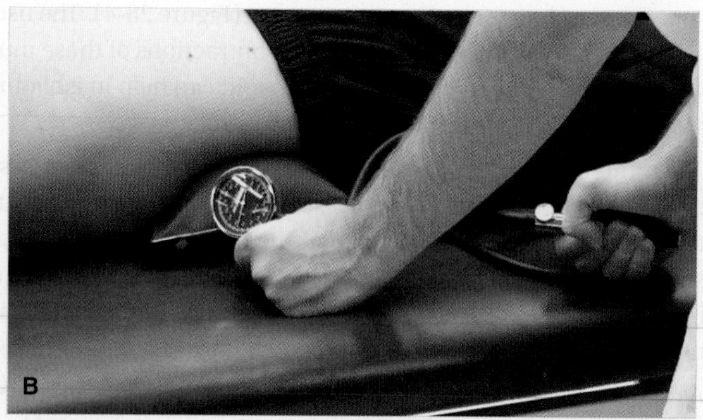

Figure 28-7

The stabilizer pressure biofeedback unit can be used as an indirect method of measuring correct activation of the spinal segment stabilization coactivation contraction. The stabilizer is inflated to 40 mm Hg pressure and placed under the patient's (**A**) abdomen or (**B**) back. The patient should be instructed to contract the transversus in a way that does not make the pressure in the cuff start to rise or fall.

segment stabilization, but gives the patients an outside feedback source to keep them more focused on the exercise.[36,69]

6. This can be followed with trunk inclination exercises in which the patients maintain a neutral lumbopelvic position and incline their trunk in different positions away from the vertical alignment and hold in positions of forward-lean to side-lean for specific time periods (Figures 28-8 and 28-9). This is first done in the sitting position. As control, strength, and endurance increase, the positions can become more exaggerated and the holding times longer.
7. Return the patient to a structured progressive resistive core exercise program (see Chapter 15). The incorporation of the segmental spinal stabilization coactivation contraction as the precursor to each exercise is the goal at this point in returning the patient to functional activity.
8. The therapist should teach this technique both as an exercise and as a behavior. The exercises should be taught and monitored in an individual session with opportunity for feedback and correction. The patients must also use this skill in the functional things they do every day. The patients are asked to trigger this spinal segment control skill in response to daily tasks, postures, pains, and certain movements (Figure 28-10*A* and *B*). As their pain is controlled, the coactivation contraction should be incorporated into activities of daily living.

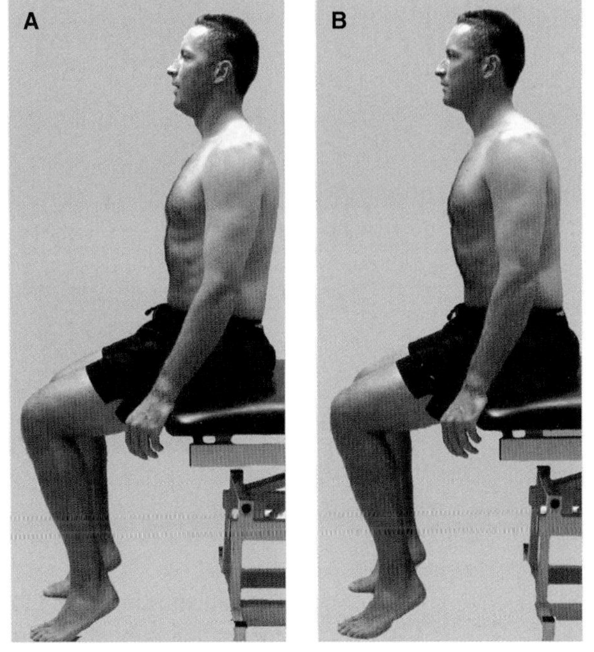

Figure 28-8 **Trunk inclination exercise**

The patient finds a comfortable neutral spine position and coactivates the transversus abdominis and lumbar multifidi to provide the segmental spinal stabilization.

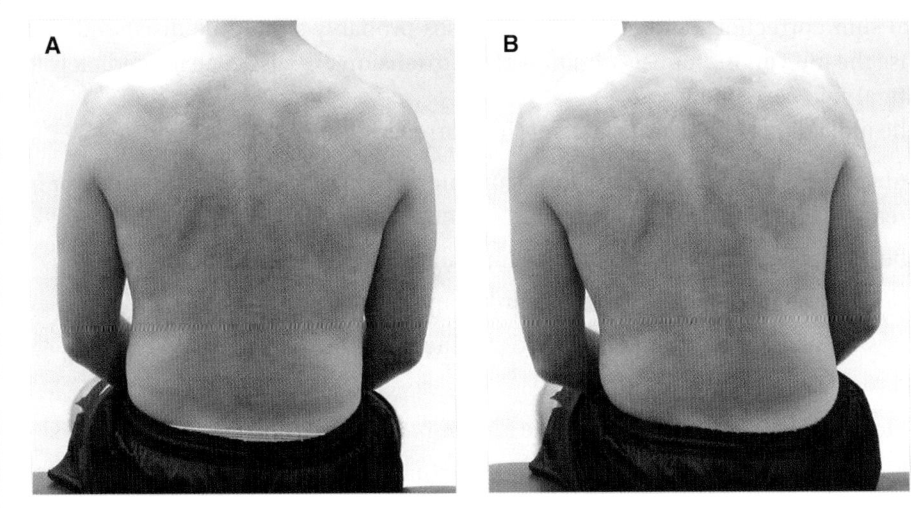

Figure 28-9

The patient challenges his or her spinal segment control by leaning away from the vertical position while holding the neutral spine position for 10 seconds.

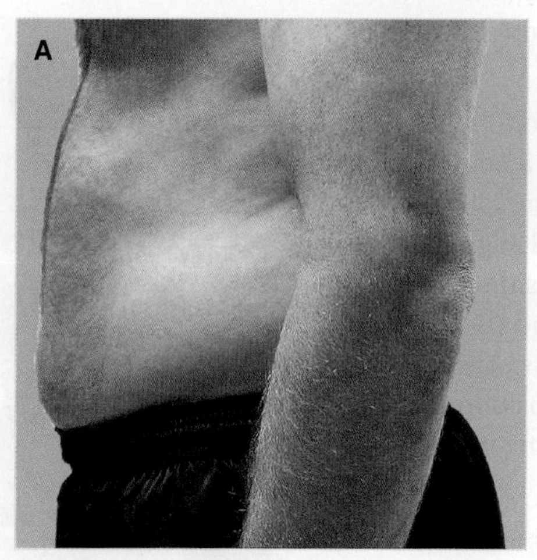

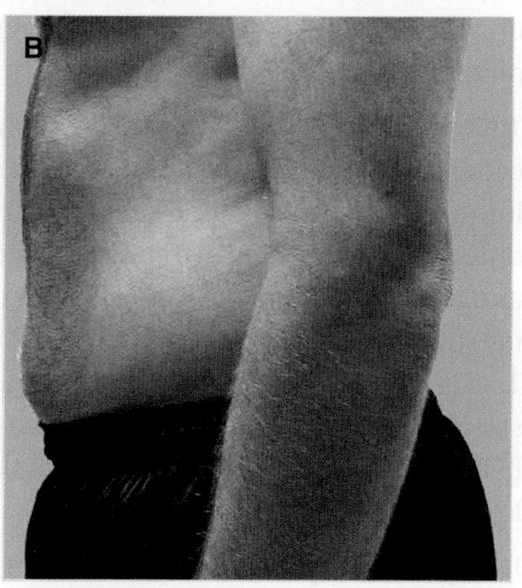

Figure 28-10

The patient is instructed to become posture savvy by frequently using the coactivation contraction throughout the patient's day. The coactivation thereby becomes a subconscious movement pattern the patient incorporates into all the patient does.

Segmental spinal stabilization is complementary for all forms of treatment and different pathologies. This exercise program can be incorporated and started at the same time as other therapies. The different forms of therapy summate, and the patient improves more quickly and maintains the gains in range and strength achieved with other therapies. Spinal segment control may also decrease pain and give the patient a measure of control to use in minimizing painful stress through the injured tissues.

Lateral Shift Corrections

Lateral shift corrections and extension exercises probably should be discussed together because the indications for use are similar, and extension exercises will immediately follow the lateral shift corrections.

The indications for the use of lateral shift corrections are as follows:[82]

- Subjectively, the patient complains of unilateral pain reference in the lumbar or hip area.
- The typical posture is scoliotic with a hip shift and reduced lumbar lordosis.
- Walking and movements are very guarded and robotic.
- Forward bending is extremely limited and increases the pain.
- Backwards bending is limited.
- Side bending toward the painful side is minimal to impossible.
- Side bending away from the painful side is usually reasonable to normal.
- A test correction of the hip shift either reduces the pain or causes the pain to centralize.
- The neurologic examination may or may not elicit the following positive findings:
    - Straight-leg raising may be limited and painful, or it could be unaffected.
    - Sensation may be dull, anesthetic, or unaffected.

- Manual muscle test may indicate unilateral weakness of specific movements, or the movements may be strong and painless.
- Reflexes may be diminished or unaffected.[50]

The patient will be assisted by the therapist with the initial lateral shift correction. The patient is then instructed in the techniques of self-correction. The lateral shift correction is designed to guide the patient back to a more symmetrical posture. The therapist's pressure should be firm and steady and more guiding than forcing. The use of a mirror to provide visual feedback is recommended for both the therapist-assisted and self-corrected maneuvers. The specific technique guide for therapist-assisted lateral shift correction is as follows (Figure 28-11):

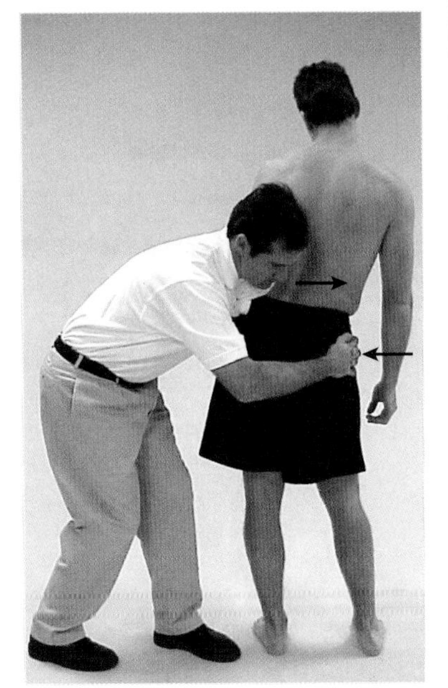

Figure 28-11 **Lateral shift correction exercise**

Emphasis is on pulling the hips, not on pushing the ribs.

1. Prepare the patient by explaining the correction maneuver and the roles of the patient and the therapist.
    a. The patient is to keep the shoulders level and avoid the urge to side bend.
    b. The patient should allow the hips to move under the trunk and should not resist the pressure from the therapist but allow the hips to shift with the pressure.
    c. The patient should keep the therapist informed about the behavior of the back pain.
    d. The patient should keep the feet stationary and not move after the hip shift correction until the standing extension part of the correction is completed.
    e. The patient should practice the standing extension exercise as part of this initial explanation.
2. The therapist should stand on the patient's side that is opposite the patient's hip shift. The patient's feet should be a comfortable distance apart, and the therapist should have a comfortable stride stance aligned slightly behind the patient.
3. Padding should be placed around the patient's elbow, on the side next to the therapist to provide comfortable contact between the patient and the therapist.
4. The therapist should contact the patient's elbow with the shoulder and chest, with the head aligned along the patient's back. The therapist's arms should reach around the patient's waist and apply pressure between the iliac crest and the greater trochanter (see Figure 28-11).
5. The therapist should gradually guide the patient's hips toward the therapist. If the pain increases, the therapist should ease the pressure and maintain a more comfortable posture for 10 to 20 seconds, and then again pull gently. If the pain increases again, the therapist should again lessen the pull and allow comfort. Then the therapist should instruct the patient to actively extend gently, pushing the back into and matching the resistance supplied by the therapist. The goal for this maneuver is an overcorrection of the scoliosis, reversing its direction.
6. Once the corrected or overcorrected posture is achieved, the therapist should maintain this posture for 1 to 2 minutes. This procedure may take 2 to 3 minutes to complete, and the first attempt may be less than a total success. Repeated efforts 3 to 4 minutes apart should be attempted during the first treatment effort before the therapist stops the treatment for that episode.
7. The therapist gradually releases pressure on the hip while the patient does a standing extension movement (Figure 28-16). The patient should complete approximately 6 repetitions of the standing extension movement, holding each for 15 to 20 seconds.

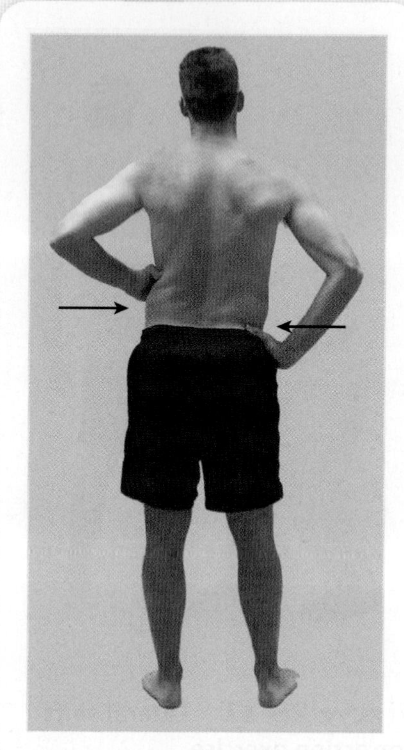

Figure 28-12 **Hip shift self-correction**

The patient can use a mirror for visual feedback as they apply the gentle guiding force to correct their hip shift posture. The patient uses one hand to stabilize themselves at the rib level and uses the other hand to guide the hips across to correct their alignment. This position is held for 30 to 45 seconds, and then the patient is instructed to go into the standing extension position for 5 to 6 repetitions, holding the position for 20 to 30 seconds.

8. Once the patient moves the feet and walks even a short distance, the lateral hip shift usually will recur, but to a lesser degree. The patient then should be taught the self-correction maneuver (Figure 28-12). The patient should stand in front of a mirror and place one hand on the hip where the therapist's hands were and the other hand on the lower ribs where the therapist's shoulder was.
9. The patient then guides the hip under the trunk, watching the mirror to keep the shoulders level and trying to achieve a corrected or overcorrected posture. He/she should hold this posture for 30 to 45 seconds and then follow with several standing extension movements as described in step 7 (see Figure 28-16).[50]

Extension Exercises

The indications for the use of extension exercise are as follows:

- Subjectively, back pain is diminished with lying down and is increased with sitting. The location of the pain may be unilateral, bilateral, or central, and there may or may not be pain radiating into either or both legs.
- Forward bending is extremely limited and increases the pain, or the pain reference location enlarges as the patient bends forward.
- Backwards bending can be limited, but the movement centralizes or diminishes the pain.[1]
- The neurologic examination is the same as outlined for lateral shift correction.[50,51]

The efficacy of extension exercise is theorized to be from 1 or a combination of the following effects:

- A reduction in the neural tension.
- A reduction of the load on the disk, which, in turn, decreases disk pressure.
- Increases in the strength and endurance of the extensor muscles.
- Proprioceptive interference with pain perception as the exercises allow self-mobilization of the spinal joints.

Hip shift posture has previously been theoretically correlated to the anatomical location of the disk bulge or nucleus pulposus herniation. Creating a centralizing movement of the nucleus pulposus has been the theoretical emphasis of hip shift correction and extension exercise. This theory has good logic, but research on this phenomenon has not been supportive.[63] However, in explaining the exercises to the patient, the use of this theory may help increase the patient's motivation and compliance with the exercise plan.

End-range hyperextension exercise should be used cautiously when the patient has facet joint degeneration or impingement of the vertebral foramen borders on neural structures. Also, spondylolysis and spondylolisthesis problems should be approached cautiously with any end-range movement exercise using either flexion or hyperextension.

Figures 28-13 to 28-20 are examples of extension exercises. These examples are not exhaustive but are representative of most of the exercises used clinically.

The order in which exercises are presented is not significant. Instead, each therapist should base the starting exercises on the evaluative findings. Jackson, in a review of back

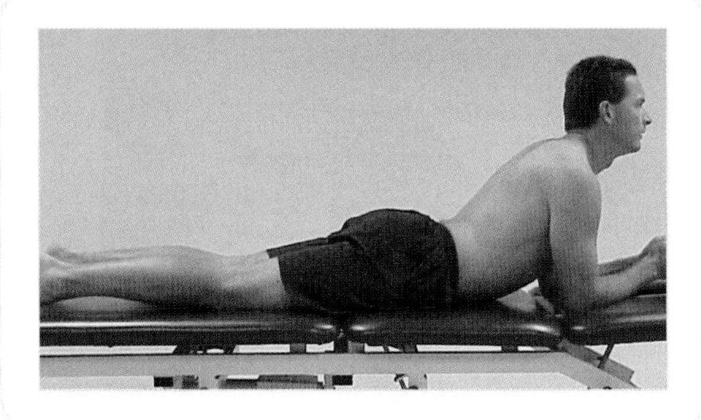

Figure 28-13 Prone extension on elbows

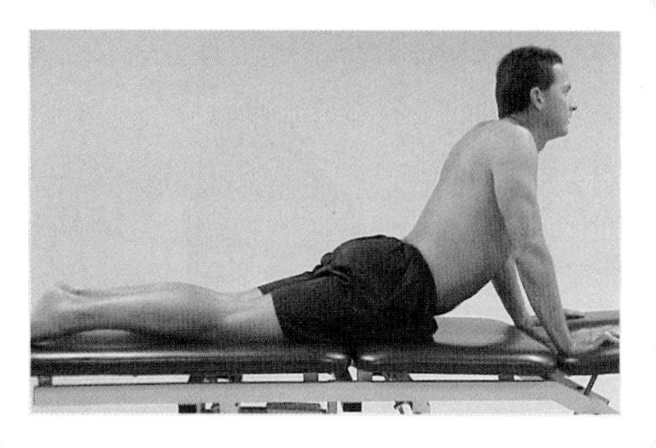

Figure 28-14 Prone extension on hands

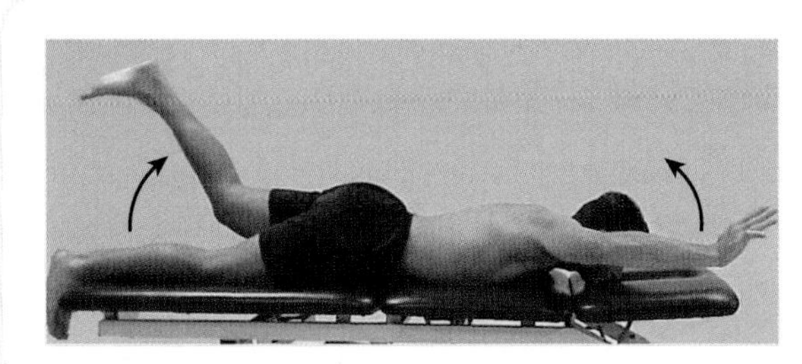

Figure 28-15 Alternate arm and leg extension

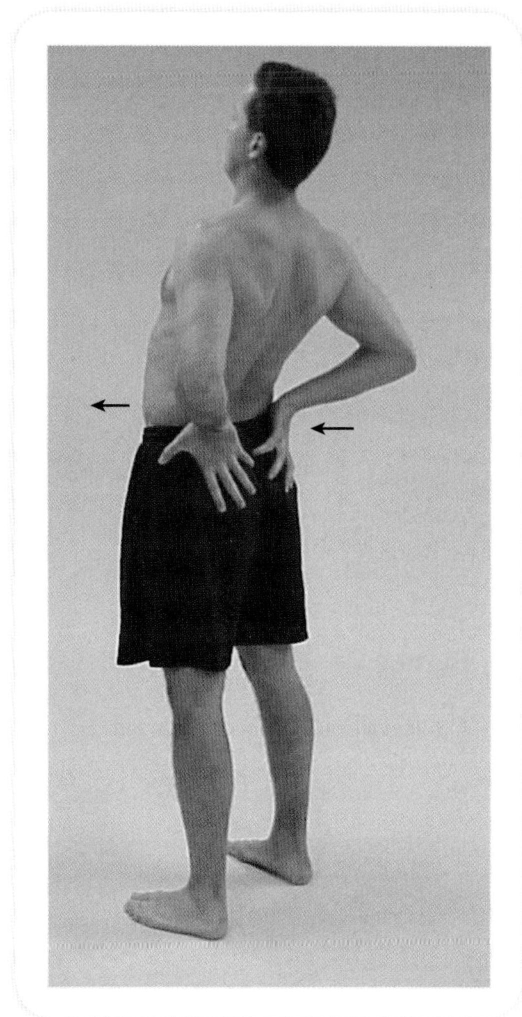

Figure 28-16 Standing extension

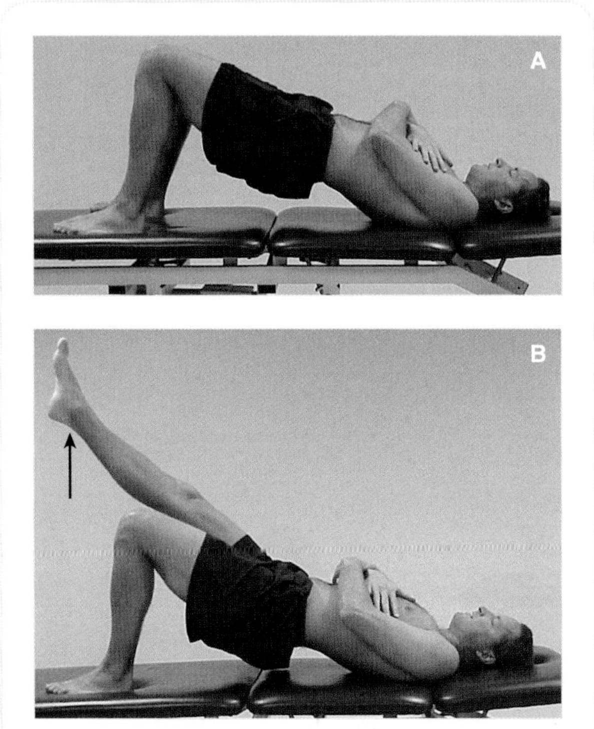

Figure 28-17 Supine hip extension—butt lift or bridge

A. Double-leg support. **B.** Single-leg support.

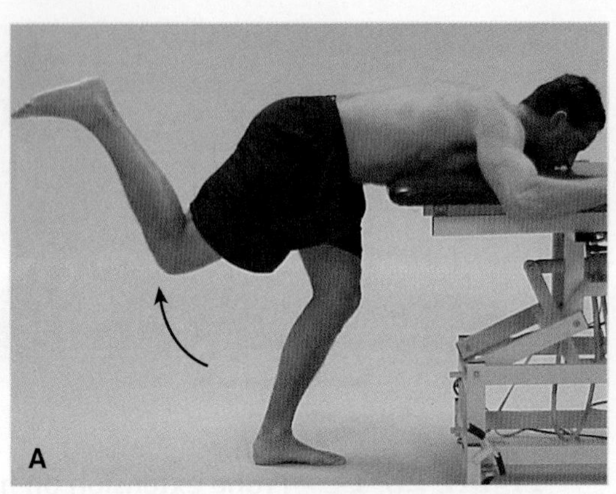

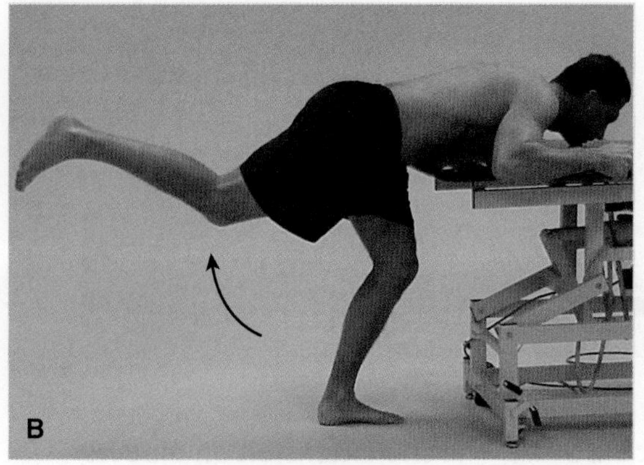

Figure 28-18 **Prone single-leg hip extension**

A. Knee flexed. **B.** Knee extended.

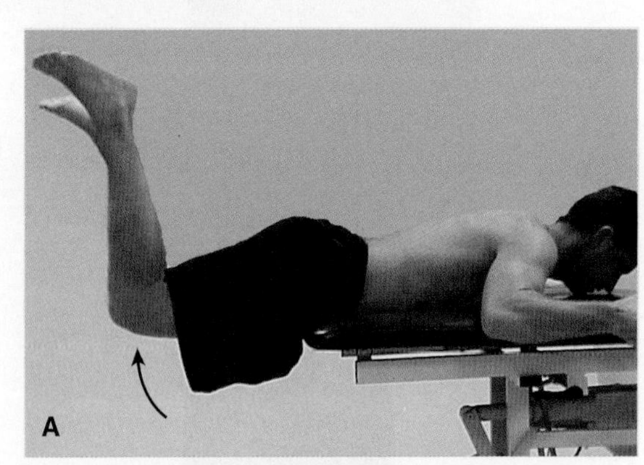

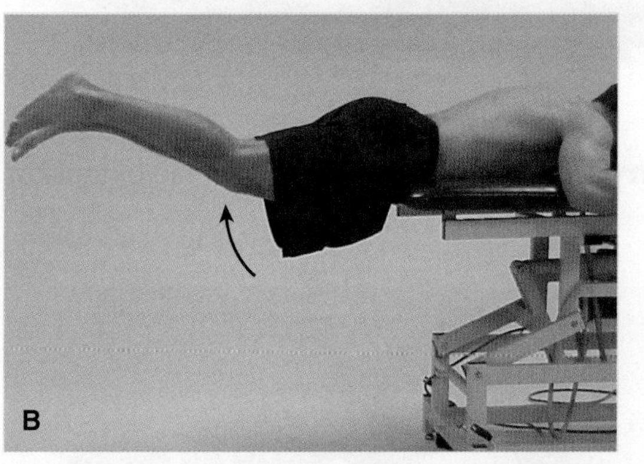

Figure 28-19 **Prone double-leg hip extension**

A. Knees flexed. **B.** Knees extended.

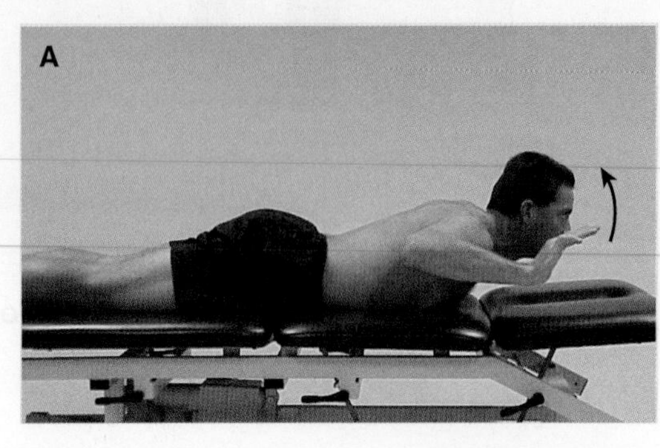

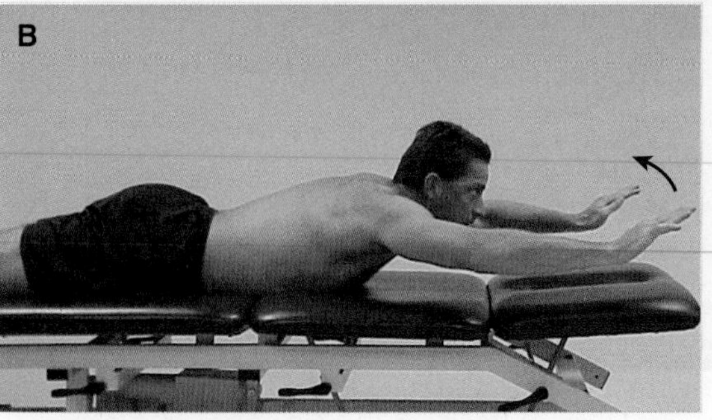

Figure 28-20 **Trunk extension—prone**

A. Hands near head. **B.** Arms extended—superman position.

exercise, stated, "no support was found for the use of a preprogrammed flexion regimen that includes exercises of little value or potential harm and is not specific to the current needs of the patient, as determined by a thorough back evaluation." The review also included a report of Kendall and Jenkin's study, which stated that one-third of the patients for whom hyperextension exercises had been prescribed worsened.[31]

Flexion Exercises

The indications for the use of flexion exercises are as follows:

- Subjectively, back pain is diminished with sitting and is increased with lying down or standing. Pain is also increased with walking.
- Repeated or sustained forward bending eases the pain.
- The patients' lordotic curve does not reverse as they forward bend.
- The end range of sustained backwards bending is painful or increases the pain.
- Abdominal tone and strength are poor.

In his approach, Saal elaborates on the thought that "No one should continue with one particular type of exercise regimen during the entire treatment program."[73] We concur with this and believe that starting with one type of exercise should not preclude rapidly adding other exercises as the patient's pain resolves and other movements become more comfortable.

The efficacy of flexion exercise is theorized to derive from 1 or a combination of the following effects:

- A reduction in the articular stresses on the facet joints.
- Stretching to the thoracolumbar fascia and musculature.
- Opening of the intervertebral foramen.
- Relief of the stenosis of the spinal canal.
- Improvement of the stabilizing effect of the abdominal musculature.
- Increasing the intraabdominal pressure because of increased abdominal muscle strength and tone.
- Proprioceptive interference with pain perception as the exercises allow self-mobilization of the spinal joints.[39]

Flexion exercises should be used cautiously or avoided in most cases of acute disk prolapse and when a laterally shifted posture is present. In patients recovering from disk-related back pain, flexion exercise should not be commenced immediately after a flat-lying rest interval longer than 30 minutes. The disk can become more hydrated in this amount of time, and the patient would be more susceptible to pain with postures that increase disk pressures. Other, less stressful exercises should be initiated first and flexion exercise done later in the exercise program.[50]

Figures 28-21 to 28-31 show examples of flexion exercises. Again these examples are not exhaustive, but are representative of the exercises used clinically.

Joint Mobilizations

The indications for the use of joint mobilizations are as follows:

- Subjectively, the patient's pain is centered around a specific joint area and increases with activity and decreases with rest.
- The accessory motion available at individual spinal segments is diminished.

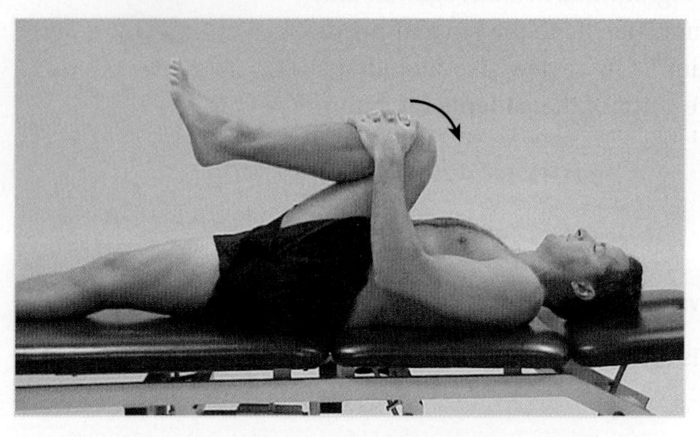

Figure 28-21 **Single knee to chest**

Stretch holding 15 to 20 seconds. Alternate legs.

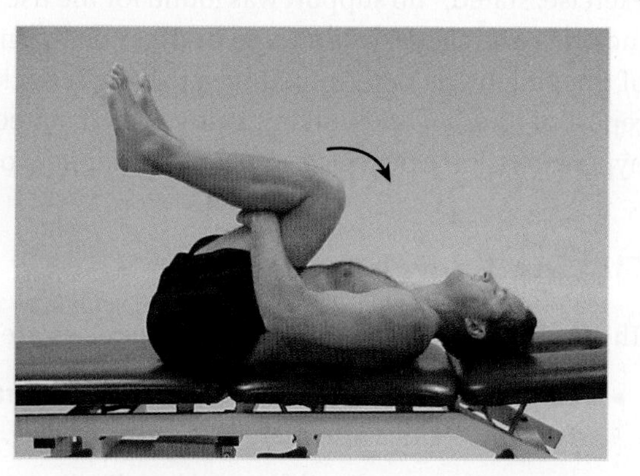

Figure 28-22 **Double knee to chest**

A. Stretching—holding posture 15 to 20 seconds.
B. Mobilizing—using a rhythmic rocking motion within a pain-free range of motion.

- Passive range of motion is diminished.
- Active range of motion is diminished.
- There may be muscular tightness or increased fascial tension in the area of the pain.
- Back movements are asymmetrical when comparing right and left rotation or side bending.
- Forward and backward bending may steer away from the midline.

The efficacy of mobilization is theorized to be from 1 or a combination of the following effects:

- Tight structures can be stretched to increase the range of motion.
- The joint involved is stimulated by the movement to more normal mechanics, and irritation is reduced because of better nutrient–waste exchange.
- Proprioceptive interference occurs with pain perception as the joint movement stimulates normal neural firing whose perception supersedes nociceptive perception.

Mobilization techniques are multidimensional and are easily adapted to any back pain problem. The mobilizations can be active or passive or assisted by the therapist. All ranges (flexion, extension, side bending, rotation, and accessory) can be incorporated within the

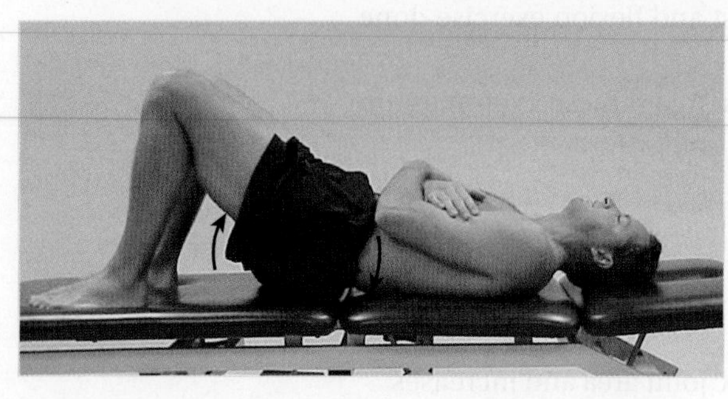

Figure 28-23 **Posterior pelvic tilt**

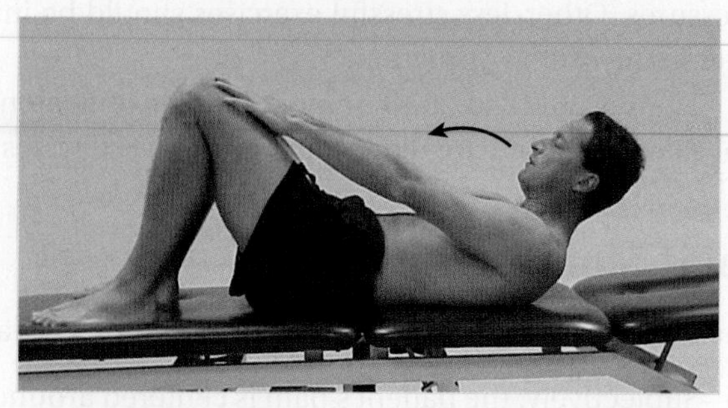

Figure 28-24 **Partial sit-up**

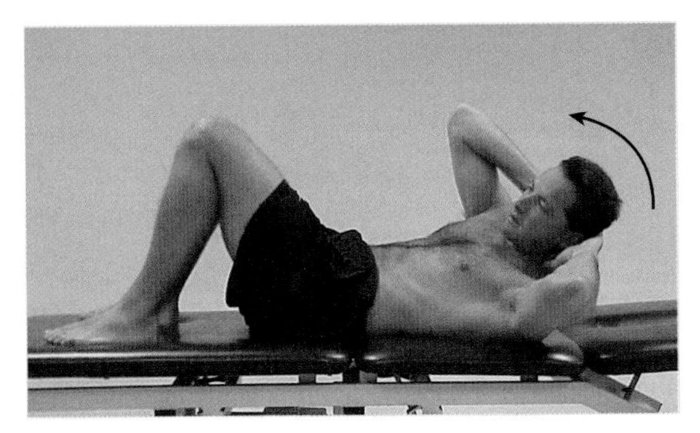

Figure 28-25 Rotation partial sit-up

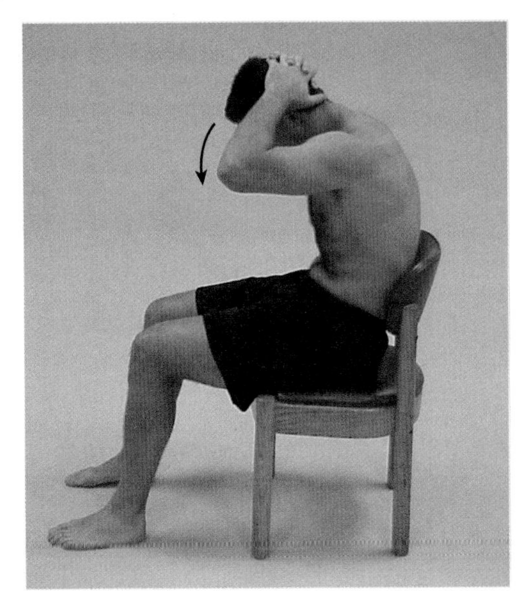

Figure 28-26 Slump sit stretch position

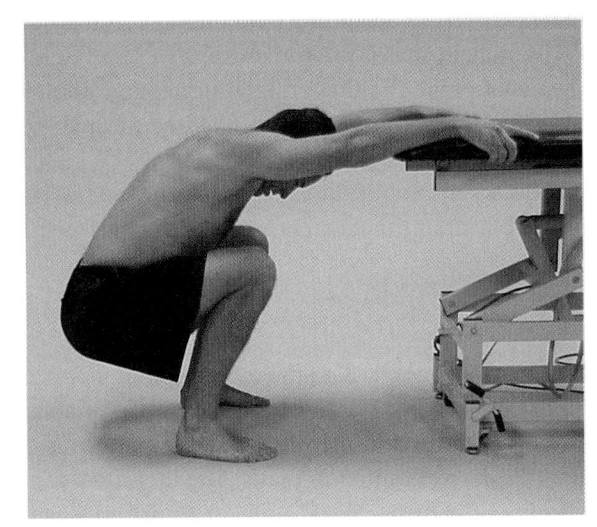

Figure 28-27 Flat-footed squat stretch

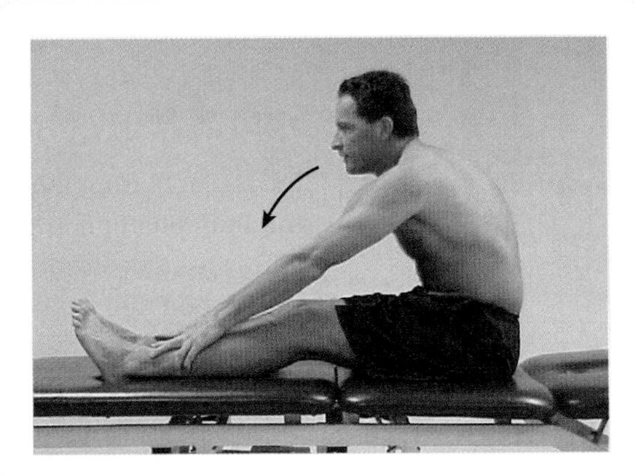

Figure 28-28 Hamstring stretch

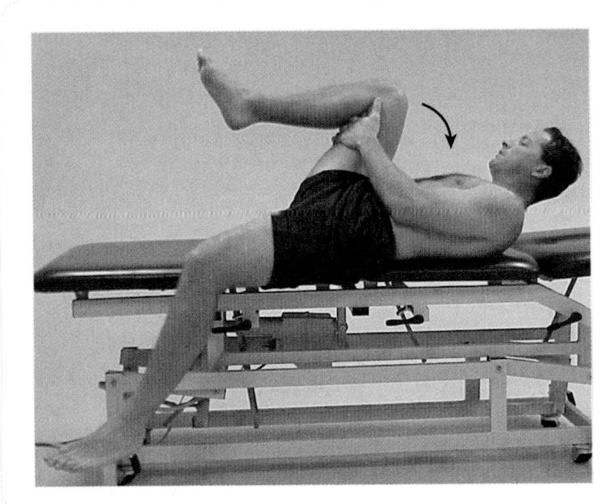

Figure 28-29 Hip flexor stretch

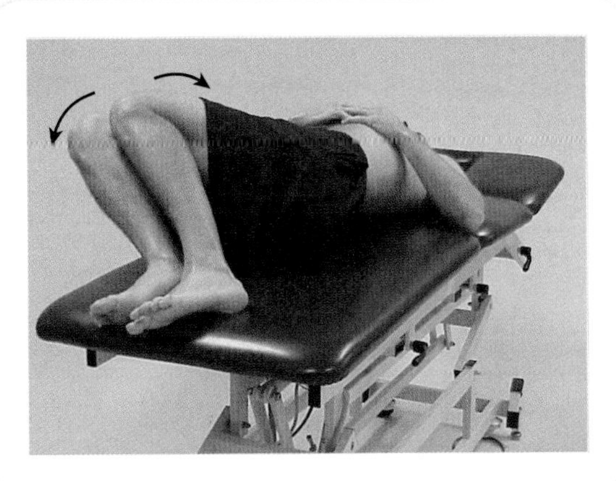

Figure 28-30 Knee rocking side to side

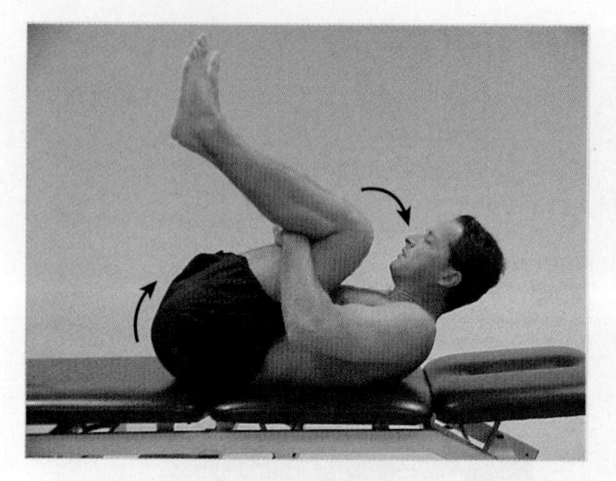

Figure 28-31 Knees toward chest rock

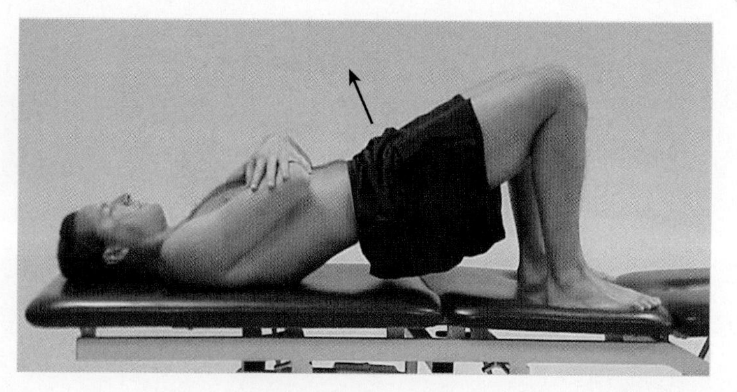

Figure 28-32 Supine hip lift-bridge-rock

exercise plan. The mobilizations can be carried out according to Maitland's grades of oscillation, as discussed in Chapter 13. The magnitude of the forces applied can range from grade 1 to grade 4, depending on levels of pain. The theory, technique, and application of the therapist-assisted mobilizations and manipulation are best gained through guided study with an expert practitioner.[46]

Figures 28-30 to 28-38 show the various self-mobilization exercises.

Figures 13-36 to 13-45 show joint mobilizations that can be used by the therapist.

Spinal Joint Manipulation

The research from the mid-1990s through 2000 has clarified the role of spinal mobilization and manipulation in the overall scheme of back and neck rehabilitation. Treatment algorithms have evolved and the role of mobilization and manipulation techniques is better understood and is taking its rightful place in rehabilitation plans. The literature supports manipulation for the short-term benefits of pain relief and quicker return to functional activities.[26] Long-term results show no detriment to this approach when compared to other specific treatment plans. The reverse, however, is true. When manipulation is not included

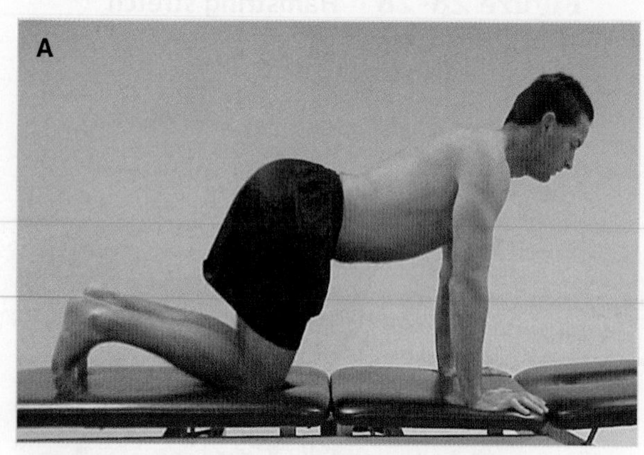

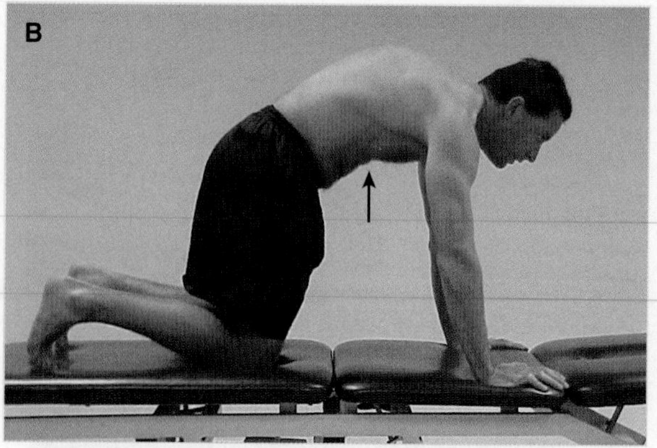

Figure 28-33 Pelvic tilt or pelvic rock

A. Swayback horse. **B.** Scared cat.

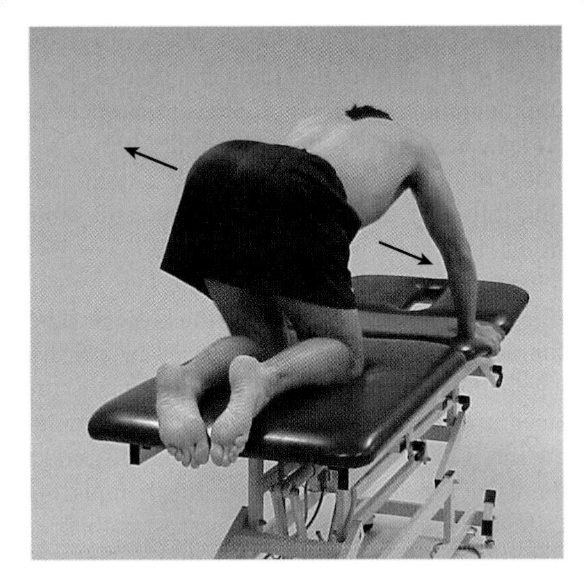

Figure 28-34 Kneeling—dog-tail wags

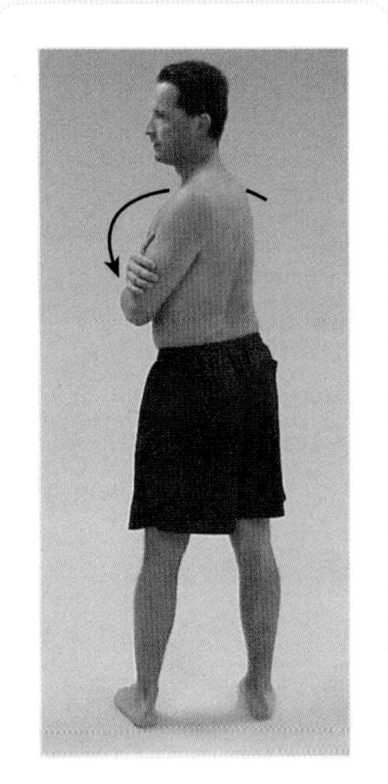

Figure 28-35 Sitting or standing rotation

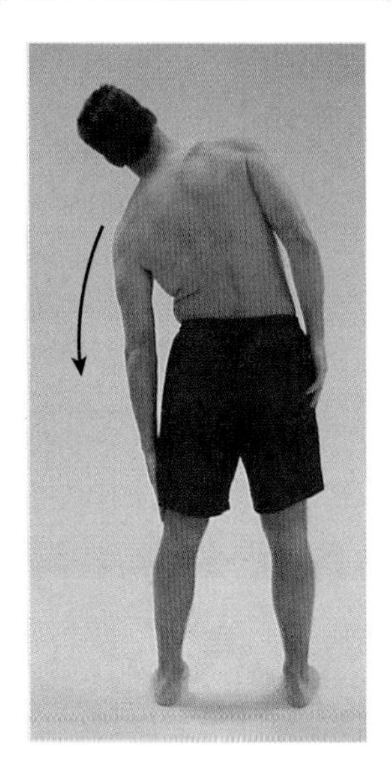

Figure 28-36 Sitting or standing side bending

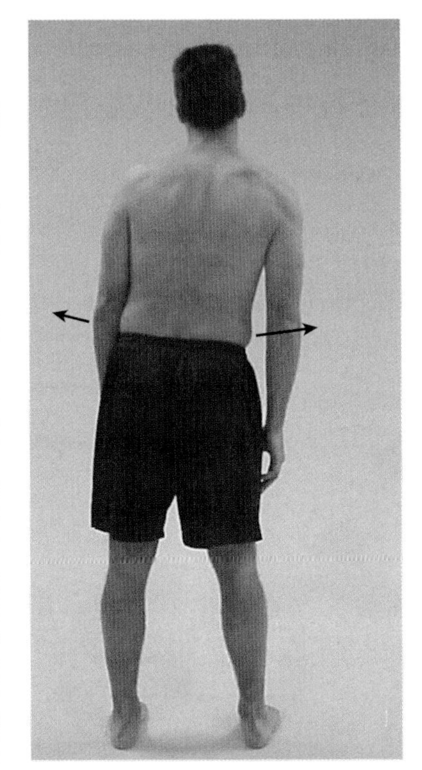

Figure 28-37 Standing hip-shift side to side

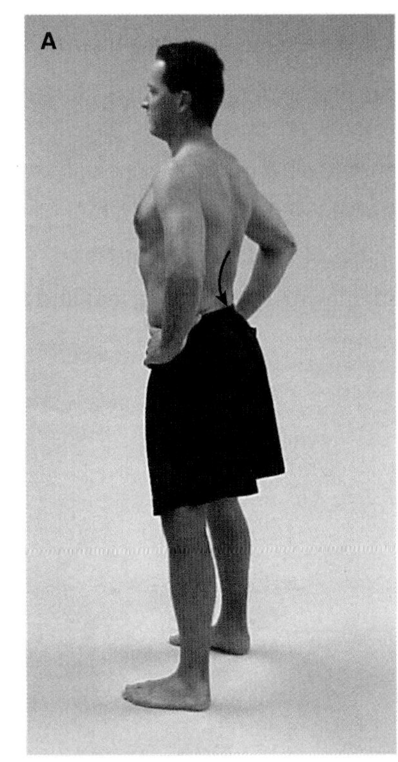

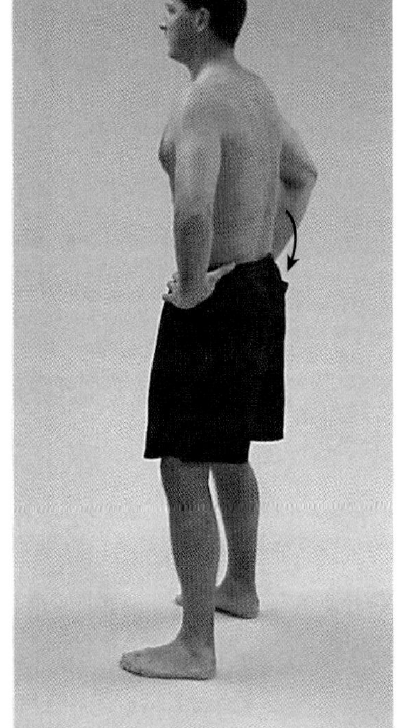

Figure 28-38 Standing pelvic rock

A. Butt out. **B.** Tail tuck.

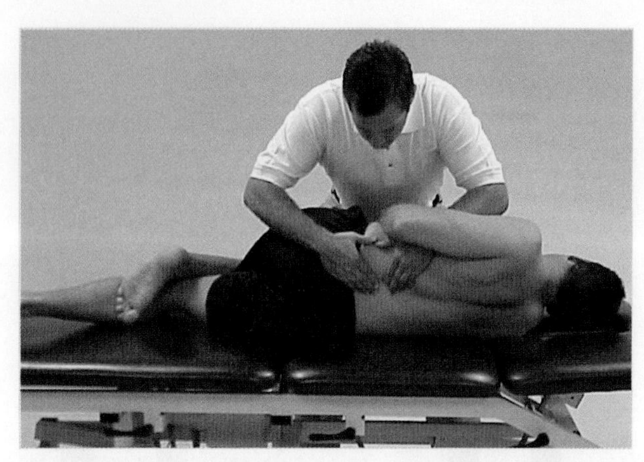

Figure 28-39

Various side-lying and back-lying positions can be used to both stretch and mobilize specific joints in the lumbar area.

in a population that would benefit, the pain and loss-of-function symptoms last longer and can worsen.[10] This makes the case for including greater use of spinal manipulation in rehabilitation plans than might have previously been used by therapists.[10,14,22,24,26]

The techniques used are shared among osteopathic, physical therapy, chiropractic, and athletic training disciplines, with theoretical rationales for use and matching certain techniques to certain evaluative findings varying between groups. The basic technique is simple and can be learned and used by any therapist from the undergraduate student to the most experienced practitioner. Figures 28-39, 28-58, and 28-59 show the basic positioning for the therapist and the patient. Once the positioning is set, the therapist delivers a high velocity, low-amplitude thrust mobilization to the lumbar spine or innominate that creates a sudden perturbation of the general lumbar and sacroiliac region. Although there is often an associated popping sound attributed to a cavitation of 1 or more of the facet joints, the success of the treatment and pain relief mechanisms are not attributed to this sound. The pain relief effect of the manipulation is poorly understood but the action mechanism will likely be multimodal and will include the afferent input to the central nervous system and its effect on the endogenous pain control systems.[4,5,15,16,25,40,65,66,71] The increased use of a technique adds to increased skill in performance and security with that particular technique.

The indications for joint manipulation in the lumbar spine and pelvis are as follows:[26]

- Subjectively, the patient's pain is limited to the low back and hip area and does not radiate below the knee.
- The symptoms have a recent onset, less than 16 days since onset.
- One lumbar segment is thought to be hypomobile.
- One hip has limited internal rotation.
- The patient will score low on a fear and avoidance to physical activity and work questionnaire.[87]

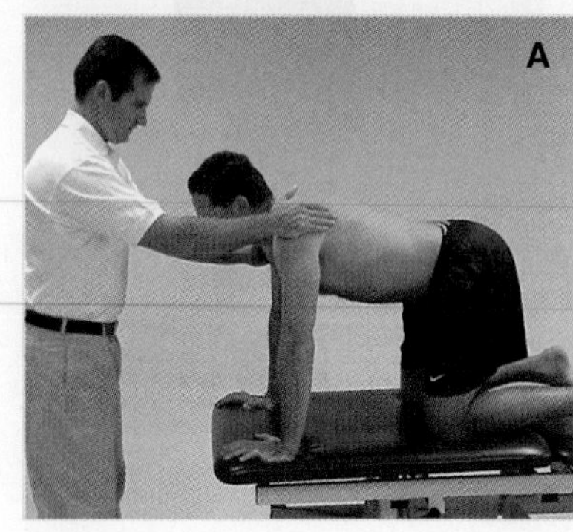

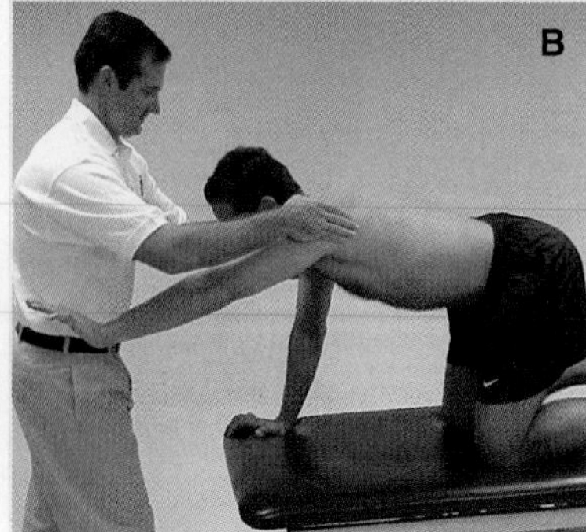

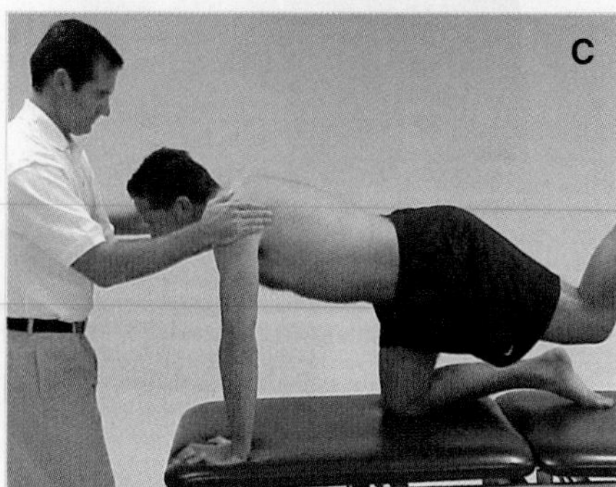

Figure 28-40

Weight shifting and stabilization exercises should progress from (**A**) quadrupeds, to (**B**) triped, to (**C**) biped.

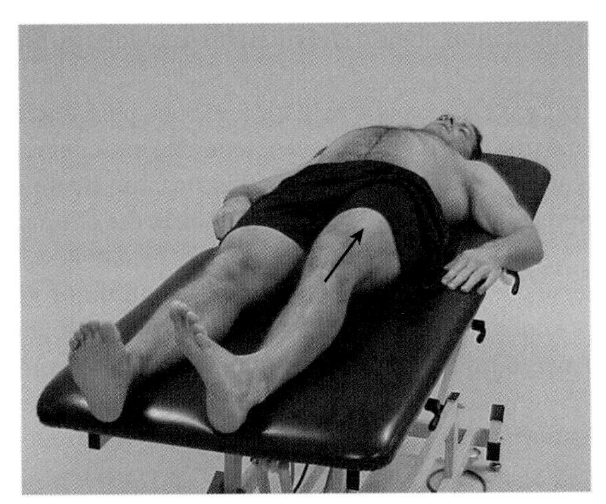

Figure 28-41 Back-lying—hip-hike shifting

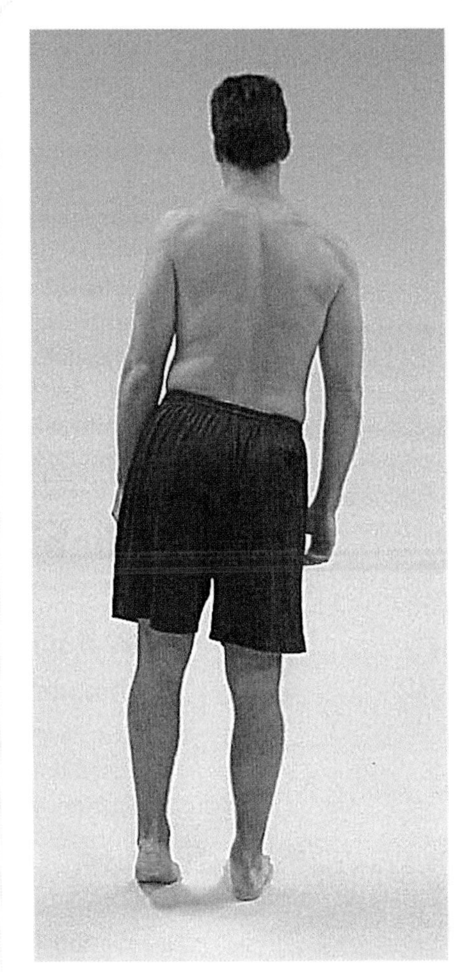

Figure 28-42 Standing hip hike

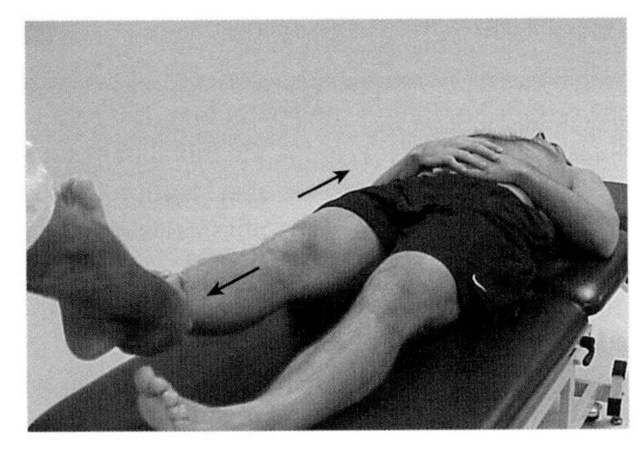

Figure 28-43 Back-lying—hip-hike resisted

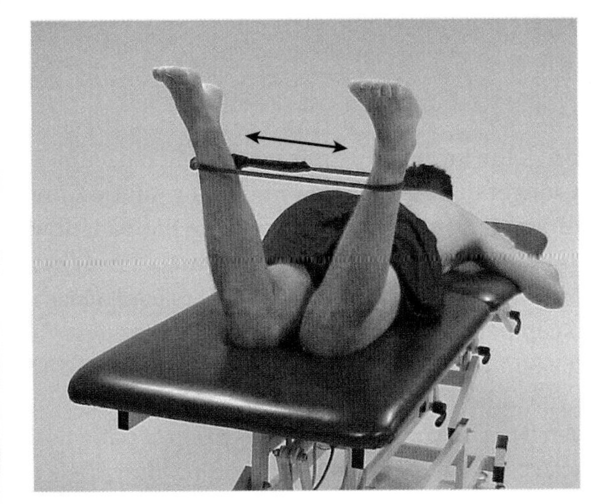

Figure 28-44 Prone-lying hip internal rotation with elastic resistance

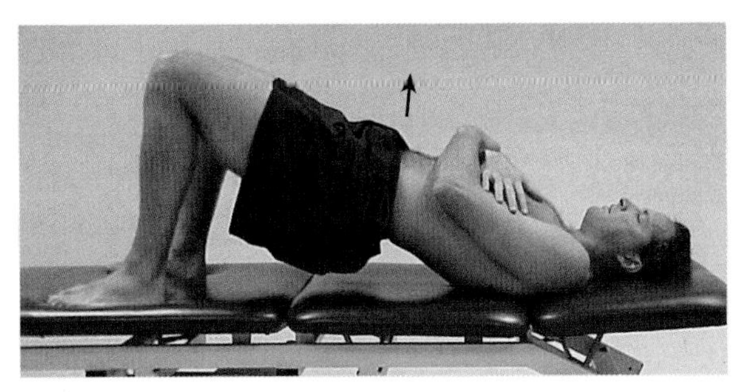

Figure 28-45 Hip-lift bridges

The athletic population should have a high proportion of low back pain patients that meets this clinical prediction rule. Manipulation should definitely be included in their rehabilitation plan.

Therapists are usually entry-level caregivers for patients with low back pain and are well positioned to use manipulation in the first treatments aimed at reducing back pain and increasing function.[14,21,22,23] If the patient has only 3 of the above findings, the treatment results might not be as good, but including manipulation would still be worth the effort and would not be contraindicated.

The side effects and potential adverse events are frequently used as contraindication to lumbar spinal manipulation but in fact are unproven and in most studies the complaints are musculoskeletal in nature and consist of mild pain, stiffness, and guarding of movements. These changes are usually self-limiting and do not affect the long-term outcome of the patient. The risk for serious complications (disk herniation, cauda equina syndrome) is very low.[8,9,23,72]

Rehabilitation Techniques for Low Back Pain

Low Back Pain

Pathomechanics

In most cases, low back pain does not have serious or long-lasting pathology. It is generally accepted that the soft tissues (ligament, fascia, and muscle) can be the initial pain source. The patient's response to the injury and to the provocative stresses of evaluation is usually proportional to the time since the injury and the magnitude of the physical trauma of the injury. The soft tissues of the lumbar region should react according to the biologic process of healing, and the time lines for healing should be like those for other body parts. There is little substantiation that injury to the low back should cause a pain syndrome that lasts longer than 6 to 8 weeks. Pain avoidance and fear mechanisms are issues that also play a big role in return to activity and require some inclusion in the rehabilitation plan.[17,70,73]

Injury Mechanism

Back pain can result from 1 or a combination of the following problems: muscle strain, piriformis muscle or quadratus lumborum myofascial pain or strain, myofascial trigger points, lumbar facet joint sprains, hypermobility syndromes, disk-related back problems, or sacroiliac joint dysfunction.[6]

Rehabilitation Concerns

Acute Versus Chronic Low Back Pain The low back pain that most often occurs is an acute, painful experience rarely lasting longer than 3 weeks. As with many injuries, therapists often go through exercise or treatment fads in trying to rehabilitate the patient with low back pain. The latest fad might involve flexion exercise, extension exercise, joint mobilization, dynamic muscular stabilization, abdominal bracing, myofascial release, electrical stimulation protocols, and so on.[3] To keep perspective, as therapists select exercises and modalities, they should keep in mind that 90% of people with back pain get resolution of the symptoms in 6 weeks, regardless of the care administered.[73,87]

There are patients who have pain persisting beyond 6 weeks. This group of patients will generally have a history of reinjury or exacerbation of previous injury. They describe a low back pain that is similar to their previous back pain experience.

These patients are experiencing an exacerbation or reinjury of previously injured tissues by continuing to apply stresses that may have created their original injury. This group of patients needs a more specific and formal treatment and rehabilitation program.[17,73]

There are also people who have chronic low back pain. This is a very small percentage of the population that suffers from low back pain. The difference between the patient with an acute injury or reinjury and a person with chronic pain has been defined by Waddell. He states, "Chronic pain becomes a completely different clinical syndrome from acute pain."[87] Acute and chronic pain not only are different in time scale, but are fundamentally different in kind. Acute and experimental pains bear a relatively straightforward relationship to peripheral stimulus, nociception, and tissue damage.[41]

There may be some understandable anxiety about the meaning and consequences of the pain, but acute pain, disability, and illness behavior are generally proportionate to the physical findings. Pharmacologic, physical, and even surgical treatments directed to the underlying physical disorder are generally highly effective in relieving acute pain. Chronic pain, disability, and illness behavior, in contrast, become increasingly dissociated from their original physical basis, and there may be little objective evidence of any remaining nociceptive stimulus. Instead, chronic pain and disability become increasingly associated with emotional distress, depression, failed treatment, and adoption of a sick role. Chronic pain progressively becomes a self-sustaining condition that is resistant to traditional medical management. Physical treatment directed to a supposed but unidentified and possibly nonexistent nociceptive source is not only understandably unsuccessful, but may also cause additional physical damage. Failed treatment may both reinforce and aggravate pain, distress, disability, and illness behavior.[54-57]

Rehabilitation Progression

A discussion of the rehabilitation progression for the patient with low back pain can be much more specific and meaningful if treatment plans are lumped into 2 stages. Stage I (acute stage) treatment consists mainly of the modality treatment and pain-relieving exercises. Stage II treatment involves treating patients with a reinjury or exacerbation of a previous problem. The treatment plan in stage II goes beyond pain relief, strengthening, stretching, and mobilization to include trunk stabilization and movement training sequences and to provide a specific, guided program to return the patient to functional activity.[73,74]

Stage I (Acute Stage) Treatment Modulating pain should be the initial focus of the therapist. Progressing rapidly from pain management to specific rehabilitation should be a primary goal of the acute stage of the rehabilitation plan. The most common treatment for pain relief in the acute stage is to use ice for analgesia. Rest, but not total bed rest, is used to allow the injured tissues to begin the healing process without the stresses that created the injury.[18] If the patient fits the clinical prediction rules for spinal manipulation, this should be initiated as soon as the patient can tolerate the positioning.[23]

Along with rest, during the initial treatment stage, the patient should be taught to increase comfort by using the *appropriate* body positioning techniques described previously, which may involve (a) lateral shift corrections (see Figure 28-11); (b) extension exercises (see Figures 28-13 to 28-20); (c) flexion exercises (see Figures 28-21 to 28-31); (d) self-mobilization exercises (see Figures 13-46 and 13-47); or (e) spinal manipulation (see Figure 28-39 and Figure 28-58). Segmental spinal stabilization exercise should be initiated concurrently with these other exercises. Outside support, in the form of corsets and the use of props or pillows to enhance comfortable positions, also needs to be included in the initial pain-management phase of treatment.[73,87] The patient should also be taught to avoid positions and movements that increase any sharp, painful episodes. The limits of these movements and positions that provide comfort should be the initial focus of any exercise.

The patient should be encouraged to move through this stage quickly and return to activity as soon as range, strength, and comfort will allow. The addition of a supportive corset during this stage should be based mostly on patient comfort. We suggest using an eclectic approach to the selection of the exercises, mixing the various protocols described according to the findings of the patient's evaluation. Rarely will a patient present with classic signs and symptoms that will dictate using one variety of exercise.

Stage II (Reinjury Stage) Treatment In the reinjury or chronic stage of back rehabilitation, the goals of the treatment and training should again be based on a thorough evaluation of the patient. Identifying the causes of the patients' back problems and recurrences is very important in the management of their rehabilitation and prevention of reinjury. A goal for this stage of care is to make the patients responsible for the management of their back problem. The therapist should identify specific problems and corrections that will help the patients better understand the mechanisms and management of their problem.[73]

Specific goals and exercises should be identified about the following:

- Which structures to stretch.
- Which structures to strengthen.
- Incorporating segmental spinal stabilization and abdominal bracing into the patient's daily life and exercise routine.
- Progression of core stabilization exercises.
- Which movements need a motor learning approach to control faulty mechanics.[73]

Stretching The therapist and the patient need to plan specific exercises to stretch restricted groups, maintain flexibility in normal muscle groups, and identify hypermobility that may be a part of the problem. In planning, instructing, and monitoring each exercise, adequate thought and good instruction must be used to ensure that the intended structures get stretched and areas of hypermobility are protected from overstretching.[36] Inadequate stabilization will lead to exercise movements that are so general that the exercise will encourage hyperflexibility at already hypermobile areas. Lack of proper stabilization during stretching may help perpetuate a structural problem that will continue to add to the patient's back pain.

In the therapist's evaluation of the patient with back pain, the following muscle groups should be assessed for flexibility.[37]

- Hip flexors
- Hamstrings
- Low back extensors
- Lumbar rotators
- Lumbar lateral flexors
- Hip adductors
- Hip abductors
- Hip rotators

Strengthening There are numerous techniques for strengthening the muscles of the trunk and hip. Muscles are perhaps best strengthened by using techniques of progressive overload to achieve specific adaptation to imposed demands (the SAID principle). The overload can take the form of increased weight load, increased holding time, increased repetition load, or increased stretch load to accomplish physiologic changes in muscle strength, muscle endurance, or flexibility of a body part.[19]

The treatment plan should call for an exercise that the patient can easily accomplish successfully. Rapidly but gradually, the overload should push the patient to challenge the muscle group needing strengthening. The therapist and the patient should monitor continuously for increases in the patient's pain or recurrences of previous symptoms. If those changes occur, the exercises should be modified, delayed, or eliminated from the rehabilitation plan.[39,73]

Core Stabilization Core stabilization training, dynamic abdominal bracing, and finding neutral position all describe a technique used to increase the stability of the trunk (see Chapter 15). This increased stability will enable the patient to maintain the spine and pelvis in the most comfortable and acceptable mechanical position that will control the forces of repetitive microtrauma and protect the structures of the back from further damage. Core muscular control is 1 key to giving the patients the ability to stabilize their trunk and control their posture. Abdominal strengthening routines are rigorous, and the patient must complete them with vigor. However, in their functional activities, the patients need to take advantage of their abdominal strength to stabilize the trunk and protect the back.[31,47,75]

Richardson et al focus attention on motor control of the transversus abdominis and lumbar multifidi in various positions.[34,73] Once this control is established, different positions and movements are added. As the vigor of the exercise is progressively increased, the patient will incorporate the more global muscles in stabilizing the patient's core (see Chapter 15). Then the patient moves into the functional exercise progression with the spinal segment stabilization as the base movement in core stabilization, which is needed to perform functionally.[73] The concept of increasing trunk stability with muscle contractions that support and limit the extremes of spinal movement is important.

Basic Functional Training The patients must be constantly committed to improving body mechanics and trunk control in all postures in their activities of daily living. The therapist needs to evaluate the patients' daily patterns and give them instruction, practice, and monitoring on the best and least stressful body mechanics in as many activities as possible.

The basic program follows the developmental sequence of posture control, starting with supine and prone extremity movement while actively stabilizing the trunk. The patient is then progressed to all fours, kneeling, and standing (Figure 28-40).

Emphasis on trunk control and stability is maintained as the patient works through this exercise sequence.[31,49,73]

The most critical aspect for developing motor control is repetition of exercise. However, variability in positioning, speed of movement, and changes in movement patterns must also be incorporated. The variability of the exercise will allow the patients to generalize their newly learned trunk control to the constant changes necessary in their movements. The basic exercise, transversus abdominis and lumbar multifidi coactivation, is the key. Incorporating this stabilization contraction into various activities helps reinforce trunk stabilization and returns trunk control to a subconscious automatic response.

The use of augmented feedback (electromyography, palpation, ultrasound imagery, pressure gauges) of the transversus abdominis and lumbar multifidi contractions may be needed early in the exercise plan to help maximize the results of each exercise session supervised by the therapist. The therapist should have the patient internalize this feedback as quickly as possible to make the patient apparatus-free and more functional. With augmented feedback, it is recommended that the patient be rapidly and progressively weaned from dependency on external feedback.

Advanced Functional Training Each activity that the patient is involved in becomes part of the advanced exercise rehabilitation plan. The usual place to start is with the patient's strength and conditioning program. Each step of the program is monitored, and emphasis is placed on spinal segmental stabilization for even the simple task of putting the weights on a bar or getting on and off exercise equipment. Each exercise in its strength and conditioning program should be retaught, and the patients be made aware of its best mechanical position and the proper stabilizing muscular contraction. The strength program is patient-specific, attempting to strengthen weak areas and improve strength in muscle groups needed for better function.[73]

The patients should be taught to start their stabilizing contractions before starting any movement. This presets their posture and stabilization awareness before their movement takes place. As the movement occurs, they will become less aware of the stabilization contraction as they attempt to complete an exercise.

They might revert to old postures and habits, so feedback is important.

Each patient is different, not only with the individual back problem but also with the abilities to gain motor skill and to overcome the fear and avoidance associated with chronic back pain.[87] Patients differ in degree of control and in the speed at which they acquire these new skills of core stabilization.

Reducing stress to the back by using braces, orthotics, shoes, or comfortable supportive furniture (beds, desks, or chairs) is essential to help the patients minimize chronic or overload stresses to their back. The stabilization exercise should also be incorporated into their activities of daily living.[59] Use of a low back corset or brace may also make the patient more comfortable (Figure 28-56).

Criteria for Return

For most low back problems the stage I treatment and exercise programs will get the patients back into their activities quickly. If the pain or dysfunction is pronounced or the problem becomes recurrent, an in-depth evaluation and treatment using stage I and stage II exercise protocols will be necessary. The team approach, with patient, doctor, and therapist working together, will provide the comprehensive approach needed to manage the patient's back problem. Close attention to and emphasis on the patient's progress will provide both the patient and the therapist with the encouragement to continue this program.

Muscular Strains

Injury Mechanism

Evaluative findings include a history of sudden or chronic stress that initiates pain in a muscular area during the workout. There are 3 points on the physical examination that must be positive to indicate the muscle as the primary problem. There will be tenderness to palpation in the muscular area and the muscular pain will be provoked with contraction and with stretch of the involved muscle.

Rehabilitation Progression

The treatment should include the standard protection, ice, and compression. Ice may be applied in the form of ice massage or ice bags, depending on the area involved. An elastic wrap or corset would protect and compress the back musculature. Additional modalities include pulsed ultrasound for a biostimulative effect and electrical stimulation for pain relief and muscle reeducation. The exercises used in rehabilitation should make the involved muscle contract and stretch, starting with very mild exercise and progressively increasing the intensity and repetition loads. In general this would include active extension exercises such as hip lifts (see Figures 28-17 to 28-19), alternate arm and leg, hip extension (see Figure 28-15), trunk extension (see Figure 28-20), and quadratus hip shift exercises (Figures 28-41 to 28-43). A good series of abdominal spinal segmental stabilization and core stabilization exercises would also be helpful (see Figures 28-23 and 28-24). Stretching exercises might include the following: knee to chest (see Figures 28-21 and 28-22), side-lying leg hang to stretch the hip flexors (see Figure 28-29), slump sitting (see Figure 28-26), and knee rocking side to side (see Figure 28-30).

Criteria for Return

Initially, the patients may wish to continue to use a brace or corset, but they should be encouraged to do away with the corset as their back strengthens and their performance returns to normal.[19,39]

Piriformis Muscle Strain

Pathomechanics

Piriformis syndrome was discussed in detail in Chapter 23. The piriformis muscle refers pain to the posterior sacroiliac region, to the buttocks, and sometimes down the posterior or posterolateral thigh. The pain is usually described as a deep ache that can get more intense with exercise and with sitting with the hips flexed, adducted, and medially rotated. The pain gets sharper and more intense with activities that require decelerating medial hip and leg rotation during weight bearing.[7]

Tenderness to palpation has a characteristic pattern, with tenderness medial and proximal to the greater trochanter and just lateral to the posterior superior iliac spine (PSIS). Isometric abduction in the sitting position produces pain in the posterior hip buttock area, and the movement will be weak or hesitant. Passive hip internal rotation in the sitting position will also bring on posterior hip and buttock pain.[61]

Rehabilitation Progression

Rehabilitation exercises should include both strengthening and stretching.[7,61] Strengthening exercises should include prone lying hip internal rotation with elastic resistance (Figure 28-44), hip-lift bridges (Figure 28-45), hand-knee position fire hydrant exercise (Figure 28-46), side-lying hip abduction straight-leg raises (Figure 28-47), and prone hip extension exercise (Figure 28-48).

Stretching exercises for the piriformis include back-lying legs-crossed hip adduction stretch (Figure 28-49), back-lying with the involved leg crossed over the uninvolved leg, ankle to knee position, pulling the uninvolved knee toward the chest to create the stretch (Figure 28-50), contract-relax-stretch with elbow pressure to the muscle insertion during the relaxation phase (Figure 28-51).[42,78,81] This can also be done in the sitting position with the same mechanics, but the patient leans over at the waist and brings the chest toward the knee.

Quadratus Lumborum Strain

Pathomechanics

Pain from the quadratus lumborum muscle is described as an aching, sharp pain located in the flank, in the lateral back area, and near the posterior sacroiliac region and upper buttocks. The patient usually describes pain on moving from sitting to standing, standing for long periods, coughing, sneezing, and walking. Activities requiring trunk rotation or side bending aggravate the pain. The muscle is tender to palpation near the origin along the lower ribs and along the insertion on the iliac crest. Pain

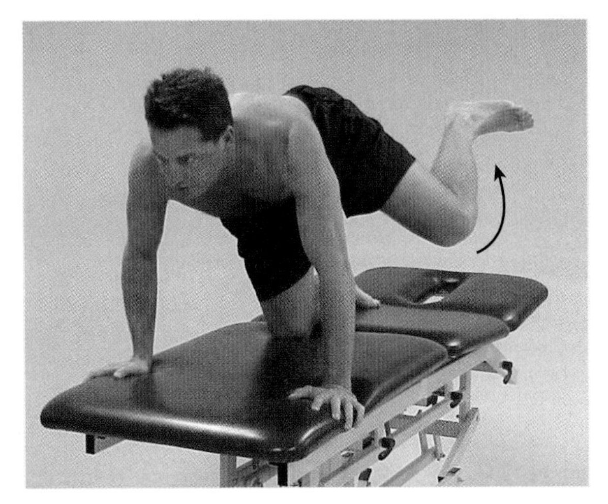

Figure 28-46 Hand-knee position—fire hydrant exercise

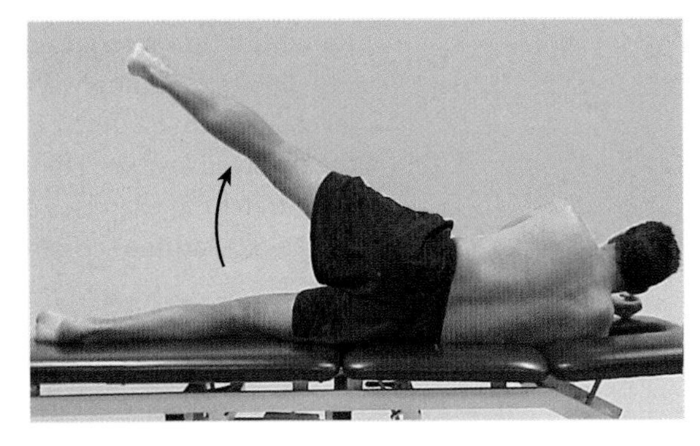

Figure 28-47 Side-lying hip abduction straight-leg raises

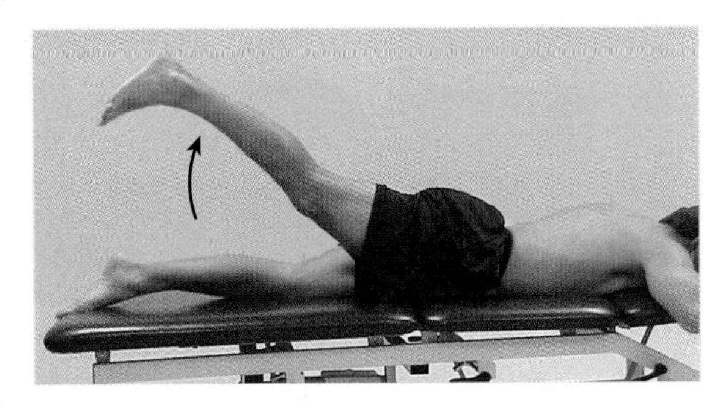

Figure 28-48 Prone hip extension exercise

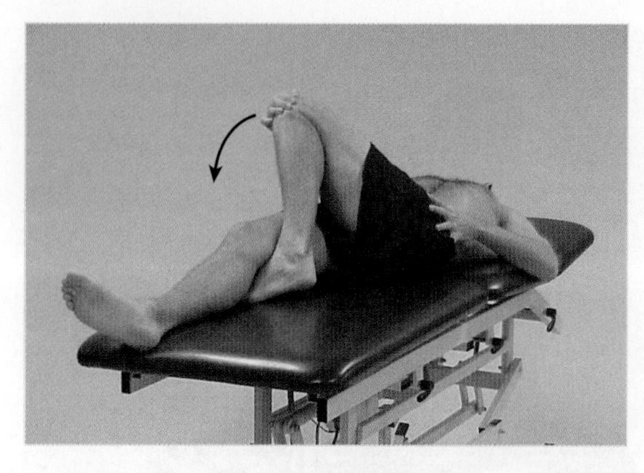

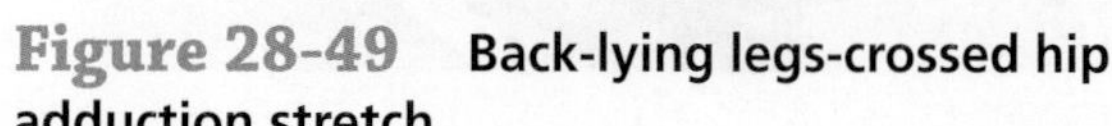

Figure 28-49 **Back-lying legs-crossed hip adduction stretch**

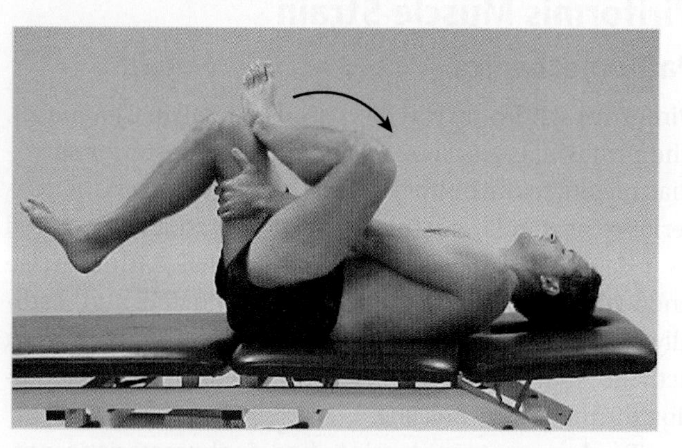

Figure 28-50 **Self piriformis stretch**

will be aggravated on side bending, and the pain will usually be localized to one side. For example, with a right quadratus problem, side bending right and left would provoke only right-side pain. Supine hip-hiking movements would also provoke the pain.

Rehabilitation Progression

Rehabilitation strengthening exercise should include back-lying hip-hike shifting (Figure 28-54), standing with 1 leg on elevated surface and the other free to move below that level, hip-hike on the free side (Figure 28-55), and back-lying hip-hike resisted by pulling on the involved leg (see Figure 28-43).

Stretching exercises should include side-lying over a pillow roll leg-hand stretch (Figure 28-52), supine self-stretch with legs crossed (Figure 28-53), hip-hike exercise with hand

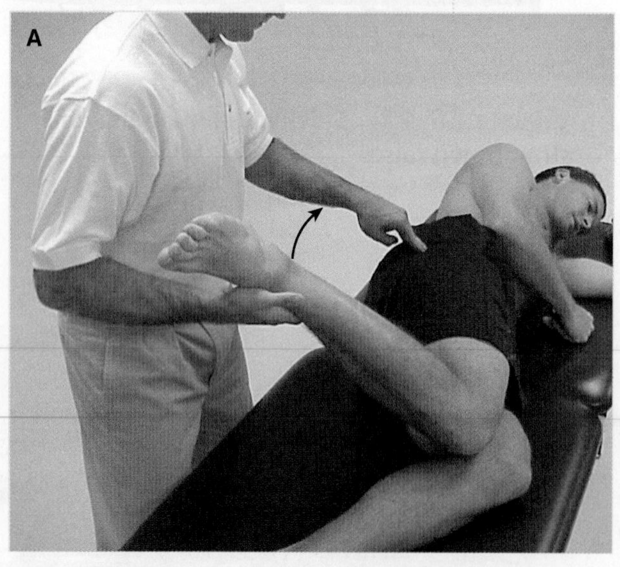

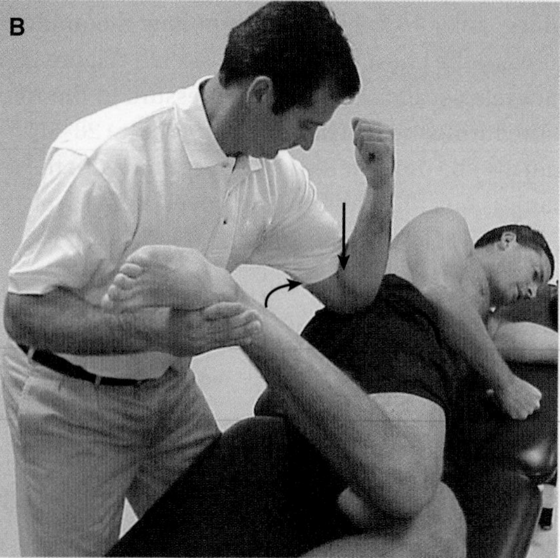

Figure 28-51 **Piriformis stretch using elbow pressure**

A. Start-contract. **B.** Relaxation-stretch.

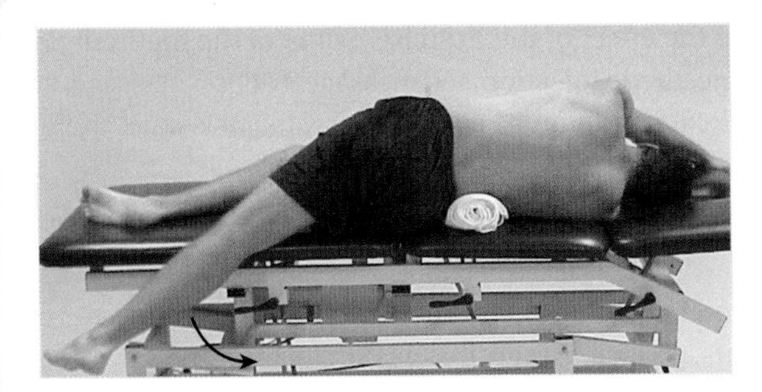

Figure 28-52 Side-lying stretch over pillow roll

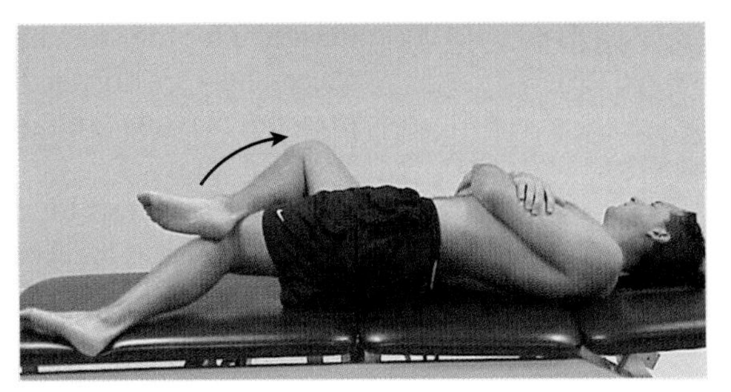

Figure 28-53 Supine self-stretch—legs crossed

pressure to increase stretch (see Figure 28-54), and standing one leg on a small book stretch (see Figure 28-55).[89]

Myofascial Pain and Trigger Points

Pathomechanics and Injury Mechanism

The above examples of muscle-oriented back pain in both the piriformis and quadratus lumborum could also have a myofascial origin. The major component in successfully changing myofascial pain is stretching the muscle back to a normal resting length. The muscle irritation and congestion that create the trigger points are relieved and normal blood flow resumes, further reducing the irritants in the area. Stretching through a painful trigger point is difficult.

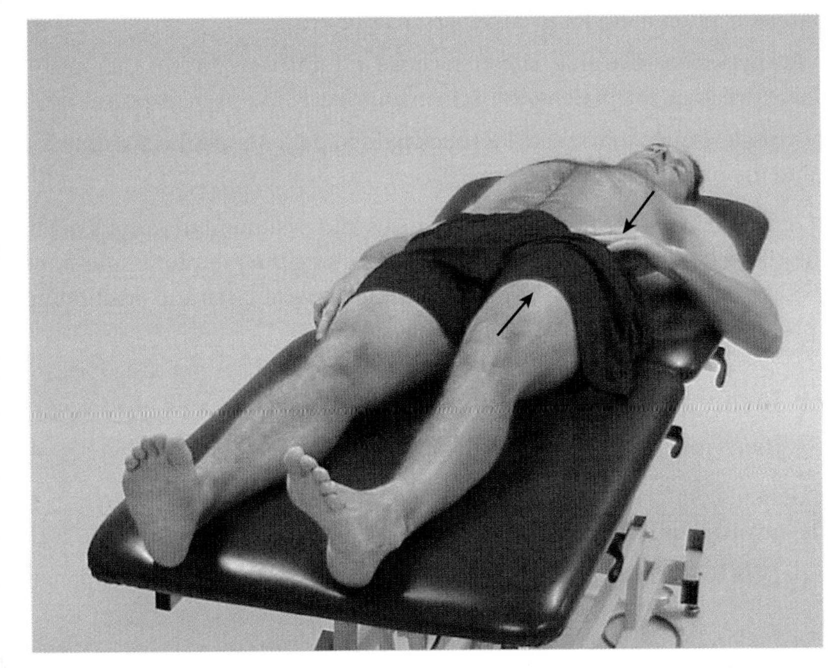

Figure 28-54 Hip-hike exercise with hand pressure

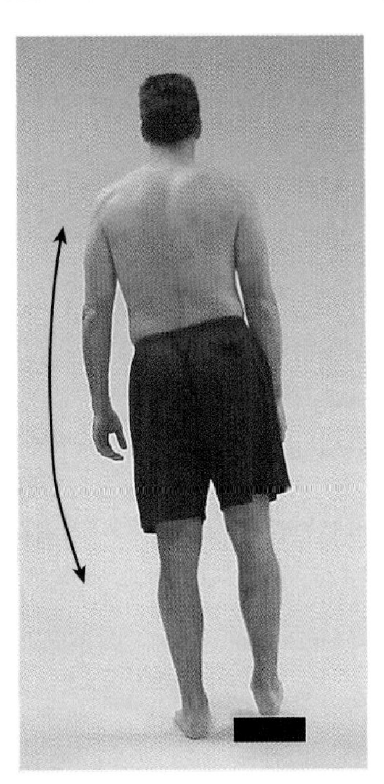

Figure 28-55 Standing 1-leg-up stretch

A variety of comfort and counterirritant modalities can be used preliminarily to, during and after the stretching, enhance the effect of the exercise. Some of the methods used successfully are dry needling, local anesthetic injection, ice massage, friction massage, acupressure massage, ultrasound electrical stimulation, extracorporeal shock wave therapy, and cold sprays.[38]

The indications for treating low back pain with myofascial stretching and treatment techniques are as follows[38]:

1. Subjectively, muscle soreness and fatigue from repetitive motions are common antecedent mechanisms. Patients are also susceptible as fatigue and stress overload specific muscle groups. There may be a history of sudden onset during or shortly after an acute overload stress, or there may be a gradual onset with repetitive or postural overload of the affected muscle. The pain may be an incapacitating event in the case of acute onset, but it may also be a nagging, aggravating type of pain with an intensity that varies from an awareness of discomfort to a severe unrelenting type of pain. The pain location is usually a referred pain area remote from the actual myofascial trigger point. These trigger points can be present but quiescent until they are activated by overload, fatigue, trauma, or chilling. These points are called *latent trigger points.* This deep, aching pain can be specifically localized, but the patient is not sensitive to palpation in these areas. This pain can often be reproduced by maintaining pressure on a hypersensitive myofascial trigger point.
2. Passive or active stretching of the affected myofascial structure increases pain.
3. The stretch range of muscle is restricted.
4. The pain is increased when the muscle is contracted against a fixed resistance or the muscle is allowed to contract into an extremely shortened range. The pain in this case is described as a muscle cramping pain.
5. The muscle may be slightly weak.
6. Trigger points may be located within a taut band of the muscle. If taut bands are found during palpation, explore them for local hypersensitive areas.
7. Pressure on the hypersensitive area will often cause a "jump sign"; as the therapist strums the sensitive area, the patient's muscle involuntarily jumps in response.
8. The primary muscle groups that create low back pain in patients are the quadratus lumborum and the piriformis muscles.[42,78,79,81]

Simons and Travell devoted 2 volumes to the causes and treatment of various myofascial pains.[78,79] They have done a very thorough job of describing the symptoms and signs of each area of the body, and they give very specific guidance on exercises and positioning in their treatment protocols.

Rehabilitation Technique

Myofascial trigger points may be treated using the following steps:

1. Position the patient comfortably but in a position that will lead the patient to stretching the involved muscle group.
2. Caution the patient to use mild progressive stretches rather than sudden, sharp, hard stretches.
3. Hot pack the area for 10 minutes, and follow with an ultrasound and electrical stimulation treatment over the affected muscle.
4. Use an ice cup, and use 2 to 3 slow strokes starting at the trigger point and moving in 1 direction toward the pain reference area and over the full length of the muscle.

5. Begin stretching well within the patient's comfort. A stretch should be maintained for a minimum of 15 seconds. The stretch should be released until the patient is comfortable again. The next stretch repetition should then be progressively more intense if tolerated, and the position of the stretch should also be varied slightly. Repeat the stretch 4 to 6 times.
6. Hot pack the area, and have the patient go through some active stretches of the muscle.
7. Refer to Simons and Travell's manual for specific references on other muscle groups.[42,78,79]
8. Soft-tissue mobilization and positional release techniques are used to treat and resolve trigger points (see Chapter 8). Therapeutic eccentric active massage has shown some clinical success. In this technique, the muscle for fascia associated with the identified trigger point is actively contracted to its shortest possible length. Using a small amount of lubricant, the active trigger point is compressed with a firm steady pressure. The therapist provides resistance to the shortened muscle, and the patient is instructed to continue to resist, but also allow the eccentric lengthening of the muscle to occur in a smooth, controlled manner. As the muscle lengthens under the compressive massage, the trigger point is compressed and the irritants in the area are dispersed over a greater area. This helps the pain decrease, and the muscle begins to function more normally.

The first repetition is usually uncomfortable for the patient. Subsequent repetitions are more comfortable and the patient can control the contraction better. Six to 8 repetitions are used for each trigger point treated. This technique is empirically based, and research studies are needed to establish their validity.

Lumbar Facet Joint Sprains

Pathomechanics and Injury Mechanism

Sprains may occur in any of the ligaments in the lumbar spine. However, the most common sprain involves lumbar facet joints. Facet joint sprain typically occurs when bending forward and twisting while lifting or moving some object. The patients will report a sudden acute episode that caused the problem, or they will give a history of a chronic repetitive stress that caused the gradual onset of a pain that got progressively worse with continuing activity. The pain is local to the structure that has been injured, and the patient can clearly localize the area. The pain is described as a sore pain that gets sharper in response to certain movements or postures. The pain is located centrally or just lateral to the spinous process areas and is deep.

Local symptoms will occur in response to movements, and the patient will usually limit the movement in those ranges that are painful. When the vertebra is moved passively with a posterior anterior or rotational pressure through the spinous process, the pain may be provoked.

Rehabilitation Progression

The treatment should include the standard protection, ice, and compression as mentioned previously. Both pulsed ultrasound and electrical stimulation could also be used similarly to the treatment of muscle strains but localized to the specific joint area.

Joint mobilization using posterior–anterior glides (see Figure 13-36) and rotational glides (see Figures 13-38 and 13-39) should help reduce pain and increase joint nutrition. The patient should be instructed in segmental spinal stabilization exercises using transversus abdominis and lumbar multifidi coactivation and good postural control (see Figures 28-3 to 28-10). Strengthening exercises for abdominals (see Figures 28-23 to 28-25) and back extensors (see Figures 28-17 to 28-20) should initially be limited to a pain-free range. Stretching in all ranges should start well within a comfort range and gradually increase until trunk movements reach normal ranges. Patients should be supported with a corset or range-limiting brace, which should be used only temporarily until normal strength, muscle control, and pain-free range are achieved.[19,45,46,83,84] It is important to guard against the development of postural changes that might occur in response to pain.

Hypermobility Syndromes (Spondylolysis/Spondylolisthesis)

Pathomechanics

Hypermobility of the low back may be attributed to spondylolysis or spondylolisthesis. Spondylolysis involves a degeneration of the vertebrae and, more commonly, a defect in the pars interarticularis of the articular processes of the vertebrae.[52] This condition is often attributed to a congenital weakness, with the defect occurring as a stress fracture. Spondylolysis might produce no symptoms unless a disk herniation occurs or there is sudden trauma such as hyperextension. Commonly spondylolysis begins unilaterally. However, if it extends bilaterally, there may be some slipping of one vertebra on the one below it. A spondylolisthesis is considered to be a complication of spondylolysis often resulting in hypermobility of a vertebral segment.[21] Spondylolisthesis has the highest incidence with L5 slipping on S1.[52]

Injury Mechanism

Movements that characteristically hyperextend the spine are most likely to cause this condition.[52]

Rehabilitation Concerns

The patients usually have a relatively long history of feeling "something go" in their back. They complain of a low back pain described as a persistent ache across the back (belt type). This pain does not usually interfere with their workout performance, but is usually worse when fatigued or after sitting in a slumped posture for an extended time. The patients may also complain of a tired feeling in the low back. They describe the need to move frequently and get temporary relief of pain through self-manipulation. They often describe self-manipulative behavior more than 10 times a day. Their pain is relieved by rest, and they do not usually feel the pain during exercise. On physical examination, the patient usually will have full and painless trunk movements, but there may be a wiggle or hesitation in forward bending at the midrange. On backwards bending, movement may appear to hinge at 1 spinal segment. When extremes of range are maintained for 15 to 30 seconds, the patient feels a lumbosacral ache. On return from forward bending, the patient will use thigh climbing to regain the neutral position. On palpation there may be tenderness localized to 1 spinal segment.[52,64]

Rehabilitation Progression

Patients with this problem will fall into the reinjury stage of back pain and may require extensive treatment to regain stability of the trunk. The patient's pain should be treated symptomatically. Initially, bracing and occasionally bed rest for 1 to 3 days will help reduce pain. The major focus in rehabilitation should be on segmental spinal stabilization exercises that control or stabilize the hypermobile segment (see Figures 28-3 to 28-10). Progressive trunk-strengthening exercises, especially through the midrange, should be incorporated. Core stabilization exercises that concentrate on transversus abdominis behavior and endurance should also be used (see Chapter 15).[33,34,36,48,60,62,67-69] The patient should avoid manipulation and self-manipulation as well as stretching and flexibility exercises. Corsets and braces are beneficial if the patient uses them only for support during higher-level activities and for short (1- to 2-hour) periods to help with pain relief and fatigue (see Figure 28-56).[31,73] Hypermobility of a lumbar vertebrae may make the patient more susceptible to lumbar muscle strains and ligament sprains. Thus it may be necessary for the patient to avoid vigorous activity. The use of a low back corset or brace might also make the patient more comfortable (see Figure 28-56).[32]

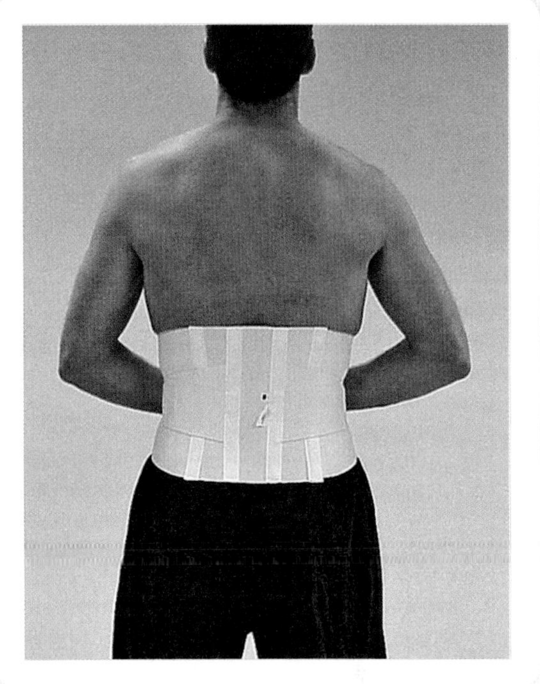

Figure 28-56 A lower-lumbar corset or brace

Disk-Related Back Pain

Pathomechanics

The lumbar disks are subject to constant abnormal stresses stemming from faulty body mechanics, trauma, or both, which, over a period of time, can cause degeneration, tears, and cracks in the annulus fibrosus.[13] The disk, most often injured, lies between the L4 and L5 vertebrae. The L5-S1 disk is the second most commonly affected.[80]

Injury Mechanism

The mechanism of a disk injury is the same as that for the lumbosacral sprain—forward bending and twisting that places abnormal strain on the lumbar region.[77] The movement that produces herniation or bulging of the nucleus pulposus may be minimal, and associated pain may be significant. Besides injuring soft tissues, such a stress may herniate an already degenerated disk by causing the nucleus pulposus to protrude into or through the annulus fibrosis. As the disk progressively degenerates, a prolapsed disk may develop in which the nucleus moves completely through the annulus. If the nucleus moves into the spinal canal and comes in contact with a nerve root, this is referred to as an extruded disk. This protrusion of the nucleus pulposus may place pressure on the spinal cord or spinal nerves, causing radiating pains similar to those of sciatica, as occurs in piriformis syndrome. If the material of the nucleus separates from the disk and begins to migrate, a sequestrated disk exists.[80]

Rehabilitation Concerns

Patients will report a centrally located pain that radiates unilaterally or spreads across the back. They may describe a sudden or gradual onset that becomes particularly severe after they have rested and then tried to resume their activities. They may complain of tingling or numb feelings in a dermatomal pattern or sciatic radiation.[76] Forward bending and sitting postures increase their pain. Patients' symptoms are usually worse in the morning on first arising and get better through the day. Coughing and sneezing may increase their pain.[80]

On physical examination, the patient will have a hip-shifted, forward-bent posture. On active movements, side bending toward the hip shift is painful and limited. Side bending away from the shift is more mobile and does not provoke the pain. Forward bending is very limited and painful, and guarding is very apparent. On palpation, there may be tenderness around the painful area. Posterior–anterior pressure over the involved segment increases the pain. Passive straight-leg raising will increase the back or leg pain during the first 30 degrees of hip flexion. Bilateral knee-to-chest movement will increase the back pain. Neurologic testing (strength, sensory reflex) may be positive for differences between right and left.[80]

REHABILITATION PLAN

TREATMENT OF DISK-RELATED BACK PAIN

INJURY SITUATION A 31-year-old mother was attempting to put her 2-year-old daughter in the child restraint seat of her minivan. After picking the child up, she bent forward and twisted to get the child into the seat and felt immediate intense pain in her low back and down the back of her right leg. Her right leg gave way and she collapsed to the floor with back and right-leg pain. She was referred to a therapist for evaluation and treatment by a family practice physician.

Functionally she was very guarded and stiff looking. On forward bending, she was very guarded and used compensating movement patterns to move from sit to stand or standing to lying down. Lumbar spine forward bending and right straight-leg raising provoked central back pain that radiated into her right posterior thigh. Backwards bending provoked central pain and was restricted at 50% of normal range. Sitting knee extension movement with the right leg provoked central pain and posterior thigh pain when the knee flexion angle reached 60 degrees. Dorsiflexion at the ankle and chin to chest movement increased this pain. Posterior–anterior mobilizations to the sacrum and the L5 spinous process increased central back pain and caused some shooting pain down the right leg. On manual muscle test, trunk extension was strong and painless. Left hip extension and left hip internal rotation and external rotation were strong but provoked right posterior leg pain. A sensory check demonstrated normal feeling over both lower extremities. On palpation, she was nontender over all major structures.

PHASE ONE Acute Phase

GOALS: Decrease pain, encourage rest, maintain spinal segment stability, and create safe, pain-free movement behaviors that minimize the stress on the disk complex.

Estimated Length of Time (ELT): Days 1 to 3

The patient was treated with 3 days of relative bed rest. She was encouraged to work on spinal segment stability exercises, knees toward chest, and knee-rocking mobilizations while in a flat-lying position (supine, side-lying, or prone). Multiple bouts of the 90/90 position and prone-on-elbows position were used for their positional traction benefit. Activities of daily living were kept to a necessary level—remain at home, avoid sitting posture. Standing and walking for brief periods (less than 10 minutes) were allowed. The physician prescribed analgesic and antiinflammatory medications.

PHASE TWO Intermediate Phase

GOALS: Decrease pain, encourage motion. Encourage rest positions that enhance centralization of the disk nucleus and provide optimum nourishment for the disk complex.

Rehabilitation Progression

The patient should be treated initially with pain-reducing modalities (ice, electrical stimulation, rest). The therapist should then use the lateral shift correction (see Figure 28-11), followed by a gentle extension exercise (see Figure 28-16). The patient is then sent home with the following rest and home-exercise program.

The patient must commit to resting in a flat-lying position three to four times a day for 20 to 30 minutes. During that time the patient can use some prone press-up extension exercises, holding the stretched position for 15 to 20 seconds for each repetition (see Figures 28-13 and 28-14). Another recommended pain-relieving position is the 90/90 position—90 degrees of hip flexion and 90 degrees of knee flexion (Figure 28-57). Both of these exercises provide very mild traction to the lumbar spine that enhances the centralization and nourishment effect of the flat-lying position on the disk, which, in turn, leads to decreased pain and increased function. Segmental spinal stabilization exercises can also be incorporated into the rest positions and may be used concurrently with other modalities (see Figures 28-3 to 28-10).[85]

The goal is to reduce the disk protrusion and restore normal posture. When posture, pain, and segmental spinal control return to normal, the core stabilization exercises should be emphasized and progressed. The patient may recover easily from the first episode, but if repeated episodes occur, the patient should start on the reinjury stage of back rehabilitation.

When the patient changes positions—sit to stand or lying to stand—the patient should do a lateral shift self-correction (see Figures 28-12 and 28-16), followed by a segmental

Estimated Length of Time (ELT): Day 4 to Week 4

After 3 days, the patient was encouraged to come to the physical therapy clinic for treatment, once a day. The above activities were preceded with the comfort modalities of hot packs and electrical stimulation. Spinal segment stabilization was reassessed, and the patient started on the beginning-level core stability exercises. The patient was instructed to be flat-lying for 20 to 30 minutes 4 times daily and to continue to minimize time spent in sitting postures. At 1 week, the patient was encouraged to walk for conditioning and movement purposes, starting with 10 minutes and working up to 30 minutes. The walking was followed by flat-lying and positional traction periods of 20 to 30 minutes. The core stability exercises were gradually progressed to continue to challenge strength and endurance as the pain became more manageable. At 3 weeks, more functional exercises were included. Squats, balance activities, and light weight lifting (no axial loading) were begun. Flat-lying postures, 4 times daily, were encouraged. At 4 weeks, the patient was instructed to gradually increase sitting times, guided by comfort.

PHASE THREE Advanced Phase

GOALS: Maximize core stability strength and endurance, retrain functional movement patterns to include spinal segment and core stability, return normal flexibility and strength to lower extremities, and encourage good mechanics in activities of daily living.

Estimated Length of Time (ELT): Week 5 to 6 Months

The patient was reevaluated, and specific flexibility and strengthening problems were identified. Tight muscle groups were stretched 3 or 4 times a day, weak muscle groups were isolated and progressively strengthened. Spinal segment stability and core stability were stressed with more challenging exercises. Normal strength and conditioning exercises were encouraged, but technique was monitored closely and the patient was encouraged to use spinal segment stability coactivation patterns in every exercise. Functional activities of daily living drills were begun, with the patient being encouraged to incorporate spinal segment coactivation patterns into her motor planning for each drill.

Criteria for Return to Function

1. The patient demonstrates good spinal segment control in the physical therapy clinic.
2. The patient has normal flexibility and strength in her lower extremities.
3. Functional performance test scores are at least 90% of previous baseline scores.
4. The patient tolerates 1 to 1.5 hours of exercise with no symptoms.
5. The patient demonstrates in exercises that she can perform the activities of daily living with no noticeable compensatory movement patterns.

spinal coactivation contraction (see Figures 28-8 to 28-10). Some gentle flexion exercises, low back corsets, and heat wraps may make the patient more comfortable.

If the disk is extruded or sequestrated, about the only thing that can be done is to modulate pain with electrical stimulation. Flexion exercises and lying supine in a flexed position may help with comfort. The use of a low back corset or brace may also make the patient more comfortable (see Figure 28-56). Sometimes the symptoms will resolve with time, but if there are signs of nerve damage, surgery may be necessary.[85]

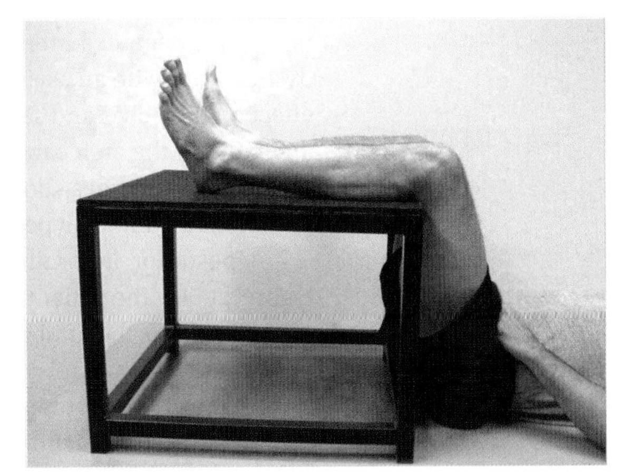

Figure 28-57 **The 90-90 position**

The patient is positioned back-lying with hips flexed to 90 degrees and knees supported at 90 degrees by stool or pillows.

Sacroiliac Joint Dysfunction

Pathomechanics and Injury Mechanism

A sprain of the sacroiliac joint may result from twisting with both feet on the ground, stumbling forward, falling backwards, stepping too far down and landing heavily on one leg, or forward bending with the knees locked during lifting.[45] Activities involving unilateral forceful movements are the usual activities associated with the onset of pain. Any of these mechanisms can produce stretching and irritation of the sacroiliac, sacrotuberous, or sacrospinous ligaments.[48]

Rehabilitation Concerns

The patient will report a dull, achy back pain near or medial to the PSIS, with some associated muscle guarding. The pain may radiate into the buttocks or posterior lateral thigh. The patient may describe a heaviness, dullness, or deadness in the leg or referred pain to the groin, adductor, or hamstring on the same side. The pain may be more noticeable during the stance phase of walking, on stair climbing, and rolling in bed.[89]

Side bending toward the painful side will increase the pain. Straight-leg raising will increase pain in the sacroiliac joint area after 45 degrees of hip motion. On palpation, there may be tenderness over the PSIS, medial to the PSIS, in the muscles of the buttocks, and anteriorly over the pubic symphysis. The back musculature will have increased tone on 1 side.[27,37,70]

If a sacroiliac joint is stressed and reaches an end-range position in rotation, the joint can become dysfunctional as pain, mechanical form-closure locking, and/or muscle guarding create hypomobility at the joint. This hypomobility is usually temporary, and often spontaneous repositioning will occur. This allows the pain to go away and muscle guarding to disappear. With the joint back to normal alignment, function returns to normal.[37,70]

When normal alignment does not spontaneously return, treatment efforts should initially mobilize or manipulate the joints and then work on spinal segment stabilization to maintain and improve sacroiliac joint stability. These exercises, along with core stability training are the key to preventing recurrences. The therapist should consider sacroiliac dysfunction as a problem with pelvic stability rather than mobility.[37,68]

Rehabilitation Progression

Recent studies of sacroiliac joint testing cast severe doubt on our ability to recognize the postural asymmetries that have been associated with directionally specific techniques.[27,37,70] The treatment of sacroiliac dysfunction has been grounded in the empiricism of doing techniques that reduce pain. Postural asymmetries have given the therapist a starting point for directionally specific techniques, but the instruction in deciding on appropriate technique is to try one and, if the outcome is not satisfactory, move on to the next technique, which may be biomechanically opposite to the first technique.[19,48] Empirically, these mobilizations have been used for many years and have demonstrated a good effect on sacroiliac dysfunctions with an asymmetry of the pelvis and pain. Each technique has about the same effect on the pelvis and sacroiliac joints because the joints are part of an arch, and forces at any point in the arch can be translated throughout the structure to the affected part of the arch. These stretches should be used only at the beginning stage of treatment to free the joint from the initial hypomobility.[89]

A posterior innominate rotation may be used to treat sacroiliac dysfunction (see Figure 28-58). The patient is positioned with legs and trunk moved toward the side of the low ASIS. This locks the lumbar spine so that the mobilization effect will be primarily at the sacroiliac joint. The therapist stands on the side away from the low ASIS and rotates the patient's trunk toward the therapist. The patient is instructed to breathe and relax as the therapist overpressures the rotation to take up the slack. The lower hand contacts the low ASIS and mobilizes or manipulates the innominate into posterior rotation.[64]

The therapist should also mobilize the sacroiliac joint using stretching positions 1 and 2 or the anterior–posterior sacroiliac joint rotation stretch to correct the postural asymmetry (Figures 28-59 and 28-60).[11-13,30,88] The stretch exercise should be done in 2 or 3 bouts a day, 3 or 4 repetitions each time, holding the stretch position for 20 to 30 seconds. Spinal segment stability exercises are utilized after each stretching bout (see Figures 28-4 to 28-10).[68] These stretches should not be continued longer than 2 or 3 days. The spinal

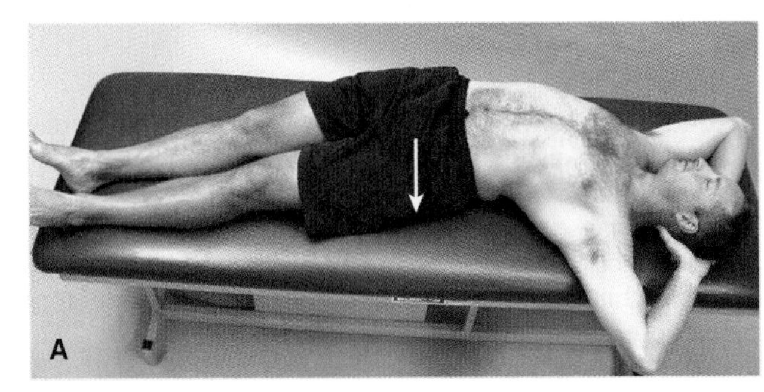

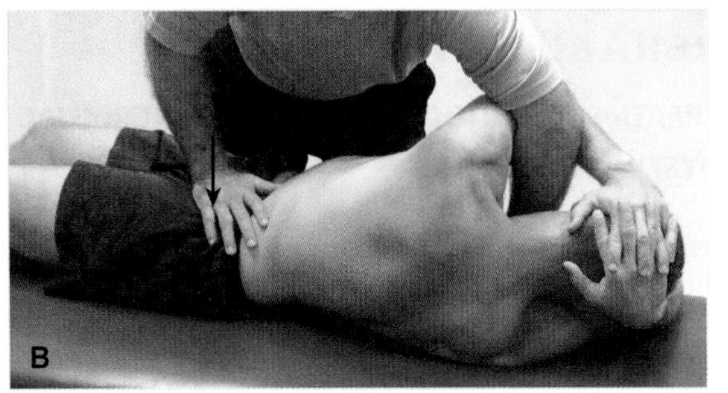

Figure 28-58 **Posterior innominate rotation**

A. Starting position. **B.** Mobilization position.

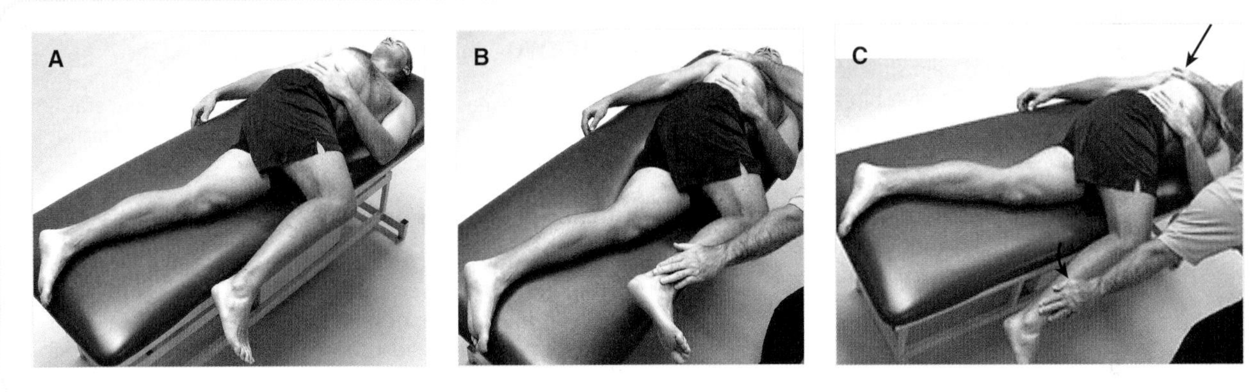

Figure 28-59 **Sacroiliac stretch, position 1**

A. Starting position. **B.** Position for isometric resistance. **C.** Stretch position.

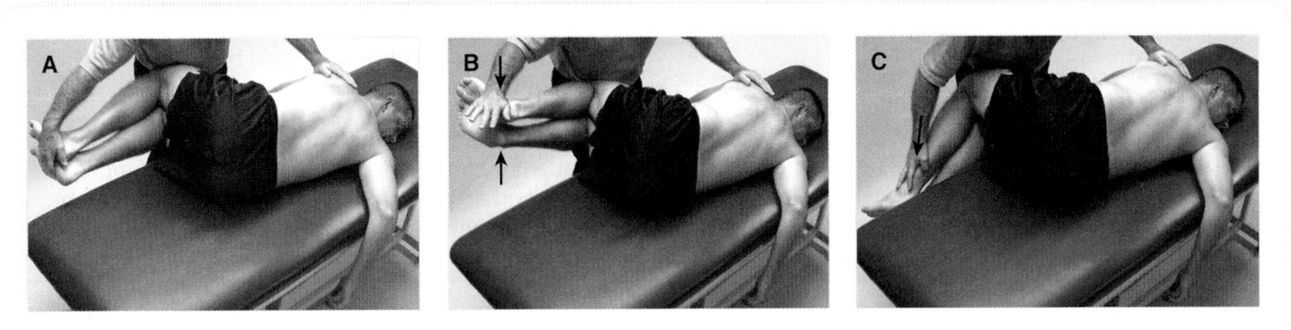

Figure 28-60 **Sacroiliac stretch, position 2**

A. Starting position. **B.** Position for isometric resistance. **C.** Stretch position.

REHABILITATION PLAN

TREATMENT PROTOCOL TO CORRECT SACROILIAC DYSFUNCTION

INJURY SITUATION A 47-year-old male was crossing an intersection when he stepped off the curb onto his left foot and misjudged the height. He felt immediate sharp pain in his low back. He was referred to physical therapy for evaluation and treatment. The patient complained of mild pain and a stiff-tight feeling in his left groin area, with hip flexion and adduction, increasing his discomfort. His previous medical history was unremarkable for hip, sacroiliac, or muscle problems, and he was in excellent physical condition with no other injuries at this time.

Functionally, the patient walked with a reduced stride length on the left, which produced a mild limp. Walking produced some mild left groin pain, and stair climbing increased this pain in his left groin. Range of motion was assessed. Lumbar spine range was full in all ranges, but side-bending left and backward bending created pain in the left sacroiliac region. Holding the backward bent position created some left groin pain similar in nature to the pain that occurred initially. Passive hip range of motion was full in all ranges, with mild groin pain provoked on the end range of flexion, abduction, and internal rotation. On manual muscle test, hip flexion and abduction were strong but produced pain in the left groin similar in nature to the presenting pain. Right and left straight-leg raise tests were positive for left groin pain. Bilateral knees-to-chest test was full-range and painless, as were the stress test of iliac approximation, iliac rotation, and posterior–anterior spring test. On palpation, there was mild tenderness along the left sacroiliac joint and over the left gluteus medius just lateral to the PSIS (posterior superior iliac spine). The hip abductors, hip flexors, and hamstring muscles were nontender but had increased tone.

PHASE ONE Acute Phase

GOALS: Modulate the pain, stretch, and strengthen the sacroiliac joint to return them to a more symmetric position.

Estimated Length of Time (ELT): Days 1 to 3

The patient was treated with stretching to bring his sacroiliac joints into symmetric positions. Spinal segment stabilization was initiated along with beginning core stabilization exercises (hip-lift bridges, isometric hip adduction ball squeezes). The left groin and sacroiliac area were treated with ice. The patient was instructed to repeat stretching and the strengthening exercises 3 times a day. He was also given analgesic medicine to make him more comfortable.

On day 2, stretching was continued and the stretching exercise load was increased by adding repetitions. A stretching program was begun for the hip abductors, hip internal rotators, hip flexors, and hamstrings. His usual weight-lifting session was modified to a nonweightbearing program. His conditioning workout was done on the exercise bike and in the pool. Hot packs were applied to the adductor area preliminary to the exercise and stretching programs. The sacroiliac area was treated with ice and electrical stimulation at a moderate sensory intensity.

On day 3, stretching was discontinued. Strengthening was increased with the addition of elastic resistance to hip abduction and adduction. Functional exercises were initiated, including line walking, minisquats, and side shuffle with tubing resistance. Modalities remained the same.

PHASE TWO Intermediate Phase

GOALS: Increase spinal segment awareness, core stabilization strength, return to functional exercises, and return to practice and play status.

Estimated Length of Time (ELT): Days 4 to 7

Pain modalities were continued. Stretching exercises to the left hip abductors, flexors, and internal rotators were continued. Strengthening exercises continued with increased repetitions, resistance, and difficulty. Hot packs and electrical stimulation were continued, as were the spinal segment and core stabilization exercises.

PHASE THREE Advanced Phase

GOALS: Maintain spinal segment strength, increase core strength, and return to normal exercise routines.

Estimated Length of Time (ELT): Day 8 to 6 Weeks Postinjury

Pain modalities should be used if needed. Tight muscle groups should continue to be stretched two or three times a day. Strengthening routines should become more challenging but not more time-consuming.

Criteria for Return to Function
The patient demonstrates that he can perform functional activities and activities of daily living with no noticeable compensatory movements.

segmental stabilization exercises are continued to try to create the behaviors that stabilize the sacroiliac joints and strengthen the muscles that support the joint. The exercises should be progressed to include more core stabilization and functional training, leading to return to sports. Corsets and pelvic stabilizing belts are also helpful during higher-level activities and/or if the patient is having problems with recurrences (see Figure 28-56).[64]

Sacroiliac stretch positions 1 and 2 that will help realign the patients' pelvis when they are having sacroiliac dysfunction. Position 1 (see Figure 28-59) and position 2 (see Figure 28-60) stretches can be done in both right side-lying and left side-lying positions. The starting position of the position-1 stretch is side-lying with the upper hip flexed 70 to 80 degrees and the knee flexed approximately 90 degrees (see Figure 28-59). The patient's trunk is then rotated toward the upper side as far as is comfortable. The patient is instructed to lift the top leg into hip abduction and internal rotation, and resist the therapist for 5 seconds. The patient is instructed to breathe and exhale as the therapist gently overpressures the trunk rotation. The patient is then instructed to relax the hip and leg and allow the leg to drop toward the floor. As the patient relaxes, the therapist applies a gentle overpressure to the foot and takes up the slack as the patient allows the hip and leg to drop further to the floor.

In the position 2 stretch (see Figure 28-60), the patient is positioned on either the right or left side. The patient is side-lying with the trunk rotated so that the lower arm is behind the hip and the upper arm is able to reach off the table toward the floor. Both knees and hips are flexed to approximately 90 degrees. The patient's knees are supported on the therapist's thigh. The therapist also supports the feet in this stage of the stretch.

Before beginning the stretch component of the position 2 stretches, the therapist provides isometric resistance to lifting both legs toward the ceiling, holding the contraction for 5 seconds. The patient is instructed to exhale while relaxing the legs and allowing them to drop toward the floor. The therapist adds a light pressure to the feet and shoulder blade area to guide the stretch and take up slack. The therapist holds the patient in a comfortable maximum stretch for 20 to 30 seconds.

SUMMARY

1. The low back pain that patients most often experience is an acute, painful experience of relatively short duration that seldom causes significant time loss from practice or competition.
2. Regardless of the diagnosis or the specificity of the diagnosis, a thorough evaluation of the patient's back pain is critical to good care.
3. Back rehabilitation may be classified as a 2-stage approach. Stage I (acute stage) treatment consists mainly of the modality treatment and pain-relieving exercises. Stage II treatment involves treating patients with a reinjury or exacerbation of a previous problem. In patients meeting the clinical prediction rule for being included in a manipulation treatment group, spinal manipulation should be initiated early in stage I.
4. Segmental spinal stabilization and core exercise should be included in the exercise plan of every patient with back pain.
5. The types of exercises that may be included in the initial pain management phase include the following: lateral shift corrections, extension exercises, flexion exercises, mobilization exercises, and myofascial stretching exercises.
6. It is suggested that the therapist use an eclectic approach to the selection of exercises, mixing the various protocols described according to the findings of the patient's evaluation.
7. Specific goals and exercises included in stage II should address which structures to stretch, which structures to strengthen, incorporating segmental spinal stabilization into the patient's daily life and exercise routine, and which movements need a motor learning approach to control faulty mechanics.
8. The rehabilitation program should include functional training that may be divided into basic and advanced phases.

9. Back pain can result from 1 or a combination of the following problems: muscle strain, piriformis muscle or quadratus lumborum myofascial pain or strain, myofascial trigger points, lumbar facet joint sprains, hypermobility syndromes, disk-related back problems, or sacroiliac joint dysfunction.
10. Cervical pain can result from muscle strains, acute cervical joint lock, ligament sprains, and various other problems.

REFERENCES

1. Adams MA, May S, Freeman BJC, Morrison HP, Dolan P. Effects of backward bending on lumbar intervertebral discs. *Spine (Phila Pa 1976)*. 2000;25(4):431-437.
2. Barr KP, Griggs M, Cadby T. Lumbar stabilization. *Am J Phys Med Rehabil*. 2005;84(6):473-480.
3. Beattie P. The use of an electric approach for the treatment of low back pain: a case study. *Phys Ther.* 1992;72(12):923-928.
4. Beffa R, Mathews R. Does the adjustment cavitate the targeted joint? An investigation into the location of cavitation sounds. *J Manipulative Physiol Ther.* 2004;27(2):1-5.
5. Bialosky JE, George SZ, Bishop MD. How spinal manipulative therapy works: why ask why? *J Orthop Sports Phys Ther.* 2008;38(6):293-295.
6. Binkley J, Finch E, Hall J, et al. Diagnostic classification of patients with low back pain: Report on a survey of physical therapy experts. *Phys Ther.* 1993;73(3):138-155.
7. Broadhurst N. Piriformis syndrome: correlation of muscle morphology with symptoms and signs. *Arch Phys Med Rehabil.* 2004;85(12):2036-2039.
8. Cagnie B, Vinck E, Beerneart A, Cambier D. How common are side effects of spinal manipulation and can these side effects be predicted? *Man Ther.* 2004;9:151-156.
9. Childs JD, Flynn TW, Fritz JM. A perspective for considering the risks and benefits of spinal manipulation in patients with low back pain. *Man Ther.* 2006;11:316-320.
10. Childs JD, Fritz JM, Flynn TW, et al. A clinical prediction rule to identify patients with low back pain most likely to benefit from spinal manipulation: a validation study. *Ann Intern Med.* 2004;141(12):920-928.
11. Cibulka M. The treatment of the sacroiliac joint component to low back pain: a case report. *Phys Ther.* 1992;72(12):917-922.
12. Cibulka M, Delitto A, Koldehoff R. Changes in innominate tilt after manipulation of the sacroiliac joint in patients with low back pain: an experimental study. *Phys Ther.* 1988;68(9):1359-1370.
13. Cibulka M, Rose S, Delitto A, et al. Hamstring muscle strain treated by mobilizing the sacroiliac joint. *Phys Ther.* 1986;66(8):1220-1223.
14. Cleland JA, Fritz JM, Whitman JM, Childs JD, Palmer JA. The use of a lumbar spine manipulation technique by a physical therapist in patients who satisfy a clinical prediction rule: a case series. *J Orthop Sports Phys Ther.* 2006;36(4):209-214.
15. Colloca CJ, Keller TS, Gunzburg R. Neuromechanical characterization of in vivo lumbar spinal manipulation. Part II: neurophysiologic response. *J Manipulative Physiol Ther.* 2003;26(9):579-591.
16. Colloca CJ, Keller TS, Gunzburg R. Biomechanical and neurophysiological responses to spinal manipulation in patients with lumbar radiculopathy. *J Manipulative Physiol Ther.* 2004;27(1):1-15.
17. DeRosa C, Porterfield J. A physical therapy model for the treatment of low back pain. *Phys Ther.* 1992;72(4):261-272.
18. Deyo R, Diehl A, Rosenthal M. How many days of bed rest for acute low back pain? A randomized clinical trial. *N Engl J Med.* 1986;315:1064-1070.
19. Donley P. Rehabilitation of low back pain in patients: the 1976 Schering symposium on low back problems. *Athl Train.* 1977;12(2):65-69.
20. Ebenbichler GR, Oddsson LI, Kollmitzer J, Erim Z. Sensory-motor control of the lower back: Implications for rehabilitation. *Med Sci Sports Exerc.* 2001;33(11):1889-1898.
21. Erhard R, Bowling R. The recognition and management of the pelvic component of low back and sciatic pain. *J Am Phys Ther Assoc.* 1979;2(3):4-13.
22. Erhard RE, Delitto A, Chibulka MT. Relative effectiveness of an extension program and a combined program of manipulation and flexion and extension exercise in patients with acute low back pain. *Phys Ther.* 1994;74(12):1093-1100.
23. Flynn TW. Move it and move on [editorial]. *J Orthop Sports Phys Ther.* 2002;32(5):193.
24. Flynn TW. There's more than one way to manipulate a spine [editorial]. *J Orthop Sports Phys Ther.* 2006;36(4):199.
25. Flynn TW, Childs JD, Fritz JM. The audible pop from high-velocity manipulation and outcome in individuals with low back pain. *J Manipulative Physiol Ther.* 2006;29(1):40-45.
26. Flynn T, Fritz J, Whitman J, et al. A clinical predication rule for classifying patients with low back pain who demonstrate short-term improvement with spinal manipulation. *Spine (Phila Pa 1976).* 2002;27(24):2835-2843.

27. Freburger JK, Riddle DL. Using published evidence to guide the examination of the sacroiliac joint region. *Phys Ther.* 2001;81(5):1135-1143.
28. Friberg O. Clinical symptoms and biomechanics of lumbar spine and hip joint in leg length inequality. *Spine (Phila Pa 1976).* 1983;8(6):643-650.
29. Frymoyer J. Back pain and sciatica: medical progress. *N Engl J Med.* 1988;318(5):291-300.
30. Grieve G. The sacroiliac joint. *Physiotherapy.* 1976;62:384-400.
31. Grieve G. Lumbar instability: Congress lecture. *Physiotherapy.* 1982;68(1):2-9.
32. Herman M. Spondylolysis and spondylolisthesis in the child and adolescent patient. *Orthop Clin North Am.* 2003;34(3):461-467.
33. Hides JA, Richardson CA, Jull GA. Multifidus muscle recovery is not automatic after resolution of acute, first-episode low back pain. *Spine (Phila Pa 1976).* 1996;21(23):2763-2769.
34. Hodges PW, Richardson CA. Inefficient muscular stabilization of the lumber spine associated with low back pain. *Spine (Phila Pa 1976).* 1996;21(22):2640-2650.
35. Hodges PW, Richardson CA. Contraction of the abdominal muscles associated with movement of the lower limb. *Phys Ther.* 1997;77(2):132-144.
36. Hodges PW. *Science of Stability: Clinical Application to Assessment and Treatment of Segmental Spinal Stabilization for Low Back Pain.* Course Handbook and Course Notes, September, Northeast Seminars, Durham, NC: 2002.
37. Hooker DN. *Evaluation of the lumbar spine and sacroiliac joint: What, why, and how?* Paper presented at the N.A.T.A. National Convention, Los Angeles, CA: 2001.
38. Huguenin L. Myofascial trigger points: the current evidence. *Phys Ther Sport.* 2004;5(1):2-12.
39. Jackson C, Brown M. Analysis of current approaches and a practical guide to prescription of exercise. *Clin Orthop Relat Res.* 1983;179:46-54.
40. Jull G, Moore A. Are manipulative therapy approaches the same? Editorial. *Man Ther.* 2002;7(2):63.
41. Lederman E. The fall of the postural-structural-biomechanical model in manual and physical therapies: exemplified by lower back pain. *CPDO Online J.* 2010;1-14.
42. Lewit K, Simons D. Myofascial pain: relief by postisometric relaxation. *Arch Phys Med Rehabil.* 1984;65(8):452-456.
43. Lindstrom I, Ohlund C, Eek C, et al. The effect of graded activity on patients with subacute low back pain: a randomized prospective clinical study with an operant-conditioning behavioral approach. *Phys Ther.* 1992;72(4):279-290.
44. MacDonald DA, Moseley GL, Hodges PW. The lumbar multifidus: does the evidence support clinical beliefs? *Man Ther.* 2006;11:254-263.
45. Maigne R. Low back pain of thoracolumbar origin. *Arch Phys Med Rehabil.* 1980;61(9):391-395.
46. Maitland G. *Vertebral Manipulation.* 5th ed. London, UK: Butterworth; 1990.
47. Mapa B. An Australian programme for management of low back problems. *Physiotherapy.* 1980;66(4):108-111.
48. McGrath M. Clinical considerations of sacroiliac joint anatomy: a review of function, motion and pain. *J Osteopath Med.* 2004;7(1):16-24.
49. McGraw M. *The Neuromuscular Maturation of the Human Infant.* New York, NY: Hafner; 1966.
50. McKenzie R. Manual correction of sciatic scoliosis. *N Z Med J.* 1972;76(484):194-199.
51. McKenzie R. *The Lumbar Spine: Mechanical Diagnosis and Therapy.* New Zealand: Lower Hutt; 1981.
52. McNeely M. A systematic review of physiotherapy for spondylolysis and spondylolisthesis. *Man Ther.* 2003;8(2):80-91.
53. Moseley GL, Nicholas MK, Hodges PW. A randomized controlled trial of intensive neurophysiology education in chronic low back pain. *Clin J Pain.* 2004;20(5):324-330.
54. Moseley GL. Is successful rehabilitation of complex regional pain syndrome due to sustained attention to the affected limb? A randomized clinical trial. *Pain.* 2005;114:54-61.
55. Moseley GL, Flor H. Targeting cortical representations in the treatment of chronic pain: a review. *Neurorehabil Neural Repair.* 2012;26(6):646-652.
56. Moseley L. Unraveling the barriers to reconceptualization of the problem in chronic pain: the actual and perceived ability of patients and health professionals to understand the neurophysiology. *J Pain.* 2003;4(4):184-189.
57. Moseley GL. Widespread brain activity during an abdominal task markedly reduced after pain physiology education: fMRI evaluation of a single patient with chronic low back pain. *Aust J Physiother.* 2005;51:49-52.
58. Norris CM. Spinal stabilization. *Physiotherapy.* 1995;81(2):61-79.
59. Norris CM. Spinal stabilization. *Physiotherapy.* 1995;81(3):127-146.
60. O'Sullivan PB, Twomey LT, Allison GT. Evaluation of specific stabilizing exercise in the treatment of chronic low back pain with radiologic diagnosis of spondylolysis or spondylolisthesis. *Spine (Phila Pa 1976).* 1997;22(24):2959-67.
61. Papadopoulos E. Piriformis syndrome. *Orthopedics.* 2004;27(8):797-799
62. Pizzutillo PD, Hummer CD. Nonoperative treatment for painful adolescent spondylolysis or spondylolisthesis. *J Pediatr Orthop.* 1994;9(5):538-540.
63. Porter R, Miller C. Back pain and trunk list. *Spine (Phila Pa 1976).* 1986;11(6):596-600.
64. Prather H. Sacroiliac joint pain: practical management. *Clin J Sport Med.* 2003;13(4):252-255.
65. Price DD, Milling LS, Kirsch I, Duff A, Montgomery GH, Nicholls SS. An analysis of factors that contributes to the magnitude of placebo analgesia in an experimental paradigm. *Pain.* 1999;83:147-156.

66. Puentedura EJ, Louw A. A neuroscience approach to managing athletes with low back pain. *Phys Ther Sport.* 2012;13(3):123-133.

67. Rantanen J, Hurme M, Falck B, et al. The lumbar multifidus muscle five years after surgery for a lumbar intervertebral disc herniation. *Spine (Phila Pa 1976).* 1993;18(5):568-574.

68. Richardson CA, Snijders CJ, Hides JA, Damen L, Pas MS, Storm J. The relationship between the transverses abdominis muscles, sacroiliac joint mechanics, and low back pain. *Spine (Phila Pa 1976).* 2002;27(4):399-405.

69. Richardson C, Jull G, Hodges P, Hides J. *Therapeutic Exercise for Spinal Segmental Stabilization in Low Back Pain.* Sydney, Australia: Churchill Livingstone; 1999.

70. Riddle D, Freburger J. Evaluation of presence of sacroiliac joint region dysfunction using a combination of tests: a multicenter intertester reliability study. *Phys Ther.* 2002;82(8):772-781.

71. Ross JK, Bereznick DE, McGill SM. Determining cavitation location during lumbar and thoracic spinal manipulation: is spinal manipulation accurate and specific? *Spine (Phila Pa 1976).* 2004;29(13):1452-1457.

72. Rubinstein SM. Adverse events following chiropractic care for subjects with neck or low back pain: Do the benefits outweigh the risks? *J Manipulative Physiol Ther.* 2008;31(6):461-464.

73. Saal J. Rehabilitation of football players with lumbar spine injury. *Phys Sportsmed.* 1988;16(9):61-68.

74. Saal J. Rehabilitation of football players with lumbar spine injury. *Phys Sportsmed.* 1988;16(10):117-125.

75. Saal J. Dynamic muscular stabilization in the nonoperative treatment of lumbar pain syndromes. *Orthop Rev.* 1990;19(8):691-700.

76. Saal JA, Saal JS. Nonoperative treatment of herniated lumbar intervertebral disk with radiculopathy: an outcome study. *Spine (Phila Pa 1976).* 1989;14(4):431-437.

77. Santilli V, Beghi E, Finucci S. Chiropractic manipulation in the treatment of acute back pain and sciatica with disc protrusion: a randomized double-blind clinical trial of active and simulated spinal manipulations. *Spine J.* 2006;6:131-137.

78. Simons D, Travell J. *Myofascial Pain and Dysfunction: The Lower Extremities.* Baltimore, MD: Lippincott Williams & Wilkins; 1998.

79. Simons D, Travell J. *Myofascial Pain and Dysfunction: The Trigger Point Manual.* Baltimore, MD: Lippincott Williams & Wilkins; 1998.

80. Solomon J. Discogenic low back pain. *Crit Rev Phys Rehabil Med.* 2004;16(3):177-210.

81. Steiner C, Staubs C, Ganon M, et al. Piriformis syndrome: pathogenesis, diagnosis, and treatment. *J Am Osteopath Assoc.* 1987;87(4):318-323.

82. Tenhula J, Rose S, Delitto A. Association between direction of lateral lumbar shift, movement tests, and side of symptoms in patients with low back pain syndrome. *Phys Ther.* 1990;70(8):480-486.

83. Threlkeld A. The effects of manual therapy on connective tissue. *Phys Ther.* 1992;72(12):893-902.

84. Twomey L. A rationale for treatment of back pain and joint pain by manual therapy. *Phys Ther.* 1992;72(12):885-892.

85. Verrills P. Interventions in chronic low back pain. *Aust Fam Physician.* 2004;33(6):421-426, 447-448.

86. Waddell G. Clinical assessment of lumbar impairment. *Clin Orthop Relat Res.* 1987;221:110-120.

87. Waddell G. A new clinical model for the treatment of low-back pain. *Spine (Phila Pa 1976).* 1987;12(7):632-644.

88. Walker J. The sacroiliac joint: a critical review. *Phys Ther.* 1992;72(12):903-916.

89. Warren P. Management of a patient with sacroiliac joint dysfunction: a correlation of hip range of motion asymmetry with sitting and standing postural habits. *J Man Manip Ther.* 2003;11(3):153-159.

Videos are available at www.accessphysiotherapy.com. Subscription is required.

29

Rehabilitation Considerations for the Older Adult

Jolene L. Bennett and Michael J. Shoemaker

OBJECTIVES

After completion of this chapter, the physical therapist should be able to do the following:

- Describe the facets of the normal aging process in terms of successful aging.
- Identify and apply common principles for managing older patients/clients with orthopedic disorders.
- Describe system changes that occur predictably with aging, inactivity and disease.
- Describe musculoskeletal injuries common to the geriatric population and the related treatment principles.
- Discuss and describe key elements of the history and physical examination for the rehabilitation of the older patient/client that may differ from younger patient/client populations.
- Understand the importance of rehabilitation for targeted functional outcomes and maintenance of functional independence in the geriatric population.

Rehabilitative care of older adults has evolved into a specialty area of practice for many clinicians. Geriatrics, or the care of the older adult, is based on the recognition that the aging process causes the body to respond differently to injury, disease, and medical care than when it was younger. The field of geriatrics continues to gain attention as a result of the rapid growth of this segment of the population and its predicted socioeconomic impact in the present century.

Traditionally, demographers have used the age of 65 years to delineate an individual reaching "old age." Reasons for this delineation include established social practices, such as retirement from work, and eligibility for benefits such as Social Security and Medicare. This segment of the population is growing steadily, both in absolute numbers and in proportion to the total population. A tremendous increase in the number of individuals reaching "old age" is projected to occur during the next 40 to 50 years. In 1900, there were 3 million persons aged 65 years and older in the United States, representing 4% of the total population. In 1988, the number of persons age 65 years and older grew to 31.6 million or 12.7% of the total population.[76] It is estimated that in 2030, more than 70 million individuals will be older than the age of 65 years, representing nearly 20% of the population.[81] This dramatic growth is a result of the large cohorts born during the post-World War II "baby boom" that will be reaching old age, and the improved survivorship in all age cohorts, especially those regarded as the oldest-old at 85+ years. The number of older adults age 85 years or older is predicted to triple in number by 2014.[14] Since the mid-19th century, life expectancy in the United States has nearly doubled, from 40 years to almost 80 years,[73] because of both medical and scientific breakthroughs and improved health habits. However, for the first time in history, life expectancy at birth has the potential to decline as a result of the effects of widespread, chronic diseases associated with obesity.[65] Thus, the United States may be faced with a large number of older adults with a greater amount of comorbidity.

The ability to move is a prerequisite to functional independence, and functional independence is considered to be a large contributor to quality of life with aging. Pain and musculoskeletal impairments can lead to disability among older Americans, and at least 39% of Medicare enrollees have at least 1 health-related activities of daily living (ADL) disability[17] and 47% report a difficulty with walking.[75] Given the projected increase in the number of older adults, the greater severity of comorbidity, and the expected prevalence of movement dysfunction, physical therapists have a critical role in helping older adults age successfully.

Orthopedic care of older adults requires the clinician to utilize a unique perspective that is different from that used when caring for younger adults. The impact of pain and musculoskeletal impairment on function is often underreported and incorrectly attributed to normal aging, and multiple comorbidities require careful consideration for providing safe and effective care. This chapter provides a perspective from which to view the older adult patient/client, in addition to specific considerations for the orthopedic rehabilitation of older adults.

Key Components of Geriatric Assessment

The following key components of geriatric assessment represent concepts unique to the older adult that should be considered when examining and developing an intervention plan for the older adult. Pain and impairments associated with musculoskeletal conditions such as osteoarthritis can have significant effects on functional status, quality of life, and the ability to continue to live independently in the community if the presenting clinical problem is not comprehensively addressed by the physical therapist. Table 29-1 presents the respective historical and examination data that should be considered for each key assessment component.

Table 29-1 History and Examination Strategies to Address Key Components of the Assessment of Older Adults

Assessment Component	History or Examination Strategy
Physiologic reserve capacity and preclinical decline	Utilize impairment- and performance-based measures with normative values • Timed Up and Go • Timed chair rise • Stair-climbing test • Six-minute walk test Ask about task modification: time to complete, compensatory strategy, or decreased frequency
Frailty	In the history and examination, consider: • Gait speed • Grip strength • Changes in activity level • Self-reported exhaustion/fatigue • Weight loss
Differentiating between the effects of aging vs. disuse vs. disease	Consider the impairments noted during the examination in light of the patient/client's clinical course and medical history
Polypharmacy	Review the medication list and be alert to common side effects and signs/symptoms not consistent with the known medical history
System-specific considerations: Cardiovascular	Screen for risk factors of cardiovascular disease Measurement of vital signs at rest and during exercise Assess for symptoms of vascular claudication Consider risk of thromboembolic disease
Pulmonary	Assess for appropriate respiratory response to exercise
Sensory	Assess sensory function and organization (sensory testing, vision screening, balance performance with conflicting sensory information) Ask about fall history and ability to rise from the floor
Neuropsychological	Screen for dementia (MMSE or SLUMS) Screen for depression (GDS)
Musculoskeletal	Screen for risk factors of osteoporosis

GDS, Geriatric Depression Scale; MMSE, Mini-Mental State Examination; SLUMS, St. Louis University Mental Status Examination.

Physiologic Reserve Capacity

Nearly all body systems demonstrate age-related changes, resulting in a reduced physiologic reserve and reduced capacity to respond to stress. Thus, older persons may require greater time to recover from exercise or acute medical illness, or they may be more susceptible to a decline in functional status. As physiologic reserve decreases, there is a threshold below which a decline in function becomes evident.[18] For example, combined quadriceps strength of approximately 300 N is required to perform a sit-to-stand without the use of the upper extremities.[31] Strength below this threshold results in impaired functional performance in sit-to-stand activities such as toileting. Another example can be found with peak oxygen consumption. Lower aerobic reserve capacity is associated with a reduced ability to complete ADL's such as housework, and an aerobic capacity of less than 20 $mL \cdot kg^{-1} \cdot min^{-1}$ is associated with a decline in community ambulation.[25]

Examination of the older adult should consider performance on functional-based tests compared to established age-related norms in order to identify clinically relevant reductions in physiologic reserve, and interventions should be provided as appropriate (Table 29-2).

The timed up-and-go test measures the time it takes to stand from a standard armchair, walk 3 meters, return to the chair, and sit. Thresholds that distinguish between levels of independence with ADL include: independence (<20 seconds), assistance with ADL (>30 seconds), and varying levels of independence (20 to 29 seconds).[68] The timed up-and-go test has also been used to assess fall risk, but has not consistently been demonstrated to be sensitive in detecting those patients who are predisposed to falling.

The timed chair rise is a measure of functional mobility and lower-body strength. Several versions of the test have been studied, including the time required to perform 5 sit-to-stand repetitions (17-inch high armless chair, no use of the upper extremities), or how many repetitions can be performed in 30 seconds.[45,46]

The 6-minute walk test has been used as a measure of exercise tolerance and endurance across a wide variety of musculoskeletal, neuromuscular, and cardiopulmonary conditions. The patient/client is instructed to walk as far as possible in 6 minutes, and vital sign response is typically monitored for heart rate, blood pressure, oxygen saturation, and perceived exertion.[4]

Comfortable gait speed is a measure of walking ability and balance. Gait speeds of less than 0.56 m/s in frail older adults have been associated with an increased risk of recurrent falls,[82] and speeds less than 0.6 m/s are strongly associated with poorer health status.[77] Comfortable gait speed can be measured over a 10-meter distance with 5 additional meters before and after the 10-meter course to allow for acceleration and deceleration.

Although grip strength is not a performance-based functional test, well-established, age-related normative data exist.[28,41,42,60,85] Additionally, grip strength is closely associated with other functional measures, development of disability, and mortality,[11,12] and also serves as a key measure for identifying frailty as discussed below.

Preclinical Disability

Given that a marked loss of physiologic reserve in one system can result in functional loss, partial loss of physiologic reserve in multiple systems may result in a change in functional status, and may be evident before a person presents to a clinician with a complaint of functional limitation or disability.[20] Preclinical disability is a clinically detectable decline in physical function, characterized by increased time to complete a task, modification of a task, or a decreased frequency of task performance.[35,37] Consequently, a patient/client may report that she only goes shopping once every 2 weeks because it is too fatiguing, or that she occasionally must use the powered cart. This patient/client may not recognize these subtle changes in task performance as being important enough to report to a health care provider, however, she might demonstrate a decline in gait speed and timed up-and-go performance that indicates the potential for continued decline in function over time. It is, therefore, important to make determinations about risk of incipient functional decline based on objective measurement(s) rather than based on patient/client self-report,[9,13,84] and to initiate interventions as early as possible to prevent further decline.

Table 29-2 Age-Related Normative Values for Functional Performance Measures

	Age Mean (Std Dev) [Std Error]		
	60-69	70-79	80-89
Timed up and go (sec)			
Male[a]	8 (2)	9 (3)	10 (1)
Female[a]	8 (2)	9 (2)	11 (3)
Combined[b]	7.24 [.17]	8.54 [.17]	
30-Second timed chair rise (reps)			
Male[c]	15.8 (4.4)	14.3 (4.2)	11.8 (4.3)
Female[c]	14 (3.75)	12.7 (3.7)	10.8 (4.1)
Combined[d]	14 (2.4)	12.9 (3.0)	11.9 (3.6)
5-Repetition timed chair rise (seconds)			
Male[e]	12.7 [.24]	13.4 [.29]	14.7 [.25]
Female[e]	13.2 [.22]	14.2 [.29]	16.58 [.30]
6-Minute walk test (meters)			
Male[a]	572 (92)	527 (85)	417 (73)
Female[b]	538 (92)	471 (75)	392 (85)
Male[c]	597 (90)	534 (104)	457 (120)
Female[c]	536 (85)	483 (97)	406 (113)
Comfortable gait speed (m/s)			
Male[a]	1.59 (.24)	1.38 (.23)	1.21 (.18)
Female[a]	1.44 (.25)	1.33 (.22)	1.15 (.21)

[a]Steffen TM, Hacker TA, Mollinger L. Age- and gender-related test performance in community-dwelling elderly people: six-minute walk test, berg balance scale, timed up and go, and gait speeds. *Phys Ther.* 2002;82:128-137.
[b]Isles RC, Low Choy NL, Steer M, Nitz JC. Normal values of balance tests in women aged 20-80. *J Am Geriatr Soc.* 2004;52:1367-1372.
[c]Rikli RE, Jones CJ. Functional fitness normative scores for community-residing older adults, aged 60-94. *J Aging Phys Act.* 1999;7:162-181.
[d]Jones CJ, Rikli RE, Beam WC. A 30 s chair stand test as a measure of lower body strength in community-residing older adults. *Res Q Exerc Sport.* 1999;70:113-117.
[e]Ostechega Y, Harris TB, Hirsch R, et al. Reliability and prevalence of physical performance examination assessing mobility and balance in older persons in the US: data from the Third National Health and Nutrition Examination Survey. *J Am Geriatr Soc.* 2000;48:1136-1141.

Frailty

In contrast to preclinical disability, it is also important to identify patients/clients who are frail, as these individuals are at high risk for a variety of adverse health outcomes, including imminent nursing home placement, surgical complications, hospitalization, and death.[50] The definition of frailty is currently under debate, although a commonly accepted definition

is the presence of any 3 of the following 5 characteristics: slow gait speed, impaired grip strength, self-reported decline in activity level, self-reported exhaustion or generalized fatigue, and unintentional weight loss.[36,50] Physical therapists are uniquely positioned to identify most of these characteristics, provide appropriate rehabilitative interventions, and make appropriate medical referrals.

Differentiation Between the Effects of Aging, Inactivity, and Disease

The diagnostic process used by physical therapists includes confirming or refuting hypotheses that attempt to explain why a particular patient/client presents with movement dysfunction. In the older adult, the history and physical examination must differentiate between the effects of aging, inactivity, and disease and the underlying impairments and functional limitations that result in movement dysfunction. Mild impairments in range of motion (ROM) may be a result of increased stiffness associated with aging that occurs in the tendinous or ligamentous structures around a joint. They may also be a result of chronic inactivity and reduced demand on a particular joint for full ROM. It is also possible that an acute immobilization contributed to the disuse of a particular joint. Additionally, ROM impairments may be caused by a pathologic process within the joint or periarticular tissues. In the older adult, pronounced effects of aging, increased likelihood of multiple disease states, and greater susceptibility to the effects of inactivity all require careful differentiation during the examination.

Polypharmacy

Older persons are more likely to have a number of medical problems and are likely taking many medications. An excessive number of prescribed medications is known as *polypharmacy*. Additionally, it should be noted that older patients/clients often take different medications prescribed by different physicians, which may contribute to polypharmacy. It has been reported that 87% of older patients/clients are taking at least 1 prescription medication and 3 over-the-counter drugs each day.[63] There is a linear relationship between the number of drugs taken and the increased potential for adverse drug reactions.[40] Approximately 19% of hospital admissions of older persons are attributable to drug reactions.[40] Increased sensitivity to drug effects can be a consequence of changes in drug absorption with age, the number of drugs taken simultaneously, or failure of health care providers to take into account the proper way to prescribe and administer drugs to geriatric patients/clients.

Although there are many potential adverse outcomes of polypharmacy, some are of particular interest to those who treat geriatric patients and clients. The effects of drugs—particularly benzodiazepines, barbiturates, and antidepressants—are among the risk factors associated with falls.[54] Even if the individual does not suffer a serious fall, the threat of a fall is often enough to cause one to limit activity, which results in deconditioning and functional decline. Delirium, a temporary change in attention and consciousness, may be mistaken for dementia (a permanent loss of intellectual abilities), when in fact it may be attributable to drug sensitivity. Confusion is especially common when drug reactions occur in someone with pre-existing mild dementia. A person suffering from a mild adverse drug reaction that goes undetected for months may experience a gradual reduction in self-care skills and independence. Patients/clients experiencing musculoskeletal complaints often are chronic users of nonsteroidal antiinflammatory drugs, which can cause gastric bleeding. Narcotics may result in oversedation and loss of functional ability.[56]

The primary care physician should regularly monitor all medications taken by older adults. The physician needs to know what drugs the patient/client is taking so that the physician can eliminate duplications and generally be aware of and avoid adverse effects of drug interactions. A thorough history of the older adult seeking rehabilitation services should include a list of current medications. One should consider adverse reactions when evaluating acute changes in functional ability and mentation. Patients/clients and families should be instructed to keep all medications in the original containers, never mix several drugs in one bottle, and throw away what is no longer in use.

System Changes with Aging, Inactivity, and Disease

Cardiovascular System

With age, there is a decrease in maximal heart rate, a mild decrease in stroke volume, and reduced arteriovenous O_2 difference that contribute to a reduction in maximal oxygen consumption (VO_{2max}) by approximately 5% to 15% per decade after age 25.[69] Activity level, however, can either mitigate or exacerbate this loss. Older adult subjects have demonstrated gains in VO_{2max} comparable to younger subjects when placed on an exercise or training program. Acute inactivity, such as that which occurs with hospitalization, can account for drastic reductions in VO_{2max}. Increased blood viscosity (from fluid loss and subsequent increase in hematocrit) and venous stasis increase the risk of thromboembolic disease. Cardiac diseases, such as coronary artery disease and the sequelae of myocardial infarction and cardiomyopathy, will greatly reduce VO_{2max}. Peripheral arterial vascular disease can substantially reduce walking tolerance through muscle ischemia and claudication pain.[69]

The impact of these changes on function is of great concern. First, with a reduction in activity tolerance, there is a tendency in older adults for further activity curtailment, resulting in further deconditioning and exacerbation of disease. Following hospitalization, older patients/clients may sustain a significant decline in function. Up to 35% of older patients/clients admitted to acute care demonstrated a decline in ADL by discharge.[23] Those patients/clients with cardiovascular disease and a history of inactivity are at a much greater risk of an adverse event during exercise; therefore, careful consideration, screening, and monitoring must occur to ensure safety during a rehabilitation program.

In a direct access setting, physical therapists must be able to screen for risk factors of cardiovascular disease, perform and interpret a cardiovascular history, and safely account for cardiac disease by modifying exercise programs and making appropriate referrals to other practitioners. Because of the high prevalence of cardiovascular disease in older adults, it is essential that physical therapists in orthopedic practice screen for and assess cardiovascular comorbidities in *each* patient/client encounter. Table 29-3 highlights modifiable and non-modifiable risk factors for cardiovascular disease. The American Heart Association (adapted by Brooks)[15,33] has guidelines for risk classification and vital sign monitoring during exercise, and should be strongly considered when initiating or progressing exercise in an older adult with known risk factors for cardiovascular disease (Table 29-4).

Table 29-3 Risk Factors for Cardiovascular Disease

Risk Factors
Modifiable Risk Factors
Age >55 years for males, >65 years for females
Stress
Smoking
Hypertension
Hyperlipidemia
Physical inactivity
Nonmodifiable Risk Factors
Age
Family history
Male gender
Other Risk Factors
Diabetes Mellitus
Obesity

Table 29-4 Risk Classification for Exercise Training and Vital Sign Monitoring

American Heart Association Risk Classification	Stress Test or Physician Clearance	Vital Sign Monitoring
A1	No	At rest during initial exam.
A2	Yes	At rest and during exercise on initial exam only.
A3	Yes	At rest and during exercise on initial exam; consider periodic monitoring.
B	Yes	At rest and during exercise until safety established, and whenever intensity is increased.
C	Yes	At rest and during exercise throughout the episode of care.
D	Yes	Exercise for conditioning purposes not recommended. Monitor vital signs at rest and during changes in functional activity level.

Class A1: Nonelderly with no symptoms or risk factors.
A2: Elderly patients with less than 2 cardiovascular risk factors.
A3: Elderly patients with more than 2 risk factors.

Class B: Known cardiovascular disease but stable and without resting ischemia or angina.
History of mild heart failure; compensated, stable.
Appropriate vital sign response with activity.
Only mild dyspnea, fatigue, or palpitations with normal, higher level activities (New York Heart Classes I and II).

Class C: Inappropriate vital sign response to activity/exercise.
Moderate to significant dyspnea, fatigue, or palpitations with low levels of activity (New York Heart Classes III and IV).
Known ischemia during exercise testing.

Class D: Unstable ischemia/angina at rest.
Severe valvular stenosis or regurgitation.
Heart failure that is not compensated.
Uncontrolled arrhythmias.

Deep vein thrombosis is another potentially fatal cardiovascular disease that requires consideration by the orthopedic physical therapist. Patients/clients undergoing orthopedic surgery with subsequent immobilization of a limb are at particularly high risk for deep vein thrombosis. The popular Homan sign is of little clinical value, as it has been demonstrated to have sensitivity of less than 50%. Wells et al[71,83] developed clinical decision rules that can be particularly useful in assessing likelihood of the presence of deep vein thrombosis (Table 29-5).

Pulmonary System

Age-related changes in the pulmonary system include reduced chest wall compliance, decreased lung elasticity, and increased peripheral chemoreceptor sensitivity to respond to respiratory acidosis.[69] These changes, however, do not account for limitations in exercise tolerance. Therefore, dyspnea not explained by previous medical history, especially in the absence of a recent cardiac work-up, requires physician referral.

Table 29-5 **Clinical Decision Rule Developed by Wells and Colleagues to Predict Likelihood of Peripheral Deep Vein Thrombosis**

Active cancer (within 6 months of diagnosis or palliative care)	1
Paralysis, paresis, or recent plaster immobilization of lower extremity	1
Recently bedridden ≥3 days or major surgery within 4 weeks of application of clinical decision rule	1
Localized tenderness along distribution of the deep venous system[a]	1
Entire lower-extremity swelling	1
Calf swelling ≥3 cm compared with asymptomatic lower extremity[b]	1
Pitting edema (greater in the symptomatic lower extremity)	1
Collateral superficial veins (nonvaricose)	1
Alternative diagnosis as likely or greater than that of deep vein thrombosis[c]	2

Score interpretation:
0: probability of proximal lower-extremity deep vein thrombosis (PDVT) of 3% [95% confidence interval (CI) 1.7% to 5.9%]
1 or 2: probability of PDVT of 17% (95% CI 12% to 23%)
3: probability of PDVT of 75% (95% CI 63% to 84%)

[a]Tenderness along the deep venous system is assessed by firm palpation in the center of the posterior calf, the popliteal space, and along the area of the femoral vein in the anterior thigh and groin.
[b]Measured 10 cm below tibial tuberosity.
[c]Most common alternative diagnoses are cellulitis, calf strain, and postoperative swelling.

Inactivity, especially bed rest, can have significant impact on pulmonary function, primarily as a result of mismatches in ventilation and perfusion, reduced alveolar ventilation, and increased susceptibility to airway closure and secretion retention.

Pulmonary diseases are most responsible for ventilatory limitations that affect exercise tolerance in the older adult. Diseases such as emphysema and chronic bronchitis comprise the diagnoses known as chronic obstructive pulmonary diseases. Restrictive diseases, including pulmonary fibrosis, may also account for dyspnea and limited exercise tolerance in the older adult.[69]

The impact of these age-, inactivity-, and disease-related changes in the pulmonary system on function often results in the downward spiral of activity-curtailment and further deconditioning because of dyspnea. These patients/clients may also have complaints about fatigue. Patients with pulmonary disease are also more susceptible to recurrent infections and disease exacerbation, leading to frequent hospitalization and associated functional decline.

Because cardiac disease is frequently present as a comorbidity in patients/clients with lung disease, the aforementioned discussion regarding risk factors and monitoring is applicable. Additionally, positioning during physical therapy interventions is a consideration, as the supine position without an elevated head can result in dyspnea. Because of a significant reduction in exercise tolerance, frequent rest breaks, as well as cueing to increase respiratory depth and decrease respiratory rate, may be needed. Breath holding should be avoided, and coordination of breathing with movement should be encouraged.

Sensory Systems

Maintaining an upright posture requires adequate sensory input regarding the body's position in space. Somatosensory, visual, and vestibular information comprise the 3 main sensory systems involved in balance and postural control. Because falls pose such a significant concern for the older adult, often resulting in orthopedic injuries, having an understanding of how age and disease can impact these sensory systems is important for physical therapists managing older patients/clients with orthopedic dysfunction.

Age-related changes in somatosensation include diminished touch, vibration, and proprioception senses.[24] Age-related changes in vision include decreased visual acuity, contrast sensitivity, dark adaptation, and depth perception.[24] Age-related changes in the vestibular system include reduced sensory hair cells and neurons, which reduces sensitivity to movement and position.[24] Any of these changes alone should not account for clinically significant declines in performance. However, when combined with either significant age-related change in multiple systems or disease in 1 or more of the sensory systems, these changes can contribute to impaired balance and increased fall risk.

Somatosensory diseases such as peripheral polyneuropathy associated with diabetes can contribute to increased fall risk and decreased stability, especially on nonlevel surfaces and when walking in dark or low-light conditions. Common diseases affecting vision include macular degeneration, cataracts, and glaucoma. If the treatment room has windows, make sure the sunlight is not directly in the patient/client's eyes. The patient/client should sit with his or her back to the window and the clinician should have the daylight shining on the clinician's face to enhance the visual contrast for the patient/client. Reduced visual function results in difficulty maintaining balance on un-level surfaces, and can markedly impair the ability to maintain balance in the presence of vestibular disease. Vestibular diseases such as vestibular neuritis, Ménière disease, and perilymphatic fistula will greatly reduce the ability to maintain balance and stability in low-light conditions, nonlevel surfaces, or in the presence of impaired vision or somatosensation.

Screening for sensory impairment contributions to impaired balance is necessary to develop optimal compensatory strategies, designing an appropriate balance retraining program, or to facilitate referral to a specialized balance center or other appropriate practitioner. Furthermore, obtaining a patient/client's fall history is an essential element to the geriatric history, especially for those orthopedic problems that are the result of a fall or that may contribute to impaired balance and gait disturbances. Orthopedic foot problems, lower-extremity weakness, and gait disturbances are consistently found to increase fall risk. Persons with 1 or more falls in the preceding 6 months are at an elevated risk for future falls.[72,74] Asking about ability to rise from the floor without assistance is not only an indicator about general mobility; need for instruction in floor transfers can be determined as well.

Auditory changes with age include high frequency hearing loss, reduced speech discrimination, and reduced filtering of background noise.[24] A variety of disease processes can further reduce conductive and/or sensorineural hearing function. Clinicians need to make an extra effort to speak directly to the patient/client, enunciate clearly, vary the volume of speech as necessary, reduce background noise, and utilize visual and tactile cues to augment communication.

Dementia and Depression

Dementia

Age-related declines in cognitive function are relatively minimal compared to changes that occur due to pathology such as Alzheimer disease and vascular dementia, and the

Table 29-6 **Strategies for Providing Intervention to Cognitively Impaired Elderly**

- *Simplify* instructions, cues (verbal, visual, and tactile), programs, environment.
- *Explain* in simple terms, in a consistent manner, with frequent repetition.
- *Slow down* speech, pace of session.
- *Avoid change*—maintain consistency of therapist, environment, program.
- *Accept the patient's reality*—in patients with severe dementia, to the extent practicable, do not correct the patient's perception of time, location, and purpose.
- *Educate and support the family*—include family, if willing, in education on treatment plan, and home exercise programs. Also be ready to confront denial in the patient and family about the patient's cognitive impairments. Encourage seeking out support groups, respite care, etc.

dementia that occurs with increasing age. Acute changes in cognitive function (delirium) do have an element of reversibility, but can often contribute to additional, persistent changes.[56]

The functional impact of cognitive decline is great, and leads to increasing dependence on others in order to remain in the community, and is highly associated with nursing home placement. Additionally, cognitive-related ADL changes and loss of function are diagnostic features of dementia.[26]

Detection of cognitive decline and initiation of referral for further work-up is important so that reversible causes can be ruled out, patient/caregiver education can begin, and referral to appropriate resources can be made to minimize the impact on function. Of particular concern to the orthopedic physical therapist is to ensure that instruction in precautions and home exercise programs be presented simply in order to ensure retention and follow-through.[56] Table 29-6 provides strategies to help with this.

Screening for dementia can be accomplished using the Mini-Mental State Examination[34] or the St. Louis University Mental Status Examination.[78] Both instruments provide thresholds that can help determine severity of impairment and need for medical referral.

Depression

Up to 18% of older adults experience depression, and depression is closely associated with physical disability, chronic pain, and cognitive decline.[39] It is essential that symptoms of depression be recognized and that appropriate referrals be made, especially given the multiple treatment options that are available, including medication, psychotherapy, and family therapy. In the older adult, depression is primarily manifested via physical rather than emotional symptoms.[64] This places the physical therapist in a key position to help with early detection of symptoms of depression and the subsequent need for referral.

The impact of depression on function cannot be overstated. Those with persistent symptoms of depression have been shown to have up to a 5-fold increase in functional disability over time, and depression has been shown to negatively impact rehabilitation gains and functional status during inpatient rehabilitation.[55,83] Depression can also impact cognitive functioning, and is considered to be a cause of reversible dementia.

Physical therapists may suspect depression in patients/clients with overt or preclinical functional decline, especially in the absence of any change in medical status. Symptoms of depression also may be suspected in patients/clients who are having trouble with concentration, retention of home exercise programs, or other signs of cognitive decline.

Additionally, probing questions about stressors, changes, or losses may help with determining whether depressive symptoms are contributing to the observed cognitive and functional decline.

The Geriatric Depression Scale is available in both 30- and 15-item formats.[2,87] Thresholds for both formats are available to indicate the possible presence of depression that can guide medical referral.

Musculoskeletal System

The biologic and mechanical behaviors of all of the musculoskeletal soft tissues—including skeletal muscle, articular cartilage, intervertebral disks, tendons, ligaments, and joint capsules—are altered with age.

Skeletal Muscle

Loss of skeletal muscle mass with age is well documented. Muscle size decreases an average of 30% to 40% over a lifetime and affects the lower extremities more than the upper extremities.[38] This decrease in muscle mass is a direct result of a reduction in both muscle fiber size and number that occurs with advancing age and is largely attributed to progressive inactivity and sedentary lifestyles.[38] Fiber loss appears to be more accelerated in type II muscle fibers, which decrease from an average of 60% in sedentary young men to below 30% after the age of 80 years.[53] Type II fibers have approximately twice the intrinsic strength per unit area, and twice the velocity of contraction, of type I fibers, and are used primarily in activities requiring power such as sprinting or strength training and are not stimulated by normal ADL.

Strength Changes

With reduced muscle mass comes a reduction in muscle force production, strength, and aerobic fitness—frequently hallmarks of advancing age. Strength loss may begin slowly around the age of 50 years and becomes more rapid with advancing age. Strength loss correlates with mass loss until advanced age, at which time fiber atrophy may not account fully for the observed strength loss, suggesting a possible neural influence. Loss of muscle strength with age is attributed to muscle fiber loss, muscle fiber atrophy, and denervation of muscle fibers.[67]

Strength Training

Exercise intensity has been shown to be the most important variable for improving strength and function in the older adult.[16] High-intensity strength training (60% to 80% of one's 1-repetition maximum) has been shown to be safe and result in significant gains in muscle strength, size, and functional mobility even in the most frail older adult.[16] Improvements in lower-extremity strength positively impacts mobility and independence with ADL. Sedentary individuals should begin exercise programs at lower initial levels and progressively increase intensity as tolerance allows. Individuals with arthritic joints may not tolerate large compressive forces across the joints and will require modifications in exercise position and intensity. It is also important to incorporate exercises that work on retraining the easily atrophied type II fibers. Exercises incorporating quicker, more explosive actions are also necessary to prepare the older adult patient for real life situations such as tripping on an obstacle and losing their balance. These explosive and reactive type of exercises must be modified for each patient/client's level of function and progress as tolerated, taking safety into consideration with each task.

Articular Cartilage

Morphologic changes in articular cartilage with age include a reduced number of chondrocytes, decreased rates of collagen and elastin synthesis, altered composition of fibril types, and reduced water content. Dehydrated cartilage may have a reduced ability to dissipate forces across the joint, leading to increased susceptibility to mechanical failure.[1] With aging and increased wear and tear, cartilage may break down, beginning with fibrillation and eventually leading to sclerosis of subchondral bone and continued cartilage degeneration. Some degree of mechanical breakdown seems to be part of the normal aging process, but severe destruction of cartilage and subchondral bone involvement leads to osteoarthritis (OA), which is the most common form of joint disease in the United States. OA can lead to significant impairments in joint function and marked disability, leading to eventual joint replacement. Rehabilitation efforts should include reduction of pain, elimination of joint stress, maintenance of joint ROM, maintenance of strength and endurance, and improvement in functional independence.[66]

Tendon, Ligament and Joint Capsule

The most prevalent symptom of changes in periarticular connective tissue is loss of extensibility, which results in subsequent reduction in joint motion. Changes in structure and function may occur as a result of normal aging and from disuse and inactivity. In addition, the tensile properties of some ligament–bone complexes show a decline in tensile stiffness and ultimate load to failure with increasing age.[86] Degenerative changes in dense fibrous tissues may result in spontaneous or low-energy-level ruptures of the rotator cuff of the shoulder, the long head of the biceps, the posterior tibial tendon, patellar ligament, and Achilles tendon; they also may lead to sprains of joint capsules and ligaments, including those of the spine. Care should be taken with explosive, high-energy activities and loading of joints in the older individual, especially when initiating an exercise program in a previously sedentary person.

Bone

Bone mineral density is defined as bone mineral content relative to the area or volume of bone in the site of measurement and is expressed as g/cm^2, with 2 g/cm^2 considered a normal value. Strength of bone and ability to withstand compressive and tensile forces is related to bone mineral density. Bone mineral density reductions are known to occur with age and disuse, as are the strength properties of bone. Throughout life, women may lose as much as 35% to 40% of cortical bone and 50% to 60% of trabecular bone.[27] Men lose slightly less bone with age. Reduction of bone mineral density below 1 g/cm^2 is considered below the fracture threshold and increases the risk of osteoporotic-related fractures.

Osteoporosis

Osteoporosis is a generalized disease of bone in which there is a marked decrease in the amount of bone. The World Health Organization defines osteoporosis as a decrease in bone mineral density of more than 2.5 standard deviations below the mean as compared to young

Table 29-7 Risk Factors for Developing Osteoporosis

- Age (over 50 years)
- Genetic factors
  - Sex (women > men)
  - Race (white > black)
  - Family history
  - Body type (small frame > large frame)
- Postmenopause
- Nutritional factors
  - Low body weight
  - Low dietary intake of calcium
  - High alcohol consumption
  - Eating disorders
  - High caffeine consumption
- Lifestyle factors
  - Immobilization/inactivity
  - Cigarette smoking
- Medical factors
  - Early menopause
  - Medication use: corticosteroids, antacids, anticoagulants
  - Menstrual cycle disorders

normals. Postmenopausal osteoporosis is caused by a decrease in estrogen and results in rapid bone loss 5 to 7 years following the onset of menopause. Women in this group have a high incidence of vertebral body fractures with subsequent postural changes, loss of body height, and persistent pain and loss of function. Advancing age is among the risk factors for developing osteoporosis (Table 29-7). Age-related osteoporosis occurs equally in men and women ages 70 years and greater, and manifests mainly in hip and vertebral fractures. Fractures of the proximal humerus, proximal tibia, pelvis, and metatarsal bones are also common. It may be prudent to assume that even asymptomatic older adults may have a reduction in bone mineral density, as reduced bone mineral density of as much as 30% may be present before being evident on plain radiographs. Exercise and mechanical stress to the bone, along with estrogen replacement and increased calcium consumption, have been well documented as preventative for the development and progression of osteoporosis.[52] Weightbearing and strengthening exercises have been shown to maintain bone density and reduce the incidence of osteoporosis-related fractures.[52] A consistent program of walking may be adequate for the lower extremities and spine, but upper-extremity resistance exercises should also be performed. For the older individual, safety and fall prevention during exercise are important concerns. The therapist should be creative in designing exercises that stress the skeletal system while ensuring safety of the patient/client.

Many patients/clients who receive physical therapy have medical conditions that require long-term corticosteroid use. Corticosteroids assist in the management of inflammatory and autoimmune illnesses. Unfortunately, long-term corticosteroid use results in a significant decrease in bone density. Bone density for patients/clients treated with corticosteroids for periods of 5 years is 20% to 40% less than density for nontreated control subjects.[70] Clinicians need to be aware of their patients/clients' use of corticosteroids because exercise and activity protocols for these patients/clients may need to be modified in order to prevent fractures from occurring.

Aging Spine

As noted above, the bone density changes of the spine are significant and a normal part of aging. Other structures that undergo significant aging changes within the spine include the ligaments of the spine, the intervertebral discs, and the zygapophyseal joints. As noted above, the aging ligaments of the spine are no different than other ligaments in the body, and they also diminish in tensile strength. This loss in tensile strength combined with loss of trunk musculature strength may lead into spinal instability. The ligamentum flavum thickens with aging and it has been demonstrated that there is a 50% increase in thickness in persons older than 60 years of age.[80] The thickened ligamentum flavum occupies valuable space within the spinal canal and with extension of the spine this ligament can cause spinal cord compression because it causes narrowing of the canal. This spinal canal narrowing is also exacerbated in the older adult patient/client by the usual aging process of osteophyte development. Lumbar stenosis is a common diagnosis among the older adult.

The intervertebral disc also undergoes significant changes with aging. The greatest changes occur at the nucleus pulposus and the transitional region between the nucleus pulposus and the annulus fibrosis. Dehydration of the nucleus pulposus starts to occur by the age of 40 years and the gelatinous nucleus pulposus becomes firm. The disc becomes stiffer and this stiffness plays a role in the decreased overall spinal ROM noted in the older adult. With aging, fissures and cracks begin to appear in the disc and disc herniation may progress with increased flexion loads to the spine while performing ADL with poor body mechanics and sustained sitting postures that are common in the older patient/client. The aging discs' ability to distribute force is also altered with these physiologic changes, and thus greater load is placed on the vertebral bodies, zygapophyseal joints, and spinal ligaments. The zygapophyseal joints undergo a degenerative process that is typical of synovial joints and degeneration of the articular cartilage is noted particularly in the cervical and lumbar spines.[58] Spinal disorders may progress into decreased mobility because of pain and lower-extremity weakness, and with decreased mobility comes the other functional deficits noted in previous sections. It is important for the physical therapist to thoroughly evaluate the aging client to determine if the pain is musculoskeletal, neurogenic, vascular, or systemic in origin. The aging process causes dysfunction in all of these systems and any one of these systems may be the cause of spine pain. The treatment program must look at the total body and include lower-extremity strengthening and flexibility exercise to provide a foundation that allows the aging client to perform proper body mechanics. Trunk stabilization exercises must also be incorporated, but the clinician may need to alter the position of treatment to accommodate areas of weakness or stiffness in the older adult patient/client.

Fractures in the Older Adult

Fractures are a common occurrence in older adults and are of both medical and socioeconomic importance. Approximately 250,000 individuals older than the age of 65 years experience a hip fracture in the United States each year.[79] Hip fractures alone have an associated mortality rate as high as 50%. Other common fracture sites include the proximal humerus, distal radius, and the vertebral bodies. There are many reasons for the increased incidence of fractures in the older adult, but the 2 primary risk factors are osteoporosis and falls. Therefore, interventions for fractures in the older adult should also include measures to prevent osteoporosis and reduce the risk for falls. Once a fracture has occurred, the clinician must work toward the restoration of preinjury levels of function, mobility, and self-care.

Fractures of the Proximal Humerus

Fractures of the proximal humerus account for approximately 4% to 5% of all fractures.[10] Their incidence rises dramatically beyond the fifth decade of life and occurs more frequently among women than among men. Existing osteoporosis is a major risk factor for proximal humeral fractures in the senior population. The most common mechanism of injury is a fall on an outstretched hand from standing height or lower. Fractures of the proximal humerus sustained in this manner are usually through the surgical neck and are nondisplaced or minimally displaced. When the mechanism involves a direct blow to the shoulder (as in a fall to the side without a protective response), the fracture pattern is usually much more complex.

Classification

Approximately 85% of fractures at the proximal humerus are nondisplaced or minimally displaced.[21] The remaining 15% exhibit various fracture patterns. Neer developed the most commonly used classification system for these fractures (Table 29-8). The Neer system classifies fractures according to the number of parts or fracture fragments and the degree of angulation (or malalignment) of the parts. To be classified as displaced or angulated, the

Table 29-8 Neer Classification System for Humerus Fractures

Category	Description
1-Part	Nondisplaced or minimally displaced
2-Part	1 Part displaced > 1 cm or angulated > 45°
3-Part	2 Parts displaced and/or angulated from each other, and from the remaining part
4-Part	4 Parts displaced and/or angulated from each other
Fracture dislocation	Displacement of the humeral head from the joint space with fracture

part must be displaced at least 1 cm or angulated at least 45 degrees.[22] The 4 important parts that may be displaced or angulated are the head (at the level of the surgical neck or anatomic neck), the greater and lesser tuberosities, and the shaft. With fracture of either of the tuberosities, the pull of the attached muscles likely will cause displacement of the fracture fragments. Fractures at the level of the anatomic neck frequently cause interruption of blood supply to the humeral head and may result in avascular osteonecrosis.

Treatment

Many methods of treatment of proximal humeral fractures have been proposed through the years. The disability that results from proximal humeral fracture is usually the result of lost ROM and the development of a frozen shoulder. Shoulder ROM can be lost by angular deformity of the proximal humerus, injury to the rotator cuff, or the development of arthrofibrosis secondary to prolonged immobilization.[22] The treatment goal for patients/clients with a proximal humeral fracture is a united fracture with pain-free function. To achieve this goal, reasonable restoration of the normal anatomy and early rehabilitation are needed. Fortunately, the majority of proximal humeral fractures are nondisplaced or minimally displaced and can be satisfactorily treated with conservative measures. The arm is immobilized with a sling until pain and discomfort decrease. Active exercises for the elbow, wrist, and fingers should begin immediately to avoid stiffness and disability in these noninjured joints. Initial immobilization and early motion has been continually described as having a high degree of success because most proximal humeral fractures are minimally displaced. Because adhesive capsulitis is a frequent complication after fractures of the proximal humerus, early motion exercises should begin as soon as tolerated. Typically, active-assisted exercises can begin about 1 week after the injury. The patient/client should wear the sling during periods of activity (such as walking) or when sleeping until the soft callus has stabilized the fracture fragments (usually 3 to 4 weeks after injury). The patient/client may remove the sling while exercising or when inactive (such as resting in a chair). Attention should also be given to scapular stabilization exercises. The function of these muscles is important for normal scapulohumeral rhythm. As the fracture healing approaches a clinical union, strengthening exercise with external resistance should be added to the overall program (Table 29-9).

Displaced Humeral Fractures

Displaced fractures are difficult to treat by closed reduction. Even if closed reduction of the "2-part" and more severe fracture is successful, the rehabilitation program may need to be scaled back to avoid redisplacement. This is especially important if the pull of the muscle

Table 29-9 Exercise Guidelines for Proximal Humerus Fractures

Problem	Exercise	Time Line
Maintain or improve ROM	Assisted ROM (wand, wall climbs, pendulum) Passive Overhead stretching (overhead pulley)	End of inflammatory stage (usually 1 week)
Restore strength	Submaximal isometrics	No risk of fragment displacement, usually immediate
	Full active ROM against gravity	X-ray evidence of union, usually 6 weeks
	External resistance/isotonics	Ability to perform full active ROM against gravity, X-ray evidence of union, usually 6 weeks
Maximize function	Touch top of head, back of neck, low back	Assisted—evidence of callus Unassisted—X-ray evidence of union, usually 6 weeks

attachments displaced one of the tuberosities. Fractures classified as 2-part and above have a greater likelihood of operative reduction and internal fixation to achieve stable fixation.[21]

For patients/clients who are undergoing open reduction with internal fixation, the postoperative goals remain the same as with non-displaced fractures: early return to function and avoiding the development of adhesive capsulitis. Because of the numerous types of fracture patterns and different surgical fixations, exercise guidelines must be individualized and modified as needed. In some cases, the surgeon will be confident that the internal fixation is stable and the patient/client may progress through the exercise program more rapidly. In other cases, pace of the rehabilitation program will be slower secondary to comminution, osteoporosis, or damage to the vascular supply. Each of these may compromise stability and/or delay healing.

Fractures of the Distal Radius

Fractures of the distal radius are one of the most common fractures encountered in orthopedics. These fractures constitute 15% of all fractures that result in emergency room visits.[30] The older adult has an increased number of distal radius fractures for 2 reasons. The first is related to the fragility of the bone secondary to postmenopausal osteoporosis. The second is related to the increased incidence of falls in the older adult as compared to younger individuals. As with proximal humeral fractures in older persons, the usual mechanism of injury is a fall on an outstretched arm.

Classification

No universally accepted classification of distal radius fractures has been developed to date. To be considered a distal radius fracture, the fracture must have occurred within 3 cm of the radiocarpal joint.[59] The Colles fracture is the most common type of distal radius fracture and is by definition a dorsally angulated and displaced fracture of the radial metaphysis within 2 cm of the articular surface.[30] Comminution of the fracture is most common in the older adult. Because of the fracture fragment displacement, the majority of these fractures require some type of reduction to ensure anatomic alignment. Most Colles fractures are managed by closed reduction and cast fixation. Open reduction with internal fixation, external fixators, or percutaneous pins and plaster may be used for severe cases with displacement. A Smith fracture, conversely, is a volar angulated and displaced metaphyseal fracture that may be intraarticular, extraarticular, or part of a fracture dislocation.[30] This type of fracture usually occurs from a fall onto the dorsum of the hand. A Smith fracture is often very unstable and may result in significant disability after it has healed. Carpal tunnel syndrome and reflex sympathetic dystrophy are potential complications of Smith fracture.

Treatment

General principles for exercise and treatment are similar for both types of distal radial fracture. Nondisplaced fractures are treated nonoperatively. A short arm cast is usually applied and the fracture immobilized for 3 to 4 weeks. If at that time there is radiographic evidence of healing and the fracture site is minimally tender, a removable splint is applied until the area is nontender. Overall, the most important rehabilitation consideration is early ROM. Full active ROM exercises for all nonimmobilized joints of the upper extremity should begin as soon as the fracture has been stabilized. This is most important for the glenohumeral joint in order to prevent the development of adhesive capsulitis. Although the cast should end at the proximal palmar crease to allow motion of the metacarpal phalangeal joints, sometimes the cast limits motion, nonetheless. Therefore, it is important to move the metacarpal phalangeal joints as much as the cast will allow. The patient/client should also perform active exercises of the remaining thumb and finger joints. Strict compliance with active ROM exercises several times a day will minimize loss of function during the immobilization period.

Typically, all immobilization is removed at about 6 weeks postinjury and ROM and strengthening exercises for the immobilized joints are initiated at this time. Emphasis should be on restoring motion in wrist extension, forearm supination, thumb opposition, and finger metacarpal phalangeal joint flexion. Restoring wrist extensor and grip strength exercises is very important to restore function of the hand and wrist.

With displaced fractures, surgical fixation is usually required.[30] Types of surgical fixation include pins in plaster, percutaneous pinning, external fixation, and open reduction with internal fixation. Postreduction care will parallel that of nondisplaced fractures.

Fractures of the Proximal Femur

Fractures of the proximal femur are common problems for the older population and are one of the most potentially devastating injuries in the older adult. The incidence of hip fracture increases after the age of 50 years and then doubles for each decade beyond 50 years of age.[48] More than 200,000 hip fractures occur in the United States each year, and the current mortality rate 1 year after hip fracture in older adult patients/clients ranges from 12% to 36%.[48] Mortality is higher than for age-matched individuals without hip fractures, with the highest mortality rates occurring in institutionalized patients/clients. After 1 year, mortality rates return to that of age- and sex-matched controls.[48]

Osteoporosis is a common predisposing factor for hip fractures. As many as 7% of hip fractures may occur spontaneously.[48] The most common mechanism for injury is a fall producing a direct blow over the greater trochanter. Following fracture, disability and functional dependence are common. Therefore, the overall goal of the treatment is to return the patient/client to the preinjury level of function.

Classification

The 3 common classifications of femoral neck fractures are those based on (a) anatomic location of the fracture, (b) direction of the fracture angle, and (c) displacement of the fracture fragments. With regard to anatomic location, surgeons divide fractures of the proximal femur into 3 groups. Femoral neck fractures are located from just below the articular surface to just superior to the intertrochanteric area. Intertrochanteric fractures are located between the greater and lesser trochanters. Subtrochanteric fractures occur in the proximal shaft below the level of the lesser trochanters. For patients/clients older than the age of 65 years, 95% of hip fractures are in the femoral neck or the intertrochanteric regions.[48]

Treatment

It is generally accepted that surgical management, followed by early mobilization, is the treatment of choice for hip fractures in the older adult.[48] Historically, nonoperative management resulted in an excessive rate of medical morbidity and mortality as well as malunion and nonunion in displaced fractures. The overall goal of treatment for fracture of the proximal femur is to return the patient/client to the preinjury level of function as quickly and as safely as possible. Age, cognitive impairment, and coexisting morbidities may impact the level of independence the patient/client is able to achieve. The therapist should develop the postoperative care on an individual basis in consultation with the physician. Because of the high degree of variability in fracture patterns and postoperative fracture stability, ongoing communication is essential to developing a safe and effective rehabilitation program.

Physical therapy should begin on the first postoperative day. Patients/clients who receive more than 1 physical therapy treatment session per day are more likely to regain functional independence and return home.[43] The treatment program should include ROM and strengthening exercises, training in transfers and gait with an assistive device, and training in functional activities such as ADL. The exercise program should increase in intensity and difficulty until the day of discharge. Some surgeons have recommended restricted weight bearing until the fracture has healed, whereas others have shown that unrestricted weight bearing can be started immediately without detrimental effects in the presence of stable internal fixation. Biomechanical data have shown that non-weightbearing ambulation places significant stresses across the hip as a result of muscular contraction at the hip and knee.[48] Gait training with an assistive device should begin on the first postoperative day. Distance should be advanced and stair training introduced over the next couple of days. Ideally, the patient/client should be able to ambulate well enough to negotiate the indoor home environment by the time of discharge. Weight bearing as tolerated with a walker is appropriate for the majority of femoral neck and intertrochanteric fracture patients/clients treated with operative reduction and internal fixation or prosthetic replacement.

Cemented fixation of prosthetic replacements allows immediate full weight bearing, whereas biologic growth fixation may delay full weight bearing for 6 to 12 weeks. Biologic growth fixation is thought to have a lower fixation failure rate than cemented fixation and is preferable in younger, more active individuals. For older individuals who are at risk for greater morbidity and mortality after fracture, the early weightbearing status afforded by cemented fixation may be desirable. Because there is a greater likelihood of instability and healing complications with subtrochanteric fractures, patients/clients with this type of fracture may require a longer period of protected weight bearing. The patient/client should advance to a cane and eventually eliminate the assistive devices when fracture healing and safety considerations permit.

During the first few weeks of fracture healing, emphasis should focus on active or active-assistive ROM exercises with gravity eliminated, progressing to full active motion exercises against gravity as soon as allowed by adequate fracture healing. It is important that the patient/client begin the exercise program as tolerated on the first postoperative day. The exercise program should be designed to help prepare the patient/client for functional activities. Patients/clients should perform the exercises in the supine, sitting, and standing positions. It is important for the patient/client to be able to move the operated limb through a full ROM against gravity in order to perform simple ADL, such as bed mobility and transfers. In most cases following operative reduction and internal fixation, there is no restriction of the ROM activities. In contrast, patients/clients who undergo prosthetic replacement of the femoral head will likely be restricted in the amounts of hip flexion (less than 90 degrees), adduction (0 degrees), and internal rotation (0 degrees) allowed in the early postoperative period because of hip dislocation risk. Exercises should progress in intensity each day until the patient/client can move and control the limb independently. After some healing has occurred (3 to 4 weeks), external resistance may be added, provided the patient/client's strength is good enough to achieve full ROM against gravity without assistance. Pain during resistance exercise may indicate that the exercise is too intensive and should be monitored by the therapist. Restoring hip-abductor and knee-extensor strength are critical for ambulatory function after hip fracture and should receive particular attention.

Total Joint Arthroplasty

Hip, knee, and shoulder arthroplasty are increasingly common procedures. Replacement of damaged cartilage surfaces with artificial weightbearing materials has enabled surgeons to dramatically improve function and relieve pain in many patients/clients. OA is the precursor to most total joint replacements and it is estimated that the prevalence of OA in the United States will increase from 43 million in 1997 to 60 million in 2020.[19] Medical advances have allowed total joint replacements of the hip and knee to become much less invasive in the last few years and depending on the type of fixation immediate weight bearing of some degree is possible. The large volume of information on this topic does not allow for an in-depth discussion on this topic to occur in this chapter.

Consensus in the research does indicate that therapeutic exercise is the treatment modality of choice for preoperative and the postoperative care following total joint arthroplasties.[66] Regarding the initial evaluation either a before and after elective surgery situation, it is important to determine the presurgical functional status of the patient/client. Items that are key to know include the patient/client's ambulation status, ROM of the involved joint, functional tasks such as walking tolerance, the need for upper extremity assist of an arm chair to stand from sitting, and the ability to navigate stairs and outdoor items such as curbs. During this interview process with the patient/client, it is essential to determine the personal goals of the patient/client and what constitutes success in the patient/client's eyes. The patient/client struggling with OA has learned how to compensate to accomplish walking and other ADL, and these patterns of movement have become natural to the patient/client. It is important during the rehabilitation process to identify these compensation patterns and work with the patient/client to modify these movement patterns to promote a return to normal and efficient movement. Astenphen et al[6] evaluated patients/clients with mild knee OA and patients/clients with severe knee OA and compared their gait with asymptomatic individuals and determined that both OA groups demonstrated increased midstance knee adduction moments, decreased peak knee flexion moments, decreased peak hip adduction moments and decreased peak hip extension moments as compared to the control group. The severe OA group also demonstrated significant kinematic differences at the hip knee and ankle joints. Many other studies have also demonstrated that knee OA patients/clients reduce the knee extension moments and decrease their walking speed and stride length to accommodate to the pain.[8,44,47,51] It is important during the later stages of rehabilitation after a total knee or hip replacement that these kinematic deficits be addressed, and exercises should focus on minimizing knee adductor moments and work on hip extension and knee extension during the stance to toe off phases of gait. This may be hard to normalize because the patient/client has been so used to compensating for the pain and ROM restrictions, but it needs to be addressed to regain the full higher-level function that the patient/client desires. Another biomechanical component that is frequently present is a leg-length asymmetry that may be structural or functional. Correcting this may involve building a temporary or permanent heel lift or shoe insert to accommodate the asymmetry.

When dealing with hip and knee replacements, ROM is always a key component of the rehabilitation process. It is essential to regain as much ROM as possible to accommodate functional tasks. Patients/clients undergoing hip replacements will have ROM restrictions initially and regaining hip ROM seems to be less of a challenge than the patients/clients undergoing knee replacement. It is essential to regain full active knee extension following surgery and sufficient knee flexion to accommodate functional tasks. The usual expectation for active knee flexion following surgery would range from 110 to 120 degrees.[62] Overall lower-extremity strength is another essential component of full recovery from joint replacement surgery. Many studies demonstrate that quadriceps strength is lowest in the patients/clients with knee OA who score the highest on the Western Ontario and McMaster Universities Arthritis Index (WOMAC), which demonstrates the most severe symptoms. Research also illustrates that the quadriceps strength decreases by 50% to 60% of the preoperative status just 1 month postsurgery.[7,61] If the overall quadriceps strength is deficient prior to surgery and then decreases even more after surgery, it is imperative that the rehabilitation program include many exercises and other modalities to increase quadriceps strength in the closed-chain position. Strengthening the other lower-extremity muscle groups, including the gluteals and hip abductors, calf muscle group, and hamstrings, is also important in order to complete the full rehabilitation program. Each of these muscle groups are needed to allow proper gait patterns, transfer from sit to stand and into and out of a car, ascend and descend stairs, and perform functional activities such as squatting; all of which are needed for efficient movement. All functional tasks require balance and proper proprioception/neuromuscular control in order to ensure efficient movements. Concepts regarding balance retraining interventions are discussed in the following section, and need to be adapted as appropriate for an individual's weightbearing status and weightbearing tolerance.

Intervention Considerations for Older Adults

Interventions for most musculoskeletal conditions in the older adult are similar to those utilized in a younger adult; however, there are several important considerations when providing interventions for older adults.

Patient/Client-Related Instruction

Patient/client-related instruction must account for the aforementioned sensory system impairments with regard to vision (eg, larger print for education materials) and hearing (eg, slower, well-articulated speech), as well as increased repetition and inclusion of a caregiver for those with cognitive impairment. The key to successful treatment of any dysfunction is the ability and desire of the patient/client to follow through with the prescribed exercise program provided by the treating clinician. Through years of experience in treating the older adult patient/client, we have found that using an analogy of a car and comparing it to the aging process of the human body is an excellent way to improve adherence, especially with regard to prevention-related interventions. We all desire to drive a luxury automobile that is powerful, smooth, efficient, quiet, and reliable. This can also be said about our human body. As we age, individual systems of the body, not unlike the systems of the automobile, can become deficient and affect the overall performance of the entire car. An example of this may be when the strength and flexibility of the lower extremities are diminished (eg, worn shocks and suspension system of the car), the articular surfaces of the joints may be more susceptible to degeneration and damage (wear and tear on the tires). Similar examples can be found using this human body and car analogy (Table 29-10).

Table 29-10 Similar Examples to the Car Analogy Using the Human Body

Car System	Body System
Shock and suspension system	Muscle strength and flexibility
Tires	Articular cartilage and joints
Engine	Cardiovascular and muscular endurance
Air filter and exhaust system	Pulmonary system
Car frame	Skeletal system
Fluids (gas, oil, coolant, etc.)	Hydration and nutrition

Therapeutic Exercise

The deleterious effects of immobility are well documented. Because of the summative effects of aging on multiple systems, fatigue, reduction in sensory information, fear of falling, and effects of accumulated disease processes, many older adults experience a gradual reduction in activity level over time. This decreased activity sets up a vicious cycle of disuse and loss of function. Loss of muscle mass, demineralization of bone, diminished cardiopulmonary function, and loss of neuromuscular control have been directly related to lack of physical activity. Disuse exacerbates the aging process and negatively impacts physiologic reserve in the face of disease and injury. Participation in a regular exercise program has proven to be an effective intervention/modality to reduce or prevent functional declines associated with aging. Regular exercise can also provide a number of psychological benefits related to preserved cognitive function, alleviation of depression symptoms, and behavior and an improved concept of personal control and self-efficacy.

Participation in a regular exercise program is an effective intervention/modality to reduce/prevent a number of functional declines associated with aging. Older individuals, who are well into the eighth and ninth decades of life, respond to both endurance and strength training. Regular exercise and physical activity contribute to a healthier, independent lifestyle with associated improved functional capacity and quality of life. Rehabilitation following injury or illness should include education regarding the benefits of physical activity and instruction for the implementation of and safe participation in a lifelong exercise program.

Endurance Training

Endurance training in the older adult is not different than in the younger adult, although there are some special considerations. First, it is important to appropriately screen the older adult for risk factors related to cardiovascular disease and adverse cardiovascular events during exercise as previously outlined. This is critical to selecting which patient/client/client is appropriate for endurance training, determining whether lower intensities are required, determining whether physician referral and clearance is needed, and determining whether closer vital sign monitoring is needed. However, in the absence of increased risk or significant comorbidity, the healthy older adult is able to perform aerobic training at similar intensities as younger adults (Figure 29-1). Training intensities up to 80% of maximum heart rate can be safely tolerated in appropriately selected individuals.[3] It should be noted that individuals on beta blocker medications for high blood pressure and/or cardiovascular disease will have a blunted heart rate response to exercise, and exercise training intensity should dictated based upon rating of perceived exertion (Table 29-11) (Figure 29-2).

Strength Training

Similar to endurance training, strength training in the appropriately selected older adult is not different than in younger adults (Figures 29-3*A* and *B*). An appropriate screening process, as previously outlined, is critical, and in those individuals without significant contraindications, higher training intensities may be utilized. In fact, strength training results in a dose–response dependent manner as younger individuals, with the greatest strength gains occurring with high (>80% of 1 repetition maximum) intensity training.[32,57] The safety and efficacy of strength training in the older adult is well-established.[57] With regard to specificity of training, attention should be given to the specific mode of exercise that most closely resembles the functional deficit for which the strength training is being used[57] to ensure that strength gains translate into improved function (Figure 29-4).

Additionally, functional training such as inclusion of variable speed, repeated functional tasks like sit-to-stand, multidirectional stepping and walking, squatting, and reaching may result in similar strength gains as a usual strength training group, but with the additional benefit

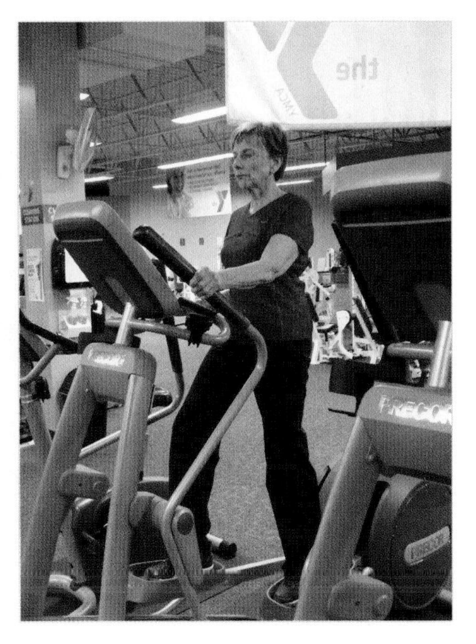

Figure 29-1 **The elliptical training machine, an excellent choice for aerobic exercise in the geriatric population because it is weight-bearing, but low impact**

Table 29-11 **Rating of Perceived Exertion**

This is a scale for effort, exertion, leg fatigue, or breathlessness (whichever symptom is the most limiting for you). The number 0 represents no effort, exertion, leg fatigue, or breathlessness. The number 10 represents the strongest or greatest effort, exertion, leg fatigue, or breathlessness that you have ever experienced. Select a number that represents your perceived level of effort, exertion, leg fatigue, or breathlessness.	
0	Nothing at all
0.5	very, very slight (just noticeable)
1	very slight
2	slight (light)
3	moderate
4	somewhat severe
5	severe (heavy)
6	
7	very severe
8	
9	
10	very, very severe (almost max)

Adapted from: Borg GAV. Psychophysical bases of perceived exertion. *Med Sci Sports Exerc.* 1982;14(5):377-381.

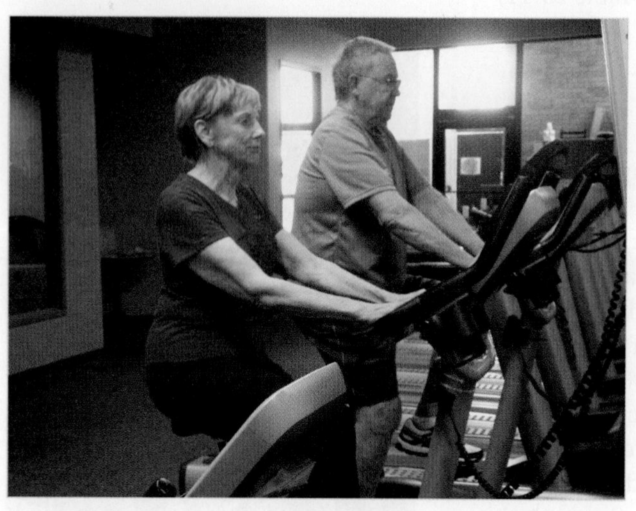

Figure 29-2

Stationary bicycling, an alternative low impact choice for aerobic exercise in the geriatric population. The bicycle is also good for range of motion in the hips and knees.

of greater changes in gait, balance, and coordination (Figure 29-5).[29,49]

Balance Retraining

Requisite to functional mobility is maintenance of the center of gravity over the base of support, which is accomplished through multiple afferent, central processing, and efferent pathways. The primary afferent pathways include the visual system, the vestibular system and proprioception. Central processing pathways generate a variety of strategies for maintaining and recovering balance depending on the context and the disturbance and the environmental and task demands; the motor and musculoskeletal responses must be activated to main upright balance. These motor responses are classified as the ankle strategy, hip strategy, and stepping strategy. If the disturbance in balance is small, then the ankle strategy is the primary protective response, where the feet remain planted on the ground and the body moves above the ankle joints. The flexor muscles at the feet begin the ankle strategy response, progressing upward using sequentially more proximal movers. If larger forces disturb the center of gravity, the hip strategy is used to maintain balance; where the feet remain planted but the hips flex and then quickly extend back to neutral to regain balance. The muscles activated first during the hip strategy are the abdominals and quadriceps and then muscles are recruited caudally. If the balance perturbation is larger than the ankle and

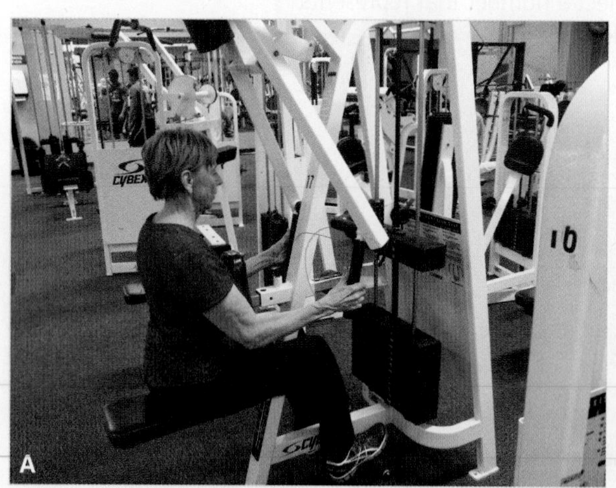

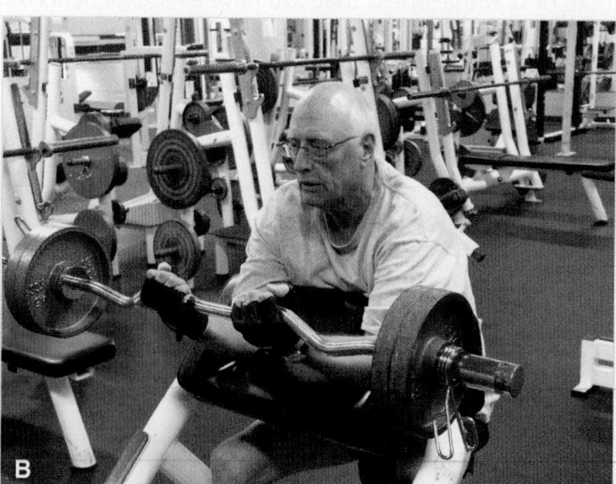

Figure 29-3

A. A senior performing seated resistance training of the upper extremities and postural stabilizers in a seated position. Caution must be used to ensure proper trunk stability and posture during this exercise. **B.** A senior performing seated resistance training of the upper extremities. Caution must be used to avoid postural compensations or the use of momentum during this exercise.

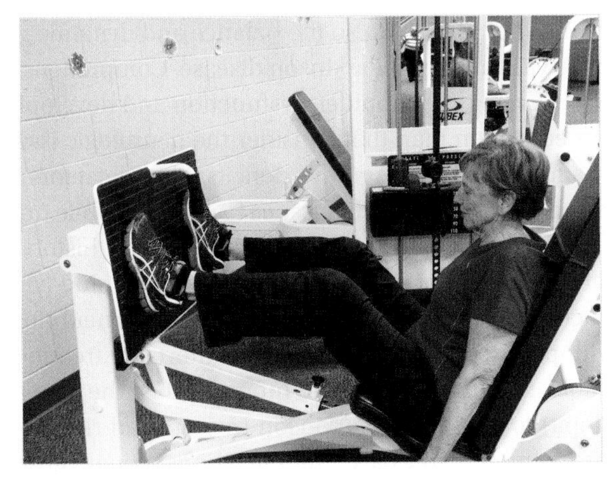

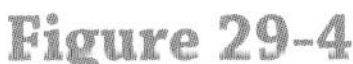

Figure 29-4

A senior performing closed chain, partial weight-bearing strengthening of the lower extremities, important for maintaining functional independence in sit to stand and other ADLs.

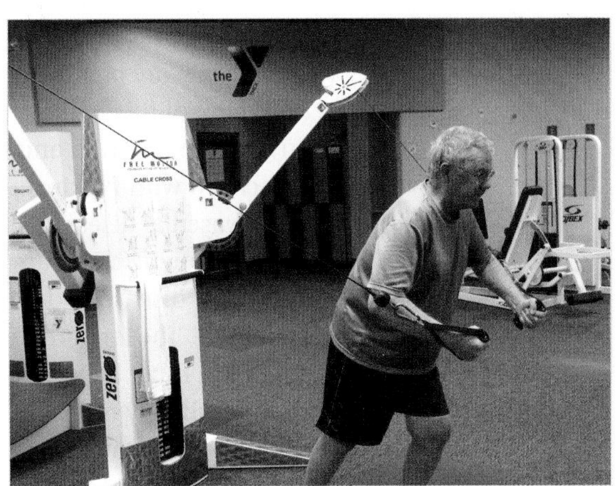

Figure 29-5

A senior performing standing resistance training for the upper extremities. Caution must be used to promote proper technique, and avoid substitution or postural compensations during this exercise.

hip strategies can "manage" then the motor response is a corrective step, stumble, or hop in order to regain the center of gravity over the base of support. All of these strategies can be anticipatory or reactive in nature, and both depend on adequate musculoskeletal function to prevent a fall. These motor responses can be improved with many different exercises and these exercises should be a part of every exercise program involving the older orthopedically involved patient/client. Additionally, balance exercises should include functional tasks such as backwards and side-stepping, stepping up to a curb, stepping around and over obstacles, walking on uneven terrain, and changing gaze and head position during walking.

Case Example

The following is an example of the principles discussed in this chapter applied to the treatment of an older individual with comorbidities and a typical orthopedic condition. A 75-year-old male presents to an outpatient orthopedic clinic with a diagnosis of adhesive capsulitis of the shoulder. The patient/client reports the mechanism of injury was when he stumbled on a throw rug at home and fell onto the floor with the force directly on his shoulder. This injury occurred approximately 4 weeks prior and now his shoulder is stiff, painful, and weak. The patient/client's primary complaint is that he cannot move his arm enough to put on his shirt without help from his wife, reach his back pocket, or put on his seatbelt. The patient/client reports he had a contusion in the deltoid region that has now resolved and he had X-rays and a MRI that ruled out any fractures or rotator cuff tears. His medical history includes an 11-year history of Parkinson disease with no other remarkable comorbidities noted. His age, gender, and history of hypertension were noted as risk factors for cardiovascular disease.

Based on the history, the physical therapist has 2 different issues that must be considered. The patient/client has the orthopedic injury that started as a hematoma and has developed into a soft-tissue restriction as a result of patient/client-induced immobilization secondary to pain and fear of hurting his shoulder more with activity. Another issue the clinician must consider is the effect of Parkinson disease on the patient/client's balance and gait, which may have been the underlying cause of the fall. The examination process must evaluate both the movement dysfunction of the shoulder and also the balance and dynamic gait deficits that are present because of the 11-year history of Parkinson disease. Comprehensive treatment of this patient/client includes treating the shoulder dysfunction and developing an exercise program and patient/client education plan that consider the neurologic issues associated with Parkinson disease, which can include cognitive deficits, his risk factors for cardiovascular disease, and his gait and balance deficits. Other issues to consider while treating this patient/client are the postural changes that have occurred with this long history of Parkinson disease and its effect on various treatment positions, such as supine, side-lying, and prone. The forward head and thoracic kyphosis that typically accompany this neurologic condition must be accommodated with pillows so as to facilitate a comfortable treatment posture when lying on the treatment table. It is also important to monitor when the patient/client takes his medication (eg, levodopa) to control his Parkinson tremors and rigidity. It would be advantageous to perform the joint and soft-tissue mobilizations along with the active exercises during the timeframe when the body is at its most relaxed state. The clinician will have difficulty making therapeutic gains and could put the patient/client at risk of injury if the clinician performs manual therapy techniques to the shoulder when the rigidity of the muscles is at its highest. The patient/client should be able to tell the clinician at which time in the medication cycle he feels his muscles are the most relaxed, which is the desirable time for treatment. Gait and balance training should be included, and vital sign monitoring during the initial exercise session and during increases in exercise intensity should be considered.

The above example illustrates the challenges present when treating the older adult patient/client in an orthopedic setting. The older adult patient/client will frequently present with a "simple" orthopedic injury that is compounded with other comorbidities. The physical therapist must consider the big picture and evaluate multiple systems to determine what functional deficits are present at the orthopedic injury site (such as shoulder in above example) and how the aging process and comorbidity affect the overall functional status of the patient/client. Treatment plans must incorporate exercises for both local and global deficits detected in the evaluation process.

SUMMARY

1. The field of geriatrics will continue to grow as the population ages. As life expectancy increases, rehabilitation of the physically disabled older adult will become an increasingly essential component of overall geriatric care.
2. The aging process affects multiple systems in the body and has a direct impact on the rehabilitation of acute and chronic musculoskeletal conditions common in the older adult.
3. Orthopedic conditions are commonly experienced by the older population. Fractures commonly occur and are often the result of osteoporosis and falls. When articular cartilage damage is severe or there is chronic joint pain, hip, knee, and shoulder arthroplasty are increasingly common procedures specifically designed to provide patients/clients with dramatically improved lifestyle and function.
4. Examination and evaluation of older adults must focus on determining the relative contributions from aging, inactivity, and disease on reduced physical functioning.
5. Emphasis in the rehabilitation program should be placed upon the importance of physical activity in preventing injury and minimizing functional decline. Rehabilitation providers must be aware of the special needs that this population has in order to facilitate the development of effective rehabilitation interventions.

REFERENCES

1. Abyad A, Boyer JT. Arthritis and aging. *Curr Opin Rheumatol.* 1992;4:153-159.
2. Almeida OP, Almeida SA. Short versions of the geriatric depression scale: a study of their validity for the diagnosis of a major depressive episode according to ICD-10 and DSM-IV. *Int J Geriatr Psychiatry.* 1999;14:858-865.
3. American College of Sports Medicine. *Guidelines for Exercise Testing and Prescription.* 5th ed. Baltimore, MD: Williams & Wilkins; 1995:1-373.
4. American Thoracic Society, Board of Directors. ATS statement: guidelines for the six-minute walk test. *Am J Respir Crit Care Med.* 2002;166:111-117.
5. Arnett SW, Laity JH, Agrawal SK, Cress ME. Aerobic reserve and physical functional performance in older adults. *Age Ageing.* 2008;37:384-389.
6. Astenphen JL, Deluzio KJ, Caldwell GE, et al. Biomechanical changes at the hip, knee and ankle joints during gait are associated with knee osteoarthritis severity. *J Orthop Res.* 2008;26:332-341.
7. Bade MJ, Kohrt WM, Stevens-Lapsley JE. Outcomes before and after total knee arthroplasty compared to healthy adults. J Orthop Sports Phys Ther. 2010;40: 559-567.
8. Baliunas AJ, Hurtwitz DE, Ryals AB, et al. Increased knee joint loads during walking are present in subjects with knee osteoarthritis. *Osteoarthritis Cartilage.* 2002;10:573-579.
9. Bean JF, Olveczky DD, Klely DK, LaRose SI, Jette AM. Performance-based versus patient-reported physical function: what are the underlying predictors? *Phys Ther.* 2011;91:1804-1811.
10. Bigliani LU, Craig EV, Butters KP. Fractures of the shoulder. In: Rockwood CA, Green DP, Bucholz RW, eds. *Fractures in Adults.* Philadelphia, PA: Lippincott; 1991.
11. Bohannon RW. Dynamometer measurements of hand-grip strength predict multiple outcomes. *Percept Mot Skills.* 2001;93:323-328.
12. Bohannon RW. Hand grip dynamometry predicts future outcomes in aging adults. *J Geriatr Phys Ther.* 2008;31(1):3-10.
13. Brach JS, VanSwearingen JM. Identifying early decline of physical function in performance-based and self-report measures. *Phys Ther.* 2002;82:320-328.
14. Brock DB, Guralnik JM, Brody JA. Demography and epidemiology of aging in the United States. In: Schneider EL, Rowe JW, eds. *Handbook of the Biology of Aging.* 3rd ed. San Diego, CA: Academic Press; 1990.
15. Brooks G. Physical therapy associated with primary prevention, risk reduction, and deconditioning. In: DeTurk WE, Cahalin LP, Guccione AA, eds. *Cardiovascular and Pulmonary Physical Therapy.* New York, NY: McGraw-Hill; 2004.
16. Buchner DM. Understanding variability in studies of strength training in older adults: a meta-analytic perspective. *Top Geriatr Rehabil.* 1993;8:1-21.
17. Burge R, Dawson-Hughes B, Solomon DH, Wong JB, Tosteson A. Incidence and economic burden of osteoporosis-related fractures in the United States, 2005-2025. *J Bone Miner Res.* 2007;22:465-475.
18. Cahalin LP. The six-minute walk test predicts peak oxygen uptake and survival in patients with advanced heart failure. *Chest.* 1996;110:325-332.
19. Centers for Disease Control and Prevention. Arthritis prevalence and activity limitations—United States. *MMWR Morb Mortal Wkly Rep.* 1994;43:433-438.
20. Chandler JM, Duncan PW. Balance and falls in the elderly: issues in evaluation and treatment. In: Guccione AA, ed. *Geriatric Physical Therapy.* St. Louis, MO: Mosby; 1993.
21. Connolly JF. Fractures of the upper end of the humerus. In: Connolly JF, ed. *Deplama's Management of Fractures and Dislocations: An Atlas.* 3rd ed. Philadelphia, PA: WB Saunders; 1981:686-738.
22. Cornell CN, Schneider K. Proximal humerus. In: Koval KJ, Zuckerman JD, eds. *Fractures in the Elderly.* Philadelphia, PA: Lippincott; 1998.
23. Covinsky KE, Palmer RM, Fortinsky RH, et al. Loss of independence in activities of daily living in older adults hospitalized with medical illnesses: Increased vulnerability with age. *J Am Geriatr Soc.* 2003;51:451-458.
24. Craik RL. Sensorimotor changes and adaptation in the older adult. In: Guccione AA, ed. *Geriatric Physical Therapy.* St. Louis, MO: Mosby; 1993.
25. Cress ME, Meyer M. Maximal voluntary and functional performance levels needed for independence in adults aged 65 to 97 years. *Phys Ther.* 2003;83:37-48.
26. Daiello LA, Micca JL, Newsome RJ. *Optimal Care of the Patient with Dementia: From Independent Living to Assisted Living.* Paper presented at the American Society of Consultant Pharmacists Annual Meeting and Exhibition, Anaheim, CA, 2002.
27. Deal CL. Osteoporosis: prevention, diagnosis, and management. *Am J Med.* 1997;102:35S-39S.
28. Desrosiers J, Bravo G, Hebert R, Dutil E. Normative data for grip strength of elderly men and women. *Am J Occup Ther.* 1995;49:637-644.
29. De Vreede PL, Samson MM, Van Meeteren NLU, Duursma SA, Verhaar HJJ. Functional-task exercise versus resistance strength exercise to improve daily function in older women: a randomized, controlled trial. *J Am Geriatr Soc.* 2005;53:2-10.
30. Dinowitz MI, Koval KJ. Distal radius. In: Koval KJ, Zuckerman JD, eds. *Fractures in the Elderly.* Philadelphia, PA: Lippincott; 1998.
31. Eriksrud O, Bohannon RW. Relationship of knee extension force to independence in sit-to-stand

performance in patients receiving acute rehabilitation. *Phys Ther.* 2003;83:544-551.

32. Fatouros IG, Kambas A, Katrabasas, et al. Resistance training and detraining effects on flexibility performance in the elderly are intensity dependent. *J Strength Cond Res.* 2006;20:634-642.
33. Fletcher GF, Balady GJ, Amsterdam EA, et al. Exercise standards for testing and training: a statement for healthcare professionals from the American Heart Association. *Circulation.* 2001;104:1694-1740.
34. Folstein MF, Folstein SE, McHugh PR. "Mini-mental state" a practical method for grading the cognitive state of patients for the clinician. *J Psychiatr Res.* 1975;12:189-198.
35. Fried LP, Starer DJ, King DE, Lodder F. Preclinical disability: hypotheses about the bottom of the iceberg. *J Aging Health.* 1991;3:285-300.
36. Fried LP, Tangen CM, Walston J, et al; Cardiovascular Health Study Collaborative Research Group. Frailty in older adults: evidence for a phenotype. *J Gerontol A Biol Sci Med Sci.* 2001;56:M146-M156.
37. Fried LP, VanDoorn C, O'Leary JR, Tinetti ME, Drickamer MA. Preclinical mobility predicts incident mobility disability in older women. *J Gerontol A Biol Sci Med Sci.* 2000;55:M43-M52.
38. Gallagher D, Visser M, DeMeersman RE. et al. Appendicular skeletal muscle mass: effects of age, gender, and ethnicity. *J Appl Physiol.* 1997;83:229-239.
39. Greerlings SW, Twish JW, Beekman AT, et al. Longitudinal relationship between pain and depression in older adults: sex, age, and physical disability. *Soc Psychiatry Psychiatr Epidemiol.* 2002;37:23-30.
40. Grymonpre RE, Mitenko PA, Sitar DS, et al. Drug associated hospital admissions in older medical patients. *J Am Geriatr Soc.* 1998;36:1092-1098.
41. Gunther CM, Burger A, Rickert M, Crispin A, Schulz CU. Grip strength in healthy Caucasian adults: reference values. *J Hand Surg Am.* 2008;33A:558-565.
42. Hanten WP, Chen WY, Austin AA, et al. Maximum grip strength in normal subjects from 20-64 years of age. *J Hand Ther.* 1999;12:193-200.
43. Hoenig H, Rubenstein LV, Sloane R, et al. What is the role of timing on the surgical and rehabilitative care of community dwelling older persons with acute hip fracture? *Arch Intern Med.* 1997;157:513-520.
44. Hurtwitz DE, Ryals AB, Case JP, et al. the knee adduction moment during gait in subjects with knee osteoarthritis is more closely correlated with static alignment than radiographic disease severity, toe out angle and pain. *J Orthop Res.* 2002;20:101-107.
45. Isles RC, Low Choy NL, Steer M, Nitz JC. Normal values of balance tests in women aged 20-80. *J Am Geriatr Soc.* 2004;52:1367-1372.
46. Jones CJ, Rikli RE, Beam WC. A 30-s chair-stand test as a measure of lower body strength in community-residing older adults. *Res Q Exerc Sport.* 1999;70:113-117.
47. Kaufman KR, Hughes C, Morrey BF, et al. Gait characteristics of patients with knee osteoarthritis. *J Biomech.* 2001;34:907-915.
48. Koval KJ, Zuckerman JD. Hip. In: Koval KJ, Zuckerman JD, eds. *Fractures in the Elderly.* Philadelphia, PA: Lippincott; 1998.
49. Krebs DE, Scarborough DM, McGibbon CA. Functional vs. strength training in disabled elderly outpatients. *Am J Phys Med Rehabil.* 2007;86:93-103.
50. Lacas A, Rockwood K. Frailty in primary care: a review of its conceptualization and implications for practice. *BMC Med.* 2012;10:4.
51. Landry SC, Mckean KA, Hubley-Kozey CL, et al. Knee biomechanics of moderate OA patients measured during gait at a self-selected and fast walking speed. *J Biomech.* 2007;40:1754-1761.
52. Lane JM. Osteoporosis: medical prevention and treatment. *Spine (Phila Pa 1976).* 1997;22:32-37.
53. Larsson L, Sjodin B, Karlsson J. Histochemical and biochemical changes in human skeletal muscle with age in sedentary males, age 22-65 years. *Acta Physiol Scand.* 1978;103:31-39.
54. Leipzig RM, Cumming RG, Tinetti ME. Drugs and falls in older people: a systematic review and meta-analysis. *J Am Geriatr Soc.* 1999;47(1):30-50.
55. Lenze EJ, Schulz R, Martire LM, et al. The course of functional decline in older people with persistently elevated depressive symptoms: longitudinal findings from the Cardiovascular Health Study. *J Am Geriatr Soc.* 2005;53:569-575.
56. Lewis CB, Bottomly JM. *Geriatric Physical Therapy: A Clinical Approach.* Norwalk, CT: Appleton & Lange; 1994.
57. Mayer F, Scharhag-Rosenberger F, Carlsohn A, Cassel M, Muller S, Scharhag J. The intensity and effects of strength training in the elderly. *Dtsch Arztebl Int.* 2011;108:359-364.
58. McKenzie R, May S. *The Lumbar Spine Mechanical Diagnosis and Therapy*, Vol. 1. Waikane, New Zealand: Spinal Publications; 2004.
59. Melton LJ, Thamer M, Ran NF, et al. Fractures attributable to osteoporosis: report from the National Osteoporosis Foundation. *J Bone Miner Res.* 1997;12:16-23.
60. Mitsionis G, Pakos EE, Stafilas KS, Paschos N, Papkostas T, Beris AE. Normative data on hand grip strength in a Greek adult population. *Int Orthop.* 2009;33:713-717.
61. Mizner RL, Petterson SC, Stevens JE, et al. Early quadriceps strength loss after total knee arthroplasty: the contributions of muscle atrophy and failure of voluntary muscle activations. *J Bone Joint Surg Am.* 2005;87:1047-1053.
62. Mizner RL, Petterson SC, Stevens JE, et al. Preoperative quadriceps strength predicts functional ability one year after total knee arthroplasty. *J Rheumatol.* 2005;32:153-1539.
63. Moellar JF, Mathiowetz NA. *Prescribed Medicines: A Summary of Use and Expenditures for Medicare*

Beneficiaries. Pub. no. PHC 89-3448. Rockville, MD: U.S. Department of Health and Human Services; 1989.

64. Mulsant BH, Ganguli M. Epidemiology and diagnosis of depression in late life. *J Clin Psychiatry*. 1999;60(Suppl 20): 9-15.

65. Olshanky SJ, Passaro DJ, Hershow RC, et al. A potential decline in life expectancy in the United States in the 21st century. *N Engl J Med*. 2005;352:1138-1145.

66. Ottawa Panel evidence-based clinical practice guidelines for therapeutic exercises and manual therapy in the management of osteoarthritis. *Phys Ther.* 2005;85:907-971.

67. Phillips SK, Bruce SA, Newton D, et al. The weakness of old age is not due to failure of muscle activation. *J Gerontol*. 1992;47:M45-M49.

68. Podsiadlo D, Richardson S. The timed up and go: a test of basic mobility in frail elderly persons. *J Am Geriatr Soc.* 1995;43:17-23.

69. Protas EJ. Physiological change and adaptation to exercise in the older adult. In: Guccione AA, ed. *Geriatric Physical Therapy*. St. Louis, MO: Mosby; 1993.

70. Reid IR. Glucocorticoid-induced osteoporosis: assessment and treatment. *J Clin Densitom*. 1998;1:65-73.

71. Riddle DL, Wells PS. Diagnosis of lower-extremity deep vein thrombosis in outpatients. *Phys Ther.* 2004;84:729-735.

72. Schmid MA. Reducing patient falls: a research-based comprehensive fall prevention program. *Mil Med.* 1990;155:202-207.

73. Shrestha LB. *Life Expectancy in the United States*. CRS Report for Congress, 2006.

74. Shumway-Cook A, Baldwin M, Polissar NL, et al. Predicting the probability of falls in community-dwelling older adults. *Phys Ther.* 1997;77:812-819.

75. Shumway-Cook A, Ciol MA, Yorkston KM, Hoffman JM, Chan L. Mobility limitations in the medicare population: prevalence and sociodemographic and clinical correlates. *J Am Geriatr Soc.* 2005;53:1217-1221.

76. Shumway-Cook A, Patla AE, Stewart A, et al. Environmental demands associated with community mobility in older adults with and without mobility disabilities. *Phys Ther.* 2002;82:670-681.

77. Stedenski S, Perera S, Wallace D, et al. Physical performance measures in the clinical setting. *J Am Geriatr Soc.* 2003;51:314-322.

78. Tariq S, Tumosa N, Chibnall J, Perry M, Morley JE. Comparison of the Saint Louis University mental status examination and the mini-mental state examination for detecting dementia and mild neurocognitive disorder; a pilot study. *Am J Geriatr Psychiatry*. 2006;14:900-910.

79. Tibbitts GM. Patients who fall: how to predict and prevent injuries. *Geriatrics.* 1996;51:24-31.

80. Twomey L, Taylor J. Age changes in the lumbar spine and intervertebral canals. *Paraplegia*. 1988;26:238-249.

81. United States Census Bureau 2004. *US Interim Projections by Age, Sex, Race, and Hispanic*. Available at http://www.census.gov/population/www/projections/usinterimproj/natprojtab02a.pdf. Last accessed June 13, 2012.

82. VanSwearingen JM, Paschal KA, Bonino P, et al. Assessing recurrent fall risk of community-dwelling, frail older veterans using specific tests of mobility and the physical performance test of function. *J Gerontol A Biol Sci Med Sci*. 1998;53:M457-M464.

83. Webber AP, Martin JL, Harker JO, et al. Depression in older patients admitted for postacute nursing home rehabilitation. *J Am Geriatr Soc.* 2005;53:1017-1022.

84. Weiss CO, Wolff JL, Egleston B, Seplaki CL, Fried LP. Incident preclinical mobility disability (PCMD) increases future risk of new difficulty walking and reduction in walking activity. *Arch Gerontol Geriatr.* 54:e329-e333, 2012.

85. Werle S, Goldhahn J, Drerup 's, Simmen BR, Sprott H, Herren DB. Age- and gender-specific normative data of grip and pinch strength in a healthy adult Swiss population. *J Hand Surg Eur Vol*. 2009;34:76-84.

86. Woo SL, Hollis JM, Adams DJ, et al. Tensile properties of the human femur-anterior cruciate ligament-tibia complex. The effects of specimen age and orientation. *Am J Sports Med*. 1991;19:217-225.

87. Yesavage JA, Brink TL, Rose TL, et al. Development and validation of a geriatric depression screening scale: a preliminary report. *J Psychiatr Res*. 1982; 17(1):37-49.

30

Considerations for the Pediatric Patient

Steven R. Tippett

OBJECTIVES

After completion of this chapter, the physical therapist should be able to do the following:

- Describe common macrotraumatic and microtraumatic musculoskeletal injuries occurring in the skeletally immature patient.
- Describe selected congenital, acquired, and musculoskeletal pathologies seen in active skeletally immature patients.
- Apply basic rehabilitation principles governing the care and prevention of macrotraumatic and microtraumatic musculoskeletal injuries in the skeletally immature patient.
- Differentiate between categories of growth plate fractures.
- Describe physiologic considerations unique to the active skeletally immature patient.
- Describe special psychological considerations for the skeletally immature athlete.
- Describe participation guidelines for the skeletally immature athlete.

Growing musculoskeletal tissue is innately predisposed to specific injuries that vary greatly from the injuries sustained by their skeletally mature counterparts, yet more and more youngsters are sustaining injuries that years ago primarily occurred in the skeletally mature athlete.[1,19,39] Many injuries that occur in youth sports today can be attributed to the increased volume of participation by youngsters in a variety of competitions that are scheduled by adults.[18]

This chapter briefly describes common macrotraumatic and microtraumatic injuries sustained by the young patient, along with basic principles that govern the treatment of these injuries. Macrotraumatic injuries occur as a result of a single, supramaximal loading of bone, ligament, muscle, or tendon. Common youth macrotraumatic injuries that are discussed include epiphyseal and avulsion fractures. Microtraumatic injuries, on the other hand, result from submaximal loading that occurs in a cyclic and repetitive fashion. Common microtraumatic injuries that occur in the immature musculoskeletal system that are presented include osteochondroses and traction apophysites. Special concerns unique to the immature musculoskeletal system that do not fall neatly into the macrotraumatic or microtraumatic categories also are presented. Finally, physiologic and psychological issues unique to the youth patient also are presented.

Macrotraumatic Musculoskeletal Injuries

Epiphyseal Fractures

Growing bone is the weak musculoskeletal link in the young athlete. Physical demands resulting in muscle strain or ligament sprain in the skeletally mature patient may result in epiphyseal plate injury in the young patient. The epiphyseal plate or growth plate is divided into zones differentiated from one another by their structure and function. Beginning at the growth area of long bone and progressing in the direction of mature long bone, the 4 regions of the growth plate are the reserve zone, proliferative zone, hypertrophic zone, and bony metaphysis. The reserve zone produces and stores matrix; the proliferative zone also produces matrix and is the site for longitudinal bone cell growth. The hypertrophic zone is subdivided into the maturation zone, degenerative zone, and zone of provisional calcification. It is within the hypertrophic zone that matrix is prepared for calcification, and it is here that the matrix is ultimately calcified.[48]

Injury to the growth plate can occur when stress or tensile loads placed upon bone exceed mechanical strength of the growth plate–metaphysis complex. Two factors that impact epiphyseal plate injury are (a) the ability of the growth plate to resist failure and (b) the forces applied to bone or the stresses induced in the growth plate. Based upon results from animal studies, it has been determined that the weakest region of the growth plate is the hypertrophic zone. The hypertrophic zone is susceptible to injury because of the low volume of bone matrix and high amount of developing immature cells in this region.[48]

The majority of epiphyseal fractures are caused by high-velocity injuries. Although growth plate fractures certainly result from youth sporting activities, a detailed description of all epiphyseal plate fractures is beyond the scope of this chapter. A brief description of the Salter-Harris classification of growth plate fractures, along with some of the more common epiphyseal plate fractures in sports, however, is warranted.

The Salter-Harris classification of growth plate fracture consists of 5 types of fractures and is based upon the relationship of the fracture line to the growing cells of the epiphyseal plate as well as the mechanism of injury (Figure 30-1). Type I fractures are caused by shearing forces in which there is complete separation of the epiphysis without fracture through bone. These fractures are most commonly seen in very young people when the epiphyseal plate is relatively thick. Type II fractures are the most common type of growth plate fractures and result from shearing and bending forces. In the type II fracture, the line of separation traverses a variable distance along the epiphyseal plate and then makes its way through a segment of the bony metaphysis that results in a triangular-shaped metaphyseal fragment. Type II fractures usually occur in an older child who has a thin epiphyseal plate. Type III fractures usually result from shearing forces and result in intraarticular fractures from the joint surface to the deep zone of the growth plate and then along the growth plate to its periphery. Type IV fractures are intraarticular and also result from shearing forces. These fractures extend from the joint surface through the epiphysis across the entire thickness of the growth plate and then through a segment of the bony metaphysis. Type V fractures are caused by a crushing mechanism and are relatively uncommon.[31]

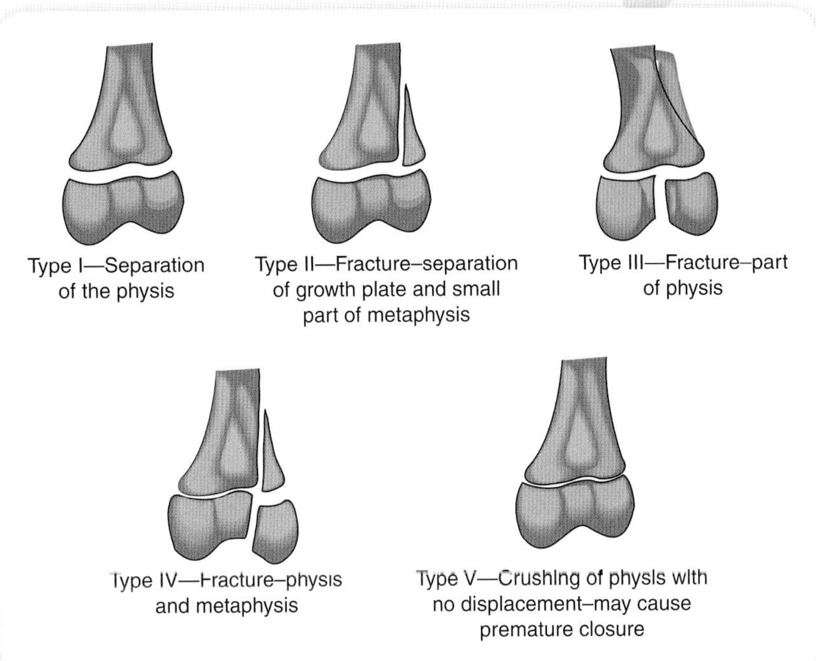

Figure 30-1 Growth plate fractures according to the Salter-Harris classification

A. Type I. **B.** Type II. **C.** Type III. **D.** Type IV. **E.** Type V.

Salter-Harris type III fractures warrant special mention. These fractures are typically limited to the distal tibial epiphysis.[48] Injury to the proximal tibial epiphysis or distal femoral epiphysis may result from valgus loading of the knee, which is frequently encountered in contact and collision sports. The clinician cannot rely solely on radiographic examination to confirm this type of injury. In a series of 6 high school athletes (5 playing football, 1 playing soccer), all injured by a valgus load, routine anterior-posterior and lateral radiographs did not demonstrate Salter-Harris type III fractures of the distal femoral epiphysis. Oblique radiographs with femoral rotation, crosstable lateral views demonstrating fat in the joint, or aspiration of a hemarthrosis with fat in the aspirate help to confirm growth plate fracture with an intraarticular component.[62] A thorough ligamentous examination with careful palpation skills is required to help differentiate joint line opening from epiphyseal plate opening.

Other common epiphyseal fractures seen in children involve the medial epicondyle and the bones of the hand. The medial epicondyle epiphyseal fracture is the most common elbow fracture seen in the young patient. From a macrotraumatic standpoint, epiphyseal fracture of the medial epicondyle is frequently the childhood counterpart of elbow dislocation in the adult and is typically caused by hyperextension and valgus loading.[1] Epiphyseal plate fractures of the medial epicondyle are typically Salter-Harris type I or II, although types III and IV injuries have also been reported. Medial epicondyle fractures typically result in the epicondyle being displaced inferiorly and possibly trapped in the elbow joint.[45] As the medial epicondyle serves as the attachment of the elbow and wrist flexors, avulsion fractures of the medial epicondyle also occur and are discussed later in the chapter in the section entitled "Avulsion Fractures".

Epiphyseal fractures in children are more common in the hand than in other long bones of the upper extremity.[53] As a result, care must be taken by the parent, coach, or health care professional not to simply disregard finger injuries as simply a "jammed finger." Growth plate fractures in the hand usually involve the proximal and middle phalanges of the border digits. The most common epiphyseal plate fracture in the skeletally immature hand is a Salter-Harris type II at the base of the proximal phalanx of the little finger.[54]

The term *Little League shoulder* is used to describe an epiphyseal fracture of the proximal humeral epiphysis that typically occurs in the young baseball pitcher.[13] Although this injury can be macrotraumatic in nature, as distraction forces across the physis can approach one-half the athlete's body weight,[20] the condition is thought to be a consequence of repetitive microtrauma. Fractures of the proximal humeral epiphysis are usually Salter-Harris type I or II. Radiographs demonstrate widening of the proximal humeral physis, and to a lesser degree may demonstrate lateral metaphyseal fragmentation, along with demineralization or sclerosis of the proximal humeral metaphysis. It should be noted that as the humerus adapts with increased retroversion, the majority of these youngsters remain asymptomatic as the condition evolves.[34,37] Avoiding all throwing until the patient is asymptomatic is vital in the treatment of this condition. Most patients are able to safely return to throwing with symptoms despite abnormal radiographs.[14]

Avulsion Fractures

As is the case with growing bone, much of the information regarding growing muscle is also based on animal studies. Although the physiology of the growth plate allows for bone growth, muscle does not inherently possess a specific structural site to allow for adaptation. It is clear that muscle adaptation does occur in order to accommodate for skeletal growth or as a response to therapeutic stretching exercise following periods of immobilization with muscle tissue in a shortened position. Based upon animal studies, it appears that a change in muscle length results from changes within the actual muscle belly itself and/or an increase in tendon length. In the skeletally immature animal model, change in muscle length occurs via changes in the length of both muscle and tendon. Research involving mature animals, on the other hand, indicates an increase in muscle length that occurs primarily through elongation of the muscle belly.[21]

When changes in muscle length do not match the changes in long-bone growth, tensile loads placed within the muscle predispose the youngster to injury. Contractile unit injury from voluntary contraction or passive stretch can be exacerbated as a result of inadequate muscle length. Injuries can range from various degrees of muscle strain to situations where the bony attachment of the muscle fails prior to muscle damage. Common sites of avulsion fracture in the lower extremity include the anterosuperior iliac spine (ASIS), anteroinferior iliac spine (AIIS), ischial tuberosity, and the base of the fifth metatarsal. As forces across the joints of the lower extremity from running, jumping, and kicking exceed most forces across the upper extremity, avulsion fractures of the lower extremity outnumber avulsion fractures of the upper extremity. Stresses across the shoulder and elbow of the young throwing athlete, however, are sufficient enough to result in avulsion of the medial humeral epicondyle and proximal humerus.

Lower Extremity

Anterosuperior Iliac Spine

Avulsion of the ASIS is caused by a contraction or stretch of the sartorius. The sartorius is the longest muscle in the body and crosses the anterior hip and proximal medial knee joints. The growth center at the ASIS appears between the ages of 13 and 15 years and fuses to the pelvis between the ages of 21 and 25 years (Tables 30-1 and 30-2).[43] Excessive force from the pulling of the sartorius with the hip in extension and knee in flexion may result in an avulsion of the ASIS. Positions of hip extension combined with knee flexion seen in the trail leg during sprinting and hurdling can predispose these athletes to ASIS avulsion fracture. When the growth center does avulse from the bony origin on the pelvis, displacement of the avulsed fragment is uncommon.[53]

Table 30-1 Maturation of Bones of the Arm and Shoulder

Bone	Maturation Timetable
Clavicle, sternal epiphysis	Closure years 18 to 24
Acromion	Closure years 18 to 19
Coracoid	Closure years 18 to 21
Subcoracoid	Closure years 18 to 21
Scapula, vertebral margin, and inferior angle	Closure years 20 to 21
Glenoid cavity	Closure year 19
Humerus, head, center, and lesser tuberosities	Fuse together years 4 to 6; fuse to shaft at years 19 to 21 in males, years 18 to 20 in females
Humerus, capitulum, lateral epicondyle, and trochlea	Fuse together at puberty; fuse to shaft at year 17 in males, year 14 in females
Olecranon	Closure years 15 to 17 in males, years 14 to 15 in females
Radius, head	Closure years 13 to 17 in males, years 14 to 15 in females
Radial tuberosity	Closure years 14 to 18
Ulna, distal epiphysis	Closure year 19 in males, year 17 in females
Styloid of ulna	Closure years 18 to 20
Radius, distal epiphysis	Closure year 19 in males, year 17 in females
Styloid process, radius	Closure variable
Lunate	Appears year 4
Navicular	Appears year 6
Pisiform	Appears year 12
Triquetrum	Appears years 1 to 2
Hamate	Appears month 6
Capitate	Appears month 6
Trapezoid	Appears year 4
Trapezium	Closure year 5
Metacarpal I, epiphysis	Closure years 14 to 21
Metacarpals II to IV, epiphysis	Closure years 14 to 21
Proximal phalanx I, epiphysis	Closure years 14 to 21
Distal phalanx I, epiphysis	Closure years 14 to 21

Table 30-2 Maturation of Bones of the Leg and Hip

Bone	Maturation Timetable
Pelvic bones	Fuse at puberty
Iliac crest	Closure year 20
Femur, head	Closure years 17 to 18 in males, years 16 to 17 in females
Greater trochanter	Closure years 16 to 17
Lesser trochanter	Closure years 16 to 17
Femur, distal epiphysis	Closure years 18 to 19 in males, year 17 in females
Proximal epiphysis	Closure years 18 to 19 in males, years 16 to 17 in females
Tibial tuberosity	Closure year 19
Fibula, proximal epiphysis	Closure years 18 to 20 in males, years 16 to 18 in females
Fibular malleolus	Closure years 17 to 18
Distal epiphysis	Closure years 17 to 18
Calcaneus, epiphysis	Closure years 12 to 22
Tarsus	Completion variable
Metatarsals I to V, epiphysis	Closure year 18 in males, year 16 in females
Metatarsals, heads	Closure years 14 to 21
Proximal phalanges I to V, epiphysis	Closure year 18
Middle phalanges II to V, epiphysis	Closure year 18
Distal phalanges	Closure year 18, beginning proximally

Anteroinferior Iliac Spine

Avulsion of the AIIS is caused by a stretch or contraction of the rectus femoris. The AIIS serves as the site of the direct (anterior, or straight) head of the rectus femoris. As is the case with ASIS avulsions, activities involving hyperextension of the hip combined with knee flexion can also result in AIIS avulsion. The growth center at the AIIS appears between the ages of 13 and 15 years and fuses at approximately 16 to 18 years.[43] As a result of earlier ossification, avulsion fractures at the AIIS are less frequent than avulsion fractures involving the ASIS. Athletes involved in running, jumping, and kicking sports usually sustain AIIS avulsion fractures.[29] When avulsion occurs, displacement of the bony muscle origin is rare because the tensor fascia lata, inguinal ligament, and an intact reflected (posterior) head of the rectus femoris (which originates at the superior rim of the acetabulum) all serve to prevent significant AIIS displacement.[53]

With both ASIS and AIIS avulsion fractures, the youngster is typically able to remember a specific event and usually unable to continue participation.[7] The patient demonstrates weakness of the involved muscle as evidenced by resisted hip flexion. In the avulsed ASIS, resisted hip flexion with the external rotation may be useful in the physical assessment. Point tenderness of the ASIS or AIIS is virtually always present. Swelling, if present, may be minimal, and there is minimal if any ecchymosis noted. Transfers from sit to supine are usually guarded and may require assistance from the patient's upper extremities or the contralateral lower extremity. Assuming a prone position may be uncomfortable. Passive stretch into complete knee flexion may or may not produce pain. Passive stretch of the hip into extension with simultaneous knee flexion may increase symptoms. Gait is typically antalgic with increased trunk flexion during stance, decreased hip flexion during swing-through, and decreased hip extension during late stance.[60]

Peroneals

Inversion ankle sprains are sustained frequently by patients of all ages in a wide variety of sport- and nonsport-related activities. As the patient inverts the ankle, stresses can be placed through the evertor muscle group, either by passive stretch or by active contraction to pull the foot back into eversion or by both. Excessive forces generated by the peroneus brevis may result in avulsion of its insertion at the base of the fifth metatarsal. Avulsion fracture of the base of the fifth metatarsal typically results in point tenderness along with weakness of resisted ankle eversion, especially when resisted at the athlete's available end-range inversion. Resisted eversion may or may not cause pain. Passive inversion of the ankle typically increases pain at the bony insertion. Swelling may be present, but occurs distal to the traditional location of swelling seen in ankle sprains. Ecchymosis, if present, typically does not arise until a few days following injury.[60]

Ischial Tuberosity

Avulsion of the hamstring origin at the ischial apophysis was first described in the mid-1850s, and it occurs with greater frequency than avulsions on the anterior aspect of the pelvis.[53] Growth centers in this region appear between the ages of 15 and 17 years and fuse to the ilia between the ages of 19 and 25 years.[42,53] Athletes with an avulsion fracture of the ischial tuberosity typically demonstrate discomfort with prolonged sitting. Assessment of hamstring length at 90 degrees of hip flexion will often show inadequate flexibility bilaterally, with more limitation on the involved side that is usually accompanied by pain. There may or may not be weakness with resisted knee flexion, but there is usually weakness noted with resisted or nonresisted prone active hip extension. There is typically minimal, if any, ecchymosis in the area, and swelling is usually not apparent.[60]

Anterior Cruciate Ligament Injury in the Young Athlete

Although the diagnosis and management principles governing injuries to the anterior cruciate ligament are found in Chapters 24 and 31, a few thoughts specific to this injury in the skeletally immature athlete is warranted. As is the case with many lower-extremity macrotraumatic injuries, sprains of the anterior cruciate ligament in young athletes is the norm rather than the exception. Although young athletes may avulse the anterior cruciate from the bony insertion, many still tear the ligament in the midsubstance and require reconstruction.

Reconstruction of the anterior cruciate ligament in the skeletally immature knee does pose problems not encountered when the distal femoral epiphysis has closed.

Standard practice involves transepiphyseal reconstruction with hamstring allograft versus extraarticular reconstruction.[2,25] Prompt surgical intervention (within 12 weeks) to the anterior cruciate ligament-deficient young athlete is paramount, as evidence demonstrates a delay in reconstruction can result in increased meniscal injuries and intraarticular chondral injury.[33] A successful return to sports after reconstruction can be expected, and many young athletes continue their careers into college.[52] Many studies have evaluated the impact of a variety of programs intended to "prevent" anterior cruciate injuries, but the success of these varied programs is mixed, and few programs specifically focus on skeletally immature athletes.[17,40]

Upper Extremity

A medial epicondyle epiphyseal fracture is the most common elbow fracture seen in the young patient (Figure 30-2).[3] As discussed previously, this injury may occur as a result

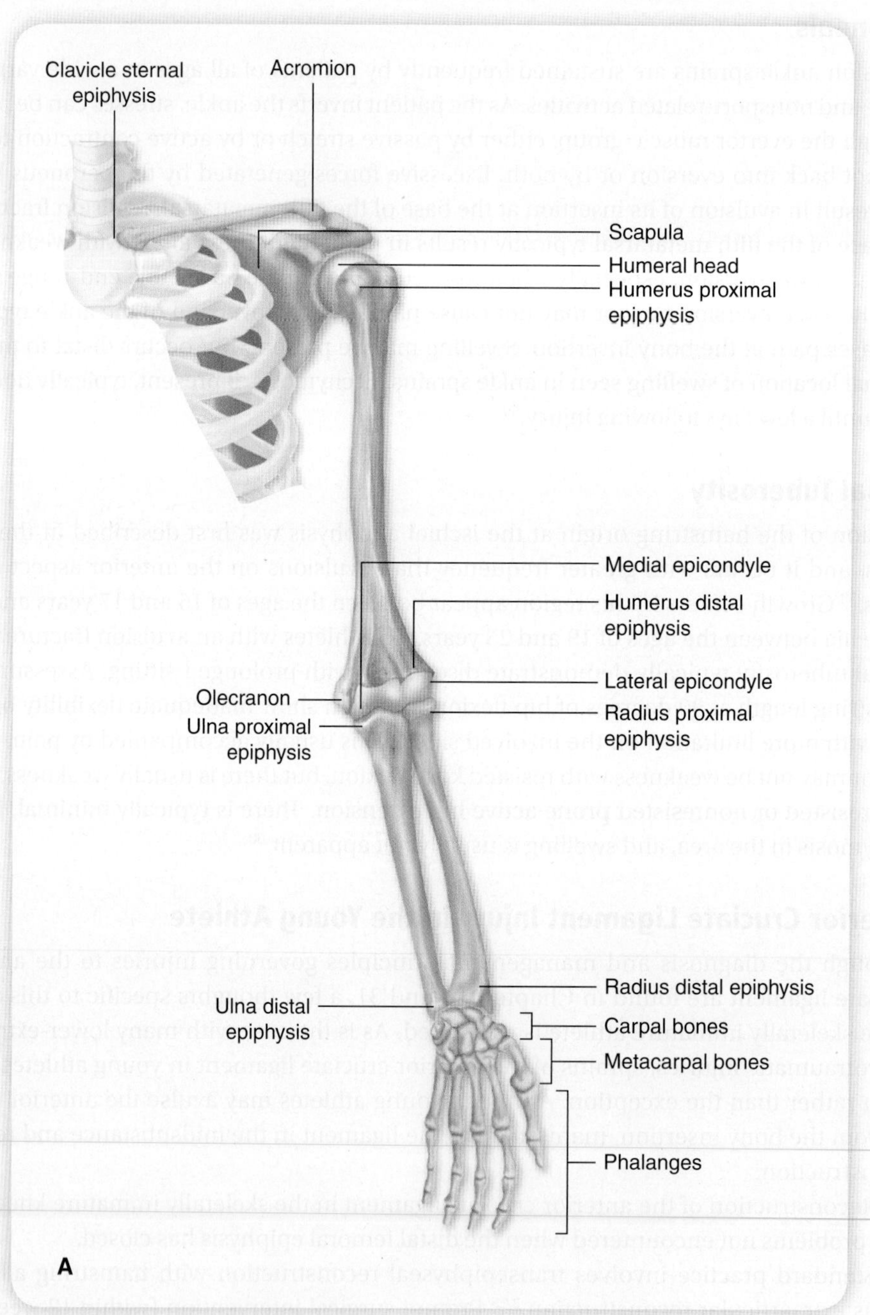

Figure 30-2 Location of upper extremity epiphyses

A. Upper-extremity ossification and epiphyseal plate closure.
B. Lower-extremity ossification and epiphyseal plate closure.

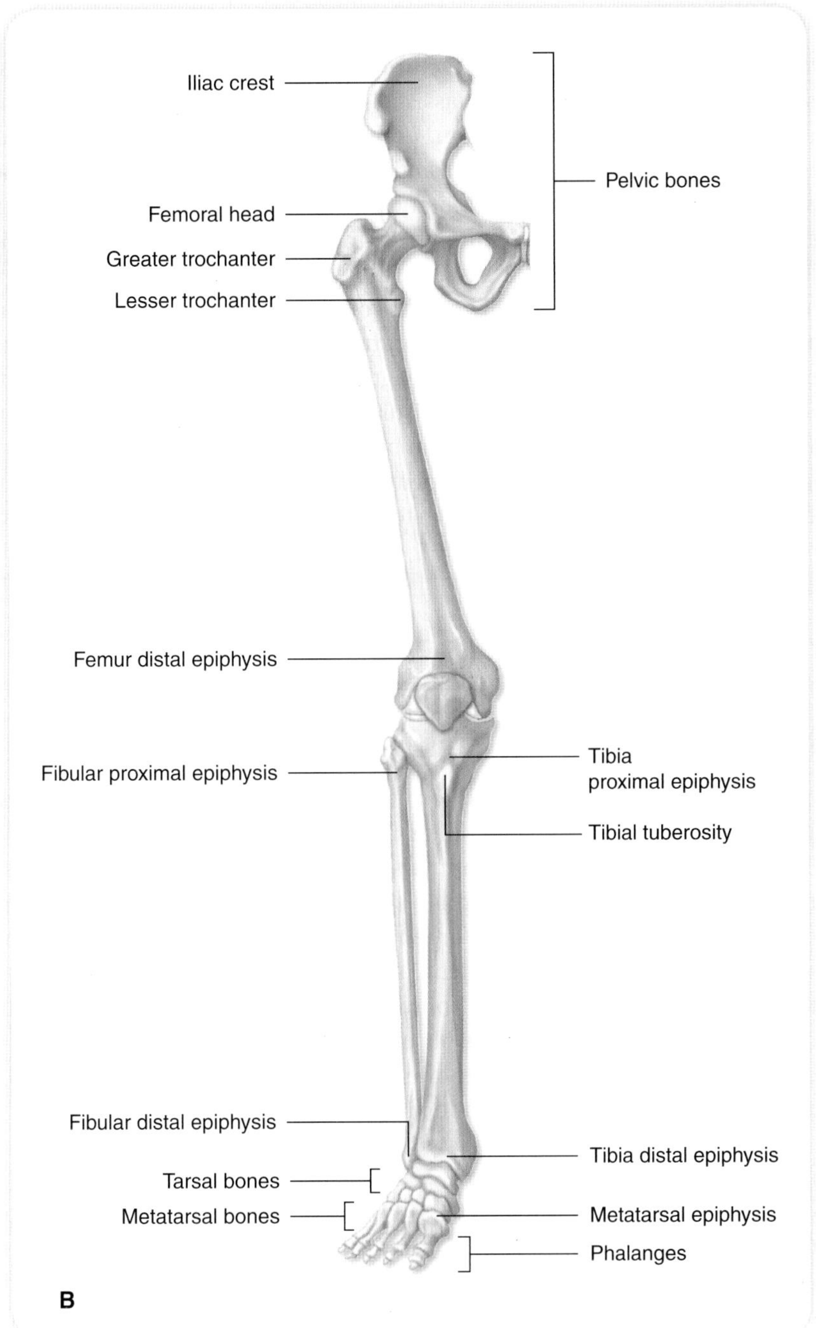

Figure 30-2 ***(Continued)***

of a macrotraumatic hyperextension or valgus injury. The medial epicondyle serves as the attachment site of the forearm flexor/pronator group, and as such can also be a location for avulsion fracture. This type of injury is typically caused by valgus loading during the acceleration phase of the throwing mechanism. Avulsion of the triceps attachment at the olecranon has also been reported. This condition has been observed to result in separated ossification centers that persist into adulthood with subsequent olecranon nonunion.[26]

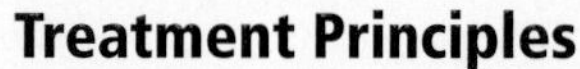

Treatment Principles

Conservative treatment of all avulsion fractures mimics that of a severe muscle strain. In fractures involving the lower extremity, assisted gait is a must until weightbearing activities are pain free and without substitution. Compression of the area in the form of elastic wraps or neoprene sleeves may provide warmth and minimize discomfort experienced with activities of daily living and early rehabilitation efforts. Modalities to minimize pain and facilitate healing are indicated early in the treatment regimen. Once inflammation from the initial injury has subsided, gentle single-joint stretching exercises can begin. Two-joint stretching exercises should begin only after 1-joint stretches are pain free. Submaximal single-joint strengthening exercises can begin when pain free. Strengthening efforts should be preceded by warm-up activities, and strengthening exercises should also be followed by stretching of the involved muscle. When isolated 2-joint strengthening efforts are tolerated without difficulty, the young athlete can be allowed to return to a functional progression program.[60] Avulsion injuries of the upper extremity must be treated with rest until the youngster is asymptomatic. A gradual return to throwing sports through a supervised functional progression program is vital.

Microtraumatic Injuries

Apophysitis

The apophysis of growing bone differs from the epiphysis of skeletally immature bone. The apophysis is an independent center of ossification that does not contribute to the longitudinal length of a long bone. An apophysis, however, does contribute to the structure and form of mature long bone by serving as a site of tendinous or ligamentous attachment. It is the role of the apophysis as the site for tendinous attachment that enters the picture of overuse injuries seen in the growing patient. At skeletal maturity, the apophysis fuses to its site of attachment to its respective long bone. Prior to skeletal maturity, however, traction placed upon an apophysis from an inflexible musculotendinous unit may result in apophyseal inflammation and delayed fusion to the long bone. Traction apophysitis commonly occurs at the tibial tubercle, calcaneus, and iliac crest.

Lower Extremity

Repetitive loading activities of the lower extremities in combination with muscle-tendon length insufficiency can yield traction forces through apophyseal centers that result in inflammation of the apophysis. Young patients involved in running, jumping, and kicking activities are inherently predisposed to large traction forces through apophyseal centers, especially during a growth spurt. These traction apophysites are typically self-limiting, but cases that do not respond to traditional conservative measures may require short-term immobilization to assist in eliminating pain and inflammation.

Calcaneal Apophysitis (Sever Disease) Sever disease is a traction apophysitis of the growth center of the calcaneus. Sever disease typically affects youngsters 8 to 13 years of age, with the peak incidence occurring at age 11 years in young females and at age 12 years in young males.[32,49] Sever disease frequently affects youngsters involved in outdoor fall sports following a dry summer that results in dry, hard ground. Soccer, football, and even band participants, especially early in the season, are commonly diagnosed with Sever disease.[60] Young soccer players who routinely participate on artificial surfaces may also experience symptoms consistent with Sever disease.[32] Spikes or other shoes lacking in adequate shock absorption and forefoot support, or shoes with broken-down heel counters, contribute to the incidence of Sever disease.

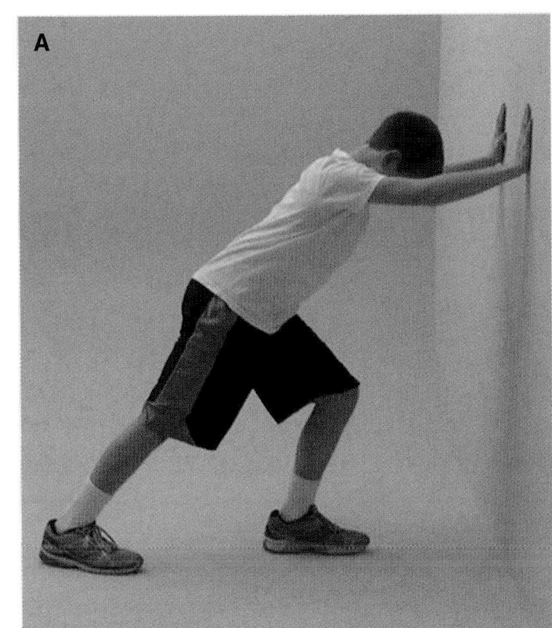

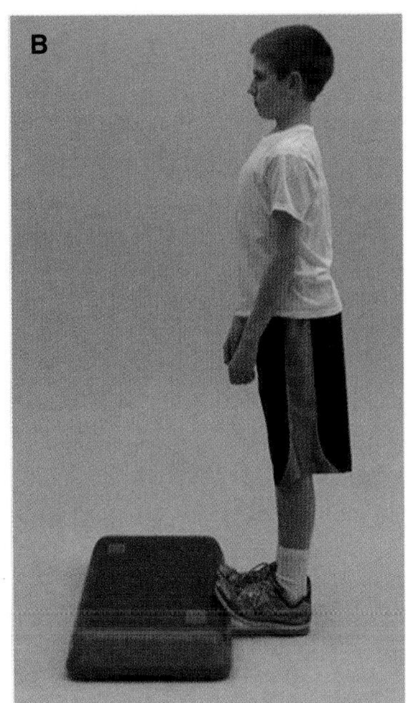

Figure 30-3

A. Front knee should be flexed for soleus stretching, back knee should be straight for gastrocnemius stretching, and heels should remain on the floor. **B.** Standing on a slantboard (see also Figure 30-4) at the point of a discernable stretch for 10 minutes can be incorporated into a home stretching program.

Sever disease is characterized by pain and point tenderness at the posterior calcaneus near the insertion of the Achilles tendon. Local signs of inflammation may be present in acute cases. Swelling at the calcaneal apophysis also may be present, but this is an exception rather than the rule. Patients with tight calves, internal tibial torsion, forefoot varus, a dorsally mobile first ray, weak dorsiflexors, and genu varus may be more susceptible to Sever disease.

Treatment of Sever disease should focus on establishing normal flexibility of the gastrocnemius-soleus muscle group (Figures 30-3 and 30-4). Calf stretching should include exercises with the knee extended and the knee flexed. Just as importantly, stretching in a weightbearing position should be performed with the correction of any rearfoot-to-lower-leg or forefoot-to-rearfoot abnormality. Orthotic intervention may be a consideration in the treatment of Sever disease and may range from temporary heel lifts or heel cups to more sophisticated custom fit orthotics to correct biomechanical abnormalities. Dorsiflexion strengthening exercises along with foot intrinsic strengthening may also help manage symptoms.[60]

Tibial Tubercle Apophysitis (Osgood-Schlatter Disease) Initially described in 1903, Osgood-Schlatter disease (OSD) is commonly seen in active and nonactive youngsters alike.[29] Like all traction apophysitises, the condition is usually self-limiting, but because of its prevalence and the ominous name, parents and young patients may mistakenly expect a poor prognosis. This is not to downplay the potential longstanding problems that can arise when the condition is not adequately diagnosed and treated.

Development of the tibial apophysis begins as a cartilaginous outgrowth. Secondary ossification centers appear with subsequent progression to an epiphyseal phase when

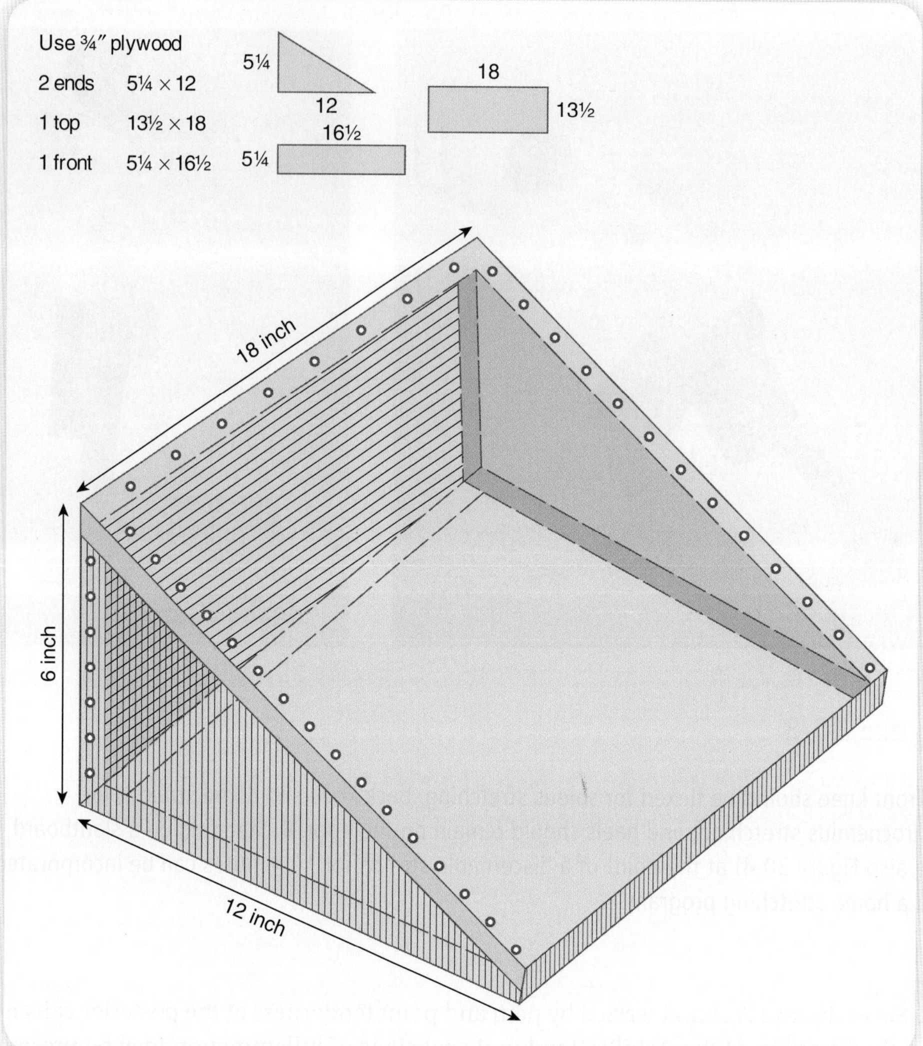

Figure 30-4 Directions for fabricating a slantboard to facilitate gastrocnemius-soleus stretching

the proximal tibial physis closes and the tibial apophysis fuses to the tibia.[23] Calcification of the apophysis begins distally at the average age of 9 years in females and 11 years in males. Fusion of the apophysis to the tibia can take place via several ossification centers and occurs, on average, at age 12 years in females and 13 years in males.[29] There is a normal transition from distal fibrocartilage to proximal fibrous tissue at the tibial apophysis. Fibrous tissue is more readily able to withstand the high tensile loads involved with athletic activities than the weaker cartilage of the secondary ossification center. Microavulsions can occur through the area of bone and cartilage at the secondary ossification center, resulting in the potential for the development of separate ossicles, which can be a source of prolonged pain or reinjury.[29] Complications of OSD are few, but in addition to the formation of an accessory ossicle, patellar subluxation (secondary to patella alta), patella baja, nonunion of the tibial tubercle, and genu recurvatum have been reported.[27,31,66]

The diagnosis of OSD is not a clinical challenge. Symptoms are typically unilateral, although up to 25% of cases can be bilateral in nature.[23] There may or may not be a history of injury. Traditional literature reveals that OSD affects more young males than females; however, recent evidence suggests no significant difference between male and female involvement.[60] The youngster typically complains of aching around the tibial tubercle that is increased during or following jumping, climbing, or kneeling activities. The tibial tubercle may be reddened, raised, or tender to palpation. Symptoms are usually confined to the tibial tubercle and typically not present at the superior or inferior patellar poles or the patellar tendon; however, patellofemoral tenderness may be present.[53] Tenderness at the cartilaginous junction of the patella and patellar tendon at the inferior patellar pole is indicative of Sinding-Larsen-Johansson disease.[55,56] Findings on radiography (especially if only performed unilaterally) are often misleading, as it is difficult to differentiate between abnormal fragmentation from normal centers of ossification. Radiographs, however, may reveal soft-tissue swelling. Some athletes with OSD also have patella alta, and some authors have noted a link between patients with OSD and Sever disease.[29]

Treatment of OSD should emphasize a judicious stretching program. Inadequate quadriceps flexibility is virtually always present. The shortened muscle group combined with the ballistic nature of quadriceps activity in jumping sports are at the heart of OSD. Overzealous stretching of the quadriceps, however, may increase the pull on the tibial tubercle and only serve to increase symptoms. Stretching of the quadriceps should begin prone, stressing an increase in quadriceps length at the knee joint only. A bolster under the hips may be required to place the muscle on slack at the hip joint. All stretching must be accompanied by a pull within the quadriceps muscle belly, not at the tibial tubercle. Two-joint stretching exercises should be instituted when adequate muscle length is established at the knee without an increase in tibial tubercle tenderness (Figure 30-5). Quadriceps weakness is frequently not a major concern in this patient population; many of these youngsters have excellent quadriceps recruitment with no atrophy. Chronic cases, however, will result in quadriceps atrophy. Pain-free isometrics or low-load and high-repetition knee extension

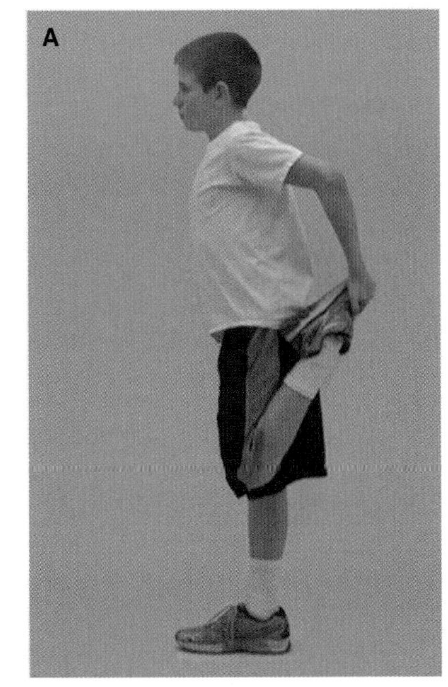

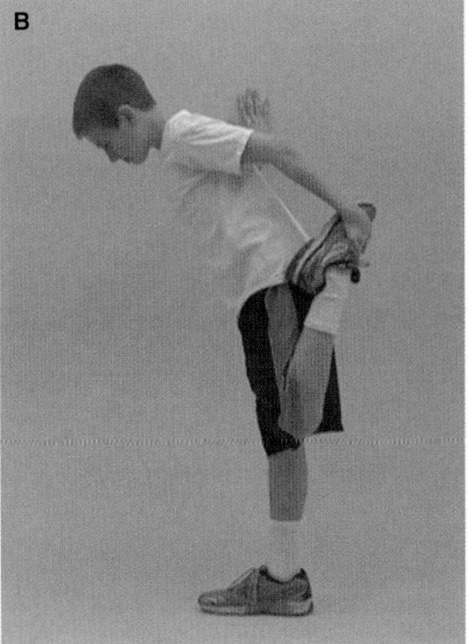

Figure 30-5 Quadriceps stretching

A. Proper technique. **B.** Improper technique with excessive trunk flexion.

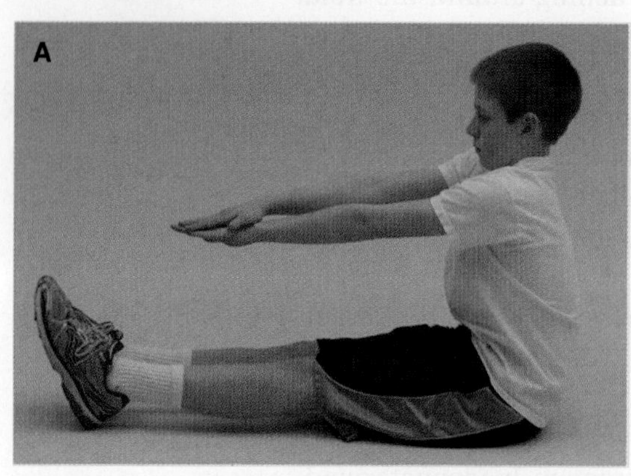

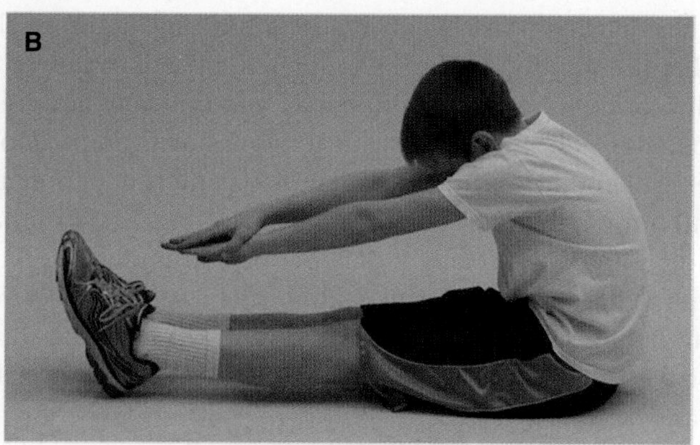

Figure 30-6 Long-sitting hamstring stretching

A. Proper technique. **B.** Improper technique with excessive thoracolumbar flexion.

exercise may be incorporated if quadriceps atrophy is noted. Progressive resistive exercises of the quadriceps must be used judiciously, as they may only serve to increase pain at the tibial tubercle. As tight hamstrings require increased quadriceps force to overcome the tight posterior structures, hamstring exercises must be included in the comprehensive program to manage OSD (Figures 30-6 and 30-7). If competing in a contact or collision sport, young athletes with OSD should be fitted with a protective pad to minimize the risks of blunt trauma to the area. When the tibial tubercle area is inflamed, even when the athlete is not participating, protective padding should also be considered to minimize the incidence of the inadvertent blunt trauma encountered in activities of daily living.[60]

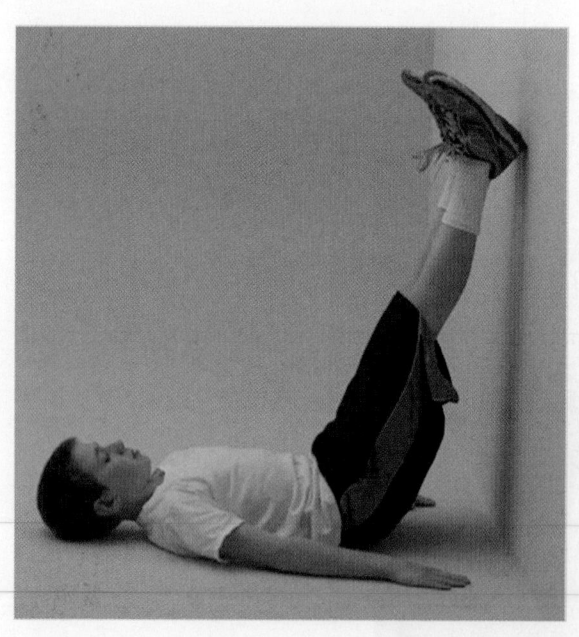

Figure 30-7 Wall stretch hamstring stretching

The youngster should maintain full knee extension and keep the buttocks on the floor. As hamstring flexibility improves, the youngster should ultimately be able to place the heels, backs of the knees, and buttocks against the wall.

Iliac Apophysitis

Iliac apophysitis is a condition typically seen in the older youngster involved in running sports. Active patients between the ages of 14 and 16 years are usually the prime candidates for iliac apophysitis.[15] The ossification center of the iliac crest appears anterolaterally and advances posteriorly until it reaches the posterior iliac spine. The average age of closure is 16 years in boys and 14 years in girls, but closure may be delayed up to 4 additional years.[28] The gluteus medius originates on the ilium just inferior to the iliac crest and is another muscle that may contribute to iliac apophysitis. The gluteus medius helps to maintain pelvic symmetry for single-leg stance activities during running and hopping. Inflammation of the iliac apophysis is thought to be from a repetitive pull of the abdominal musculature at its insertion on the iliac crest.[43] During physical activities, the abdominal muscles serve as trunk stabilizers and accessory muscles of respiration. Although most commonly seen as an overuse apophysitis, incomplete avulsion fractures of the iliac apophysis have been reported from sudden contraction of the abdominals with a quick change in direction while running.

Patients who experience iliac apophysitis usually demonstrate exquisite point tenderness along the iliac crest, which is typically unilateral and located along the anterior one-half of the iliac crest. Seated or standing lateral trunk flexion away from the side of involvement is usually uncomfortable. Weakness or pain with resisted hip abduction, oblique abdominal muscular activity, and pain or compensation with hopping on the involved leg may also be present. A complete lower-extremity biomechanical examination may be indicated to determine structural or compensatory leg length inequality that may contribute to iliac apophysitis.

Treatment of iliac apophysitis should center on regaining normal flexibility of the iliotibial band, the abdominals, and gluteus medius. The patient at the outset of a flexibility program typically tolerates 2-joint stretching of the iliotibial band with the knee extended (Figure 30-8). The traditional Ober test position, along with variations, is efficient stretching activity, but often accompanied by substitution of excessive hip flexion, trunk flexion, or rotation. Seated lateral flexion away from the side of involvement, progressed to standing lateral flexion, which is then progressed to standing lateral flexion with arms extended overhead, is a good stretching progression. Prone press-ups with rotation and lateral flexion may also be incorporated into the stretching program.[60]

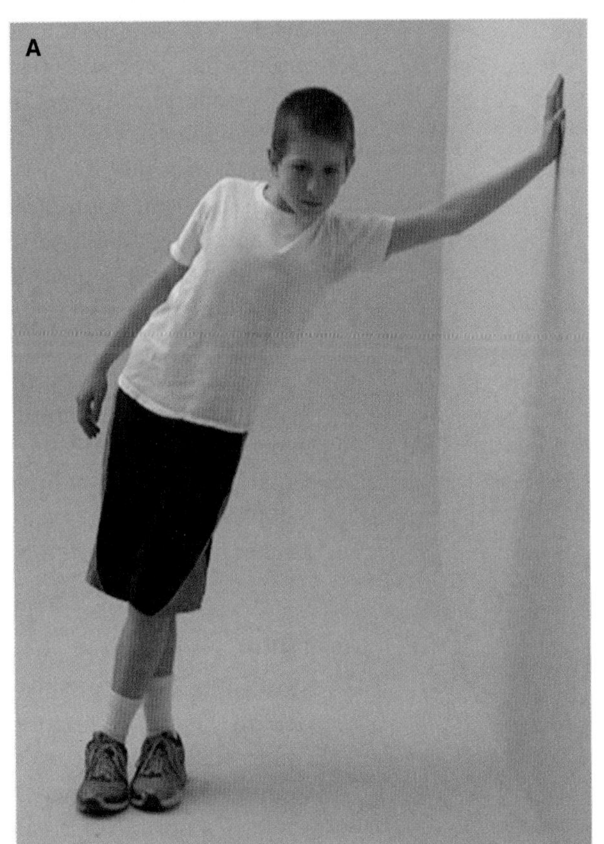

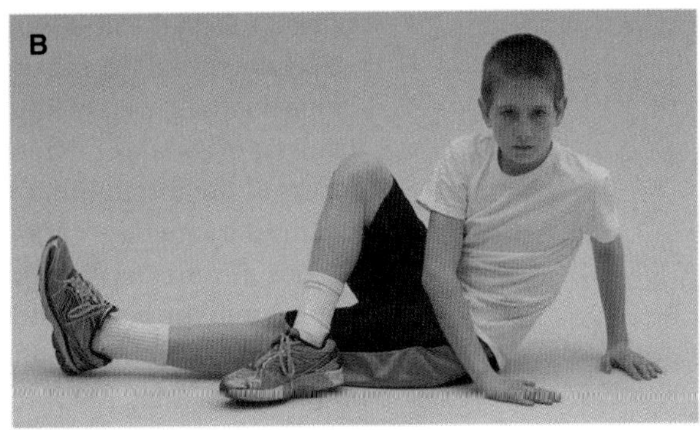

Figure 30-8

A. Standing iliotibial band stretching. The uninvolved leg is crossed over in front of the involved leg and the youngster leans the hips toward the wall. **B.** Side-lying iliotibial band stretching. Lying on the involved side with feet, hips, and shoulders in a straight alignment, the athlete pushes up onto extended elbows.

Fifth Metatarsal Apophysitis (Iselin Disease) Out of many traction apophysites that affect the young patient, Iselin disease is the most rarely encountered. The insertion of the peroneus brevis may be irritated by activities requiring fine foot control as in the case of dancers and gymnasts. Patients with abnormal relationships between the forefoot and rearfoot may be predisposed to Iselin disease. A tight gastrocnemius-soleus complex or weak dorsiflexors may also contribute to apophysitis at the base of the fifth metatarsal.[51]

Upper Extremity

As previously noted, the elbow is subjected to large forces during the throwing mechanism. These forces are especially problematic in baseball pitchers and catchers, as well as young tennis players.[30] In the skeletally immature patient, these forces may result in shoulder and/or elbow injury. Much has been done to explore the reasons for shoulder and elbow injury in the throwing youngster. In regards to the youth baseball pitcher, the previously held notion that throwing the curve ball at an early age was the primary cause in developing elbow problems. Recent work, however, demonstrates that the velocity of throwing and the number of pitches contribute to a much greater extent than the type of pitch.[47] The American Orthopaedic Society for Sports Medicine does recommend age-appropriate introduction to a variety of pitches with the fastball only from age 8 years followed by the introduction of a changeup at age 10 years, the curve at age 14 years, and other offspeed pitches following after that.[30] To minimize the risk of overuse injury, various organizations have proposed guidelines to limit throwing in the developing arm. The American Academy of Orthopaedic Surgeons recommends limiting pitching to no more than 4 to 10 innings per week and 60 to 100 pitches per game.[30] Little League Baseball recommends age-specific pitch counts, as well as suggested rest periods between throwing.[5] Knowledge of and adherence to the pitch count recommendations are inconsistent.[18,35] Measures to consider regarding the prevention of overuse injuries in children include preparticipation exams, ensuring appropriate parental supervision and coaching, recognizing sport readiness, avoiding training errors, delaying single-sport specialization, allowing for adequate rest and recovery, and avoiding overscheduling.[16,36]

Although these guidelines are an important step in preventing upper-extremity overuse injury, they are only part of the story. Many youngsters participate in organized baseball programs that are not officially affiliated with Little League. These youngsters may not have guidelines to regulate how much an individual can pitch. These guidelines also do not apply to batting practice and often are not considered when youngsters pitch in tournament play. Finally, the number of innings may not be the best indicator to use, as an inning in baseball played by 9- to 12-year-olds ranges from 4 to 50 pitches per inning, and the number of pitches per pitching outing ranges from 4 to 100.[4]

Spine

Most spine injuries involve the muscles, ligaments, and intervertebral disks. These injuries are usually self-limiting and rarely result in significant neurologic compromise.[59] Two conditions of the osseous structures of the spine, however, do involve the young patient: spondylolysis and spondylolisthesis. Spondylolysis is a bony defect in the pars interarticularis, a portion of the neural arch located between the superior and inferior articular facets. Physical forces encountered by youngsters involved in physical activities play a significant role in the development of spondylolysis. Activities that involve repetitive loading, especially with the lumbar spine in extension/hyperextension, such as ballet, gymnastics, diving, football, weight lifting, and wrestling, have been implicated in spondylolysis. Spondylolysis originates in children between the ages of 5 and 10 years, and most frequently occurs at the fifth lumbar vertebra, with the fourth lumbar vertebra being involved second most frequently.[42] Many youngsters with spondylolysis remain asymptomatic for long periods of time and are not diagnosed until later in their skeletal development. Radiographs from the lateral and oblique views are required in order to visualize the fracture in its entirety along the longitudinal plane. Positive radiograph findings include asymmetry of the neural arch, inferior apophyseal joint, and posterior elements with rotation of the spinous process away from a unilateral spondylolytic lesion. CT scan and bone scan with single-photon emission computed tomography can aid in the radiologic diagnosis and staging of spondylolysis.[41] A common finding in patients with spondylolysis (symptomatic or asymptomatic) is hamstring spasm.[58] The etiology of this hamstring spasm is thought to be caused by either a postural reflex to stabilize the L5-S1 segment or to nerve root irritation.[27,41,42,58]

Spondylolisthesis is a condition in which a vertebra slips anterior to the vertebra immediately below it. Spondylolisthesis most frequently takes place between the fifth lumbar and first sacral vertebrae, although the condition can occur at more than one spinal segment. The superior border of the inferior vertebra is divided into quarters, and the slip is described in terms of the width that the superior vertebra slips anteriorly in relation to the vertebra below it. A grade 1 spondylolisthesis is an anterior slip of 25% or less of the vertebral width; a grade 2 slip is up to 50% of the vertebral width; a grade 3 spondylolisthesis is a slip up to 75% of the vertebral width; and a grade 4 is a complete anterior slip. Spondylolisthesis is classified as degenerative, traumatic, pathologic, or isthmic. It is the isthmic classification that typically involves the young patient. In the isthmic category of spondylolisthesis, it is debatable whether a bilateral spondylolysis is a precursor for slippage and resultant instability of a spinal segment.

Treatment of spondylolysis and spondylolisthesis centers on healing of the bony defect and decreasing the patient's symptoms. Treatment depends upon the physician's personal preference and ranges from relative rest without a brace to 23 hours of bracing. When bracing is used, the brace is typically a rigid custom-fit lumbar spinal orthosis designed to keep the youngster out of extension. In addition to activity modification, hamstring stretching is an integral part of the treatment program.

Special Considerations

Musculoskeletal Considerations

Some conditions involving the young patient may actually be congenital in nature, but do not cause symptoms until the youngster becomes physically active in youth sports or physical education classes. Conditions such as these have unknown etiologies; some clearly have genetic predispositions, whereas others may be traced to excessive activity. Musculoskeletal conditions that are discussed here include tarsal coalition, Legg-Calvé-Perthes disease (LCPD), slipped capital femoral epiphysis (SCFE), osteochondroses, and patellofemoral pain syndrome.

Tarsal Coalition

Persistent ankle and foot pain in the young patient in conjunction with recurrent ankle sprains could possibly be a result of an underlying tarsal coalition. A tarsal coalition is an abnormal fusion between tarsal bones in the rearfoot or midfoot caused by a failure of bony segmentation. The most common tarsal coalitions occur between the calcaneus and navicular, the talus and the navicular, or the talus and calcaneus. Most tarsal coalitions present clinically in patients between the ages of 8 and 16 years, with anywhere from 50% to 60% of tarsal coalitions occurring bilaterally. There is familial predisposition in some cases of tarsal coalition.[51] As coalitions can be fibrous, cartilaginous, or osseous, radiographs of the foot are many times interpreted as being unremarkable. Bone scan and CT scan may be of benefit in those cases where radiographs fail to demonstrate pathologic findings. Stretching and strengthening of extrinsic and intrinsic ankle musculature may help to minimize motion and strength losses. A custom made or off-the-shelf orthosis may also help to minimize symptoms.[36]

Legg-Calvé-Perthes Disease

LCPD is an avascular necrosis of the femoral head thought to be caused by an occlusion of the blood supply to the femoral head from excessive fluid pressure resulting from an inflammatory or traumatic synovial effusion of the hip joint. LCPD typically involves active youngsters between the ages of 3 and 11 years and is found 4 times more frequently in young boys than in young girls. LCPD is usually unilateral, although 15% of youngsters have bilateral involvement.[49] Youngsters diagnosed with LCPD may or may not be able to recall a history of trauma, but LCPD should be ruled out in any male athlete younger than 12 years of age

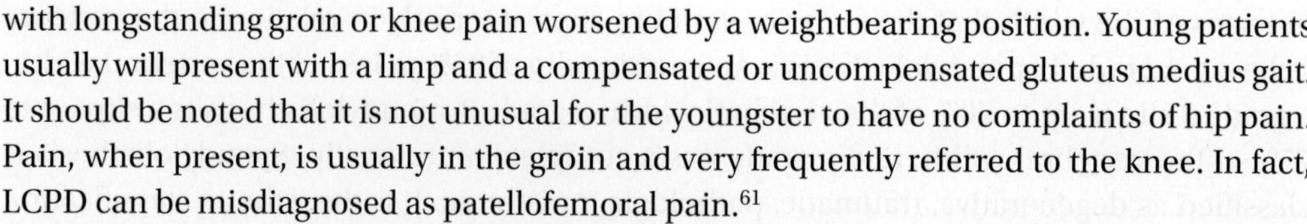

with longstanding groin or knee pain worsened by a weightbearing position. Young patients usually will present with a limp and a compensated or uncompensated gluteus medius gait. It should be noted that it is not unusual for the youngster to have no complaints of hip pain. Pain, when present, is usually in the groin and very frequently referred to the knee. In fact, LCPD can be misdiagnosed as patellofemoral pain.[61]

Slipped Capital Femoral Epiphysis

SCFE, although rare, is a condition that may not manifest itself until a youngster becomes involved in sports activities. SCFE involves boys twice as often as girls and typically occurs between 10 and 15 years of age during a period of rapid growth.[53,64] A suspected causative factor is a potential hormonal imbalance; consequently, SCFE should be suspected in youngsters who are tall and thin or short and obese who complain of longstanding thigh, groin, or knee pain. Progressive cases of SCFE may result in a varus deformity with concomitant external rotation.

There are also other conditions that may result in groin pain or pain around the pelvis that may be manifested after a macrotraumatic event. Musculoskeletal conditions include hernia, avulsion fracture of the lesser trochanter, iliopectineal bursitis/tendinitis (snapping hip), abdominal muscle strain, congenital dislocation of the hip, septic arthritis, and toxic synovitis. Nonmusculoskeletal differential diagnoses as a source of acute or persistent hip pain include leukemia and neuroblastoma.[48] Other potential causes of hip pain are bone tumor, appendicitis, pelvic inflammatory disease, hemophilia, arterial insufficiency, and sickle cell anemia.[22]

Osteochondroses

Osteochondrosis and osteochondritis are 2 distinctly different pathologic entities. Osteochondrosis is typically a self-limiting disorder that involves a secondary epiphyseal center or pressure epiphysis at the end of a long bone or a primary epiphyseal center of a small bone.[57] Osteochondrosis involves degeneration or avascular necrosis with resultant regeneration or recalcification and typically does not demonstrate bony fragmentation.[8,57] Osteochondritis, on the other hand, is an inflammation of the subchondral bone and articular cartilage. Osteochondritis dissecans involves resultant fragmentation of articular cartilage within the joint. Many of the osteochondroses have their origins in chronic, repetitive trauma. The pathology and subsequent prognosis of osteochondrosis and osteochondritis of immature bone differ from that of mature bone.

Juvenile osteochondritis dissecans (JOCD) of the knee can be a devastating condition if not diagnosed and treated early. Although ischemia, genetic predisposition, and abnormal ossification are theoretical causes of JOCD,[24] growing evidence suggests that microtrauma to the immature knee over the course of months and years is the primary cause of JOCD.[9,10] The majority of JOCD lesions involve the medial femoral condyle, and most lesions occur on the weightbearing surface. The site of JOCD pathology is subchondral bone, not articular cartilage.[11] Many lesions go undiagnosed or misdiagnosed. In a series of 192 patients, 80% had symptoms for more than 15 months and 90% had symptoms for longer than 8 months.[9] Symptoms center around an insidious onset of knee pain, with or without effusion, and knee pain that is increased with weightbearing activities and typically reduced with rest. Youngsters with JOCD are usually involved in year-round physical activity, or participate in more than 1 sport with little, if any rest, between sporting seasons. Successful treatment is based upon accurate diagnosis, staging of the activity of the lesion, the ability of the lesion to heal, and subsequent nonoperative or operative intervention. Conservative treatment centers around minimizing weightbearing and shear forces, activity modification, stretching of inflexible hamstrings and calves that serve to increase joint reaction forces, and appropriate quadriceps strengthening exercises initiated and progressed on an individual basis.

Another common site of osteochondrosis involves the elbow of a growing patient. Osteochondrosis of the capitellum of the elbow is called Panner disease. Panner disease is typically seen in young throwing athletes who complain of chronic dull aching in the elbow joint. Point tenderness at the lateral elbow is common, as is a subtle loss of elbow extension.[8] As the condition progresses, the loss of extension can be more pronounced and accompanied by a loss of pronation and supination. Initially, rest and activity modification is important and should be followed by a range of motion and strengthening program along with a supervised functional progression program to return to throwing.

Patellofemoral Pain

Patellofemoral pain is frequently encountered in many physical therapy clinics. Symptoms in youngsters are comparable to their adult counterparts. Dull peripatellar aching, pain with stairs or prolonged sitting, giving way of the knee, and pseudolocking episodes in extension are classic signs of patellofemoral involvement. Treatment is symptomatic and should include pain-free quadriceps strengthening; hamstring, calf, and iliotibial band stretching; correction of biomechanical abnormalities; activity modification; bracing; and screening for signs of hyperelasticity that may indicate patellofemoral joint instability.

Growing Pains

Prior to closing out the description of various microtaumatic concerns in the youngster, the clinician should also be made aware of the significance of the diagnosis of growing pains. It is not uncommon for the physical therapist to receive a referral to address various musculoskeletal issues in a growing child with the chief complaint of pain. The referring practitioner may lack sufficient knowledge in musculoskeletal examination principles to provide an adequate clinical impression. Because the presenting chief complaint in an active child can be pain, a clinical diagnosis of growing pains is made. Growing pains is a misnomer as the process of growing should not be painful and the majority of children who truly have growing pains do not experience symptoms during growth spurts. The diagnosis of growing pains should never be taken at face value by the therapist.

When present, growing pains are typically seen in younger children. Pain is usually in the thighs, calves, or shins and is bilateral. It is usually present during the evening or at night, and there is usually no morning stiffness. The youngster does not typically limp on the involved lower extremity. In cases where pain is located in areas other than the lower extremities, when pain is accompanied by morning stiffness, a limp, malaise, recurrent fever, and/or night sweats, further examination is indicated as opposed to accepting the clinical impression of growing pains at face value.

Physiologic Considerations

The youngster's cardiovascular response to exercise is related to the size of the youngster.[65] Children demonstrate a double sigmoid growth pattern from birth to adulthood. There is a rapid gain in growth in infancy and early childhood that slows down during middle childhood. The second rapid increase in growth occurs during adolescence. The peak height velocity is defined as the maximum rate of growth in stature and occurs in girls from 10.5 to 13 years, but may start as early as 9 years or as late as 15 years. Peak height velocity of boys occurs from 12.5 to 15 years, but may start as early as 10 years or as late as 16 years.[48]

As the youngster's heart is smaller than that of the mature adult, its capacity as a reservoir for blood is also smaller. Children, therefore, have a lower stroke volume at all levels of exercise.[65] The exercising youngster compensates for this lower stroke volume with an increased heart rate. As is seen in the adult, the youngster's systolic blood pressure rises during exercise, but the child's elevation in systolic blood pressure is less than that seen in the adult.[65] The red blood cell count for young boys and girls are similar with comparable abilities to carry oxygen to exercising organs. After menarche, however, females demonstrate lower blood volume and fewer red blood cells, with a resultant decreased oxygen-carrying capacity. Thus, young girls typically demonstrate a mean blood pressure lower than that seen in young boys.[50]

As the child's thoracic cavity is smaller than that of the mature adult, the child demonstrates a smaller vital capacity than the adult and also shows an elevated respiration rate as compared to the mature adult.[6,65] As the child matures, the ability to perform work (both aerobic and anaerobic) increases.[4,6,49,65] After menarche, girls have a slightly lower oxygen uptake per kilogram of body weight but are similar to boys per kilogram of lean body weight.[21,28] The maximum oxygen uptake is similar in young boys and girls until approximately 12 years of age. Males continue to demonstrate an increase until 16 to 18 years of age, with females failing to show significant gains after 12 to 14 years of age.[5,63] Young boys and girls have similar proportions of slow-twitch and fast-twitch muscle fiber. Strength differences between the genders are minimal when strength is expressed relative to fat-free weight. Both young boys and young girls have been shown to be able to safely participate in strength-training programs.[8,10,26,38]

Independent of gender, the young athlete typically does not tolerate prolonged periods of heat exposure; therefore, care must be taken when the youngster participates in sports in a hot and humid environment. A child has a greater surface area-to-mass ratio than does the typical adult, resulting in a greater transfer of heat into their young bodies. The child also has a higher production of metabolic heat per kilogram of body weight as compared to adult counterparts, which serves to further challenge the young thermoregulatory system.[4,6,49,65]

Psychological Considerations

To this point, the chapter has presented many physical and physiologic characteristics that constitute the unique challenges to evaluating and treating youth injuries. Before concluding this chapter, however, another vital area must also be discussed—the unique psychological demands placed upon young athletes, especially those involved in intense competition and training.

There are many benefits to physical activity in the youngster (Table 30-3).[12] There are many differences, however, between free-flowing play and organized sports. Organized sports, fortunately or unfortunately, carry the obligatory win or lose connotations of competition and also involve adults who coach and train the youngster as well as adults who interpret and enforce the rules that govern competition. The adverse effect of adult influences upon the young athlete is but one potential negative psychological aspect of youth sport participation.

Participation in organized sport can be taken to an extreme. Intensive participation can be described in terms of frequency and/or intensity. Examples of intensive participation include the ice skater or gymnast who trains daily for hours and competes all year round for years on end. Other examples include the multisport athlete who trains and competes on a daily basis all year round. This intensive participation places significant physical demands on the

Table 30-3 Benefits of Physical Activity in Children

Physical
Increased maximal aerobic power and general stamina
Control of body mass and fat reduction
Increased muscle strength and endurance
Increased range of motion
Decreased blood lipid levels
Improved ventilatory efficiency
Increased oxygen consumption
Psychological
Feelings of competency and mastery
Personal self-esteem
Engaging in enjoyable behavior
Achieving desired goals
Gaining admiration of others
Safe training in risk-taking behavior
Satisfaction in achievement
Feeling of working toward a goal
Peer group interaction
Awareness of, and adherence to, rules
Personal role definition

Table 30-4 Potential Negative Aspects of Intensive Youth Sport Participation

- Children are not permitted to be children.
- Children are denied important social contacts and experiences.
- Children are victims of a disrupted family life.
- Children may experience impaired intellectual development.
- Children are exposed to excessive psychological/physiologic stress.
- Children may become so involved with sport that they become detached from society.
- Children may face a type of abandonment upon completion of their athletic career.

body, demands that may result in serious overuse or stress-failure injury. Just as the young body grows to accept greater physical demands, so does the young mind. Intensive participation places many demands on the youngster, some of which may be unrealistic. As this relates to intense competition, research demonstrates that a child's cognitive ability to develop a mature understanding of the competition process does not occur until the age of 12 years. It is not until between the ages of 10 and 12 years that children develop the capacity to comprehend more than just one other viewpoint. Finally, after the age of 12 years, the youngster can readily adopt a team perspective.[30,44]

Table 30-4 identifies the negative psychological aspects of intense youth sport participation. Psychological issues may also enter the picture when rehabilitating youth sport participants involved in intense competition and training. Risk factors for psychological complications in the injured child include stress in the family, high-achieving siblings, over- or underinvolved parent(s), a paradoxical lack of leisure in athletic activity, self-esteem that is reliant on athletic prowess, and a narrow range of interests beyond athletics.[32,46]

This chapter provided an overview of the unique physical and psychological issues that affect youth sport participants. The rehabilitation professional evaluating and treating the young athlete must be cognizant of these unique features. Evaluation and treatment principles must reflect the special circumstances that present in the youth athlete.

SUMMARY

1. Pediatric patients are not miniature adults and should not be treated as such.
2. There are many proposed benefits of strength training in children and adolescents, including increased strength, power, endurance, and neuromuscular skill.
3. Current evidence indicates that there are no contraindications to strength-based exercises in young patients.
4. Children and adolescents should not be allowed to exercise to exhaustion or train without supervision.
5. A high index of suspicion for epiphyseal injury should be used when examining young patients after traumatic injuries. Immature bone is susceptible to damage at the growth plates.
6. Apophyseal injuries occur uniquely in the growing child or adolescent, and are due to traction placed on the bony apophysis by the musculotendinous unit that inserts there.
7. There are many excellent physical and psychosocial benefits to sport participation in children and adolescents.

REFERENCES

1. Agricola R, Bessems JH, Ginai AZ, Heijboer MP. The development of cam-type deformity in adolescent and young male soccer players. *Am J Sports Med.* 2012;40:1099.
2. Anderson AF, Anderson CN. Transepiphyseal anterior cruciate ligament reconstruction in pediatric patients: surgical technique. *Sports Health.* 2009;1:76.
3. Andrish JT. Upper extremity injuries in the skeletally immature athlete. In: Nicholas JA, Hershman EB, eds. *The Upper Extremity in Sports Medicine.* St. Louis, MO: Mosby; 1990:673.
4. Axe MJ, Snyder-Mackler L, Konin JG, Strube MJ. Development of a distance-based interval throwing program for Little League-aged athletes. *Am J Sports Med.* 1996;24:594.
5. Bar-Or O. The prepubescent female. In: Shangold M, Mirkin G, eds. *Women and Exercise.* 2nd ed. Philadelphia, PA: Davis; 1994:240-251.
6. Bar-Or O. *Pediatric Sports Medicine for the Practitioner: From Physiologic Principles to Clinical Applications.* New York, NY: Springer-Verlag; 1983.
7. Best TM. Muscle-tendon injuries in young athletes. *Clin Sports Med.* 1995;14:669.
8. Bianco AJ. Osteochondritis dissecans. In: Morrey BF, ed. *The Elbow and Its Disorders.* Philadelphia, PA: Saunders; 1985:254.
9. Cahill BR. Treatment of juvenile osteochondritis of the knee. *Sports Med Arthroscopy Rev.* 1994;2:65.
10. Cahill BR, moderator. *Proceedings of the Conference on Strength Training and the Pubescent.* Chicago, IL: American Orthopaedic Society for Sports Medicine; 1988.
11. Cahill BR. Treatment of juvenile osteochondritis dissecans and osteochondritis dissecans of the knee. *Clin Sports Med.* 1985;4:367.
12. Cahill BR, Pearl AJ. *Intensive Participation in Children's Sports.* Champaign, IL: Human Kinetics; 1993.
13. Cahill BR, Tullos HS, Fain RH. Little League shoulder. *Sports Med.* 1974;2:150.
14. Carson WC, Gasser SI. Little Leaguer's shoulder: a report of 23 cases. *Am J Sports Med.* 1998;26:575.
15. Clancy WG. Running. In: Reider B, ed. *Sports Medicine: The School-Aged Athlete.* Philadelphia, PA: Saunders; 1991:632.
16. DiFiori JP. Evaluation of overuse injuries in children and adolescents. *Curr Sports Med Rep.* 2010;9:372.
17. DiStafano LJ, Blackburn JT, Marshall SW, Guskiewicz. Effects of an age-specific anterior cruciate ligament injury prevention program on lower extremity biomechanics in children. *Am J Sports Med.* 2011;39:949.
18. Fazarale JJ, Magnussen RA, Pedroza AD, Kaeding CC. Knowledge of and compliance with pitch count recommendations: a survey of youth baseball coaches. *Sports Health.* 2012;4:202.
19. Fleisig GS, Weber A, Hassell N, Andrews JR. Prevention of elbow injuries in youth baseball pitchers. *Curr Sports Med Rep.* 2009;8:250.
20. Frush TJ, Lindenfeld, TN. Peri-epiphyseal and overuse injuries in adolescent athletes. *Sports Health.* 2009;1:201.
21. Garrett WE, Best TM. Anatomy, physiology, and mechanics of skeletal muscle. In: Simon SS, ed. *Orthopaedic Basic Science.* Rosemont, IL: American Academy of Orthopaedic Surgeons; 1994.
22. Goodman CG, Snyder TE. *Differential Diagnosis in Physical Therapy.* 2nd ed. Philadelphia, PA: Saunders; 1995.
23. Graf BK, Fujisaki CK, Reider B. Disorders of the patellar tendon. In: Reider B, ed. *Sports Medicine: The School-Aged Athlete.* Philadelphia, PA: Saunders; 1991:355.
24. Graf BK, Lange RH. Osteochondritis dissecans. In: Reider B, ed. *Sports Medicine: The School-Aged Athlete.* Philadelphia, PA: Saunders; 1991.
25. Hui C, Roe J, Ferguson D, Walter A. Outcome of anatomic transphyseal anterior cruciate ligament reconstruction in Tanner stage 1 and 2 patients with open physes. *Am J Sports Med.* 2012;40:1093.
26. Ireland ML, Andrews JR. Shoulder and elbow injuries in the young athlete. *Clin Sports Med.* 1988;7:473.
27. Jakob RP, Von Gumppenberg S, Engelhardt P. Does Osgood–Schlatter disease influence the position of the patella? *J Bone Joint Surg Br.* 1981;63:579.
28. Kemper HC. Exercise and training in childhood and adolescence. In: Torg JS, Welsh RP, Shephard RJ, eds. *Current Therapy in Sports Medicines* 2. Toronto, Canada: Decker; 1990.
29. Kujala UM, Kvist M, Heinonen O. Osgood-Schlatter's disease in adolescent athletes: retrospective study of incidence and duration. *Am J Sports Med.* 1985;13:239.
30. Kramer DE. Elbow pain and injury in young athletes. *J Pediatr Orthop.* 2010;S7.
31. Lancourt JE, Cristini JA. Patella alta and patella infera: their etiological role in patellar dislocation, chondromalacia, and apophysitis of the tibial tubercle. *J Bone Joint Surg Am.* 1975;57:1112.
32. Larkin J, Brage M. Ankle, hindfoot, and midfoot injuries. In: Reider B, ed. *Sports Medicine: The School-Aged Athlete.* Philadelphia, PA: Saunders; 1991:365.
33. Lawrence JT, Argawal N, Ganley TJ. Degeneration of the knee joint in skeletally immature patients with a diagnosis of an anterior cruciate ligament tear: is there harm in delay of treatment? *Am J Sports Med.* 2011;39:2582.
34. Leonard J, Hutchinson MR. Shoulder injuries in skeletally immature throwers: review and current thoughts. *Br J Sports Med.* 2010;44:306.
35. Little League Baseball, Inc. Williamsport, PA.
36. Luke A, Lazaro RM, Bergeron MF, Keyser L. Sports-related injuries in youth athletes: is overscheduling a risk factor? *Clin J Sport Med.* 2011;21:307.

37. Murachovsky J, Ikemoto, RY, Nascimento GP, Bueno RS. Does the presence of proximal humerus growth plate changes in young baseball pitchers happen only in symptomatic athletes? An x-ray evaluation of 21 young baseball pitchers. *Br J Sports Med.* 2010;44:90.
38. National Strength and Conditioning Association. Position paper on prepubescent strength training. *Natl Strength Train J.* 1985;7:27.
39. Neale T. Use of Tommy John surgery for young elbows on the rise. *MedPage Today.* http://www.medpagetoday.com/Orthopedics/Orthopedics/10573.
40. Noyes FR, Barber Westin SD. Anterior cruciate ligament injury prevention training in female athletes: a systematic review of injury reduction and results of athletic performance tests. *Sports Health.* 2012;4:36.
41. O'Leary PF, Boiardo RA. The diagnosis and treatment of injuries of the spine in athletes. In: Nicholas JA, Hershman EB, eds. *The Lower Extremity and Spine in Sports Medicine.* 3rd ed. St. Louis, MO: Mosby; 1995:1171.
42. Outerbridge AR, Micheli LJ. Overuse injuries in the young athlete. *Clin Sports Med.* 1995;14:503.
43. Paletta GA, Andrish JT. Injuries about the hip and pelvis in the young athlete. *Clin Sports Med.* 1995;14:59.
44. Passer MW. Determinants and consequences of children's competitive stress. In: Smoll FL, Magill RA, Ash MJ, eds. *Children in Sport.* 3rd ed. Champaign, IL: Human Kinetics; 1988.
45. Peterson HA. Physeal fractures. In: Morrey BF, ed. *The Elbow and Its Disorders.* Philadelphia, PA: Saunders; 1985:222.
46. Pillemer FG, Micheli LJ. Psychological considerations in youth sports. *Clin Sports Med.* 1988;7:679.
47. Ray T. Youth baseball injuries: recognition, treatment, and prevention. *Curr Sports Med Rep.* 2010;9:294.
48. Roemmich JN, Rogol AD. Physiology of growth and development: its relationship to performance in the young athlete. *Clin Sports Med.* 1995;14:483.
49. Salter RB. *Textbook of Disorders and Injuries of the Musculoskeletal System.* 2nd ed. Baltimore, MD: Lippincott Williams & Wilkins; 1983.
50. Sanborn CF, Jankowski CM. Physiological considerations for women in sport. *Clin Sports Med.* 1994;13:315.
51. Santopietro FJ. Foot and foot-related injuries in the young athlete. *Clin Sports Med.* 1988;7:563.
52. Shelbourne DK, Sullivan AN, Bohard K, Gray T. Return to basketball and soccer after anterior cruciate ligament reconstruction in school-aged athletes. *Sports Health.* 2009;1:236.
53. Sim FH, Rock MG, Scott SG. Pelvis and hip injuries in athletes: anatomy and function. In: Nicholas JA, Hershman EB, eds. *The Lower Extremity and Spine in Sports Medicine.* 3rd ed. St. Louis, MO: Mosby; 1995:1025.
54. Simmons BP, Lovallo JL. Hand and wrist injuries in children. *Clin Sports Med.* 1988;7:495.
55. Smith AD, Tao SS. Knee injuries in young athletes. *Clin Sports Med.* 1995;14:650.
56. Stanitski CL. Anterior knee pain syndrome in the adolescent. *J Bone Joint Surg Am.* 1993;75:1407.
57. Stanitski CL. Combating overuse injuries: a focus on children and adolescents. *Phys Sportsmed.* 1993;21:87.
58. Stinson JT. Spondylolysis and spondylolisthesis in the athlete. *Clin Sports Med.* 1993;12:517.
59. Tall RL, DeVault W. Spinal injury in sport: Epidemiologic considerations. *Clin Sports Med.* 1993;12:441.
60. Tippett SR. Lower extremity injuries in the young athlete. *Orthop Phys Ther Clin N Am.* 1997;6:471.
61. Tippett SR. Referred knee pain in a young athlete: a case study. *J Orthop Sports Phys Ther.* 1994;19:117.
62. Torg JS, Pavlov H, Morris VB. Salter–Harris type-III fracture of the medial femoral condyle occurring in the adolescent athlete. *J Bone Joint Surg Am.* 1981;63:586.
63. Van De Loo DA, Johnson MD. The young female athlete. *Clin Sports Med.* 1995;14:687.
64. Waters PM, Millis MB. Hip and pelvic injuries in the young athlete. *Clin Sports Med.* 1988;7:513.
65. Woodall WR, Weber MD. Exercise response and thermoregulation. *Orthop Phys Ther Clin N Am.* 1998;7:1.
66. Zimbler S, Merkow S. Genu recurvatum: a possible complication after Osgood-Schlatter disease. *J Bone Joint Surg Am.* 1984;66:1129.

31

Considerations for the Physically Active Female

Barbara J. Hoogenboom, Teresa L. Schuemann, and Robyn K. Smith

OBJECTIVES

After completion of this chapter, the physical therapist should be able to do the following:

- Recognize/identify the general anatomic, physiologic, and neuromuscular differences that exist between genders.
- Develop an understanding of common gender differences that predispose the female athlete to development of patellofemoral dysfunction.
- Identify characteristics that may contribute to increased susceptibility of the female to anterior cruciate ligament (ACL) injury, including mechanism of injury, intrinsic factors, extrinsic factors, and combined factors.
- Identify typical muscular activation and timing patterns, as well as the kinematics and joint position of the lower extremity during performance of physical tasks by females.
- Educate physically active females, coaches, and other sports medicine personnel regarding prevention of ACL injuries, including proper cutting and jumping techniques and neuromuscular reeducation/strengthening of the lower extremity.
- Prescribe a lower-extremity reactive neuromuscular training exercise program for the physically active female to aid in ACL injury prevention.
- Identify possible sequelae to ACL injury and rehabilitation.

(continued)

OBJECTIVES *(continued)*

- Utilize the concept of "envelope of function" to minimize adverse effects of musculoskeletal injury and subsequent rehabilitation.
- Understand the importance of incorporating core strengthening into an exercise program of the physically active female.
- Identify the potential stresses and risks that occur in the shoulder joint complex as a consequence of softball windmill pitching.
- Prescribe an exercise program specific to the windmill softball pitcher.
- Understand the potential stresses to the shoulder complex during freestyle swimming and identify which musculature is at greatest risk for fatigue and subsequent impingement.
- Develop a comprehensive rehabilitation program for the swimmer with a shoulder injury.
- Develop a general understanding of most common injuries sustained by female gymnasts and identify potential risks involved in the excessive training at an early age common among female gymnasts.
- Acknowledge the implications that excessive, early training may have on hormonal and growth processes in the young female athlete.
- Describe the components of the female triad to enable prevention, identification, and treatment of these components as a member of a multidisciplinary medical team.
- Educate physically active females in proper exercise guidelines when planning for, during, and after pregnancy with a thorough knowledge of the physiologic changes that occur during this unique time.

The visibility of the athletic female, which has grown dramatically over the past century, is now established throughout the world. At the beginning of the century, in 1902, the modern Olympic Games were founded, but women were excluded from participation. At that time, women's sports were considered to be "against the laws of nature."[212] In 1972, Title IX of the Educational Assistance Act was passed. This was a pivotal point in the history of the United States regarding female participation in sports and exercise. Title IX states that "no person in the U.S. shall, on the basis of sex, be excluded from participation in, be denied the benefits of, or be subject to discrimination under any educational program of action receiving federal financial assistance" [212, p. 841] After Title IX, a 600% increase was seen in all levels of women's athletic participation.[211] Women and girls of all ages and abilities are participating in sports in record high numbers. In fact, 43.2% of collegiate athletes[5] and approximately 46% of Olympic athletes[3] were female as of publication of this text.

Participation in sports by girls and women continues to grow. The National Federation of State High School Associations has collected data on sports participation across the United States since 1971.[6] In its most recent school year report, the National Federation of State High School Associations reports 7,692,520 scholastic (high school aged participants) (both male and female), the greatest number of participants ever. Likewise, the total number of females participating set an all time high with 3,207,533 participants.[6] Basketball remains the most popular high school sport for girls in the United States, with almost 18,000 participants, followed by track and field/cross country, volleyball, softball, and soccer.[6]

Studies by the National Collegiate Athletic Association (NCAA) describe a 10% increase in participation across athletic programs for women from 1989 to 1993.[24] The greatest single rise in female participants of 21.18% occurred during the 1982-1983 school year, as compared to a 5.85% increase in male participants.[6] The NCAA reports that more than 100,000 women participate in intercollegiate sports each year; in fact, this number is fast approaching 200,000.[5] The most recently available participation report indicates that 195,657 women participated in collegiate sports (43.2% of all participants), with the greatest number participating in soccer, followed by track and field, softball, and basketball. Currently, women play in a wide variety of sports, play at many levels, are offered the opportunity not only to participate but also to gain monetary reimbursement (scholarship and professional salaries) and media acclaim. As participation and notoriety has increased, so has the need to understand the injuries being sustained by female athletes.

With the increase in women's participation in sport came an increased injury incidence among female athletes.[43] It was common, even 15 years ago, for a female athlete to receive different treatment than a male with an identical injury. For example, women runners who complained of tendonitis were often told to stop running, whereas men were given a specific treatment protocol that combined rest with activity. This is no longer commonplace. No longer are male athletes predominant recipients of rehabilitation. Active females are being rehabilitated as frequently as active males. There has been some suggestion that females are more susceptible to athletic injury than males[176]; however, current literature indicates that injury patterns are more sport-specific than gender-specific.[212,249] Nonetheless, there are several types of injuries, which seem to be more prevalent in the female athlete. Such injuries are of increasing concern to the sports medicine specialist.

One heavily researched area in the sports medicine arena is the increased rate of anterior cruciate ligament (ACL) injury among females when compared to males.[212,237,270] Female athletes have a 4 to 6 times higher incidence of ACL injuries compared to their male counterparts.[133,206] Other injuries found to be frequent among female athletes include patellofemoral pain syndrome, spondylosis and spondylolithesis, stress fractures, bunions, and shoulder pain.[16,32,43,80,85,158,229,252] The reasons for the high frequencies of these types of injuries in females remain elusive but have been receiving more attention in the last decade. The media, medical, and rehabilitation communities have brought female ACL injuries and the female athlete triad to the forefront of attention (see later section "The Female Athlete Triad"). A discussion regarding basic gender differences serves as a basis for further discussion of injuries common to representative, individual sports, as well as other considerations regarding the active female.

Gender Differences

Physiologic Strength Differences

Gender differences between females and males are evident in strength, aerobic capacity, and endurance. These differences become pronounced after puberty. Prepubertal boys and girls have similar strength, and when corrected for lean body mass, and their $\dot{V}O_2$ max is also similar.[250,256] Endurance performance is just slightly better in boys than in girls before puberty. However, these differences may be a result of social rather than biologic constraints, including the possibility of fewer role models for girls, less opportunities, and different training programs.[212,256] At puberty, these gender-related discrepancies are exaggerated because of both anatomical and physiologic differences. This time period seems to be a time when female athletes are particularly at risk, as a result of the hormonal, biomechanical, and functional performance changes that occur.[109,252]

Skeletal muscle physiology in men and women does not differ significantly.[251] Testosterone and androstenedione are the androgenic hormones that are most important in muscle fiber development. There is a variance in resting testosterone levels, but the average for females is between one-tenth and one-half the blood levels of males. Consequently, men have greater potential for strength and power development related to testosterone levels alone. When considering estrogen levels, women have higher levels than men, and this hormone interferes with muscular development as a result of its role in increasing body fat stores. After puberty, women typically have less lean body mass than men, especially in the lower body, because of increased estrogen levels, and subsequent fat body mass increases.[88] Average body fat for a sedentary college-age woman is 23% to 27%, whereas for a college-age man it is 15% to 18%. It is typical for some athletes (especially runners, gymnasts, and ballet dancers) to demonstrate lower body fat percentages because of the performance and appearance demands of their sports. These two physiologic hormonal differences (body fat and blood hormone levels) help to explain why muscle mass is predictably lower in women than in men.[88,275]

Strength can be examined in 2 different ways. Absolute strength is the maximum amount of weight one can lift (e.g. 50 lb). Relative strength relates this maximal amount to an individual's muscle mass (e.g. 80 lb of muscle mass can lift 50 lb).[141] Men appear to demonstrate larger *absolute* strength gains as a consequence of larger cross-sectional muscle fiber size. However, the actual number of muscle fibers is similar between genders. When examining *relative* gains in strength, studies show that women and men achieve similar results while undergoing identical weight-training programs.[141,196] "Because muscle cross-sectional area (muscle fiber size multiplied by the number of muscle fibers) is directly related to the ability to produce force, individuals who have larger muscles are able to lift more weight."[196, p. 4] Table 31-1 provides examples of this conclusion.

When comparing strength to lean body mass (body weight without fat) or cross-sectional area, women are about equal to men and are equally capable of developing strength *relative* to total muscle mass.[196] Gender is irrelevant in the ability of a muscle to produce force.[196] Holloway and Baechle[141] were unable to show significant gender differences in adaptations to resistance training, except for the amount of muscle hypertrophy. Absolute strength gains are a result of the combination of muscle hypertrophy and neuromuscular recruitment. When diet is unchanged during a resistance training program, the average woman responds with a decrease in intramuscular and subcutaneous fat stores, and little change in limb circumference (less hypertrophy than males) mostly owing to lower testosterone levels and smaller muscle fiber size.[141,196,212] True muscle hypertrophy is less visible in females, but improved muscular definition is evident.[196]

Table 31-1 Relative Versus Absolute Strength in Female Versus Male Athletes

Female soccer player 125 lb	With 15% body fat = 106 lb lean body mass Absolute strength = 150 lb squat Relative strength = 150/106 = 1.4
Male soccer player 155 lb	With 12% body fat = 136.5 lb lean body mass Absolute strength = 185 lb squat Relative strength = 185/136.5 = 1.4

Note: Equal *relative strength* but greater *absolute strength* in demonstrated by the male soccer player.

Dore et al[88] found that males and females exhibited similar cycling peak power until age 14 years. At age 14 years, loosely considered to be the transition to puberty, males demonstrated higher cycling peak power. Males had higher lean leg volume than females. As age increased, where there were similar lean leg volumes, males still showed greater cycling peak power. Conclusions were twofold: (a) the sex-related difference can be explained by the difference in body composition, specifically there is a lower limb fat increase in girls, whereas there is an increased lean body mass in boys; and (b) the question of the possibility that differences in neuromuscular activation exist, which could play a role in peak muscle performance.[88] Neuromuscular differences are examined more thoroughly later in this chapter, in the section entitled "Neuromuscular Differences".

So far, no evidence exists to suggest that women should undergo strength training any differently than men. "Assuming equal nutrition, the rate and degree of improvement in strength should be equal between genders. Significant gains in muscle strength and endurance can be achieved by use of a training program 3 to 4 days a week."[196, p. 5] Once either gender has reached a high level of competitiveness and muscularity, changes in muscle mass and fiber content is minimal.[17] However, women do show lower proportions of their total lean body mass in their upper body, contributing to gender strength differences that are greater in the upper body than in the lower body. Nevertheless, hypertrophy and absolute strength differences evident between genders occur as a result of the physiologic changes that occur at puberty.[196]

Anatomical Differences

Anatomical differences are also a reason for variance in strength. Men and women's bodies respond differently to similar weight training programs as a result of anatomical differences. These differences include women are 3 to 4 inches shorter; are 25 to 30 lb lighter; have 10 to 15 lb (8% to 10%) more body fat; have 40 to 45 fewer pounds of fat-free weight (bone, muscle, organs); have less muscle mass supported by narrower shoulders; and have shorter extremities.[196] "All these factors combined give men a mechanical advantage over women, which enables them to handle more weight and generate more power."[196, p. 3] Broader shoulders tend to benefit males in developing muscular strength in the upper body, whereas wider pelvises seem to benefit females in developing lower body strength. Men with broader shoulders have a higher center of gravity than women with wider pelvises, giving men a superior mechanical advantage for gaining upper-body mass.[196] Thus, as previously stated, the largest difference in absolute strength in females versus males is found in the upper body as compared to the lower body.[141]

Structural differences have been noted between genders in both the upper and lower extremities. In the upper body, structural differences include narrower shoulders, shorter arm lengths, decreased muscle fiber, and total muscle cross-sectional area, and according to some authors, increased carrying angle of the forearm.[196,250] When examining structural differences of the lower extremity between genders, multiple factors affect alignment. Women have greater amounts of static external knee rotation, greater active internal hip rotation, greater interacetablular distance, and increased hip width when normalized to femoral length than men.[65] These factors contribute to greater knee valgus (genu valgum) angles in women. The structural combination of increased hip adduction and rotation, femoral anteversion, and genu valgum may explain the larger quadriceps (Q) angle and rotational positioning of the lower extremity in women than in men (Figures 31-1 and 31-2). The average Q angle for men is 13 degrees and for women it is 18 degrees,[61] but measurement of the Q angle is examiner dependent and can be erratic. Lower-extremity structural differences may play a factor in lower-extremity injuries in the active female.[65] Structural differences related to ACL injury are discussed in greater detail later in this chapter, in section entitled "Intrinsic Factors".

Patellofemoral Dysfunction

As previously mentioned, the larger Q angle found in females has been identified as a predisposing factor to patellofemoral dysfunction, which plagues many active females regardless of sport or age. Anterior knee pain is one of the most common sources of complaint among female athletes.[41] Most patellofemoral dysfunction can be categorized as mechanical or inflammatory, with the rare exceptions of tumors, regional pain syndrome, and referred pain patterns.[147] For the active female, patellofemoral dysfunction should be thoroughly evaluated to determine whether instability, malalignment, tracking abnormalities (either of the patella itself or the femur underneath it), compression forces, or motor control issues contribute to the anterior knee discomfort. Appropriate patellar mobility should include sufficient superior glide with active quadriceps contraction, as well as equal medial and lateral glide.[235] Increased patellar lateral glide indicates abnormal laxity and instability when correlated with a positive apprehension test that simulates instances of patellar subluxation or dislocation.[147,235] Patellar instability is a mechanical cause of anterior knee pain and occurs more frequently in females than in males.[147] The active female is more susceptible to patellar instability secondary to the anatomical alignment and muscular strength differences already described. However, contemporary thinking supports more a biomechanical and motor control approach to both the genesis and treatment of patellofemoral syndromes and anterior knee pain.[54] Treatment of patellar instability and other patellofemoral diagnoses have been discussed in much greater detail in Chapter 24.

Alignment observation should include not only Q-angle measurements but also determination of tibial torsion, foot position, and leg-length discrepancies. Malalignment may include superior or inferior position of the patella, medial or lateral patellar glide, rotation, or tilt. Abnormal positions of the patella may include 1 or a combination of these factors.[190] Common patellar malalignment patterns include "grasshopper" or "squinting" patella. A complete evaluation of muscular balance, including both flexibility and strength of the hip, pelvis, and thigh musculature, directs treatment to minimize these suboptimal patterns.[190] McConnell patellar taping[191] or the use of kinesiotape applications[29] may provide proprioceptive input to affect patellar tracking and muscular recruitment. These interventions provide symptomatic relief in many patients, which allows for a conservative rehabilitation program to be completed.[191]

A static Q-angle measurement is not as helpful as the same measurement before and during an activity such as a minisquat to determine if the Q angle increases, demonstrating lack of optimal motor control.[147] Patellar tracking should be assessed to ensure normal position of the patella within the trochlear groove throughout knee motion. An example of abnormal patellar tracking is a J sign, when the examiner observes the patella jump laterally (at approximately 30 degrees of flexion) as the knee moves from flexion into extension and is associated with patellofemoral symptoms.[178,235] Conservative management of patellar tracking abnormalities, especially in the adolescent female athlete, should be the rule[147] and should be addressed systematically after a thorough evaluation of the muscle imbalance for flexibility and strength. Neuromuscular training to address recruitment patterns of both proximal and thigh musculature, core stability, and balance deficits are elaborated upon later in this chapter. Techniques to be discussed have applicability with the rehabilitation program for most biomechanical causes of anterior knee pain.

This discussion of patellofemoral dysfunction illustrates the increased predisposition to this injury complaint of the physically active female based on the gender differences in anatomy and strength. A subsequent review of the neuromuscular differences precedes the discussion of another widespread knee injury that is more common in female than in male athletes.

Neuromuscular Differences

When comparing genders, research supports differences in dynamic neuromuscular control of lower limb biomechanics.[129,130,133,218,295] Neuromuscular control is a combination of proprioception and the muscular systems' response to the proprioceptive input. Imbalances in quadriceps-to-hamstring ratios, differences in jump-landing positions, weakness in proximal hip musculature, higher landing forces, and lower gluteus maximus electromyographic (EMG) activity during landing are all reported in females when compared to males.[132,145,295] Noyes et al[218] conducted research using the drop-jump test with both male and female athletes that measured the distance between the hips, knees, and ankles in the coronal plane during landing. Findings revealed no significant difference between male and female subjects in mean knee and ankle separation distance during the landing and takeoff phases. Significant differences between male and female athletes were shown in knee and ankle separation during the prelanding phase only (the 3 phases include takeoff, prelanding, and landing). However, after a 6-week Sportsmetrics neuromuscular training program[128] (Appendix A), female athletes had statistically greater knee and ankle separation distances than those of males in all 3 phases of the jump-land sequence.[207]

Hewett et al[130] went beyond the coronal plane and measured a drop jump-landing task in females with 3-dimensional motion analysis. Data were gathered on athletes prior to sports participation. Athletes who had injured their ACL demonstrated significantly higher knee abduction angles (knee valgus) at initial contact and increased maximal limb displacement than did those who were uninjured. Peak vertical ground reaction force corresponded with knee abduction angle. The greater the abduction angle, the greater the ground reaction force in ACL-injured athletes but not in uninjured athletes. Athletes who sustained ACL injuries "demonstrated significant increases in dynamic lower extremity valgus and knee abduction loading before sustaining their injuries compared to uninjured controls."[130, p. 497] Maximum knee flexion angle at landing was 10.5 degrees less in injured than in noninjured athletes. These differences suggest decreased neuromuscular control or alternative strategies for function in the lower extremity of females as evidenced by biomechanical differences observed.[12,30]

Coactivation of the quadriceps and hamstrings is an important protective mechanism at the knee joint for protection against not only excessive anterior shear forces but also knee abduction and dynamic lower-extremity valgus forces.[34] Female athletes have lower hamstring-to-quadriceps-strength ratios than males during isokinetic testing at 300 degrees per second.[129] When the hamstrings are underrecruited, relative overrecruitment of the quadriceps may result. This recruitment strategy used by females may directly limit the potential for balanced muscular cocontraction, which aids in protecting ligaments.[130] It has also been postulated that males may use a protective mechanism involving the hamstrings, considered to resist anterior tibial translation, to counteract high-peak landing forces. Females tend to contract their quadriceps first in response to an anterior tibial translation, which provides additional anterior translation, whereas males responded by contracting their hamstrings first, thereby limiting the anterior translation. With these findings, it is suggested that females tend to be "ligament-dominant" in their joint strategies, whereas males demonstrate more "muscle-dominant" joint strategies.[133]

Greater knee abduction angles during jump-stop unanticipated cutting activity were also described by Ford et al.[105] Females demonstrated greater knee abduction angles (knee valgus) at initial contact than their male counterparts. Greater knee abduction angles support the concept of ligament dominance rather than muscular control to absorb the ground reaction force during sporting maneuvers. In such a movement strategy, the athlete is allowing the ground reaction force to control the direction of motion of the knee joint, which, in turn, causes the ligaments to take up a disproportionate amount of force.[105]

Proximal hip musculature activation is also found to differ between genders. Zazulak et al[295] reported that female athletes demonstrated less activity of the gluteus maximus

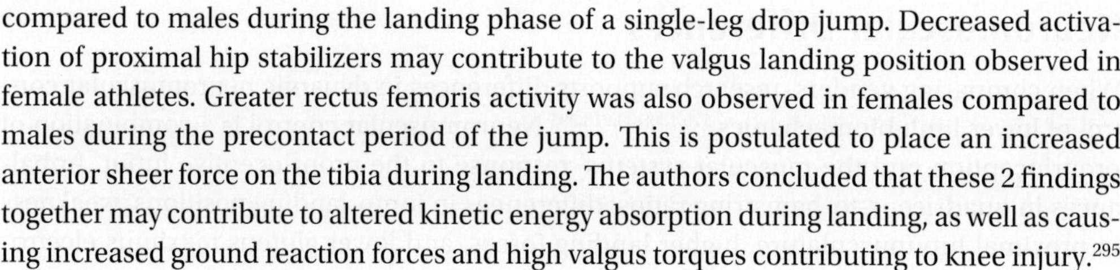

compared to males during the landing phase of a single-leg drop jump. Decreased activation of proximal hip stabilizers may contribute to the valgus landing position observed in female athletes. Greater rectus femoris activity was also observed in females compared to males during the precontact period of the jump. This is postulated to place an increased anterior sheer force on the tibia during landing. The authors concluded that these 2 findings together may contribute to altered kinetic energy absorption during landing, as well as causing increased ground reaction forces and high valgus torques contributing to knee injury.[295]

Female sex hormones may also have significant effects on neuromuscular control. Estrogen has both direct and indirect effects on the neuromuscular system. During the ovulatory phase, there is a slowing of muscle relaxation. Throughout the menstrual cycle, estrogen levels fluctuate radically. Fluctuating hormone status has profound effects on muscle function,[253] tendon and ligament strength, and the central nervous system.[133] Hormonal influences on neuromuscular control is discussed further in the ACL section of this chapter. Clearly, neuromuscular patterning and performance is affected by many factors.

Anterior Cruciate Ligament Injuries

With higher participation rates of females at all levels, increased sport-related injuries were expected; however, what was unexpected was the disproportionate number of knee ligament injuries that occur. The most serious injury that has risen to the forefront of attention is injury to the ACL of females. A pattern of disproportionately high ACL injury rates in females, compared to their male athlete counterparts, was identified. For example, during the 1989-1990 intercollegiate basketball season, the NCAA Injury Surveillance System data showed that female athletes injured their ACLs 7.8 times more often than males,[228] and this trend continues. Sports that appear to have high risk, at all levels of play, involve jumping, rapid deceleration, and cutting maneuvers. Sports such as soccer, basketball, volleyball, team handball, and gymnastics have been identified as high-risk sports for the female athlete.[24,25,44,63,71,87,103,115,127,132,171,180,195,222,247,261,296,298] In fact, more than 30,000 serious knee injuries in female athletes at the high school and intercollegiate levels are projected to occur yearly in the United States.[125]

The costs of ACL injuries are dramatic, not only financially (medical and rehabilitation services) but also in terms of long-term consequences, such as concurrent injury (such as articular cartilage or meniscus), lost playing time, lost scholarships, and increased potential for long-term posttraumatic osteochondral degeneration and disability.[112,119,289] According to Ireland,[148,150] even in the era where prevention has been deemed important, females continue to experience a higher rate of injury to the ACL than their male counterparts. What is especially troubling is that even as years have passed and female athletes begin sports play earlier, train harder, and receive improved training and coaching, their injury rate has not declined.[150] Therefore, the present focus remains less on reporting injury statistics and hypothesizing about potential causes and continues in the era of prevention. Prevention of ACL injuries in the female athlete has become a priority for the sports medicine, rehabilitation, and research communities.

Mechanisms of Injury

As more women and girls participate in sports, much attention has been given to understanding the mechanisms of ACL injuries. Many authors have described 2 mechanisms of injury: contact and noncontact.[24,25,146,218] Approximately 30% of all ACL injuries are classified as contact injuries, and the remaining 70% are not related to direct contact and classified as noncontact.[119] Some authors have reported that as many as 75% of sports-related injuries to the ACL are via noncontact mechanisms.[219] Contact injuries are easily discerned from the clinical history surrounding the injury and typically occur during contact sports like football and rugby. In contrast, the mechanisms and activities that are involved in noncontact ACL injuries are less apparent and vary between sports. Sports that are at high risk for, and incur, many noncontact ACL injuries are those classified as noncontact or collision sports such as basketball, soccer, volleyball, gymnastics, and team handball.[23,25,31,111,150,283]

Early writing by Henning in the late 1980s influenced much of the current thinking about the mechanisms of noncontact ACL injuries.[119] After studying injuries incurred by female basketball players over a 10-year time span, Henning concluded that the 3 most common mechanisms of injury were[119]:

- Planting and cutting (29% of all injuries)
- Straight-knee landings (28% of all injuries)
- One-step stop with the knee hyperextended (26% of all injuries)

Henning concluded that prevention and skill development (especially in the female athlete) must incorporate the *opposite* of the previously mentioned motor behaviors, including:

- The accelerated rounded turn, performed off a flexed knee
- Bent knee landings
- The 3-step stop

These motor behaviors are addressed more thoroughly later in the chapter in the section on prevention and training.

Subsequently, many mechanisms have been described for contributing to noncontact injuries, including sudden forceful twisting motions with the foot planted,[194] planting/sidestepping/cutting maneuvers,[77] "out of control play,"[119, p. 142] landing,[49,103] and deceleration maneuvers.[119] Video analysis of ACL injuries that occurred during the play of basketball and soccer demonstrated that women were injured most commonly when landing from a jump and when they suddenly stopped running.[119] It is very interesting to note that women and girls have been shown to perform landing and cutting activities with more erect posture than men, and therefore place themselves at greater risk for ACL injury.[119] Video analysis of actual ACL injuries demonstrated that the position of the lower limb at the time of injury is often knee flexion less than 30 degrees, a position of knee valgus, and external rotation of the foot relative to the knee (Figure 31-3).[49,119,128]

Postural and positional variations in motor skills, when combined with greater valgus alignment and increased quadriceps activation, may further increase the possibility of injury for the female athlete.[132] Total positional control of the lower extremity is important, both in terms of flexion/extension and varus/valgus. Low flexion angles (commonly described as less than 45 degrees flexion) increase the anterior strain on the ACL when active quadriceps contractions occur. The quads act as the ACL antagonist and add to the anterior/posterior straight plane load sustained by the ACL. Likewise, increased varus/valgus positioning of the lower extremity adds torque to the knee that challenges the ACL in its derotational function. Factors to explain the position of the lower extremities of females during landing may include deficits in proximal muscle strength and endurance as well as neuromuscular skill factors.

Finally, related to impact during landing, current research suggests that strategies differ in females as compared to males. This may be a result of biomechanical factors, poorer muscle strength and/or neuromuscular control, or insufficient strategies for shock absorption, as previously discussed.[169] Dufek and Bates[94] examined the relationship between landing forces and injury stating that many injuries that occur during jumping sports occur during landing. Male athletes appear to employ different mechanisms to compensate for high landing forces than do females.[129,132] Markolf et al[186] demonstrated that muscular contraction can decrease both the varus and valgus laxity of the knee when landing. Jumping and landing are addressed in greater detail in a later section entitled "Knee Kinematics and Landing Characteristics".

In summary, although women do sustain contact mechanism ACL injuries, the vast majority appears to occur by noncontact mechanisms. According to the Hunt Valley Consensus conference,[119] "The common at-risk situation for noncontact ACL injuries appears to be deceleration, which occurs when the athlete cuts, changes direction, or lands from a jump."[119, p. 149]

Although many studies offer strong support for noncontact mechanisms of injury as prevalent in the female athlete,[25,118,180,207,208,279] Ireland maintains that the "true incidence of noncontact ACL injuries and the actual numbers of athletes affected are difficult to determine."[150, p. 150] The discrepancy between ACL injury rates by sex and mechanism of injury, at all levels of sport participation, remains a hot topic in sports medicine. Fortunately, neuromuscular control, balance, and motor skill training all appear to be critical modifiable factors associated with injury prevention.

Factors Related to Anterior Cruciate Ligament Injury in the Female Athlete

Why women continue to sustain 2 to 8 times more ACL injuries than their male counterparts continues to be an unanswered question for researchers in many disciplines. Clearly, injuries to the ACL occur as a result of complex interactions of anatomical, biomechanical, neuromuscular, hormonal, and environmental factors. Various factors have been suggested to explain these differences and are categorized by many authors as intrinsic (factors that are not controllable) and extrinsic (factors that are controllable).[22,24,118,124,146,150] More recently, a third category of factors, described as "both" or partially controllable has been described by Ireland (Table 31-2).[150]

Intrinsic Factors

Intrinsic or noncontrollable factors have been described as hormonal effects of estrogen, inherent ligamentous laxity present in females, and other anthropometric differences in men and women, such as lower-extremity alignment, notch width, and ACL size.

Table 31-2 **Summary of Factors Suggested to Contribute to ACL Injury in Female Athletes**

Intrinsic Factors	Extrinsic Factors	Combined Factors
Lower-extremity alignment • Q angle/pelvic width • Varus/valgus of the knee (see Figures 31-2 and 31-10) • Foot alignment Hyperextension Physiologic rotatory laxity ACL size Notch size and shape Hormonal influences Inherited skills/coordination	Strength Endurance Shoes/footwear Motivation	Proprioception • Balance • Position sense Neuromuscular control Muscular firing order Kinematics of movement (See Figures 31-4, 31-5, 31-8, and 31-10*A*, *B*) Acquired skills • Sport-specific motor programs

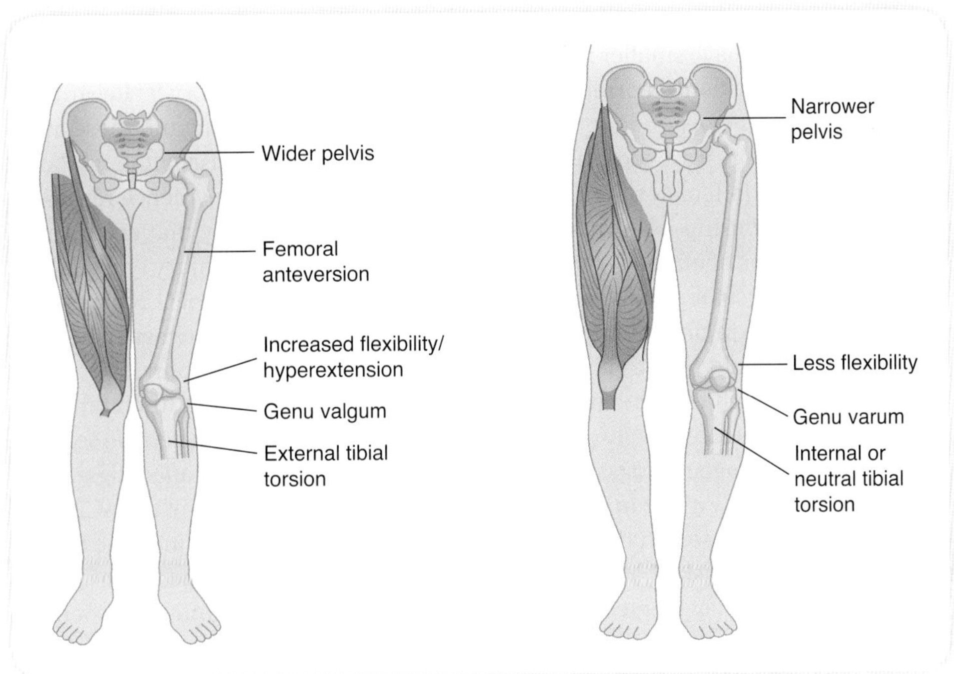

Figure 31-1 Structural differences between men and women

Women (*left*) typically exhibit a wider pelvis, femoral anteversion greater tibial external rotation, and genu valgum. (Reproduced from Griffin LY. *Rehabilitation of the Injured Knee*. St. Louis, MO: Mosby-Year Book; 1995, with permission from Elsevier.)

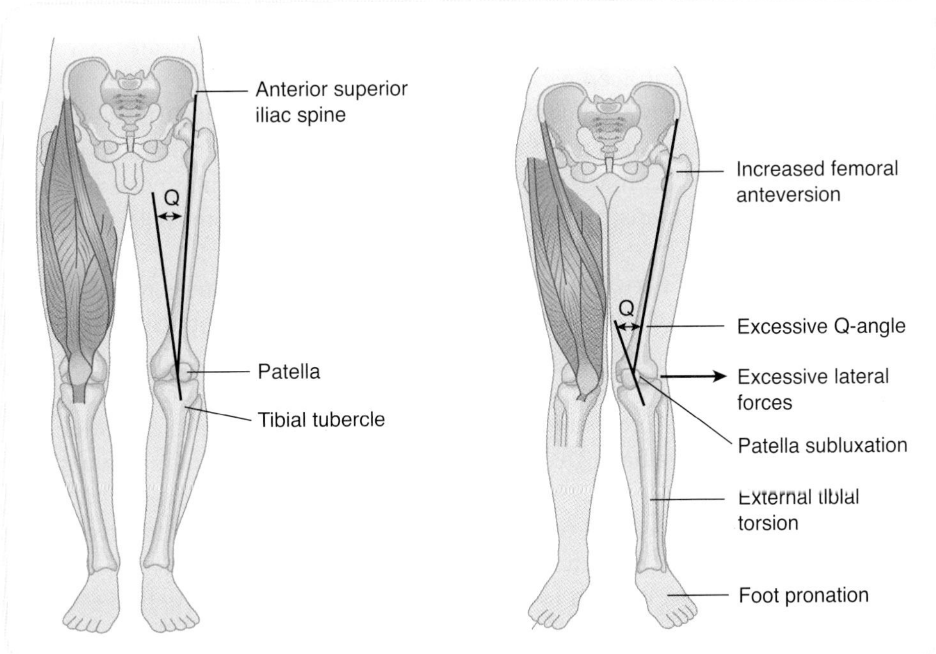

Figure 31-2 Gender differences in Q angle

Women (*right*) exhibit a greater Q angle, increased external tibial torsion, and femoral anteversion. (Reproduced from Griffin LY. *Rehabilitation of the Injured Knee*. St. Louis, MO: Mosby-Year Book; 1995, with permission from Elsevier.)

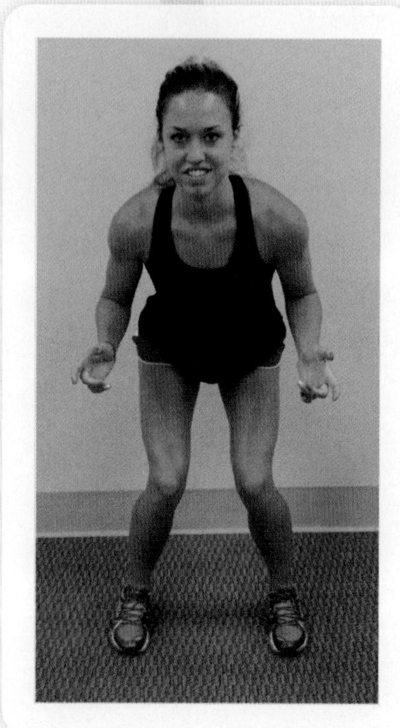

Figure 31-3 Typical position of ACL injury

Note that knee valgus, foot external rotation, and knee flexion are less than 30 degrees.

Investigation regarding notch width and ACL size has demonstrated females to have smaller notches and smaller ACLs than males[22,144,269,279]; however, the evidence correlating this with injury is contradictory.[133] Regardless, there is little or no opportunity for reasonable intervention, and these areas have been researched less in the last several years. Likewise, although laxity is greater in females than in males,[248] there is conflicting evidence regarding the relationship of laxity to injury. Exercise-induced laxity that occurs after 30 minutes of athletic activity may play a role in ligament injury and relate to neuromuscular protective training.[272] Finally, investigations of Q angle in relationship to injury demonstrate that injury rate differences between males and females could not be accounted for by the differences in anatomy.[118]

Research efforts have been dedicated to understanding the interaction between female sex hormones and ACL injuries. Because the female sex hormones estrogen, progesterone, and relaxin are cyclical and affect ligaments, they may play a role in fluctuation in both strength and laxity of the ACL.[133,289] Conflicting research evidence exists as to what portion of the menstrual cycle is the most "risky,"[25,26,288,289] and whether the effects of hormones (estrogen, especially) may be greater than just on the ligament itself and may extend to changes in motor skill.[133,236] Originally, the ovulatory phase was described as the time during which most injuries occurred.[289] More recently, Slauterbeck and Hardy[263] found that many injuries occurred around menses. In their most recent work, Wojtys et al[288] described that more ACL injuries than expected (43%) occurred during the ovulatory phase (in all females) and fewer injuries than expected occurred during the luteal phase (34%). The distribution of injury by phases was different for those women who were taking oral contraceptives, with only a trend toward more injuries in the ovulatory phase (29%), and fewer injuries than expected during the follicular phase (14%), demonstrating the potential for some protection offered by use of oral contraceptives. Möller-Neilson and Hammer[199] also reported decreased injury rates in women who used oral contraceptives.

The effects of hormones may extend beyond their effect on the ACL itself. Evidence suggests that the neuromuscular system may be significantly affected by the fluctuating milieu of female sex hormones.[133,166] Estrogen may have effects on neuromuscular patterning and performance throughout the menstrual cycle, but seems to decrease motor skills in the premenstrual phase.[175,236]

Clearly, the relationship between female hormones and ACL injuries remains controversial, not only in terms of susceptibility of ligaments to injury but also in terms of mechanism and location of action. It is not clear whether hormones influence muscle function and motor skills,[236] the neuromuscular system,[133,175,230] or cerebral/central nervous system function.[165,236,288] Interestingly, over the last several decades, suggestions for control of intrinsic factors have been given, such as notchplasty and hormonal manipulation for protection of the ACL in females. These examples were not received with much zeal by the medical community and were never accepted as reasonable interventions. Most in sports medicine agree that to reduce the number of ACL injuries sustained by the female athlete, attention must be paid to factors that are modifiable,[150] such as extrinsic or combination factors.

Extrinsic Factors

Extrinsic or controllable factors are parameters such as leg strength (both total absolute strength and hamstrings/quadriceps ratios), muscle recruitment order, muscle reaction time, playing style, training/preparation, coaching/conditioning, skill acquisition, and surfaces of play.[146,150,290]

Generation of muscular force is a key element in providing dynamic stability about joints. The inability to control external forces may result in injury to the static structures providing stability to that joint. The inherent physiologic differences in muscle mass and hormonal levels of testosterone between males and females make it predictable that males will always be stronger than females. If body mass is accounted for and subjects of similar activity levels are compared, does this inequality still exist?

Huston and Wojtys[145] tested this hypothesis using isokinetic testing and concluded that athletic females and a control group of females were both statistically weaker in quadriceps and hamstrings muscle strength at 60 degrees per second, as compared to their male counterparts. Other researchers have also documented that women have less muscle strength in the quadriceps and hamstrings than men, even when normalized for body weight.[122] Anderson et al[22] also tested the quadriceps and hamstrings isokinetically at 60 and 240 degrees per second and found similar results. With corrections for body mass, the male athletes generated greater peak torque, greater work, and average power outputs than the female athletes for both quadriceps and hamstrings ($p < 0.05$).[22] Knapik et al[158] determined that female athletes with a hamstring muscle group more than 15% weaker than the other side were 2.5 times more likely to sustain a lower-extremity injury. They also reported that this side-to-side imbalance in hamstring strength existed in 20% to 30% of female athletes.

Previous research illustrates the importance of hamstring strength and endurance in acting as an agonist to the ACL for dynamic knee joint stability.[22,90,145,247] The hamstring muscles have been shown to be protective of the ACL because of their ability to shield the ACL from excessive anterior shear and strain. If the hamstrings are to effectively counteract the torque produced by the quadriceps, they must demonstrate a certain percentage of strength as compared to the quadriceps they are opposing. Knapik[157] also reported that athletes with a hamstring-to-quadriceps ratio of less than 0.75 were 1.6 times more likely to be injured. Isokinetic testing by Moore and Wade[200] revealed that hamstring-to-quadriceps ratios in females were significantly lower than those in males at 60, 180, and 300 degrees per second. Huston also determined that females had hamstring-to-quadriceps ratios in the 0.40 range.[145] Eccentric hamstrings-to-quadriceps ratio was also significantly weaker in female athletes as compared to male athletes.[202] It has been hypothesized that hamstring-to-quadriceps ratios lower than 0.60 may predispose an athlete to ACL injury.[131]

As indicated previously, strength deficits in the female athlete are evident and may play a role in predisposing the female to an ACL injury. If strength may play a role, how does the endurance mode of these muscles play a role in knee stability and injury vulnerability? A study conducted by Rozzi et al[247] demonstrated that both males and females had a decrease in the ability to detect joint motion moving into the direction of extension, an increase in the onset time of contraction for the medial hamstring and lateral gastrocnemius muscles in response to landing a jump, and an increase in the electromyogram of the first contraction of the vastus medialis and lateralis muscles while landing a jump when fatigued.[234] Research by Zhou et al[297] has shown electromechanical delay of the knee extensors to increase by 147% after muscular fatigue. Nyland et al[220] looked at the effects of eccentric work-induced hamstring fatigue on sagittal and transverse plane knee and ankle biodynamics and kinetics during a running, crossover cut, or directional change. They determined that hamstring fatigue created decreased dynamic transverse plane knee control demonstrated by increased knee internal rotation during heel strike. Peak ankle plantarflexion moment and decreased knee internal rotation magnitude during the propulsion phase of the cutting maneuver when fatigued is believed to represent a compensatory attempt for knee dynamic stability from the gastrocnemius and soleus.[220] Wojtys et al[290] also demonstrated the effect of fatigue on knee joint stability. When the quadriceps and hamstrings were exercised to a point of fatigue, there was resultant increase in tibial movement, causing increased vulnerability to ACL injury.[290]

Combined Factors

More recently, combined or partially controllable factors have been suggested as those that have contributions inherent to the individual (intrinsic factors) combined with those that are more extrinsic in nature and, therefore, able to be modified.[145] Examples of combined factors are proprioception and neuromuscular control. Both of these factors are affected by an individual's genetic makeup, but can be taught, to some extent, by structured programs to address their areas of deficiency.[119,129,131,132]

Proprioception has been defined as the culmination of all neural inputs originating from joints, tendons, muscles, and associated deep-tissue proprioceptors. These inputs into the central nervous system result in the regulation of reflexes and motor control.[131] The body receives proprioceptive information by three separate systems. They include the visual system, the vestibular system, and the peripheral mechanoreceptors. When discussing injuries to the ACL, the role of the mechanoreceptors has been the primary focus in the literature. Researchers agree that the ACL does contain mechanoreceptors, but if the central nervous system has a decreased sensory feedback from the knee, there is a decreased ability to stabilize the knee joint dynamically. This places the knee at risk for injury, either microtrauma or macrotrauma.[140] Following injury to the capsuloligamentous structures, it is thought that a partial deafferentation of the joint occurs as the mechanoreceptors become disrupted. This partial deafferentation, which is secondary to injury, may be related to either direct or indirect injury. Direct trauma effects would include disruption of the joint capsule or ligaments, whereas posttraumatic joint effusion or hemarthrosis[154] can illustrate indirect effects.

Whether a direct or indirect cause, the resultant partial deafferentation alters the afferent information into the central nervous system and, therefore, the resulting reflex pathways to the dynamic stabilizing structures. These pathways are required by both the feed-forward and feedback motor control systems to dynamically stabilize the joint. A disruption in the proprioceptive pathway will result in an alteration of position and kinesthesia.[36,262] Barrett[38] showed an increase in the threshold to detection of passive motion in a majority of patients with ACL rupture and functional instability. Corrigan,[73] who also found diminished proprioception after ACL rupture, confirmed this finding. Diminished proprioceptive sensitivity has also been shown to cause giving way or episodes of instability in the ACL-deficient knee.[51] Rozzi et al[248] tested proprioception by measuring knee-joint kinesthesia as the threshold to detection of passive motion while moving either the direction of knee flexion or extension. The study determined that females took significantly longer than the males to detect joint motion moving in the direction of knee-joint extension implicating the hamstrings as deficient in proprioception. Injury to the capsuloligamentous structures not only reduces the joint's mechanical stability but also diminishes the capability of the dynamic neuromuscular restraint system. Therefore, any aberration in joint motion and position sense will impact both the feed-forward and feedback neuromuscular control systems. Without adequate anticipatory muscle activity, the static structures may be exposed to insult unless the reactive muscle activity can be initiated to contribute to dynamic restraint.

The reader is referred to the previous section on gender differences to review the various neuromuscular control factors that vary from female to male. In reference to the female athlete and ACL injuries, the following specific variables will be examined: the muscle firing patterns of the lower extremity with physical tasks, the timing of those muscular responses, and the kinematics and joint position of the lower extremity during activity.

Muscular Activation and Timing Patterns

In a study conducted by Huston and Wojtys,[145] different muscular firing patterns were illustrated between females (control and athlete group) and males (control and athlete group). They tested muscular response to anterior translation of the tibia using EMG recordings during a relaxed response to movement and a voluntary muscle contraction response to movement. All 4 groups recruited the gastrocnemius muscle first in the relaxed response to anterior translation of the tibia. The spinal level of muscle firing pattern was gastrocnemius-hamstring-quadriceps for all groups, but as the translation of the tibia continued in the relaxed response phase of the testing, female athletes relied more on quadriceps activity than on hamstrings to stabilize their knee. The predominant muscle recruitment order of the male athletes and both control groups was the hamstring-quadriceps-gastrocnemius muscle pattern. In contrast, the female athletes recruitment pattern was quadriceps-hamstring-gastrocnemius. During the voluntary muscle contraction response, the female athletes demonstrated the same response as the female controls and both male groups. This pattern was hamstring-quadriceps-gastrocnemius. These results support the concept of "quadriceps dominance" in female athletes in terms of muscular recruitment.

With respect to the muscle reaction time in this study, no significant differences were found at the spinal cord level for the quadriceps and hamstrings; however, the male and female athletes produced significantly faster gastrocnemius muscle responses compared to the two control groups. In the intermediate phase of the relaxed response testing and the voluntary response to tibial translation, there was no significant difference for all muscles between all 4 groups. When testing muscular strength and time to reach this peak force utilizing isokinetic testing, Huston and Wojyts[145] found no differences in time-to-peak torque for knee extension at 60 and 240 degrees per second for all groups. Significant differences did exist between male and female athletes for hamstring time-to-peak torque at 60 and 240 degrees per second. The female athletes were statistically significantly slower than the male athletes and minimally slower than the female control group, although this difference was not statistically significant.[145] Contrary to Huston and Wojyts, Rozzi et al[248] did not find sex differences in the time-to-peak torque tested isokinetically for either hamstrings or quadriceps. This same study did find significantly greater EMG peak amplitude of the lateral hamstrings for the female athletes when landing from a jump on 1 leg. The authors stated that this finding may be related to the idea that female athletes possess inherent joint laxity and the hamstrings must activate at a higher level to provide stability to the joint.[248]

The latency period between sensory feedback and dynamic movement is known as electromechanical delay and has been shown to be shorter in males compared to females, thus allowing superior efficiency of dynamic stabilization in males.[170]

DeMont et al[86] studied the muscular activity before foot strike in various functional activities for ACL-deficient subjects, ACL-reconstructed subjects, and a control group, and compared involved to uninvolved legs of each subject. All subjects were female. The tasks consisted of downhill walking, running, hopping, and landing from a step. Different bilateral activation of vastus medialis obliques occurred with downhill walking and running activities for the ACL-deficient group. The ACL-deficient group also showed a significant increase in vastus lateralis activation during running and landing when compared bilaterally and also when compared to ACL reconstructed and control group subjects. Activation of the lateral gastrocnemius was lower in downhill walking and higher in the landing task in the ACL-deficient group also. The ACL-reconstructed group showed significant differences between the involved and uninvolved limb in the lateral gastrocnemius for the hop. These side-to-side differences for the ACL-deficient and ACL-reconstructed groups, and group differences between ACL-deficient and control groups, suggest that the females with an ACL-deficient knee use unique strategies involving the vastus medialis obliques, vastus lateralis, and lateral gastrocnemius, and these muscles need to be addressed in the rehabilitation process. A similar study performed by Swanik et al[274] demonstrated ACL-deficient subjects to exhibit greater peak activity (as measured by isometric electromyography) in the medial hamstring in comparison with the ACL-reconstructed group and greater peak activity in the lateral hamstring than the control group during running. During landing from a step, the ACL-deficient group demonstrated significantly less isometric EMG activity in the vastus lateralis when compared to the control group. These findings suggest the importance of the hamstrings in controlling anterior tibial translation and rotation, as well as their possible role in inhibition of the quadriceps in an effort to dynamically stabilize the knee in the ACL-deficient knee.

For dynamic stabilization to occur at the knee, many muscles are involved that directly pass around the joint as well as other muscles that are distally and proximally positioned but play a role in controlling the forces at the knee. Baratta et al[34] investigated muscular coactivation patterns at the knee. Subjects consisted of nonathletes, recreational athletes, and highly competitive athletes, and EMG data were collected during an isokinetic strength test. High-performance athletes with hypertrophied quadriceps had inhibitory effects on the coactivation of the hamstrings compared to the recreational athletes. They also determined that athletes who routinely exercised their hamstrings demonstrated inhibited quadriceps and had coactivation patterns similar to those of the nonathletes. Muscular balance is key to efficient dynamic joint stabilization.

Muscle stiffness is important to stability of the knee and demonstrated when muscles surrounding the knee contract, offering the joint increased contact force and decreased joint mobility. Markolf et al[186] reported that nonathletes could increase varus and valgus knee stiffness 2 to 4 times with isometric contraction of the hamstrings and quadriceps. Athletes in the same study were able to increase their joint stiffness by a factor of 10 with the same isometric contraction. Bryant and Cooke[56] demonstrated gender differences in knee stiffness in a study in 1988. When testing varus and valgus stiffness, females rotated at the tibia 66% more than the males and were 35% less stiff. Another study that looked at gender differences in the anterior-posterior plane of motion determined a significant difference in females, and males, ability to stiffen the knee joint. Men were able to increase their joint stiffness by 4 times, whereas the females were only able to stiffen their joint by 2 times.[146] The exact mechanism of knee stiffness is not completely understood, although a study by Such et al determined that lower-extremity muscle mass had the largest influence on the stiffness properties of the knee.[273]

Knee Kinematics and Landing Characteristics

As noted in the previous section on the mechanisms of injury, it is well documented in the literature that most of the ACL injuries occur when landing from a jump or during deceleration and pivoting. It has been documented that the quadriceps exerts its maximum anterior sheer force when the knee flexion angles are the smallest (20 to 25 degrees flexion), which places a measurable strain on the ACL.[260] Eccentric activation of the quadriceps at high velocities present during athletic movements may produce too much force for the static and dynamic stabilizers of the knee to resist, thus allowing injury to occur. EMG studies demonstrate eccentric quadriceps muscle activation during such activities as running, cutting, and landing from a jump to be more than 2 times greater than maximum voluntary contraction.[119] It has also been documented in the literature that there is a significant difference in how males and females perform the previously noted movement patterns.

Malinzak et al[179] were one of the first research groups to investigate these kinematic gender differences. EMG and 3-dimensional kinematic analyses of cutting and running were obtained from male and female athletes. Females demonstrated significantly less knee flexion, increased knee valgus, and decreased hip flexion than males during both of these movement patterns. Females also had greater quadriceps and lower hamstring activation levels especially at heel strike.[144] Colby et al[72] investigated 4 different cutting maneuvers in males and females using 2-dimensional video analyses and electromyography and had similar results as Malinzak et al.[179] The average knee flexion angle was 22 degrees for each cutting maneuver. Quadriceps activity was 161% of the maximum voluntary isometric contraction as compared to 14% of the maximum voluntary isometric contraction for hamstring activity.[72] This further demonstrates the "quadriceps/-dominant" state and how weak hamstrings or hamstring/quadriceps muscular imbalances present in female athletes could contribute to their susceptibility for ACL injuries.

Lephart et al[170] also investigated strength and lower-extremity kinematics during landing. Single-leg landing and forward hop tasks were studied using electromyography and force plates with female basketball, volleyball, and soccer players, and matched male subjects. This study also tested strength of the quadriceps and hamstrings via isokinetic testing. The following results were all significant at the level of $p < 0.05$. For single-leg landing, females had greater hip internal rotation, less knee flexion, and less lower-leg internal rotation. The females also had significantly less time to maximum angular displacement of knee flexion. During the forward hop task, females had less knee flexion, less lower-leg internal rotation, and more time to maximum angular displacement for hip internal rotation and less time to maximum angular displacement for knee flexion. There were no significant difference for vertical ground reaction force variable for both landing and hopping tasks. Isokinetic testing revealed significant lower peak torque to body weight for knee extension and flexion ($p < 0.05$). Overall, the females landed in a more valgus position and with less knee flexion, thus less time for absorption of the impact forces. The weakness demonstrated in the quadriceps and hamstrings may also play a role in the landing kinematics.[170]

In a follow-up study to Malinzak, Chappel et al[64] hypothesized that female recreational athletes would have increased proximal anterior tibial shear force, knee extension moment, and knee valgus moment while performing forward, backward, and vertical stop-jumps. The results of this study are similar to those of previous studies. Women exhibited greater proximal tibia anterior shear force than did men during the landing phase of all jumps. All subjects exhibited greater proximal tibia anterior shear force during the landing phase of the backward stop-jump task than during the other 2 stop-jumps. Women also exhibited greater valgus and extensor moments than did the males for all 3 stop-jumps.

Ground reaction force differences during landing are an interesting kinematic variable to examine between males and females. Dufek and Bates[94] examined landing forces and pointed out that higher landing forces had a positive relationship with injury occurrence. Hewett et al[132] examined the results of a neuromuscular training program and determined that the training program resulted in significant decreases in peak landing forces and decreases in valgus-varus moments at the knee. They indicated that the valgus-varus moments at the knee served as significant predictors of peak landing forces. This same study demonstrated that the males' landing forces were an average of 2 bodyweights greater than the females, yet they have lower rate of serious injury. It has been hypothesized that high landing forces by the males are dissipated through increased knee flexor activity at the instant of landing and greater angular knee flexion at landing. Both of these strategies may allow males to dissipate ground reaction forces more efficiently.

The previously mentioned studies have all looked intimately at the knee joint. But what effects do the trunk, hip, and ankle have on the kinematics of the knee joint? Bobbert and van Zandwijk[48] described, in their research, the knee being "slaved" to the moment produced at the hip. It has been theorized that, because most females have weak hip extensors, they use the iliopsoas for trunk control over their hips and land in a more erect posture and have greater extensor moments at the knee. Decreased trunk flexion also decreases maximal quadriceps and hamstrings activation, thus decreasing dynamic stabilization directly at the knee joint. Observation of videotapes of ACL injuries has demonstrated that two-thirds of the injuries occurred when the center of gravity appeared behind the knee. Another theory regarding this variable is that during upright landings, the rectus femoris may act as a hip stabilizer and pull the trunk forward. This powerful contraction by the rectus femoris may also produce a large tibia anterior shear force. More research needs to be performed to prove or disprove these theories, but trunk and hip control appear essential to efficient athlete maneuvers and should be part of all prevention and rehabilitation programs.

In summary of the extrinsic and combined factors that may predispose the female athlete for higher incidence of ACL injuries, the following items were revealed:

1. Females are weaker in their quadriceps and hamstrings as compared to males.
2. Females have a lower hamstring-to-quadriceps ratio as compared to males.
3. When both men and women are fatigued, the stability of the knee joint is compromised.
4. ACL-deficient subjects have decreased proprioception.
5. Females are slower to detect proprioception as measured by detection of passive movement in the direction of knee extension as compared to males.
6. Females use more of a quadriceps-hamstring-gastrocnemius muscle firing pattern in response to anterior tibia translation and males use more hamstring-quadriceps-gastrocnemius pattern.
7. Females are slower to reach peak torque for the hamstring group as compared to males.
8. Females have a longer electromechanical delay between stimulus and action as compared to males.
9. Females demonstrate a decrease in muscle stiffness and thus decreased ability to stabilize knee joint as compared to males.
10. Females demonstrate the following patterns when landing from a jump or decelerating
    a. Decrease in knee flexion
    b. Increase in knee valgus (see Figure 31-3)
    c. Increase in hip internal rotation (see Figure 31-3)
    d. Decrease in trunk and hip flexion

Assessment and Screening

As noted previously, many research studies have focused on determining the exact cause of the higher frequency of ACL injuries in females as compared to males. Although much time has been spent on this subject, no definitive intrinsic, extrinsic, or combined factors have been identified as strong predictors of ACL injuries. A study by Arendt et al,[25] published in 1999, set out to determine potential patterns that cause ACL injuries by using the NCAA Injury Surveillance System. The conclusions of this study stated that common noncontact ACL injuries mechanism were pivoting or landing from a jump. They found no comorbidity or illness patterns. The injured athletes were experienced, with many years of sports participation before and during high school. Hyperextension was the only physical examination feature that could possibly be linked to ACL injuries. Females were more likely to be injured just prior to or just after their menses and not midcycle.[25] Because of the multifactorial presentation of this injury, the sample size for such a study must be quite large to be predictive. These authors stated that their project was to be viewed as a pilot study and hoped it would stimulate more research in this area. Subsequently, many researchers have attempted to formulate skill-related tasks and functional assessments that could accurately predict the risk of ACL injury.

Based on this information, should the clinician working with these athletes conduct a screening process in an attempt to identify those athletes at risk and thereby institute prevention programs to minimize the incidence of ACL injuries among their athletic teams? Current research and practical knowledge do not offer a single valid and reliable screening tool, although some evidence exists that a examining a set of variables (body mass, tibial length, knee valgus, knee flexion during landing, and hamstring-to-quadriceps ratio) may assist in the prediction of athletes prone to high loads during landing.[206] Most clinicians do not have access to the technology and equipment necessary to examine balance, proprioception, kinesthesia, neuromuscular patterns, or kinematic analysis of forces and angles. This does not mean the clinician cannot look at the athlete with simple functional testing. Strength and muscular endurance can be examined either isokinetically or with one repetition maximum testing. Functional tests, such as single-leg and tandem stance balancing, can screen for basic proprioception deficits, and single-leg hop tests, vertical jump, and the tuck jump assessment can assist in grossly examining explosive power of the lower extremity and dynamic stability at the hips and knees. Observing joint positions and landing characteristics from a jump, both visually and with simple video analysis, is an easy thing for the clinician to do. Incorrect technique or motor performance deficits that can be identified can then be corrected to enhance physical performance and possibly lower injury risk, especially for the female athlete.

Injury prevention programs have been developed and tested based on the previous information with the goal of enhancing physical performance and decreasing injury occurrence among female athletes. The authors of this chapter believe that addressing the previously stated deficits common to female athletes can only enhance their physical performance and as a result may decrease the risk of ACL injury. Both high-tech screening and low-tech (clinical) screening procedures are important. When a deficit is identified, it should be addressed, and only good things can come from any education or improvement that occurs.

Prevention and Exercise Considerations

As noted previously, the research indicates some possible areas where females and males differ in their muscle physiology, biomechanics, hormonal levels, joint stability, joint kinematics, proprioception, and skill level in athletics. Which of these factors are controllable and what has the research determined as the best approach for injury prevention? That is the question we all ask ourselves. Although this topic of injury prevention for ACLs has received much attention lately, it is not a new topic. Henning was investigating this idea in the early 1980s, and after a 10-year study of ACL injuries in female basketball players, he formulated a prevention program based on altering the "quad-cruciate interaction."[119] As previously mentioned, Henning concluded that the most common mechanisms of injury to the ACL were planting and cutting, straight-leg landing, and 1-step stop with the knee hyperextended.[119] His prevention program consisted of activities to eliminate or minimize these mechanisms. Henning proposed using an accelerated rounded turn off a bent knee instead of the pivot-and-cut movement pattern. He also emphasized drills that worked on landing on a bent knee and a 3-step stop with the knee bent. The common thread in all the drills was the bent knee position. It has also been illustrated in research studies discussed in the previous sections of this chapter that females do land from jumps with a straight-leg position and have excessive valgus knee position with landing and cutting movements during sports (see Figures 31-3 and 31-7*B*). Both of these positions put the females at risk for an ACL injury. Henning's prevention program did show some success in decreasing ACL injuries (89% decrease). Although his program did have its limitations, it was an admirable start in addressing this problem and provided impetus for modern prevention programs.

Proprioception deficits in ACL-injured and ACL-reconstructed patients is well documented. So, it only seems natural to look at this component and incorporate it into a prevention program. Caraffa et al[60] did just this in developing their 5-phase proprioceptive program that progressed the athlete through increasingly difficult skills using different balance boards. The study showed a statistically significant decrease in ACL injuries in semi-professional and amateur soccer players for the exercise program versus the control group of skill-matched soccer players. The study received criticism for not being randomized and for flaws in program standardization, but it can be looked at as a pilot study and a plausible approach to developing a prevention program incorporating proprioception training.

In the mid-1990s, Hewett et al[132] conducted a seminal study to determine the effect of jump training on landing mechanics and lower-extremity strength in 11 female athletes involved in jumping sports. Vertical jump height, isokinetic muscle strength, and force analysis testing were performed prior to and after the training program for the female athletes and a group of male athletes. The jump program was performed over a 6-week period and was performed on alternate days, 3 days a week. During the jumping program, 4 basic techniques were emphasized:

1. Correct posture with spine erect, shoulders back, and body alignment of shoulders over knees throughout the jump. Control of the trunk over the body is important.
2. Jumping straight up with no excessive side-to-side or forward-backward movement.
3. Soft landings, including toe-to-heel rocking and bent knees.
4. Instant muscular recoil for preparation for the next jump.

See Appendix A for details of the *Jump-Training Program*.[132]

The results of the training program for the female group revealed peak landing forces decreased 22%, knee varus-valgus moments decreased approximately 50%, and hamstring-to-quadriceps peak torque ratios increased 26% on the nondominant side and 13% on the dominant side. Hamstring power increased by 44% with training on the dominant side and 21% on the nondominant side. Mean vertical jump height also increased by 10%. Multiple regression analysis revealed that varus-valgus moments were significant predictors of peak landing forces.[132]

The results of this study led the researchers to continue with a follow-up project with this jump-training program. Hewett et al[129] developed a prospective research study to determine the effect of this same jump-training program on the incidence of knee injury in female athletes. They monitored 2 groups of female athletes; 1 group performed the jump-training program and 1 group did not. A group of untrained male athletes were also used for comparison. The groups were monitored throughout the high school soccer, volleyball, and basketball seasons. Results of this study revealed that the untrained female athletes had a 3.6 times higher incidence of knee injury than trained female athletes ($p < 0.05$) and 4.8 times higher incidence than male athletes ($p < 0.03$). The incidence of knee injury in trained female athletes was not significantly different from that in the untrained male athletes.[129] The results of this early, innovative study indicated that a plyometric training program may have a positive effect in reducing incidence of female ACL injuries. The authors of this study acknowledged several limitations to their study. It was not a randomized, double-blind study, and there were not equal numbers of each type of sports participant in each group. Conclusions from this study indicate that the plyometric training program decreased the magnitude of varus-valgus moments at the knee and improvement in hamstring-to-quadriceps strength ratio. As noted previously, many researchers believe that these 2 lower-extremity variables, as well as trunk motion, play a strong role in ACL injury in female athletes.[106,132,216] However, it should be noted that the results from contemporary research suggest that a prevention program must train roughly 89 female athletes in order to prevent 1 ACL injury when applied generally to a group.[206]

An interesting fact to note about many of these prevention programs is the component of *educating* the athlete about how to correctly perform landing or cutting tasks. Henning developed a teaching tape consisting of examples of noncontact ACL injuries followed by illustrations of the recommended drills done in the gym as well as on the playing field. He stated that young athletes are more receptive to technique modification and called it "improved player technique skills."[119] Ettlinger et al[101] stated that ACL injuries in alpine skiers could be reduced as much as 60% by using standardized training programs before the ski season. The subjects were trained to avoid high-risk behavior, recognize potentially dangerous situations, and to respond quickly whenever these conditions were encountered. Hewett et al[132] used verbal cueing to encourage proper jumping and landing techniques. Such phrases as "on your toes," "straight as an arrow," "light as a feather," "shock absorber," and "recoil like a spring" were all used to illustrate proper technique. Similarly, Myer et al used the tuck jump assessment task and both verbal and visual feedback during the task to fine-tune and attempt to correct jumping and landing strategies.[205] The authors of this chapter also use 3 words beginning with the letter *L* to instruct athletes in correct performance of all motor skills: *L*ow, *L*ight, and (in) *L*ine. These cues refer to low, flexed knee landings and transitions, softness and quietness during landings; and parallel thighs during activity, respectively. This pneumonic is also referred to as L^3.

Another important study by Onate et al[224] reported the importance of feedback and educating the athletes in proper technique performance. They looked at the effects of augmented feedback versus sensory feedback on the reduction of jump-landing forces. The augmented feedback group received information on how to land softer via video and verbal analysis, the sensory feedback group was asked to use the experience with their baseline jumps to land softer, and the control groups were given no extraneous feedback on how to land softer. The subjects in the augmented feedback had significantly reduced peak vertical ground reaction force as compared to the sensory feedback and control groups.[224] All clinicians and researchers must remember that even though you may have the perfect prevention program, if your subjects do not understand the movement pattern and technique you are asking them to perform, it is all for naught.

Myer et al[204] examined a comprehensive neuromuscular training program to study the effects on lower-extremity biomechanics and improved performance in the female athlete's vertical jump, single-leg hop, speed, bench press, and squat. As previously discussed, multiple research studies have been carried out examining the positive effects of a plyometric or jump-training program; however, this study combined plyometrics with core strengthening, balance training, interval speed training, and resistance training.[204] Fifty-three female athletes involved in basketball, volleyball, or soccer participated. Forty-one subjects were assigned to the training group and 12 to the control group. Pretesting was conducted 1 week before the training program and posttesting 4 days after the final training session. The athletes received feedback on biomechanical analysis and correct technique before and after training sessions. The 90-minute training sessions were held 3 days a week (Tuesday, Thursday, and Saturday). Table 31-3 provides a breakdown of the training sessions. Subjects trained for 6 weeks, while control subjects did not change their normal exercise program. Results demonstrated statistically significant improvements compared to their pretrained values in vertical jump height, single-leg hop distance, sprint speed, bench press maximum, and squat maximum for the trained group. Knee flexion range of motion (ROM) during landing from a box jump was significantly increased. Varus and valgus torques were significantly lower for the right knee and showed a trend toward decrease valgus torque in the left knee. The control group showed no increase in any of the previously measured parameters over a 6-week period.[204] This study supports the benefits of a comprehensive exercise approach when treating the female athlete. A combination of plyometrics, core strengthening, balance training, upper- and lower-body strengthening, speed training, and, very importantly, education on technique proves to be valuable in improving athletic

Table 31-3 Neuromuscular Training Program Schedule

Tuesday	Thursday	Saturday
• 30-minute plyometric station • 30-minute strength station • 30-minute core-strengthening and balance station	• 30-minute plyometric station • 30-minute speed station • 30-minute strengthening and balance station	• 45-minute speed station • 45-minute strength station

Developed by Myer et al.[204]

performance, as well as in decreasing potentially dangerous variables in knee biomechanics when running and jumping.[106]

Mandelbaum et al[182] performed a recent prospective study similar to thc previous studies to examine prevention of ACL tears in the female athlete. The authors developed a community-based program named the "Prevent Injury and Enhance Performance Program," which was created specifically for female soccer players between the ages of 14 and 18 years. This program consists of basic warm-up activities, stretching techniques for the trunk and lower extremities, strengthening exercises, plyometric activities, and soccer-specific agility drills. The program also places heavy emphasis on proper landing technique. This training program was implemented to address the feed-forward mechanism as described previously. The specific goal was to improve the athlete's ability to anticipate external forces or loads to stabilize the knee joint, protecting the inherent structures.[182]

Results of this study using the "Prevent Injury and Enhance Performance Program" were impressive in reducing ACL injury in soccer players. Analysis of data from the first year of the study revealed an 88% overall reduction in ACL injury compared to the control group followed by a 74% reduction of ACL injury during the second year of the study. The authors concluded that prophylactic training focusing on developing neuromuscular control of the lower extremity through strengthening exercises, plyometrics, and sports-specific agilities drills "may address the proprioceptive and biomechanical deficits that are demonstrated in the high-risk female athletic population."[182, p. 1008] These researchers and others continue to study the "Prevent Injury and Enhance Performance Program" with a variety of populations.

Exercise Considerations

When designing an exercise program for any athlete, and especially the female athlete, the authors of this chapter like to use the lower-extremity reactive neuromuscular training sequence described in Table 31-4. The basic premise of the exercise sequence is to begin with a stable base of support in a closed-chain position. Then, progress with resistance and perturbations from resistance or trunk and upper-extremity movements. When the athlete becomes proficient with the exercises performed with a stable base, the base is then narrowed and an environment of instability is created.

The progression repeats with an unstable base of support. Sport-specific training is added next with the goal of neuromuscular control becoming a natural, noncognitive, adaptation to the movement patterns required by the sport. The following are some ideas we have developed based on our clinical experience, as well as being creative with the exercise progression.

Table 31-4 Lower-Extremity Reactive Neuromuscular Training, From Less to More Difficult (Top—Less Difficult, Bottom—Most Difficult)

Description of Activity	Examples	Figure Demonstrating[a]
Stable base, bilateral lower extremities	Partial squats, step down and hold	None
Unstable base, bilateral lower extremities	Wobble boards, foam rollers	None
Stable base, unilateral lower extremity	Single-limb stance, unilateral squats star diagram, contralateral LE tubing ("steamboats")	Figures 31-5 and 31-6*A* and *B*
Unstable base, unilateral lower extremity	Wobble boards, foam rollers, minitramp	Figure 31-7*A* and *B*
Stable base, with added UE/trunk challenges	Squat positions with ball throws, perturbations	None
Unstable base, with added UE/trunk challenges	Wobble boards, foam rollers, DynaDiscs, with ball throws, perturbations	Figures 31-8 and 31-9
Jump/landing sequence from stable base	Jump/land on gym floor, Jump/land from minimal elevation (stair, mat)	None
Jump/landing sequence from unstable base	Jump/land from mini-tramp	Figure 31-10*A* and *B*
Jump/landing sequence with distractions	Jump/land with twists, external resistance, passing balls	None

LE, lower extremity; UE, upper extremity.
[a]See Figures 31-6 to 31-10.

Based on the previous descriptive information about female neuromuscular and functional strategies, how does the rehabilitation professional gets the females to bend their knees, avoid the valgus knee position, and get their gluteal region down with the trunk flexed to minimize the potential risk of knee injury? We propose that you make the athlete's exercise program focus on these exact positions (see Figure 31-11).

Strengthening the quadriceps and hamstrings in the flexed trunk and knee position can be performed with simple wall sits, step-down position with a static hold (see Figures 31-4 and 31-5) and progress into closed-chain squats in a protected position using the Smith Squat Rack. The key part of this squat is to note that the athlete never fully extends knee and works in a range of 30 to 90 degrees of knee flexion and uses the bench as her spotter. This is the position we want her to assume when performing sports, so we must train her muscles in this position. What about powerlifting techniques for females, such as the power clean or snatch? The purpose of these powerlifting movements should not be for brute strength but rather for quick footwork and bent knee position with trunk stabilization. Female athletes often do not do the simple squat technique performed by most males in all levels of sports. Proper technique for free-weight lifting is the key, and lighter-weight body bars are optimal for learning, rather than the heavy 45-lb standard weightlifting bars. The Smith squat machine is also useful for early control of the bar during squats and other upper extremity lifts. Treadmill retro uphill walking in a knee-flexed position is also effective for working the quadriceps in an optimal position. If the hamstrings are to be active when the trunk is flexed, then they also need to be strengthened in a flexed trunk position such as seated open-chain resisted knee flexion. Another way to work the gluteals and

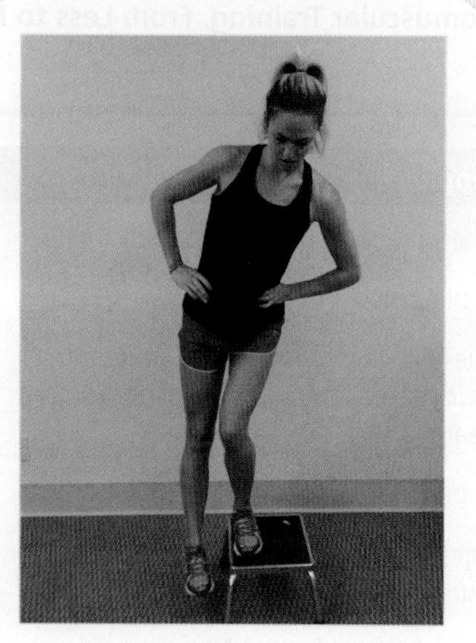

Figure 31-4 Example of a unilateral stable base exercise

Note the incorrect valgus and internal rotation. Training must be done with the lower extremity in proper alignment.

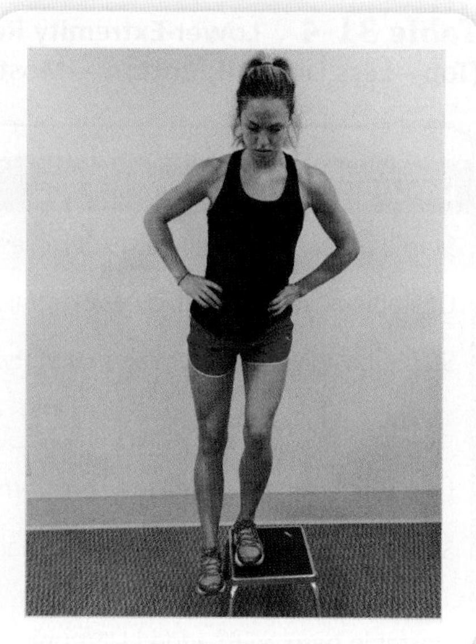

Figure 31-5 Better stance lower-extremity position

Subjects must be corrected and coached to work in excellent lower-extremity alignment. Note that this can also be done in mirror for visual feedback and corrections.

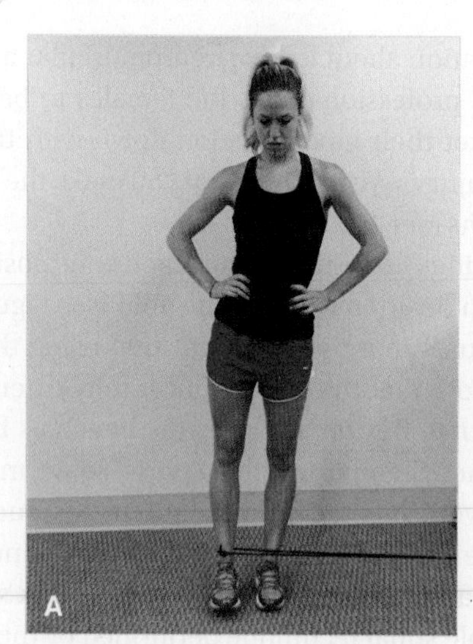

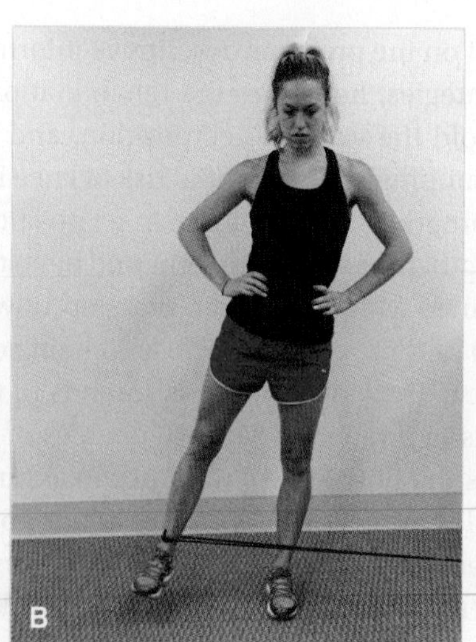

Figure 31-6

Single limb stance hip abduction/adduction with elastic resistance to offer perturbation. AKA "Steamboats" (**A**) Start position (**B**) Finish position.

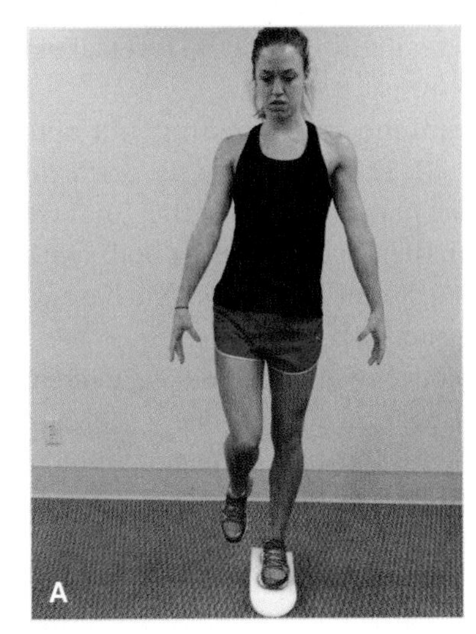

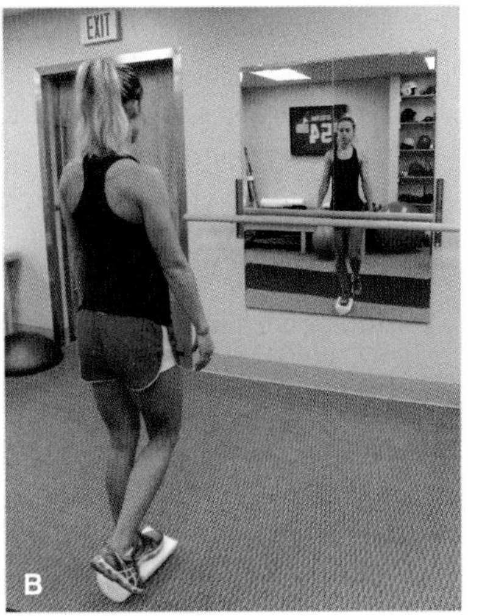

Figure 31-7

A. Unstable surface (1Ž2 foam roll) balance activity. **B.** Same activity with use of mirror for visual feedback on lower extremity positioning during the task.

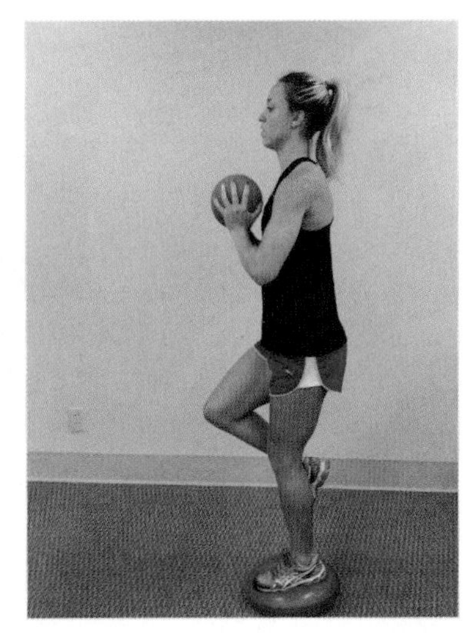

Figure 31-8

Subject, on DynaDisc/unstable base on DynaDisc (unstable base, 1 lower extremity) throwing a ball to/from another person for distraction/balance perturbation.

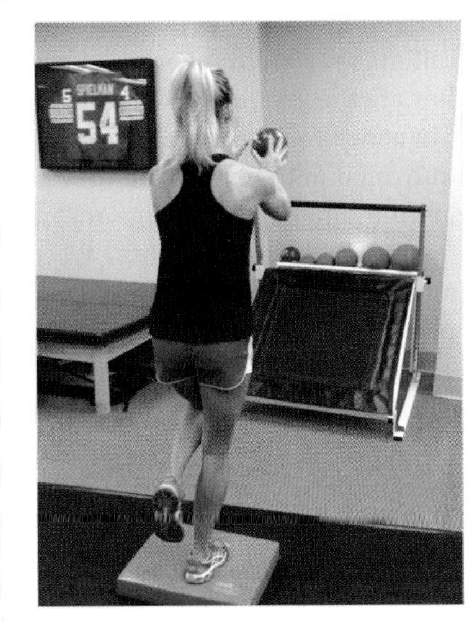

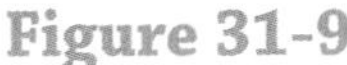

Figure 31-9

Unstable base, unilateral lower extremity exercise, with distraction/perturbation technique of ball throw/catch.

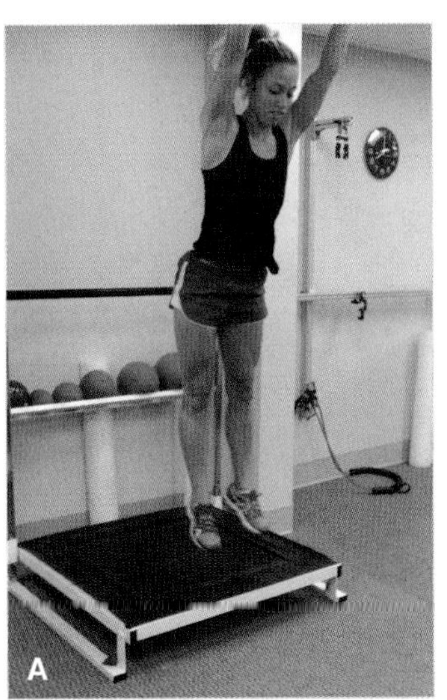

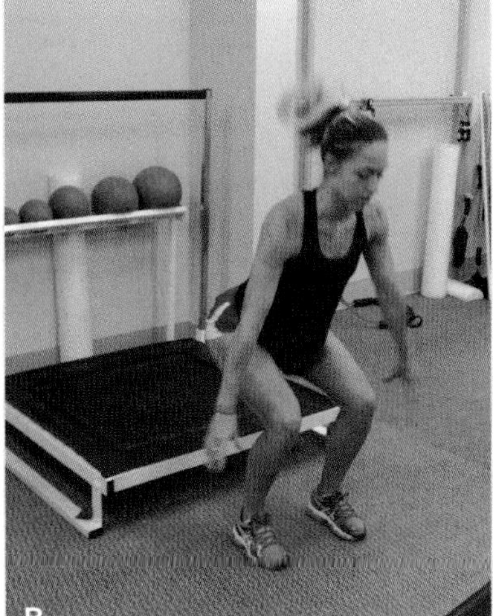

Figure 31-10 **Dynamic jump/land training**

Subject shown airborne after jumping off minitramp (**A**). Subject landing from jump (**B**). During exercise training, stress correct lower extremity position and "soft landing."

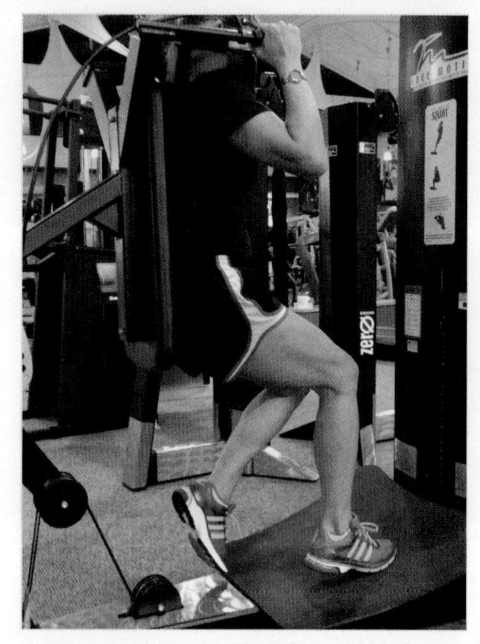

Figure 31-11

Single limb plantar flexion, training the plantar flexors in the "down low" position.

hamstrings in a closed-chain trunk flexed position is to do a semi-squat uphill walking lunge on a treadmill. This is the reversal of the retro uphill squat walk.

Another possibility is to combine strengthening and neuromuscular retraining. In Figure 31-12, the athlete is performing a unilateral, closed-kinetic chain partial squat on the Total Gym, using a DynaDisc under her foot, thereby performing both types of exercise concurrently. This is an example of an unstable base used during a unilateral strengthening activity.

Muscular fatigue slows electromechanical delay, decreases knee stability, and compromises proprioception.[220,247] Muscular fatigue will happen to all athletes if they compete at an intense level, so the athlete must be trained to have a stable knee even when fatigued. Fatiguing the athlete and then *carefully* working on proprioception, cutting and deceleration maneuvers, and proper landing position from a jump are possible techniques for training, although controversial.

When the big picture of total-body positioning is examined, attention must be paid to the joints distal and proximal to the knee joint. Often the ankle and its role as the first link of the chain to absorb the forces and then stabilize the base of support are forgotten. Adequate motion of the talocrural and the subtalar joints must be present for normal landings to occur. The gastrocnemius and soleus have a role in posterior stabilization of the knee joint and need to be strengthened in the position in which they must excel: knee and trunk flexion (see Figure 31-11). In the study by Huston and Wojtys,[145] the gastrocnemius was the first muscle to respond to tibia anterior translation in the relaxed position. An intriguing thought is that maybe the foot and calf muscles are the key to knee stability, as they are the first line of defense for all closed-chain activities. The trunk and hips are the joints proximal to the knee, and they possess the most muscular mass and thus the most potential for efficient body control. We call this concept "The Butt and Gut" and believe firmly in its role in proficient movement patterns for all joints of the body. Females are usually weaker in their gluteal muscles and lack some trunk control with high-level sports movements. Emphasis on hip rotators, hip extensors, transverse abdominals, and hip adductors strength and endurance should be part of every athlete's fitness program. With strong hip and trunk muscles, the landing and running characteristics of genu valgus, hip internal rotation, straight knee position at foot impact, and erect trunk position should be minimized and possibly eliminated.[105,130,133]

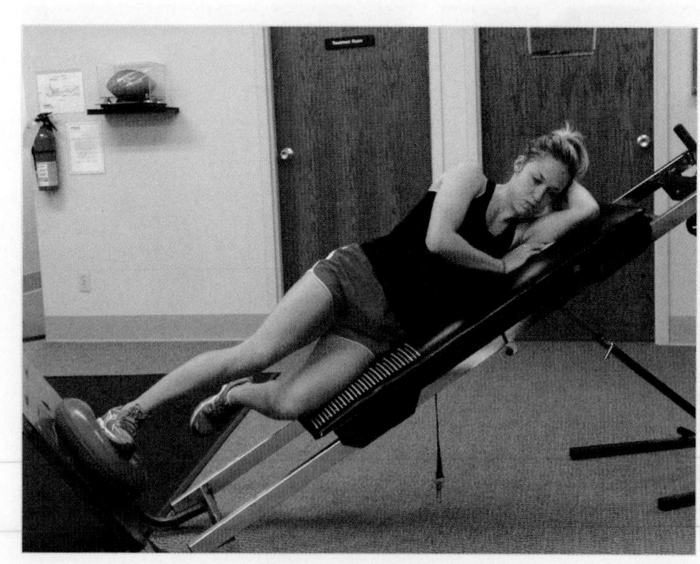

Figure 31-12 **Use of DynaDisc on Total Gym for strength training**

Single-leg partial squats with an unstable surface. Close attention is paid to the position and alignment of the lower extremity. Foot position shown could be improved.

Educating your athletes in proper movement patterns is the key to success for injury prevention. As noted previously, research shows that visual and verbal cueing enhances the performance of proper technique in the quest for optimal position of the body for injury prevention and efficient, powerful sports movements. Simple video can be used to record an athlete during a movement or task, allow the athlete to see what they look like performing the task, and identify what improvements could be made and what the goal is regarding proper technique.

Excellent clinicians frequently review the literature and then think of bold, creative ways to exercise their patients based on the positions that make the female athlete vulnerable to ACL injury. Although ACL reconstructive surgery provides excellent, predictable outcomes in most cases, and rehabilitation after ACL reconstruction has become standard physical therapy practice, no reconstructed knee is as good as an uninjured knee. In the world of ACL injuries in female athletes, the mother's old quote "an ounce of prevention is worth a pound of cure" rings true.

Sequelae from Anterior Cruciate Ligament Injury

We refer the reader to Chapter 24 for a complete analysis of the information regarding evaluation and treatment of the female athlete (or any athlete) suffering an ACL injury. Prevention of this debilitating injury cannot be more emphasized with the growing concerns that have been raised among the sports medicine community regarding the early degenerative changes after a knee injury and specifically following an ACL injury.[81,82,98,114,244,246] Curl et al reviewed more than 30,000 knee arthroscopies with a variety of patient ages and reported chondral injuries in 63% of these patients, with an average of 2.7 articular cartilage injuries per knee.[79] Bone bruises, most common in the lateral compartment, are observed in 80% of MRI studies following ACL tear.[198] At the time of surgery, 9% of all ACL injured patients have documented acute cartilage defects. This same population demonstrates a 19% incidence of articular cartilage defects at 9-year follow-up.[246] This significant increase in cartilage defects demonstrates that stabilization of the knee through ACL reconstruction does not eliminate the risk of degenerative changes in the articular cartilage.[13,14] In fact, many current studies indicate that despite reconstruction of the injured ACL, patients will develop osteoarthritis within 5 years after surgery. In a systematic review conducted by Oiestad et al, the authors reported that up to 13% of those with isolated ACL injuries and 24% to 48% of those with ACL plus other concomitant knee injuries experienced demonstrable osteoarthritis within 10 years, lower than some of the reports in the literature.[223] Whether this is a result of subclinical or unrecognized osteochondral or meniscal injury concomitant with the ACL injury or the reconstructive surgery is unknown.

Numerous studies show good-to-excellent results following ACL reconstructive surgery with reference to stability, normal knee mobility, normalized strength, and return to previous level of activity.[10,28,81,82,143,153,185,221,258,266] Work completed by Daniels et al was the first to document concern regarding early degenerative changes in knees that had stability restored with an ACL reconstruction in 5-year[80] and 10-year follow-up studies.[81] At 5- to 20-year follow-up, patients post-ACL reconstruction demonstrate up to a 50% increase in radiographic changes associated with arthritis compared to the contralateral, uninjured knee.[229] Concern regarding such degenerative changes was expressed by Gilquist who wrote that these surgeries resulted in "giving the patient enough security to go back to strenuous sports and then [ruin] the knee."[114] This concern is valid, but one must consider the concept of joint function and define "full" function.

Dye describes the knee joint as a mechanical engineering model with a complex, metabolically active system for transmission of forces among the femur, tibia, fibula, and patella,

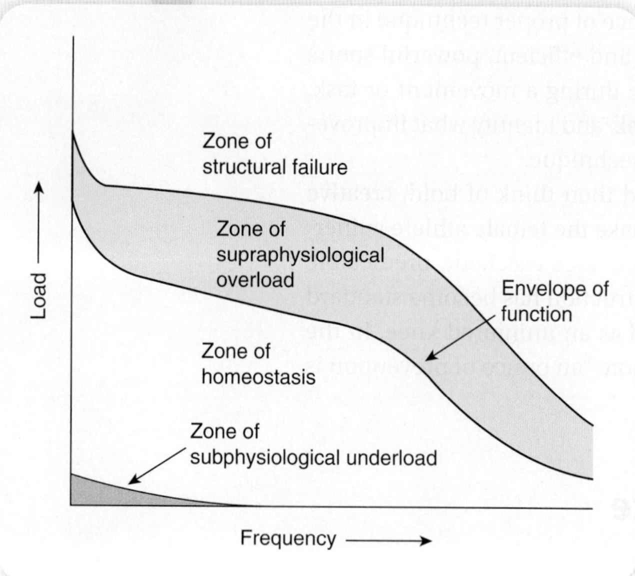

Figure 31-13 **Envelope of function**

with cruciate ligaments acting as linkages, articular cartilage and menisci as weightbearing entities and force absorbers, and muscles as force generators and absorbers.[98] In our view, the concept of musculoskeletal function includes the capacity not only to generate, transmit, absorb and dissipate loads but also to maintain tissue homeostasis while doing so.[97]

This statement beautifully illustrates our belief that joint function is not truly attained unless the system can escape from tissue destruction or degeneration while completing a desired level of functional activity. Dye presents the concept of "envelope of function,"[96] which is the safe zone of loading that a system can maintain normal homeostasis as illustrated in a load distribution curve (see Figure 31-13). Below this safe zone is the subphysiologic loading zone, causing loss of tissue homeostasis secondary to decreased loading, which results in such injuries as osteopenia and muscular atrophy. Above the "envelope of function" is a zone of structural failure with loads great or frequent enough to cause actual failure of an element of the system, such as a meniscal or ACL tear. The zone that is immediately above the envelope of function, the zone of supraphysiologic load, represents loads at a force or frequency that cause a disruption of the tissue homeostasis before failure, that is, stress fractures or articular cartilage degeneration.

This concept of "envelope of function" correlates nicely with the Wolff law that states cyclical loading of the cartilage and bone results in increased strength and durability of these structures and ultimately the musculoskeletal system. However, excessive loading results in degradation of the cartilage microstructure and arthritic changes.[181] Maintaining activity within the "envelope of function" results in maintenance of tissue homeostasis and the ability to strengthen the musculoskeletal system, while exceeding this physiologic loading and moving into the "supraphysiologic loading zone" with increased intensity, duration, or frequency of activity results in degradation of the system and disruption of tissue homeostasis. Sports medicine personnel involved in the orthopedic medical care of a female athlete should adhere to the principle of remaining in the zone of homeostasis as defined by the current status of the joint involved. Defining this zone is a difficult task after completing the rehabilitation following an orthopedic injury such as an ACL tear and surgical reconstruction. The challenge of attaining a level of activity (loading) of the injured joint to allow tissue building, such as muscular hypertrophy, without entrance into the zone of supraphysiologic loading (overloading) that could affect articular cartilage degeneration or meniscal irritation, requires extreme care in planning with respect to activity intensity, duration, and frequency. Determining such a zone also requires excellent communication between the surgeon and the rehabilitation professional regarding any preexisting conditions and surgical findings. Astute observation of the sports medicine specialist for signs of inflammation with a prescribed rehabilitation program and allowed functional/sporting activities is necessary to ensure proper physiologic loading.

The physically active female may be at greater risk than her male counterparts for articular cartilage degeneration and concerns. Gender difference in the knee joint size and greater valgus alignment may result in a greater stress concentration in the lateral and patellofemoral compartments of the female's knee. MRI studies of the human knee demonstrate that females have significantly less cartilage thickness and volume than age-matched males.[68] Articular cartilage has a complicated organization of hyaline cartilage with an extracellular matrix composed principally of type II collagen and sparsely distributed chondrocytes. Animal studies also document lower levels of proteoglycan and collagen in the cartilage of female rats. Considering the increased incidence of ACL injury in females versus males and the female articular cartilage basic science, chondral injury concerns are well founded.

Core Stabilization for the Female Athlete

The common prerequisite for participation and success in all types of sports is a strong and stable core of the human body. Control of balance in upright posture and stability of the segments of the spine are required not only for activities of daily living but also for high-level sports activity.[100] This stability enables athletes to transmit forces from the earth through the kinetic chain of the body and ultimately propel the body or an object using the limbs.[74] The concept of core stabilization of the trunk and pelvis as a prerequisite for movements of the extremities was described biomechanically in 1991.[52] Subsequently, core stabilization has become a major trend, both in treatment of injuries and in training regimes used to enhance athletic performance and prevent injury.

Many terms and rehabilitation programs are associated with the concept of core stability, including lumbar stabilization, dynamic stabilization, motor control (neuromuscular) training, neutral spine control, muscular fusion, and trunk stabilization.[12] The core has been conceptually described as either a box or a cylinder[241] because of its anatomical and structural composition. The abdominals create the anterior and lateral walls; the paraspinals and gluteals form the posterior wall, while the diaphragm and pelvic floor create the top and bottom of the cylinder, respectively (Figure 31-14). Additionally, hip girdle musculature reinforces and supports the bottom of the cylinder. Envisioning this cylindrical system helps to understand its function as that of a dynamic muscular support system, described by some authors as the powerhouse, engine, or a "muscular corset that works as a unit to stabilize the body and spine, with and without limb movement."[12, p. S86]

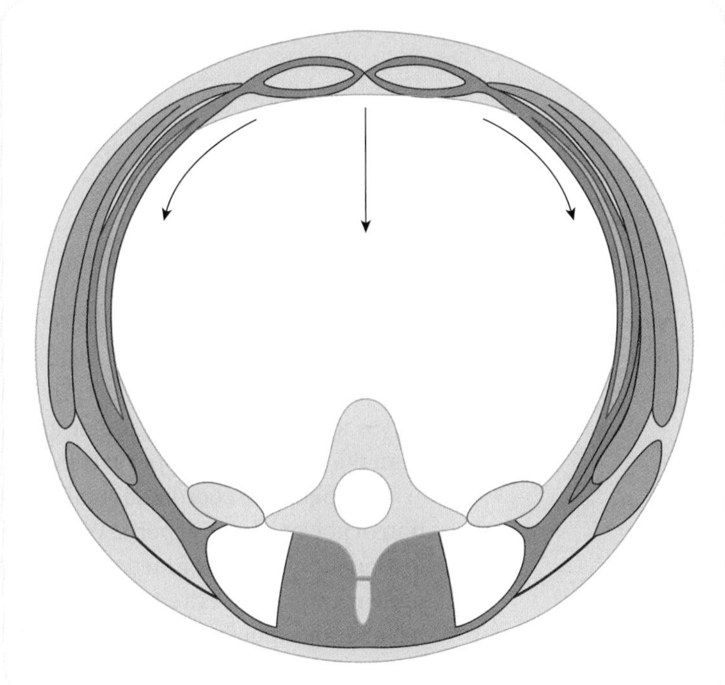

Figure 31-14 Anatomic cylinder of trunk

The muscle contraction of "drawing in" of the abdominal wall with an isometric contraction of the lumbar multifidus. The interrelationship and the interaction between these 2 muscles and the fascial system can be appreciated, and the figure illustrates how they can work together to give spinal support. (Reproduced, with permission, from Richardson C, Jull G, Hodges P, Hides J. *Therapeutic Exercise for Spinal Segmental Stabilization in Low Back Pain: Scientific Basis and Clinical Approach*. Edinburgh, UK: Churchill Livingstone; 1999.)

Proximal stability for distal mobility is a commonly understood principle of human movement. It was originally described by Knott and Voss[159] and applied in the concepts associated with proprioceptive neuromuscular facilitation. Nowhere is the concept of dynamic proximal stability more important than in sports. Without proximal control of the core, athletes could not use the lower extremities to propel the body in running and jumping or use the upper extremities to support or propel the body (in activities such as gymnastics and

Table 31-5 Examples of Core Demands, Kinetic Chain Relationships, and Outcomes of Specific Sporting Tasks

Sporting Activity	Core Demands	Kinetic Chain Relationships	Outcome
Windmill softball pitch	Rotational and flexion/extension stability, acceleration, and deceleration of trunk	Transmission of forces from ground to LEs through trunk to UE to ball	Velocity, location, rotation of pitched ball (55 to 70 mph); delivery of various types of pitches (drop, rise, breaking ball, etc)
Gymnastics: vault event	Rotational and flexion/extension stability; power with punch from horse	Transmission of forces from horse to UEs through trunk to propel body in airborne positions	Conversion of horizontal energy to vertical; speed, position, and trajectory of body through space
Tennis serve	Rotational and flexion/extension stability; acceleration and deceleration of trunk	Transmission of forces from ground to LEs through trunk to UE through racquet to ball	Velocity, location, spin of served ball (80 to 120 mph); delivery of various types of serves
Swimming: butterfly stroke	Flexion/extension stability	Transmission of forces from UEs to trunk to LEs to team with butterfly kick	Efficient propulsion of body through water, avoid excess trunk flexion and extension
Volleyball serve	Rotational and flexion/extension stability; acceleration and deceleration of trunk	Transmission of forces from ground to LEs through trunk to UE to ball	Velocity, location, rotation of served ball; various types of spins and serves (floater, topspin)

LE, lower extremity; UE, upper extremity.

swimming), or to manipulate, use, and throw objects (such as throwing a shot put or softball, or using a tennis racquet). The core is in the middle of the human kinetic chain and serves a link between the upper and lower extremities. This allows for transfer of energy from the lower to the upper extremities and vice versa.

Strength and coordination of the core musculature is vital to performance and generation of power in many sports. When the core is functioning optimally, muscles elsewhere in the kinetic chain also function optimally allowing the athlete to produce strong, functional movements of the extremities (Table 31-5).[65,156] Even small alterations in the kinetic chain have serious repercussions throughout other portions of the kinetic chain and thus on skills that are based upon efficient utilization of the entire chain.[156] Therefore, without proper stabilization and dynamic concentric and eccentric control of the trunk during athletic tasks, the extremities or "transition zones" between the core and extremities can be overstressed (ie, hip and rotator cuff).

A wide variety of movements are associated with sport performance; therefore, athletes must possess sufficient strength and dynamic motor control of the core in all 3 planes of movement (transverse, frontal, sagittal).[167] Core stability is vital to athletic performance and especially important for the female athlete. In a study of male and female runners, females were found to have greater hip adduction, hip internal rotation, and tibial external rotation movements during the stance phase of running. Ferber et al[102] believe that gender differences in lower-extremity kinematics place greater demands on the core musculature of female athletes. Additionally, core stability may even be more vital for the female athlete as a result of her overall decreased total extremity strength as compared to her age-matched male participant.[65] Documented differences in proximal strength measures in female athletes suggest that females may have a less-stable base upon which torque and force can be generated or resisted. This "lack of core stability" is a possible contributor to lower-extremity injury.[119,149] Although important energy has been devoted to prevention of ACL and other knee injuries in the female athlete, the sports physical therapist must broaden his/her focus to the body as a whole and include core strengthening activities as a part of preparatory training for all female athletes.

Reviewing and considering the anatomy of the core allows the sports physical therapist to best understand principles of injury and rehabilitation (refer to Chapter 15). Stability of the core requires both passive (offered by bony and ligamentous structures) and dynamic stiffness (offered by coordinated muscular contractions). A spine without the contributions of the muscular system is unable to bear essential compressive loads and remain stable.[187] Anatomists have known for decades that a compressive load of as little as 2 kg causes buckling of the lumbar spine in the absence of muscular contractions.[201] Likewise, significant microtrauma of the lumbar spine occurs with as little as 2 degrees of rotation, demonstrating the vital stabilizing function of the muscles of the lumbar spine.[110,116] Core stabilization is important not only for protection of the lumbar spine but also to resist the reactive forces produced by moving limbs that are transmitted to the spine and other muscles of the core.[193]

Contemporary research has illuminated the roles of two important local muscle groups: the transversus abdominis (TA)[75,136,137,139] and the multifidus.[134,287] The TA—deepest of the abdominal muscles—uses its horizontal fiber alignment and attachment to the thoracolumbar fascia to increase intraabdominal pressure, thereby making the core cylinder as a whole more stable. Although increased intraabdominal pressure is associated with the control of spinal flexion forces and a decrease in load on the extensor muscles,[278] it is probable that the TA is most important in its ability to assist in intersegmental control[240] by offering "hooplike" cylindrical stresses to enhance stiffness and limit both translational and rotational movement of the spine.[100,192] Bilateral contraction of the TA performs the movement of "drawing in of the abdominal wall"[258] and does not produce spinal movement. The TA is active throughout the movements of both trunk flexion and extension, suggesting a unique stabilizing role during dynamic movement, different from the other abdominal muscles.[75,76,193] Also, EMG evidence suggests that the more internal muscles of the trunk (TA and internal obliques) behave in an anticipatory or feed-forward manner to provide proactive control of spinal stability during movements of the upper extremities,[137,138] regardless of the direction of limb movements.[138] This is important to remember when treating the athlete whose sport is heavily reliant on the upper extremity such as softball, swimming, gymnastics, and volleyball.

Mechanisms of Injury to the Core

Many potential mechanisms of injury exist for the athlete. Cholewicki et al[66] suggest that a common factor for injury to athletes may be the inability to generate sufficient core stability to resist external forces imposed upon the body during high-speed events. Other authors suggest a deficient endurance of the trunk stabilizing musculature that predisposes the athlete to traumatic forces over time,[241] and motor control deficits and imbalances of the local muscles (TA and multifidus) and the global musculature (rectus abdominis and erector spinae) that occur during performance of functional activities. A weak core could result in inefficient movements, altered postures, and an increased potential for both macro- and microtraumatic injury.[65]

Two examples of microtraumatic injuries that occur in the female athlete are spondylolysis and spondylolisthesis. The athletic population is more prone to these

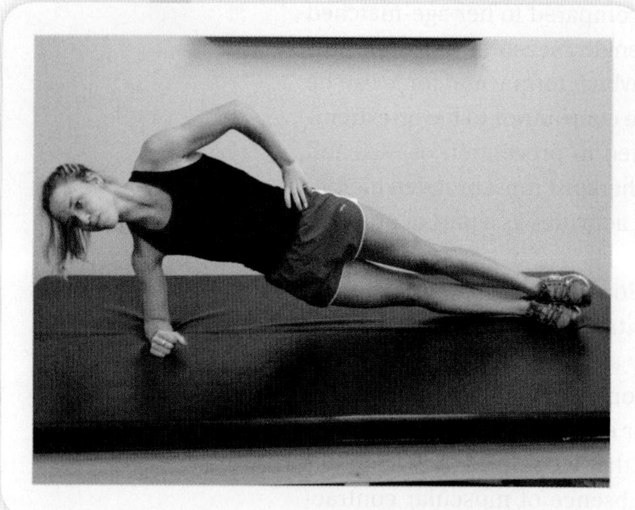

Figure 31-15 Example of side-bridging

conditions and more likely to be symptomatic from these injuries. Spondylolytic microfracture of the pars is believed to happen as a result of shear forces occurring during repetitive flexion and extension.[275] Athletes with high rates of this type of microtraumatic injury include gymnasts,[99] divers, figure skaters, swimmers who perform the butterfly stroke,[275] and volleyball players,[99] as a result of extreme extension/flexion reversals in trunk posture demanded by these sports. In fact, gymnasts younger than age 24 years have 4 times greater incidence of spondylolysis than the general female population.[275] Microtraumatic injuries may occur from muscular imbalances or uncontrolled shear forces acting on the spine,[123,275] or because of lack of muscular control and stabilization offered by the core stabilizers. Sports, such as golf, diving, and softball, have the potential for microtraumatic injury to the core to be induced similarly, but related to extremes of rotation, often in combination with extension. Careful assessment of motor strategies and subsequent corrective movement retraining by the sports physical therapist may be a key to prevention of many microtraumatic injuries.

Leetun et al[167] found that male athletes had statistically greater core stability scores on tests of hip abduction, hip external rotation, and the side bridge when compared to female athletes (Figure 31-15).[167] Athletes who experienced injury to the core (spine/hip/thigh), knee or ankle, and foot during an athletic season demonstrated lower core stability measures than those who did not.[167] Again, this leads the sports physical therapist to consider core strength, endurance, and motor performance training as a possible intervention for prevention of injury, especially for the female athlete.

Rehabilitation and Treating the Core

Simple, reliable, and objective clinical test procedures for dynamic motor control of the core are not readily available. Clinically, therapists utilize manual muscle tests that examine isometric holding of muscles, some positional holding tests (the plank or side plank) for endurance in isometric positions, and pressure biofeedback to assess the ability of a patient to hold the core stable during some dynamic tasks. A clinical test for the multifidus was devised that involves the activation of the multifidus at various segments under the palpating finger of a therapist.[241] This is performed in the prone position using the command "gently swell out your muscles under my fingers without using your spine or pelvis. Hold the contraction while breathing normally," [241, p. 116] including side-to-side comparison to assess for segmental activation or inhibition. For many excellent examples of core strengthening exercises, refer to Chapter 15. To make these exercises more specific to your female athlete, incorporate these concepts while performing training programs for other regions. For example, for a swimmer, the therapist may have the athlete lie prone on a swiss ball while performing Thera-Band movements mimicking the pull-through phase. The ball introduces an unstable base to challenge the core muscles.

Knowledge and application of core stabilization will benefit female athletes in all sports at all levels by improving performance, increasing athleticism, and decreasing the potential for injury to the spine and extremities. To provide an optimal, comprehensive exercise program for all female athletes, functional core exercises should be implemented into the female athlete's sports-specific program.

Special Considerations Concerning the Shoulder in the Active Female

Shoulder Laxity

Are women more prone to shoulder injuries? This question does not have ample research to be answered conclusively. Most studies do not separate shoulder injuries by gender or separate general injuries from specific ones. In 2001, Sallis et al[249] compared sports injuries in men and women and failed to show a significant difference in overall injury rate. However, these authors reported that in all sports, women reported a higher rate of hip and shoulder injuries. A significant difference was found with a higher rate of shoulder injuries in female swimmers compared to their male counterparts. Yet, the training for female and male swimmers differed greatly, so it is difficult to draw any specific conclusion.[249] The training regimen, their structural build, and/or presence of laxity may have predisposed the athletes to overuse injuries. Conclusions are unable to be drawn, until more controlled, specific research is carried out.

Other studies have described differences in various injuries between genders. Kroner and Lind[162] found no difference in shoulder dislocations between genders. All shoulder dislocations were recorded over a 5-year period in an area within a population of 253,753 athletes. Of this population, 53.3% of shoulder dislocations occurred in males and 46.7% occurred in females. However, a notable difference occurred between the age group where the peak incidence occurred. Males were 21 to 30 years old, and females were 61 to 80 years old. The injury in the older age group was typically caused by a fall on an outstretched arm.[162]

A high incidence of shoulder impingement is reported in female softball players[286] and both genders of volleyball players.[32,53] The shoulder was also the most commonly injured upper-extremity joint in both genders during alpine skiing.[254]

Clinical experience might suggest that women in general are more flexible and demonstrate increased laxity of their joints when compared to men. Are women more at risk for shoulder injuries because of laxity? First, it is important to describe the difference between laxity and instability. Laxity is not synonymous with instability. Laxity is the physiologic motion that allows for normal ROM. Instability is the abnormal *symptomatic* motion that results in pain, subluxation, or dislocation.[55]

There are many general joint laxity tests in literature, the most well known are those by Carter and Wilkinson,[62] which have been modified by Beighton[42] (Table 31-6 and

Table 31-6 Generalized Joint Laxity Tests

Carter and Wilkinson	Beighton et al
1. Passive thumb apposition to forearm	**1.** Passive hyperextension of small finger >90
2. Passive finger hyperextension so finger parallel to forearm	**2.** Passive thumb apposition to forearm
3. Elbow hyperextension >10 degrees	**3.** Elbow hyperextension >10 degrees
4. Knee hyperextension >10 degrees	**4.** Knee hyperextension >10 degrees
5. Excessive ankle dorsiflexion and foot eversion	**5.** Trunk flexion, knee extension, and palms flat on floor

Source: Adapted from Brown GA, Tan JL, Kirkley A. The lax shoulder in females. Issues, answers, but many more questions. *Clin Orthop Relat Res.* 2000;372:110-122.

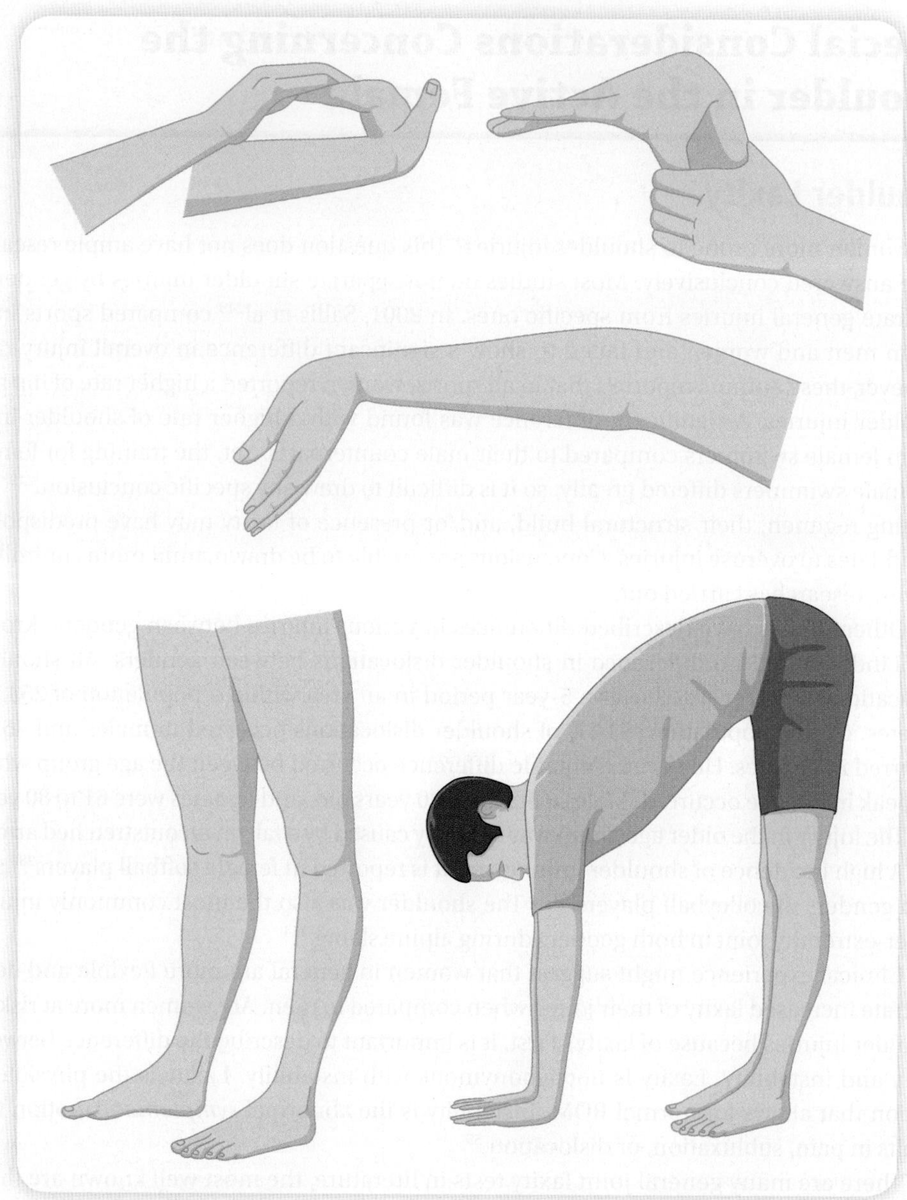

Figure 31-16

Hypermobility screening maneuvers, as developed by Carter and Wilkinson and modified by Beighton et al.

Figure 31-16). These tests examine ROM at the trunk (single test) and knees, fingers, thumbs, and elbows bilaterally and assigns a point system (0 to 9; a score greater than 5 = diagnosed as hypermobile). Other hypermobility tests have not been proven reliable and valid. Consequently, many studies found in literature regarding general laxity differences between genders are not valid. Of the studies in literature, only 1 utilized the 0 to 9 Beighton scale examining generalized mobility in adolescents.[83] The authors reported that of 264 adolescent athletes, 22% of all females and 6% of all males tested were generally "hypermobile." However, it would be incorrect to conclude from this study that generalized laxity correlates with shoulder laxity. The astute clinician can and should recall the structural and physiologic differences between the genders and take into account clinical experience in order to rehabilitate the female athlete's shoulder in a multifaceted way.

Softball, swimming, and gymnastics are 3 sports that emerge when considering the female athlete. There is a high incidence of injury in both genders when considering softball/baseball, swimming, and gymnastics. Softball is discussed separately because of the difference in the pitching delivery and the differences in rules regarding number of allowable pitches. Swimming is discussed separately because of the extreme high numbers of shoulder injuries that occur in female swimmers. Finally, the sport of gymnastics is described in relationship to its injury potential in females.

Shoulder Injuries in the Windmill Softball Player

Little research has focused on softball pitching biomechanics or injury rates sustained by pitchers. Yet, softball was the team sport with the greatest participation in the United States in 1995. In 1996, Plummer[234] reported softball as one of the fastest growing sports for women at the college and high school levels. In fact, in the most recent school year data, softball was the high school sport with the fourth greatest female participation rate, following only basketball, outdoor track and field, and volleyball.[6] When comparing the sport of softball to baseball, it is very similar in many demands and functional tasks. Although the softball playing field is smaller, the reaction time for a batter is directly comparable to baseball. The biggest difference between baseball and softball exists in pitching. The softball mound is flat instead of elevated as in baseball. The distance from home plate to the pitching rubber is 40 ft for youth softball and 60 ft 6 in for baseball. A baseball weighs 5 oz in comparison to a softball that weighs 6¼ to 7 oz.[37] The delivery of the pitch also differs significantly between the windmill pitch in fast-pitch softball and the overhand release in baseball or general overhead throwing. Similar musculature is used, but in a very different order and with different mechanics (see Figure 31-17),[286] with the biceps being more active in the softball pitching motion (38% maximum voluntary isometric contraction) than the overhead throwing motion (19% maximum voluntary isometric contraction).[243,259]

In a review of the existing literature, only 4 studies have addressed female softball injury incidence and prevalence. Results suggested that 63% to 80% of all injuries were in the upper extremity and 37% to 50% of the pitchers studied had a time-loss injury in 1 season.[135,257,274,286] Furthermore, there were 5.6 injuries per 1000 athlete exposures in softball compared to 4.0 injuries per 1000 athlete exposures in baseball, 63% of which involved the shoulder. Marshall et al described overuse of the shoulder as among the most common injury in female collegiate softball players.[188] Based upon these statistics and clinical experience, it would seem prudent to investigate injury prevention strategies.[286]

Likewise, there are only 2 published studies on windmill pitching biomechanics, as compared to numerous studies on baseball pitching biomechanics. In these studies, it is reported that shoulder distraction forces are similar to those found in overhand pitching. Barrentine et al[37] reported that maximum distraction stresses at the shoulder (98% body weight) were reached at 77% of the delivery phase and maximum compressive force at the elbow (70% body weight) occurred at the end of the delivery phase. The difference between baseball and softball pitching is the phase of pitching during which the distraction forces occur, and the position of the humerus during the pitch. In windmill pitching, maximum distraction forces at the shoulder occur during acceleration, whereas maximum shoulder distraction forces for baseball occur during windmill pitching. Shoulder distraction forces occur when the humerus is in a slightly flexed position while controlling internal rotation and elbow extension during acceleration, before ball release. Notably, centrifugal

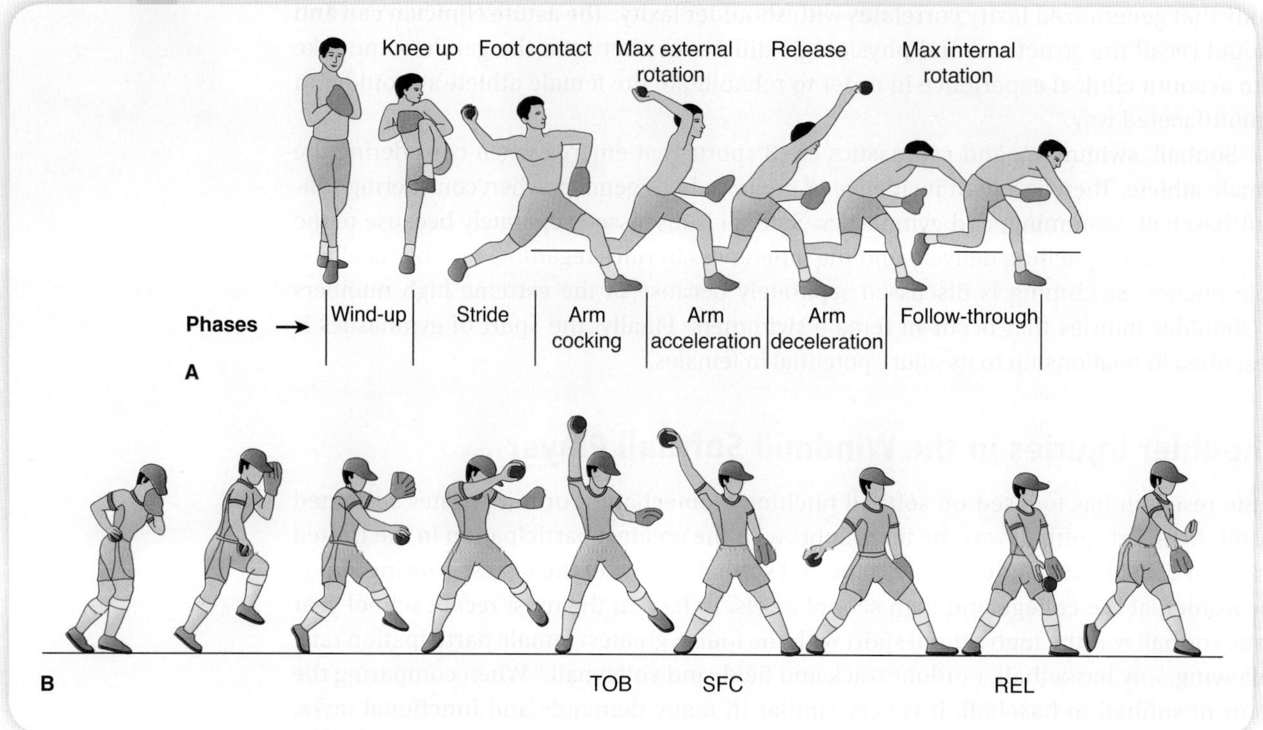

Figure 31-17 Six phases of pitching a baseball (A) and three named phases of pitching a softball (B)

REL, ball release; SFC, stride foot contact; TOB, top of the backswing. (A. Reproduced, with permission, from Fleisig GS, Andrews JR, Dillman CJ, Escamilla RF. Kinematic and kinetic comparison between baseball pitching and football passing. *J Appl Biomech.* 1996;12:207-224; and **B.** Reproduced, with permission, from Werner SL, Guido JA, McNiece RP, Richardson JL, Delude NA, Stewart GW. Biomechanics of youth windmill softball pitching. *Am J Sports Med.* 2005;33(4):553.)

distraction force on the glenohumeral joint is accentuated because the elbow remains in full extension during most of the circumduction motion. For overhand pitching, maximum shoulder distraction forces occur when the humerus is rotated internally and horizontally adducted while maintaining a position of abduction during deceleration after ball release. The biceps labrum complex and the rotator cuff are both at risk for overuse injury at these phases. Conversely, medial elbow injuries are reported less frequently in softball pitching compared to baseball, likely because of the small amount of varus torque produced during the windmill motion.[37]

It is interesting that a softball pitcher may pitch any number of consecutive innings and games, while baseball pitchers are carefully monitored and often restricted in number of pitches and innings they are allowed to throw. Softball pitchers can throw 1200 to 1500 pitches in a 3-day period as compared to 100 to 150 for baseball. A reason for this seems related to the traditional belief that softball windmill pitching forces were much less in the shoulder and elbow than that of the baseball pitch.[286] This is may be true for the amount of varus torque at the elbow, but not for the distraction forces at the shoulder.

Werner et al[286] studied the biomechanics of 53 female windmill pitchers, ages ranging from 11 to 19 years. Statistically significant different ranges of motion were found, including greater shoulder external rotation and decreased internal rotation in the dominant arm. What remains unknown is whether these ROM differences are a result of the windmill biomechanics or the concurrent demands of overhand throwing, which is also a big part of softball. Elbow-carrying angle and hyperextension were found to be similar bilaterally.

Maximum elbow and shoulder distraction forces were 46% body weight and 94% body weight, respectively.

This study along with the study conducted by Barrentine et al[37] show that the compressive forces at the elbow and the distraction forces at the shoulder are similar to baseball pitchers. Thus, allowing softball pitchers to throw an unlimited number of pitches is subjecting them to potential forces of sufficient amplitude to cause overuse injuries. With such high magnitude of shoulder distraction stress and rapid deceleration of the humerus near ball release, the posterior rotator cuff is at high risk for injury, as is the biceps labrum complex, because of the combination of shoulder distraction stress and elbow extension torque.[286] With overuse, eccentric muscle loading of the posterior muscle girdle can cause stretching of these muscles allowing dynamic anterior instability of the humeral head.[41] When rehabilitating softball pitchers, it is important for the clinician to understand the stresses and forces present during pitching. Educating coaches and athletic trainers regarding these findings is also necessary for injury prevention. An important implementation for windmill pitching injury prevention may be to establish a pitch count as is traditional in baseball.

Rehabilitation and Return to Play

It is important to know the demands of the sport of softball for efficient rehabilitation. The game requires the same demands of baseball for the overhead throw, hitting, running, cutting, quick bursts of acceleration and deceleration, sliding, and catching. The difference in rehabilitation occurs with the differences in the demands of pitching compared to baseball pitching. In the windmill pitch, the pectoralis major is an important contributor to the power of the pitch and also acts as a stabilizer against anterior forces. The subscapularis helps the pectoralis major in its role as a stabilizer. The serratus anterior is a scapulohumeral synchronizer.[177] The teres minor is also found to be very active in decelerating the humerus. These muscles should be highlighted in the rehabilitation program along with the standard return-to-throwing rehabilitation.

Core strengthening is also a key factor in return to play for the softball player. The demands on the core during throwing and hitting cannot be ignored. The transfer of energy from the ground through the limbs to core must provide a stable base for the upper extremities to function properly.[142]

Consequently, rehabilitation and return to play for the windmill softball pitcher may include some variations to the typical softball or baseball rehabilitation program that does not require the windmill motion in the athlete's return to playing. As with any overhead athlete, it will be important to restore a balance of stability and mobility in the shoulder, with a strong, stable core. It is also important to strengthen scapular stabilizers as one would in any overhead athlete rehabilitation program. For the windmill pitcher, it may be more effective to include specific functional activities highlighting the demands of the pitch when acute pain and inflammation have subsided. Functional exercises that the authors of this chapter like to use are summarized in Table 31-7 with Figures 31-18 to 31-33 to demonstrate the techniques. These exercises are functional and windmill-pitch specific.

The trunk rotation with a bicep curl (see Figure 31-18) mimics the motion required in the trunk and arm near and at ball release. The Thera-Band provides resistance for trunk facilitation/control while the weight in the hand provides concentric and eccentric strengthening for the shoulder extensors/flexors and biceps.

The step-up with ipsilateral arm raise and contralateral hip extension (see Figure 31-20) synchronously fires the latissimus dorsi and hip extensors. At the beginning of the pitch delivery, the dominant leg remains in a closed chain, neutral hip position. The hip then travels into extension, which is mimicked in the step up. During the first 25% of the pitch delivery phase, the latissimus dorsi is very active.

Table 31-7 Sample Functional Exercises for Return-to-Windmill Pitching

Exercise	Muscles Affected	Targeted Pitching Phase Cycle
Trunk rotation with biceps curl (see Figure 31-18)	Trunk and hip rotators Biceps	End of SFC to REL
Lawn mower with external rotation (see Figure 31-19)	Scapular retractors Teres minor	SFC to REL
Step up/arm lift/hip extension (see Figure 31-20)	Hip extensors Latissimus dorsi	First 25% of pitch delivery (up to TOB)
Chest press on swiss ball with serratus punches (see Figure 31-21)	Core stabilizers Pectoralis major Serratus anterior	Pectoralis major is a key muscle in power of entire pitch cycle and stabilizes against anterior sheer forces
Step up with hip ER/IR (see Figure 31-22)	Hip extensors Hip internal rotators Hip external rotators Quadriceps and hamstrings	Beginning of windup to TOB (with ER movement of the exercise) At REL (with IR movement of the exercise)
"Full can" in tall kneeling on DynaDisc or BOSU ball (see Figure 31-23)	Core stabilizers Shoulder ER	SFC → REL
Physioball deceleration throw with therapist (see Figure 31-24)	Concentric and eccentric training of biceps Shoulder flexors/extensors Trunk/hip rotators	Just after SFC → REL
Lunging with military press (see Figure 31-25)	LE—Quadriceps, hamstrings, hip extensors, and rotators UE—Shoulder external rotators, deltoids, latissimus dorsi Core stabilizers	No specific phase
Push-up plus progression (see Figure 31-26)	Pectoralis major Serratus anterior Triceps	Pectoralis and serratus active through entire cycle
Shoulder IR with Thera-Band sitting on swiss ball (see Figure 31-27)	Shoulder internal rotators (subscapularis) Core stabilizers	Beginning → SFC

ER, external rotation; IR, internal rotation; LE, lower extremity; REL, ball release; SCF, stride food contrast; TOB, top of backswing; UE, upper extremity.

The chest press on a Physioball with serratus punch (see Figure 31-21) challenges the core, as it has to stabilize the trunk on the ball while strengthening the pectoralis major, which is a key muscle in the power of the pitch and a major stabilizer against anterior sheer forces. Although not positionally correct for the softball pitch, this exercise incorporates the serratus anterior, which is important to strengthen as the scapula must provide a strong, stable base.

The step-up with closed-chain hip external and internal rotation (see Figure 31-22) trains the hip and core in the similar motions the hip passes through from beginning of wind up (step-up phase), before and during stride foot contact (hip external rotation), and at delivery phase when the pelvis is closing and the hip goes into internal rotation.

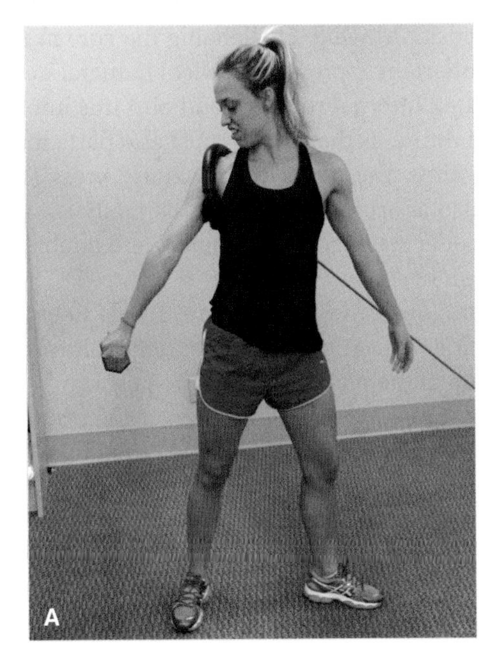

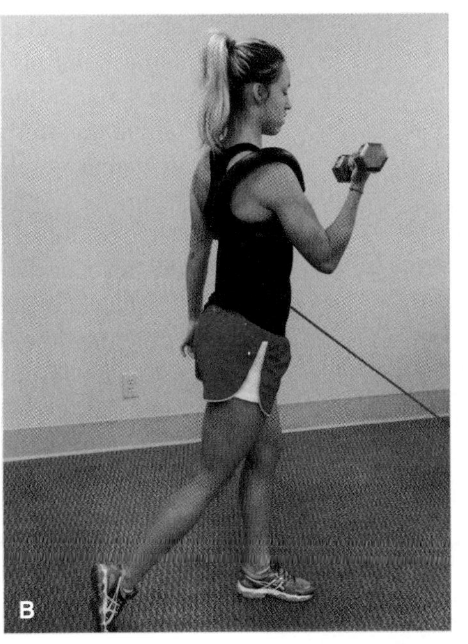

Figure 31-18 **Trunk rotation with biceps curl**

A. Start in stride stance facing sideways, front foot pointing forward, back foot pointing sideways with Thera tubing wrapped around waist and secured at shoulder (to resist rotation). **B.** Weight in dominant/pitching hand. Perform a bicep curl while rotating trunk forward.

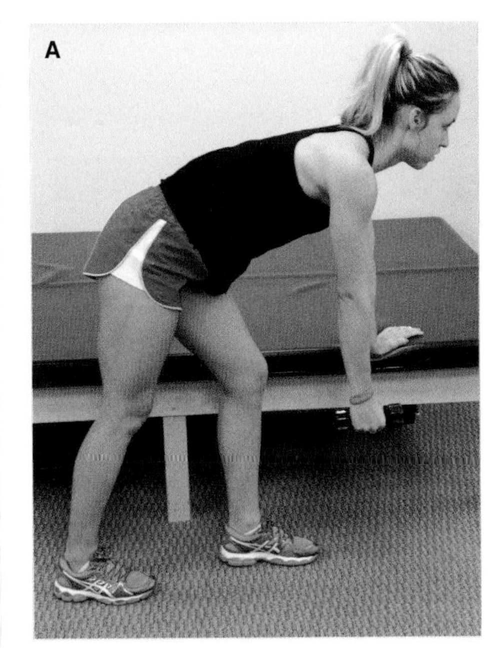

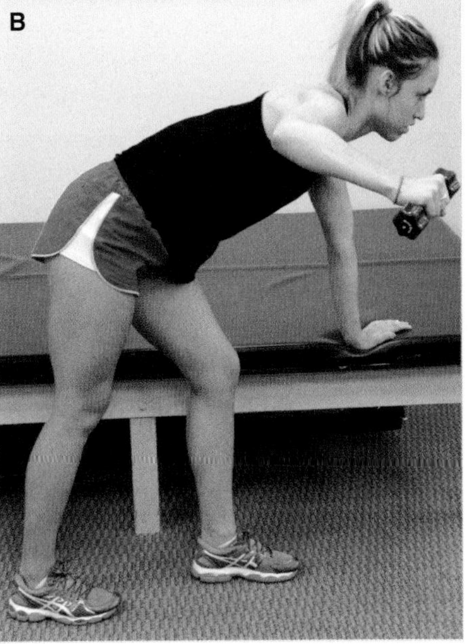

Figure 31-19 **Lawn Mower with external rotation**

A. Stance, forward flexion at waist with weight in hand. **B.** Retract scapula like a rowing motion, adding external rotation at the end.

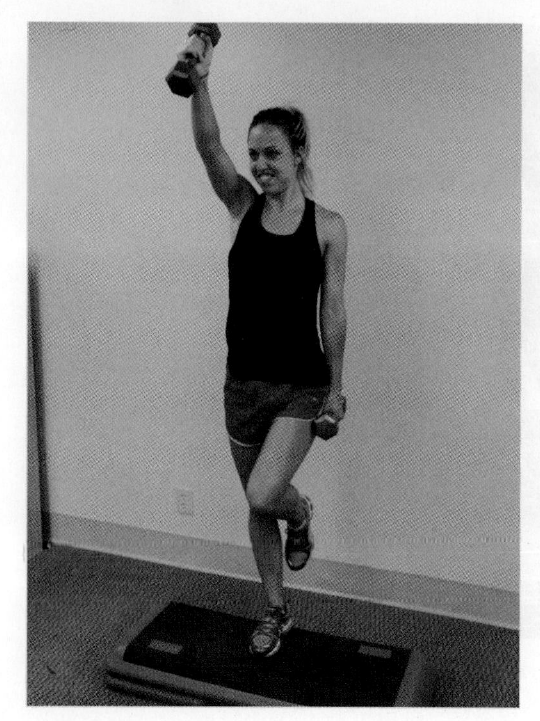

Figure 31-20 **Step up/arm lift/hip extension**

Step onto step with dominant leg (right for right-handed pitcher) and lift ipsilateral arm into flexion with weight while left leg raises into hip extension.

In Figure 31-23, the athlete is strengthening the shoulder elevators (full can position) while challenging the core at the same time. This is important to provide excellent humeral steering, balance the strong internal rotators, and also it is important in the overhead throw, as the pitcher must also participate in defensive plays. Thus, the lunge with military press (see Figure 31-25) can also assist in trunk/lower extremity control while overhead shoulder stability is maintained, and double as the top of backswing movement.

Plyoball deceleration throw (see Figure 31-24) helps to strengthen the shoulder concentrically and eccentrically mimicking the last portion of the pitching cycle. The push-up "with a plus" exercise (see Figure 31-26) is important as the pectoralis and the serratus anterior are muscles active throughout the entire pitching cycle.

Return to pitching should be gradual with a progression of percent effort as well as number of pitches. Refer to Appendix B for a return-to-windmill pitching program. A return-to-throwing program is also included in Appendix C. The return-to-throwing guidelines should be modified to the specific athlete. Is she an exclusive pitcher who only needs to make shorter overhand throws to the bases? Or does she also play another position when not pitching, that is, outfield or infield? This should be a factor in the decision making regarding the final distance at which the softball player performs the throwing program. For example, an exclusive pitcher is not going to need to spend time at the 120 ft and 150 ft stage; more time would be focused on specific windmill exercises and shorter overhand throwing.

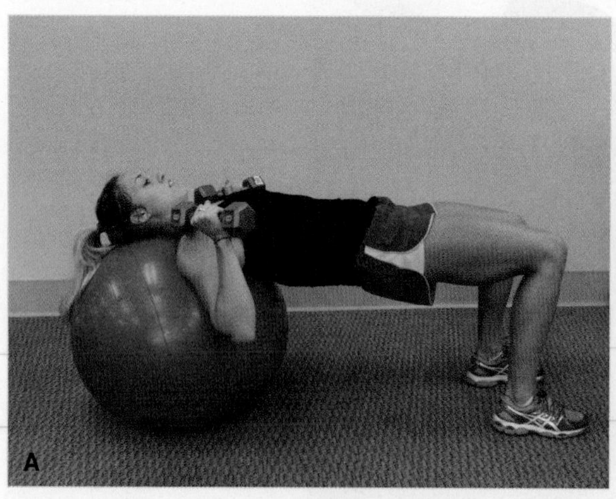

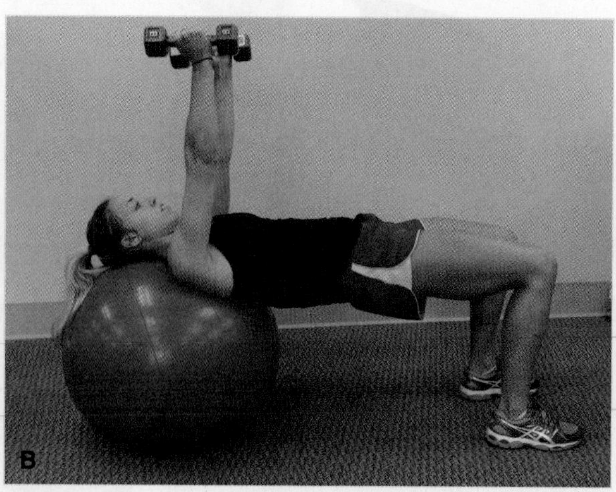

Figure 31-21 **Chest press on Physioball with serratus punch**

A. Lie on back over ball, feet shoulder width apart, dumbbells in both hands. Start with elbows bent, weights at chest.

B. Straighten elbows pressing weights together, at the end of the motion add scapular protection.

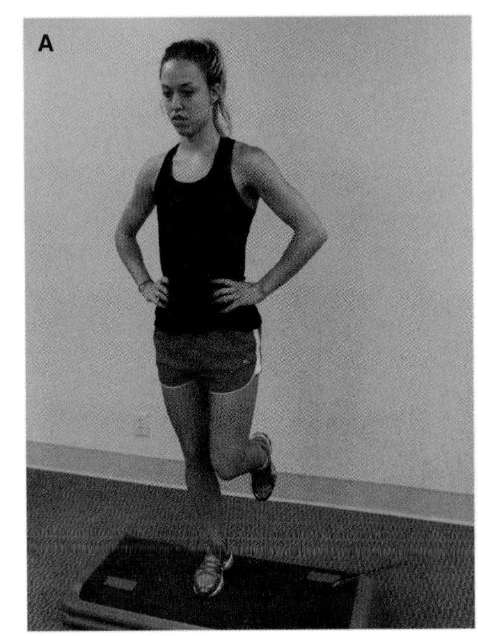

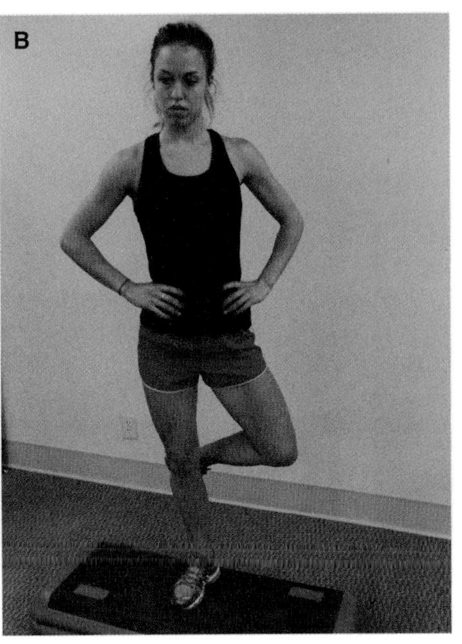

Figure 31-22 **Step up with closed chain external rotation/internal rotation**

Step up onto step with dominant leg, keep other leg in slight hip flexion with knee flexion (**A**). Slowly rotate into internal rotation and external rotation on dominant leg. (**B**, external rotation shown.)

More research is needed in the area of windmill pitching as well as educating coaches and players in the potential risk of injury with overuse. Clearly, current research is showing forces at the shoulder to be much higher than once believed. The active female can perhaps decrease the risk of suffering from an overuse shoulder injury by following pitch guidelines closer to that of a baseball pitcher and performing a windmill-specific exercise routine.

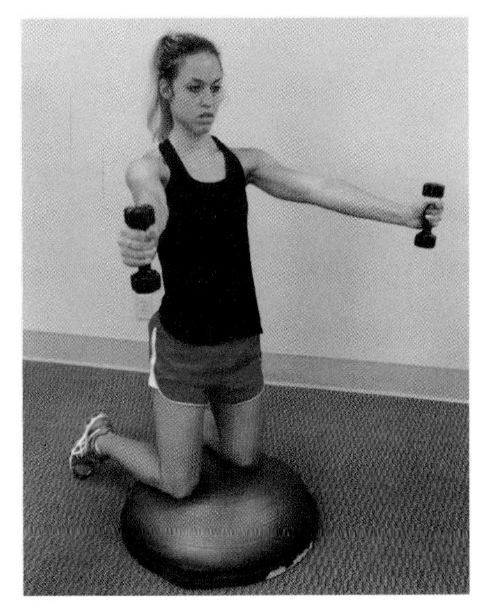

Figure 31-23 **Full can, tall kneeling on DynaDisc or BOSU ball**

Start in tall kneeling position on balance challenging surface. Raise weight at 45-degree angle with thumbs up, within comfort range. Emphasize good trunk alignment throughout exercise.

Shoulder Injuries in Female Swimmers

There is insufficient research to conclusively report that female swimmers actually sustain shoulder injuries at a higher rate than male swimmers. Most studies are not gender specific when injuries to the upper extremity are reported.[15,231,285,291,292] It is evident, however, that differences exist between males and females in anatomy, upper-body strength, and laxity, as previously discussed. Therefore, with high numbers of shoulder injuries reported in swimming,[285] it is important for the sports medicine personnel to understand the demands and risks that the sport imposes.

Swimming has become a very popular recreational and competitive athletic activity. Triathlons are becoming increasingly popular as well, and swimming is 1 of the 3 components. Ninety percent of complaints by swimmers that are significant enough to seek medical attention pertain to the shoulder.[285] Sport-specific

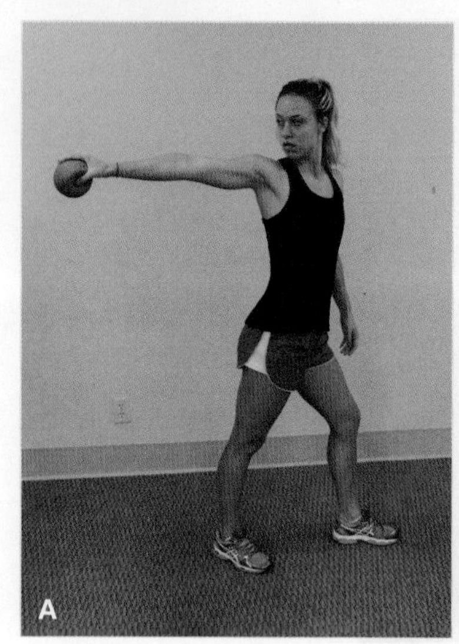

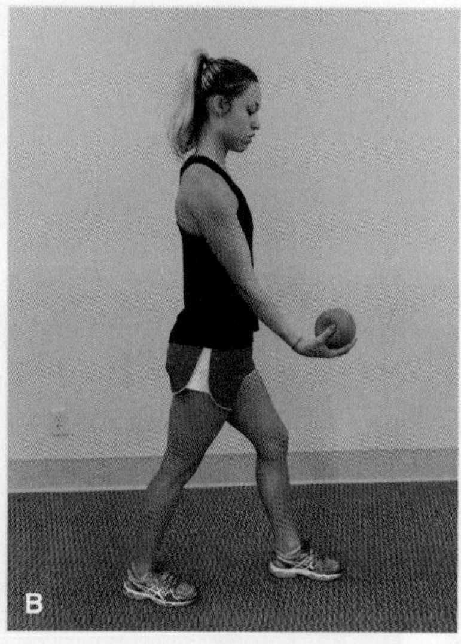

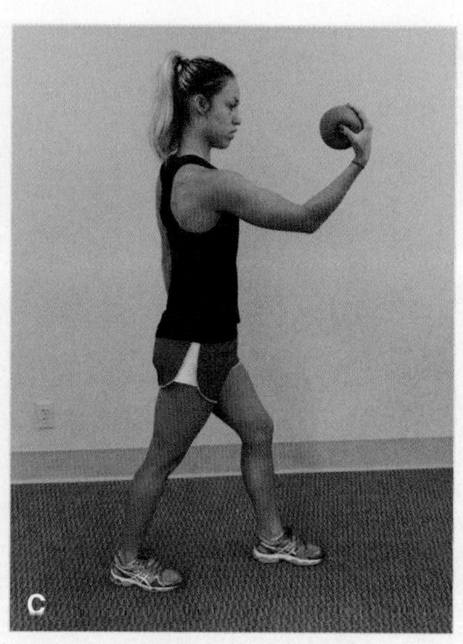

Figure 31-24 **Plyoball deceleration throw with therapist**

Standing in stride stance facing sideways, horizontally abduct the shoulder and extend the elbow. Therapist tosses Plyoball; athlete catches (**A**) while simultaneously rotating pelvis forward and bringing ball through (**B**), flexing the shoulder and elbow (mimicking delivery and follow through) (**C**); then reverse the same motion and athlete tosses back to therapist with shoulder and elbow extended (ie, reverse sequence from C→B→A). Focuses on concentric and eccentric training. Have athlete mimic her delivery as much as possible.

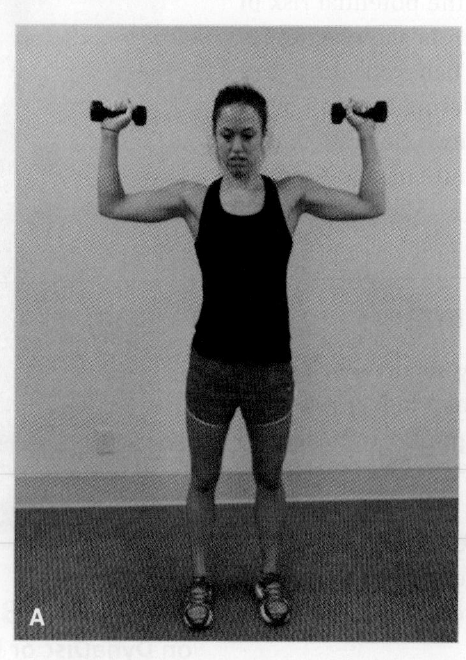

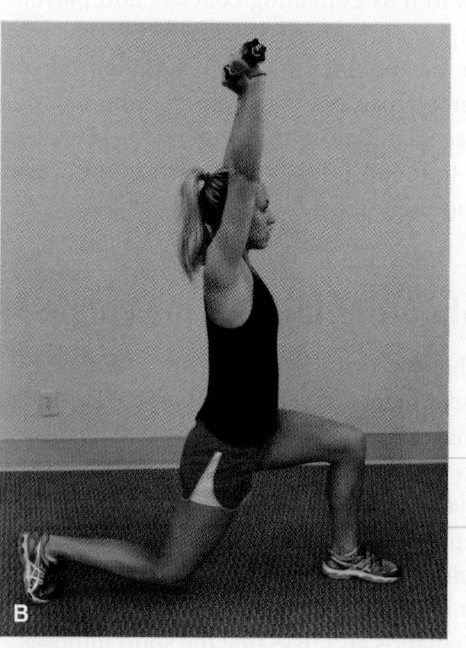

Figure 31-25 **Lunging with military press**

A. Start with legs straight, elbows bent, hands shoulder height. Raise arms overhead, extending elbows; as arms raise overhead, perform lunge. **B.** Return to starting position.

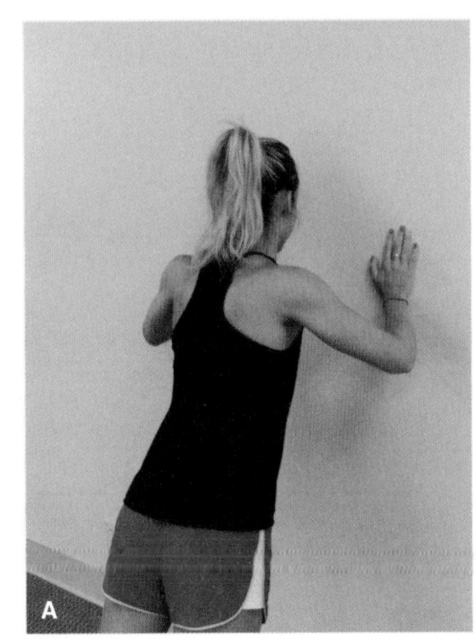

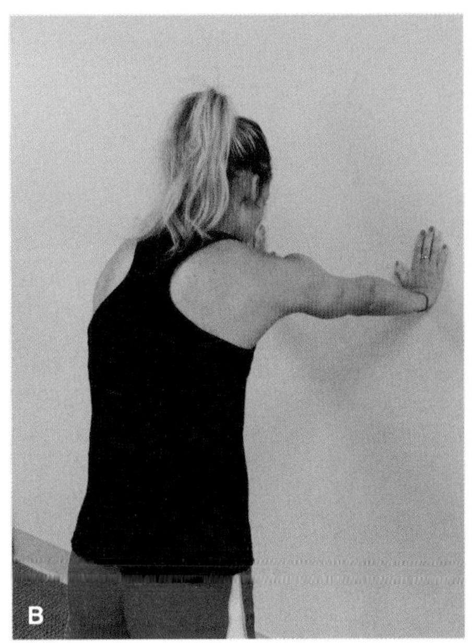

Figure 31-26 **Wall push-up "plus"**

A. Hands shoulder width apart, flex elbows as lower down to wall. **B.** Extend elbows and at end of exercise add an extra push (plus) into scapular protraction. Progression: at wall, at table, on floor, hands on wobble board or BOSU ball, feet on Physioball, hands on floor. Note poor trunk positioning on left.

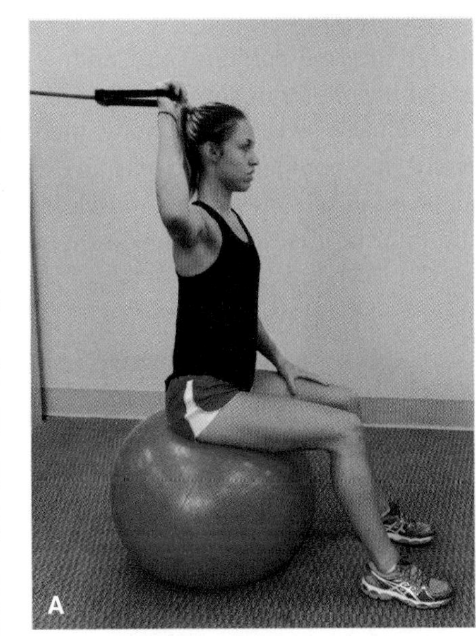

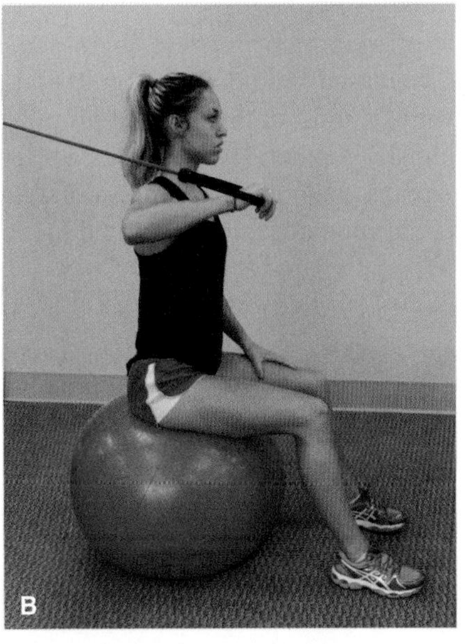

Figure 31-27 **Thera-Band shoulder internal rotation on Physioball**

While sitting on Physioball and facing away from door, grasp Thera-Band at shoulder height. In the 90/90 position (**A**), pull band forward into internal rotation (**B**). May also train external rotators by facing wall and pulling opposite direction.

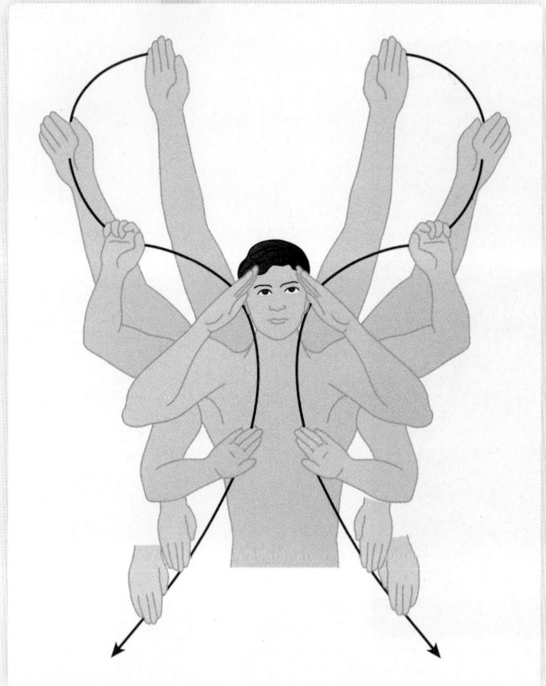

Figure 31-28 **The S-shaped curve in pull-through**

(Adapted from Pink M, Perry J, Browne A, Scovazzo ML, Kerrigan J. The normal shoulder during freestyle swimming. An electromyographic and cinematographic analysis of twelve muscles. *Am J Sports Med.* 1991;19:574.)

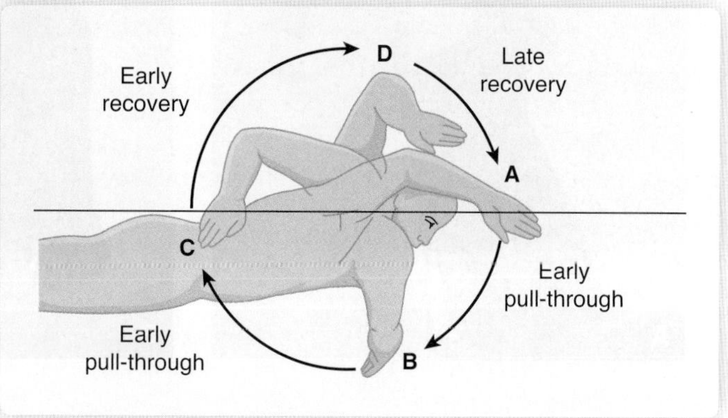

Figure 31-29 **Phases of the freestyle swimming stroke cycle**

(Adapted from Pink M, Perry J, Browne A, Scovazzo ML, Kerrigan J. The normal shoulder during freestyle swimming. An electromyographic and cinematographic analysis of twelve muscles. *Am J Sports Med.* 1991;19:569-576.)

demands of swimming include increased shoulder internal rotation and adduction strength, increased shoulder ROM, and endurance of the shoulder complex. During the freestyle stroke, most of the forward propulsion is produced by the upper body, the legs help minimally (Figures 31-34 and 31-35). Specifically, the shoulder adductors and extensors (pectoralis major and latissimus dorsi) should be assessed. These same muscles produce internal rotation. Increases in adduction and internal rotation can lead to muscle

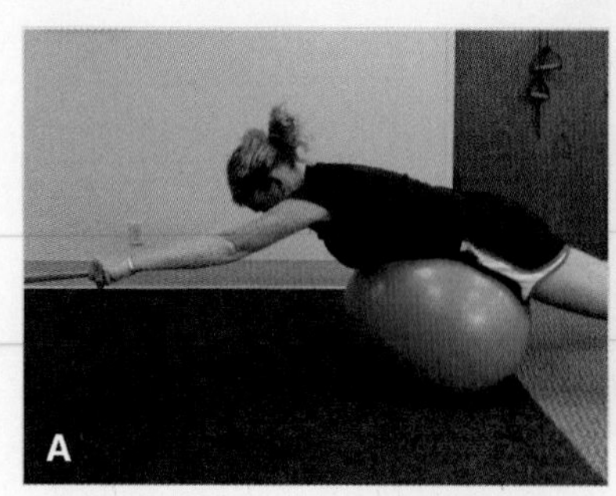

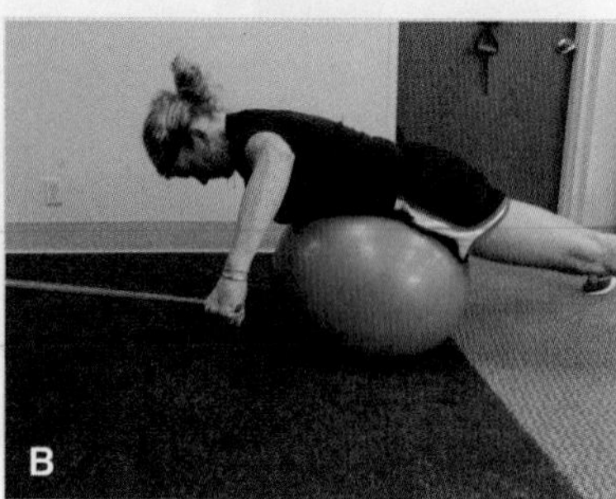

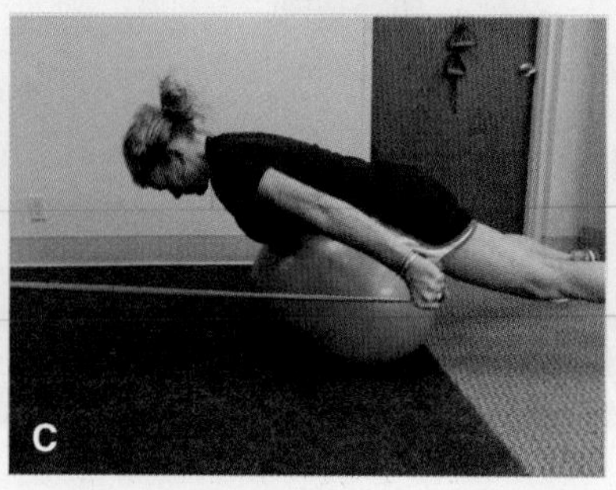

Figure 31-30 **Prone swimming exercise on ball**

A. Start position. **B.** Internal rotation or during pull through. **C.** Finish position. Note: performing this exercise prone on the ball increases sport position specificity and demands on the core musculature.

imbalances, which can reduce glenohumeral stability and provide optimal conditions for impingement. Freestyle is used 80% of the time during the swimmer's training, regardless of what stroke the athlete uses competitively.[15] Therefore, impingement poses a potential problem to all swimmers.

As mentioned previously, swimming requires shoulder ROM greater than that of nonswimmers in order to excel. This increased motion allows for longer stroke length, which directly correlates to a swimmer's speed. Although the increased ROM is beneficial to performance, it can be detrimental to glenohumeral stability. Excessive ROM produces capsuloligamentous laxity, which decreases the force produced by the rotator cuff muscles to provide stability.[285]

The third specific demand includes the incredible endurance necessary of the rotator cuff and scapular stabilizers. The teres minor, infraspinatus, and subscapularis are rotator cuff muscles that fire continuously through the swimming cycle. The scapular stabilizer that also fires continuously is the serratus anterior. These muscles are at risk for fatigue with resultant possibilities of impingement or instability/subluxation of the shoulder. The repetitive nature of swimming predisposes the participant to overuse injury from microtrauma and mechanical primary impingement. This can ultimately lead to instability, rotator cuff fatigue, and resultant secondary impingement.[15] Swimmers average 8000 to 20,000 m of training per day and may practice twice a day, with no rest days in between. This subjects the shoulder complex to an incredibly high number of stroke repetitions. An average competitive swimmer may swim 10,000 m per day. Thus, an athlete who swims 20 cycles per 50 m (estimated for the average swimmer), completes 4000 repetitions per shoulder, every day.[15]

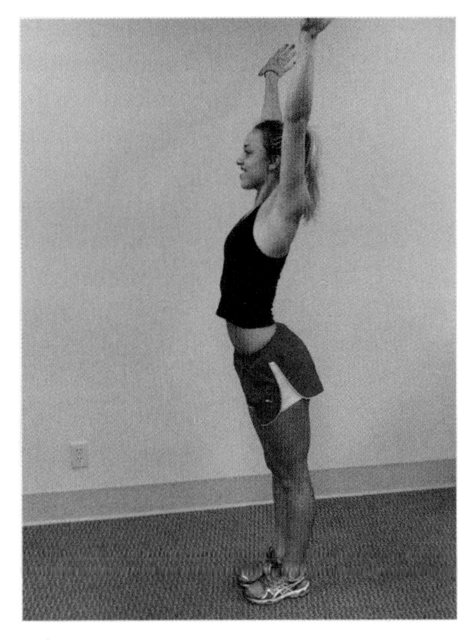

Figure 31-31

Typical gymnast pose before/after routines and landing jumps/tumbling moves. Note excessive lumbar lordosis.

Unpublished data from Centinela Hospital Medical Center Biomechanics Laboratory report that swimmers exhibited a higher incidence of positive Hawkins test than positive Neer tests for shoulder impingement.[232] The Hawkins test analyzes compression of the rotator cuff tendons under the acromion, whereas the Neer test analyzes the pinching of the rotator cuff undersurface on the anterosuperior glenoid rim. This may indicate that swimmers tend to display more problems with compression of the cuff tendons under the acromion rather than undersurface tears. EMG studies reveal swimmers with painful shoulders have altered muscle-firing patterns when compared to swimmers with no shoulder pain. The serratus anterior has decreased muscle activity and the rhomboids have increased activity from the nonpainful shoulders, during mid pull through. If the serratus anterior is not functioning properly to aid in scapular upward rotation and protraction, then the acromion would also lack upward rotation placing the swimmer at risk for compression of the cuff tendons under the acromion.

Interestingly, the rhomboids are an antagonist muscle to the serratus anterior. When the serratus anterior fatigues, there is no other muscle that can help produce the same action. The antagonist muscle is called upon to help stabilize the scapula creating a disturbance in the synchrony of normal scapular rotation during propulsion.

As previously noted, the serratus anterior and subscapularis fire continuously throughout the freestyle stroke. The serratus anterior is firing continuously to provide a stable base for the humerus, and the subscapularis is firing caused by the humerus being in predominately internal rotation throughout the stroke. These 2 muscles are susceptible to injury because of fatigue.[232]

In a similar example, the same research documented that the subscapularis (an internal rotator) had decreased muscle activity and the infraspinatus (an external rotator) is

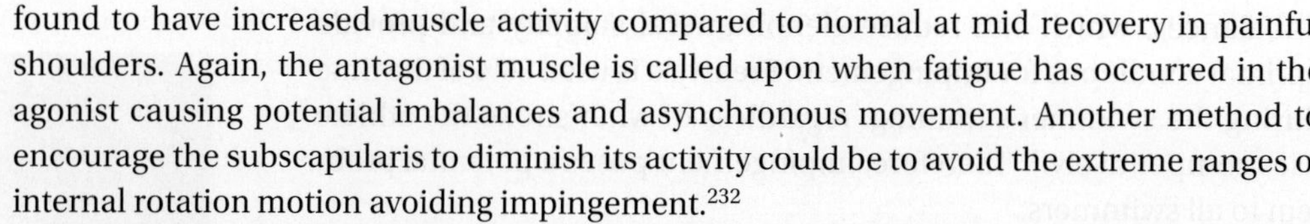

found to have increased muscle activity compared to normal at mid recovery in painful shoulders. Again, the antagonist muscle is called upon when fatigue has occurred in the agonist causing potential imbalances and asynchronous movement. Another method to encourage the subscapularis to diminish its activity could be to avoid the extreme ranges of internal rotation motion avoiding impingement.[232]

Three-dimensional videography was used by Yanai and Hay[292] to determine when, during the swimming motion, the shoulder experienced impingement. During the front crawl in swimming, on average, impingement occurred during 24.8% of the stroke time. However, each subject monitored experienced impingement in some cycles and not others. This suggests that stroke technique may play a factor in susceptibility to impingement.[292] Some studies show that between 50% and 70% of the time, shoulder pain was reported during pull through;[78,242] others, however, report impingement occurs more often during the recovery stage.[291,292] During early pull-through, the pectoralis major and the teres minor are highly active, with their activity peaking at mid pull-through. The teres minor is the prime contributor to maintaining humeral head congruency in the glenoid because of its insertion closer to the axis of rotation than the pectoralis. In painful shoulders, the most notable difference during pull-thorough was decreased muscle activity of the serratus anterior.[232]

The hand entry position during freestyle stroke is also reported to be a frequent point of pain in swimmers.[291] During hand entry and forward reach, the upper trapezius, rhomboids, and serratus anterior are all active to form a force couple to properly position the glenoid fossa. The supraspinatus and the anterior and middle deltoid are also active to abduct and flex the humerus as the hand reaches forward in the water. Without the supraspinatus, the deltoid proper firing of predisposes the humeral head to excessive movement within glenoid fossa.[232]

Rehabilitation and Return to Swimming

Shoulder rehabilitation for these female swimmers should be multifaceted. Great emphasis should be placed on restoring normal ROM, strength, and endurance based on the evaluative findings. Table 31-8 lists the typical signs and symptoms of possible causes of

Table 31-8 Typical Signs and Symptoms and Possible Causes of Swimmer's Shoulder

Signs and Symptoms	Possible Cause
Postural deformities of rounded shoulders and thoracic kyphosis	Tightness of the pectoralis minor
Weakness of the posterior cuff muscles and scapular stabilizers	Weakness can be a result of strength imbalances between the anterior and posterior muscles secondary to the demands of the sport and to stretch weakness
Limited internal rotation and excessive external rotation ROM	Tightness of the posterior capsule or posterior cuff muscles which causes a shift in the available ROM
Decay of normal scapulothoracic rhythm	Tightness of the anterior chest musculature and weakness of the scapular stabilizers

Source: Adapted from Allegrucci M, Whitney SL, Irrgang JJ. Clinical implications of secondary impingement of the shoulder in freestyle swimmers. *J Orthop Sports Phys Ther.* 1994;20(6):313.

swimmer's shoulder. Exercises should incorporate trunk and hip movements along with both scapular and glenohumeral neuromuscular retraining. Core stability should also be emphasized in the shoulder rehabilitation program as it needs to provide a stable base for the athlete to propel their body forward.

Range of Motion

Flexibility and mobilization techniques should reflect the findings from the evaluation. Importance should be given to restore normal ROM without compromising stability. The most typical restrictions are found in the posterior portion of the glenohumeral joint capsule or tightness of the posterior rotator cuff muscles.[285] Swimmers, in general, tend to spend more time stretching their anterior capsule. This results in loss of internal rotation and horizontal adduction. Horizontal adduction may be improved by stabilizing the scapula on the thorax while crossing the arm over the chest. This can be performed at 90 degrees of shoulder flexion and above to address all portions of the cuff. Posterior capsule flexibility is improved by flexing the shoulder to 90 degrees and providing a downward force on the flexed elbow.

Internal rotation ROM, rather than external rotation, at the end range of abduction proves to be important for swimmers. This motion is most important during the late recovery stage of the freestyle stroke. Internal rotation should be stretched at 90 degrees, 135 degrees, and at end-range abduction in stretches assisted by the therapist or utilizing self-stretches such as the "sleeper stretch." External rotation stretching should still be carried out if it is lacking. Other important muscles to check for normal flexibility include the pectoralis major and minor, upper trapezius, levator scapulae, biceps, triceps, and serratus anterior. Swimming strokes do not happen in a straight cardinal plane of motion; during the arm cycle, there are multiple combinations of movements taking place.[15] A flexibility program can be creatively structured with this in mind.

Strength and Endurance Training

Development of a strength and endurance training program should focus on restoring normal balance to the anterior and posterior shoulder musculature. It also should focus on restoring equilibrium between scapular and humeral movements. It is important to remember that increased adduction and internal rotation strength is unavoidable in swimmers. To avoid muscular imbalance, emphasis on rotator cuff exercises with importance on external rotation strength is beneficial.[285] The 3 primary considerations in a strengthening program are (a) isolate the rotator cuff and scapular muscles, (b) implement endurance-based exercises, and (c) include sports-specific functional exercises.[15] Table 31-9 provides primary considerations and rationale for developing a strengthening program for swimmers.

Female swimmers appear to be highly susceptible to secondary impingement as a consequence of flexibility, strength, and muscular endurance factors discussed earlier. Please refer to Chapter 20 for details on primary and secondary impingement. Table 31-10 provides basic guidelines for progression of treatment for swimmer's shoulders with 2-degree impingement. The initial goal in the rehabilitation program is to establish a stable scapular base and strengthen the rotator cuff muscles in a neutral position.[255] Phase II introduces exercises up to 90 degrees. In Phase III, overhead exercises can be initiated with functional training. Phase IV is gradual return to athletic activity, progressing in speed and distance.[15] Most swimming programs emphasize only upper-extremity strengthening and function. Challenging core stability during some upper-extremity exercises is beneficial to the athlete. Swimming is a chain of events involving the arms, trunk, and legs together. Focusing solely on the shoulder complex fails to address all areas of the kinetic chain vital to swimming efficiency and performance.

Table 31-9 Considerations and Rationale in a Strengthening Program for Swimmers

Primary Considerations	Rationale
Isolation of the rotator cuff and scapulohumeral muscles (correctly train prime movers/stabilizers, not antagonists)	EMG studies demonstrate cuff muscles act independent of each other during the stroke cycle
Muscular endurance, high repetitions of specific exercises (sprint, middle-distance, or long-distance swimmer—should reflect in number of repetitions given)	Swimming involves excessive repetition and muscular endurance; 3 sets of 10 repetitions are inadequate
Sports-specific function	Exercises specific to the swimmers stroke and body postures help return to sport as efficiently and quickly as possible

Table 31-10 Basic Guidelines for Progression of Treatment for Swimmer's Shoulders with a 2-Degree Impingement

Phase I

Modalities PRN for pain control

Address ROM losses

Rotator cuff strengthening at 0 degrees abduction, with towel support

- Side lying ER
- Thera-Band ER/IR
- Thera-Band ER/IR isometric "step-always"

Scapulothoracic muscle in neutral

- Shrugs
- Prone arm raise at 0 degree abduction
- Scapular retraction (row)
- Prone ball roll (for lower trap)
- Prone ball stabilization on floor

Aerobic conditioning

- Bike
- Kicking in water

Phase II (0 to 90)

Rotator cuff strengthening

- Prone ER
- Thera-Band ER
- Prone arm raise with ER at 90 degrees abduction, progress to 120 degrees abduction
- Elevation in scapular plane (full can)

Scapulothoracic exercises

- Scapular protraction (supine on ball progress to standing using Thera-Band with shoulder at 90 degrees, and in a weightbearing position on one-half foam roller)
- Stabilization exercises
  - Bilateral → unilateral
  - Add dynamic resistance
  - Progress to stabilizing on a ball

Table 31-10 Basic Guidelines for Progression of Treatment for Swimmer's Shoulders with a 2-Degree Impingement *(Continued)*

• Push-up "plus" progression   ▪ Wall → table → modified (on knees) → regular Axial humeral muscles • Flexion • Abduction in the plane of the scapula (challenge core on BOSU ball in tall kneeling) • Lat pull-down • Chest press (challenge core stability by laying supine on ball) • Bench press Proprioception • Active and passive matching Aerobic conditioning • Upper body ergometer • Rower • Kicking in water
Phase III—Functional training

Full range flexion and abduction strengthening
Combined movement patterns
• Proprioceptive neuromuscular facilitation D1 and D2 (Thera-Band, Bodyblade, manual, Plyoball)
Stroke-specific exercise
• Simulation of pull-through and reverse pull-through with Thera-Band (prone on swiss ball to challenge core at same time) (see Figure 31-30)
• Simulation of recovery:
  1. Prone horizontal abduction with ER
  2. Prone horizontal adduction with IR at 160 degrees abduction
  3. Thera-Band-resisted ER at 30 degrees of abduction progressing to 90 degrees of abduction
Plyometric exercises
Swim bench (if available)

ER, external rotation; IR, Internal rotation.

Source: Adapted and modified from Allegrucci M, Whitney SL, Irrgang JJ. Clinical implications of secondary impingement of the shoulder in freestyle swimmers. *J Orthop Sports Phys Ther.* 1994;20(6):316.

Proprioception and Functional Training

Retraining joint proprioception in freestyle swimmers, and all athletes, is important. Are differences seen in swimming stroke patterns with painful shoulders intentional changes to avoid pain, or caused by inadequate feedback from joint receptors from capsular damage? Multiple studies have shown proprioceptive deficits in subjects with glenohumeral joint multidirectional instability.[35,47,89] However, no studies specific to symptomatic swimming athletes are available. Proprioception is derived from both conscious and unconscious components, as was previously described in detail in other chapters. Making the athlete consciously aware of humeral and scapular position during strength training and swimming may help to improve conscious proprioception. However, only conscious training is not enough, unconscious neuromuscular output is also vital to athletic performance. Training unconscious proprioceptive awareness can be carried out with plyometric training.[15]

Plyometric training is used to not only enhance power and explosiveness but may also help improve "synchrony of movement that is needed for the swimming stroke." [15, p. 315]

Progression of an upper-extremity plyometric training program for swimmers should include progressing the degree of shoulder abduction (starting in more neutral positions increasing to overhead); progressing the weight of the medicine ball; and increasing speed, repetitions, and difficulty.

Closed-chain exercises can be useful in rehabilitation of the swimmer because they mimic how the body is pulled over the arms during pull through, while engaging the trunk and core muscles for stabilization.[15] For example, in Phase III, a Thera-Band can be used to provide resistance mimicking the pull through phase while the athlete is prone over a Physioball (see Figure 31-30). This forces the core muscles to stabilize the athlete's body as her arm is going through a specific motion. During this exercise, it is important to keep the shoulder at 90 degrees of abduction to ensure proper mechanics and avoid impingement. Internal obliques are also important muscles to strengthen because of the rotation required at the trunk for the swimmer to body roll during freestyle. If core muscles are weak or lack endurance, they will not provide a stable base for the upper extremities. As discussed in several contexts, but especially important in the swimmer, a weak core can be a contributing factor in a shoulder injury.[119,149]

Throughout the rehabilitation program, it is feasible for the athlete to continue swimming with use of swimming aids (ie, kickboard held under the body), modification of yardage, and altered rest time. This active rest concept is dependent on the severity and nature of shoulder injury and should be athlete and injury specific. For example, an impingement injury caused by fatigue of the posterior cuff muscles may still respond positively to treatment in conjunction with a significant decrease in yardage and increase in rest time before swimming again to avoid fatigue. It is vital to educate both the coach and swimmer that at the first sign of shoulder pain the athlete is to stop swimming.[15]

In conclusion, freestyle swimmers can present with signs and symptoms of either instability or impingement, or a combination of both. The rotator cuff provides stability at the glenohumeral joint and can therefore be a source of pain or disability when instability or impingement occurs. It is essential to provide the optimum environment for the rotator cuff to work effectively by balancing adequate stability with the appropriate mobility in the shoulder complex. Accordingly, for an efficient and effective rehabilitation program, clinicians must have knowledge of the sport-specific skills that are required. Finally, creativity in designing the rehabilitation program to incorporate the core with upper-extremity activities and meet the swimmers' demands (sprinter, middle, or long-distance swimmer) is essential as well.[15]

Considerations in the Female Gymnast

The final sport for special consideration in regard to the female athlete is gymnastics. Gymnastics is important to consider because of its high potential for micro- and macrotraumatic injuries, as well as the vulnerability of its athletes to body image issues that are elaborated upon in the female athlete triad section. Certainly, similar considerations may exist in sports not mentioned; however, it is beyond the scope of this chapter to attempt to cover all sports in which women participate.

Multiple injuries occur in gymnasts of all ages and ability levels, whether recreational or competitive. Women's gymnastics involves 4 apparatuses: beam, floor exercise, vault, and uneven bars. Men's gymnastics involves 6 apparatuses: floor exercise, rings, parallel bars, pommel horse, vault, and high bar. The demands of this sport include the need for great flexibility, incredible strength, balance, and explosive power. Competitive gymnastics requires intensive training with a large time commitment, usually beginning at a young age. The average junior elite gymnast (age 10 to 14 years) spends more than 5 days per week training, for a total of approximately 25 hours a week.[57] Such demand on a young body is not without penalty. The period of rapid growth, which occurs in adolescence, causes the young gymnast to be more susceptible to injury than the postpubescent gymnast.[57] Questions also arise in regards to the possibility of stunted or inhibited growth during these vital years of development and maturation.[58,277,284]

Recently, a Gymnastics Functional Measurement Tool was developed and studied by Sleeper et al.[264] This field-based assessment tool was found to correlate with United States Gymnastics competitive level of the athletes and allows sports practitioners to reliably examine and score performance in 10 important physical tasks necessary for participation in gymnastics. Such a sport-specific test battery may assist the clinician to determine readiness for participation in gymnastics and risk for potential injury.

Gymnasts sustain a large variety of injuries. Caine et al[57] followed 50 competitive gymnasts over a 1-year period tracking injuries. The most commonly injured regions in the body by order of frequency were (a) the lower extremity (63.7%), particularly the ankle and knee; (b) the upper extremity (20.4%), particularly the wrist; (c) and the spine and trunk (15.2%), particularly the lower back. These findings are consistent with other multiple studies conducted.[33,57,172,252,271] Gymnasts were most likely to injure themselves on the floor exercise (35.4%), followed by the balance beam (23.1%), the uneven bars (20%), and, lastly, the vault (13.8%). The remaining 7.7% of injuries were placed under “other,” pertaining to possible warm-up or conditioning periods. The distribution between sudden onset and gradual onset of injury was 44.2% and 55.8%, respectively. Clearly traumatic as well as overuse injuries occur in this sport.

Female gymnasts of today are shorter, lighter, and mature later than their predecessors 30 years earlier. Increased magnitude and intensity of training at an early age has become standard. The question arises whether these external characteristics are a result of self-selection for gymnastics or a result of inadequate nutrition for the level of activity during this crucial period of development.[58] Studies suggest that the shorter femoral leg length seen in female gymnasts may be a result of the repetitive compressive stress causing premature closure of femoral and tibial epiphyses.[58,59,183,276] A short-term longitudinal study by Mansfield and Emans[183] reported that gymnasts advance through puberty without a normal pubertal growth spurt. Catchup growth does occur once the gymnast retires from the sport or significantly reduces training[58]; however, it is questionable whether adequate growth and normal height are eventually achieved. Longitudinal studies of 1 set of triplets and 2 sets of twins (one gymnast, other one(s) not) reveal significantly later onset of menarche when compared to their nongymnast sibling. In the set of triplets, energy expenditure exceeded energy intake by 600 kcal and the gymnast had lower body weight and percent body fat compared to her siblings.[58]

Lower levels of hormones and decreased serum growth factors have also been identified in gymnasts. Serum leptin is involved in the regulation of energy intake and energy expenditure. Leptin is secreted by adipocytes and binds to an appetite-stimulating neuropeptide, which produces neurons in the hypothalamus. Leptin levels increase with food intake and decrease during periods of starvation. Low body fat levels have been linked to low levels of leptin. A decline in leptin levels has an effect on the secretion of gonadotropins and sex steroids, which may be a factor in delayed menarche and amenorrhea leading to the female athlete triad, which is discussed in detail later in this chapter.[284]

Some additional noteworthy considerations in the sport of gymnastics include (a) gymnasts do not wear any type of supportive shoe while training and competing, making it difficult to correct faulty biomechanics at the foot with any type of orthosis; (b) the typical postural salute to judges, and landing of jumps and dismounts, is a hyperlordotic position of the lumbar spine, potentially contributing to trunk instability problems (see Figure 31-31); (c) gymnastics, unlike many sports, has a significant amount of skills and activities performed with the upper extremities in a closed-chain position; and (d) gymnasts jump and land from various heights with twisting and rotational components. With these factors in mind, focus should be placed on balancing strength and flexibility to help correct faulty biomechanics or structural faults; emphasis placed on core strength and stability and education of gymnasts should occur regarding ideal trunk posturing at the beginning and end of routines. Likewise, education on proper jumping and landing must be an integral part of training and rehabilitation. Refer to the section "Anterior Cruciate Ligament Injuries" earlier in this chapter for more detail on jumping and landing.

Of additional concern are the body image requirements and subsequent disorders common in the sport of gymnastics potentially leading to inadequate caloric intake.[58,59,277] Educating the coaches, gymnast, and rehabilitation staff in regard to the female athlete triad potential risks of osteoporosis and stress fractures, as well as stunted growth patterns, is important.

The Female Athlete Triad

Historical Perspective and Evolution

The female athlete triad (Triad) was first described by Rosemary Agostini, MD, Barbara Drinkwater, PhD, Aurelia Nattiv, MD, and Kimberly Yeager, MD, MPH, in the early 1990s.[1,50,96,213,214] The Triad (see Figure 31-32) was used to describe the connection between 3 independent clinical disorders: eating disorders, amenorrhea, and osteoporosis. Continued research and discussion among sports medicine professionals in varied disciplines led to the American College of Sports Medicine publishing the first *Female Athlete Triad Position Statement* in 1997.[96] The purpose of the position statement was to provide direction for identification, prevention, and treatment of these individual, yet connected, medical disorders in this specialty population.[8,19,213,215]

Evolution of this original concept has continued. Classification of eating disorders such as anorexia nervosa (AN),[209] bulimia nervosa (BN), and eating disorders not otherwise specified (EDNOS) were the severe forms of nutritional deficit that were observed. Because a minority of female athletes fit the diagnostic criteria for any of these diseases,

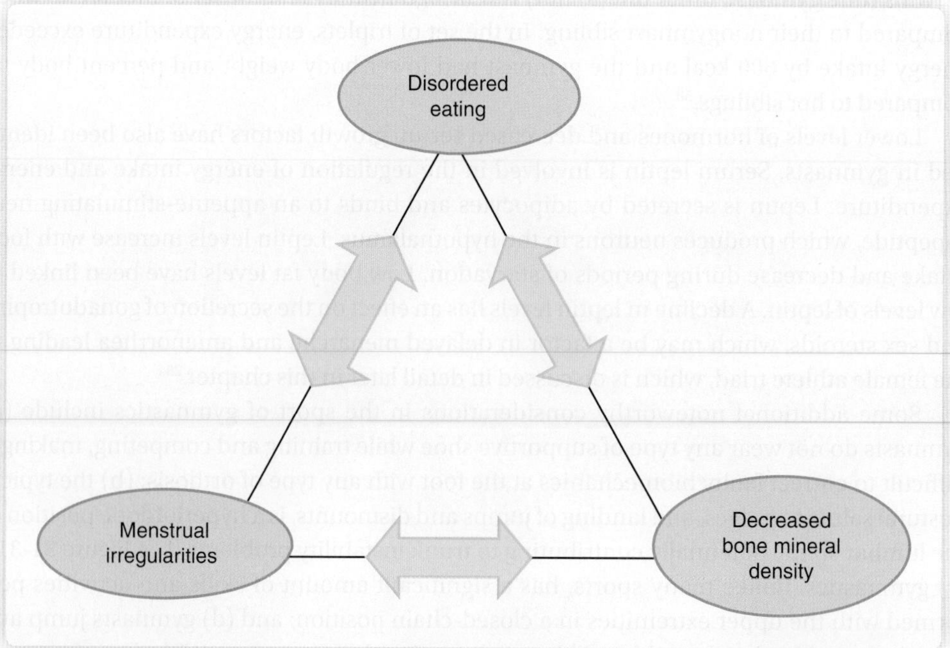

Figure 31-32 **The female athlete triad, as first described in 1997**

the term eating disorders has been expanded to include the concept of *disordered eating* patterns that encompasses a wide range of harmful nutritional strategies associated with the other factors of the Triad.[21,215] Osteoporosis (identified in the original Triad description) has been modified to include osteopenia and the less-severe forms of bone loss more commonly seen in females screened and diagnosed with the Triad. Discussion also ensued regarding the expansion of amenorrhea to include menstrual irregularities and other reproductive dysfunctions that are associated with but independent of amenorrhea. These other dysfunctions are intermittently seen in association with other components of the Triad, and include oligomenorrhea, anovulation, and altered luteal phase length.[213, 215] The revised and updated Triad describes the interaction and coexistence of eating disorders/disordered eating behavior, menstrual irregularities, and decreased BMD.[215]

Further evolution has established a spectrum concept for each of the independent yet interrelated components. The current concept of the Triad refers to the interrelationship between energy availability, menstrual function, and BMD. Each of these components is described and illustrated as a spectrum in the publication of the revised position statement by the American College of Sports Medicine in 2007.[215] Each spectrum ranges from the healthiest state to the unhealthiest state of a female athlete in each of these components (see Figure 31-33).

Components

Energy Availability

There is a very important relationship between the amount of calories consumed and the amount of calories expended for any athlete. The spectrum of energy availability ranges from low energy availability with or without an eating disorder to optimal energy availability. Optimal energy availability defined as the appropriate balance of calories; or simply stated: calories taken in versus calories expended. Energy availability is critical for optimal

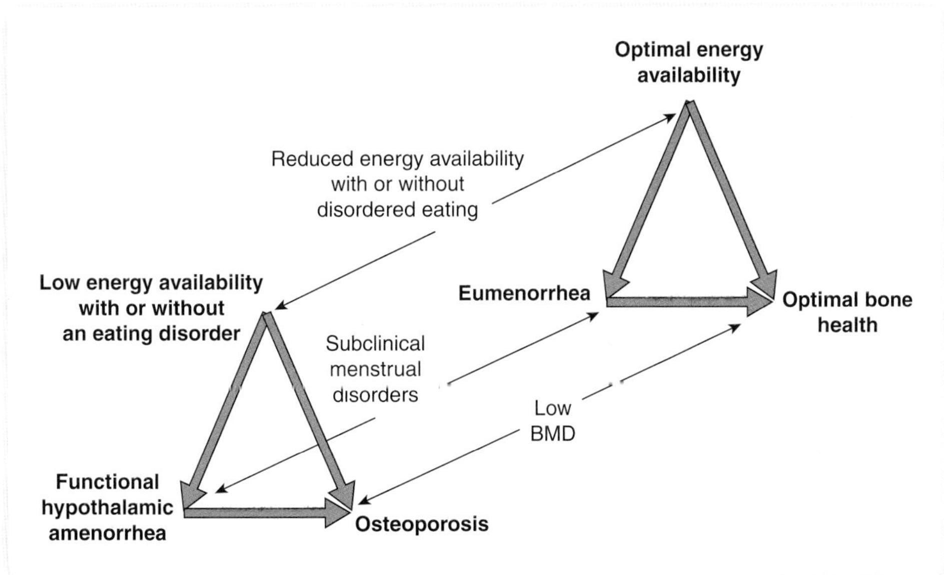

Figure 31-33 The female athlete triad, as described in 2007

Note the spectra between "optimal health" and "poor health" in the 3 components of the triad.

performance, maintenance of body composition, and prevention of health problems.[23] For the female athlete, the prevention of health problems includes:

- establishing and maintaining normal menstruation[39,215]
- preservation of a strong immune system[213]
- building and repairing muscle tissue and bone[23,39]

A "negative energy balance" resulting from a sustained negative calorie balance (intake less than output) can be a result of many factors, ranging in decreasing severity from a clinically diagnosed eating disorder to the elimination of a food group, for example, dairy or meat from the diet, to inadvertently not eating enough to keep up with a sudden or unexpected increase in a training schedule. The internal and external pressures to achieve athletic success, attain a body composition of unreasonably low body fat percentage, and/or achieve or maintain unrealistically low body weight often lead to disordered eating patterns and occasionally to clinical eating disorders.[11,18-21,39,40]

Clinical eating disorders include AN, BN, and EDNOS.[39] Each of these disorders have specific diagnostic criteria that are established (Tables 31-11 to 31-13). AN represents the extreme of voluntary starvation with severe caloric restriction and an altered self-image, viewing oneself as overweight when in reality being as much as 15% below of ideal body weight. The prevalence of AN is 0.5% to 1% in adolescent and young adult women as compared to 2% to 4% with BN.[23] BN is characterized by a "binge and purge" eating behavior. Binging occurs as a result of physiologic hunger followed by purging to eliminate the caloric intake.[23] The purging behavior takes a multitude of forms including vomiting, laxative use, diuretic use, enemas, and excessive exercise.[11,19,21,39,40,117,126,152] Physiologic and psychological problems resulting from this purging behavior include fluid and electrolyte imbalances, dehydration, acid-base imbalances, cardiac arrhythmia, the enlargement of the parotid glands, erosion of tooth enamel, gastrointestinal disorders, low self-esteem, anxiety, depression, and reported cases of suicide.[19,21,39,40,45,50]

Table 31-11 Diagnostic Criteria for Anorexia Nervosa (AN)

A. Refusal to maintain body weight at or above a minimally normal weight for age and height. Weight loss leading to maintenance of body weight <85% of that expected; or failure to make expressed weight gain during period of growth, leading to body weight <85% of that expected.
B. Intense fear of gaining weight or becoming fat, even though underweight.
C. Disturbance in the way in which one's body weight or shape is experienced; undue influence of body weight or shape on self-evaluation; or denial of the seriousness of the current low body weight.
D. In postmenarchal females, amenorrhea, i.e., the absence of at least 3 consecutive menstrual cycles. A female is considered to have amenorrhea if her periods occur only following hormone administration.

Specify type:

Restricting type: During the episode of anorexia nervosa, the person does not regularly engage in binge eating or purging behavior, i.e., self-induced vomiting or misuse of laxatives or diuretics.

Binge eating/purging type: During the episode of anorexia nervosa, the person regularly engages in binge eating or purging behavior, i.e., self-induced vomiting or misuse of laxatives or diuretics.

Data from DSM-IV, American Psychiatric Association, 1994.

Table 31-12 Diagnostic Criteria for Eating Disorder Not Otherwise Specified (EDNOS)

A. For females, all of the criteria for AN are met, except the individual has regular menses.
B. All criteria for AN are met except that, despite significant weight loss, the person's current weight is in the normal range.
C. All criteria for BN are met except that the binge eating and inappropriate compensatory mechanisms occur at a frequency of less than 2 per week for a duration of less than 3 months.
D. Regular use of inappropriate compensatory behavior by an individual of normal body weight after eating small amounts of food (self-induced vomiting after consumption of 2 cookies).
E. Repeatedly chewing and spitting out, but not swallowing, large amounts of food.
F. Binge-eating disorder: recurrent episodes of binge eating in the absence of the regular use of inappropriate compensatory behaviors characteristic of BN.

Data from DSM- IV, American Psychiatric Association, 1994.

The EDNOS diagnosis includes those individuals who meet every other criteria for AN except amenorrhea/oligomenorrhea or decreased body weight or those individuals who demonstrate all other criteria for BN with a decreased frequency or duration of the purging behavior. This additional category, EDNOS may lead to better detection and treatment of those female athletes who exhibit the criteria for AN but paradoxically maintain "normal"

Table 31-13 Diagnostic Criteria for Bulimia Nervosa (BN)

A. Recurrent episodes of binge eating. An episode of binge eating is characterized by both of the following:
   1. Eating, in a discrete period of time, e.g., within any 2-hour period, an amount of food that is definitely larger than most people would eat during a similar period of time and under similar circumstances, **and**
   2. A sense of lack of control over eating during the episode, e.g., a feeling that one cannot stop eating or control what or how much one is eating.
B. Recurrent inappropriate compensatory behavior in order to prevent weight gain, such as self-induced vomiting; misuse of laxatives, diuretics or other medications; fasting; or excessive exercise.
C. The binge eating and inappropriate compensatory behaviors both occur, on average, at least twice a week for 3 months.
D. Self-evaluation is unduly influenced by body shape and weight.
E. The disturbance does not occur exclusively during episodes of anorexia nervosa.

Specify type:
Purging type: The person regularly engages in self-induced vomiting or the misuse of laxatives or diuretics.
Non-purging type: The person uses other inappropriate compensatory behaviors, such as fasting or excessive exercise, but does not regularly engage in self-induced vomiting or the misuse of laxatives or diuretics.

Data from DSM- IV, American Psychiatric Association, 1994.

body weight because of the increased lean body mass.[19,21,40] Despite the many strides that have been made in the classification of disordered eating, there are a plethora of unhealthy eating behaviors that elude the AN, BN, or EDNOS diagnoses and result in a negative energy balance.

It is difficult to estimate the number of female athletes who demonstrate disordered eating or unhealthy eating habits. Several different surveys have been developed in an attempt to identify collegiate female athletes with disordered eating behaviors. The prevalence of eating disorders ranged from 6% to 60%, depending upon the tool used, how the tool was administered, the athletic population, and the defining criteria.[11,21,39,40,45,50,213,215,226] There are many reasons for this wide range of those classified as disordered eaters. Many athletes consider disordered eating patterns normal and harmless. Others deny disordered eating patterns on standard questionnaires. Many studies referenced to assess the prevalence of eating disorders use questionnaires that assess symptoms of eating disorders without an assessment by a trained clinician or a screening tool that confirms defined disordered eating patterns.[152] In 2004, the National Eating Disorder Screening program screened more than 16,000 students and 59% scored positive for symptoms of an eating disorder.[50] Reinking et al[239] determined that disordered eating patterns were not significantly different in athletes versus nonathletes in a collegiate setting. However, there was a greater disposition of disordered eating patterns in lean versus nonlean athletes.[239] At least 1 confounding factor of this study was that there was a requirement at this university that all athletes take a nutrition class. Although some authors have shown that nutritional knowledge does change eating patterns in athletes,[293,294] other studies question whether knowledge is easily translated into action in female athletes.[238] Such studies remain valuable, but lead to a wide range of prevalence in research reports, as well as lack of consensus about the role of education on affecting eating behaviors.

There are several theories as to why disordered eating patterns occur, including incorrect popular perceptions, biologic factors, and psychological reasons. Many attribute the evolution of these unhealthy eating patterns to the overwhelming desire to be thin.[9,11,19,21,245] Specifically with athletes, this desire is often held in conjunction with the desire to win at all costs.[50] Many female athletes think and are told that “thinner is better.” There is a perception among athletes, coaches, and the media that thinner athletes are faster, stronger, and more powerful. Biologic imbalances in neurotransmitters (serotonin, norepinephrine, and melatonin) have been suggested as an etiology for eating disorders.[39,40] Psychological contributing factors include poor coping skills leading to poor stress management, insufficient family support, sexual and/or physical abuse, and low self-esteem.[40] Struggling with many changes in their bodies, adolescent female athletes are particularly at risk for development of disordered eating patterns that may be the stepping stone for the other components of the Triad. Early detection with knowledge of the warning signs of eating disorders is key (see Table 31-14).

Menstrual Function

The spectrum of menstrual function is another component of the Triad and ranges from functional hypothalamic amenorrhea to eumenorrhea. Eumenorrhea is defined as regular menstrual cycles at intervals near the median interval for young adult women.[213] In young adult women, menstrual cycles recur at a median interval of 28 days, which varies with a standard deviation of 7 days.[213] Menstrual irregularities include primary amenorrhea, secondary amenorrhea, oligomenorrhea, and suppressed luteal phase (luteal phase deficiency) and anovulation.[91,174] Amenorrhea is defined as the absence of menstrual bleeding and is classified as either primary or secondary. Primary amenorrhea refers to absence of menstrual bleeding by the age of 16 years even though other female sex characteristics are apparent *or* by age 14 years in the absence of sexual development. Secondary amenorrhea

Table 31-14 Warning Signs of Eating Disorders[11,17,21]

Aneroxia Nervosa (AN)	Bulimia Nervosa (BN)
Physical signs • Significant weight loss unrelated to medical illness • Fat and muscle atrophy • Amenorrhea • Dry hair and skin • Cold, discolored hands and feet • Decreased body temperature • Cold intolerance • Lightheadedness • Decreased ability to concentrate • Bradycardia • Lanugo (fine, baby hair)	***Physical signs*** • Swollen parotid glands • Face and extremity edema • Sore throat and chest pain • Fatigue • Bloating, abdominal pain • Diarrhea or constipation • Menstrual irregularities • Callous formation or scars on knuckles (Russell's sign) • Erosion of dental enamel
Behaviors • Severe reduction in food intake • Excessive denial of hunger • Compulsive and/or excessive exercising without signs of fatigue or weakness • Peculiar, ritualistic patterns of food handling • Intense fear of weight gain	***Behaviors*** • Exhibits much concern about weight • Eating patterns that alternate between purging and fasting • Depression, guilt, and/or shame especially following a binge

is defined as the cessation of the menstrual cycle for at least 3 months after the initiation of menstruation.[50] Amenorrhea, as defined by the International Olympic Committee, means fewer than 2 menstrual cycles per year.[3] The main difference between primary and secondary amenorrhea is that in the latter at least 1 menstrual cycle did occur, indicating that the reproductive chain, including the hypothalamus, pituitary gland, ovaries, and uterus, successfully completed at least 1 cycle.[91,107,213] With secondary amenorrhea, this chain became disrupted and is not functioning normally.

The normal physiology of menstruation is a complex, coordinated interaction of hormonal and organ involvement occurring in a cyclical manner.[11,50,109,121,251] The menstruation cycle is divided into 3 phases: the follicular phase, during which the egg matures; the ovulatory phase, during which the egg is released; and the luteal phase, in which the uterine lining prepares for the implantation of the fertilized ovum. If implantation does not occur, then the uterine lining is sloughed and menstrual bleeding begins.[109,121] The hypothalamus produces and secretes gonadotropin-releasing hormone (GnRH) regularly. This stimulates the intact and functioning pituitary gland to produce luteinizing hormone and follicle-stimulating hormone. Luteinizing hormone and follicle-stimulating hormone stimulate the ovaries for maturation and release of oocytes (eggs). The ovaries cyclically produce estrogen and progesterone that stimulate the endometrium (uterine lining) to develop and the cyclical withdrawal of estrogen and progesterone result in menstrual shedding of the uterine lining. This ultimately leads to menstrual bleeding from a normal uterus with an unobstructed tract to the external genetalia.[109,121] This well-coordinated, yet complicated, cycle of events may be disrupted anywhere along this process, demonstrating that there are many reasons for the onset

Table 31-15 Causes of Amenorrhea[28,73]

Pregnancy Abnormalities of the reproductive tract Ovarian failure Pituitary tumors
Hypothalamic amenorrhea Chronic anovulation Polycystic ovarian disease Exercise-associated amenorrhea

of amenorrhea.[109,121] Pregnancy and hypothalamic amenorrhea are the 2 most common reasons for the cessation of menstrual cycles. One subset of hypothalamic amenorrhea has been described as "exercise-related" or "athletic" amenorrhea.[50,265] Determining the diagnosis of athletic amenorrhea is one of exclusion of all the other possible causes, requiring an extensive evaluation by a physician with experience and expertise with athletic women. It should be noted that cessation of menstruation is *not* a normal consequence of athletic participation or training for sport (see Table 31-15).[174]

The loss of menstrual cycling coincident with exercise has long been recognized by professional dancers, athletes, coaches, and the medical profession.[11,50] The etiology, prevalence, and treatment of athletic amenorrhea are not completely known and agreed upon to date. In the early 1970s, it was proposed that low body fat and weight were the cause of this cessation of menstrual bleeding. This hypothesis has since been refuted and other factors have been postulated and are currently under investigation. These factors include the physical stress of exercise, increased endogenous opioids from exercise, and overall energy availability based on the "energy balance" discussed previously.[40,50,84,174,213] All of these factors are postulated to directly affect the production and release of GnRH from the hypothalamus.

The prevalence of amenorrhea again is difficult to accurately assess because some female athletes and coaches welcome the cessation of menstrual bleeding. This condition indicates to these athletes and coaches that sufficient training rather than a problem is occurring, so medical workup is not even considered. It is reported that 10% to 20% of vigorously exercising women are amenorrheic as compared to 5% of the general population when pregnant women are excluded.[187] The prevalence of amenorrheic elite runners and professional ballet dancers rises as high as 40% to 50%.[50,92,93,161,164,187,216] The dangers of prolonged amenorrhea include reversible loss of reproductive capacity and possibly irreversible bone loss. The long-term consequences of adolescent amenorrhea are yet to be fully understood and determined.

Oligomenorrhea is defined as menstrual cycles greater than 36 days or having less than 8 menses per year.[95,213] This may result from anovulation, which results from low levels of both estrogen and progesterone *or* normal estrogen production but low levels of progesterone.[213] Female athletes with luteal suppression often present with irregular menses. This component of the Triad still emphasizes amenorrhea, but an expanded view of the Triad includes all of these menstrual irregularities. Detection of menstrual irregularities are often attempted by interview or via a completed self-questionnaire by the female athlete. The preparticipation screening process is an ideal time to assess for these irregularities and appropriately refer to a medical expert such as a physician with experience and expertise with athletic women for a thorough evaluation.

Bone Mineral Density

The final component of the Triad is the BMD spectrum, ranging from osteoporosis to optimal bone health. Osteoporosis is currently the most common bone disease in the United States, affecting more than 25 million Americans to date.[7,108,163,210] The definition per the Consensus Development Conference on Osteoporosis is a disease characterized by low bone mass, microarchitectural deterioration of bone tissue leading to enhanced skeletal fragility, and an increased risk for fracture.[210] Measures of BMD with dual-energy X-ray absorptiometry (DEXA)[26] are used to diagnose osteoporosis and osteopenia with diagnostic criteria that have been established for postmenopausal women.[34] Figure 31-34 is a DEXA scan of a female athlete. Unfortunately, there are no similar diagnostic criteria that have been established for premenopausal women to date.[155,210,215,225]

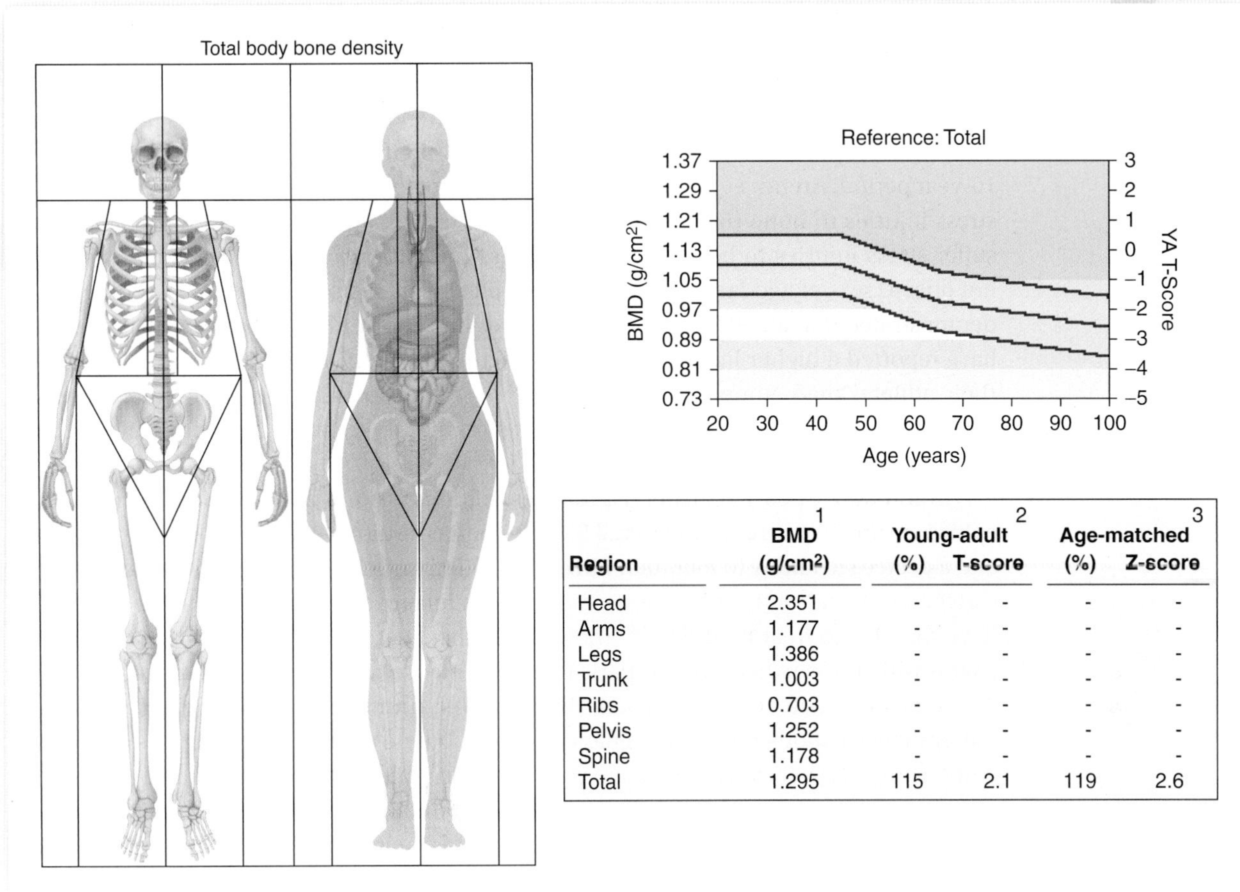

Region	1 BMD (g/cm²)	2 Young-adult (%)	T-score	3 Age-matched (%)	Z-score
Head	2.351	-	-	-	-
Arms	1.177	-	-	-	-
Legs	1.386	-	-	-	-
Trunk	1.003	-	-	-	-
Ribs	0.703	-	-	-	-
Pelvis	1.252	-	-	-	-
Spine	1.178	-	-	-	-
Total	1.295	115	2.1	119	2.6

Figure 31-34 DEXA Scan for individual with normal bone density

There are 2 types of bones: cortical bone, which is tightly compacted plates of bone, and trabecular or spongy bone, which is made up of bone spicules separated by spaces in a honeycomb fashion.[70,93,95] The peripheral skeleton (long bones) is comprised predominantly of cortical bone. This bone is less susceptible to changes in reproductive hormones than the trabecular bone. The axial skeleton (pelvis, vertebral column, and ends of the long bones) is comprised mostly of trabecular bone. These aspects of our skeleton are more susceptible to changes in reproductive hormones reflecting the predominant location of bony changes that occur with both menopause and exercise-induced amenorrhea.[70,215] BMD is determined by the ratio of osteoclastic (resorption) and osteoblastic (remodeling) activity. Weightbearing activities directly stimulate osteoblastic activity according to the Wolff law. Sex hormones, estrogen and testosterone, also favor osteoblastic activity with peak bone growth noted during puberty. The opposite effect of rapid bone loss is seen at menopause with the loss of estrogen. Estrogen also plays a role by limiting osteoclastic activity, thus improving the absorption of calcium at the gastrointestinal level and decreasing elimination of calcium at the renal level.[70,95] Other factors affecting BMD include genetics, smoking, alcohol consumption, cortisol levels, and nutrition.[34,36] Calcium and vitamin D consumption is critical for proper bone health. Calcium is necessary for bone remodeling, but the amount of calcium absorbed is dependent upon an adequate amount of vitamin D.[23,104,108,217]

Abnormalities in bone homeostasis have been documented in female athletes with both premature osteoporosis,[72,108] scoliosis,[45,108,282] and fractures, including premature osteoporotic[84,91] and stress fractures of various locations [91,92,108,151] All athletes have cyclic stresses creating an increased rate of osteoclastic activity followed by osteoblastic activity. If adequate rest or time is not given, an imbalance preventing adequate new bone to be laid down occurs, resulting in a progressive weakening and fracture of the involved bone.[108] This phenomenon occurs more frequently in female athletes, resulting in stress injuries to the bone. In a retrospective review of medical records of a Division I college institution over a 10-year period, Arendt et al[23] demonstrated that female distance runners suffered the most stress injuries to bone (6.4%). Across all sports, female athletes were 2 times as likely to suffer stress injuries to bone as male athletes. The authors attributed this increased rate not only to sex-related factors but also BMD, menstrual history, and diet.[113] Another study demonstrated that athletes with stress fractures had a lower bone density.[203] Other studies have reported a higher incidence of stress fractures among amenorrheic and oligomenorrheic athletes than eumenorrheic athletes.[23,189,216] Menstrual irregularities and decreased BMD certainly are not seen in every case of stress injury to bone, but both may place the athlete at higher risk.[92]

In addition to being at higher risk for stress injuries to bone, athletes with menstrual difficulties are unlikely to reach their total BMD potential resulting in an overall lower peak BMD and a decreased ability to maintain BMD over a lifetime because of lower levels of estrogen. Outcomes of studies regarding bone loss are pessimistic regarding the ability to reverse the lower BMD with treatment.[93,113,189] There are studies that report an increase in serial BMD results with amenorrheic counterparts resuming menses, but the levels remain below their eumenorrheic-matched counterpart. Amenorrheic runners using hormone replacement therapy have demonstrated maintenance of BMD, but no gains.[165] These studies collectively demonstrate the necessity to educate young female athletes in the importance of adequate nutrition, including calories, calcium and vitamin D intake, regular menses, and appropriate training levels, including weightbearing activities for their maturity level.

Interaction Between the Components of the Female Triad

The 3 components of the Triad have been presented and described as independent medical conditions, and now the link between them is detailed. The possible theories behind athletic amenorrhea were mentioned previously. The observations that both amenorrheic athletes had decreased body fat and individuals with AN had low body fat led to the hypothesis that altered body composition was not only correlated but causative. Loucks et al completed research matching amenorrheic and eumenorrheic (normal menstruation) athletes for body fat and found that menstruation status was independent of this variable.[173] Another study concluded that the only difference between the groups (amenorrheic vs. eumenorrheic) with such matched athletes was the negative energy balance that occurred with training in the amenorrheic group.[197] These studies indicate that it is the negative energy balance of caloric intake versus expenditure rather than body fat stores that is linked to the condition of amenorrhea.

Another theory to explain exercise-induced amenorrhea was that the physical stress of the exercise increased the levels of cortisol that were capable of disrupting the menstrual cycle. Again, both amenorrheic athletes and individuals diagnosed with AN demonstrated elevated cortisol levels with corresponding decreased levels of GnRH. As discussed previously in the section on amenorrhea, decreased levels of GnRH can result in exercise-induced amenorrhea. Cortisol has another role in the body as well with the regulation of plasma glucose and is released not only in response to physical stress of exercise but also with decreased levels of plasma glucose. The difficulty lies in separating these roles and determining whether high levels of cortisol disrupts the normal hormonal cascade by suppressing GnRH levels resulting in amenorrhea because of the physical stress of exercise or the decreased plasma levels of glucose. Loucks et al demonstrated that the hormonal cascade changes seen in luteinizing hormone could be normalized in females receiving dietary supplementation, highlighting once again the important role of nutrition (positive energy balance) with intense exercise.[174]

"Negative energy balance" as the cause of exercise-induced amenorrhea has been supported in the research.[11,84,120] Two studies demonstrate that a combination of exercise training and caloric restriction in animals and humans results in amenorrhea with reversal upon an increase in caloric intake.[174,197] This further supports the existence of a direct relationship between daily energy availability and the hormonal cascade controlling the menstrual cycle.[1,2,173,174,197] These articles may explain why female athletes with similar body composition and training intensity have varied menstrual status including amenorrhea, oligomenorrhea, and eumenorrhea (normal menstrual cycling). It is not directly the exercise intensity that causes the change in the hormonal cascade controlling menstruation, but rather, the sustained negative energy balance in those female athletes not taking in enough calories for the energy expended during training. Interventions subsequently should include increased caloric intake in order to attain a positive energy balance in combination with other interventions to target restoration of normal bone metabolism. More specific intervention strategies will be discussed later in this chapter.

The interactions of the disordered eating patterns resulting in the negative energy balance and osteopenia should also be elaborated on. Unhealthy eating behaviors with diagnosed clinical eating disorders (AN, BN, EDNOS) and subclinical eating disorders can rapidly cause an inadequate intake of calcium, vitamin D, and vitamin K, resulting in decreased building blocks for osteoblastic activity to increase overall BMD and allow for normal bone homeostasis during sports participation. As discussed previously, the window of opportunity to reach peak bone mass occurs prior to the third decade of life and is most important in adolescence. These correspond with the same time that disordered eating patterns are most prevalent and the time that many female athletes are competing at high levels, with high training intensities, durations, and frequency. Failure to reach optimum BMD during this time secondary to inadequate nutrition may not be reversible.[213]

Additional interactions between menstrual irregularities and osteopenia are also evident. Some of these interactions with the multifactorial role of estrogen with normal bone metabolism and the ability to achieve peak BMD as it is related to secondary amenorrhea have already been discussed. The condition known as hypoestrogenemia lacks well-designed studies specifically addressing the effect of delaying menarche as a result of premenarchal training. Premenarchal training in a number of sports has been correlated with delayed menarche, but this does not imply causation.[107,161] A retrospective study with college gymnasts suggests that delayed menarche is associated with increased risk of scoliosis, stress fractures, and low peak BMD.[184] These patterns start to demonstrate the serious and long-term implications of triad interactions and the synergistic nature of the component spectrums. Each of the components of the Triad exist on a continuum of severity, thus the interactions between the components falls in a spectrum of severity as well. Early detection of the components greatly assists with the treatment of each component, as well as the interactions that may be present.

Screening

Preparticipation screenings provide an excellent opportunity to identify the components of the Triad. Appendices D and E are examples of screening questionnaires for information gathering regarding eating habits, menstrual history, and bone health. More extensive questionnaires and surveys regarding eating habits and menstrual history can be included should preliminary screening indicate a need. Additional resources can be found in Appendix F.

Menstrual history is often used for predicting bone density.[91,165] In addition, Drinkwater has demonstrated a linear relationship between the degree of bone loss and the degree of menstrual dysfunction.[91,92] Any abnormalities with menstrual cycle detected in the medical history section should be noted and discussed with the primary care or team physician in order to facilitate further studies to confirm bone density. It has been recommended that any female athlete with history of clinical eating disorders, amenorrhea, or oligomenorrhea for more than 3 months have further study to determine bone density. Similarly, documented history of stress fractures may indicate further study. History of stress fractures, especially of the femoral neck, sacrum, or pelvis (cancellous bone), is increasingly concerning secondary to a recent study that found that female athletes with a stress fracture in cancellous bone are more likely to have osteopenia than athletes who sustain a stress fracture in cortical bone such as the tibia or metatarsal.[164] Increasing access, ease, and affordability of DEXA scans have facilitated the ability to confirm a suspicion of bone density problems.

Logistically, implementing these screening tools works nicely in sports preparticipation screening. It is the experience of the authors and documented by other medical professionals that information regarding eating habits and beliefs, self-image, and menstrual history is more accurately gathered when there is a trained medical professional interviewing the female athlete rather than the use of tools that require self-administration.[39,40,126] Many athletes with problems in these areas suffer guilt and shame regarding their behaviors and are skilled at hiding their actions, but most will provide honest and accurate answers to direct and nonjudgmental questioning. It is important to make clear that the information gathered will be held in confidence and will be used for the athlete's benefit. Questionnaires such as found in Appendix D or a combination of established questionnaires (see Appendix E) may also be used outside the preparticipation screening environment for any female athlete suspected of having the Triad.

A recent study indicated that there is a lack of confidence in members of the sports medicine team regarding screening and successfully identifying athletes with eating disorders.[94] One hundred and seventy-one athletic trainers who worked at NCAA Divisions IA and IAA institutions completed a survey that examined college athletic trainers' confidence in helping female athletes who have eating disorders. Less than 33% felt confident in asking an athlete if she had an eating disorder and only 25% felt confident identifying a female athlete with an eating disorder, although virtually all of them (91%) had dealt with a female athlete with an eating disorder and (93%) thought that increased attention to preventing eating disorders among collegiate female athletes was necessary. Less than half worked at an institution that provided training or education on eating disorders to them. The authors of that study recommended that athletic programs develop and implement eating disorder policies, as well as provide education on prevention of eating disorders, to increase confidence of athletic trainers in identifying and supporting a female athlete with an eating disorder.[94]

It is sometimes difficult to be confident in our skill at screening athletes for the components of the Triad because of the difficulty in differentiating healthy and unhealthy dedication to excellence in sport. Distinguishing between healthy and unhealthy eating and exercising behaviors is one challenge for the sports medicine team. In addition to keeping in mind the set criteria for the 3 types of clinical eating disorders, there are other characteristics that have been outlined to distinguish between women developing components of the Triad and athletic women. Athletes remain goal-directed in training with good and improving exercise tolerance and efficient body metabolism. Athletes have well-developed muscles, a body composition with normal fat store levels, and an unimpaired body image. Athletes with or developing components of the Triad have poor to decreasing exercise tolerance and a distorted body image. Body metabolism has dropped resulting in signs such as dry skin, cold intolerance, and decreasing muscle size and development.[11,120] Consideration of these additional factors may assist in improving the confident detection of athletes with components of the triad and facilitate referral for early intervention.

Prevention and Treatment

The ongoing concern about the onset of each of these conditions and the interrelated nature of these conditions with female athletes has led to education and legislative efforts to decelerate the growth of this entity. In 1993, the Eating Disorders Information and Education Act was incorporated into the Women's Health Equity Act.[11,45,152] From this act, the National Eating Disorder screening program was activated on college campuses throughout the United States, not only to enhance the screening and treatment for the Triad but also to accelerate the prevention programs for each of these components.[40,50,70,152] As the American College of Sports Medicine's position statement stated a call to action and medical professionals began to intervene in the screening, prevention, and treatment of this growing entity, efforts have continued and have significantly accelerated with the establishment of this act and program. One study compared 149 female varsity athletes with 209 female controls (nonathletes) from 2 NCAA Division I universities to assess eating habits and behaviors, as well as alcohol consumption and drinking behaviors. The results showed that problem eating and drinking behaviors existed in both groups but not at different rates as previously demonstrated. The authors concluded, "this finding may be the result of coach, athletic trainer, and peer-group counseling at these 2 schools or a general trend for lower rates of unhealthy behaviors among female athletes."[120] Sundgot-Borgen found that education to coaches and athletes had a positive effect on the prevention of disordered eating patterns.[267] In 2002, the formation of the Female Athlete Triad Coalition, a nonprofit 501(c)(3) organization, represents key medical, nursing, athletic, and sports medicine groups, as well as concerned individuals who come together to promote optimal health and well-being for female athletes and active girls and women. Ongoing educational efforts for all concerned parties to prevent the Triad and promote optimal health and well-being for female athletes and active girls and women.[1,8]

Nevertheless, we are far from attaining the goal of maximal prevention of this entity. Other studies have addressed the confidence of medical professionals in screening, preventing, and helping female athletes with nutrition, disordered eating, and menstrual dysfunction.[40,45,126] Beals surveyed NCAA Division I athletic programs and found that education about menstrual dysfunction and eating disorders was made available to athletes in 73% of the participating programs; only 61% of these schools made this education available to the coaches, and less than 41% of schools made this education a requirement of either the athletes or coaching staffs. Of the respondents, only 35% believed that the menstrual dysfunction screening and 26% that the eating disorders screening was successful.[39] When female collegiate cross-country runners were screened about nutritional knowledge, several specific areas of deficient nutritional knowledge were identified. These areas of deficient nutritional knowledge included vitamin supplementation, the necessity for fat in the body and diet, the necessity of a calcium source in the diet, the recommended amount of calcium, and appropriate sources of it. The authors noted that those athletes that completed a nutrition course in college scored significantly higher overall, indicating appropriate nutritional knowledge might lead to better nutritional choices.[294]

Providing accurate information regarding sports nutrition is essential for athletes. Good nutritional information is often addressed in the context of avoiding poor health implications, which often will not motivate an athlete to make the necessary dietary improvements. Optimizing performance with appropriate body composition and aiding recovery following increased training or injury may serve as better motivators.[215] Proper nutrition is a significant determinant of athletic performance. Hawley et al reports, "no single factor plays a greater role in optimizing performance than diet."[126] A good place to start in the provision of sound nutritional advice is the revised Food Pyramid (see Figure 31-35) developed by the United States Department of Agriculture.[280] Ongoing

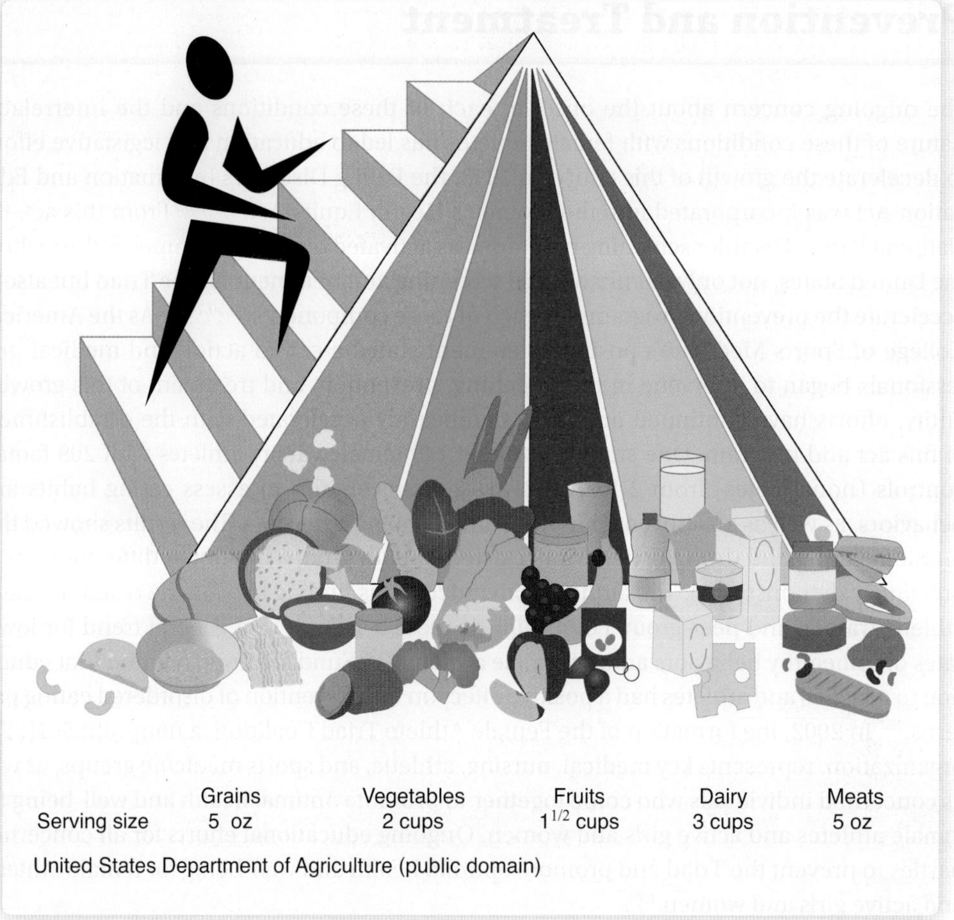

Figure 31-35 **MyPyramid—updated version of the Food Guide Pyramid**[4]

research has led to its development and continued revision. Modifications and additions to the original pyramid illustration have been completed to include a reorganization of the essential food groups, size, and portion information for each of these groups, the necessity of hydration and exercise for a healthy lifestyle, and the ability to further tailor the recommendations depending on your sex, age, and activity level.[152,280] The pyramid can provide the basics for nutrition. Additionally, the U.S. government has provided a simple graphic called "MyPlate" that is helpful regarding the general composition of a healthy diet displayed on a plate (Figure 31-36). To build on these basics, further guidance regarding appropriate body composition, iron intake, calcium intake,[217] fat consumption, and possible supplementation is necessary.

Other strategies to be implemented for prevention of the Triad include education of athletes, parents, and coaches on sound training techniques including limitations of total training hours for adolescents and elimination of weight determinations and body fat level standards by coaches. Education of these same individuals about the Triad, including predisposing factors, warning signs, and implications, can be completed. Other educational goals should include the elimination of myths such as amenorrhea is normal, rest is not needed, and that food is the enemy. Promotion of healthy attitudes, such as food is the fuel that provides the nutrients necessary to optimize performance, as well as healthy body images of female athletes, will continue to assist in the prevention of the triad. These strategies and others can be explored to assist female athletes to realize that thinner is not better, her chosen sport does not have an ideal weight that must be attained, and a healthy balance of calories consumed must be maintained with the energy expended in order to optimize athletic performance.[1,11,18,21,45]

Treatment of the components of the Triad should be in the hands of a multidisciplinary team including but not limited to team physicians, sports physical therapists,[227] certified athletic trainers,[281] sports dieticians, sports psychologists, and coaches. Treatment of disordered eating patterns needs to resolve the psychosocial factors, stabilize medical conditions, and establish healthy eating patterns. Sundgot-Borgon found that cognitive behavioral therapy, in addition to nutritional counseling, was more beneficial in the treatment of female athletes with disordered eating patterns than nutritional therapy alone.[268] Nutritional counseling should include the necessity of balancing caloric intake with the caloric expenditure of training to attain a positive energy balance.[11,21,39,70] The attainment of a positive energy balance is also key to treating menstrual irregularities.[213,215] After identification of the underlying cause of menstrual irregularities, the focus will be to treat this and establish normal menstrual function.[213,215] Optimizing calcium and other micronutrient and macronutrient intake as well as modification of a training regime to ensure this positive energy balance is the first step.[70,117,215] Continued medical supervision to observe the effect of these changes is necessary and possible intervention with hormone replacement is decided upon an individual basis.[57] Once again, attaining a positive energy balance with adequate calcium intake and resumption of normal menstruation is important to treating a female athlete with bone density loss.[163] Exercise modification may be necessary to establish a bone homeostasis favorable to osteoclastic activity with exercise prescription for appropriate weight bearing and resistive exercise. These recommendations, as well as pharmacologic treatment, are based on the individual's data and risk profile. The National Osteoporosis Foundation has established guidelines[210] for pharmacologic treatment of postmenopausal women, but these guidelines cannot be readily utilized for the younger female athlete. Further study and research is needed in this area. The multidisciplinary team led by a qualified medical professional should coordinate efforts for treatment of the individual components of the Triad, subsequently ending the cascade into the interdependent relationship between these components with the root of this treatment being the establishment of a "positive energy balance" for each athlete. Appendix F provides additional sources of information regarding the Triad.

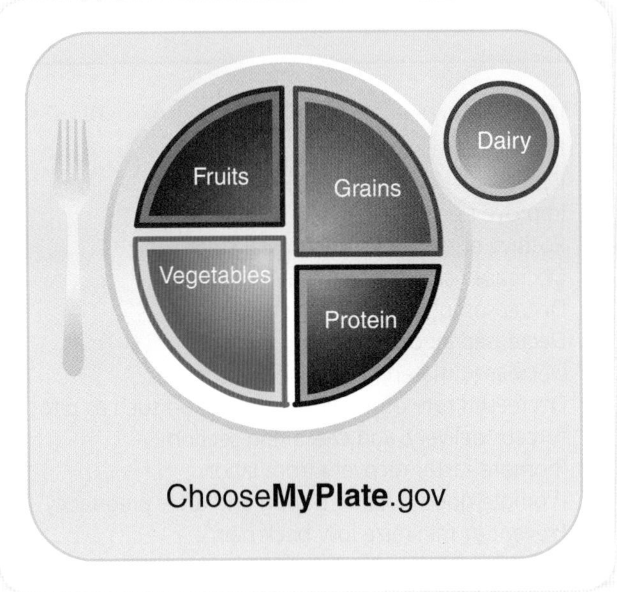

Figure 31-36 **MyPlate graphic**

This graphic simply illustrates excellent eating related to meal composition on a plate.

Pregnancy in the Physically Active Female

The physically active female enjoys many benefits from the exercise she regularly completes. Pregnancy does not change these benefits but does present special challenges for the female athlete as she plans and manages her pregnancy (Table 31-16). The main challenge is exercising at a level that safeguards the health of both the mother and fetus.[27] There are physiologic changes to the cardiovascular, respiratory, and musculoskeletal system that need to be understood and considered in order to decide a safe level of exercise throughout the pregnancy. Knowledge of these physiologic changes and the consequences of exercise and training on the course of pregnancy, labor, and delivery should provide guidance

Table 31-16 Exercise Benefits during Pregnancy

- Increase or maintain aerobic fitness
- Increase cardiac reserve
- Increased tolerance for physical work
- Improve sleep
- Positive effect on psychological state
- Decrease risk of gestational diabetes
- Decreases in total mood disturbance
- Decreased labor time
- Decreased maternal pain perception
- Decreased rate of medical intervention such as pitocin, forceps delivery, and caesarean section
- Promote faster recovery from labor
- Promote good posture during and after pregnancy
- Prevent or minimize low back pain
- Prevent excessive "fat" weight gain
- Prevention of gestational diabetes

for the medical provider of the physically active female to establish guidelines that ensure her and the fetus's safety throughout gestation.

More physicians are encouraging females to remain active during their pregnancies. Adopting a new exercise routine or significantly increasing the intensity of the present exercise routine is not recommended at this time of considerable physiologic change.[28] Known physiologic changes to the cardiovascular system include substantial increases in blood volume up to 50% by the end of pregnancy. This increase occurs first in the plasma volume causing a dilutional anemia in the first and second trimester. The blood volume increase continues in the third trimester with the red cell mass increasing so the anemia is partially corrected.[69] This blood volume expansion results in greater oxygen-carrying capacity, but concurrently increases cardiac work. In highly conditioned athletes, this blood volume increase is greater than in sedentary females.[67] Additional cardiovascular changes include increased stroke volume, cardiac output, and resting pulse by 10 to 15 beats per minute. These increases may help to ensure adequate blood flow to the uterus during exercise, as well as dissipation of heat.[67] Blood pressure usually falls during pregnancy reaching its lowest levels in midpregnancy. Increased circulation to the uterus, kidneys, skin, and breasts occurs and is accompanied by a reduction in venous tone. With this reduction and the increasing size of the uterus decreasing venous return to the heart especially in the supine position, supine hypotension can occur.[67] This is the basis for the recommendation to avoid supine exercise after the first trimester.[18]

When exercising, the female athlete has increases in pulse rate, cardiac output, and blood pressure.[18] The pregnant athlete experiences these same increases to a lesser degree. With these increases, the increased blood flow goes primarily to the working muscles and results in some shunting of blood from the uterus and developing fetus.[67] This observation has raised concern of risk to the fetus with intense and/or prolonged exercise, but evidence for such concern is lacking.[28,67] Respiratory system changes may help to alleviate the ultimate result of the blood shunting that occurs.

Respiratory system changes occurring during pregnancy include increased tidal volume, minute ventilation, and oxygen consumption, as well as decreased residual volume and functional residual capacity. The ultimate result is an unchanged overall vital capacity; however, the pregnant woman may experience shortness of breath because of an increased sensitivity to carbon dioxide driving increased ventilation and lower blood levels of carbon dioxide and slightly more alkaline pH.[233] These biochemical changes have a safeguarding effect for the fetus by increasing placental gas exchange and preventing fetal acidosis.[67] Pregnant women are just as efficient in achieving increased levels of oxygen consumption during exercise as nonpregnant women,[67] but changes in maternal oxygenation are amplified in the fetus. Because anaerobic exercise results in relative maternal hypoxia and acidosis, it is recommended that prolonged anaerobic exercise be avoided. On the other hand, aerobic exercise in pregnant subjects has been shown to result in greater increases in minute ventilation than nonpregnant women. This hyperventilation helps protect the fetus from hypoxia or changes in pH with aerobic exercise.[67]

Changes in the musculoskeletal system of the pregnant, active female result in significant postural, gait, and balance changes. The pregnant female's center of gravity moves forward, often driving an increased lumbar lordosis with a resultant stretch weakness of the core stabilizers.[67] Ligamentous laxity increasing the mobility of all joints especially the pelvis resulting in maternal "waddling" in late pregnancy and a frequent complaint of low back pain as the weight increases with resultant increased forces on the vertebral column. Pelvic or abdominal support devices made especially for the pregnant female can help support the growing abdominal weight as well as stabilization of the pelvis as relaxin becomes more prevalent prior to delivery. Secondary to these musculoskeletal concerns of ligamentous laxity causing increased propensity to falling and increased torque on already lax ligaments, a pregnant women may want to consider swimming, stationary cycling, stair-climbing apparatus, or a treadmill to minimize the risk of falling and to decrease forces on taxed joints.[67]

The effects of exercise on pregnancy outcomes have been studied with reference to fetal development, fetal growth, metabolic status of the fetus, and labor. It is known that high maternal core temperature is associated with fetal development problems, such as neural tube defects, early in gestation. Many of the physiologic changes during pregnancy help to keep maternal temperature lower with or without exercise, but additional precautions especially in the first trimester should be taken to ensure a near normal maternal temperature during exercise sessions.[18,28,67] Historically, it has been a concern that exercising during pregnancy would cause decreased fetal growth and low birth weight. It has been found that women who begin pregnancy underweight have a greater risk of delivering an underweight or preterm newborn. Because female athletes may be underweight at the start of a pregnancy, this finding would include this population. If there is attention and care given to nutrition and appropriate weight gain before or at the initiation of the pregnancy, this concern can be minimized.[66] There is also evidence to demonstrate that if moderate exercise continues throughout pregnancy and does not exceed prepregnancy levels, there is no compromise of fetal growth.[18,67] However, it has been shown that pregnant women who exercise intensely deliver approximately 1 week earlier than those who are sedentary or exercise moderately. This early delivery subsequently causes a relatively low birth rate because of the average 100-g difference in birth weight and decreased body fat deposition in the earlier-delivered baby as compared to full-term babies. Recent reports confirm that exercise during pregnancy has little effect on the acute status of the fetus when mother and unborn baby are healthy.[28,65,67] Fetal heart rate and oxygenation remain normal with intense exercise during the third trimester up to labor.[18,67] Actual labor and delivery are improved by regular exercise throughout pregnancy with less necessary medical intervention, less forceps delivery, cesarean sections, shorter labor with faster dilation, 50% less transition time, and less pushing time to delivery.[67]

Based on the current research, the American Academy of Obstetricians and Gynecologists published the most recent guidelines for exercise in pregnancy and postpartum, recognizing the safety and benefits of exercise throughout pregnancy.[18] These guidelines encourage the physically active female to continue exercising throughout pregnancy, with special attention given to adequate weight gain, preventing hyperthermia, and avoiding injury. The guidelines give specific recommendations regarding adequate nutrition, highlighting that pregnancy requires an additional 300 kcal per day in order to maintain metabolic homeostasis, cautioning exercising pregnant women to ensure an adequate caloric intake. Additional instructions encourage strict adherence to contraindications to exercise, such as pregnancy-induced hypertension, preterm rupture of membranes, preterm labor during the prior or current pregnancy, incompetent cervix/cerclage, persistent second- or third-trimester bleeding, and intrauterine growth retardation.[16] These recommendations suggest, for the first time, a possible role for exercise in the prevention of gestational diabetes. Furthermore, the recommendations promote exercise for sedentary women and those with medical or obstetric complications, but only after medical evaluation and clearance. In summary, the physically active female can safely continue athletic pursuits and/or exercise throughout her pregnancy with some considerations regarding intensity and contact.

SUMMARY

1. For more than a decade, female athlete participation has significantly risen at all levels including high school, collegiate, and Olympics.[3,5,6] The benefits for the female to remain physically active continue to outweigh the costs.[19,46,160,168] An awareness of the gender differences enables the sports medicine specialist to develop prevention, training, and rehabilitation programs that will effectively minimize the cost of remaining physically active throughout the female's life span in a variety of sport endeavors.
   - Anatomical, strength, and neuromuscular differences exist between female and male athletes. These differences should be understood and acknowledged during examination and treatment of female athletes.
   - ACL injuries continue to be prevalent among female athletes.
   - ACL injuries in female athletes are multifactorial. Some factors can be modified, while others cannot. Contemporary prevention and rehabilitation focus on neuromuscular strategies for movement.
   - Core stability is vital for athletic performance by all athletes. Female athletes should address the core during rehabilitation after injury as well as during performance training.
   - The athletically active female has many unique issues including laxity, sport-specific potential for injury (softball pitching, swimming, gymnastics), and the Triad.
   - Specific protocols are included for rehabilitation of the athletic female who participates in softball and swimming.
   - Progressive reactive neuromuscular training for lower extremity and core stabilization is important. A sample progression is included.
   - The Triad is an important condition about which the sports medicine provider must be knowledgeable in order to provide screening, education, and appropriate referral.
   - The physically active female can safely participate in activity during pregnancy, following the medical guidelines such as those prescribed by American College of Obstetricians and Gynecologists.

REFERENCES

1. The Female Athlete Triad Coalition. http://www.femaleathletetriad.org. Accessed August 15, 2012.
2. National Eating Disorder Screening Program. http://www.mentalhealthscreening.org. Accessed on August 1, 2012.
3. Olympic Movement. http://www.olympic.org. Accessed December 12, 2012.
4. United States Department of Agriculture. My Pyramid: Steps to a Healthier You. http://www.mypyramid.gov. Accessed June 1, 2011.
5. National Collegiate Athletic Association. http://www.ncaa.org. Accessed December 15, 2012.
6. National Federation of High School Associations. http://www.nhfs.org. Accessed on December 12, 2012.
7. National Osteoporosis Foundation. Physician's Guide: Impact and Overview. http://www.nof.org/osteoporsis/stats.htm. Accessed on October 20, 2004.
8. International Olympic Committee. http://www.olympic.org/uk/organisation/commissions/women. Accessed January 15, 2012.
9. Office on Women's Health, U.S. Department of Health and Human Services. http://www.womanhealth.gov. Accessed August 15, 2012.
10. Aglietta P, Bruzzi R, D'Andria P, Zaccherotti G. Long-term study of anterior cruciate ligament reconstruction for chronic instability using the central one-third patellar tendon and a lateral extraarticular tenodesis. *Am J Sports Med.* 1992;20:28-45.
11. Agostini, R. Women in sports. In: Mellion MB, Walsh JM, Shelton G, eds. *The Team Physician's Handbook.* Philadelphia, PA: Hanley & Belfus; 1990:179-188.
12. Akuthota V, Nadler SF. Core strengthening. *Arch Phys Med Rehabil.* 2004;85(Suppl 1):S86-S92.

13. Alford JW, Cole BJ. Cartilage restoration, Part 1. *Am J Sports Med.* 2005;33(2):295-132.
14. Alford JW, Cole BJ. Cartilage restoration, Part 2. *Am J Sports Med.* 2005;33(3):443-460.
15. Allegrucci M, Whitney SL, Irrgang JJ. Clinical implications of secondary impingement of the shoulder in freestyle swimmers. *J Orthop Sports Phys Ther.* 1994;20(6):307-318.
16. Almeida SS, Trone DW, Leone DM, et al. Gender differences in musculoskeletal injury rates: A function of symptom reporting? *Med Sci Sports Exerc.* 1995;31: 1807-1812, 1995.
17. Always SE, Gummbt WH, Stray-Gundersen J, et al. Effects of resistance training on elbow flexors of highly competitive bodybuilders. *J Appl Physiol.* 1992;72:1512-1521.
18. American College of Obstetricians and Gynecologists. Exercise during pregnancy and the postpartum period. *ACOG Technical Bulletin 189.* Washington, DC: ACOG; 1994.
19. American College of Sports Medicine. *Exercise Management for Persons with Chronic Diseases and Disabilities.* Champagne, IL: Human Kinetics; 1997.
20. American Physical Therapy Association. *Guide to Physical Therapy Practice.* 2nd ed. Alexandria, VA: American Physical Therapy Association; 2001.
21. American Psychiatric Association. *Diagnostic and Statistical Manual of Mental Disorders-IV.* Washington, DC: American Psychiatric Press; 1994.
22. Anderson AF, Dome DC, Gautam S, et al. Correlation of anthropometric measurements, strength, anterior cruciate ligament size, and intercondylar notch characteristics to sex differences in anterior cruciate ligament tear rates. *Am J Sports Med.* 2001;29(1):58-66.
23. Arendt E, Agel J, Heikes C, Griffiths H. Stress injuries to bone in college athletes. *Am J Sports Med.* 2003;31(6):959-968.
24. Arendt E, Dick R. Knee injury patterns among men and women in collegiate basketball and soccer. *Am J Sports Med.* 1995;23(6):694-701.
25. Arendt EA, Agel J, Dick R. Anterior cruciate ligament injury patterns among collegiate women. *J Athl Train.* 1999;34:86-92.
26. Arendt EA, Bershadsky B, Agel J. Periodicity of non-contact anterior cruciate ligament injuries during the menstrual cycle. *J Gend Specif Med.* 2002;5:19-26.
27. Artal R. Exercise and pregnancy. *Clin Sports Med.* 1992;11:363-77.
28. Artal R, O'Toole M. Guidelines of the Ametican College of Obstetricians and Gynecologists for exercise during pregnancy and the postpartum period. *Br J Sports Med.* 2003;37(1):6-12.
29. Aytar A, Ozunlia N, Surenkok O, Bultaci G, Oztop P, Karatas M. Initial effects of Kinesotape in patients with patellofemoral pain syndrome: A randomized double-blind study. *Isokinet Exerc Sci.* 2011;19(2):135-142.
30. Bach BR, Jones GT, Sweet FA, Hager CA. Arthroscopy-assisted anterior cruciate ligament reconstruction using patellar tendon substitution. Two- to four-year follow-up results. *Am J Sports Med.* 1994;22:758-767.
31. Backx FJG, Beijer HJM, Bol E. Injuries in high-risk persons and high-risk sports. *Am J Sports Med.* 1991;19:124-130.
32. Bahr R, Reeser JC. Injuries among world-class professional beach volleyball players. *Am J Sports Med.* 31(1), 2003.
33. Bak K, Kalms SB, Olesen S, et al. Epidemiology of injuries in gymnastics. *Scand J Med Sci Sports.* 1994;4:148-154.
34. Baratta R, Solomonow M, Zhou BH. Muscular coactivation: The role of the antagonist musculature in maintaining knee stability. *Am J Sports Med.* 1988;16:113-122.
35. Barden JM, Balyk R, Raso JV, et al. Dynamic upper limb proprioception in multidirectional shoulder instability. *Clin Orthop.* 2004;420:181-189.
36. Barrack RL, Lund PJ, Skinner HB. Knee joint proprioception revisited. *J Sport Rehabil.* 1994;3:18-42.
37. Barrentine S, Fleising G, Whiteside J, et al. Biomechanics of windmill softball pitching with implications about injury mechanisms at the shoulder and elbow. *J Orthop Sports Phys Ther.* 1998;28:405-415.
38. Barrett DS. Proprioception and function after anterior cruciate reconstruction. *J Bone Joint Surg Br.* 1991;73B:833-837.
39. Beals KA, Manore MM. The prevalence and consequences of subclinical eating disorders in female athletes. *Int J Sport Nutr.* 1994;4:175-195.
40. Beals KA. Eating disorder and menstrual dysfunction screening, education and treatment programs. *Phys Sportsmed.* 2003;31(7):33-38.
41. Beck X, Wildermuth BP. The female athlete's knee. *Clin Sports Med.* 1985;4(2):345-366.
42. Beighton PH, Horan FT. Dominant inheritance in familial generalized articular hypermobility. *J Bone Joint Surg Br.* 1970;52:145-147.
43. Beim G, Stone DA. Issues in the female athlete. *Orthop Clin North Am.* 1995;26(3):443-451.
44. Bjordal JM, Amly F, Hannestad B, Strand T. Epidemiology of anterior cruciate ligament injuries in soccer. *Am J Sports Med.* 1997;25:341-345.
45. Black DR, Larkin LJS, Coster DC, Leverenz LJ, Abood DA. Physiologic screening test for eating disorders/disordered eating among female collegiate athletes. *J Athl Train.* 2003;38(4):286-297.
46. Blair SN, Goodyear NN, Gibbons LW, Cooper KH. Physical fitness and incidence of hypertension in healthy normotensive men and women. *JAMA.* 1984;252:487-490.
47. Blasier RB, Carpenter JE, Huston LJ. Shoulder proprioception. Effect of joint laxity, joint position, and direction of motion. *Orthop Rev.* 1994;23:45-50.
48. Bobbert MF, van Zandwijk JP. Dynamics of force and muscle stimulation of human vertical jumping. *Med Sci Sports Exerc.* 1999;31:303-310.
49. Boden BP, Dean GS, Feagin JA, Garrett WE. Mechanisms of anterior cruciate ligament injury. *Orthopedics.* 2000;23(6):573-578.

50. Bolen JD. Differentiating healthy from unhealthy behaviors in active and athletic women. In: Agostini R, ed. *Medical and Orthopedic Issues of Active and Athletic Women.* Philadelphia, PA: Hanley & Belfus; 1994: 102-107.
51. Borsa PA, Lephart SM, Kocher MS, et al. Functional assessment and rehabilitation of shoulder proprioception for glenohumeral instability. *J Sports Rehabil.* 1994;3:84-104.
52. Bouisset S. Relationship between postural support and intentional movement: Biomechanical approach. *Arch Int Physiol Biochem Biophys.* 1991;99:77-92.
53. Briner WW, Benjamin HJ. Volleyball injuries: Managing acute and overuse disorders. *Phys Sportsmed.* 1999;27(3):48-56.
54. Brody LT, Thein JM. Nonoperative treatment for patellofemoral pain. *J Orthop Sports Phys Ther.* 28(5):33634, 1998.
55. Brown GA, Tan JL, Kirkley A. The lax shoulder in females. Issues, answers, but many more questions. *Clin Orthop Relat Res.* 2000;372:110-122.
56. Bryant JT, Cooke TD. Standardized biomechanical measurement of varus-valgus stiffness and rotation in normal knees. *J Orthop Res.* 1988;6:863-870.
57. Caine D, Cochrane B, Caine C, et al. An epidemiologic investigation of injuries affecting young competitive female gymnasts. *Am J Sports Med.* 1989;17(6): 811-820.
58. Caine D, Lewis R, O'Connor P, et al. Does gymnastics training inhibit growth of females? *Clin J Sport Med.* 2001;11(4):260-270.
59. Caine D, Lindner K. Overuse injuries of growing bones: The young female gymnast at risk? *Phys Sportsmed.* 1985;13:51-54.
60. Caraffa A, Cerulli G, Projetti M, et al. Prevention of anterior cruciate ligament injuries in soccer. A prospective controlled study of proprioceptive training. *Knee Surg Sports Traumatol Arthrosc.* 1996;4(1):19-21.
61. Carson W, James S, Larson R, et al. Patellofemoral disorders: Physical and radiographic evaluation. *Clin Orthop.* 1984;185:165-185.
62. Carter C, Wilkinson J. Persistent joint laxity and congenital dislocation of the hip. *J Bone Joint Surg Br.* 1964;46:40-45.
63. Chandy TA, Grana WA. Secondary school athletic injury in boys and girls: A three-year comparison. *Phys Sportsmed.* 1985;13(3):106-111.
64. Chappell JD, Bing Y, Kirkendall DT, et al. A comparison of knee kinetics between male and female recreational athletes in stop-tasks. *Am J Sports Med.* 2002;30(2):261-267.
65. Chmielewski T, Ferber R. Rehabilitation considerations for the female athlete. In: Andrews JR, Harrelson GL, Wilk KE, eds. *Physical Rehabilitation of the Injured Athlete.* 3rd ed. Philadelphia, PA: Saunders-Elsevier; 2004: 315-328.
66. Cholewicki J, Simons APD, Radebold A. Effects of external trunk loads on lumbar spine stability. *J Biomech.* 2000;33:1377-1385.
67. Christian JS, Christian SS, Stamm CA, McGregor JA. Pregnancy, physiology and exercise. In: Ireland ML, Nattiv A, eds. *The Female Athlete.* Philadelphia, PA: Saunders; 2002:185-190.
68. Cicuttini F, Forbes A, Morris K, Darling S, Bailey M, Stuckey S. Gender differences in knee cartilage volume as measured by magnetic resonance imaging. *Osteoarthritis Cartilage.* 1999;7:265-271.
69. Clapp JF. A clinical approach to exercise during pregnancy. *Clin Sports Med.* 1994;13:443-458.
70. Clark N. *Sports Nutrition Guidebook.* Brookline, MA: Sportsmed Brookline; 1997.
71. Cohen AR, Metzl JD. Sports-specific concerns in the young athlete: Basketball. *Pediatr Emerg Care.* 2000,16(6).462-468.
72. Colby S, Francisco A, Yu B, et al. Electromyographic and kinematic analysis of cutting maneuvers. *Am J Sports Med.* 2000;28(2):234-240.
73. Corrigan JP, Cashman WF, Brady MP. Proprioception in the cruciate deficient knee. *J Bone Joint Surg Br.* 1992;74:247-250.
74. Cresswell AG, Oddson L, Thorstensson A. The influence of sudden perturbations on trunk muscle activity and intraabdominal pressure while standing. *Exp Brain Res.* 1994;98:336-341.
75. Cresswell AG, Thorstensson A. Change in intra-abdominal pressure, trunk muscle activation and force during isokinetic lifting and lowering. *Eur J Appl Physiol.* 1994;68:315-321.
76. Cresswell AG. Responses of intra-abdominal pressure and abdominal muscle activity during dynamic trunk loading man. *Eur J Appl Physiol.* 1993;66:315-320.
77. Cross MJ, Gibbs NJ, Grace JB. An analysis of the sidestep cutting maneuver. *Am J Sports Med.* 1989;17:363-366.
78. Cuillo JV, Stevens GC. The prevention and treatment of injuries to the shoulder in swimming. *Sports Med.* 1989;7:182-204.
79. Curl WW, Krone J, Gordon ES, Rushing J, Smith BP, Poehling GG. Cartilage injuries: A review of 31,516 knee arthroscopies. *Arthroscopy.* 1997;13:456-460.
80. Dahm D. The shoulder and upper extremities. In: Sweden N, ed. *Women's Sports Medicine and Rehabilitation.* Gaithersburg, MD: Aspen Publishers; 2001:7-17.
81. Daniel DM, Fithian DC, Stone ML, et al. A ten-year prospective outcome study of the ACL-injured patient. *Orthop Trans.* 1996-1997;20:700-701.
82. Daniel DM, Stone ML, Dobson BE, et al. Fate of the ACL-injured patient. A prospected outcome study. *Am J Sports Med.* 1994;22:632-666.
83. DeCoster LC, Vailas JC, Lindsay RH, et al. Prevalence and feature of joint hypermobility among adolescent athletes. *Arch Pediatr Adolesc Med* 1997;151:989-992.

84. DeCourcey B. Dedication or destruction? How disordered eating can affect athletes. *NATA News.* 10-13, February 2005.
85. DeHaven KE, Linter DM. Athletic injuries: Comparison by age, sport and gender. *Am J Sports Med.* 1986;14(3):218-224.
86. DeMont RG, Lephart SM, Giraldo JL, et al. Muscle preactivity of anterior cruciate ligament—deficient and reconstructed females during functional activities. *J Athl Train.* 1999;34(2):115-120.
87. DiBrezzo R, Oliver G. ACL injuries in active girls and women. *J Phys Educ Recreation Dance.* 2000;71(6):24-27.
88. Dore E, Martin F, Ratel S. Gender differences in peak muscle performance during growth. *Int J Sports Med.* 2005;26:274-280.
89. Dover GC, Kaminski TW, Meister K, et al. Assessment of shoulder proprioception in the female softball athlete. *Am J Sports Med.* 2003;31(3):431-437.
90. Draganich LF, Vahey JW. An in vitro study of anterior cruciate ligament strain induced by quadriceps and hamstring forces. *J Orthop Res.* 1990;8:57-63.
91. Drinkwater BL, Bruemmer B, Chestnut CH III. Menstrual history as a determinant of current bone density in young athletes. *N Engl J Med.* 1984;311:277.
92. Drinkwater BL, Nilson K, Chestnut CH III. Bone mineral content of amenorrheic and eumenorrheic athletes. *N Engl J Med.* 1984;311:277.
93. Drinkwater BL, Nilson K, Chestnut CH III. Bone mineral density after resumption of menses in amenorrheic athletes. *JAMA.* 1986;256(3):380-382.
94. Dufek JS, Bates BT. Biomechanical factors associated with injury during landing in jumping sports. *Sports Med.* 1991;12(5):326-337.
95. Dugowson CE, Drinkwater BL, Clark JM. Nontraumatic femur fracture in oligomenorrheic athlete. *Med Sci Sports Exerc.* 1991;23:1323-1325.
96. Dye SE, Chew MH. Restoration of osseious homeostasis after anterior cruciate ligament reconstruction. *Am J Sports Med.* 1993;21:748-750.
97. Dye SE, Wojtys EM, Fu FH, Fithian DC, Gilquist J. Factors contributing to function of the knee joint following injury or reconstruction of the anterior cruciate ligament. *J Bone Joint Surg Am.* 1998;80(9):1380-1391.
98. Dye SE. The knee as a biologic transmission with an envelope of function. A theory. *Clin Orthop.* 1996;325:10-18.
99. Dyrek DA, Micheli LJ, Magee DJ. Injuries to the thoracolumbar spine and pelvis. In: Zachazewski JE, Magee DJ, Quillen WS, eds. *Athletic Injures and Rehabilitation.* Philadelphia, PA: Saunders; 1996:465-484.
100. Ebenbichler GR, Oddsson LIE, Kollmitzer J, Erim Z. Sensory-motor control of the lower back: Implications for rehabilitation. *Med Sci Sports Exerc.* 2001;33(11):1889-1898.
101. Ettlinger CF, Johnson RJ, Shealy JE. A method to help reduce the risk of serious knee sprains incurred in alpine skiing. *Am J Sports Med.* 1995;23:531-537.
102. Ferber RI, Davis M, Williams DS. Gender differences in lower extremity mechanics during running. *Clin Biomech (Bristol, Avon).* 2003;18:350-357.
103. Ferretti A, Papandrea P, Conteduca F, Mariana PP. Knee ligament injuries in volleyball players. *Am J Sports Med.* 1992;20:203-207.
104. Food Nutrition Board. *Recommended Dietary Allowances.* Washington, DC: National Academy of Sciences; 2010.
105. Ford KR, Myer GD, Toms HE, et al. Gender differences in the kinematics of unanticipated cutting in young athletes. *Med Sci Sports Exerc.* 2005;37(1):124-129.
106. Ford KR, Shapiro R, Myer GD, van den Bogert AJ, Hewett TE. Longitudinal sex differences during landing in knee abduction in young athletes. *Med Sci Sports Exerc.* 2010;42(10):1923-1931.
107. Frisch RE, Gotz-Welbergen AV, McArthur JW, et al. Delayed menarche and amenorrhea of college athletes in relation to age of onset of training. *JAMA.* 1999;282:637-645.
108. Ganong WF. Hormonal control of calcium metabolism & the physiology of bone. *Medical Physiology.* Norwalk, CT: Appleton & Lange; 1985:326-337.
109. Ganong WF. The gonads: Development and function of the reproductive system. *Medical Physiology.* Norwalk, CT: Appleton & Lange; 1985:370-382.
110. Gardner-Morse M, Stokes I. The effect of abdominal muscle coactivation on lumbar spine stability. *Spine (Phila Pa 1976).* 1998;23:86-92.
111. Garrick JG, Requa RK. Girls sports injuries in high school athletics. *JAMA.* 1978;239:2245-2248.
112. Gelber AC, Hochberg MC, Mead LA, et al. Joint injury in young adults and risk for subsequent knee and hip osteoarthritis. *Ann Intern Med.* 2000;133:321-328.
113. Georgious EK, Ntalles K, Papageorgiou A, et al. Bone mineral loss related to menstrual history. *Acta Orthop Scand.* 1989;60:192-194.
114. Gilquist J. Repair and reconstruction of the ACL: Is it good enough? *Arthroscopy.* 1993;9:68-71.
115. Gomez E, DeLee JC, Farney WC. Incidence of injury in Texas girls' high school basketball. *Am J Sports Med.* 1996;24:684-687.
116. Gracovetsky S, Farfan H, Helleur C. The effect of the abdominal mechanism. *Spine (Phila Pa 1976).* 1985;10:317-324.
117. Grandjean AC, Reimers KJ, Ruud J. Nutrition. In: Ireland ML, Nattiv A, eds. *The Female Athlete.* Philadelphia, PA: Saunders; 2002:81-89.
118. Gray J, Taunton JE, McKenzie DC, et al. A survey of injuries to the anterior cruciate ligament of the knee in female basketball players. *Int J Sports Med.* 1985;6:314-316.
119. Griffin LY, Agel J, Albohm MJ, et al. Noncontact anterior cruciate ligament injuries: Risk factors and strategies for prevention. *J Am Acad Orthop Surg.* 2000;8(3):141-150.
120. Gutgessell ME, Moreau KL, Thompson DL. Weight concerns, problem eating behaviors, and roblem drinking

behaviors in female collegiate athletes. *J Athl Train.* 2003;38(1):62-66.

121. Guyton AC. *Textbook of Medical Physiology.* 12th ed. Philadelphia, PA: Saunders; 2011.
122. Hakkinen K, Kraemer WJ, Newton RU. Muscle activation and force production during bilateral and unilateral concentric and isometric contractions of the knee extensors in men and women at different ages. *Electromyogr Clin Neurophysiol.* 1997;37:131-142.
123. Hall CM. Therapeutic exercise for the lumbopelvic region. In: Hall CM, Thein-Brody L, eds. *Therapeutic Exercise, Moving Toward Function.* 2nd ed. Philadelphia, PA: Lippincott Williams & Wilkins; 2005:349-401.
124. Harner CD, Paulos LE, Greenwald AD. Detailed analysis of patients with bilateral anterior cruciate ligament injuries. *Am J Sports Med.* 1994;22:37-43.
125. Harrer MF, Hosea TM, Berson L, et al. The gender issue: Epidemiology of knee and ankle injuries in high school and college players. Proceedings of the 65th Annual meeting of the American Academy of Orthopedic Surgeons. New Orleans, LA, March 19-23, 1998. Abstract 260.
126. Hawley JA, Dennis SC, Lindsay FH, Noakes TD. Nutritional practices of athletes: Are they suboptimal? *J Sports Sci.* 1995;13:S75-S81, 1995.
127. Haycock CE, Gillette JV. Susceptibility of women athletes to injury: Myth vs. reality. *JAMA.* 1976;236(2):163-165.
128. Hewett TE, Torg JS, Boden BP. Video analysis of trunk and knee motion during non-contact anterior cruciate ligament injury in female athletes. Lateral trunk and knee abduction motion are combined components of the injury mechanism. *Br J Sports Med.* 2009;43:417-422.
129. Hewett TE, Lindenfeld TN, Riccobene JV, et al. The effect of neuromuscular training on the incidence of knee injury in female athletes. *Am J Sports Med.* 1999;27(6):699-705.
130. Hewett TE, Myer GD, Ford KR, et al. Biomechanical measures of neuromuscular control and valgus loading of the knee predict anterior cruciate ligament injury risk in female athletes: A prospective study. *Am J Sports Med.* 2005;33(4):492-501.
131. Hewett TE, Paterno MV, Myer GD. Strategies for enhancing proprioception and neuromuscular control of the knee. *Clin Orthop Relat Res.* 2002;402:76-94.
132. Hewett TE, Stroupe AL, Nance TA, et al. Plyometric training in female athletes: Decreased impact forces and increased hamstring torques. *Am J Sports Med.* 1996;24(6):765-773.
133. Hewett TE. Neuromuscular and hormonal factors associated with knee injuries in female athletes. *Sports Med.* 2000;29(5):313-327.
134. Hides JA, Stokes MJ, Saide M, Jull GA, Cooper DH. Evidence of lumbar multifidus muscle wasting ipsilateral to symptoms in patients with acute/subacute low back pain. *Spine (Phila Pa 1976).* 1994;19:165-172.
135. Hill JL, Humphries B, Weidner T, Newton RU. Female collegiate windmill pitchers: Influences to injury incidence. *J Strength Cond Res.* 2004;18(3):426-431.
136. Hodges PW, Butler JE, McKenzie D, Gandevia SC. Contraction of the human diaphragm during postural adjustments. *J Appl Physiol.* 1997;505:239-248.
137. Hodges PW, Richardson CA. Delayed postural contraction of transverse abdominis in low back pain associated with movement of the lower limb. *J Spinal Disord.* 1998;1:46-56.
138. Hodges PW, Richardson CA. Feedforward contraction of transverse abdominis is not influenced by the direction of arm movement. *Exp Brain Res.* 1997;114:362-370.
139. Hodges PW. Is there a role for transversus abdominis in lumbo-pelvic stability? *Man Ther.* 1999;4(2):74-86.
140. Hoffman M, Schrader J, Koceja D. An investigation of postural control in postoperative anterior cruciate ligament reconstruction patients. *J Athl Train.* 1999;34(2):130-136.
141. Holloway JB, Baechle TR. Strength training for female athletes: A review of selected aspects. *Sports Med.* 1990;9:216-228.
142. Hoogenboom BJ, Bennett JL. *Core Stabilization for the Female Athlete. SPTS Female Athlete Home Study Course.* Indianapolis, IN: The Sports Physical Therapy Section; 2004.
143. Howell SM, Taylor MA. Brace-free rehabilitation, with early return to activity, for knees reconstructed with double-looped semitendinosus and gracilis graft. *J Bone Joint Surg Am.* 1996;78:814-825.
144. Huston LJ, Greenfield ML, Wojtys EM. Anterior cruciate ligament injuries in the female athlete. *Clin Orthop Relat Res.* 2000;372:50-63.
145. Huston LJ, Wojtys EM. Neuromuscular performance characteristics in elite female athletes. *Am J Sports Med.* 1996;24(4):427-436.
146. Hutchinson MR, Ireland ML. Knee injuries in female athletes. *Sports Med.* 1995;19:288-301.
147. Hutchinson MR, Williams RI, Ireland ML. In: Ireland ML, Nattiv A, eds. *The Female Athlete.* Philadelphia, PA: Saunders; 2002:387-419.
148. Ireland ML, Wall C. Epidemiology and comparison of knee injuries in elite male and female United States basketball athletes [abstract]. *Med Sci Sports Exerc.* 22:S82, 1990.
149. Ireland ML, Willson JD, Ballantyne BT, Davis IM. Hip strength in females with and without patellofemoral pain. *J Orthop Sports Phys Ther.* 2003;33:637-651.
150. Ireland ML. Anterior cruciate ligament injury in female athletes: Epidemiology. *J Athl Train.* 1999;34(2):150-154.
151. Johnson AW, Weiss CB, Stento K, Wheeler D. An atypical cause of low back pain in the female athlete. *Am J Sports Med.* 2001;29(4):498-508.
152. Johnson MD, Disordered eating. In: Agostini R, ed. *Medical and Orthopedic Issues of Active and Athletic Women.* Philadelphia, PA: Hanley & Belfus; 1994:141-151.
153. Johnson RJ, Eriksson E, Haggmark T, Pope MH. Five- to ten-year follow-up evaluation after reconstruction of the anterior cruciate ligament. *Clin Orthop.* 1984;183:122-140.

154. Kennedy JC, Alexander IJ, Hayes KC. Nerve supply to the human knee and its functional importance. *Am J Sports Med.* 1982;10:329-335.

155. Khan KM, Liu-Ambrose T, Sran MM, et al. New criteria for female athlete triad syndrome? As osteoporosis is rare, should osteopenia be among the criteria for defining the female athlete triad syndrome? *Br J Sports Med.* 2002;36: 10-13.

156. Kibler WB. Determining the extent of the deficit. In: Kibler WB, Herring SA, Press JM, eds. *Functional Rehabilitation of Sports and Musculoskeletal Injuries.* Gaithersberg, MD: Aspen; 1998:16-20.

157. Knapik JJ, Bauman CL, Jones BH. Preseason strength and flexibility imbalances associated with athletic injuries in female collegiate athletes. *Am J Sports Med.* 1991;19(1):76-81.

158. Knapik JJ, Sharp MA, Canham-Chervak M, et al. Risk factors for training-related injuries among men and women in basic combat training. *Med Sci Sports Exerc.* 2001;33:946-954.

159. Knott M, Voss D. *Proprioceptive Neuromuscular Facilitation: Patterns and Techniques.* New York, NY: Harper & Row; 1968.

160. Kohl, HW, LaPorte RE, Blair SN. Physical activity and cancer. An epidemiological perspective. *Sports Med.* 1988;6:222-237.

161. Koutedakis Y, Jamurtas A. The dancer as a performing athlete: Physiological considerations. *Sports Med.* 2004;34(10):651-661.

162. Kroner K, Lind T, Jensen J. The epidemiology of shoulder dislocations. *Arch Orthop Trauma Surg.* 1989;108(5):288-290.

163. Lane JM. Osteoporosis. In: Ireland ML, Nattiv A, eds. *The Female Athlete.* Philadelphia, PA: Saunders; 2002: 249-258.

164. Lavienja A, Braam JLM, Knapen MHJ, Geusens P, Brouns F, Vermeer C. Factors affecting bone loss in female endurance athletes. *Am J Sports Med.* 2003;31(6):889-895.

165. Lebrun CM. The effect of the phase of the menstrual cycle and the birth control pill in athletic performance. *Clin Sports Med.* 1994;13(2):419-441.

166. Lebrun CM. Effects of the menstrual cycle and birth control pill on athletic performance. In: Agostini R, ed. *Medical and Orthopedic Issues of Active and Athletic Women.* Philadelphia, PA: Hanley & Belfus; 1994:78-91.

167. Leetun DT, Ireland ML, Willson JD, Ballantyne BT, Davis IM. Core stability measures as risk factors for lower extremity injury in athletes. *Med Sci Sports Exerc.* 2004;36(6):926-934.

168. Leon AS, Connett J, Jacobs DR, Rauramaa R. Leisure-time physical activity levels and risk of coronary heart disease and death. The multiple risk factor intervention trial. *JAMA.* 1987;258:2388-2395.

169. Lephart SM, Abt JP, Ferris CM. Neuromuscular contributions to anterior cruciate ligament injuries in females. *Curr Opin Rheumatol.* 2002;14:168-173.

170. Lephart SM, Rerris CM, Riemann BL, Myers JB, Fu FH. Gender differences in strength and lower extremity kinematics during landing. *Clin Orthop Relat Res.* 2002;401:162-169.

171. Lindenfeld TN, Schmitt DJ, Hendy MP, et al. Incidence of injury in indoor soccer. *Am J Sports Med.* 1994;22: 364-371.

172. Linder KJ, Caine DJ. Injury patterns of female competitive club gymnasts. *Can J Sport Sci.* 1990;15(4):254-261.

173. Loucks AB, Horvath SM, Feedson PS. Menstrual status and validation of body fat prediction in athletics. *Hum Biol.* 1994;56:383-392.

174. Loucks AB, Verdun M, Heath EM. Low energy availability, not stress of exercise, alters LH pulsatility in exercising women. *J Appl Physiol.iol.J Appl Physiol.* 1998;84:37-46.

175. Loucks J, Thompson H. Effects of menstruation on reaction time. *Res Q.* 1968;39:407-408.

176. Lutter JM. A 20-year perspective: What has changed? In: Pearl AJ, ed. *The Athletic Female.* Champaign, IL: Human Kinetics; 1993:1-8.

177. Maffett MW, Jobe FW, Pink MM, et al. Shoulder muscle firing patterns during the windmill softball pitch. *Am J Sports Med.* 1997;25(3):369-374.

178. Magee DJ. The knee. In: *Orthopedic Physical Assessment.* 4th ed. Philadelphia, PA: Saunders; 2002:661-763.

179. Malinzak RA, Colby SM, Kirkendall DT, et al. A comparison of knee motion patterns between men and women in selected athletic tasks. *Clin Biomech (Bristol, Avon).* 2001;16:438-445.

180. Malone TR, Hardaker WT, Garrett WE, et al. Relationship of gender to anterior cruciate ligament injuries in intercollegiate basketball players. *J South Orthop Assoc.* 1993;2:36-39.

181. Mandelbaum BR, Browne JE, Fu FH, et al. Articular surface lesions of the knee. *Am J Sports Med.* 1998;26:853-861.

182. Mandelbaum BR, Silver HJ, Watanabe DS, et al. Effectiveness of a neuromuscular and proprioceptive training program in preventing anterior cruciate ligament injuries in female athletes. *Am J Sports Med.* 2005;33:1003-1010.

183. Mansfield MJ, Emans SJ. Growth in female gymnasts: Should training decrease during puberty? *J Pediatr.* 1993;122:237-240.

184. Mansfield MJ, Emans SJ. Growth and nutrient requirements at adolescence. In: Grand RJ, Sutphen JL, Dietz WH, eds. *Pediatric Nutrition. Theory and Practice.* Boston, MA: Butterworths; 1987:357-371.

185. Marcacci M, Zaffagnini S, Iacono F, Neri MP, Petitto A. Early versus late reconstruction of anterior cruciate ligament rupture. Results after five years of followup. *Am J Sports Med.* 1995;23:690-693.

186. Markolf KL, Graff-Radford A, Amstutz HC. In vivo knee stability: A quantitative assessment using an instrumented clinical testing apparatus. *J Bone Joint Surg Am.* 1978;60:664-674.

187. Marshall LA, Clinical evaluation of amenorrhea. In: Agostini R, ed. *Medical and Orthopedic Issues of Active and Athletic Women*. Philadelphia, PA: Hanley & Belfus; 1994:152-163.

188. Marshall SW, Hamsra-Wright KL, Dick R, Grove KA, Agel J. Descriptive epidemiology of collegiate female softball injuries: NCAA injury surveillance system, 1988-1989 to 2003-2004. *J Athl Train.* 2007;42(2):286-294.

189. Marx RG, Saint-Phard D, Callahan LR, et al. Stress fracture sites related to underlying bone health in athletic females. *Clin J Sport Med.* 2001;11:73-76.

190. Mascal CL, Landel R, Powers C. Management of patellofemoral pain targeting hip, pelvis, and trunk muscle function: 2 Case reports. *J Orthop Sports Phys Ther.* 2003;33(11):647-660.

191. McConnell J. The management of chondromalacia patellae: A long term solution. *Aust J Phys Ther* 1986;32(4): 215-223.

192. McGill S, Brown S. Reassessment of the role of intra-abdominal pressure in spinal compression. *Ergonomics.* 1987;30:1565-1588.

193. McGill S. *Low Back Disorders: Evidence-Based Prevention and Rehabilitation*. Champaign, IL: Human Kinetics; 2002.

194. McLean SG, Myers PT, Neal RJ, Walters MR. A quantitative analysis of knee joint kinematics during the sidestep cutting maneuver. *Bull Hosp Jt Dis.* 1989;57(1):30-38.

195. Messina DF, Farney WC, DeLee JC. Thin incidence of injury in high school basketball: A prospective study among male and female athletes [abstract]. Book of abstracts and outlines for the 24th annual meeting of the American Orthopedic Society for Sports Medicine. Vancouver, British Columbia, Canada, July 12-15, 1998. Abstract 362.

196. Meth S. Gender difference in muscle morphology. In: Swedan N, ed. *Women's Sports Medicine and Rehabilitation*. Gaithersburg, MD: Aspen; 2001:3-6.

197. Meyerson M, Gutin B, Warren MP, et al. Resting metabolic rate and energy balance in amenorrheic and eumenorrheic runners. *Med Sci Sports Exerc.* 1993;23:15-22.

198. Mink JH, Deutsch A. Occult cartilage and bone injuries of the knee: Detection, classification, and assessment with MR imaging. *Radiology.* 1989;170:823-829.

199. Möller-Neilson J, Hammer M. Sports injuries and oral contraceptive use: Is there a relationship? *Sports Med.* 1991;12:152-160.

200. Moore JR, Wade G. Prevention of anterior cruciate injuries. *J Nat Strength Cond Assoc.* 1989;2:35-40.

201. Morris JM, Lucas DM, Bressler B. Role of the trunk in stability of the spine. *J Bone Joint Surg.* 1961;43:327-351.

202. Moul JL. Differences in selected predictors of anterior cruciate ligament tears between male and female NCAA Division I collegiate basketball players. *J Athl Train.* 1998;33:118-121.

203. Myburgh KH, Hutchins J, Fataar AB, et al. Low bone density is an etiologic factor for stress fractures in athletes. *Ann Intern Med.* 1990;113:754-759.

204. Myer GD, Ford KR, Palumbo J. Neuromuscular training improves performance and lower-extremity biomechanics in female athletes. *J Strength Cond Res.* 2005;19(1):51-60.

205. Myer GD, Ford KR, Hewett TE. Tuck jump assessment for reducing anterior cruciaye ligament injury risk. *Athl Ther Today.* 2008;13(5):39-44.

206. Myer GD, Jensen BL, Ford KR, Hewett TE. Real-time assessment and neuromuscular training feedback techniques to prevent anterior cruciate ligament injury in female athletes. *Strength Cond J.* 2011;33(3):21-35.

207. Myklebust G, Maehium S, Holm I, et al. A prospective cohort study of anterior cruciate ligament injuries in elite Norwegian team handball. *Scand J Med Sci Sports.* 1998;8:149-153.

208. Myklebust G, Maehlum S, Engebretsen L, et al. Registration of cruciate ligament injuries in Norwegian top level team handball. A prospective study covering two seasons. *Scand J Med Sci Sports.* 1997;7:289-292.

209. National Association of Anorexia Nervosa and Associated Disorders. *Facts about Eating Disorders*. http://www.alltrue.net/site/adadweb.htm. Accessed October 15, 2004.

210. National Osteoporosis Foundation. *Physician's Guide: Impact and Overview.* http://www.nof.org/osteoporsis/stats.htm. Accessed October 20, 2004.

211. National Collegiate Athletic Association. *NCAA Injury Surveillance System, 1997-1998*. Overland Park, KS: NCAA; 1998.

212. Nattiv A, Arendt EA, Riehl R. The female athlete. In: Zachazewski JE, Magee DJ, Quillen WS, eds. *Athletic Injuries and Rehabilitation*. Philadelphia, PA: Saunders; 1996: 841-852.

213. Nattiv A, Callahan LR, Kelmon-Sherstinsky A. The female athlete triad. In: Ireland ML, Nattiv A, eds. *The Female Athlete*. Philadelphia, PA: Saunders; 2002:223-235.

214. Nattiv A, Yeager K, Drinkwater B, Agostini R. The female athlete triad. In: Agostini R, ed. *Medical and Orthopedic Issues of Active and Athletic Women*. Philadelphia, PA: Hanley & Belfus; 1994:169-174.

215. Nattiv A, Loucks AB, Manore MM, Sanborn CF, Sundgot-Borgen J, Warren MP. American College of Sports Medicine position stand: The female athlete triad. *Med Sci Sports Exerc.* 2007;39(10):1867-1882.

216. Nelson ME, Fisher EC, Castos PD, et al. Diet and bone status in amenorrheic runners. *Am J Clin Nutr.* 1986;43:910-916.

217. Optimal calcium intake. *NIH Consens Statement.* 1994; 12(4):1-31.

218. Noyes FR, Barber-Westin SD, Fleckenstein C, et al. The drop-jump screening test. Difference in lower limb control by gender and effect of neuromuscular training in female athletes. *Am J Sports Med.* 2005;33(2):197-207.

219. Noyes FR, Mooar PA, Mathews DS, et al. The symptomatic anterior cruciate-deficient knee. Part 1. The long term functional disability in the athletically active individual. *J Bone Joint Surg Am.* 1983;65:154-162.

220. Nyland JA, Shapiro R, Caborn DNM, et al. The effect of quadriceps femoris, hamstring, and placebo eccentric fatigue on knee and ankle dynamics during crossover cutting. *J Orthop Sports Phys Ther.* 1997;25:171-184.
221. O'Neill DB. Arthroscopically assisted reconstruction of the anterior cruciate ligament. A prospective randomized analysis of three techniques. *J Bone Joint Surg Am.* 1996;78:803-813.
222. Oliphant JG, Drawbert JP. Gender differences in anterior cruciate ligament injury rates in Wisconsin intercollegiate basketball. *J Athl Train.* 1996;31:245-247.
223. Oistad BE, Engebretsen L, Storheim K, Risberg MA. Knee osteoarthritis after anterior cruciate ligament injury: A systematic review. *Am J Sports Med.* 2009;37(3):1434-1443.
224. Onate JA, Guskiewicz KM, Sullivan RJ. Augmented feedback reduces jump landing forces. *J Orthop Sports Phys Ther.* 2001;31(9): 511-517.
225. Osteoporosis prevention, diagnosis, and therapy. *NIH Consens Statement* 2001;17:1-45.
226. Otis CL, Drinkwater B, Johnson MD, et al. American College of Sports Medicine. Position Stand: The female athlete triad. *Med Sci Sports Exerc.* 1997;29(5):i-ix.
227. Papanek PE. The female athlete triad: An emerging role for physical therapy. *J Orthop Sports Phys Ther.* 2003;33(10):594-614.
228. Pearl AJ. *The Athletic Female*. Champaign, IL: Human Kinetics; 1993.
229. Pester S, Smith PC. Stress fractures in the lower extremities of soldiers in basic training. *Orthop Rev.* 1992;21:297-303.
230. Pierson WR, Lockart A. Effect of menstruation on simple reaction and movement time. *Br Med J.* 1963;1:796-797.
231. Pink M, Perry J, Browne A, et al. The normal shoulder during freestyle swimming. *Am J Sports Med.* 1991;19:569-576.
232. Pink MM, Jobe FW. Biomechanics of swimming. In: Zachazewski JE, Magee DJ, Quillen WS, eds. *Athletic Injuries and Rehabilitation*. Philadelphia, PA: Saunders; 1996.
233. Pivarnik JM, Lee W, Spillman T, et al. Maternal respiration and blood gases during aerobic exercise performed at moderate altitude. *Med Sci Sports Exerc.* 1992;24:868-872.
234. Plummer B. *Media Guide*. Oklahoma City, OK: International Softball Federation; 1996.
235. Post WR. History and physical examination. In: Fulkerson JP, ed. *Disorders of the Patellofemoral Joint*. 4th ed. Philadelphia, PA: Lippincott Williams & Wilkins; 2004:43-75.
236. Posthuma BW, Bass MJ, Bull SB, et al. Detecting changes in functional ability in women during premenstrual syndrome. *Am J Obstet Gynecol.* 1987;156:275-278.
237. Quatman CE, Ford KR, Myer GD, Hewett TE. Maturation leads to gender differences in landing force and vertical jump performance. *Am J Sports Med.* 2006;34(5): 806-813.
238. Raymond-Barker P, Petroczi A, Questad E. Assessment of nutritional knowledge in female athletes susceptible to the female athlete triad syndrome. *J Occup Med Toxicol.* 2007;2:10.
239. Reinking MF, Alexander LE. Prevalence of disordered eating behaviors in undergraduate female collegiate athletes and nonathletes. *J Athl Train.* 2005;40(1):47-51.
240. Reinold M. Biomechanical implications in shoulder and knee rehabilitation. In: Andrews JR, Harrelson GL, Wilk KE, eds. *Physical Rehabilitation of the Injured Athlete.* 3d ed. Philadelphia, PA: Saunders-Elsevier; 2004:34-50.
241. Richardson C, Jull G, Hodges P, Hides J. Therapeutic exercise for spinal segmental stabilization in low back pain: Scientific basis and clinical approach. Edinburgh, UK: Churchill Livingstone; 1999.
242. Richardson AR, Jobe FW, Collins HR. The shoulder in competitive swimming. *Am J Sports Med.* 1980;8(3):159-163.
243. Rojas IL, Provencher MT, Bhuta S, et al. Biceps activity during windmill softball pitching. Injury implications and comparison with overhead throwing. *Am J Sports Med.* 2009;37(3):558-565.
244. Roos H, Adalberth T, Dahlberg L, Lohmander LS. Osteoarthritis of the knee after injury to the anterior cruciate ligament or meniscus: The influence of time and age. *Osteoarthritis Cartilage.* 1995;3:261-267.
245. Rosen LW, Hough DO. Pathogenic weight control behaviors of female college gymnasts. *Phys Sportsmed.* 1988;16:141-146.
246. Rosen MA, Jackson DW, Berger PE. Occult lesions documented by magnetic resonance imaging associated with anterior cruciate ligament ruptures. *Arthroscopy.* 1991;7:45-51.
247. Rozzi SL, Lephart SM, Fu FH. Effects of muscular fatigue on knee joint laxity and neuromuscular characteristics of male and female athletes. *J Athl Train.* 1999;34(2):106-114.
248. Rozzi SL, Lephart SM, Gear WS, et al. Knee joint laxity and neuromuscular characteristics of male and female soccer and basketball players. *Am J Sports Med.* 1999;27(3):312-319.
249. Sallis RE, Jones K, Sunshine S, et al. Comparing sports injuries in men and women. *Int J Sports Med.* 2001;22(6):420-423.
250. Sanborn CF, Jankowski CM. Physiologic considerations for women in sport. *Clin Sports Med.* 1994;13:315-357.
251. Sanborn CF, Jankowski CM. Gender-specific physiology In: Agostini R, ed. *Medical and Orthopedic Issues of Active and Athletic Women*. Philadelphia, PA: Hanley & Belfus; 1994:23-28.
252. Sands WA, Shultz BB, Newman AP. Women's gymnastics injuries. A 5-year study. *Am J Sports Med.* 1993;21(2):271-276.
253. Sarwar R, Niclos BB, Rutherford OM. Changes in muscle strength, relaxation rate and fatigability during the human menstrual cycle. *J Physiol.* 1996;493:267-272.

254. Schonhuber H, Leo R. Traumatic epidemiology and injury mechanisms in professional alpine skiing. *J Sports Traumatol.* 2000;22:141-158.

255. Scovazzo ML, Browne A, Pink M, et al. The painful shoulder during freestyle swimming: An electromyographic cinematographic analysis of twelve muscles. *Am J Sports Med.* 1991;19(6):577-582.

256. Shangold M, Mirkin G. *Women and Exercise: Physiology and Sports Medicine.* 2nd ed. Philadelphia, PA: FA Davis; 1994.

257. Shanley E, Rauh MJ, Michener LA, Ellenbecker TS. Incidence of injuries in high school softball and baseball players. *J Athl Train.* 2011;46(6):648-654.

258. Shelbourne KD, Klootwyck TE, Wilckens JH, DeCarlo MS. Ligament stability two to six years after anterior cruciate ligament reconstruction with autogenous patellar tendon graft and participation in accelerated rehabilitation program. *Am J Sports Med.* 1995;23:575-579.

259. Sherman RT, Thompson RA. The female athlete triad. *J Sch Nurs.* 2004;4:197-202.

260. Shoemaker SC, Adams D, Daniel DM, Woo SL. Quadriceps/anterior cruciate graft interaction: An in vitro study of joint kinematics and anterior cruciate ligament graft tension. *Clin Orthop.* 1993;294:379-390.

261. Sickles RT, Lombardo JA. The adolescent basketball player. *Clin Sports Med.* 1993;12(2):207-219.

262. Skinner HB, Wyatt MP, Hodgdon JA, Conrad DW, Barrack RL. Effect of fatigue on joint position sense of the knee. *J Orthop Res.* 1986;4:112-118.

263. Slauterbeck JR, Hardy DM. Sex hormones and knee ligament injuries in female athletes. *Am J Med Sci.* 2001;322(4):196-199.

264. Sleeper MD, Kenyon LK, Casey E. Measuring fitness in female gymnasts: The gymnastics functional measurement tool. *Int J Sports Phys Ther.* 2012;7(2);124-138.

265. Snow-Harter C. Athletic amenorrhea and bone health. In: Agostini R, ed. *Medical and Orthopedic Issues of Active and Athletic Women.* Philadelphia, PA: Hanley & Belfus; 1994:164-168.

266. Sommerlath K, Lysholm J, Gilquist J. The long-term course after treatment of anterior cruciate ligament ruptures. A 9 to 16 year follow up. *Am J Sports Med.* 1991;29:156-162.

267. Sondgot-Borgen J. The female athlete triad and the effect of preventive work. *Med Sci Sports Exerc. 1998;*33(Suppl 5):S181.

268. Sondgot-Borgen J. The long-term effect of CBT and nutritional counseling in treating bulimic elite athletes: A randomized controlled study. *Med Sci Sports Exerc.* 2001;33(Suppl 5):S97.

269. Souryal TO, Freeman TR. Intracondylar notch size and anterior cruciate ligament injuries in athletes. *Am J Sports Med.* 1993;21:535-539.

270. Squire DL. Issues specific to the preadolescent and adolescent athletic female. In: Pearl AJ, ed. *The Athletic Female.* Champaign, IL: Human Kinetics; 1993: 113-121.

271. Steele V, White J. Injury prediction in female gymnasts. *Br J Sports Med.* 1986;20:31-33.

272. Steiner ME, Grana WA, Chillag K, Schelberg-Karnes E. The effect of exercise on anterior-posterior knee laxity. *Am J Sports Med.* 1986;14:24-29.

273. Such CH, Unsworth A, Wright V, Dowson D. Quantitative study of stiffness in the knee joint. *Ann Rheum Dis.* 1975;34:286-291.

274. Swanik CB, Lephart SM, Giraldo JL, Demont RG, Fu FM. Reactive muscle firing of anterior cruciate ligament-injured females during functional activities. *J Athl Train.* 1999;34(2):121-129.

275. Swedan N. *Women's Sports Medicine and Rehabilitation.* Gaithersburg, MD: Aspen; 2001.

276. Theintz GE, Howald H, Weiss U, et al. Evidence for a reduction of growth potential in adolescent female gymnasts. *J Pediatr.* 1993;122:306-313.

277. Thomis M, Claessens AL, Lefevre J, et al. Adolescent growth spurts in female gymnasts. *J Pediatr.* 2005;146(2):239-244.

278. Thomson KE. On the bending moment capability of the pressurized abdominal cavity during human lifting activity. *Ergonomics.* 1988;31:817-828.

279. Traina SM, Bromberg DF. ACL injury patterns in women. *Orthopedics.* 1997;20:545-549.

280. United States Department of Agriculture. *MyPyramid: Steps to a Healthier You.* http://www.mypyramid.gov. Accessed May 1, 2012.

281. Vaughan JL, King KA, Cottrell RR. Collegiate athletic trainers' confidence in helping female athletes with eating disorders. *J Athl Train.* 2004;39(1):71-76.

282. Warren MP, Brooks-Gunn J, Hamilton LF, et al. Scoliosis and fractures in young ballet dancers. *N Engl J Med.* 1986;314:1348-1353.

283. Wedderkopp N, Kaltoft M, Lundgaard B. Prevention of injuries in young female players in European team handball: A prospective intervention study. *Scand J Med Sci Sports.* 1999;9:41-47.

284. Weimann E. Gender-related differences in elite gymnasts: The female athlete triad. *J Appl Physiol.* 2001;92(5):2146-2152.

285. Weldon EJ, Richardson AB. Upper extremity overuse injuries in swimming: A discussion of swimmer's shoulder. *Clin Sports Med.* 2001;20(3):423-438.

286. Werner SL, Guido JA, McNeice RL, et al. Biomechanics of youth windmill softball pitching. *Am J Sports Med.* 2005;33(4):552-560.

287. Wilke HJ, Wolf S, Claes LE, Arand M, Wiesend A. Stability increase of the lumbar spine with different muscle groups. A biomechanical in vitro study. *Spine (Phila Pa 1976).* 1995;20:192-198.

288. Wojtys EM, Huston LJ, Boynton MD, et al. The effect of menstrual cycle on anterior cruciate ligament injuries in women as determined by hormone level. *Sports Med.* 2002;30:182-188.

289. Wojtys EM, Huston LJ, Lindenfeld TN, et al. Association between the menstrual cycle and anterior cruciate ligament injuries in female athletes. *Am J Sports Med.* 1998;26:614-619.

290. Wojtys EM, Huston LJ. Neuromuscular performance in normal and anterior cruciate ligament-deficient lower extremities. *Am J Sports Med.* 1994;22:89-104.

291. Yanai T, Hay JG, Miller GF. Shoulder impingement in front-crawl swimming: I. A method to identify impingement. *Med Sci Sports Exerc.* 2000;32(1):21-29.

292. Yanai T, Hay JG. Shoulder impingement in front-crawl swimming: II. Analysis of stroking technique. *Med Sci Sports Exerc.* 2000;32 (1):30-40.

293. Yeager KK, Agostini R, Nattiv A, Drinkwater B. The female athlete triad: Disordered eating, amenorrhea, osteoporosis. *Med Sci Sports Exerc.* 1993;25:775.

294. Zawila LG, Steib CM, Hoogenboom B. The female collegiate cross-country runner: Nutritional knowledge and attitudes. *J Athl Train.* 2003;38(1):67-74.

295. Zazulak BT, Ponce PL, Straub SJ, et al. Gender comparison of hip muscle activity during single-leg landing. *J Orthop Sports Phys Ther.* 2005;35(5):292-299.

296. Zelisko JA, Noble HB, Porter M. A comparison of men's and women's professional basketball injuries. *Am J Sports Med.* 1982;10:297-299.

297. Zhou S, Carey MF, Snow RJ, Lawson DL, Morrison WE. Effects of muscle fatigue and temperature on electromechanical delay. *Electromyogr Clin Neurophysiol.* 1998;38:67-73.

298. Zillmer DA, Powell JW, Albright JP. Gender-specific injury patterns in high school varsity basketball. *J Womens Health (Larchmt).* 1992;1:69-76.

Appendix A: Jump-Training Program

This program was developed by Cincinnati Sports Medicine and is reprinted, with permission, from Hewett TE, Stroupe AL, Nance TA, Noyes FR. Plyometric training in female athletes: Decreased impact forces increased hamstring torques. *Am J Sports Med.* 1996;24:765-773.

Exercise		Repetitions or Time Intervals
Phase I: Technique	**Week 1**	**Week 2**
1. Wall jumps	20 seconds	25 seconds
2. Tuck jumps[a]	20 seconds	25 seconds
3. Broad jumps, stick landing	5 repetitions	10 repetitions
4. Squat jumps[a]	10 seconds	15 seconds
5. Double-leg cone jumps[a]	30 seconds/30 seconds	30 seconds/30 seconds
6. 180-Degree jumps	20 seconds	25 seconds
7. Bounding in place	20 seconds	25 seconds
Phase II: Fundamental	**Week 3**	**Week 4**
1. Wall jumps	30 seconds	30 seconds
2. Tuck jumps[a]	30 seconds	30 seconds
3. Jump, jump, jump, vertical jump	5 repetitions	8 repetitions
4. Squat jumps[a]	20 seconds	20 seconds
5. Bounding for distance	1 run	2 runs
6. Double-leg cone jumps[a]	30 seconds/30 seconds	30 seconds/30 seconds
7. Scissors jump	30 seconds	30 seconds
8. Hop, hop, stick landing[a]	5 repetitions/leg	5 repetitions
Phase III: Performance	**Week 5**	**Week 6**
1. Wall jumps	30 seconds	30 seconds
2. Step, jump up, down, vertical	5 repetitions	10 repetitions
3. Mattress jumps	30 seconds/30 seconds	30 seconds/30 seconds
4. Single-legged jumps for distance[a]	5 repetitions/leg	5 repetitions/leg
5. Squat jumps[a]	25 seconds	25 seconds
6. Jumping into bounding[a]	3 runs	4 runs
7. Single-legged hop, hop, stick landing	5 repetitions/leg	5 repetitions/leg

[a]Jumps to be performed on mat-type surface. This program is set up to run for 6 weeks. Jump training should be performed 3 times per week. Stretching and warm-up should be done before any jumping exercises. Stretching should also follow all jump training sessions. A 30-second rest period should follow each jump-training exercise.

Description of Jump Training Exercises

1. Wall jumps: With knees slightly bent and arms raised overhead, bounce up and down off toes.
2. Tuck jumps: From standing position, jump and bring both knees up to chest as high as possible. Repeat quickly.
3. Broad jumps stick landing: Two-footed jump as far as possible. Hold landing for 5 seconds.
4. Squat jumps: Standing jump raising both arms overhead. Land in squatting position touching both hands to floor.
5. Double-leg cone jumps: Double-leg jump with feet together. Jump side to side over cones quickly. Cones approximately 8 in high. Repeat forward and backward.
6. 180-Degree jumps: Two-footed jump. Rotate 180 degrees in midair. Hold landing 2 seconds, then repeat in reverse direction.
7. Bounding in place: Jump from one leg to the other leg straight up and down, progressively increasing rhythm and height.
8. Jump, jump, jump, vertical jump: Three broad jumps with vertical jump immediately after landing the third broad jump.
9. Bounding for distance: Start bounding in place and slowly increase distance with each step, keeping knees high.
10. Scissors kicks: Start in stride position with one foot well in front of other. Jump up, alternating foot positions in midair.
11. Hop, hop, stick the landing: Single-legged hop. Stick landing for 5 seconds. Increase distance of hop as technique improves.
12. Step, jump up, down, vertical: Two-footed jump onto 6- to 8-in step. Jump off step with 2 ft, then vertical jump.
13. Mattress jumps: Two-footed jump on mattress, tramp, or other easily compressed device. Perform side-to-side/back-to-front.
14. Single-legged jumps for distance: One-legged hop for distance. Hold landing (knees bent) for 5 seconds.
15. Jump into bounding: Two-footed broad jump. Land on single leg, then progress into bounding for distance.

Appendix B: Interval Windmill Pitching Program

This program is reprinted, with permission, from Werner SL, Guido JA, McNeice RL, Richardson JL, Delude NA, Stewart GW. Biomechanics of youth windmill softball pitching. *Am J Sports Med.* 2005;33(4):552-560.

A warm-up period, stretching, and overhand throwing should precede all steps in the program.

Warm-up

Jogging, jumping rope, etc to increase blood flow to the muscles; once a light sweat is developed, move to stretching.

Stretching

Full body stretching is important for reducing the chance of injury and for increasing mobility of all parts of the body (which allows the whole body to be used to throw, rather than just the arm).

Throwing

Overhand throwing is important to loosen the throwing arm before pitching. Throw from 30 to 60 ft until the throwing arm feels ready to pitch.

Pitching

Progress to the next step of the program once current step is accomplished is completely free of pain. Allow at least 24 hours to pass between successive steps. Each athlete progresses at a different rate. There is no optimal length of this program. Once step 14 is completed successfully, the athlete is ready to return to unrestricted windmill pitching.

Phase I

Step 1	15 pitches at 50% effort	Step 5	30 pitches at 75% effort
Step 2	30 pitches at 50% effort	Step 6	30 at 75%, 45 at 50%
Step 3	45 pitches at 50% effort	Step 7	45 at 75%, 15 at 50%
Step 4	60 pitches at 50% effort	Step 8	60 pitches at 75%

Phase II

Step 9	45 at 75%, 15 at 100%	Step 11	45 at 75%, 45 at 100%
Step 10	45 at 75%, 30 at 100%		

Phase III

Step 12	30 pitches at 75% as a warm-up, 15 change ups at 100%, 50 fastballs at 100%
Step 13	30 pitches at 75% as a warm-up, 30 change ups at 100%, 30 fastballs at 100%
Step 14	30 pitches at 75% as a warm-up, 75 pitches at 100%, mix in change ups

Appendix C: Interval Softball Throwing Program

This program is reprinted, with permission, from Werner SL, Guido JA, McNeice RL, Richardson JL, Delude NA, Stewart GW. Biomechanics of youth windmill softball pitching. *Am J Sports Med.* 2005;33(4):552-560.

Warm-up

Jogging, jumping rope, etc to increase blood flow to the muscles; once a light sweat is developed, move to stretching.

Stretching

Full body stretching is important for reducing the chance of injury and for increasing mobility of all parts of the body (which allows the whole body to be used to throw, rather than just the arm).

Throwing Mechanics

A crow-hop technique should be used in all phases of the interval-throwing program. This technique places the arm in a mechanically sound position for throwing.

Throwing

Warm-up throws should take place from 30 to 45 ft and progress to the distance indicated for the following successive phases. Progress to the next step of the program once current step is accomplished completely free of pain. Allow at least 24 hours to pass between successive steps. Each athlete progresses at [a] different rates [*sic*]. There is no optimal length of this program. Once step 11 is completed successfully, the athlete is ready to return to unrestricted overhand throwing.

45 Phase

Step 1	10 to 15 warm-up throws 25 throws at 45 ft Rest 15 minutes 10 to 15 warm-up throws 25 throws at 45 ft
Step 2	10 to 15 warm-up throws 25 throws at 45 ft Rest 10 minutes 10 to 15 warm-up throws 25 throws at 45 ft. Rest 10 minutes 10 to 15 warm-up throws 25 throws at 45 ft

60 Phase

Step 3	10 to 15 warm-up throws 25 throws at 60 ft Rest 15 minutes 10 to 15 warm-up throws 25 throws at 60 ft
Step 4	10 to 15 warm-up throws 25 throws at 60 ft Rest 10 minutes 10 to 15 warm-up throws 25 throws at 60 ft Rest 10 minutes 10 to 15 warm-up throws 25 throws at 60 ft

90 Phase

Step 5	10 to 15 warm-up throws 25 throws at 90 ft Rest 15 minutes 10 to 15 warm-up throws 25 throws at 90 ft

Step 6	10 to 15 warm-up throws 25 throws at 90 ft Rest 10 minutes 10 to 15 warm-up throws 25 throws at 90 ft Rest 10 minutes 10 to 15 warm-up throws 25 throws at 90 ft
120 Phase	
Step 7	10 to 15 warm-up throws 25 throws at 120 ft Rest 15 minutes 10 to 15 warm-up throws 25 throws at 120 ft
Step 8	10 to 15 warm up throws 25 throws at 120 ft Rest 10 minutes 10 to 15 warm-up throws 25 throws at 120 ft Rest 10 minutes 10 to 15 warm-up throws 25 throws at 120 ft
150 Phase	
Step 9	10 to 15 warm-up throws 25 throws at 150 ft Rest 15 minutes 10 to 15 warm-up throws 25 throws at 150 ft
Step 10	10 to 15 warm-up throws 25 throws at 150 ft Rest 10 minutes 10 to 15 warm-up throws 25 throws at 150 ft Rest 10 minutes 10 to 15 warm-up throws 25 throws at 150 ft
Step 11	10 to 15 warm-up throws 25 throws at 150 ft Rest 10 minutes 10 to 15 warm-up throws 25 throws at 150 ft Rest 10 minutes 10 to 15 warm-up throws 50 throws at 150 ft

Appendix D: Female Triad Screening Questionnaire[1]

1. Do you worry about your weight or body composition? Yes/No
2. Do you limit or carefully control the foods that you eat? Yes/No
3. Do you try to lose weight to meet weight or image/appearance requirements in your sport? Yes/No
4. Does your weight affect the way you feel about yourself? Yes/No
5. Do you worry that you have lost control over how much you eat? Yes/No
6. Do you make yourself vomit, use diuretics or laxatives after you eat? Yes/No
7. Do you currently or have you ever suffered from an eating disorder? Yes/No
8. Do you ever eat in secret? Yes/No
9. What age was your first menstrual period? Yes/No
10. Do you have monthly menstrual cycles? Yes/No
11. How many menstrual cycles have you had in the last year? Yes/No
12. Have you ever had a stress fracture? Yes/No

Appendix E: Female Athlete Triad In-Depth Questionnaire[1]

Please circle the response that best matches your situation.
Never = 1, Rarely = 2, Occasionally = 3, More often than not = 4, Regularly = 5, Always = 6

1. Do you want to weigh more or less than you do? 1 2 3 4 5 6
2. Do you lose weight regularly to meet weight requirements for your sport? 1 2 3 4 5 6
   How do you do it?______________________________
3. Is weight/body composition an issue for you? 1 2 3 4 5 6
4. Are you satisfied with your eating habits? 1 2 3 4 5 6
5. Do you think your performance is directly affected by your weight? 1 2 3 4 5 6
   If so how?______________________________
6. Do you have forbidden foods? 1 2 3 4 5 6
7. Are you a vegetarian? 1 2 3 4 5 6
   Since what age?______________________________
8. Do you miss meals? 1 2 3 4 5 6
   If so, how often?_______________ For what reason?_______________
9. Do you have rapid increases of decreases in your body weight? 1 2 3 4 5 6
10. What do you consider your ideal competitive weight? 1 2 3 4 5 6
11. Has anyone ever suggested you lose weight or change your eating habits? 1 2 3 4 5 6
12. Has a coach, judge, or family member ever called you fat? 1 2 3 4 5 6
13. What do you do to control your weight? 1 2 3 4 5 6
14. Do you worry if you have missed a workout? 1 2 3 4 5 6

15. Do you exercise or are you physically active as well as training for your sport? 1 2 3 4 5 6

16. Do you have stress in your life outside of sport? 1 2 3 4 5 6

What are these stresses?____________________

17. Are you able to cope with stress? 1 2 3 4 5 6

How?____________________

18. What is your family structure?____________________

19. Do you use or have you use(d) these ways to lose weight?

a. Laxatives 1 2 3 4 5 6

b. Diuretics 1 2 3 4 5 6

c. Vomiting 1 2 3 4 5 6

d. Diet pills 1 2 3 4 5 6

e. Saunas 1 2 3 4 5 6

f. Plastic bags or wrap during training 1 2 3 4 5 6

g. Other methods (please state)____________________ 1 2 3 4 5 6

Review of systems: (headaches/visual problems, galactorrhea/acne/male pattern hair distribution)

Complete history of injuries.

Nutritional analysis assessing energy balance and nutrient balance.

Appendix F: Other Sources and Screening Tools to Assess Eating Disorders and Other Components of Female Triad

1. www.alltrue.net/site/adadweb.htm—National Association of Anorexia Nervosa and Associated Disorders.
2. www.femaleathletetriad.org—The Female Athlete Triad Coalition
3. www.mentalhealthscreening.org—website of National Eating Disorder Screening Program
4. www.ncaa.org—website of the National Collegiate Athletic Association
5. www.nof.org—website for National Osteoporosis Foundation
6. www.hedc.org—Harvard Eating Disorders Center (HEDC)
7. www.womanhealth.gov—website of Office on Women's Health, U.S. Department of Health and Human Services

Developed Screening Tools for Female Triad components[21,34,40]

1. Female Athlete Screening Tool (FAST)
2. Eating Disorder Inventory (EDI)
3. Eating Disorder Inventory-2 (EDI-2)
4. Eating Disorder Exam 12.0D
5. Eating Attitudes Test (EAT)
6. Bulemia Test (BULIT)
7. Bulemia Test-Revised (BULIT-Rev)

8. Setting Conditions for Anorexia Nervosa Scale (SCANS)
9. Restrained Eating Questionnaire
10. Physiologic Screening Test
11. Diagnostic Criteria for Anorexia Nervosa, Bulimia Nervosa, and Eating Disorders not otherwise specified (*Diagnostic and Statistical Manual of Mental Disorders*, 4th Edition [DSM-IV])

Index

Page numbers followed by *f* and *t* denote figures and tables, respectively.

B

C

I

J

M

N

P

Q

R

S

T